Mechanics and Strength of Materials

to

---

*loving memory
of
my father*

Late Sri K Sivaramulu

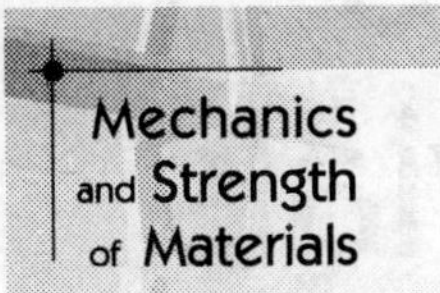

Mechanics and Strength of Materials

ISBN: 978-93-88725-64-4

First Edition: 2019

Published by Satish Kumar Jain and produced by Varun Jain for

CBS Publishers & Distributors Pvt Ltd
4819/XI Prahlad Street, 24 Ansari Road, Daryaganj, New Delhi 110 002, India.
Ph: 23289259, 23266861, 23266867   Fax: 011-23243014   Website: www.cbspd.com
e-mail: delhi@cbspd.com; cbspubs@airtelmail.in
Corporate Office: 204 FIE, Industrial Area, Patparganj, Delhi 110 092
Ph: 4934 4934   Fax: 4934 4935   e-mail: publishing@cbspd.com; publicity@cbspd.com

Branches

- **Bengaluru:** Seema House, 2975, 17th Cross, K.R. Road,
  Banasankari 2nd Stage, Bengaluru 560 070, Karnataka
  Ph: +91-80-26771678/79   Fax: +91-80-26771680   e-mail: bangalore@cbspd.com
- **Chennai:** 7, Subbaraya Street, Shenoy Nagar, Chennai 600 030, Tamil Nadu
  Ph: +91-44-26680620, 26681266   Fax: +91-44-42032115   e-mail: chennai@cbspd.com
- **Kochi:** 42/1325, 1326, Power House Road, Opposite KSEB Power House,
  Ernakulam 682 018, Kochi, Kerala
  Ph: +91-484-4059061-65   Fax: +91-484-4059065   e-mail: kochi@cbspd.com
- **Kolkata:** 6/B, Ground Floor, Rameswar Shaw Road, Kolkata-700 014, West Bengal
  Ph: +91-33-22891126, 22891127, 22891128   e-mail: kolkata@cbspd.com
- **Mumbai:** 83-C, Dr E Moses Road, Worli, Mumbai-400018, Maharashtra
  Ph: +91-22-24902340/41   Fax: +91-22-24902342   e-mail: mumbai@cbspd.com

Representatives

• **Bhopal**	0-8319310552	• **Bhubaneswar**	0-9911037372	• **Hyderabad**	0-9885175004
• **Nagpur**	0-9421945513	• **Patna**	0-9334159340	• **Pune**	0-9623451994
• **Dhaka (Bangladesh)**	01912-003485	• **Jharkhand**	0-9811541605	• **Uttarakhand**	0-9716462459

Printed at: Rashtriya Printers, Dilshad Garden, New Delhi

Mechanics and Strength of Materials

K Raghavendra MTech
Assistant Professor
Department of Mechanical Engineering
Ballari Institute of Technology and Management (BITM)
Ballari, Karnataka 583104

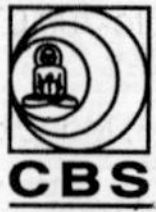

CBS Publishers & Distributors Pvt Ltd

New Delhi • Bengaluru • Chennai • Kochi • Kolkata • Mumbai
Bhopal • Bhubaneswar • Hyderabad • Jharkhand • Nagpur • Patna • Pune • Uttarakhand • Dhaka (Bangladesh)

Preface

It gives me a great satisfaction in presenting this book titled *Mechanics and Strength of Materials*, written according to the syllabus prescribed by VTU, Belagavi, for III semester students of mechanical and civil engineering. This book also serves as a reference, across allied branches of engineering and polytechnics.

The manuscript is based on the lectures delivered by me. The concepts are presented in a simple and lucid language to explain the subject, within the scope of the topics, adhered to the syllabus. In order to solve more problems, the syllabus has been split into 12 chapters, for ease of reference.

I owe my gratitude to my mother Smt B Susheela, whose blessings inspired me in bringing out this book. I am thankful to my wife Smt V Radhika, son Chi K Naga Ganesh and daughter Chi K Shanvi, for their continuous support and encouragement in preparing this book.

I express my sincere thanks to Dr Kori Nagaraj, Prof and Head, Department of Mechanical Engineering, RYME College, Ballari; Dr Yadavalli Basavaraj, Prof and Head, Department of Mechanical Engineering, BITM, Ballari; Dr Raghavendra Joshi, Professor, Department of Mechanical Engineering, BITM, Ballari, for their support and cooperation during the preparation of this manuscript.

In spite of care being taken, errors might have crept in without knowledge. I would be grateful to the readers, if they could bring to attention, the errors if any, noticed by them.

Last but not the least, I would like to thank the entire team of CBS Publishers and Distributors, New Delhi, for making all possible efforts in the publication of this book.

K Raghavendra

Contents

10. COLUMNS AND STRUTS

701–751

11. STRAIN ENERGY

752–841

MECHANICS OF MATERIALS (MOM)

Sub Code: 17ME34   **3rd Semester**

MODULE 1

Stress and Strain: Introduction, Hooke's law, Calculation of stresses in straight, Stepped and tapered sections, Composite sections, Stresses due to temperature change, Shear stress and strain, Lateral strain and Poisson's ratio, Generalized Hooke's law, Bulk modulus, Relationship between elastic constants.   **10 Hours**

MODULE 2

Analysis of Stress and Strain: Plane stress, Stresses on inclined planes, Principal stresses and maximum shear stress, Principal angles, Shear stresses on principal planes, Maximum shear stress, Mohr circle for plane stress conditions.

Cylinders: Thin cylinder: Hoop's stress, maximum shear stress, circumferential and longitudinal strains. Thick cylinders: Lames equations.   **10 Hours**

MODULE 3

Shear Forces and Bending Moments: Type of beams, Loads and reactions, Relationship between loads, shear forces and bending moments, Shear force and bending moments of cantilever beams, Pin support and roller supported beams subjected to concentrated loads and uniformly distributed constant / varying loads.

Stress in Beams: Pure bending, Curvature of a beam, Longitudinal strains in beams, Normal stresses in Beams with rectangular, circular, 'I' and 'T' cross sections, Flexure Formula, Bending Stresses, Deflection of beams (Curvature).   **10 Hours**

MODULE 4

Torsion: Circular solid and hallow shafts, Torsional moment of resistance, Power transmission of straight and stepped shafts, Twist in shaft sections, Thin tubular sections, Thin walled sections.

Columns: Buckling and stability, Critical load, Columns with pinned ends, Columns with other support conditions, Effective length of columns, Secant formula for columns.   **10 Hours**

MODULE 5

Strain Energy: Castigliano's theorem I and II, Load deformation diagram, Strain energy due to normal stresses, Shear stresses, Modulus of resilience, Strain energy due to bending and torsion.

Theories of Failure: Maximum Principal stress theory, Maximum shear stress theory.   **10 Hours**

STRENGTH OF MATERIALS (SOM)

Sub Code: 17CV32 **3rd Semester**

MODULE 1

Simple Stresses and Strain: Introduction, Definition and concept and of stress and strain. Hooke's law, Stress-Strain diagrams for ferrous and non-ferrous materials, factor of safety, Elongation of tapering bars of circular and rectangular cross sections, Elongation due to self-weight. Saint Venant's principle, Compound bars, Temperature stresses, Compound section subjected to temperature stresses, state of simple shear, Elastic constants and their relationship. **10 Hours**

MODULE 2

Compound Stresses: Introduction, state of stress at a point, General two dimensional stress system, Principal stresses and principal planes. Mohr's circle of stresses **05 Hours**

Thin and Thick Cylinders: Introduction, Thin cylinders subjected to internal pressure; Hoop stresses, Longitudinal stress and change in volume. Thick cylinders subjected to both internal and external pressure; Lame's equation, radial and hoop stress distribution. **05 Hours**

MODULE 3

Shear Force and Bending Moment in Beams: Introduction to types of beams, supports and loadings. Definition of bending moment and shear force, Sign conventions, relationship between load intensity, bending moment and shear force. Shear force and bending moment diagrams for statically determinate beams subjected to points load, uniformly distributed loads, uniformly varying loads, couple and their combinations. **10 Hours**

MODULE 4

Bending and Shear Stresses in Beams: Introduction, pure bending theory, Assumptions, derivation of bending equation, modulus of rupture, section modulus, flexural rigidity. Expression for transverse shear stress in beams, Bending and shear stress distribution diagrams for circular, rectangular, 'I', and 'T' sections. Shear centre (only concept) **06 Hours**

Columns and Struts: Introduction, short and long columns. Euler's theory; Assumptions, Derivation for Euler's Buckling load for different end conditions, Limitations of Euler's theory. Rankine-Gordon's formula for columns. **04 Hours**

MODULE 5

Torsion in Circular Shaft: Introduction, pure torsion, Assumptions, derivation of torsion equation for circular shafts, torsional rigidity and polar modulus Power transmitted by a shaft, combined bending and torsion. **07 Hours**

Theories of Failure: Introduction, maximum principal stress theory (Rankine's theory), Maximum shearing stress theory (Tresca's theory), Strain energy theory (Beltrami and Haigh), and maximum strain theory (St. Venant's theory). **03 Hours**

Syllabus Comparison

Sl. No.	Chapters	CBCS Scheme (Module system)	
		MECH	CIVIL
1.	Simple Stresses and Strains	M1	M1
2.	Stresses in Composite Sections	M1	M1
3.	Compound Stresses (Analysis of Stress and Strain)	M2	M2
4.	Thick and Thin Cylinders	M2	M2
5.	Shear Forces and Bending Moments	M3	M3
6.	Deflection of Beams	M3	**
7.	Bending Stresses in Beams	M3	M4
8.	Shear Stresses in Beams	**	M4
9.	Torsion of Circular Shafts	M4	M5
10.	Columns and Struts	M4	M4
11.	Strain energy (Energy Methods)	M5	**
12.	Theories of Failure	M5	M5

** Not applicable

Symbols used

Chapter 1

F = Load
l = Length
A = Cross-sectional area
σ = Conventional or Engineering or nominal stress (tensile or compressive)
ε = Conventional or Engineering strain
δl = Deformation
Δ = Total deformation
d = Diameter
E = Young's modulus
$\bar{\sigma}$ = True stress
$\bar{\varepsilon}$ = True strain
w = Specific weight of the bar material ($= \rho g$)
ρ = Specific mass or density of the material
R = Reactions
n = Factor of safety

Chapter 2

F = Load
l = Length
σ = Stress (tensile or compressive)
τ = Shear stress
ε = Strain
γ = Shear strain
ε_v = Volumetric strain
δl = Deformation
δ = Expansion allowance
Δ = Total deformation
V = Original volume
δV = Change in volume
α = Coefficient of thermal or linear expansion
b = Breadth
h = Depth
d = Diameter
d_o = Outer diameter
d_i = Inner diameter
μ = Poisson's ratio
E = Young's modulus
K = Bulk modulus
G = Shear modulus or modulus of rigidity
t = Increase in temperature

$\dfrac{E_1}{E_2}$ = Modular ratio

Chapter 3

F = Load
σ_x = Tensile stress acting along x axis
σ_y = Tensile stress acting along y axis
τ_{xy} = Shear stress
ϕ = Angle made by oblique plane AB
σ_n = Normal stress
τ = Tangential stress
σ_1 = Major principal stress
σ_2 = Minor principal stress
τ_{max} = Maximum shear stress
ϕ_1 = Angle of first principal plane
ϕ_2 = Angle of second principal plane
$\phi_{s\,max}$ = ϕ_{s1} = Maximum angle of shear plane/stress
$\phi_{s\,min}$ = ϕ_{s2} = Minimum angle of shear plane/stress

Chapter 4

d = Diameter of the cylinder
d_i = Inner diameter of hollow cylinder
d_o = Outer diameter of hollow cylinder
d_m = Mean diameter
t = Thickness of the cylinder
p = Internal pressure in the cylinder
L = Length of the cylinder
σ_c or σ_1 = Circumferential or hoop stress
σ_l or σ_2 = Longitudinal or axial stress
τ_{max} = Maximum shear stress
η = Efficiency of the riveted joint
μ = Poisson's ratio
δd = Change in diameter
δL = Change in length
δV = Change in volume
ϵ_l = Longitudinal strain
ϵ_c = Circumferential strain
ϵ_v = Volumetric strain
E = Young's modulus
K = Bulk modulus
G = Rigidity modulus

Chapter 5

W = Concentrated or point load
w = Uniformly distributed load per unit length
M = Bending moment
L = Length of the beam
F_n = Shear force at salient points
M_n = Bending moment at salient points

Chapter 6

W = Concentrated or point load
w = Uniformly distributed load per unit length
M = Bending moment
I = Moment of inertia
σ or σ_b = Bending stress in the layer
y or c = Distance of extreme fiber from neutral axis
c_1 = Distance of neutral axis from base or bottom layer
c_2 = Distance of neutral axis from top layer
E = Young's modulus of the material of the beam
R = Radius of curvature
EI = Flexural rigidity
Z = Section modulus
L = Length
b = Width
h = Depth
D = Diameter

Chapter 7

F = Load
M = Bending moment
I = Moment of inertia
σ or σ_b = Bending stress in the layer
y or c = Distance of extreme fiber from neutral axis
τ = Shear stress
τ_{max} = Maximum shear stress
y = Distance of fiber considered above neural axis (N.A)
$\bar{y}$ = Distance of CG of area A above N.A
c_1 = Distance of neutral axis from base or bottom layer
c_2 = Distance of neutral axis from top layer
A = Cross-sectional area
Z = Section modulus
L = Length
b = Width
h = Depth
D = Diameter

Chapter 8

W = Concentrated or point load
w = Uniformly distributed load per unit length
M = Bending moment
L = Length of the beam
σ or σ_b = Bending stress in the layer
y = Deflection
θ = Slope
E = Young's modulus of the material of the beam
I = Moment of inertia

R = Radius of curvature
EI = Flexural rigidity
Z = Section modulus

Chapter 9

d = Diameter of solid shaft
d_o = Outer diameter of hollow shaft
d_i = Inner diameter of hollow shaft

$K = \dfrac{d_i}{d_o}$ = Ratio of inner diameter to outer diameter of hollow shaft
τ = Shear stress
γ = Shear strain
G = Modulus of rigidity
T = Torsional moment of resistance or torque or twisting moment
J = Polar moment of inertia
θ = Angle of twist
L = Length of the shaft
Z_p = Polar section modulus
P = Power transmitted
N = Speed
J/r = Torsional section modulus
GJ = Torsional rigidity or stiffness of the shaft.
L_s = Length of solid shaft
L_H = Length of hollow shaft
ρ = Density of shaft material
W_H, W_s = Weight of hollow shaft and solid shaft respectively
T_H, T_s = Torque transmitted by hollow shaft and solid shaft respectively
S_H, S_s = Stiffness of hollow shaft and solid shaft respectively
q = Shear flow
A_m = Area of tube or area enclosed by the median line
s = Length or perimeter of median line
σ_D = Direct or axial stress
σ_b = Bending stress
M = Bending moment
Z = Section modulus
σ_1 = Maximum principal stress
σ_2 = Minimum principal stress
τ_{max} = Maximum shear stress

Chapter 10

F_s = Safe load
F_{cr} = Crippling or buckling load
E = Young's modulus
I = Least moment of inertia
L = Effecive length of column
d = Diameter of shaft or rod
d_o = Outer diameter of hollow shaft or rod
d_i = Inner diameter of hollow shaft or rod

$K = \dfrac{d_i}{d_o}$ = Ratio of inner diameter to outer diameter of hollow shaft or rod

k = Radius of gyration

l = Length of the column

n = Factor of safety

μ = Poisson's ratio

$\dfrac{L}{k}$ = Slenderness ratio

σ_{cr} = Crippling or buckling stress

σ_y = Yield or elastic strength of the material in tension

σ_b = Bending stress

σ_{max} = Maximum stress

y_{max} = Maximum deflection

M_{max} = Maximum bending moment

e = eccentricity

Chapter 11

F or W = Load

F_s = Shear load

Q = Fictitious or dummy load

A = Cross-sectional area

E = Young's modulus

F = Load

G = Modulus of rigidity

M = Bending moment of the beam

M_o = Fictitious or dummy moment

T = Torque

U = Strain energy

Up = Strain energy at elastic limit

h = Height through which the weight falls

l = Length

u = Strain energy density or strain energy per unit volume or resilience

u_p = Proof resilience

w = Specific weight of the material

γ = Shear strain

τ = Shear stress

ϵ = Normal strain

σ = Static stress

σ' = Impact stress

δl = Deformation

$\sigma l'$ = Deformation due to impact action

y = Static deflection

y' = Deflection of the beam due to impact

σ_b = Bending stress due to static load or weight

σ_b' = Impact stress due to bending

EI = Flexural rigidity

EA = Axial rigidity

GJ = Torsional rigidity

Chapter 12

F_s = Shear load
U_h = Hydrostatic energy
U_d = Distortion energy
σ_1 = Maximum principal stress
σ_2 = Minimum principal stress
σ_h = Hydrostatic stress or spherical or dilatational stress.
σ_D = Direct or axial stress
σ_b = Bending stress
σ_d = Working stress or design stress or allowable stress or applied stress
σ_e or σ_{yt} = Yield or elastic strength of the material in tension
σ_u or σ_{ut} = Ultimate strength of the material in tension
τ_e = Yield or elastic strength of the material in shear
τ_{max} = Maximum shear stress
E = Young's modulus
F = Load
G = Modulus of rigidity
U = Total strain energy
d = Diameter of shaft
n = Factor of safety
ε = Strain
μ = Poisson's ratio
τ = Shear stress

Simple Stresses and Strains

Chapter Outline

1.1 INTRODUCTION

The strength of a material is its ability to withstand an applied stress without failure. Strength of materials is a subject which deals with loads, deformations and the forces acting on the material. It is also known by other names such as *mechanics of solids, mechanics of materials,* and *mechanics of deformable solids.*

The principal objective of mechanics of materials is to determine the stresses, strains, and displacements in structures and their components due to the loads acting on them and to ensure that the structure used will be safe against maximum internal effects that may be produced by any combination of loading.

- ***Rigid Body:*** A rigid body is an idealization of a solid body of finite size in which deformation is neglected. In other words, the distance between any two given points of a rigid body remains constant in time regardless of external forces exerted on it.
- ***Deformable body:*** A deformable body is a physical body that deforms, meaning it changes its shape or volume while being acted upon by an external force.

1.2 LOADS

Load may be defined as the combined effect of external forces acting on a body.

- The loads may be classified as
  - a. Dead/steady loads,
  - b. Live/variable/fluctuating loads,
  - c. Inertia loads
  - d. Centrifugal loads.
- Apart from these loads may also be classified as
  - i. Tensile loads,
  - ii. Compressive loads,
  - iii. Torsional/twisting load,
  - iv. Bending loads
  - v. Shear loads.
- Further loads can also be either as
  - i. Point/concentrated load
  - ii. Distributed load.

In general,

- ***Transverse loading***: Here the forces applied are perpendicular to the longitudinal axis of a member. Transverse loading causes the member to bend and deflect from its original position, with internal tensile and compressive strains accompanying change in curvature. Transverse loading also induces shear forces that cause shear deformation of the material and increase the transverse deflection of the member.
- ***Axial loading***: Here the applied forces are collinear with the longitudinal axes of the member. These forces cause the member to either stretch or shorten.
- ***Torsional loading***: Twisting action caused by a pair of externally applied equal and oppositely directed couples acting on parallel planes or by a single external couple applied to a member that has one end fixed against rotation.

1.3 STRESS

When a body is subjected to a load within the elastic limits, it develops an equal and opposite resisting force within the body. This resisting force per unit area is called stress.

$$\sigma = \frac{F}{A} \text{ MPa or N/mm}^2 \qquad \qquad \text{... (Eq. 1.1)}$$

where F = Force acting on the member or body (Newton)
A = Cross sectional area (mm^2)

The stresses are of the following types:

- ***Tensile stress:*** is the stress state caused by an applied load that tends to elongate the material in the axis of the applied load, in other words the stress caused by pulling the material. Due to this the length of the member increases, while its cross section decreases, as shown in **Fig. 1.1(a).**

  The strength of structures of equal cross sectional area loaded in tension is independent of shape of the cross section. Materials loaded in tension are susceptible to stress concentrations such as material defects or abrupt changes in geometry. However, materials exhibiting ductile behavior (most metals for example) can tolerate some defects while brittle materials (such as ceramics) can fail well below their ultimate material strength.

- *Compressive stress:* is the stress state caused by an applied load that acts to reduce the length of the material (compression member) in the axis of the applied load, in other words the stress state caused by squeezing/pushing the material. Due to this the length of the member decreases, while its cross-section increases, as shown in **Fig. 1.1(b)**.

Compressive strength for materials is generally higher than their tensile strength. However, structures loaded in compression are subject to additional failure modes dependent on geometry, such as Euler buckling.

In general the tensile and compressive stresses are referred to as normal stresses.

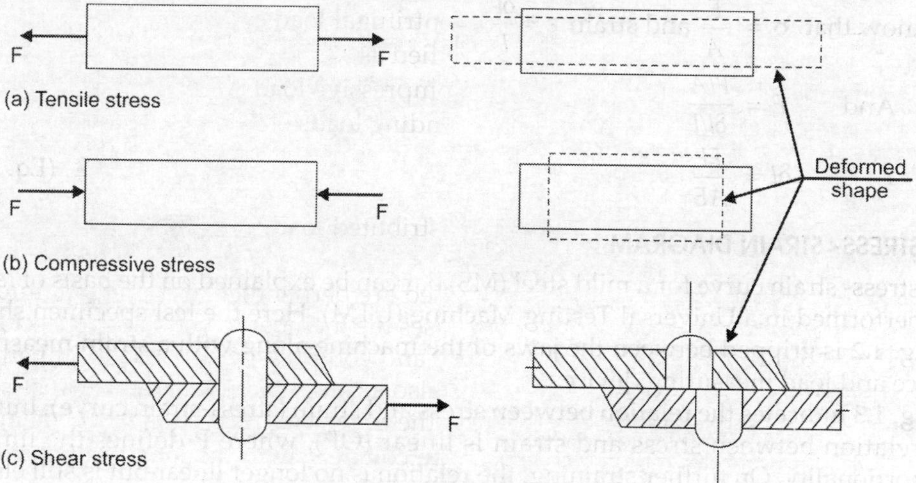

Fig. 1.1: Types of stresses

- *Shear stress (τ):* is the stress state caused by a pair of opposing forces acting along parallel lines of action through the material, in other words the stress caused by faces of the material sliding relative to one another. An example is cutting paper with scissors or stresses due to torsional loading, or a rivet subjected to tensile loading, as shown in **Fig. 1.1(c)**.

1.4 STRAIN (ε)

The deformation of a body per unit length is called strain. The deformation can be elongation/contraction.

The strains are of the following types:

- *Tensile strain:* When a body is subjected to tensile stress, the strain produced in the body is referred to as tensile strain. Due to this the length of the member increases, while its cross section decreases, as shown in **Fig. 1.1(a)**.

$$\varepsilon = \frac{\text{change in length}}{\text{original length}} = \frac{\delta l}{l} \qquad \qquad \dots \text{(Eq. 1.2)}$$

- *Compressive strain:* When a body is subjected to compressive stress, the strain produced in the body is referred to as compressive strain. Due to this the length of the member decreases, while its cross-section increases, as shown in **Fig. 1.1(b)**.
- *Shear strain:* When a body is subjected to shear stress, the strain produced in the body is referred to as shear strain.

1.5 HOOKE'S LAW

It states that, "when a body is loaded within the elastic limits, stress is directly proportional to strain".

$$\sigma \propto \varepsilon$$

$$\sigma = E \cdot \varepsilon$$

$$E = \sigma/\varepsilon \quad \text{MPa or N/mm}^2 \qquad \qquad \text{... (Eq. 1.3)}$$

E is a proportionality constant, known as Modulus of elasticity or Young's modulus

Relation between stress, strain and Young's modulus:

We know that $\sigma = \dfrac{F}{A}$ and strain $\varepsilon = \dfrac{\delta l}{l}$

And $\quad E = \dfrac{F/A}{\delta l/l}$

$$\therefore \quad \delta l = \frac{Fl}{AE} \qquad \qquad \text{... (Eq. 1.3a)}$$

1.6 STRESS- STRAIN DIAGRAM

The stress- strain curve for a mild steel (MS) bar can be explained on the basis of *tensile test* performed in a Universal Testing Machine (UTM). Here the test specimen shown in **Fig. 1.2** is gripped between the jaws of the machine along with a strain measuring device and load measuring device.

Fig. 1.3 indicates the relation between stress and strain (stress-strain curve). Initially the relation between stress and strain is linear (OP), where P defines the limit of proportionality. On further straining, the relation is no longer linear but is still elastic, i.e. the material regains its original shape and size upon the removal of applied load. The maximum load that can be applied without causing the material to undergo permanent deformation defines the elastic limit (PE). Point **A** marks the end of elastic state and initiation of plastic state, known as *upper yield point* (Y_U).

Upon further straining, there is a sudden drop in stress and then extension occurs at approximately constant stress, known as *lower yield point* (Y_L). After Y_L, stress increases with further increase in strain. This effect of the material being able to withstand greater stress despite uniform reduction in cross-sectional area is called *strain or work hardening.*

At S (design/working stress) the rate of work hardening is unable to keep pace with the rate of reduction in cross sectional area. Hence 'necking' (local strain hardening) takes place leading to fracture at B (Ultimate/fracture/breaking stress).

Fig. 1.4 indicates the failure of ductile and brittle materials. **Fig. 1.5** represents the stress-strain curve for different materials.

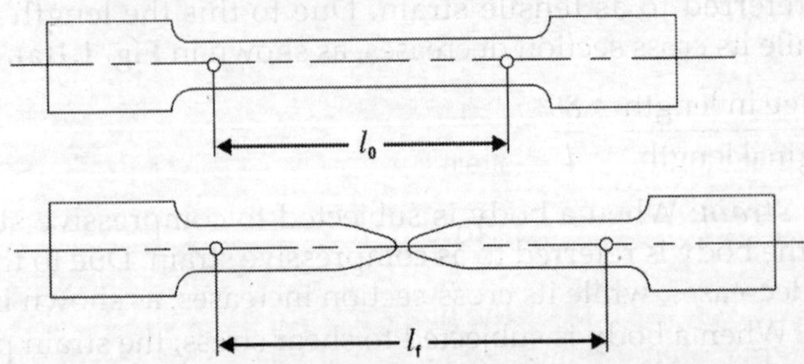

Fig. 1.2: Test specimen made of ductile

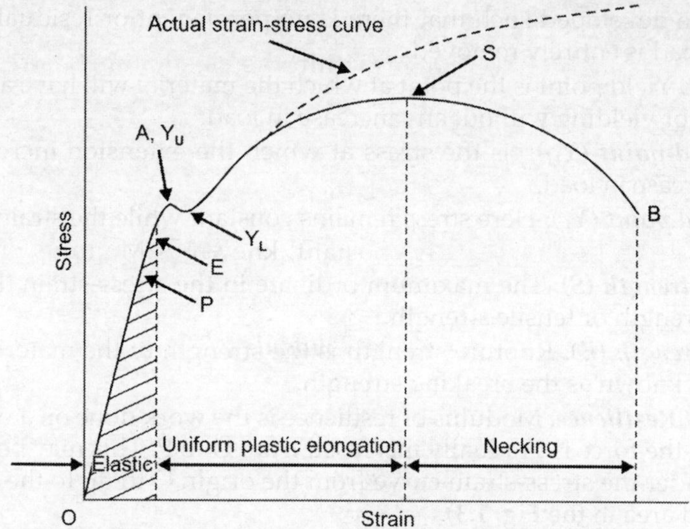

Fig. 1.3: Stress–strain curve for ductile material (MS)

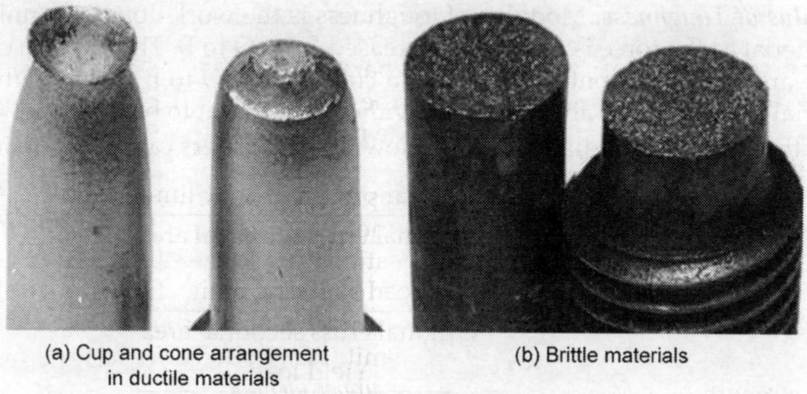

(a) Cup and cone arrangement
in ductile materials

(b) Brittle materials

Fig. 1.4: Failure of specimen

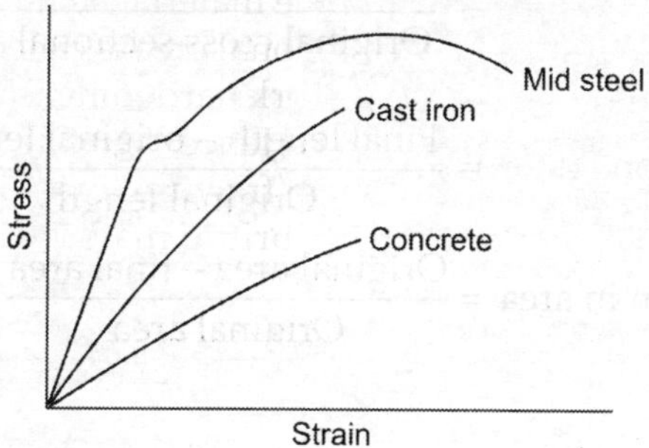

Fig. 1.5: Stress–strain curve for various materials

- *Limit of proportionality:* refers to the limit until which stress is directly proportional to strain.
- *Elastic Limit:* The elastic limit is the limit beyond which the material will no longer regains its original shape when the load is removed, or it is the maximum stress

that may be developed such that there is no permanent or residual deformation when the load is entirely removed.

- **Yield Point:** Yield point is the point at which the material will have an appreciable elongation or yielding without any increase in load.
- **Upper yield point (Y_u):** is the stress at which the extension increases without further increase in load.
- **Lower yield point (Y_L):** Here stress remains constant while the strain increases for some time.
- **Ultimate strength (S):** The maximum ordinate in the stress-strain diagram is the ultimate strength or tensile strength.
- **Rupture strength (B):** Rupture strength is the strength of the material at rupture. This is also known as the breaking strength.
- **Modulus of Resilience:** Modulus of resilience is the work done on a unit volume of material as the force is gradually increased from O to P. This may be calculated as the area under the stress-strain curve from the origin O to up to the elastic limit E (the shaded area in the **Fig. 1.3**).

  The resilience of the material is its ability to absorb energy without creating a permanent distortion.
- **Modulus of Toughness:** Modulus of toughness is the work done on a unit volume of material as the force is gradually increased from O to B. This may be calculated as the area under the entire stress-strain curve (from O to B). The toughness of a material is its ability to absorb energy without causing it to break.

From the stress- strain diagram, the following parameters can be evaluated:

- Limit of proportionality $= \dfrac{\text{Load at proportionally limit}}{\text{Original cross sectional area}}$ ... (Eq. 1.4)

- Elastic limit $= \dfrac{\text{Load at elastic limit}}{\text{Original cross sectional area}}$ ... (Eq. 1.5)

- Yield strength $= \dfrac{\text{Yield load}}{\text{Original cross sectional area}}$ ... (Eq. 1.6)

- Ultimate strength $= \dfrac{\text{Maximum tensile load}}{\text{Original cross sectional area}}$ ... (Eq. 1.7)

- Percentage elongation $= \dfrac{\text{Final length} - \text{original length}}{\text{Original length}} = \dfrac{l_f - l_o}{l_o}$ ... (Eq. 1.8)

- Percentage reduction in area $= \dfrac{\text{Original area} - \text{final area}}{\text{Original area}} = \dfrac{A_o - A_f}{A_o} \times 100$

  ...(Eq. 1.9)

1.7 FACTOR OF SAFETY (*n*)

It is defined as the ratio of ultimate stress to the working stress.

Factor of safety $n = \dfrac{\text{Ultimate stress}}{\text{Ultimate stress}} = \dfrac{\sigma_u}{\sigma_d}$ ... (Eq. 1.10a)

Ultimate stress: is the maximum stress that the material is subjected to during a test.
Working or allowable or design stress (σ_d): is defined as the maximum safe stress that the material can carry under a given load.

The allowable stress should be limited to a value not exceeding the proportional limit of the material so that Hooke's law is not invalidated. Working stress is based on yield point stress for ductile materials and ultimate strength for brittle materials.

$$n = \frac{\sigma_u}{\sigma_d} \quad \text{...used for brittle materials} \qquad \text{... (Eq. 1.10b)}$$

$$n = \frac{\sigma_y}{\sigma_d} \quad \text{...used for ductile materials} \qquad \text{... (Eq. 1.10c)}$$

1.8 MECHANICAL PROPERTIES OF MATERIALS

Following are some of the most important mechanical properties of engineering materials:

- ***Elasticity:*** is the ability of a material to regain its original shape and size, when the load causing the deformation is removed. *Example: Steel, copper, aluminium, concrete, etc.*
- ***Plasticity:*** is the property of a material which does not regain its original shape and size, when the load causing the deformation is removed.
- ***Strength:*** is the ability of a material to withstand the action of external forces.
- ***Toughness:*** is the property of a material which absorbs energy elastically before failure, i.e. to withstand elastic and plastic deformation.
- ***Stiffness or rigidity:*** is the ability of a material to resist elastic deformation.
- ***Hardness:*** is the property of a material which resists indentation/ penetration or property of a material to resist plastic deformation.
- ***Resilience:*** is the property of a material to absorb energy elastically.
- ***Ductility:*** is the property of a material of drawing it into wires. *Example: Mild steel (MS)*
- ***Brittleness:*** is the property of the material which breaks easily into pieces. *Example: Cast iron*
- ***Malleability:*** is the property of the material which can be beaten into sheets. *Example: MS, aluminium, etc.*
- ***Creep:*** refers to the slow and progressive deformation of a material with time at constant stress. .
- ***Fatigue:*** refers to the behavior of a material when subjected to fluctuating or repeated loads.
- ***Fracture:*** refers to the separation of a material into two or more parts under stress.
    - **a. *Ductile fracture:*** This occurs after extensive plastic deformation and is characterized by slow crack propagation.
    - **b. *Brittle fracture:*** This occurs by rapid propagation of a crack after little or no plastic deformation.

Apart from these, a metal should have good thermal and electrical conductivities.

- ***Thermal conductivity:*** is defined as the rate at which heat can flow through a material under the influence of a given temperature gradient.
- ***Electrical conductivity:*** It is a measure of the material's ability to accommodate the transport of an electric charge.

Other classifications of materials include:

- *Homogeneous material:* A material which has a uniform structure throughout without any flaws or discontinuities is termed a homogeneous material.
- *Non-homogeneous or inhomogeneous material:* Materials such as concrete and poor-quality cast iron will thus have a structure which varies from point to point depending on its constituents and the presence of casting flaws or impurities.
- *Isotropic material:* If a material exhibits uniform properties throughout in all directions it is said to be isotropic
- *Non-isotropic or Anisotropic material:* If a material does not exhibits uniform properties throughout in all directions it is said to be non-isotropic or anisotropic.
- *Orthotropic material:* An orthotropic material is one which has different properties in different planes.

A typical example of such a material is wood, although some composites which contain systematically orientated "inhomogeneities" may also be considered to fall into this category

1.9 DIFFERENCE BETWEEN DUCTILE AND BRITTLE MATERIALS

Sl No.	Ductile material	Brittle material
1.	Material fails by yielding. (Necking occurs before failure).	Material fails by fracture.
2.	Ductility of a material is its ability to deform when a tensile force is applied upon it. It is also referred to as the ability of a substance to withstand plastic deformation without undergoing rupture.	Brittleness, on the other hand is exactly an opposite property of ductility as it is the ability of a material to break without first undergoing any kind of deformation upon application of force.
3.	A ductile material is one with a large Percentage of elongation before failure.	Brittle material is one which is having very low percentage of elongation.
4.	If the percentage of elongation is $\geq 5\%$, the material is ductile.	If the percentage of elongation is $< 5\%$, the material is brittle.
5.	For ductile material, the ultimate tensile and compressive strength have approximately the same absolute value.	Brittle materials break suddenly under stress at a point just beyond its elastic limit. Design is based on ultimate stress.
6.	Design is based on yield strength.	Brittle materials fail due to tensile (normal) stresses and rupture occurs along a surface perpendicular to the load.
7.	Ductile materials usually fail on planes that correspond to the maximum shear stresses (45°).	
8.	Material can be drawn into wires.	Breaks into pieces.
9.	Examples: Steel, high strength alloys, aluminium, gold, etc.	Examples: Cast iron, glass, stone, etc.

1.10 TRUE STRESS AND TRUE STRAIN

- *True stress ($\bar{\sigma}$):* is defined as the ratio of instantaneous load to that of instantaneous cross-sectional area at a given instant of time. The true stress is given as

$$\bar{\sigma} = \sigma(1+\varepsilon) = \frac{F_f}{A_f}$$

... (Eq. 1.11)

- **True strain ($\bar{\varepsilon}$):** is defined as the ratio of instantaneous change in length to the instantaneous length at a given instant of time. The true strain is given as

$$\bar{\varepsilon} = \ln(1+\varepsilon) \qquad \qquad \text{... (Eq. 1.12)}$$

For volume consistency, $A_f l_f = A_o l_o$ ... (Eq. 1.13)

σ = Conventional or engineering or nominal stress = $\dfrac{F_o}{A_o}$

ε = Conventional or engineering strain

F_o = Load

F_f = Load at failure

A_o = Original cross sectional area

A_f = Final cross sectional area

- **Proof stress:** is the stress necessary to cause permanent extension equal to defined percentage (say 0.2%). Proof stress can be expressed as the stress at which the stress-strain diagram departs by a specified percentage of the gauge length from the produced straight line of proportionality. If the specified percentage is 0.2% of the gauge length, the corresponding proof stress is designated as 0.2% proof stress.

    The proof stress of a material is determined by drawing a straight line parallel to the linear portion of the stress-strain diagram from a point which is equal to the specified percentage of the strain on the gauge length as shown in **Fig. 1.6**. The intersection of this line with the stress-strain curve represents 0.2 % proof stress for the material.

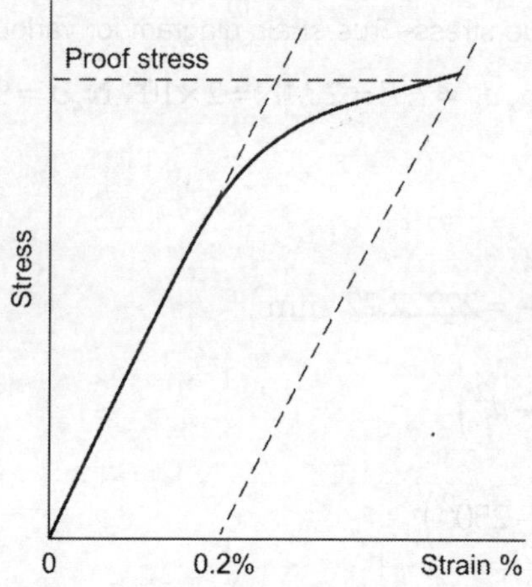

Fig. 1.6: Determination of proof stress

Fig. 1.7 Indicates true stress-true strain diagram for various materials

1. **A steel rod of 30 mm × 30 mm carries an axial load of 100 kN. Calculate the deformation of the bar if E = 2.1 GPa and length of the rod is 50 mm.**

Solution: $A = 30 \times 30 = 900$ mm^2, $F = 100$ kN, $\delta l = ?$, $E = 2.1 \times 10^5$ MPa, $l = 50$ mm.

We know that, $\delta l = \dfrac{Fl}{AE} = \dfrac{100 \times 10^3 \times 50}{900 \times 2.1 \times 10^5} = 0.0265$ mm

2. **A cast iron (C.I) column has an internal diameter of 250 mm. what should be the minimum external diameter, so that it may carry a load of 2 MN, without the stress exceeding 90 MPa.**

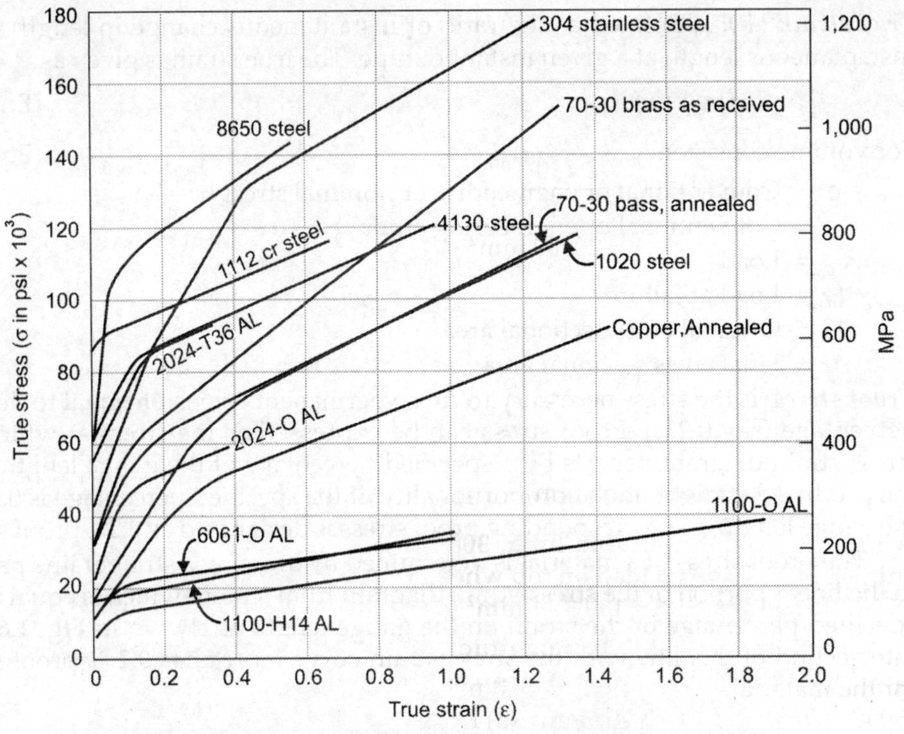

Fig. 1.7: True stress–True strain diagram for various materials

Solution: $d_i = 250$ mm, $d_o = ?, F = 2$ MN $= 2 \times 10^6$ N$, \sigma = 90$ MPa

We know that $\sigma = \dfrac{F}{A}$

i.e. $A = \dfrac{2 \times 10^6}{90} = 22222.22$ mm^2

But $A = \dfrac{\pi}{4}\left(d_o^2 - d_i^2\right)$

$$22222.22 = \dfrac{\pi}{4}\left(d_o^2 - 250^2\right)$$

$$d_o^2 = 9.08 \times 10^4 \text{ mm}^2$$

$\therefore \qquad d_o = 301.32$ mm $\simeq 302$ mm

3. **A hollow steel column of external diameter 300 mm has to support an axial load of 2 MN. If ultimate stress for steel is 400 MPa, find the internal diameter, if factor of safety is 4.**

Solution: $d_o = 300$ mm, $d_i = ? \ F = 2$ MN $= 2 \times 10^6$ N, $\sigma_u = 400$ MPa, factor of safety $n = 4$

We know that $\sigma = \dfrac{F}{A}$ ... Eq. (i)

But $n = \dfrac{\sigma_u}{\sigma_d}$

$$4 = \frac{400}{\sigma_d}$$

$$\therefore \qquad \sigma_d = \sigma = 100 \text{ MPa}$$

$$\therefore \quad \text{Eq. (i) yields...} \quad 100 = \frac{2 \times 10^6}{A}$$

$$A = 20000 \text{ mm}^2$$

Also $\quad A = \frac{\pi}{4}\left(d_o^2 - d_i^2\right)$

$$20000 = \frac{\pi}{4}\left(300^2 - d_i^2\right)$$

$$d_i^2 = 64.54 \times 10^3 \text{ mm}^2$$

$$\therefore \quad d_i = 254.05 \text{ mm} \approx 255 \text{ mm}$$

4. A hollow C.I cylinder 4 m long, 300 mm outer diameter and 50 mm thick is subjected to a central load on top when standing straight. The stress produced is 75 MN/m². Assume $E = 150$ kN/mm² and find

a. Magnitude of load   b. Longitudinal strain   c. Total decrease in length.

Solution: $l = 4$ m $= 4000$ mm, $d_o = 300$ mm, $t = 50$ mm, $\sigma = 75$ MN/m² $= 75$ N/mm², $E = 150$ kN/mm² $= 150 \times 10^3$ N/mm². (a) $F = ?$ (b) $\varepsilon = ?$ (c) $\delta l = ?$

a. *To find F:*

We know that $\quad \sigma = \dfrac{F}{A}$

$$F = \sigma A = \sigma \times \frac{\pi}{4}\left(d_o^2 - d_i^2\right) \qquad [d_i = d_0 - 2t = 300 - 2 \times 50 = 200 \text{ mm}]$$

$$= 75 \times \frac{\pi}{4}\left(300^2 - 200^2\right)$$

$$F = 2.945 \times 10^6 \text{ N}$$

b. *To find ε:* $\qquad E = \dfrac{\sigma}{\varepsilon} \Rightarrow \varepsilon = \dfrac{\sigma}{E} = \dfrac{75}{150 \times 10^3} = 0.0005$

c. *To find δl:* $\qquad \varepsilon = \dfrac{\delta l}{\varepsilon} \Rightarrow \delta l = \varepsilon l = 0.0005 \times 4000 = 2 \text{ mm}$

5. A signal is being worked by a steel wire 750 m long and 6 mm in diameter. Find the movement which must be given to the signal box end of the wire at a pull of 1.6 kN, if the movement at the signal is to be 250 mm. Take $E = 2 \times 10^5$ N/mm².

VTU – (CV) June/ July 14 – 07 Marks

Solution: $l = 750 \times 10^3$ mm, $d = 6$ mm, $F = 1.6$ kN $= 1600$ N, $E = 2 \times 10^5$ N/mm², $\delta = 250$ mm, movement $= ?$

Here total movement, $\delta = \delta + \delta l$

But $\qquad \delta l = \dfrac{Fl}{AE} = \dfrac{1600 \times 750 \times 10^3}{(\pi \times 6^2 / 4) \times 2 \times 10^5} = 212.21 \text{ mm}$

$$\therefore \quad \Delta = 250 + 212.21 = 462.21 \text{ mm}$$

6. The following results were obtained on a tensile test specimen:

Original diameter = 20 mm, gauge length = 100 mm, limit at proportionality = 82 kN, extension = 0.12 mm. The specimen yielded a load of 86 kN and maximum load withstood was 153 kN.

Calculate: a. Stress at proportionality   b. Young's modulus

  c. yield stress   d. ultimate stress

Solution: d_o = 20 mm, l_o = 100 mm, $F_\alpha = 82 \times 10^3$ N, δl = 0.12, $F_y = 86 \times 10^3$ N, $F_u = 153 \times 10^3$ N. a) σ_α = ?, b) E = ?, c) σ_y = ?, d) σ_u = ?

a. To find σ_α:

$$\sigma_a = \frac{F_\alpha}{A_o} = \frac{82 \times 10^3}{(\pi \times 20^2 / 4)} = 261 \text{ MPa}$$

b. To find E:

$$E = \frac{\sigma_\alpha}{\varepsilon} = \frac{\sigma_\alpha}{\delta l / l_o} = \frac{261}{0.12/100} = 217.51 \times 10^3 \text{ MPa}$$

c. To find σ_y:

$$\sigma_y = \frac{F_y}{A_o} = \frac{86 \times 10^3}{(\pi \times 20^2 / 4)} = 273.74 \text{ MPa}$$

d. To find σ_u:

$$\sigma_u = \frac{F_u}{A_o} = \frac{153 \times 10^3}{(\pi \times 20^2 / 4)} = 487 \text{ MPa}$$

7. For the laboratory tested specimen the following data were obtained:

Diameter of the specimen = 25 mm, length of the specimen = 300 mm, extension under the load of 15 kN = 0.045 mm, load at yield point = 127.65 kN, maximum load = 208.60 kN, neck diameter = 17.75 mm, length of the specimen after failure = 375 mm

Determine: a. Young's modulus   b. Yield point stress
  c. Ultimate stress   d. Percentage elongation
  e. Percentage reduction in area
  f. Allowable stress, taking factor of safety as 2.

VTU – June/ July 2008 – 10 Marks; [Similar: (CV) June/ July 2013 – 10 Marks]

Solution: d_o = 25 mm, l_o = 300 mm, $F_\alpha = 15 \times 10^3$ N, δl = 0.045 mm, $F_y = 127.65 \times 10^3$ N, $F_u = 208.6 \times 10^3$ N, d_f = 17.75 mm, l_f = 375 mm. a) E = ?, b) σ_y = ?, c) σ_u = ?, d) Percentage elongation = ?, e) Percentage reduction in area = ?, f) allowable stress = ?, if factor of safety $n = 2$

a. To find E:

$$E = \frac{F_\alpha l_o}{A_o \delta l} = \frac{(15 \times 10^3) \times 300}{(\pi \times 25^2 / 4) \times 0.045} = 203.72 \times 10^3 \text{ MPa}$$

b. To find σ_y:

$$\sigma_u = \frac{F_y}{A_o} = \frac{127.65 \times 10^3}{(\pi \times 25^2 / 4)} = 260.05 \text{ MPa}$$

c. To find σ_u:

$$\sigma_u = \frac{F_u}{A_o} = \frac{208.60 \times 10^3}{(\pi \times 25^2 / 4)} = 425 \text{ MPa}$$

d. Percentage elongation: Percentage elongation $\left(\dfrac{l_f - l_o}{l_o}\right) \times 100 = \left(\dfrac{375 - 300}{300}\right)$

$$\times 100 = 25\%$$

e. Percentage reduction in area: Percentage reduction in area

$$= \left(\frac{A_o - A_f}{A_o}\right) \times 100 = \left(\frac{25^2 - 17.75^2}{25^2}\right) \times 100 = 49.59\ \%$$

f. Allowable stress: Allowable or safe stress $= \dfrac{\sigma_y}{n} = \dfrac{260.05}{2} = 130.025\ \text{MPa}$

8. The tensile stress was conducted on a mild steel bar. The following data was obtained from the test:

Diameter of steel bar = 16 mm, gauge length of the bar = 80 mm, load at proportionality limit = 72 kN, extension at a load of 60 kN = 0.115 mm, load at failure = 80 kN, final gauge length of the bar = 104 mm, diameter of rod at failure = 12 mm. Determine:

a. Young's modulus   **b. Proportionality limit**

c. True breaking stress   **d. Percentage elongation.**

VTU – June/ July 2013 – 10 Marks; Dec. 14/ Jan. 15 – 08 Marks

Solution: $d_o = 16$ mm, $l_o = 80$ mm, $F_\alpha = 72 \times 10^3$ N, $F = 60 \times 10^3$ N, $\delta l = 0.115$ mm, $F_f = 80 \times 10^3$ N, $d_f = 12$ mm, $l_f = 104$ mm. a) $E = ?$, b) $\sigma_\alpha = ?$, c) $\sigma_b = ?$, d) Percentage elongation $= ?$,

a. To find E $E = \dfrac{F l_o}{A_o \delta l} = \dfrac{(60 \times 10^3) \times 80}{(\pi \times 16^2 / 4) \times 0.115} = 207.59 \times 10^3\ \text{MPa}$

b. To find $\sigma_\alpha = \dfrac{F_\alpha}{A_o} = \dfrac{72 \times 10^3}{(\pi \times 16^2 / 4)} = 358\ \text{MPa}$

c. To find $\sigma_f = \dfrac{F_f}{A_f} = \dfrac{80 \times 10^3}{(\pi \times 12^2 / 4)} = 707.36\ \text{MPa}$

d. Percentage elongation:

$$\text{Percentage elongation} \ = \left(\frac{l_f - l_o}{l_o}\right) \times 100 = \left(\frac{104 - 80}{80}\right) \times 100 = 30\%$$

9. A tensile specimen with 12 mm diameter and 50 mm gauge length reaches a maximum load of 90 kN and fractures at 70 kN. The minimum diameter at fracture is 10 mm.

Determine: **a. The engineering stress at maximum load**

b. True stress   **c. Engineering strain**   **d. True strain**

Solution: $d_o = 12$ mm, $l_o = 50$ mm, $F = 90$ kN, $F_f = 70$ kN, $d_f = 10$ mm. a) $\sigma = ?$, b) $\bar{\sigma} = ?$, c) $\varepsilon = ?$, d) $\bar{\varepsilon} = ?$

a. Engineering stress (σ) $\qquad \sigma = \dfrac{F}{A_o} = \dfrac{90 \times 10^3}{(\pi \times 12^2 / 4)} = 795.78 \text{ MPa}$

b. True stress ($\bar{\sigma}$) $\qquad \bar{\sigma} = \dfrac{F_f}{A_f} = \dfrac{70 \times 10^3}{(\pi \times 10^2 / 4)} = 891.27 \text{ MPa}$

c. Engineering strain (σ) $\qquad \varepsilon = \dfrac{\delta l}{l} = \dfrac{l_f - l_o}{l_o}$ $\qquad\qquad\qquad$ ... Eq. (i)

$$\text{But for volume consistency,} \quad A_f l_f = A_o l_o$$

$$l_f = \frac{A_o l_o}{A_f} = \frac{d_0^2 l_o}{d_f^2} = \frac{12^2 \times 50}{10^2} = 72 \text{ mm}$$

$\therefore$ Eq. (i) yields... $\qquad\qquad \varepsilon = \dfrac{72 - 50}{50} = 0.44$

d. Engineering strain $= \bar{\varepsilon} = \ln(1 + \varepsilon) = \ln(1 + 0.44) = 0.3646$

10. A 50 mm diameter forging billet is decreased in height from 125 mm to 50 mm. Determine the engineering strain and true strain in the direction of compression. Also compute final diameter after fracture.

Solution: $d_o = 50$ mm, $l_o = 125$ mm, $l_f = 50$ mm, $\varepsilon = ?$, $\bar{\varepsilon} = ?$, $d_f = ?$

a. Engineering strain (ε) $\qquad \varepsilon = \dfrac{\delta l}{l} = \dfrac{l_f - l_o}{l_o} = \dfrac{50 - 125}{125} = -0.6$

$\qquad\qquad\qquad\qquad\qquad\qquad\qquad\qquad$ (negative because compression)

b. True strain ($\bar{\varepsilon}$) $\qquad\qquad \bar{\varepsilon} = \ln(1 + \varepsilon) = \ln(1 - 0.6) = -0.916$

c. To find d_f: For volume consistency, $A_f l_f = A_o l_o$

$$A_f = \frac{A_o l_o}{l_f}$$

$$d_f^2 = \frac{d_o^2 l_o}{l_f}$$

$$\therefore \ d_f = \sqrt{\frac{50^2 \times 125}{50}} = 79.06 \text{ mm}$$

1.11 DEFORMATION IN BARS OF VARYING CROSS-SECTION

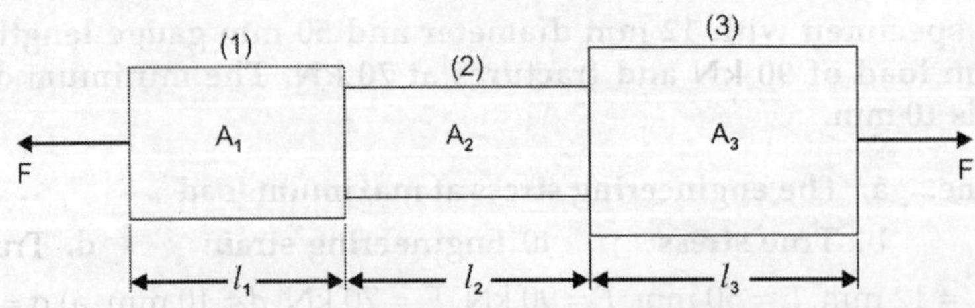

Fig. 1.8: Bars of varying cross-section

Consider a bar of varying cross section subjected to tensile load (F) as shown in **Fig. 1.8.** Here the total deformation of the bar is equal to the sum of deformations of individual sections.

$$\text{Let,} \quad F = \text{Tensile force.}$$

$$E = \text{Young's modulus of the material,}$$

$$l_1 = \text{Length of section (1),}$$

$$A_1 = \text{Area of section (1),}$$

Similarly, $l_2, A_2; l_3, A_3$ be corresponding values of sections (2) & (3) respectively.

Since, total deformation $\quad \Delta = \delta l_1 + \delta l_2 + \delta l_3 + \dots$

$$= \frac{Fl_1}{A_1 E} + \frac{Fl_2}{A_2 E} + \frac{Fl_3}{A_3 E}$$

$$\Delta = \frac{F}{E}\left[\frac{l_1}{A_1} + \frac{l_2}{A_2} + \frac{l_3}{A_3} \right] \qquad \dots \text{(Eq. 1.14)}$$

...This equation is used when the bar is made of same material (E is constant)

$$\Delta = F\left[\frac{l_1}{A_1 E_1} + \frac{l_2}{A_2 E_2} + \frac{l_3}{A_3 E_3} \right] \qquad \dots \text{(Eq. 1.15)}$$

... This equation is used when the bar is made of different materials.

11. **A steel bar is 900 mm long and has rods of diameters 40 mm and 30 mm at either ends. The length of each rod is 200 mm. The middle portion has a diameter of 15 mm for the remaining length. If the bar is subjected to an axial pull of 15 kN, find its total elongation. Take E = 200 GPa.**

Solution: $l = 900$ mm, $d_1 = 40$ mm, $d_3 = 30$ mm, $l_1 = l_3 = 200$ mm, $d_2 = 15$ mm, $l_2 = 900\text{–}400 = 500$ mm, $F = 15 \times 10^3$, N, $E = 200 \times 10^3$ MPa, $\Delta = ?$

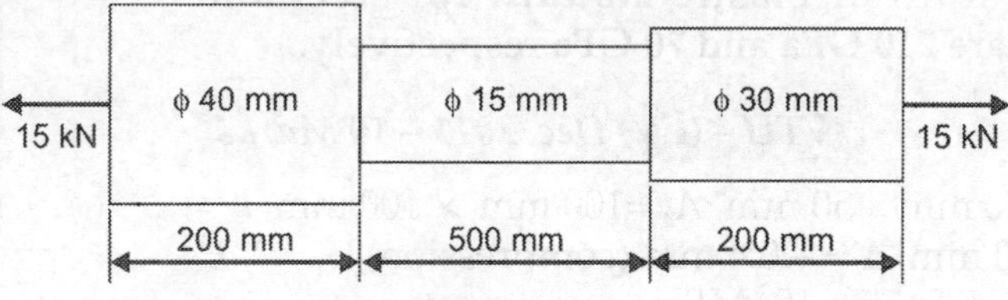

Fig. 1.9: Problem 11

Total deformation, $\qquad \Delta = \delta l_1 + \delta l_2 + \delta l_3$

Since the bar is made of same material, we have

$$\Delta = \frac{F}{E}\left[\frac{l_1}{A_1} + \frac{l_2}{A_2} + \frac{l_3}{A_3} \right]$$

$$= \frac{15 \times 10^3}{200 \times 10^3}\left[\frac{200}{(\pi \times 40^2 / 4)} + \frac{500}{(\pi \times 15^2 / 4)} + \frac{200}{(\pi \times 30^2 / 4)} \right]$$

$$\therefore \quad \Delta = 0.2454 \text{ mm}$$

12. The bar shown in Fig. 1.10 is tested in universal testing machine. It is observed that at a load of 40 kN the total extension is 0.285 mm. Determine the Young's modulus of the material.

VTU – Dec. 2012 – 09 Marks; June/ July 2016 – 07 Marks

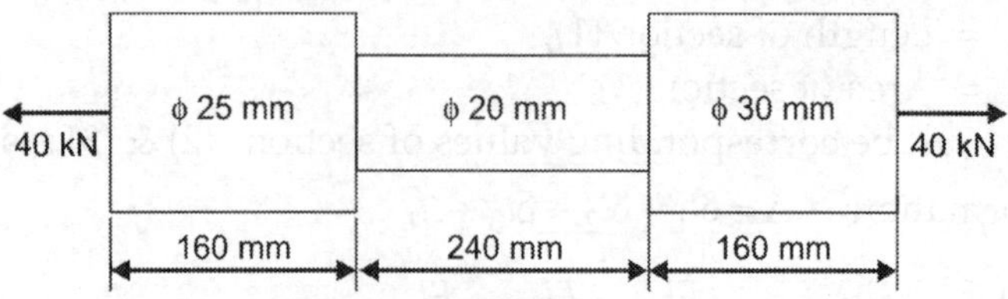

Fig. 1.10: Problem 11

Solution: $d_1 = 25$ mm, $d_2 = 20$ mm, $d_3 = 30$ mm, $l_1 = l_3 = 160$ mm, $l_2 = 240$ mm, $F = 40 \times 10^3$ N, $E = ?$, $\Delta = 0.285$ mm

Total deformation, $\Delta = \delta l_1 + \delta l_2 + \delta l_3$

Since the bar is made of same material, we have

$$\Delta = \frac{F}{E}\left[\frac{l_1}{A_1} + \frac{l_2}{A_2} + \frac{l_3}{A_3}\right]$$

$$0.285 = \frac{40 \times 10^3}{E}\left[\frac{160}{(\pi \times 25^2/4)} + \frac{240}{(\pi \times 20^2/4)} + \frac{160}{(\pi \times 30^2/4)}\right]$$

$$\therefore \quad E = 1.85 \times 10^5 \text{ MPa}$$

13. A member is formed by connecting a steel bar to an aluminium bar as shown in Fig. 1.11. Assuming that the bars are prevented from buckling sideways, calculate the magnitude of an axial force that will cause the total length of the member to decrease by 0.4 mm. The values of elastic modulli for steel and aluminium are 210 GPa and 70 GPa respectively.

VTU – (CV) Dec. 2011 – 10 Marks

Solution: $A_s = 50$ mm $\times$ 50 mm, $A_a = 100$ mm $\times$ 100 mm, $l_s = 400$ mm, $l_a = 500$ mm, $\Delta = -0.4$ mm (compression), $F = ?$, $E_s = 210 \times 10^3$ MPa, $E_a = 70 \times 10^3$ MPa

Total deformation, $\Delta = \delta l_1 + \delta l_2$

Since the bar is made of different materials, we have

$$\Delta = F\left[\frac{l_s}{A_s E_s} + \frac{l_a}{A_a E_a}\right]$$

$$-0.4 = F\left[\frac{400}{(50 \times 50) \times 210 \times 10^3} + \frac{500}{(100 \times 100) \times 70 \times 10^3}\right]$$

$$\therefore \quad F = -270.90 \times 10^3 \text{ N}$$

$$= 270.96 \text{ kN (compression)}$$

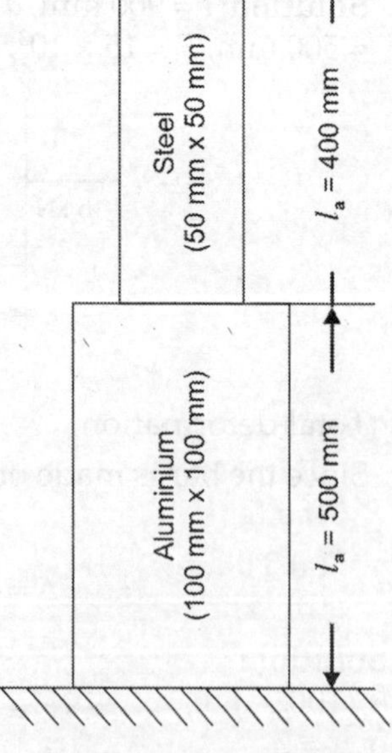

Fig. 1.11: Problem 13

14. **A steel tie rod 50 mm in diameter and 2.5 m long is subjected to a pull of 100 kN. To what length the bar should be bored centrally so that the total extension will increase by 15% under the same pull, the bore being 25 mm in diameter. Take $E = 200$ GPa.**

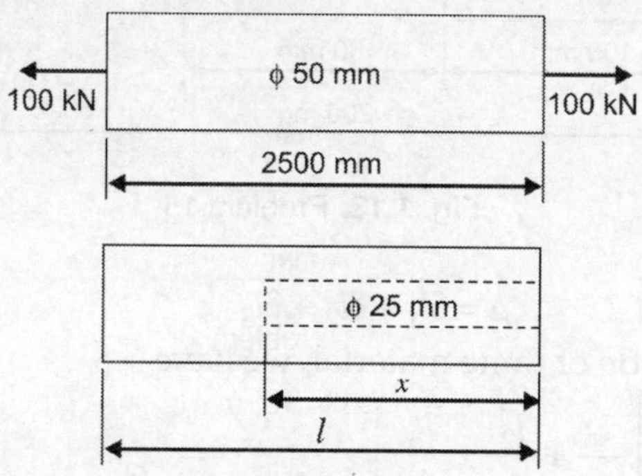

Fig. 1.12: Problem 14

Solution: $d = 50$ mm, $l = 2500$ mm, $F = 100 \times 10^3$ N, $x = ?$, bore dia $d_1 = 25$ mm, $E = 200 \times 10^3$ MPa, $\delta l = 15\% = 0.15$

a. Solid rod: $\delta l = \dfrac{Fl}{AE} = \dfrac{100 \times 10^3 \times 2500}{(\pi \times 50^2 / 4) \times 200 \times 10^3} = 0.6366$ mm.

b. Rod with bore:

Increase in elongation,
$$\Delta = 15\% \ \delta l$$
$$\Delta = 1.15 \times 0.6366 = 0.7321 \text{ mm}$$

Since the bar is made of same material, we have

$$\Delta = \frac{F}{E}\left[\frac{l_1}{A_1} + \frac{l_2}{A_2} + \frac{l_3}{A_3}\right]$$

$$0.7321 = \frac{100 \times 10^3}{200 \times 10^3}\left[\frac{2500 - x}{(\pi \times 50^2 / 4)} + \frac{x}{[\pi \times (50^2 - 25^2)/4]}\right]$$

$$1.4642 = [5.09 \times 10^{-4}(2500 - x)] + 6.79 \times 10^{-4} x$$

$$= 1.2725 + 1.79 \times 10^{-4} x$$

$$\therefore x = 1127.6 \text{ mm} = 1.12 \text{ m}$$

15. **A bar 350 mm long is 50 mm square in section for a length of 100 mm, 30 mm in diameter for a length of 60 mm and 40 mm in diameter for the remaining length. If a tensile load of 120 kN is applied to the bar, determine:**

(a) **The total elongation**

(b) **The maximum and minimum stress. Take $E = 210$ GPa.**

Solution: $A_1 = 50$ mm $\times$ 50 mm, $d_2 = 30$ mm, $d_3 = 40$ mm $l_1 = 100$ mm, $l_2 = 60$ mm $l_3 = 350 - (100 + 60) = 190$ mm, $F = 120 \times 10^3$ N, $E = 210 \times 10^3$ MPa. a) $\Delta = ?$ b) σ_{max}, $\sigma_{min} = ?$

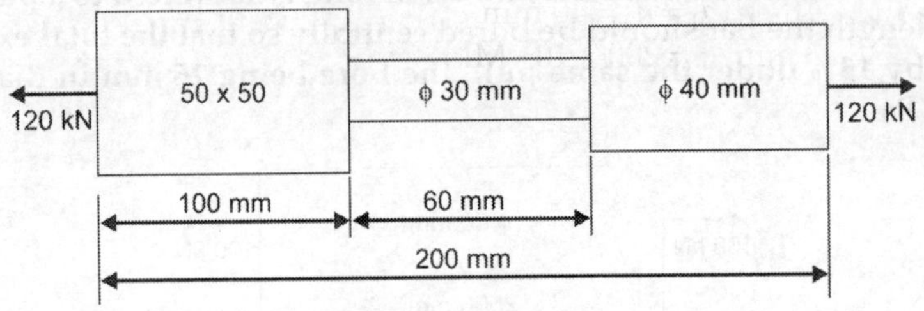

Fig. 1.13: Problem 15

a. To find Δ:

Total deformation, $\qquad \Delta = \delta l_1 + \delta l_2 + \delta l_3$

Since the bar is made of same material, we have

$$\Delta = \frac{F}{E}\left[\frac{l_1}{A_1} + \frac{l_2}{A_2} + \frac{l_3}{A_3}\right]$$

$$= \frac{120\times10^3}{210\times10^3}\left[\frac{100}{(50\times50)} + \frac{60}{(\pi\times30^2/4)} + \frac{190}{(\pi\times40^2/4)}\right]$$

$$\therefore \Delta = 0.1578 \text{ mm}$$

b. Stresses:

$$\sigma_1 = \frac{F}{A_1} = \frac{120\times10^3}{500\times50} = 48 \text{ MPa}$$

$$\sigma_2 = \frac{F}{A_2} = \frac{120\times10^3}{(\pi\times30^2/4)} = 169.76 \text{ MPa}$$

$$\sigma_3 = \frac{F}{A_3} = \frac{120\times10^3}{(\pi\times40^2/4)} = 95.49 \text{ MPa}$$

Thus $\sigma_{max} = 169.76$ MPa and $\sigma_{min} = 48$ MPa

16. **The bar shown in Fig. 1.14 is subjected to loading. Find the diameter of the middle portion if the stress there is to be limited to 100 N/mm². Also find the length of the middle portion, if the total extension of the bar is to be 0.13 mm. Take E = 200 GPa.**

VTU – (CV) Jan. 2013 – 12 Marks

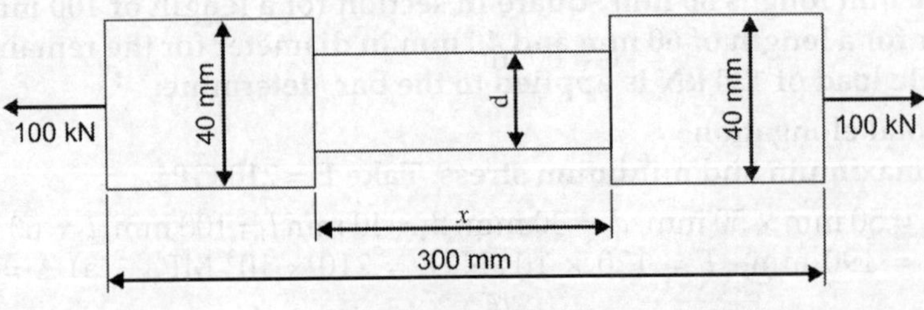

Fig. 1.14: Problem 16

Solution: $F = 100 \times 10^3$ N, $d_1 = d_3 = 40$ mm $\Rightarrow A_1 = A_3 = 1256.64$ mm^2, $l = 300$ mm, $\sigma_2 = 100$ N/mm^2, $\Delta = 0.13$ mm, $E = 200 \times 10^3$ MPa, $d_2 = ?$, $x = ?$

a. To find d_2 $\sigma_2 = \dfrac{F}{A_2}$

$$100 = \frac{100 \times 10^3}{\pi d_2^2 / 4}$$

$$d_2 = 35.68 \text{ mm}$$

b. To find x:

Since diameters are same, $\sigma_1 = \sigma_3 = \dfrac{F}{A_3} = \dfrac{100 \times 10^3}{1256.64} = 79.58$ MPa

Since the bar is made of same material, we have

$$\Delta = \delta l_{end\ portion} + \delta l_{mid\ portion}$$

$$0.13 = \left[\frac{\sigma_1 (l - x)}{E} + \frac{\sigma_2 x}{E} \right]$$

$$= \frac{1}{200 \times 10^3} [79.58 \times (300 - x) + 100x]$$

$$26000 = (23874 - 79.58x) + 100x$$

$$2126 = 20.42x$$

$$\therefore x = 104.11 \text{ mm}$$

17. **A tie bar is as shown in Fig. 1.15. If the middle portion is also of square cross section, find its size and length. The stress in the middle portion is not to exceed 140 MPa. The total extension is 0.14 mm and E = 200 GPa. Take F = 87.5 kN**

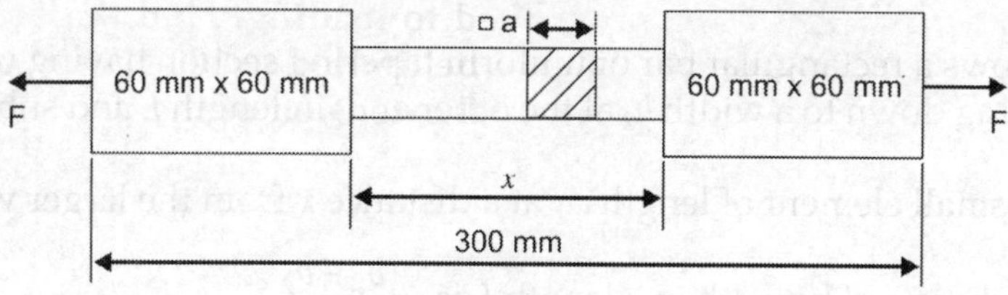

Fig. 1.15: Problem 17

Solution: $F = 87.5 \times 10^3$ N, $A_1 = A_3 = 60$ mm $\times$ 60 mm $= 3600$ mm^2, $l = 300$ mm, $\sigma_2 = 140$ N/mm^2, $\Delta = 0.14$ mm, $E = 200 \times 10^3$ MPa, $a = ?$, $x = ?$

a. To find a: $\sigma_2 = \dfrac{F}{A_2}$

$$140 = \frac{87.5 \times 10^3}{a^2} \qquad (here\ A_2 = a^2)$$

$$a = 25 \text{ mm}.$$

b. *To find* x:

Since cross section is same, $\sigma_1 = \sigma_3 = \dfrac{F}{A_3} = \dfrac{87.5 \times 10^3}{3600} = 24.31$ MPa

Since the bar is made of same material, we have

$$\delta = \delta l_{end\ portions} + \delta l_{mid\ portion}$$

$$0.14 = \left[\frac{\sigma_1(l-x)}{E} + \frac{\sigma_2 x}{E}\right]$$

$$= \frac{1}{200 \times 10^3}[24.31 \times (300-x) + 140x]$$

$$28000 = 7293 - 24.31x + 140x$$

$$20707 = 115.69x$$

$$x = 178.98 \text{ mm}$$

1.12 DEFORMATION IN BARS OF UNIFORMLY TAPERING RECTANGULAR CROSS-SECTION (BAR)

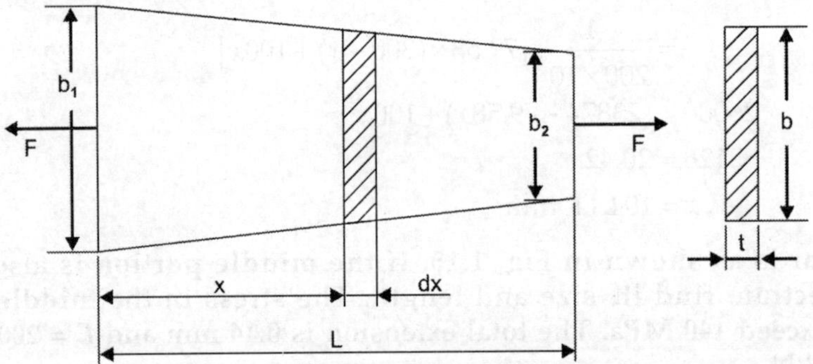

Fig. 1.16: Elongation in bar of uniform tapering rectangular c/s

Fig. 1.16 shows a rectangular bar of uniform tapering section having width b_1 at one end and tapering down to a width b_2 at the other end, in length L and subjected to axial force F.

Consider a small element of length dx at a distance x from the larger width (b_1).

The rate of change of breadth in a length L is $= \dfrac{b_1 - b_2}{L}$

Therefore width at section x is $\qquad b = b_2 - \left(\dfrac{b_1 - b_2}{L}\right)x$

$$\therefore b = b_1 - kx \text{ where } k = \left(\frac{b_1 - b_2}{L}\right) \qquad \text{... Eq. (a)}$$

The cross sectional area of the element, $\quad A = b \times t = (b_1 - kx)t \qquad$ ... Eq. (b)

We know that $\delta l = \dfrac{Fl}{AE}$

For the element under consideration, we have

$$\delta l' = \frac{F\,dx}{(b_1 - kx)tE} \qquad \text{... Eq. (c)}$$

Thus the total extension of the bar, $\delta l = \displaystyle\int_0^L \delta l'$

$$= \int_0^L \frac{F\,dx}{(b_1 - kx)\times tE}$$

$$= \frac{F}{tE}\int_{.0}^L \frac{dx}{(b_1 - kx)} = \frac{F}{tE}\left[\ln(b_1 - kx)\left(\frac{-1}{k}\right)\right]_0^L$$

$$= \frac{F}{tEk}\left[-\ln(b_1 - kx)\right]_0^L$$

$$= \frac{F}{tEk}\left\{-\ln\left[b_1 - \left(\frac{b_1 - b_2}{L}\right)x\right]\right\}_0^L \quad \text{...using Eq. (a)}$$

$$= \frac{F}{tEk}\left\{\left[-\ln\left(b_1 - \left(\frac{b_1 - b_2}{L}\right)L\right)\right] - \left[-\ln(b_1 - 0)\right]\right\}$$

$$= \frac{F}{tEk}(-\ln b_2 + \ln b_1) = \frac{F}{tEK}(\ln b_1 - \ln b_2)$$

$$\delta l = \frac{F}{tEk}\ln\left(\frac{b_1}{b_2}\right)$$

$$\therefore \delta l = \frac{FL}{tE(b_1 - b_2)}\ln\left(\frac{b_1}{b_2}\right)$$

$$\text{... (Eq. 1.16), using Eq.(a)}$$

1.13 DEFORMATION IN BARS OF UNIFORMLY TAPERING CIRCULAR CROSS-SECTION (ROD)

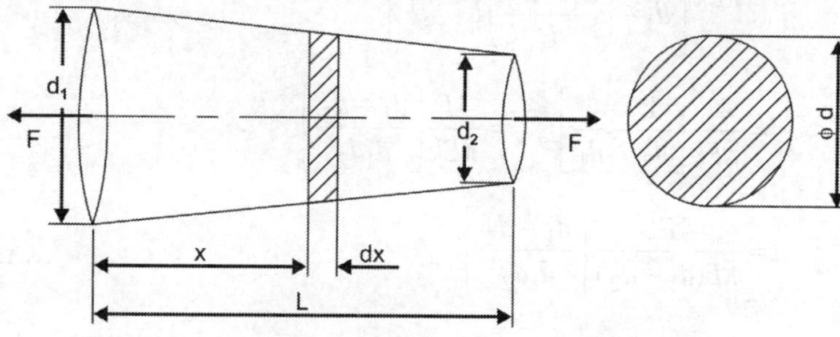

Fig. 1.17: Elongation in rod of uniform tapering circular c/s

Fig. 1.17 shows a circular rod of uniform tapering section having diameter d_1 at one end and tapering down to a diameter d_2 at the other end, in length L and subjected to axial force F.

Consider a small element of length dx at a distance x from the larger diameter (d_1).

The rate of change of diameter in a length L is $= \dfrac{d_1 - d_2}{L}$

Therefore diameter at section x is $\qquad d = d_1 - \left(\dfrac{d_1 - d_2}{L}\right) x$

$$\therefore d = d_1 - kx \quad \text{where } k = \left(\dfrac{d_1 - d_2}{L}\right) \qquad \text{... Eq. (d)}$$

The cross sectional area of the element, $A = \dfrac{\pi}{4} d^2 = \dfrac{\pi(d_1 - kx)^2}{4} \qquad$ ... Eq. (e)

We know that $\delta l = \dfrac{Fl}{AE}$

For the element under consideration, we have $\delta l' = \dfrac{F\,dx}{\left[\dfrac{\pi(d_1 - kx)^2}{4}\right] E} = \dfrac{4F\,dx}{\pi(d_1 - kx)^2\, E}$

$$\text{... Eq. (f)}$$

Thus the total extension of the bar, $\delta l = \displaystyle\int_0^L \delta l'$

$$= \int_0^L \frac{4F\,dx}{\pi(d_1 - kx)^2 \times E} = \frac{4F}{\pi E}\int_0^L (d_1 - kx)^{-2}\,dx$$

$$= \frac{4F}{\pi E}\left[\frac{(d_1 - kx)^{-1}}{(-1).(-k)}\right]_0^L = \frac{4F}{\pi Ek}\left[\frac{1}{(d_1 - kx)}\right]_0^L$$

$$= \frac{4F}{\pi Ek}\left[\frac{1}{d_1 - kL} - \frac{1}{d_1 - k(0)}\right] = \frac{4F}{\pi Ek}\left[\frac{1}{d_1 - kL} - \frac{1}{d_1}\right]$$

$$= \frac{4F}{\pi Ek}\left[\frac{1}{d_1 - \left(\dfrac{d_1 - d_2}{L}\right)L} - \frac{1}{d_1}\right] \qquad \text{... using Eq. (d)}$$

$$= \frac{4F}{\pi Ek}\left[\frac{1}{d_2} - \frac{1}{d_1}\right] = \frac{4F}{\pi Ek}\left[\frac{d_1 - d_2}{d_1 d_2}\right]$$

$$= \frac{4FL}{\pi E(d_1 - d_2)}\left[\frac{d_1 - d_2}{d_1 d_2}\right] \qquad \text{... using Eq. (d)}$$

$$\therefore \delta l = \frac{4FL}{\pi E d_1 d_2} \qquad \text{... (Eq. 1.17)}$$

If the rod is uniform, then the above (Eq. 1.17) reduces to the form,

$$\delta l = \frac{4FL}{\pi E d^2}$$

... (Eq. 1.18)

18. Determine the elongation caused by an axial load of 100 kN applied to a flat bar 20 mm thick, tapering from 120 mm to 40 mm in a length of 10 m. Take $E = 200$ GPa. Derive the expression you use.

VTU – (CV) June/ July 2009 – 08 Marks

Solution: $\delta l = ?$, $F = 100 \times 10^3$ N, $t = 20$ mm, $b_1 = 120$ mm, $b_2 = 40$ mm, $L = 10$ m $= 10000$ mm, $E = 200 \times 10^3$ MPa

We know that $\delta l = \dfrac{FL}{tE(b_1 - b_2)} \ln\left(\dfrac{b_1}{b_2}\right)$

$$= \frac{(100 \times 10^3) \times 10000}{20 \times (200 \times 10^3) \times (120 - 40)} \ln\left(\frac{120}{40}\right)$$

$$\delta l = 3.43 \text{ mm}$$

For expression, refer Art 1.12

19. If in the above problem, if the average area is used for calculating the extension, what would be the percentage error?

Solution: Percentage error $= \dfrac{\delta l - \delta l'}{\delta l} \times 100$

... Eq. (i)

But $\quad \delta l' = \dfrac{FL}{A_{avg}.E}$

... Eq. (ii)

$$A_{avg} = \frac{b_1 t + b_2 t}{2} = \frac{(120 + 40) \times 20}{2} = 1600 \text{ mm}^2$$

Eq. (ii) yields... $\delta l' = \dfrac{(100 \times 10^3) \times 1000}{1600 \times (200 \times 10^3)} = 3.13$ mm

Eq. (i) yields... Percentage error $= \left(\dfrac{3.43 - 3.13}{3.43}\right) \times 100 = 8.75\%$

20. A conical rod tapers from a diameter of 15 mm to a diameter of 40 mm in a length of 400 mm. Determine the elongation of the rod under an axial tensile load of 400 kN. Take $E = 0.2$ MN/mm².

VTU – (CV) June/ July 2013 – 04 Marks

Solution: $d_1 = 40$ mm, $d_2 = 15$ mm, $L = 400$ mm, $\delta l = ?$, $F = 400 \times 10^3$ N, $E = 0.2 \times 10^6$ N/mm²

We know that $\delta l = \dfrac{4FL}{\pi E d_1 d_2}$

$$= \frac{4 \times (400 \times 10^3) \times 400}{\pi (0.2 \times 10^6) \times 40 \times 15}$$

$$\delta l = 1.697 \text{ mm}$$

21. The diameter of a circular rod varies uniformly from $(D + a)$ to $(D - a)$. Prove that the percentage involved in finding the Young's modulus of the rod by considering it as a uniform of mean diameter is $(10a/D)^2$.

Solution:

Let $\quad d_1 = (D + a)=$ Larger diameter

$\qquad d_2 = (D - a)=$ Smaller diameter

$\qquad E =$ Young's modulus of the rod

$\qquad L =$ Length of the rod.

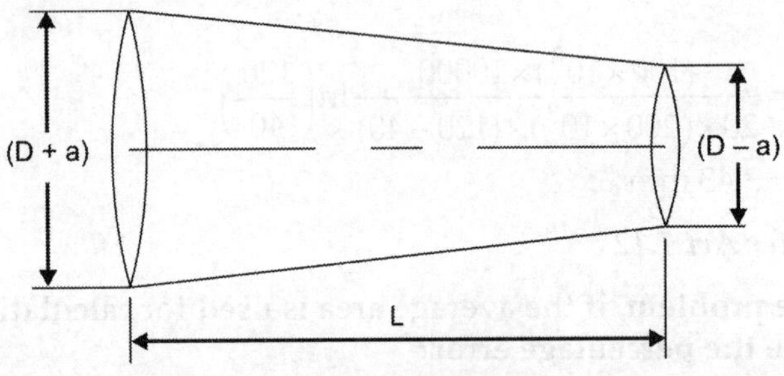

Fig. 1.18: Problem 21

We know that for a circular tapering rod, $\delta l = \dfrac{4FL}{\pi E d_1 d_2}$

$$= \frac{4FL}{\pi E (D + a)(D - a)}$$

$$= \frac{4FL}{\pi E (D^2 - a^2)}$$

$$\therefore \ E = \frac{4FL}{\pi \delta l (D^2 - a^2)}$$

Similarly for a uniform rod, $E' = \dfrac{4FL}{\pi \, \delta l \, D^2}$ $\qquad\qquad$ ... using (Eq. 1.18)

Percentage error in Young's modulus $= \left(\dfrac{E - E'}{E} \right) \times 100$

$$= \left(1 - \frac{E'}{E} \right) \times 100 = \left[1 - \frac{4FL / \pi \, \delta l D^2}{4FL / \pi \delta l (D^2 - a^2)} \right] \times 100 \qquad \text{... using Eq. (i)}$$

$$= \left[1 - \frac{(D^2 - a^2)}{D^2} \right] \times 100 = \left(\frac{D^2 - D^2 + a^2}{D^2} \right) \times 100$$

Percentage error in Young's modulus $= \left(\dfrac{10a}{D}\right)^2$

22. A 1.5 m long steel bar having uniform diameter of 40 mm for a length of 1m and in the next 0.5 m its diameter gradually reduces to 20 mm. Determine the elongation of the bar when subjected to an axial tensile load of 160 kN. Take $E = 200$ GPa.

VTU – (CV) Dec. 14/ Jan. 15 – 10 Marks

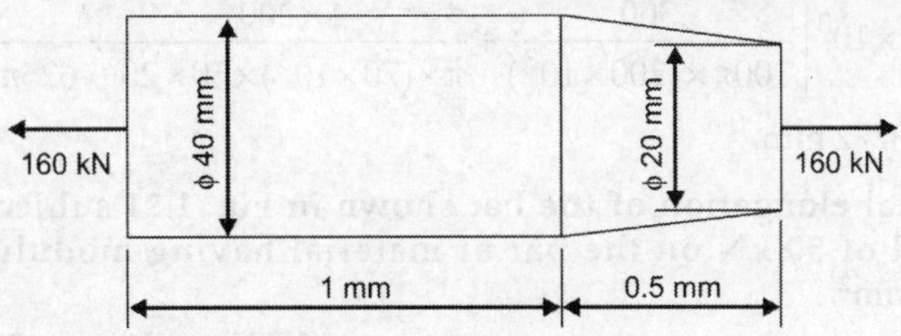

Fig. 1.19: Problem 22

Solution: $d_1 = 40$ mm, $\Rightarrow A_1 = 400\pi$ mm^2, $d_2 = 20$ mm, $\Delta = ?$, $l_1 = 1000$ mm, $l_2 = 500$ mm, $F = 160 \times 10^3$ N, $E = 200 \times 10^3$ MPa.

Total deformation, $\Delta = \delta l_1 + \delta l_2$

$$= \left[\frac{Fl_1}{A_1 E} + \frac{4Fl_2}{\pi E d_1 d_2}\right]$$

$$= \frac{F}{E}\left[\frac{l_1}{A_1} + \frac{4l_2}{\pi d_1 d_2}\right]$$

$$= \frac{160 \times 10^3}{200 \times 10^3}\left[\frac{1000}{400\pi} + \frac{4 \times 500}{\pi \times 40 \times 20}\right]$$

$$\therefore \quad \Delta = 1.273 \text{ mm}$$

23. A stepped bar is subjected to an external loading as shown in Fig. 1.20. Calculate the change in length of the bar. Take $E = 200$ GPa for steel, $E = 70$ GPa for aluminum and $E = 100$ GPa for copper.

VTU – Dec. 07/ Jan. 08 – 08 Marks; June/ July 14 – 10 Marks;
(Similar) Dec. 13/ Jan. 14 – 10 Marks

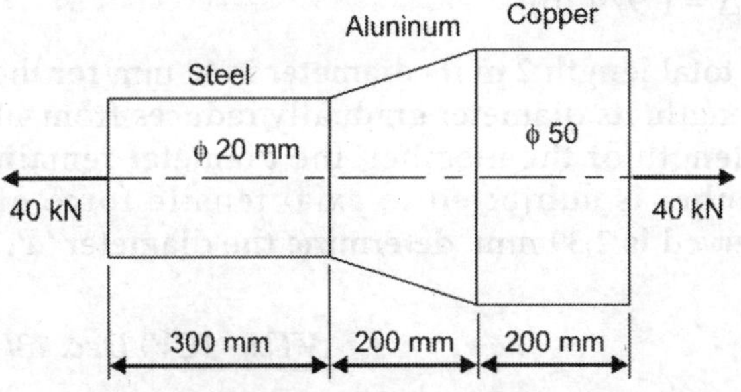

Fig. 1.20: Problem 23

Solution: $d_1 = 20$ mm, $\Rightarrow A_1 = 100\pi$ mm², $d_2 = d_3 = 50$ mm $\Rightarrow A_3 = 625\pi$ mm², $l_1 = 300$ mm, $l_2 = 200$ mm, $l_3 = 200$ mm $\Delta = ?$, $F = 40 \times 10^3$ N, $E_1 = 200 \times 10^3$ MPa, $E_2 = 70 \times 10^3$ MPa, $E_3 = 100 \times 10^3$ MPa

Total deformation, $\Delta = \delta l_1 + \delta l_2 + \delta l_3$

$$= \left[\frac{Fl_1}{A_1E_1} + \frac{4Fl_2}{\pi E_2 d_1 d_2} + \frac{Fl_3}{A_3E_3} \right] = F\left[\frac{l_1}{A_1E_1} + \frac{4l_2}{\pi E_2 d_1 d_2} + \frac{l_3}{A_3E_3} \right]$$

$$= 40 \times 10^3 \left[\frac{300}{100\pi \times (200 \times 10^3)} + \frac{4 \times 200}{\pi \times (70 \times 10^3) \times 50 \times 20} + \frac{200}{625\pi \times (100 \times 10^3)} \right]$$

$$\therefore \Delta = 0.3772 \text{ mm}$$

24. **Find the total elongation of the bar shown in Fig. 1.21 subjected to an axial tensile load of 50 kN on the bar of material having modulus of elasticity 2.1×10^5 N/mm².**

VTU – (CV) June 2012 – 06 Marks

Solution: $d_1 = 26$ mm, $\Rightarrow A_1 = 169\pi$ mm², $d_2 = d_3 = 18$ mm $\Rightarrow A_3 = 81\pi$ mm², $l_1 = 1000$ mm, $l_2 = 1200$ mm, $l_3 = 800$ mm $\Delta = ?$, $F = 50 \times 10^3$ N, $E_1 = E_2 = E_3 = 2.1 \times 10^5$ MPa

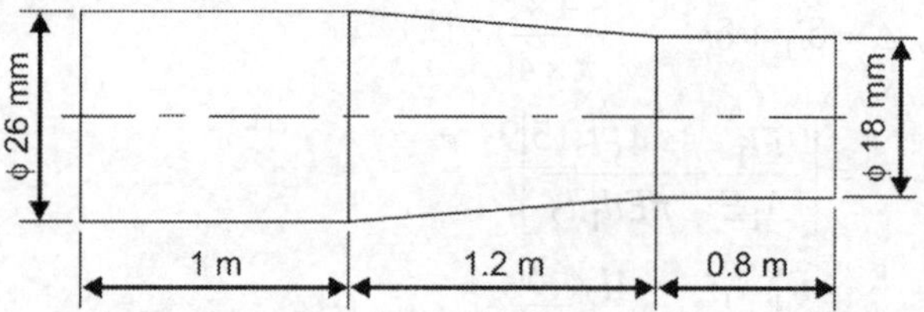

Fig. 1.21: Problem 24

Total deformation, $\Delta = \delta l_1 + \delta l_2 + \delta l_3$

$$= \left[\frac{Fl_1}{A_1E_1} + \frac{4Fl_2}{\pi E_2 d_1 d_2} + \frac{Fl_3}{A_3E_3} \right]$$

$$= \frac{F}{E}\left[\frac{l_1}{A_1} + \frac{4l_2}{\pi d_1 d_2} + \frac{l_3}{A_3} \right]$$

$$= \frac{50 \times 10^3}{2.1 \times 10^5}\left[\frac{1000}{169\pi} + \frac{4 \times 1200}{\pi \times 26 \times 18} + \frac{800}{81\pi} \right]$$

$$\therefore \Delta = 1.974 \text{ mm}$$

25. **A member is of total length 2 m its diameter is 40 mm for the first 1m length. In the next 0.5 m length, its diameter gradually reduces from 40 mm to 'd' mm. For the remaining length of the member, the diameter remains 'd' mm uniform. When this member is subjected to axial tensile force of 150 kN, the total elongation observed is 2.39 mm. determine the diameter 'd'. Assume $E = 2 \times 10^5$ N/mm².**

VTU – (CV) Dec. 13/ Jan. 14 – 10 Marks

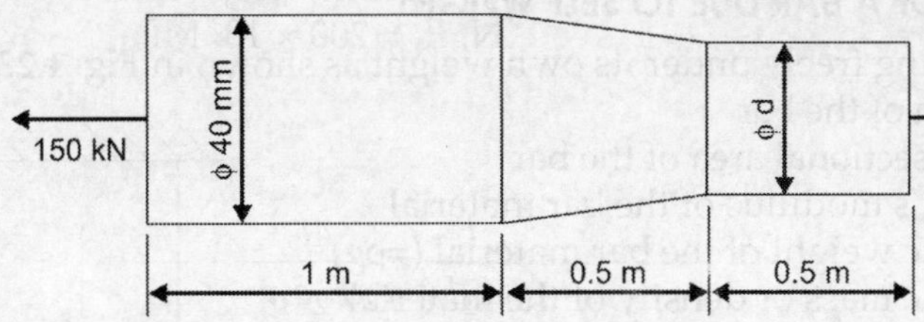

150 kN — φ 40 mm — φ d — 150 kN — 1 m — 0.5 m — 0.5 m

Fig. 1.22: Problem 25

Solution: $d_1 = 40$ mm, $\Rightarrow A_1 = 400\pi$ mm^2, $d_2 = d_3 = $ d, $l_1 = 1000$ mm, $l_2 = 500$ mm, $l_3 = 500$ mm $\Delta = 2.39$ mm, $F = 150 \times 10^3$ N, $E = 2 \times 10^5$ N/mm^2. $d = ?$

Total deformation, $\quad \Delta = \delta l_1 + \delta l_2 + \delta l_3$

$$= \left[\frac{Fl_1}{A_1 E_1} + \frac{4Fl_2}{\pi E_2 d_1 d_2} + \frac{Fl_3}{A_3 E_3} \right]$$

$$= \frac{F}{E} \left[\frac{l_1}{A_1} + \frac{4l_2}{\pi d_1 d_2} + \frac{l_1}{A_2} \right]$$

$$\frac{2.39 \times (2 \times 10^5)}{150 \times 10^3} = \left[\frac{1000}{400\pi} + \frac{4 \times 500}{\pi \times 40 \times d} + \frac{4 \times 500}{\pi \times d^2} \right]$$

$$3.186 = 0.7957 + \left[\frac{15.915}{d} + \frac{636.62}{d^2} \right]$$

$$2.3903 = \left[\frac{15.915}{d} + \frac{636.62}{d_2} \right]$$

$$2.3903 d^2 = 15.915 d + 636.62$$

$$2.3903 d^2 - 15.915\, d - 636.62 = 0$$

$$\therefore d = 19.98 \text{ mm}$$

26. Two circular rods made of same material are subjected to a pull F and are deformed by the same amount. What is the ratio of their length, if one of them has a constant diameter of 80 mm and the other tapers from 100 mm at one end to 50 mm at the other end?

Solution: $d_1 = 80$ mm $\Rightarrow A_1 = 1600\pi$ mm^2, $d_2 = 100$ mm, $d_3 = 50$ mm, $l_1 = l_2$, $\delta l_1 = \delta l_2$, $F = $ constant, $E_1 = E_2$, $l_1/l_2 = ?$

Given $\quad\quad \delta l_1 = \delta l_2$

$$\delta l_{\,const.diameter} = \delta l_{\text{taper}}$$

$$\frac{Fl_1}{A_1 E} = \frac{4Fl_2}{\pi E d_1 d_2}$$

$$\frac{l_1}{A_1} = \frac{4l_2}{\pi d_1 d_2}$$

$$\frac{l_1}{1600\pi} = \frac{4l_2}{\pi \times 100 \times 50}$$

$$\frac{l_1}{l_2} = 1.28$$

1.14 ELONGATION OF A BAR DUE TO SELF WEIGHT

Consider a bar hanging freely under its own weight as shown in **Fig. 1.23**.

Let.
l = Length of the bar
A = Cross sectional area of the bar
E = Young's modulus of the bar material
w = Specific weight of the bar material (=ρg)
ρ = Specific mass or density of the material

Consider a small section of length dy at a distance y from the free end.

The weight of the bar for a length y is $W = wAy$

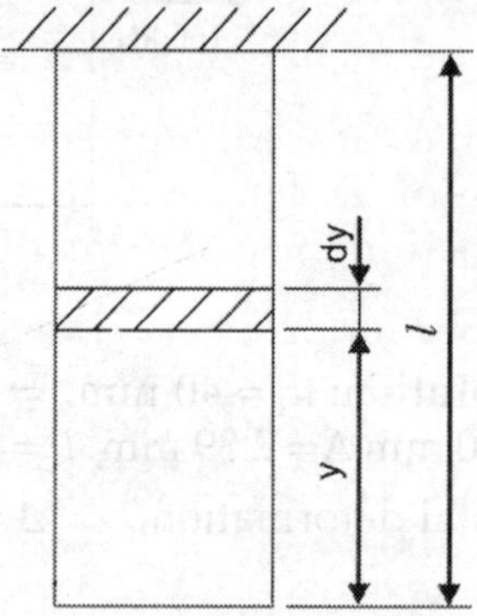

Fig. 1.23: Elongation due to self weight

Elongation of the section, $\quad \delta l' = \dfrac{Wl}{AE}$

$$= \dfrac{(wAy)\times dy}{AE}$$

$$\delta l' = \dfrac{(wy)\times dy}{E} \qquad\qquad \text{... Eq. (a)}$$

$\therefore$ Total deformation of the bar,

$$\delta l = \int_0^l \delta l'$$

$$= \int_0^l \dfrac{wy}{E}\times dy$$

$$= \dfrac{w}{E}\left[\dfrac{y^2}{2}\right]_0^l$$

$$\delta l = \dfrac{wl^2}{2E} = \dfrac{\rho g l^2}{2E} \quad (\because\ w = \rho g) \qquad\qquad \text{... (Eq. 1.19)}$$

$$\text{Or} \quad \delta l = \dfrac{Wl}{2AE} \quad (\because\ w = W/Al) \qquad\qquad \text{... (Eq. 1.20)}$$

$$W = \text{Total weight of the bar.}$$

Thus the extension produced due to self weight of a bar of uniform cross section fixed at one end and suspended vertically is equal to half the extension produced by a load equal to self weight applied at the free end.

27. **A steel wire of 6 mm diameter is used for lifting a load of 1.5 kN at its lower end, the length of the wire being 160 m. Calculate the total elongation of the wire taking $E = 2 \times 10^5$ N/mm^2 and unit weight of steel = 78 kN/m^3.**

VTU – (CV) Dec. 08/ Jan. 09 – 10 Marks

Solution: $d = 6$ mm $\Rightarrow A_1 = 9\pi$ mm^2, $F = 1500$ N, $l = 160$ m, $\Delta = ?$, $E = 2 \times 10^5$ N/mm^2, $w = 78$ kN/m^3 = 7.8×10^{-5} N/mm^3

Total elongation, $\quad \Delta = \delta l_{load} + \delta l_{self\ weight}$

$$= \dfrac{Fl}{AE} + \dfrac{wl^2}{2E}$$

$$= \frac{1.5 \times 10^3 \times (160 \times 10^3)}{9\pi \times 2 \times 10^5} + \frac{7.8 \times 10^{-5} \times (160 \times 10^3)^2}{2 \times 2 \times 10^5}$$

$$\therefore \ \Delta = 47.43 \text{ mm}$$

28. A uniform rope of length l hangs vertically. Find the extension of the first a units of the length of the rope from the top due to self weight of the rope itself. Also find the extension of the rope.

Solution: We know that the extension of the rope due to self weight is

$$\delta l = \frac{wl^2}{2E} \qquad\qquad \text{... using Eq. (1.19)}$$

Therefore extension of the rope a units from the top is $= $ *total extension $-$ extension of* $(l-a)$ *units*

$$= \frac{wl^2}{2E} - \frac{w(l-a)^2}{2E}$$

$$= \frac{w}{2E}\left[l^2 - (l-a)^2\right]$$

$$= \frac{w}{2E}\left[l^2 - (l^2 + a^2 - 2la)\right]$$

$$= \frac{w}{2E}\left[-a^2 + 2la\right] = \frac{wa}{2E}\left[2l - a\right]$$

1.15 DEFORMATION OF A BAR OF UNIFORM STRENGTH

Fig. 1.24(a) shows a bar subjected to tensile load F. For a bar to be of uniform strength, the stress intensity at any section due to external load and the weight of the portion should be constant. Consider an elementary strip of length dy at a distance y from the lower end having area of upper end as A_1 and area of lower end as A_2.

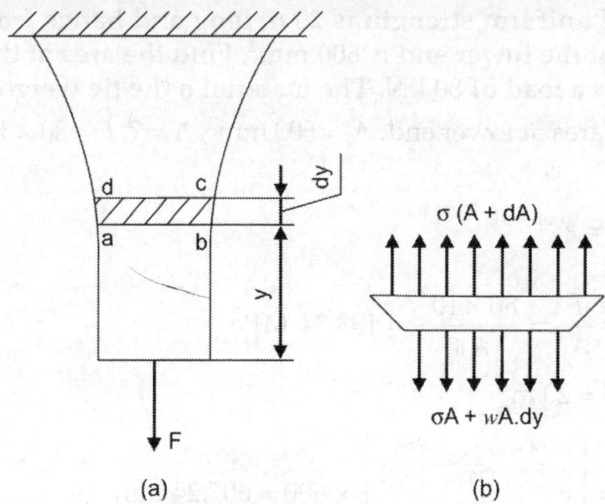

Fig. 1.24: Bar of uniform strenght

Let $\qquad A$ = Area of the strip at a distance y from the lower end (ab)

$\qquad (A + dA)$ = area at a distance $(y + dy)$ from the lower end (cd)

$\qquad\qquad w$ = specific weight of the material ($= \rho g$)

$\qquad\qquad \rho$ = specific mass or density of the material

For the strip *abcd* to be in equilibrium,

The sum of upward forces = the sum of down ward forces

i.e. $\sigma(A + dA) = \sigma A + wA\,dy$

$$\sigma\,dA = wA\,dy$$

$$\frac{dA}{A} = \frac{w\,dy}{\sigma} \qquad \qquad \text{... Eq. (i)}$$

Integrating the above equation, we have

$$\int \frac{dA}{A} = \int \frac{w}{\sigma}\,dy$$

$$\ln A = \frac{w}{\sigma}y + C_1 \qquad \qquad \text{... Eq. (ii)}$$

Where C_1 = a constant of integration.

Applying the boundary condition, @ $y = 0$, $\quad A = A_2$

Eq. (ii) yields... $\ln A_2 = C_1$

Substituting the value of C_1 in Eq. (ii), we have

$$\ln A = \frac{w}{\sigma}y + \ln A_2$$

$$\ln A - \ln A_2 = \frac{w}{\sigma}y$$

$$\ln\left(\frac{A}{A_2}\right) = \frac{wy}{\sigma}$$

$$\frac{A}{A_2} = e^{(wy/\sigma)}$$

Or $\qquad A = A_2\,e^{(\rho g y/\sigma)} \qquad \qquad \text{... (Eq. 1.21a)}$

@ $y = x$, $\quad A = A_1$

$$A_1 = A_2\,e^{(\rho g y/\sigma)} \qquad \qquad \text{... (Eq. 1.21b)}$$

29. A vertical tie of uniform strength is 20 m long and hangs from the ceiling. The area of the bar at the lower end is 600 mm². Find the area at the upper end when the tie is to carry a load of 80 kN. The material o the tie weighs 80 kN/m³.

Solution: $l = 160$ m, area at lower end, $A_2 = 600$ mm², $A_1 = ?$, $F = 80 \times 10^3$ N, $w = 80$ kN/m³ $= 8 \times 10^{-5}$ N/mm³

We know that $\quad \dfrac{A_1}{A_2} = e^{(wy/\sigma)} \qquad \qquad \text{... Eq. (i)}$

But $\qquad \sigma = \dfrac{F}{A_2} = \dfrac{80 \times 10^3}{600} = 133.34$ MPa

Also $\qquad y = l = 20$ m

Eq. (i) yields... $A_1 = \left[e^{\left(\frac{(8\times 10^{-5})\times 20000}{133.34}\right)}\right] \times 600 = 607.24$ mm²

1.16 PRINCIPLE OF SUPERPOSITION

Sometimes a body or member is subjected to a number of forces acting not only at the ends but also at intermediate points along its length as shown in **Fig. 1.25(a)**. Such a body or member can be analyzed by the application of *principle of superposition*.

According to this principle, the resulting deformation is equal to the algebraic sum of deformations caused by individual forces acting along the length of the member.

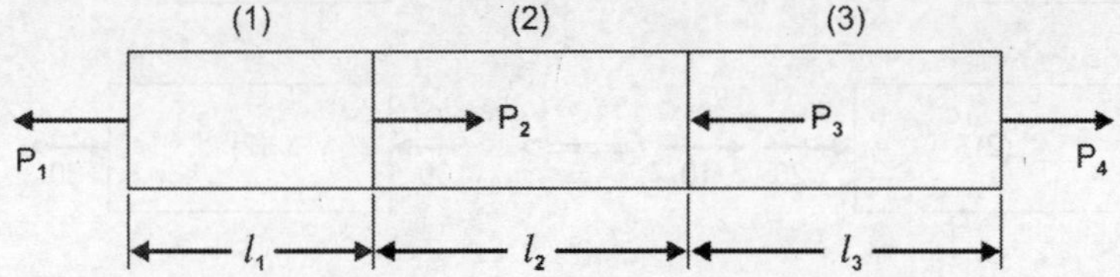

Fig. 1.25(a): Principle of superposition

Consider a body subjected to a system of forces as shown in **Fig. 1.25(a)**.

Let l_1 = length of element (1)

A_1 = area of element (1)

Similarly l_2, A_2 and l_3, A_3 be corresponding parameters for elements (2) and (3) respectively.

P_1, P_2, P_3, P_4 = forces acting on the elements (1), (2) and (3) respectively.

According to principle of superposition, $\Delta = \delta l_1 + \delta l_2 + \delta l_3$ ... (Eq. 1.22)

$$\text{Where } \delta l = \frac{Fl}{AE} \text{ and } F = \text{tensile or compressive force}$$

Based on analysis, the forces acting on individual elements are shown in **Fig. 1.25(b)**.

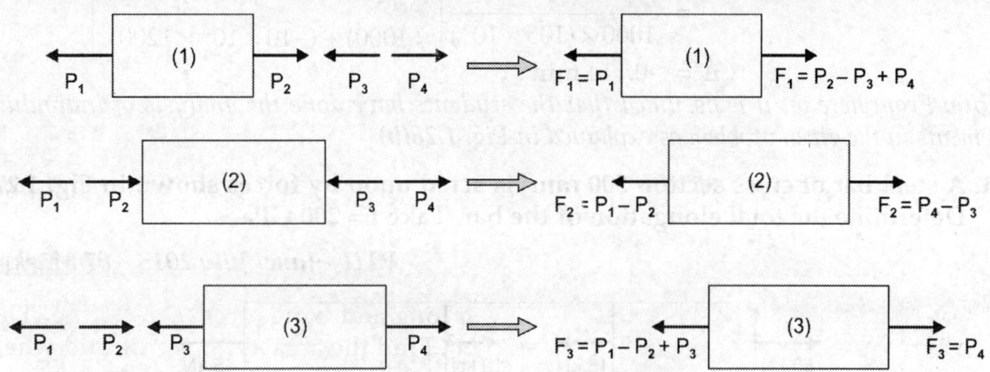

Fig. 1.25(b): Analysis of elements

30. **A brass bar having a cross sectional area of 1000 mm² is subjected to axial forces as shown in Fig. 1.26(a). Determine the total elongation of the bar if E =105 GPa.**

VTU – May/ June 2010 – 10 Marks; June/ July 2013– 10 Marks

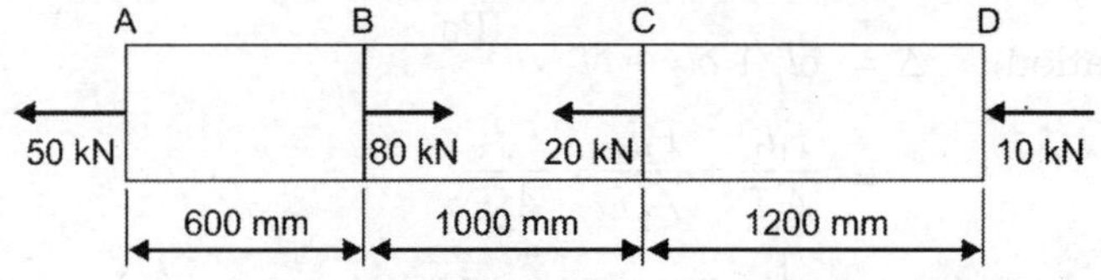

Fig. 1.26(a): Problem 30

Solution: $A = A_1 = A_2 = A_3 = 1000$ mm², $l_1 = 600$ mm, $l_2 = 1000$ mm, $l_3 = 1200$ mm, $E = 105 \times 10^3$ N/mm², $\Delta = ?$

From **Fig. 1.26(b)**, based on analysis $F_1 = 50$ kN, $F_2 = -30$ kN, $F_3 = -10$ kN

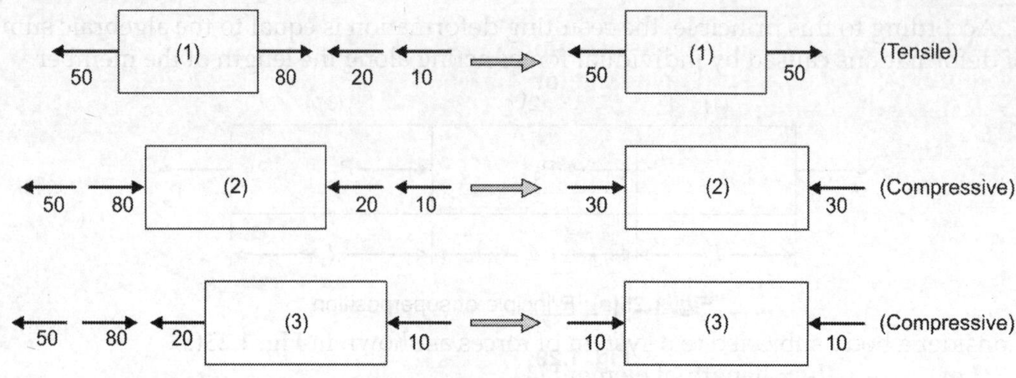

Fig. 1.26(b): Problem 30

Total deformation, $\Delta = \delta l_1 + \delta l_2 + \delta l_3$

$$= \frac{F_1 l_1}{A_1 E} + \frac{F_2 l_2}{A_2 E} + \frac{F_3 l_3}{A_3 E}$$

$$= \frac{1}{AE}\left[F_1 l_1 + F_2 l_2 + F_3 l_3\right]$$

$$= \frac{1}{1000 \times (105 \times 10^3)}\left[\begin{array}{l}(50 \times 10^3 \times 600) + (-30 \times 10^3 \\ \times\, 1000) + (-10 \times 10^3 \times 1200)\end{array}\right]$$

$\therefore \Delta = -0.114$ mm

Note: From here on it is assumed that the students have done the analysis of individual elements in the given problem as explained in **Fig. 1.26(b)**

31. A steel bar of cross section 500 mm² is acted upon by forces shown in Fig. 1.27. Determine the total elongation of the bar. Take *E*= 200 GPa.

VTU – June/ July 2013 – 07 Marks

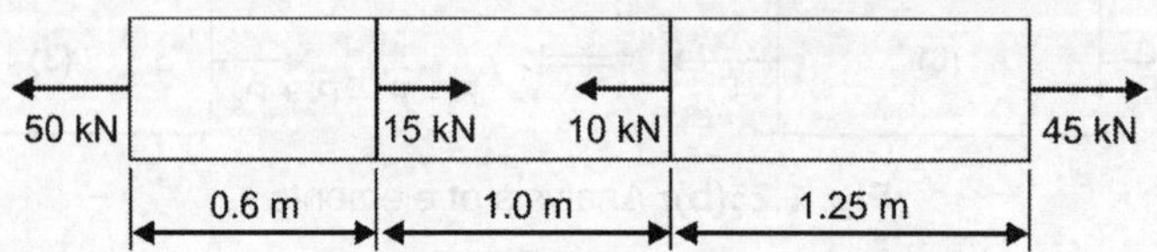

Fig. 1.27: Problem 31

Solution: $A = A_1 = A_2 = A_3 = 500$ mm², $l_1 = 600$ mm, $l_2 = 1000$ mm, $l_3 = 1250$ mm, $E = 200 \times 10^3$ N/mm², $\Delta = $?

  Based on analysis, $F_1 = 50$ kN, $F_2 = 35$ kN, $F_3 = 45$ kN

Total deformation, $\Delta = \delta l_1 + \delta l_2 + \delta l_3$

$$= \frac{F_1 l_1}{A_1 E} + \frac{F_2 l_2}{A_2 E} + \frac{F_3 l_3}{A_3 E}$$

$$= \frac{1}{AE}\left[F_1 l_1 + F_2 l_2 + F_3 l_3\right]$$

$$= \frac{1}{500 \times (200 \times 10^3)}\left[\begin{array}{c}(50 \times 10^3 \times 600) + (35 \times 10^3 \times 1000) \\ + (45 \times 10^3 \times 1250)\end{array}\right]$$

$\therefore \Delta = 1.213$ mm

32. A brass bar of uniform cross sectional area 300 mm² is subjected to a load as shown in Fig. 1.28. Find the total elongation of the bar and the magnitude of load *P* if Young's modulus is 84 GPa.

VTU – Dec. 15/ Jan. 16 – 08 Marks

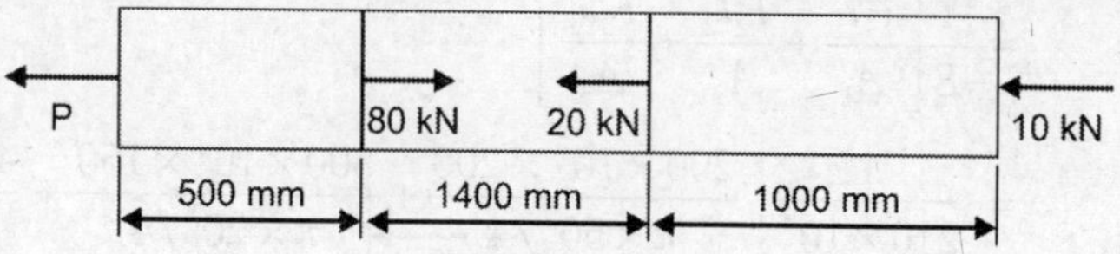

Fig. 1.28: Problem 32

Solution: $A = A_1 = A_2 = A_3 = 300$ mm², $l_1 = 500$ mm, $l_2 = 1400$ mm, $l_3 = 1000$ mm, $E = 84 \times 10^3$ N/mm², P= ?, Δ = ?

To find P:

For equilibrium, $\quad P + 20 + 10 = 80 \Rightarrow P = 50$ kN

To find Δ:

Based on analysis, $F_1 = 50$ kN, $F_2 = -30$ kN, $F_3 = -10$ kN

Total deformation, $\quad \Delta = \delta l_1 + \delta l_2 + \delta l_3$

$$= \frac{F_1 l_1}{A_1 E} + \frac{F_2 l_2}{A_2 E} + \frac{F_3 l_3}{A_3 E}$$

$$= \frac{1}{AE}\left[F_1 l_1 + F_2 l_2 + F_3 l_3\right]$$

$$= \frac{1}{300 \times (84 \times 10^3)}\left[\begin{array}{c}(50 \times 10^3 \times 500) + (-30 \times 10^3 \\ \times 1400) + (-10 \times 10^3 \times 1000)\end{array}\right]$$

$$\therefore \Delta = -1.071 \text{ mm}$$

33. Determine the deformation of a circular bar of varying cross-section subjected to forces as shown in Fig. 1.29. Take $E = 210$ kN/mm².

VTU – (CV) Dec. 15/ Jan. 16 – 08 Marks

Solution: $d_1 = 50$ mm, $d_2 = 20$ mm, $d_3 = 150$ mm, $l_1 = 200$ mm, $l_2 = 150$ mm, $l_3 = 200$ mm, $E = 210 \times 10^3$ N/mm², Δ = ?

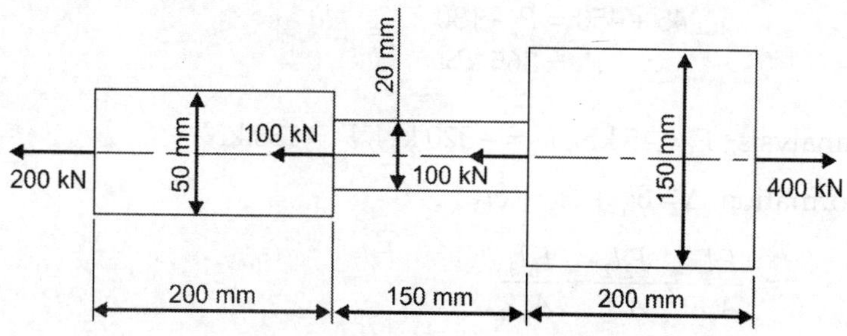

Fig. 1.29: Problem 33

Based on analysis, $F_1 = 200$ kN, $F_2 = 300$ kN, $F_3 = 400$ kN

Total deformation, $\Delta = \delta l_1 + \delta l_2 + \delta l_3$

$$= \frac{F_1 l_1}{A_1 E} + \frac{F_2 l_2}{A_2 E} + \frac{F_3 l_3}{A_3 E}$$

$$= \frac{1}{E}\left[\frac{F_1 l_1}{A_1} + \frac{F_2 l_2}{A_2} + \frac{F_3 l_3}{A_3}\right]$$

$$= \frac{1}{210 \times 10^3}\left[\frac{200 \times 10^3 \times 200}{\pi \times 50^2 / 4} + \frac{300 \times 10^3 \times 150}{\pi \times 20^2 / 4} + \frac{400 \times 10^3 \times 200}{\pi \times 150^2 / 4}\right]$$

$$\therefore \Delta = 0.801 \text{ mm}$$

34. **A member ABCD is subjected to point loads P_1, P_2, P_3 and P_4 as shown in Fig. 1.31. Calculate the force P_2 necessary for equilibrium, if $P_1 = 45$ kN, $P_3 = 450$ kN and $P_4 = 130$ kN. Determine the total elongation of the member, assuming the modulus of elasticity to be 2.1×10^5 N/mm^2.**

> *VTU – Dec. 2011 – 12 Marks; June 2012 – 08 Marks; (CV) June/ July 2013 – 10 Marks; [Similar: June/ July 2013 – 10 Marks; Dec. 2011 – 10 Marks; June/ July 2015 – 10 Marks]*

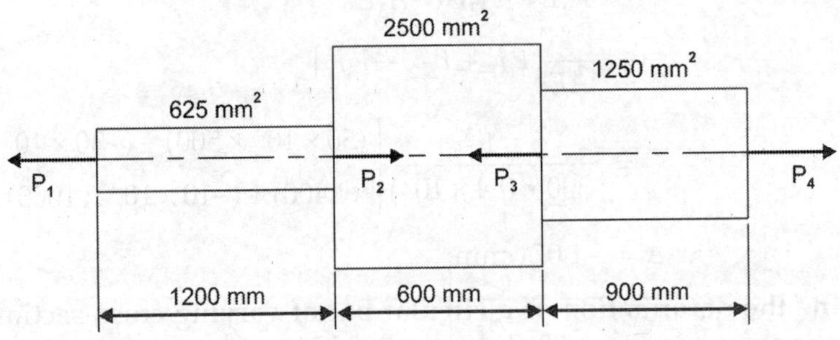

Fig. 1.31: Problem 35

Solution: $A_1 = 625$ mm^2, $A_2 = 2500$ mm^2, $A_3 = 1250$ mm^2, $l_1 = 1200$ mm, $l_2 = 600$ mm, $l_3 = 900$ mm, $P_1 = 45$ kN, $P_3 = 450$ kN, $P_4 = 130$ kN, $E = 2.1 \times 10^5$ N/mm^2, $P_2 = ?$, $\Delta = ?$

a. To find P_2:

For equilibrium, $\qquad P_1 + P_3 = P_2 + P_4$

$$45 + 450 = P_2 + 130$$

$$\therefore \quad P_2 = 365 \text{ kN}$$

b. To find Δ:

Based on analysis, $F_1 = 45$ kN, $F_2 = -320$ kN, $F_3 = 130$ kN

Total deformation, $\Delta = \delta l_1 + \delta l_2 + \delta l_3$

$$= \frac{F_1 l_1}{A_1 E} + \frac{F_2 l_2}{A_2 E} + \frac{F_3 l_3}{A_3 E}$$

$$= \frac{1}{E}\left[\frac{F_1 l_1}{A_1} + \frac{F_2 l_2}{A_2} + \frac{F_3 l_3}{A_3}\right]$$

$$= \frac{1}{2.1 \times 10^5}\left[\frac{45 \times 10^3 \times 1200}{625} + \frac{(-300 \times 10^3 \times 600)}{2500} + \frac{130 \times 10^3 \times 900}{1250}\right]$$

$$\therefore \Delta = 0.4914 \text{ mm}$$

35. A member ABCD is subjected to loads as shown in Fig. 1.30. Calculate:
   (a) Force P necessary for equilibrium
   (b) Total elongation of the bar.   Take E = 210 GN/m².

VTU – Dec. 09/ Jan. 10 – 06 Marks

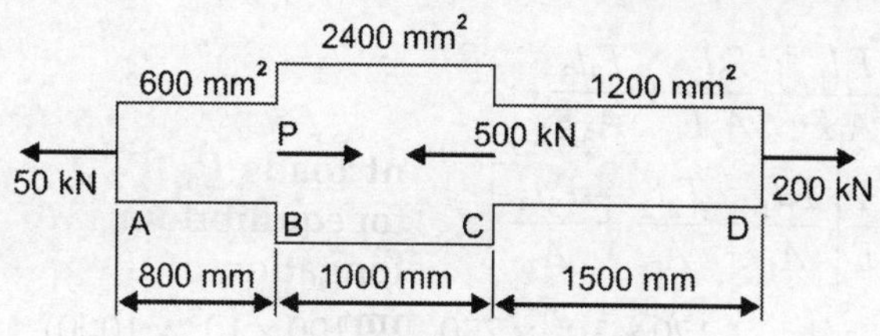

Fig. 1.30: Problem 34

Solution: A_1 = 600 mm², A_2 = 2400 mm², A_3 =1200 mm², l_1 =800 mm, l_2 = 1000 mm, l_3 =1500 mm, E = 210 × 10³ N/mm², Δ = ?

a. To find P:
   For equilibrium, $50 + 500 = P + 200 \Rightarrow P = 350$ kN
b. To find Δ:
   Based on analysis, F_1 = 50 kN, $F_2 = -300$ kN, F_3 = 200 kN

   Total deformation, $\Delta = \delta l_1 + \delta l_2 + \delta l_3$

$$= \frac{F_1 l_1}{A_1 E} + \frac{F_2 l_2}{A_2 E} + \frac{F_3 l_3}{A_3 E}$$

$$= \frac{1}{E}\left[\frac{F_1 l_1}{A_1} + \frac{F_2 l_2}{A_2} + \frac{F_3 l_3}{A_3}\right]$$

$$= \frac{1}{210 \times 10^3}\left[\frac{50 \times 10^3 \times 800}{600} + \frac{(-300 \times 10^3 \times 1000)}{2400} + \frac{200 \times 10^3 \times 1500}{1200}\right]$$

$$\therefore \Delta = 0.913 \text{ mm}$$

36. A member ABCD is subjected to point loads P_1, P_2, P_3 and P_4 as shown in Fig. 1.32. Calculate the force P_3 necessary for equilibrium, if P_1 = 120 kN, P_2 = 220 kN and P_4 = 160 kN. Determine also the net change in length of the member. Take E = 200 GN/m².

VTU – June/ July 2014 – 08 Marks

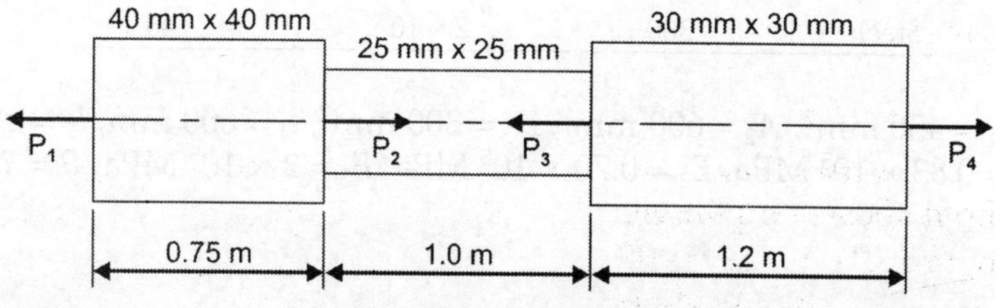

Fig. 1.32: Problem 36

Solution: $A_1 = 40 \times 40 = 1600$ mm^2, $A_2 = 25 \times 25 = 625$ mm^2, $A_3 = 30 \times 30 = 900$ mm^2, $l_1 = 750$ mm, $l_2 = 1000$ mm, $l_3 = 1200$ mm, $P_1 = 120$ kN, $P_2 = 220$ kN, $P_4 = 160$ kN, $E = 2 \times 10^5$ N/mm^2, $P_3 = ?$, $\Delta = ?$

a. To find P_2:

For equilibrium,
$$P_1 + P_3 = P_2 + P_4$$
$$120 + P_3 = 220 + 160$$
$$\therefore \quad P_2 = 260 \text{ kN}$$

b. To find Δ:

Based on analysis, $F_1 = 120$ kN, $F_2 = -100$ kN, $F_3 = 160$ kN

Total deformation, $\Delta = \delta l_1 + \delta l_2 + \delta l_3$

$$= \frac{F_1 l_1}{A_1 E} + \frac{F_2 l_2}{A_2 E} + \frac{F_3 l_3}{A_3 E}$$

$$= \frac{1}{E}\left[\frac{F_1 l_1}{A_1} + \frac{F_2 l_2}{A_2} + \frac{F_3 l_3}{A_3} \right]$$

$$= \frac{1}{2 \times 10^5}\left[\frac{120 \times 10^3 \times 750}{1600} + \frac{(-100 \times 10^3 \times 1000)}{625} + \frac{160 \times 10^3 \times 1200}{900} \right]$$

$$\therefore \Delta = 0.548 \text{ mm}$$

37. **A compound bar consisting of bronze, aluminium and steel segments is loaded axially as shown in Fig. 1.33. Determine the maximum allowable value of P, if the change in length of the bar is not to exceed 2 mm and the working stresses in each material of the bar indicated in the table below is not to be exceeded.**

VTU – Dec. 2011 – 15 Marks

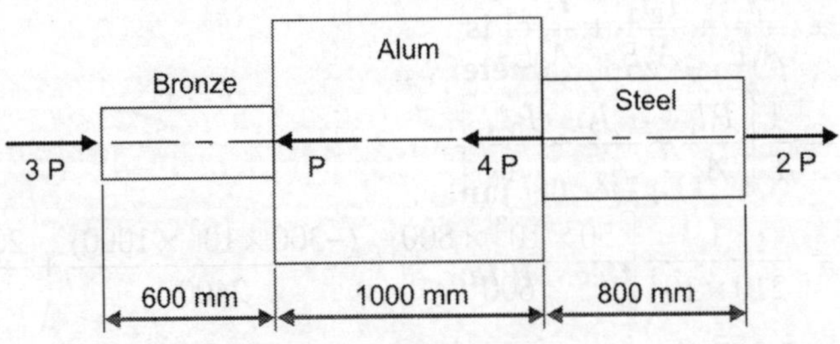

Fig. 1.33: Problem 37

Material	Area A (mm^2)	Elastic Modulus E (MPa)	Working Stress σ_w (MPa)
Bronze	450	0.83×10^5	120
Aluminium	600	0.70×10^5	80
Steel	300	2×10^5	140

Solution: $A_1 = 450$ mm^2, $A_2 = 600$ mm^2, $A_3 = 300$ mm^2, $l_1 = 600$ mm, $l_2 = 1000$ mm, $l_3 = 800$ mm, $E_1 = 0.83 \times 10^5$ MPa, $E_2 = 0.70 \times 10^5$ MPa, $E_3 = 2 \times 10^5$ MPa, $P = ?$, $\Delta = 2$ mm, stresses = ?

To find P:

Based on analysis, $F_1 = -3P, F_2 = -2P, F_3 = 2P$

Total deformation,
$$\Delta = \delta l_1 + \delta l_2 + \delta l_3 \qquad \dots \text{Eq. (i)}$$

$$\delta l_1 = \frac{F_1 l_1}{A_1 E_1} = \frac{-3P \times 600}{450 \times (0.83 \times 10^5)} = -4.82 \times 10^{-5} P$$

$$\delta l_2 = \frac{F_2 l_2}{A_2 E_2} = \frac{-2P \times 1000}{600 \times (0.70 \times 10^5)} = -4.76 \times 10^{-5} P$$

$$\delta l_3 = \frac{F_3 l_3}{A_3 E_3} = \frac{2P \times 800}{300 \times (2 \times 10^5)} = 2.67 \times 10^{-5} P$$

Eq. (i) yields...
$$2 = (-4.82 \times 10^{-5} P) + (-4.76 \times 10^{-5} P) + (2.67 \times 10^{-5} P)$$
$$\therefore \quad P = -28943.56 \text{ N}$$

To find stresses:

$$\sigma_1 = \frac{F_1}{A_1} = \frac{-3 \times (-28943.56)}{450} = 192.96 \text{ MPa}$$

$$\sigma_2 = \frac{F_2}{A_2} = \frac{-2 \times (-28943.56)}{600} = 96.48 \text{ MPa}$$

$$\sigma_3 = \frac{F_3}{A_3} = \frac{2 \times (-28943.56)}{300} = -192.96 \text{ MPa}$$

38. **A round bar with stepped portion is subjected to forces as shown in Fig. 1.34. Determine the magnitude of force P such that the net deformation in the bar does not exceed 1 mm. E for steel is 200 GPa and for aluminium is 70 GPa. Big end diameter and small end diameter of the tapering bar are 40 mm and 12.5 mm respectively.**

VTU – Dec.08/ Jan.09 – 10 Marks; June/ July 2011 – 08 Marks;
(CV) Dec. 13/ Jan. 14 – 08 Marks;
Dec. 14/ Jan. 15 – 10 Marks; June/ July 2016 – 10 Marks

Solution: $d_1 = 12.5$ mm, $d_2 = 40$ mm; $A_2 = 400$ mm², $A_3 = 200$ mm², $l_1 = 600$ mm, $l_2 = 700$ mm, $l_3 = 500$ mm, $E_1 = 70 \times 10^5$ MPa, $E_2 = E_3 = 200 \times 10^3$ MPa, $P = ?$, $\Delta = 1$ mm

To find P:

Based on analysis, $F_1 = 4P, F_2 = 2P, F_3 = 3P$

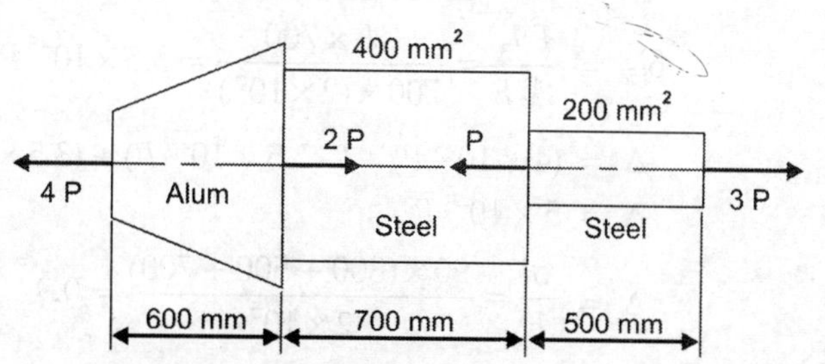

Fig. 1.34: Problem 38

Total deformation, $\Delta = \delta l_1 + \delta l_2 + \delta l_3$ ... Eq. (i)

$$\delta l_1 = \frac{4F_1 l_1}{\pi E_1 d_1 d_2} = \frac{4 \times (4P) \times 600}{\pi \times (70 \times 10^3) \times 12.5 \times 40} = 8.73 \times 10^{-5} P$$

$$\delta l_2 = \frac{F_2 l_2}{A_2 E_2} = \frac{2P \times 700}{400 \times (200 \times 10^3)} = 1.75 \times 10^{-5} P$$

$$\delta l_3 = \frac{F_3 l_3}{A_3 E_3} = \frac{3P \times 500}{200 \times (200 \times 10^3)} = 3.75 \times 10^{-5} P$$

Eq. (i) yields... $1 = (8.73 \times 10^{-5}\, P) + (1.75 \times 10^{-5}\, P) + (3.75 \times 10^{-5}\, P)$

$\therefore \quad P = 7027.41$ N

39. **A stepped bar is subjected to forces as shown in Fig. 1.35. Determine the magnitude of the force P, taking the allowable stress for the material as 90 MPa. Also find the net deformation induced in the bar. Take E = 2 × 10^5 N/mm^2.**

VTU – June 2012 – 08 Marks

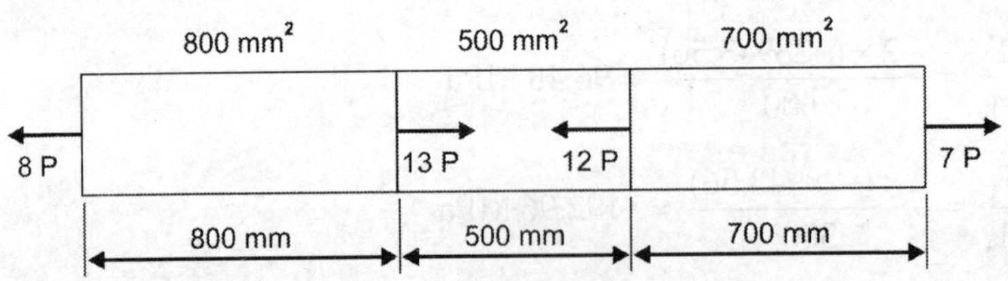

Fig. 1.35: Problem 39

Solution: $A_1 = 800$ mm², $A_2 = 500$ mm², $A_3 = 700$ mm², $l_1 = 800$ mm, $l_2 = 500$ mm, $l_3 = 700$ mm, $E = 2 \times 10^5$ N/mm², $P = ?$, $\sigma = 90$ MPa

To find P:
Based on analysis, $F_1 = 8P, F_2 = -5P, F_3 = 7P$

Total deformation, $\Delta = \delta l_1 + \delta l_2 + \delta l_3$ ... Eq. (i)

$$\delta l_1 = \frac{F_1 l_1}{A_1 E} = \frac{8P \times 800}{800 \times (2 \times 10^5)} = 4 \times 10^{-5} P$$

$$\delta l_2 = \frac{F_2 l_2}{A_2 E} = \frac{-5P \times 500}{500 \times (2 \times 10^5)} = -2.5 \times 10^{-5} P$$

$$\delta l_3 = \frac{F_3 l_3}{A_3 E} = \frac{7P \times 700}{700 \times (2 \times 10^5)} = 3.5 \times 10^{-5} P$$

$\therefore$ Eq. (i) yields... $\Delta = (4 \times 10^{-5}\, P) + (-2.5 \times 10^{-5}\, P) + (3.5 \times 10^{-5}\, P)$

$\therefore \quad \Delta = 5 \times 10^{-5} P$ ... Eq. (ii)

Also $\quad \Delta = \dfrac{\sigma l}{E} = \dfrac{90 \times (800 + 500 + 700)}{2 \times 10^5} = 0.9$ ... Eq. (iii)

Equating Eqs (ii) and (iii), we have

$$5 \times 10^{-5} P = 0.9$$
$$\therefore P = 18000 \text{ N} = 18 \text{ kN}$$

40. A steel bar of uniform cross sectional area 800 mm² is suspended vertically as shown in Fig. 1.36(a). Determine the total elongation of the bar, take $E = 200$ GPa.

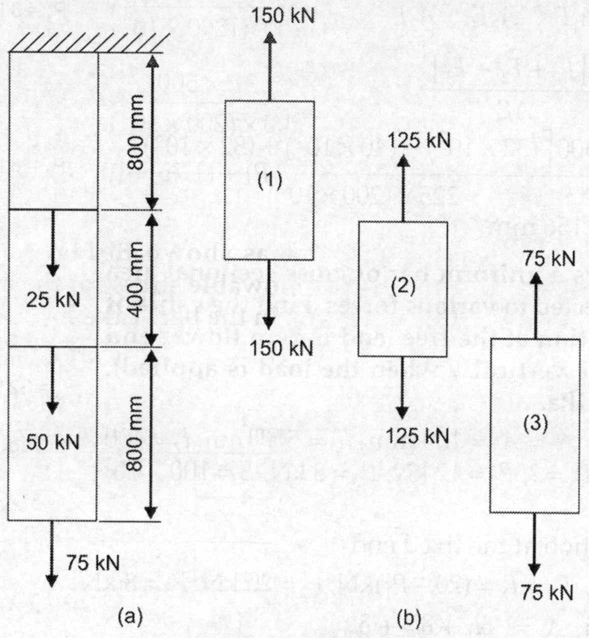

Fig. 1.36: Problem 40

Solution: $A = A_1 = A_2 = A_3 = 800$ mm², $l_1 = 800$ mm, $l_2 = 400$ mm, $l_3 = 800$ mm, $E = 200 \times 10^3$ N/mm², $\Delta = ?$

Let $R =$ be the reaction at the fixed end

From **Fig. 1.36(b)**, based on analysis, $F_1 = R = 150$ kN, $F_2 = 125$ kN, $F_3 = 75$ kN

Total deformation,

$$\Delta = \delta l_1 + \delta l_2 + \delta l_3$$

$$= \frac{F_1 l_1}{A_1 E} + \frac{F_2 l_2}{A_2 E} + \frac{F_3 l_3}{A_3 E}$$

$$= \frac{F_1 l_1 + F_2 l_2 + F_3 l_3}{AE}$$

$$= \frac{\left[(150 \times 10^3 \times 800) + (125 \times 10^3 \times 400) + (75 \times 10^3 \times 800)\right]}{800 \times 200 \times 10^3}$$

$$\therefore \Delta = 1.438 \text{ mm}$$

41. A prismatic bar is subjected to loads, P_1, P_2 and P_3 as shown in Fig. 1.37. The bar is made of steel with modulus of elasticity $E = 200$ GPa and cross sectional area $A = 225$ mm². Determine the deflection Δ at the lower end of the bar due to the applied loads.

VTU – June/ July 2009 – 10 Marks

Solution: $A = A_1 = A_2 = A_3 = 225$ mm², $l = l_1 = l_2 = l_3 = 500$ mm, $P_1 = P_2 = 8$ kN, $P_3 = 32$ kN, $E = 200 \times 10^3$ N/mm², $\Delta = ?$

Let R = be the reaction at the fixed end

Based on analysis, $F_1 = R = 32$ kN, $F_2 = 40$ kN, $F_3 = 32$ kN

Total deformation, $\Delta = \delta l_1 + \delta l_2 + \delta l_3$

$$= \frac{F_1 l_1}{A_1 E} + \frac{F_2 l_2}{A_2 E} + \frac{F_3 l_3}{A_3 E}$$

$$= \frac{l[F_1 + F_2 + F_3]}{AE}$$

$$= \frac{500\left[(32\times10^3) + (40\times10^3) + (32\times10^3)\right]}{225\times(200\times10^3)}$$

$$\therefore \quad \Delta = 1.156 \text{ mm}$$

42. Fig. 1.38 shows a uniform bar of cross sectional area 100 mm² subjected to various forces. Find the value of P_1, if deformation at the free end is zero (lower end does not move vertically when the load is applied). Take $E = 100$ GPa.

Solution: $A = A_1 = A_2 = A_3 = 100$ mm₂, $l_1 = 500$ mm, $l_2 = 400$ mm, $l_3 = 500$ mm, $P_1 = ?$, $P_2 = 12$ kN, $P_3 = 8$ kN, $E = 100 \times 10^3$ N/mm², $\Delta = 0$

Let R= be the reaction at the fixed end

Based on analysis, $F_1 = R = (20 - P_1)$kN, $F_2 = 20$ kN, $F_3 = 8$ kN

Total deformation, $\Delta = \delta l_1 + \delta l_2 + \delta l_3$

$$0 = \frac{F_1 l_1}{A_1 E} + \frac{F_2 l_2}{A_2 E} + \frac{F_3 l_3}{A_3 E}$$

$$0 = \frac{1}{AE}[F_1 l_1 + F_2 l_2 + F_3 l_3]$$

$$0 = [(20 - P_1)\times 500 + (20\times 400) + (8\times 500)]$$

$$(P_1 - 20)\times 500 = 12000$$

$$\therefore \quad P_1 = 44 \text{ kN}$$

43. Determine the magnitude of load P necessary to produce no change in length of the bar shown in Fig. 1.39. Given c/s area = 400 mm² and $E = 2 \times 105$ MPa.

VTU – Dec. 14/ Jan. 15 – 08 Marks; (CV) Dec. 10 – 08 Marks

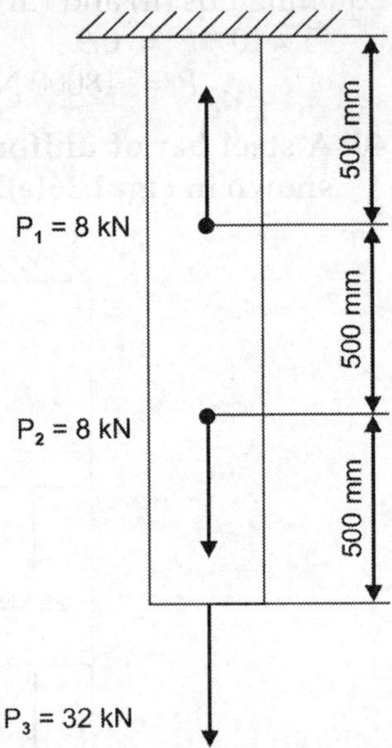

Fig. 1.37: Problem 41

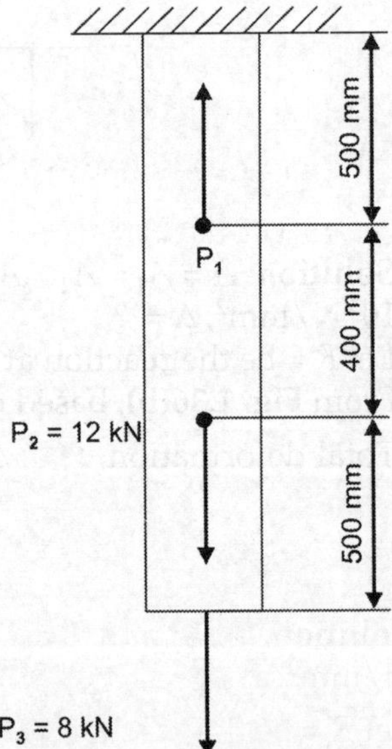

Fig. 1.38: Problem 42

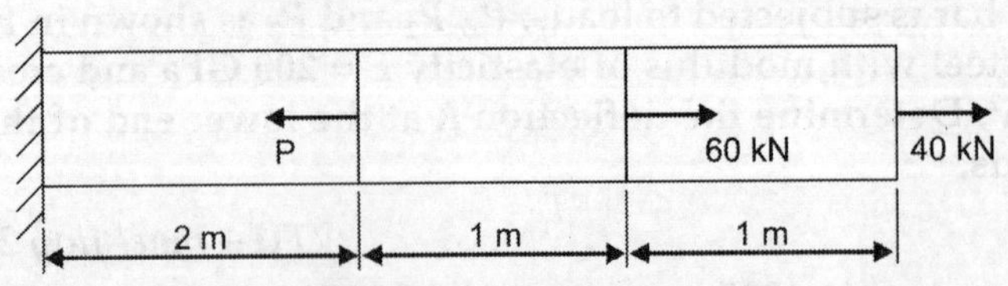

Fig. 1.39: Problem 43

Solution: $A = A_1 = A_2 = A_3 = 400$ mm^2, $l_1 = 2000$ mm, $l_2 = 1000$ mm, $l_3 = 1000$ mm, $E = 2 \times 10^5$ MPa, $\Delta = 0$, $P = ?$

Let $R =$ be the reaction at the fixed end

Based on analysis, $F_1 = R = (100 - P)$, $F_2 = 100$ kN, $F_3 = 40$ kN

To find P:

Total deformation,

$$\Delta = \delta l_1 + \delta l_2 + \delta l_3$$

$$0 = \frac{F_1 l_1}{A_1 E} + \frac{F_2 l_2}{A_2 E} + \frac{F_3 l_3}{A_3 E}$$

$$0 = \frac{1}{AE}\left[F_1 l_1 + F_2 l_2 + F_3 l_3 \right]$$

$$0 = \left\{ \left[(100 - P) \times 2000 \right] + (100 \times 1000) + (40 \times 1000) \right\}$$

$$(P - 20) \times 2000 = 140000$$

$$\therefore P = 170 \text{ kN}$$

44. **A steel rod having diameter 40 mm is loaded as shown in Fig. 1.40. Taking $E = 200$ GPa, determine:**

   (i) **The displacement at the free end.**

   (ii) **The distance x from the left hand support to a point at which the displacement is zero.**

VTU – (CV) Dec. 09/ Jan. 10 – 10 Marks

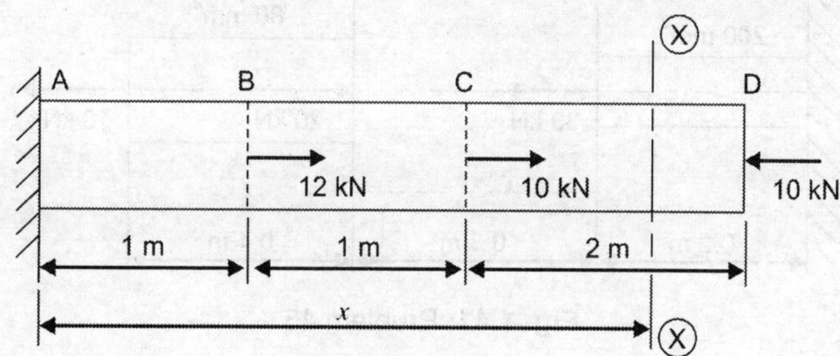

Fig. 1.40: Problem 44

Solution: $d = 40$ mm $\Rightarrow A = 1256.64$ mm^2, $l_1 = l_2 = 1000$ mm, $l_3 = 2000$ mm, $E = 200 \times 10^3$ N/mm^2. a) $\Delta = ?$ b) $x = ?$ if $\Delta = 0$

Let $R =$ be the reaction at the fixed end

Based on analysis, $F_1 = R = 12$ kN, $F_2 = 0$ kN, $F_3 = -10$ kN

   a. To find Δ:

Total deformation,

$$\Delta = \delta l_1 + \delta l_2 + \delta l_3$$

$$= \frac{F_1 l_1}{A_1 E} + \frac{F_2 l_2}{A_2 E} + \frac{F_3 l_3}{A_3 E}$$

$$= \frac{1}{AE}\left[F_1 l_1 + 0_2 + F_3 l_3 \right]$$

$$= \frac{1}{1256.64 \times (200 \times 10^3)} \left\{ \begin{array}{l} 12 \times 10^3 \times 1000) + 0 \\ + [-10 \times 10^3 \times 2000)] \end{array} \right\}$$

$$\therefore \Delta = -0.0318 \text{ mm}$$

b. To find x, when $\Delta = 0$:

Total deformation, $\quad \Delta = \delta l_1 + \delta l_2 + \delta l_3$

$$0 = \frac{F_1 l_1}{A_1 E} + \frac{F_2 l_2}{A_2 E} + \frac{F_3 l_3}{A_3 E}$$

$$= \frac{1}{AE} [F_1 l_1 + 0_2 + F_3 l_3]$$

$$= \frac{1}{1256.64 \times (200 \times 10^3)} \left\{ \begin{array}{l} (12 \times 10^3 \times 1000) + 0 + \\ [-10 \times 10^3] \times (x - 2000)] \end{array} \right\}$$

$$12 \times 10^6 = 10 \times 10^3 \times (x - 2000)$$

$$1200 = (x - 2000)$$

$$\therefore x = 3200 \text{ mm}$$

45. A stepped bar is subjected to forces as shown in Fig. 1.41. Determine the net deformation in the stepped bar. Take $E = 2 \times 10^5$ N/mm².

VTU – Jan. 2013 – 10 Marks

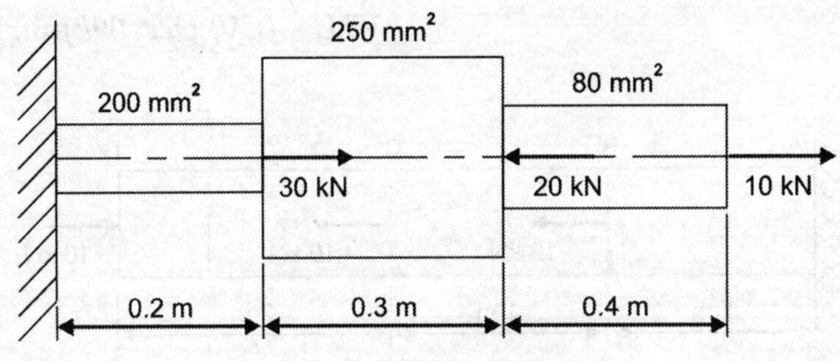

Fig. 1.41: Problem 45

Solution: $A_1 = 200$ mm², $A_2 = 250$ mm², $A_3 = 80$ mm², $l_1 = 200$ mm, $l_2 = 300$ mm, $l_3 = 400$ mm, $E = 2 \times 10^5$ N/mm², $\Delta = ?$

Let $R =$ be the reaction at the fixed end

Based on analysis, $F_1 = R = 20$ kN, $F_2 = -10$ kN, $F_3 = 10$ kN

Total deformation, $\Delta = \delta l_1 + \delta l_2 + \delta l_3$

$$= \frac{F_1 l_1}{A_1 E} + \frac{F_2 l_2}{A_2 E} + \frac{F_3 l_3}{A_3 E}$$

$$= \frac{1}{AE} \left[\frac{F_1 l_1}{A_1} + \frac{F_2 l_2}{A_2} + \frac{F_3 l_3}{A_3} \right]$$

$$= \frac{1}{2 \times 10^5} \left[\frac{20 \times 10^3 \times 200}{200} + \frac{(-10 \times 10^3 \, 300)}{250} + \frac{10 \times 10^3 \times 400}{80} \right]$$

$$\therefore \Delta = 0.290 \text{ mm}$$

46. A stepped bar is subjected to forces as shown in Fig. 1.42(a). Determine the stresses induced in different portions and the net deformation. Take $E = 200$ GPa.

VTU – May/ June 2010 – 08 Marks; (CV) May/ June 2010 – 08 Marks

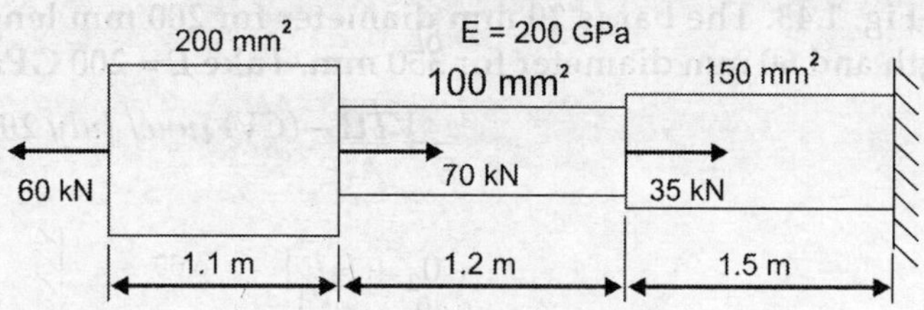

Fig. 1.42(a): Problem 46

Solution: $A_1 = 150$ mm², $A_2 = 100$ mm², $A_3 = 200$ mm², $l_1 = 1500$ mm, $l_2 = 1200$ mm, $l_3 = 1100$ mm, $E = 2 \times 10^5$ N/mm². a) stresses = ? b) Δ = ?

a. To find stresses:

Let R = be the reaction at the fixed end

From **Fig. 1.42(b)**, based on analysis, $F_1 = R = -45$ kN, $F_2 = -10$ kN, $F_3 = 60$ kN

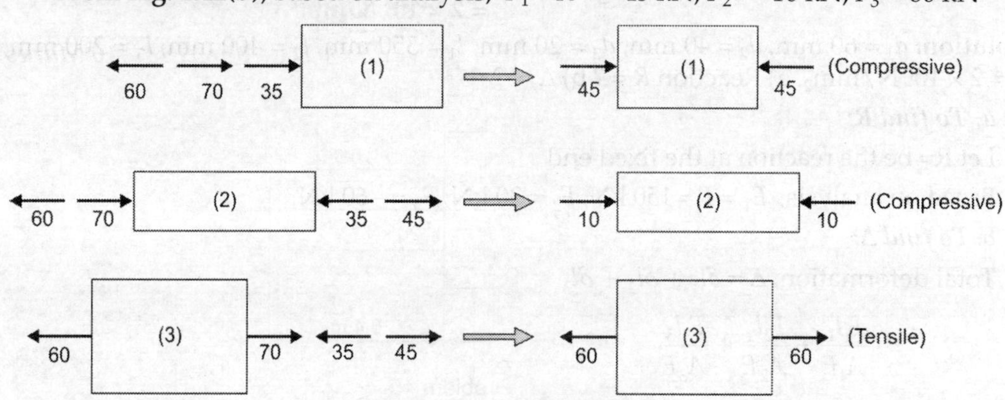

Fig. 1.42(b): Problem 46

Hence the stresses are
$$\sigma_1 = \frac{F_1}{A_1} = \frac{-45 \times 10^3}{150} = -300 \text{ MPa}$$

$$\sigma_2 = \frac{F_2}{A_2} = \frac{-10 \times 10^3}{100} = -100 \text{ MPa}$$

$$\sigma_3 = \frac{F_3}{A_3} = \frac{60 \times 10^3}{200} = 300 \text{ MPa}$$

b. To find Δ:

Total deformation,
$$\Delta = \delta l_1 + \delta l_2 + \delta l_3$$

$$= \frac{F_1 l_1}{A_1 E} + \frac{F_2 l_2}{A_2 E} + \frac{F_3 l_3}{A_3 E}$$

$$= \frac{1}{E}\left[\sigma_1 l_1 + \sigma_2 l_2 + \sigma_3 l_3\right]$$

$$= \frac{1}{2 \times 10^5}\left[(-300 \times 1500) + (-100 \times 1200) + (300 \times 1100)\right]$$

$$\therefore \ \Delta = -1.20 \text{ mm}$$

47. Calculate net change in length of the stepped bar and reaction at the support A as shown in Fig. 1.43. The bar is 20 mm diameter for 200 mm length, 40 mm for 400 mm length and 60 mm diameter for 350 mm. Take $E = 200$ GPa.

VTU – (CV) June/ July 2014 – 10 Marks

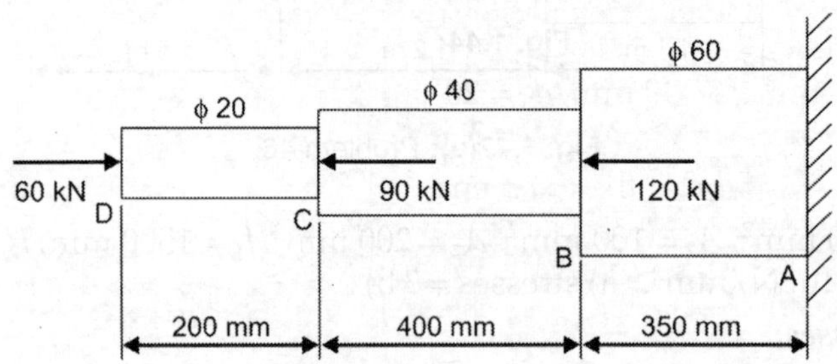

Fig. 1.43: Problem 47

Solution: $d_1 = 60$ mm, $d_2 = 40$ mm, $d_3 = 20$ mm, $l_1 = 350$ mm, $l_2 = 400$ mm, $l_3 = 200$ mm, $E = 2 \times 10^5$ N/mm$_2$. a) Reaction $R = ?$ b) $\Delta = ?$

a. To find R:

Let R= be the reaction at the fixed end

Based on analysis, $F_1 = R = 150$ kN, $F_2 = 30$ kN, $F_3 = -60$ kN

b. To find Δ:

Total deformation, $\Delta = \delta l_1 + \delta l_2 + \delta l_3$

$$= \frac{F_1 l_1}{A_1 E} + \frac{F_2 l_2}{A_2 E} + \frac{F_3 l_3}{A_3 E}$$

$$= \frac{1}{E}\left[\frac{F_1 l_1}{A_1} + \frac{F_2 l_2}{A_2} + \frac{F_3 l_3}{A_3}\right]$$

$$= \frac{4}{2 \times 10^5 \times \pi}\left[\frac{150 \times 10^3 \times 350}{60^2} + \frac{30 \times 10^3 \times 400}{40^2} + \frac{(-60 \times 10^3) \times 200}{20^2}\right]$$

$$(\because A = \pi d^2 / 4)$$

$$\Delta = 0.050 \text{ mm}$$

48. A mild steel circular bar has three segments as shown in Fig. 1.44. Find
   (a) The total elongation of the bar
   (b) The length of the middle segment to have zero elongation of the bar
   (c) The diameter of the last segment to have zero elongation of the bar.
   Take $E = 205$ GPa.

VTU – June 2012 – 10 Marks; [Similar: Dec. 2012 – 08 Marks]

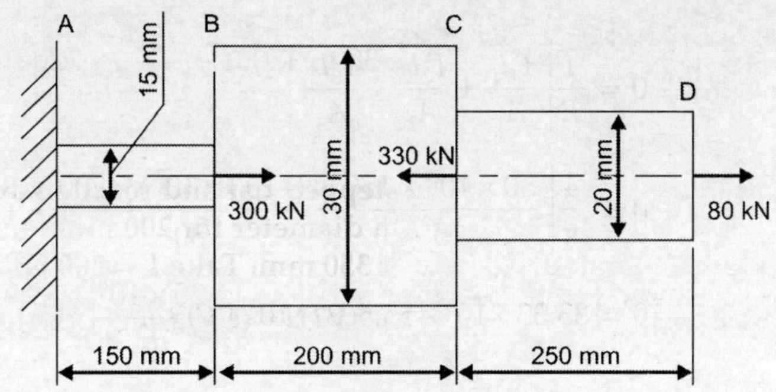

Fig. 1.44: Problem 48

Solution: $d_1 = 15$ mm, $d_2 = 30$ mm, $d_3 = 20$ mm, $l_1 = 150$ mm, $l_2 = 200$ mm, $l_3 = 250$ mm, $E = 2.05 \times 10^5$ N/mm^2. a) $\Delta = $?, b) $l_2 = $?, if $\Delta = 0$, c) $d_3 = $?, if $\Delta = 0$.

Let $R = $ be the reaction at the fixed end

Based on analysis, $F_1 = R = 50$ kN, $F_2 = -250$ kN, $F_3 = 80$ kN

a. To find Δ:

Total deformation, $\Delta = \delta l_1 + \delta l_2 + \delta l_3$

$$= \frac{F_1 l_1}{A_1 E} + \frac{F_2 l_2}{A_2 E} + \frac{F_3 l_3}{A_3 E}$$

$$= \frac{1}{E}\left[\frac{F_1 l_1}{A_1} + \frac{F_2 l_2}{A_2} + \frac{F_3 l_3}{A_3}\right]$$

$$= \frac{4}{(2.05 \times 10^5) \times \pi}\left[\frac{50 \times 10^3 \times 150}{15^2} + \frac{(-250 \times 10^3) \times 200}{30^2} + \frac{80 \times 10^3 \times 250}{20^2}\right]$$

$$\Delta = 0.1725 \text{ mm}$$

b. To find $l_2 = $?, if $\Delta = 0$:

Total deformation, $\quad \Delta = \delta l_1 + \delta l_2 + \delta l_3$

$$0 = \frac{F_1 l_1}{A_1 E} + \frac{F_2 l_2}{A_2 E} + \frac{F_3 l_3}{A_3 E}$$

$$0 = \frac{1}{E}\left[\frac{F_1 l_1}{A_1} + \frac{F_2 l_2}{A_2} + \frac{F_3 l_3}{A_3}\right]$$

$$0 = \frac{4}{\pi}\left[\frac{50 \times 10^3 \times 150}{15^2} + \frac{(-250 \times 10^3) \times l_2}{30^2} + \frac{80 \times 10^3 \times 250}{20^2}\right]$$

$$0 = 33.33 \times 10^3 - 277.77\, l_2 + 50000$$

$$277.77\, l_2 = 83330$$

$$l_2 = 300 \text{ mm}$$

c. To find $d_3 = $?, if $\Delta = 0$

Total deformation, $\quad \Delta = \delta l_1 + \delta l_2 + \delta l_3$

$$0 = \frac{F_1 l_1}{A_1 E} + \frac{F_2 l_2}{A_2 E} + \frac{F_3 l_3}{A_3 E}$$

$$0 = \frac{1}{E}\left[\frac{F_1 l_1}{A_1} + \frac{F_2 l_2}{A_2} + \frac{F_3 l_3}{A_3}\right]$$

$$0 = \frac{4}{\pi}\left[\frac{50 \times 10^3 \times 150}{15^2} + \frac{(-250 \times 10^3) \times 200}{30^2} + \frac{80 \times 10^3 \times 250}{d_3^2}\right]$$

$$0 = 33.33 \times 10^3 - 55.563 \times 10^3 + \frac{20 \times 10^6}{d_3^2}$$

$$22.22 \times 10^3 = \frac{20 \times 10^6}{d_3^2}$$

$$d_3^2 = 900 \text{ mm}^2$$

$$d_3 = 33.85 \text{ mm}$$

1.17 INDETERMINATE SYSTEMS

Till now we have dealt with problems which can be solved/analyzed by simple equation of statics alone considering the static equilibrium conditions; wherein the axial forces and reactions were obtained by the use of free body diagrams and solving the equilibrium equations known as *statistically determinate problems/structures*.

On the other hand, there are problems which cannot be solved alone by the use of static equations. Such problems or structures are referred to as *statistically indeterminate problems/structures*. In solving these problems, the deformation characteristic of the structure has to be accounted for along with the equations of static equilibrium. Thus equations that contain deformation characteristics are referred to as compatibility equations.

Referring to **Fig. 1.45(b)**, we have

For compatibility, extension of element (1) = contraction of element (2)

i.e. $\quad \delta l_1 = \delta l_2$ $\hfill$ ...(Eq. 1.23)

1.18 DIFFERENCE BETWEEN DETERMINATE AND INDETERMINATE STRUCTURES

Determinate structures	Indeterminate structures or Redundant structures
Equilibrium conditions are fully adequate to analyze the structure.	Equilibrium conditions are not adequate to analyze the structure.
Shear force and bending moment at any section is independent of the material property of the structure.	Shear force and bending moment at any section is dependent of the material property of the structure.
Shear force and bending moment at any section is independent of the cross section or moment of inertia.	Shear force and bending moment at any section depends upon the cross section or moment of inertia.
Temperature variations do not cause stresses.	Temperature variations cause stresses.
No stresses are caused due to lack of fit.	Stresses are caused due to lack of fit.
Compatibility conditions are not required to analyze the structure.	Compatibility conditions are required to analyze the structure.

49. A homogeneous rod of uniform cross section is attached to unyielding supports and carries an axial load F as shown in Fig. 1.45 (a). Determine the reactions.

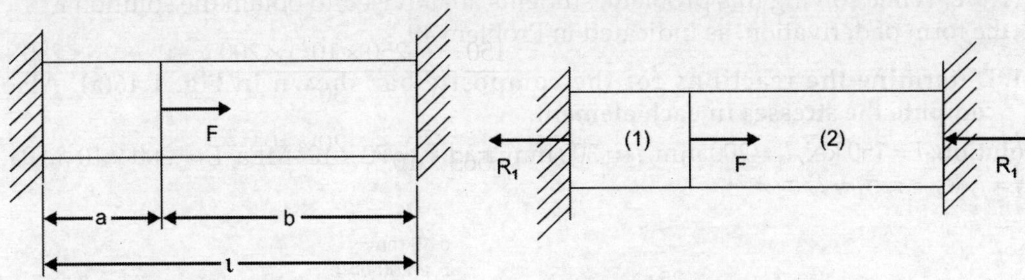

Fig. 1.45(a): Problem 49   **Fig. 1.45(b):** Problem 49

Solution: Since the bar is held between two rigid supports, the left portion (1) is subjected to tension while the right portion (2) is subjected to compression, as shown in **Fig. 1.45(b)**.

For equilibrium, $\Sigma F_H = 0$

$$R_1 + R_2 = F \qquad \qquad \text{... Eq. (i)}$$

For compatibility, extension of element (1) = contraction of element (2)

$$\text{i.e. } \delta l_1 = \delta l_2$$

$$\frac{R_1 a}{AE} = \frac{R_2 a}{AE}$$

$$R_1 a = R_2 b$$

$$\therefore \ R_1 = R_2\left(\frac{b}{a}\right) \qquad \qquad \text{... Eq. (ii)}$$

Substituting Eq. (ii) in Eq. (i), we have

$$R_2\left(\frac{b}{a}\right) + R_2 = F$$

$$R_2\left(\frac{b+a}{a}\right) = F$$

$$R_2 = \frac{Fa}{l} \qquad \qquad (\because l = a + b) \qquad \qquad \text{... Eq. (iii)}$$

$\therefore$ Eq. (ii) yields... $R_1 = \left(\dfrac{Fa}{l}\right)\left(\dfrac{b}{a}\right)$

$$\therefore \ R_1 = \frac{Fb}{l}$$

50. If in the above problem 49, $F = 450$ kN, $a = 300$ mm, $b = 200$ mm, and $E = 200$ GPa find the reactions assuming a square rod of 20 mm.

Solution: $F = 450$ kN, $a = 300$ mm, $b = 200$ mm, and $E = 200 \times 10^3$ MPa, $R_1 = ?$, $R_2 = ?$

We know that $R_1 = \dfrac{Fb}{l} = \dfrac{450 \times 200}{500} = 180$ kN $(\because l = a + b)$ ... Eq. (iii)

$$\text{Also} \quad R_2 = \frac{Fa}{l} = \frac{450 \times 300}{500} = 270 \text{ kN}$$

Note: While solving this problem, students are advised to obtain the solution in the form of derivation, as indicated in Problem 49.

51. Determine the reactions for the composite bar shown in Fig. 1.46(a). Also compute the stresses in each element.

Solution: $F = 150$ kN, $l_1 = 200$ mm, $l_2 = 300$ mm, and $E_1 = 70 \times 10^3$ MPa, $E_2 = 200 \times 10^3$ MPa, $R_1 = ?, R_2 = ?, \sigma_1 = ?, \sigma_2 = ?$

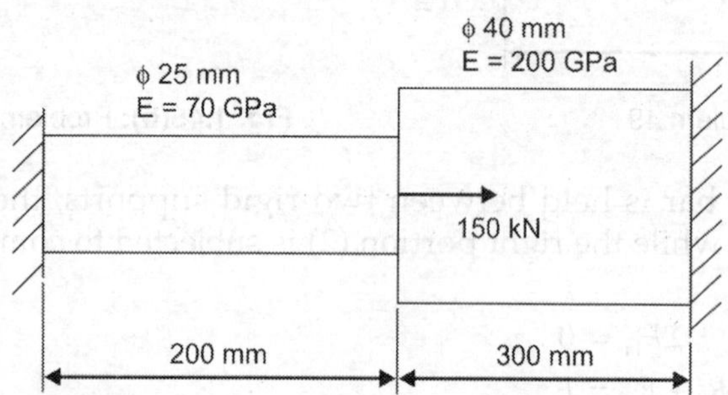

Fig. 1.46(a): Problem 51

a. To find reactions:

Based on analysis, the reactions are as shown in **Fig's. 1.46(b) & (c)** respectively.

For equilibrium, $\quad \Sigma F_H = 0$

$$R_1 + R_2 - F = 0$$
$$R_1 + R_2 = 150 \times 10^3 \text{ N} \qquad \qquad \ldots \text{Eq. (i)}$$

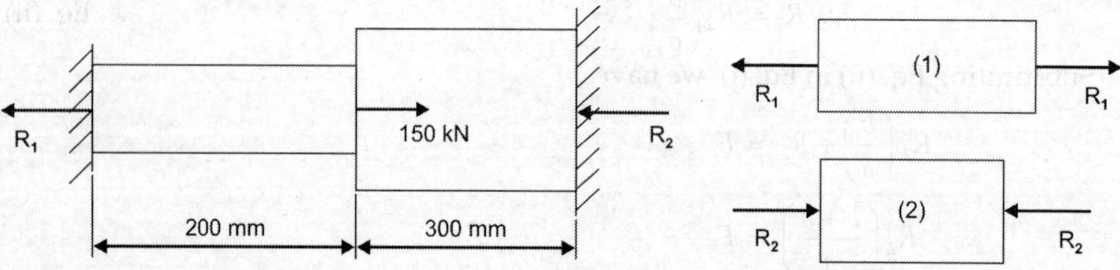

Fig. 1.46(b): Problem 51   **Fig. 1.46(c):** Problem 51

For compatibility, extension of element (1) = contraction of element (2)

$$\text{i.e. } \delta l_1 = \delta l_2$$

$$\text{i.e. } \frac{R_1 l_1}{A_1 E_1} = \frac{R_2 l_2}{A_2 E_2}$$

$$\frac{R_1 \times 200}{(\pi \times 25^2/4) \times (70 \times 10^3)} = \frac{R_2 \times 300}{(\pi \times 40^2/4) \times (200 \times 10^3)}$$

$$\therefore \quad R_1 = 0.205 R_2 \qquad \qquad \ldots \text{Eq. (ii)}$$

$\therefore$ Eq. (i) yields... $\quad 0.205 R_2 + R_2 = 150 \times 10^3$

$$\therefore \quad R_2 = 124.47 \times 10^3 \text{ N}$$

and Eq. (ii) yields... $\quad R_1 = 0.205 \times (124.47 \times 10^3)$

$$\therefore \quad R_1 = 25.52 \times 10^3 \text{ N}$$

b. To find stresses:

Stress in element (1), $\qquad \sigma_1 = \dfrac{R_1}{A_1} = \dfrac{25.52 \times 10^3}{\pi \times 25^2/4} = 52 \text{ MPa}$

Stress in element (2), $\qquad \sigma_2 = \dfrac{R_2}{A_2} = \dfrac{124.47 \times 10^3}{\pi \times 40^2/4} = 99.05 \text{ MPa}$

52. A stepped bar of steel, held between two supports as shown in Fig. 1.47(a) is subjected to loads $P_1 = 80$ kN and $P_2 = 60$ kN. Find the reactions developed at the ends A and B. Take $E = 200$ GPa.

VTU – Dec. 10 – 08 Marks

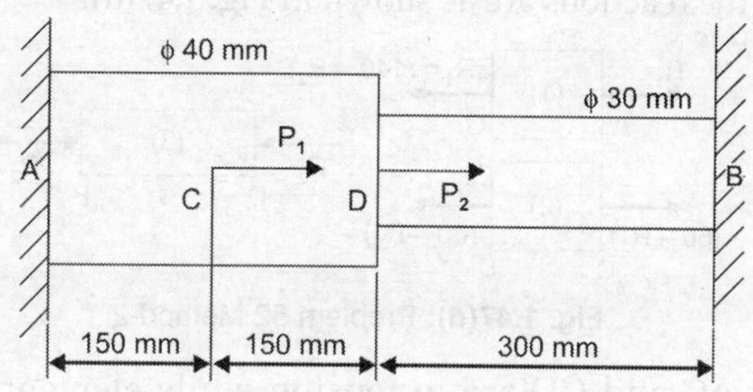

Fig. 1.47(a): Problem 52

Solution: $P_1 = 80$ kN, $P_2 = 60$ kN, $d_1 = d_2 = 40$ mm, $d_3 = 30$ mm, $l_1 = l_2 = 150$ mm, $l_3 = 300$ mm and $E_1 = E_2 = E_3 = 200 \times 10^3$ MPa, $R_A = ?$, $R_B = ?$

Method 1:

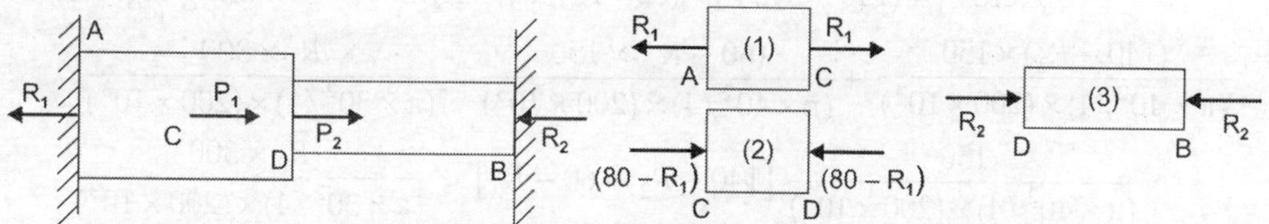

Fig. 1.47(b): Problem 52 $\qquad$ **Fig. 1.47(c):** Problem 52 Method – 1

Based on analysis, the reactions are as shown in **Fig's. 1.47(b) & (c)** respectively.

For equilibrium, $\qquad \Sigma F_H = 0$

$$R_1 + R_2 = P_1 + P_2 = 80 + 60$$
$$R_1 + R_2 = 140 \text{ kN} \qquad\qquad \text{... Eq. (i)}$$

Here element AC in tension while elements CD and DB are subjected to compression.

i.e. for compatibility, $\quad \delta l_{AC} = \delta l_{CD} + \delta l_{BD}$

$$\frac{F_1 l_1}{A_1 E_1} = \frac{F_2 l_2}{A_2 E_2} + \frac{F_3 l_3}{A_3 E_3}$$

Here $F_1 = R_1$, $F_2 = (80 - R_1)$, $F_3 = R_2$; $E_1 = E_2 = E_3 = E$ $\qquad$ *... using Fig. 1.47(c)*

$$\frac{R_1 \times 150}{(\pi \times 40^2/4) \times (200 \times 10^3)} = \frac{(80 - R_1) \times 150}{(\pi \times 40^2/4) \times (200 \times 10^3)} + \frac{R_2 \times 300}{(\pi \times 30^2/4) \times (200 \times 10^3)}$$

$$\frac{R_1 \times 150}{40^2} = \frac{(80 - R_1) \times 150}{40^2} + \frac{R_2 \times 300}{30^2}$$

$$0.09375R_1 = (80 - R_1)0.09375 + 0.34R_2$$

$$0.1875R_1 - 0.342R_2 = 7.5 \qquad \qquad \qquad \text{... Eq. (ii)}$$

Solving Eqs (i) and (ii), we have
$$R_1 = 104.58 \text{ kN} \text{ and } R_2 = 35.41 \text{ kN}$$

Method 2:

Based on analysis, the reactions are as shown in **Fig. 1.47(d)**.

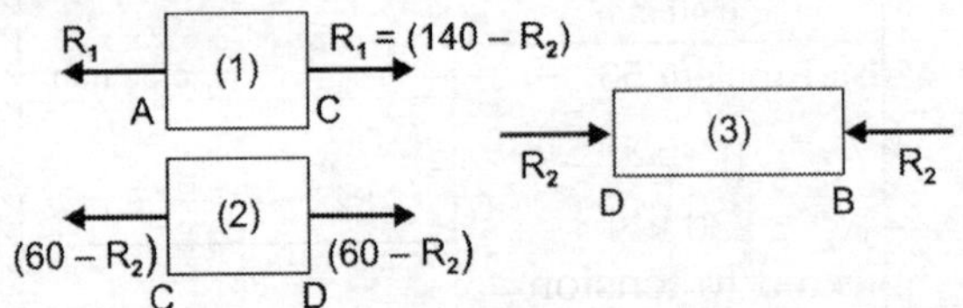

Fig. 1.47(d): Problem 52 Method-2

Here elements AC and CD are in tension while element DB is subjected to compression

i.e. for compatibility, $\quad \delta l_{AC} + \delta l_{CD} = \delta l_{BD}$

$$\frac{F_1 l_1}{A_1 E_1} + \frac{F_2 l_2}{A_2 E_2} = \frac{F_3 l_3}{A_3 E_3}$$

Here $F_1 = (140 - R_2)$, $F_2 = (60 - R_2)$, $F_3 = R_2$ $\qquad$ *... using **Fig. 1.47(d)***

$$\frac{(140 - R_2) \times 150}{(\pi \times 40^2/4) \times (200 \times 10^3)} + \frac{(60 - R_2) \times 150}{(\pi \times 40^2/4) \times (200 \times 10^3)} = \frac{R_2 \times 300}{(\pi \times 30^2/4) \times (200 \times 10^3)}$$

$$\frac{150}{(\pi \times 40^2/4) \times (200 \times 10^3)} \left[140 - R_2 + 60 - R_2\right] = \frac{R_2 \times 300}{(\pi \times 30^2/4) \times (200 \times 10^3)}$$

$$(200 - 2R_2) = 3.56 \, R_2 \quad \therefore \quad R_2 = 36 \text{ kN}$$

$\therefore$ Eq. (i) yields... $R_1 = 140 - 36 = 104$ kN

53. **A circular bar ABCD is rigidly fixed at A and B and is subjected to axial forces as shown in Fig. 1.48 (a).**

    Determine **(a) The reactions and forces in each portion of the bar.**

    (b) Displacements of points B and C. Take $E = 200$ **GPa.**

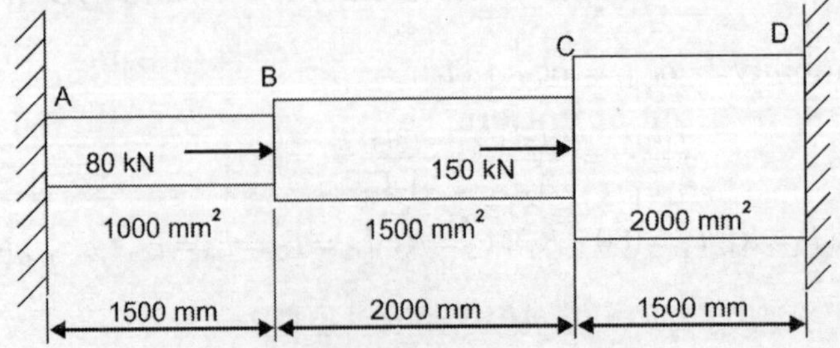

Fig. 1.48(a): Problem 53

Solution: $A_1 = 1000$ mm^2, $A_2 = 1500$ mm^2, $A_3 = 2000$ mm^2, $l_1 = 1500$ mm, $l_2 = 2000$ mm, $l_3 = 1500$ mm, $E_1 = E_2 = E_3 = 200 \times 10^3$ MPa. a) $R_A = $?, $R_B = $? b) $\delta_B, \delta_C = $?

a. To find reactions:

Based on analysis, the reactions are as shown in **Figs. 1.48(b)** & **(c)** respectively.

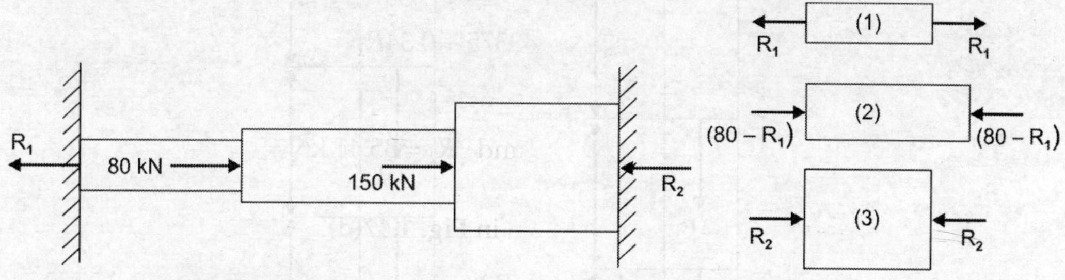

Fig. 1.48(b): Problem 53   **Fig. 1.48(c): Problem 53**

For equilibrium, $\Sigma F_H = 0$

$$R_1 + R_2 = 230 \text{ kN} \qquad \qquad \text{... Eq. (i)}$$

Here element AB is subjected to tension while elements BC and CD are subjected to compression.

i.e. for compatibility, $\delta l_{AC} = \delta l_{CD} + \delta l_{BD}$

$$\frac{F_1 l_1}{A_1 E_1} = \frac{F_2 l_2}{A_2 E_2} + \frac{F_3 l_3}{A_3 E_3}$$

Here $F_1 = R_1$, $F_2 = (80 - R_1)$, $F_3 = R_2$ ... using **Fig. 1.48(c)**

$$\frac{R_1 \times 1500}{1000 \times (2 \times 10^3)} = \frac{(80 - R_1) \times 2000}{1500 \times (2 \times 10^5)} + \frac{R_2 \times 1500}{2000 \times (2 \times 10^5)}$$

$$\frac{R_1 \times 1500}{40^2} = \frac{(80 - R_1) \times 2000}{1500} + \frac{R_2 \times 1500}{2000}$$

$$1.5 R_1 = 1.34 (80 - R_1) + 0.75 R_2$$

$$2.84 R_1 - 0.75 R_2 = 107.2 \qquad \qquad \text{... Eq. (ii)}$$

Solving Eqs (i) and (ii), we have

$$R_1 = 77.91 \text{ kN and } R_2 = 152.08 \text{ kN}$$

b. To find displacements:

At B, $\delta l_B = \delta l_{AB} = \dfrac{R_1 l_1}{A_1 E_1} = \dfrac{(77.91 \times 10^3) \times 1500}{1000 \times (2 \times 10^5)} = 0.5843$ mm

At C, $\delta l_C = \dfrac{R_2 \times 1500}{2000 \times (2 \times 10^5)} = \dfrac{(152.08 \times 10^3) \times 1500}{2000 \times (2 \times 10^5)} = 0.5703$ mm

54. Fig. 1.49(a) shows a rod of uniform section loaded axially between supports. Find the end reactions.

Solution: $l_1 = l_2 = l_3 = l/3$, $A_1 = A_2 = A_3 = A$, $= P_1 = 2P$, $P_2 = P$, $R_1 = $?, $R_2 = $?

To find reactions:

Based on analysis, the reactions are as shown in **Fig. 1.49(b).**

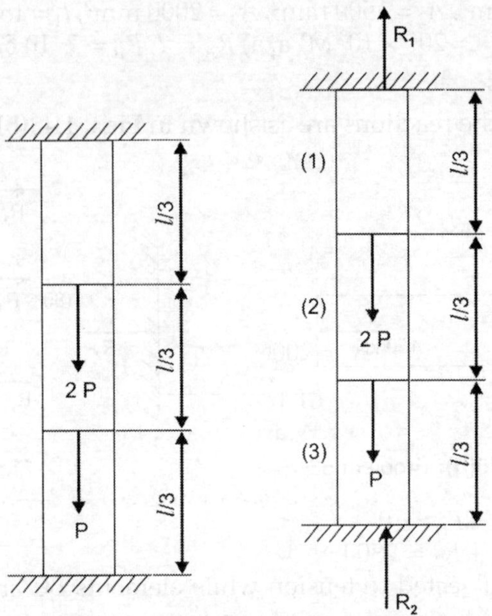

Fig. 1.49(a): Problem 54   Fig. 1.49(b): Problem 54

For equilibrium, $\Sigma F_H = 0$

$$R_1 + R_2 = 2P + P = 3P \qquad \text{... Eq. (i)}$$

Here element (1) is subjected to tension while elements (2) and (3) are subjected to compression.

i.e. for compatibility, $\delta l_1 = \delta l_2 + \delta l_3$

$$\frac{F_1 l_1}{A_1 E_1} = \frac{F_2 l_2}{A_2 E_2} + \frac{F_3 l_3}{A_3 E_3}$$

Here $F_1 = R_1$, $F_2 = (2P - R_1)$, $F_3 = R_2$

$$\frac{R_1 \times (l/3)}{AE} = \frac{(2P - R_1) \times (l/3)}{AE} + \frac{R_2 \times (l/3)}{AE}$$

$$R_1 = (2P - R_1) + R_2 \qquad \text{... Eq. (ii)}$$

$$2R_1 - R_2 = 2P$$

Solving Eqs (i) and (ii), we have

$$R_1 = 5P/3 \text{ and } R_2 = 4P/3$$

55. Fig. 1.50 shows a rod of uniform section loaded axially between supports. Find the end reactions.

Solution: $l_1 = l_2 = l_3 = l/3$, $A_1 = A_2 = A_3 = A$, $R_1 = ?$, $R_2 = ?$

To find reactions:

Based on analysis, the reactions are similar to as shown in **Fig. 1.49(b)**.

For equilibrium, $\Sigma F_H = 0$

$$R_1 + R_2 = 3000 + 1500$$

$$R_1 + R_2 = 4500 \text{ N} \qquad \text{... Eq. (i)}$$

Here element AB is subjected to tension while elements BC and CD are subjected to compression.

i.e. for compatibility, $\delta l_{AB} = \delta l_{BC} + \delta l_{CD}$

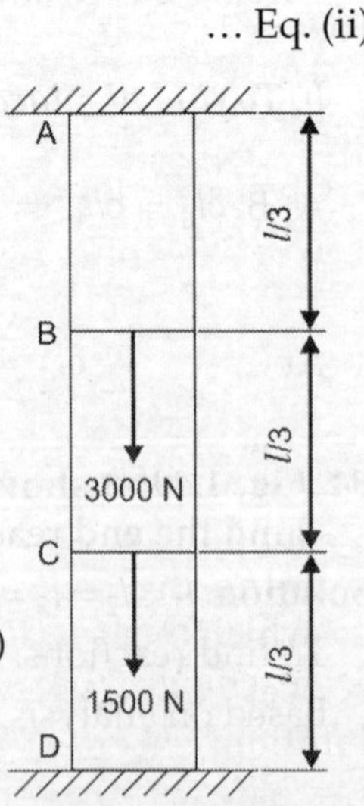

Fig. 1.50: Problem 55

$$\frac{F_1 l_1}{A_1 E_1} = \frac{F_2 l_2}{A_2 E_2} + \frac{F_3 l_3}{A_3 E_3}$$

Here $F_1 = R_1$, $F_2 = (3000 - R_1)$, $F_3 = R_2$

$$\frac{R_1 \times (l/3)}{AE} = \frac{(3000 - R_1) \times (l/3)}{AE} + \frac{R_2 \times (l/3)}{AE}$$

$$R_1 = (3000 - R_1) + R_2$$

$$2R_1 - R_2 = 3000 \qquad \text{... Eq. (ii)}$$

Solving Eqs (i) and (ii), we have

$$R_1 = 2500 \text{ N and } R_2 = 2000 \text{ N}$$

56. A vertical circular steel bar of length $3l$ fixed at both ends is loaded at intermediate sections by forces W and $2W$ as shown in Fig. 1.51. Determine the end reactions if $W = 1.5$ kN.

Solution: $l_1 = l_2 = l_3 = l$, $A_1 = A_2 = A_3 = A$, $R_1 = ?$, $R_2 = ?$

To find reactions:

Based on analysis, the reactions are similar to as shown in **Fig. 1.49(b).**

For equilibrium, $\qquad \Sigma F_H = 0$

$$R_1 + R_2 = 2W + W = 3W \qquad \text{... Eq. (i)}$$

Here element AB is subjected to tension while elements BC and CD are subjected to compression.

i.e. for compatibility, $\quad \delta l_{AB} = \delta l_{BC} + \delta l_{CD}$

$$\frac{F_1 l_1}{A_1 E_1} = \frac{F_2 l_2}{A_2 E_2} + \frac{F_3 l_3}{A_3 E_3}$$

Here $F_1 = R_1$, $F_2 = (2W - R_1)$, $F_3 = R_2$

$$\frac{R_1 \times l}{AE} = \frac{(2W - R_1) \times l}{AE} + \frac{R_2 \times l}{AE}$$

$$R_1 = (2W - R_1) + R_2$$

$$2R_1 - R_2 = 2W \qquad \text{... Eq. (ii)}$$

Solving Eqs (i) and (ii), we have

$$R_1 = 5W/3 \text{ and } R_2 = 4W/3$$

Given $W = 1.5$ kN

$$R_1 = 5W/3 = 5 \times \left(\frac{1.5}{3}\right) = 2.5 \text{ kN}$$

$$R_2 = 4W/3 = 4 \times \left(\frac{1.5}{3}\right) = 2 \text{ kN}$$

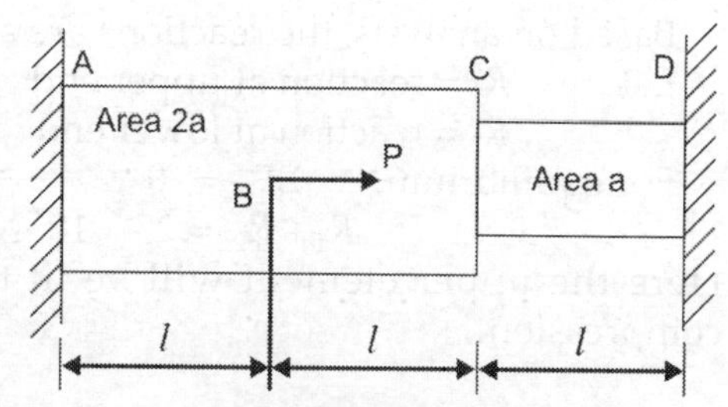

Fig. 1.51: Problem 56

57. An axially loaded bar is held between supports as shown in Fig. 1.52(a). Determine the displacement of point B at which the load P acts. Also determine the reactions at the supports.

Solution: $l_1 = l_2 = l_3 = l$, $A_1 = A_2 = 2a$, $A_3 = a$, a) $R_1 = ?$, $R_2 = ?$, b) $\delta_B = ?$

Fig. 1.52(a): Problem 57

a. To find reactions:

Based on analysis, the reactions are as shown in **Fig's. 1.52(b) & (c)** respectively.

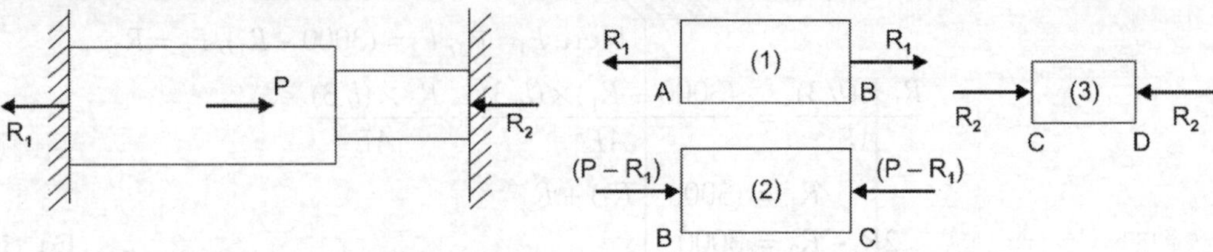

Fig. 1.52(b): Problem 56   **Fig. 1.52(c):** Problem 56

For equilibrium, $\quad \Sigma F_H = 0$

$$R_1 + R_2 = P \qquad \qquad \text{... Eq. (i)}$$

Here element AB in tension while elements BC and CD are subjected to compression.

i.e. for compatibility, $\quad \delta l_{AB} = \delta l_{BC} + \delta l_{CD}$

$$\frac{F_1 l_1}{A_1 E_1} = \frac{F_2 l_2}{A_2 E_2} + \frac{F_3 l_3}{A_3 E_3}$$

Here $F_1 = R_1$, $F_2 = (P - R_1)$, $F_3 = R_2$

$$\frac{R_1 \times l}{2aE} = \frac{(P - R_1) \times l}{2aE} + \frac{R_2 \times l}{aE}$$

$$\frac{R_1}{2} = \frac{(P - R_1)}{2} + R_2$$

$$R_1 = (P - R_1) + 2R_2$$

$$2(R_1 - R_2) = P$$

$$(R_1 - R_2) = 0.5P \qquad \qquad \text{... Eq. (ii)}$$

Solving Eqs (i) and (ii), we have

$$R_1 = \left(\frac{3P}{4}\right) \text{ and } R_2 = \left(\frac{P}{4}\right)$$

b. To find displacements:

At D, $\quad \delta l_B = \delta l_{CD} = \dfrac{R_1 l_1}{A_1 E} = \left(\dfrac{3P}{4}\right)\left(\dfrac{1}{2aE}\right) = \dfrac{3Pl}{8aE}$

58. A composite bar is as shown in Fig. 1.53(a). Determine the reactions at the support and the stresses in each bar. Take $E = 200$ GPa.

Solution: $l_1 = 1500$ mm, $l_2 = 2000$ mm, $d_1 = 8$ mm, $d_1 = 12$ mm, $P = 25$ kN, $R_1 = ?$, $R_2 = ?$, $\sigma_1 = ?$, $\sigma_2 = ?$

a. To find reactions:

Based on analysis, the reactions are as shown in **Fig's. 1.53(b) & (c)** respectively.

Let $\quad R_1$ = reaction at upper end

$\quad\quad\quad R_2$ = reaction at lower end

For equilibrium, $\quad \Sigma F_H = 0$

$$R_1 + R_2 = 25 \times 10^3 \text{ N} \qquad \qquad \text{... Eq. (i)}$$

Here the upper element will be in tension while the lower element will be in compression.

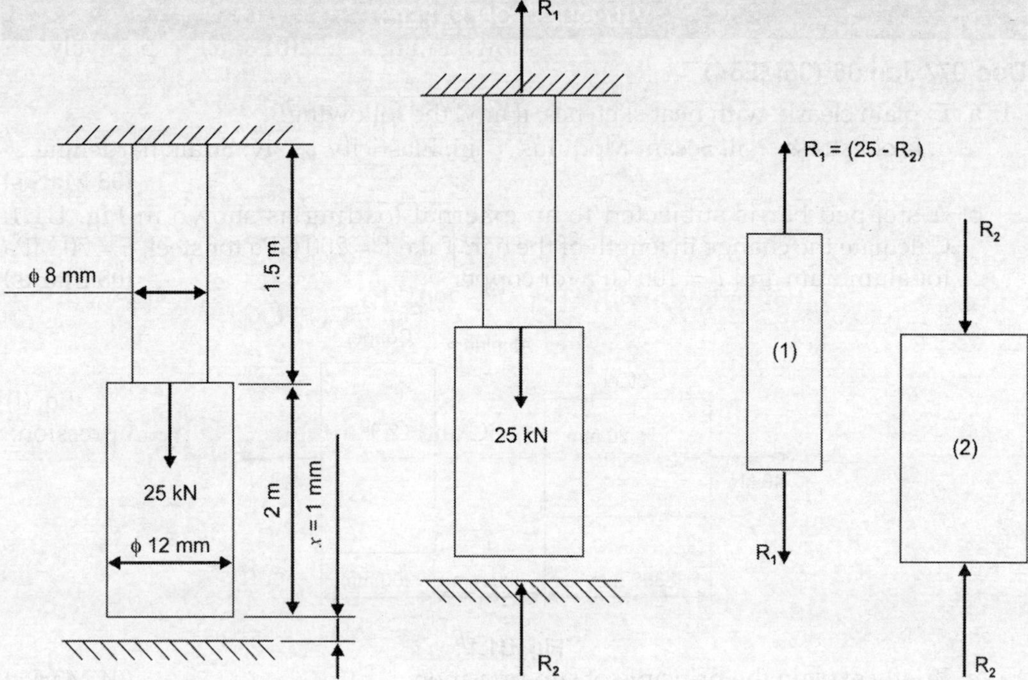

Fig. 1.53(a): Problem 58   Fig. 1.53(b): Problem 58   Fig. 1.53(c): Problem 58

i.e. for compatibility, $\quad \delta l_1 = \delta l_2 + a$
$$\delta l_1 - \delta l_2 = a$$

$$\frac{F_1 l_1}{A_1 E_1} - \frac{F_2 l_2}{A_2 E_2} = 1$$

Here $F_1 = (25 \times 10^3 - R_1)$, $F_2 = R_2$

$$\frac{(P - R_1) l_1}{A_1 E_1} - \frac{R_2 l_2}{A_2 E_2} = 1$$

$$\frac{(25 \times 10^3) \times 1500}{(\pi \times 8^2 / 4) \times (200 \times 10^3)} - \frac{R_2 \times 2000}{(\pi \times 12^2 / 4) \times (200 \times 10^3)} = 1$$

$$3.730 - (1.492 \times 10^{-4} R_2) - 8.842 \times 10^{-5} R_2 = 1$$
$$2.730 = 2.736 \times 10^{-4} R_2$$
$$R_2 = 11488.56 \text{ N}$$

$\therefore$ Eq. (i) yields ... $\quad R_1 = 25 \times 10^3 - 11488.56$
$$R_1 = 13511.44 \text{ N}$$

b. Stresses

$$\sigma_1 = \frac{R_1}{A_1} = \frac{13511.44}{(\pi \times 8^2 / 4)} = 268.78 \text{ MPa}$$

$$\sigma_2 = \frac{R_2}{A_2} = \frac{11488.56}{(\pi \times 12^2 / 4)} = 101.59 \text{ MPa}$$

Dec.07/ Jan.08 (06ME34)

1. a. Explain clearly with neat sketches, if any, the following:
   i. Proof stress   ii. Secant Modulus   iii. Elasticity   iv. Strain hardening.
   (08 Marks)

   b. A stepped bar is subjected to an external loading as shown in **Fig. U1.1.** Calculate the change in length of the bar. Take $E = 200$ GPa for steel, $E = 70$ MPa for aluminum and $E = 100$ GPa for copper. **(08 Marks)**

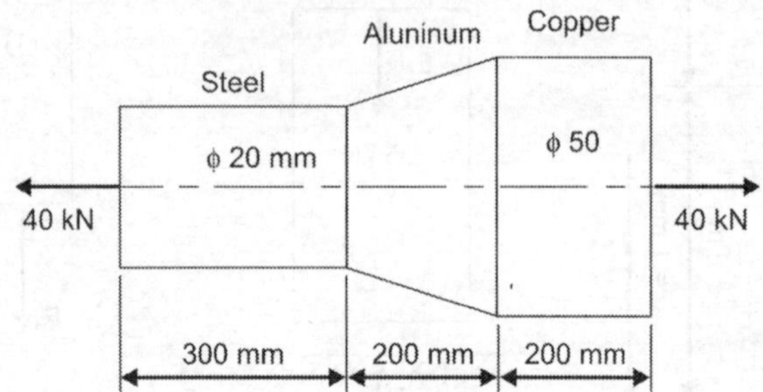

Fig. U1.1

   c. Briefly explain the principle of superposition. **(04 Marks)**

June/ July 2008 (06ME34)

2. a. Define Hooke's law, modulus of elasticity, elasticity and strain. **(04 Marks)**
   b. Derive an expression for total extension of a tapered circular bar cross section of diameter D and d, when it is subjected to an axial pull of load P. **(06 Marks)**
   c. For the laboratory tested specimen the following data were obtained:
   Diameter of the specimen = 25 mm
   Length of the specimen = 300 mm
   Extension under the load of 15 kN = 0.045 mm
   Load at yield point = 127.65 kN
   Maximum load = 208.60 kN
   Neck diameter = 17.75 mm
   Length of the specimen after failure = 375 mm
   Determine:
   i. Young's modulus   ii. Yield point stress   iii. Ultimate stress
   iv. Percentage elongation   v. Percentage reduction in area   **(10 Marks)**

Dec.08/ Jan.09 (06ME34)

3. a. Define:
   i. Poisson's ratio   ii. Bulk modulus   iii. Factor of safety
   (03 Marks)

   b. Derive an expression for total deformation of a tapering rectangular bar of cross section b_1 and b_2, when it is subjected to an axial force P. **(07 Marks)**

   c. A round bar with stepped portion is subjected to forces as shown in **Fig. U1.2.** Determine the magnitude of force P such that the net deformation in the bar does not exceed 1 mm. E for steel is 200 GPa and for aluminium is 70 GPa. Big end diameter and small end diameter of the tapering bar are 40 mm and 12.5 mm respectively. **(10 Marks)**

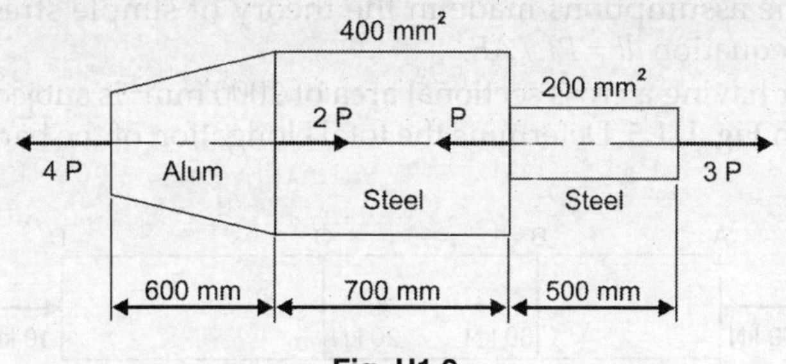

Fig. U1.2

June/July 2009 (06ME34)

4. a. Define the following terms:
     i. Elastic limit
     ii. True stress
     iii. Factor of safety
     iv. Poisson's ratio **(04 Marks)**
   b. Prove that the extension of a uniform bar due to self weight is half of the extension when the load equal to its self weight is applied at the end of the suspended bar. **(08 Marks)**
   c. A prismatic bar is subjected to loads, P_1, P_2 and P_3 as shown in **Fig. U1.3**. The bar is made of steel with modulus of elasticity $E = 200$ GPa and cross sectional area $A = 225$ mm². Determine the deflection δ at the lower end of the bar due to the applied loads. **(10 Marks)**

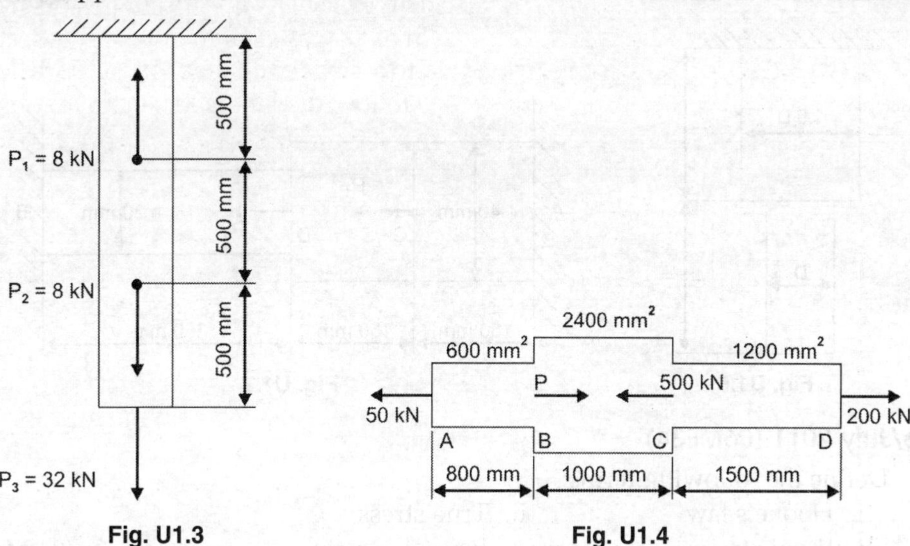

Dec. 09/Jan. 10 (06ME34)

5. a. Define: i. Stress ii. Principle of superposition **(04 Marks)**
   b. A member ABCD is subjected to loads as shown in **Fig. U1.4**. Calculate:
     i. Force P necessary for equilibrium
     ii. Total elongation of the bar. Take $E = 210$ GN/m². **(06 Marks)**

May/June 2010 (06ME34)

6. a. Explain: i. Poisson's ratio   ii. Young's modulus   **(04 Marks)**
   b. Mention the assumptions made in the theory of simple stress and strain and derive the equation $dl = PL/AE$. **(06 Marks)**
   c. A brass bar having a cross sectional area of 1000 mm^2 is subjected to axial forces as shown in **Fig. U1.5**. Determine the total elongation of the bar if $E = 105$ GPa. **(10 Marks)**

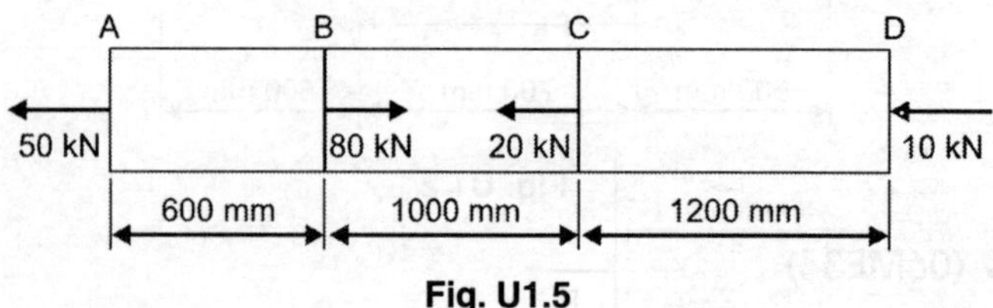

Fig. U1.5

Dec. 2010 (06ME34)

7. a. State Hooke's law. Sketch the typical stress-strain curve for aluminium. **(04 Marks)**
   b. A stepped bar having circular cross sections of diameter 1.5D and D is shown in **Fig. U1.6**. If ρ and E are the density and Young's modulus of elasticity respectively, find the extension of the bar due to self weight. **(08 Marks)**
   c. A stepped bar of steel, held between two supports as shown in **Fig. U1.7** is subjected to loads $P_1 = 80$ kN and $P_2 = 60$ kN. Find the reactions developed at the ends A and B. **(08 Marks)**

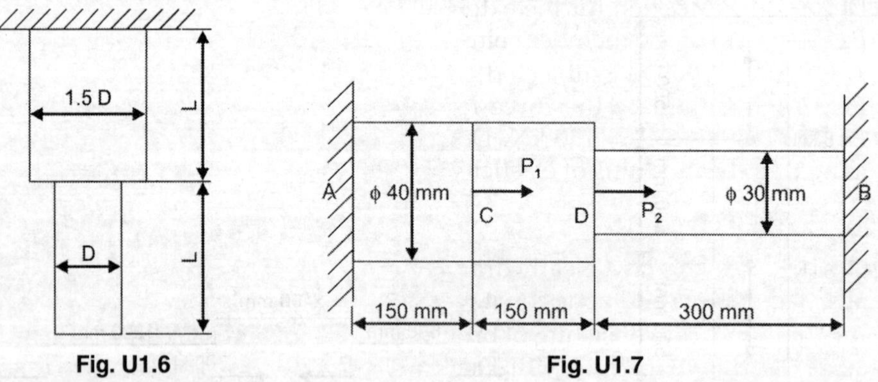

Fig. U1.6   **Fig. U1.7**

June/July 2011 (06ME34)

8. a. Define the following terms:
   i. Hooke's law   ii. True stress
   iii. Proof stress   iv. Poisson's ratio   **(04 Marks)**
   b. Derive an expression for the extension of a tapering bar whose diameter d_1 at one end tapers linearly to diameter d_2 at the other end in a length L, under an axial pull P and the elastic modulus of the material is E. **(08 Marks)**
   c. A round bar with stepped portion is subjected to forces as shown in **Fig. U1.8**. Determine the magnitude of force P such that the net deformation in the bar does not exceed 1 mm. E for steel is 200 GPa and that for aluminium is 70 GPa. Big end diameter and small end diameter of the tapering bar are 40 mm and 12.5 mm respectively. **(08 Marks)**

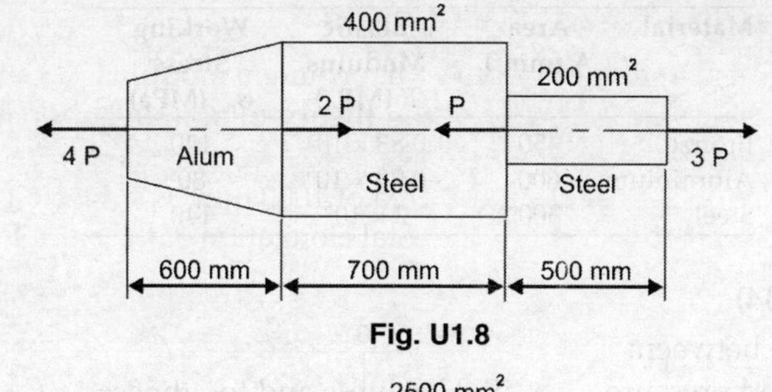

Fig. U1.8

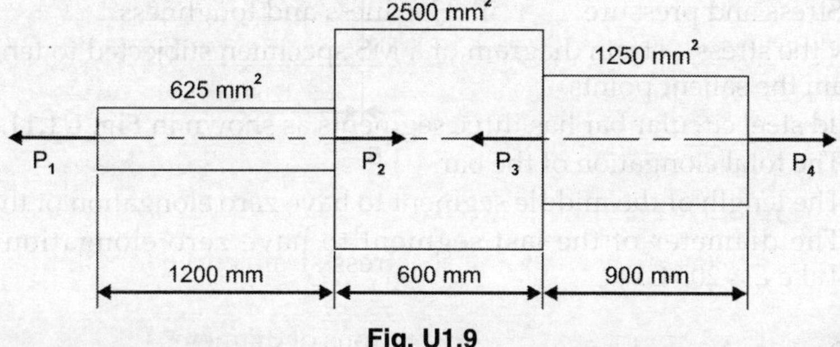

Fig. U1.9

Dec. 2011 (06ME34)

9. a. Define:
   - i. Hooke's law
   - ii. Poisson's ratio
   - iii. Elastic limit
   - iv. Modulus of rigidity. **(04 Marks)**

   b. Derive an expression for the extension of a member subjected to a tensile load P. The length of the member being L and its Young modulus is E. **(04 Marks)**

   c. A member ABCD is subjected to point loads P_1, P_2, P_3 and P_4 as shown in **Fig. U1.9**. Calculate the force P_2 necessary for equilibrium, if P_1 = 45 kN, P_3 = 450 kN and P_4 = 130 kN. Determine the total elongation of the member, assuming the modulus of elasticity to be 2.1×10^5 N/mm^2. **(12 Marks)**

Dec. 2011 (10ME34)

10. a. State the Hooke's law. Neatly draw the stress-strain diagram for steel indicating all salient points and zones on it. **(05 Marks)**

    b. A compound bar consisting of bronze, aluminium and steel segments is loaded axially as shown in **Fig. U1.10**. Determine the maximum allowable value of P, if the change in length of the bar is not to exceed 2 mm and the working stresses in each material of the bar indicated in the table below is not to be exceeded. **(15 Marks)**

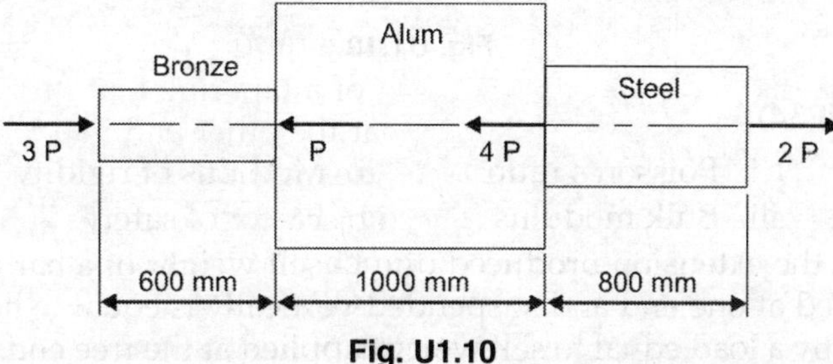

Fig. U1.10

Material	Area A (mm²)	Elastic Modulus E (MPa)	Working Stress σ_w (MPa)
Bronze	450	0.83×10^5	120
Aluminium	600	0.70×10^5	80
Steel	300	2×10^5	140

June 2012 (06ME34)

11. a. Differentiate between:
   i. Stress and pressure   ii. Hardness and toughness   **(04 Marks)**
   b. Draw the stress – strain diagram of a MS specimen subjected to tensile test and explain the salient points.   **(06 Marks)**
   c. A mild steel circular bar has three segments as shown in **Fig. U1.11.** Find
   i. The total elongation of the bar
   ii. The length of the middle segment to have zero elongation of the bar
   iii. The diameter of the last segment to have zero elongation of the bar.
   Take E = 205 GPa.   **(10 Marks)**

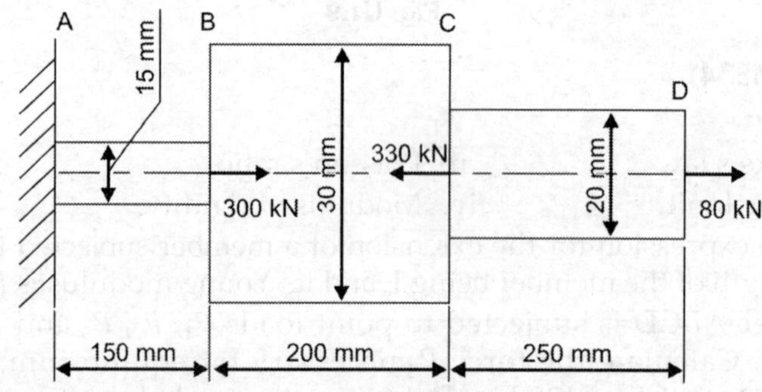

Fig. U1.11

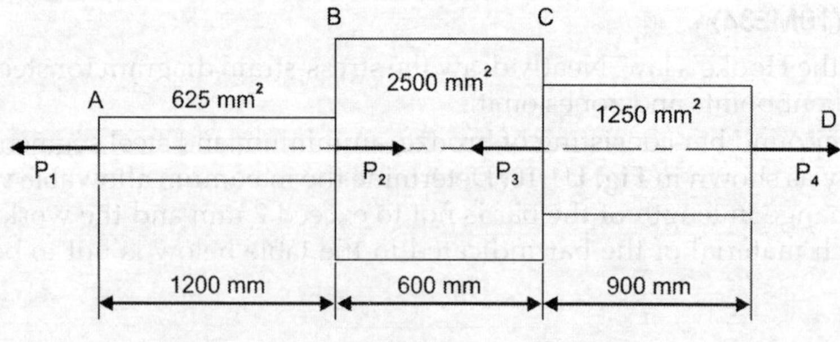

Fig. U1.12

June 2012 (10ME34)

12. a. Define: i. Poisson's ratio   ii. Modulus of rigidity
   iii. Bulk modulus   iv. Factor of safety.   **(04 Marks)**
   b. Show that the extension produced due to self weight of a bar of uniform cross section fixed at one end and suspended vertically is equal to half the extension produced by a load equal to self weight applied at the free end.   **(08 Marks)**

c. A member ABCD is subjected to point loads P_1, P_2, P_3 and P_4 as shown in **Fig. U1.12.** Calculate the force P_2 necessary for equilibrium, if $P_1 =$ 45 kN, $P_3 =$ 450 kN and $P_4 =$ 130 kN. Determine the total elongation of the member, assuming the modulus of elasticity to be 2.1×10^5 N/mm^2. **(08 Marks)**

Dec. 2012 (10ME34)

13. a. Define; i. Ductility   ii. True stress   iii. Principle of superposition

(06 Marks)

b. Determine the stresses in various segments of the circular bar shown in **Fig. U1.13.**
  i. Compute the total elongation assuming Young's modulus of steel to be 195 GPa.
  ii. Determine the length of the middle segment so that the bar length does not change under the applied loads. **(08 Marks)**

c. Derive an expression for the extension of a uniformly tapering rectangular bar subjected to axial load P. **(06 Marks)**

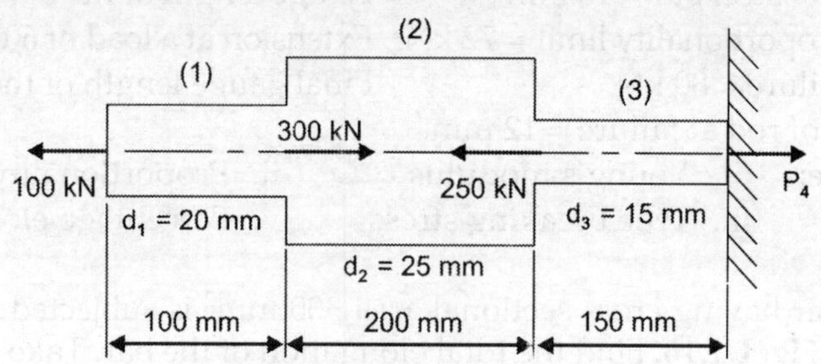

Fig. U1.13

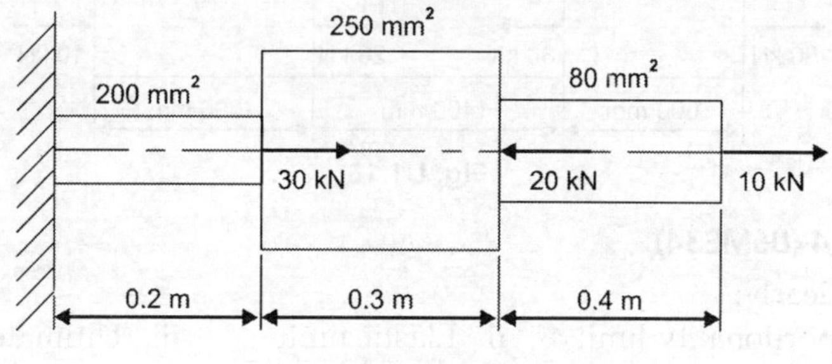

Fig. U1.14

Jan. 2013 (06ME34)

14. a. Define: i. Hooke's law   ii. True stress   iii. Factor of safety

(06 Marks)

b. Derive an expression for extension in a bar of uniform cross section fixed at one end and suspended vertically, due to self weight. **(07 Marks)**

c. A stepped bar is subjected to forces as shown in **Fig. U1.14.** Determine the net deformation in the stepped bar. Take $E = 2 \times 10^5$ N/mm^2. **(10 Marks)**

June/July 2013 (06ME34)

15. a. Define: i. Young's modulus   ii. Poisson's ratio   iii. Factor of safety.
   (05 Marks)

   b. Derive an expression for the deformation of a tapered bar of circular section, subjected to tensile load.   **(08 Marks)**

   c. A steel bar of cross section 500 mm^2 is acted upon by forces shown in **Fig. U1.15**. Determine the total elongation of the bar. Take E= 200 GPa.
   (07 Marks)

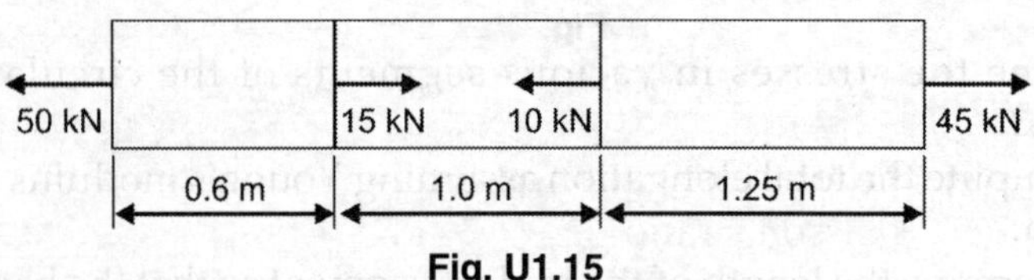

Fig. U1.15

June/July 2013 (10ME34)

16. a. The tensile stress was conducted on a mild steel bar. The following data was obtained from the test:

   Diameter of steel bar = 16 mm   Gauge length of the bar = 80 mm
   Load at proportionality limit = 72 kN   Extension at a load of 60 kN = 0.115 mm
   Load at failure = 80 kN   Final gauge length of the bar = 104 mm
   Diameter of rod at failure = 12 mm.
   Determine: i. Young's modulus   ii. Proportionality limit
              iii. True breaking stress   iv. Percentage elongation.
   (10 Marks)

   b. A brass bar having cross sectional area 300 mm^2 is subjected to axial forces as shown in **Fig. U1.16**. Find the total elongation of the bar. Take E = 84 GPa.
   (10 Marks)

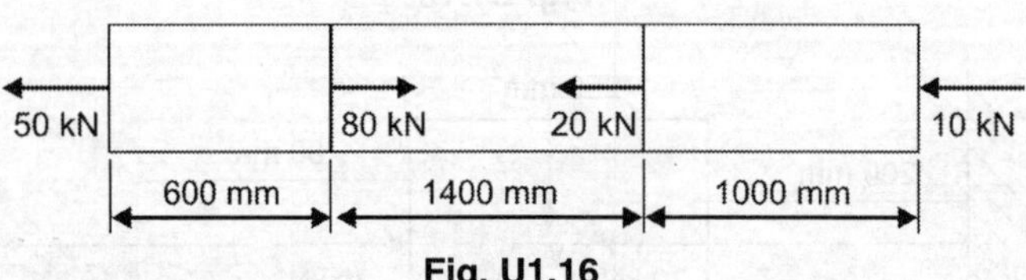

Fig. U1.16

Dec. 13/Jan. 14 (06ME34)

17. a. Explain clearly:
   i. Proportionality limit   ii. Elastic limit   iii. Ultimate stress
   (03 Marks)

   b. A rod of radius r_1 at one end tapers uniformly to a radius r_2 at the other end over a length L. It is subjected to an axial force P. Derive an expression for its change in length   **(07 Marks)**

   c. A stepped bar is subjected to external loading as shown in **Fig. U1.17**. Calculate the change in length of the bar. E = 200 GPa for steel, E = 100 GPa for copper, E = 70 GPa for aluminium.   **(10 Marks)**

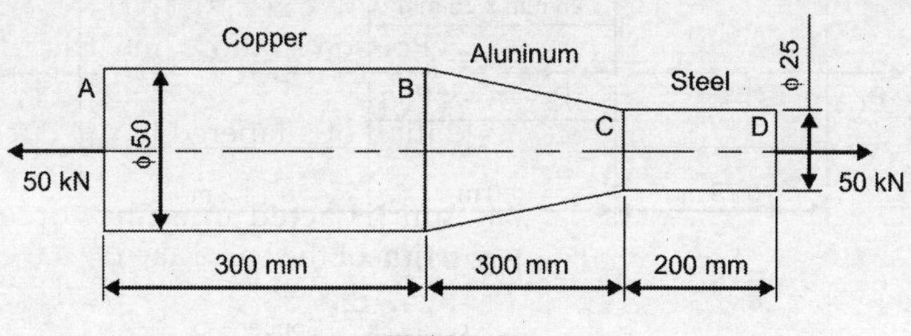

Fig. U1.17

Dec. 13/Jan. 14 (10ME34)

18. a. Define: i. True stress   ii. Factor of safety
          iii. Poisson's ratio   iv. Principle of superposition.

(04 Marks)

   b. A bar of uniform thickness t tapers uniformly from a width of b_1 at one end to b_2 at the other end, in an axial length of L. Find the expression for the change in length of the bar subjected to an axial force P. **(08 Marks)**

   c. A vertical circular steel bar of length $3l$ fixed at both ends is loaded at intermediate sections by forces W and $2W$ as shown in **Fig. U1.18**. Determine the end reactions if $W = 1.5$kN. **(08 Marks)**

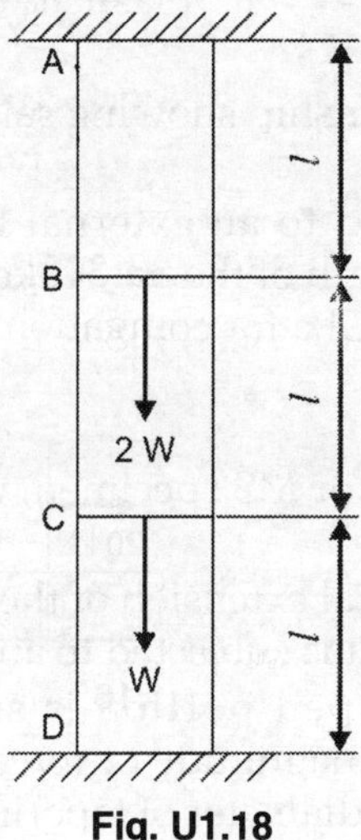

Fig. U1.18

June/July 2014 (06ME34)

19. a. Define: i. Poisson's ratio   ii. Bulk modulus
          iii. Factor of safety   iv. Principle of superposition.

(04 Marks)

   b. Distinguish between a ductile material and a brittle material. Give one example each. Draw typical stress-strain diagram for each of them indicating salient points on them. **(08 Marks)**

   c. A member is subjected to point loads P_1, P_2, P_3 and P_4 as shown in **Fig. U1.19**. Calculate the force P_3 necessary for equilibrium, if $P_1 = 120$ kN, $P_2 = 220$ kN and $P_4 = 160$ kN. Determine also the net change in length of the member. Take $E = 200$ GN/m^2. **(08 Marks)**

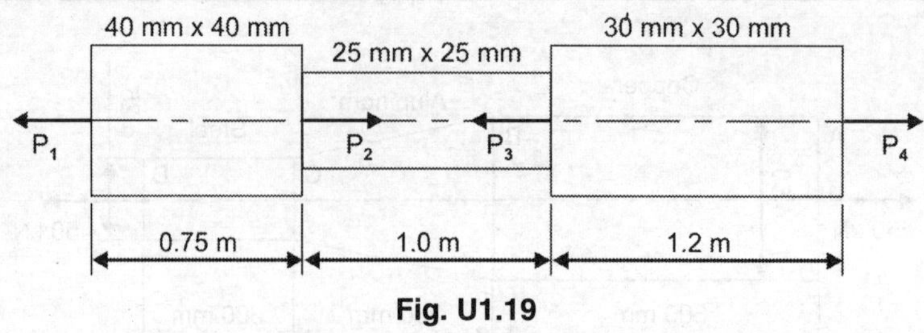

Fig. U1.19

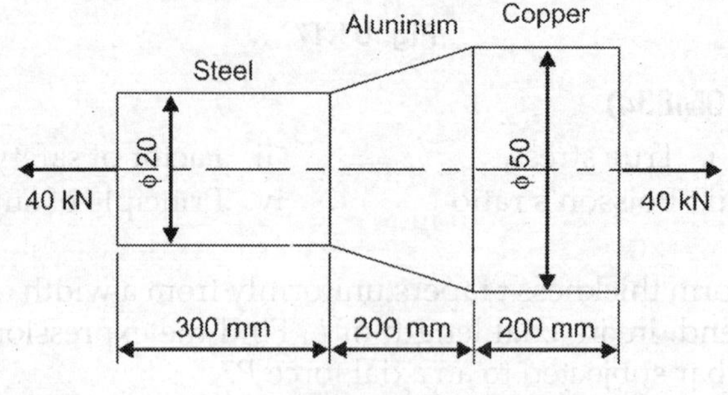

Fig. U1.20

June/July 2014 (10ME34)

20. a. Define: i. Hooke's law   ii. Elasticity   iii. Lateral strain

(04 Marks)

b. Explain stress-strain relationship showing salient points on the diagram.

(06 Marks)

c. A stepped bar is subjected to an external loading as shown in Fig. U1.20. Calculate the change in length of the bar. Take $E = 200$ GPa for steel, $E = 70$ MPa for aluminum and $E = 100$ GPa for copper. **(10 Marks)**

Dec. 14/Jan. 15 (06ME34)

21. a. Draw stress – strain curve for MS specimen, when loaded in tension and mark all salient points on it. **(04 Marks)**

b. Derive an expression for total extension of the tapered circular bar cross-section of diameter D and d when it is subjected to an axial pull of P. **(06 Marks)**

c. A round bar having stepped portion is subjected to forces as shown in **Fig. U1.21.** Determine the magnitude of force P such that the net deformation does not exceed 1 mm. The diameter of tapering section at the big and small end is 40 mm and 12.5 mm respectively. Take E for steel as 200 GPa and that for aluminum as 70 GPa. **(10 Marks)**

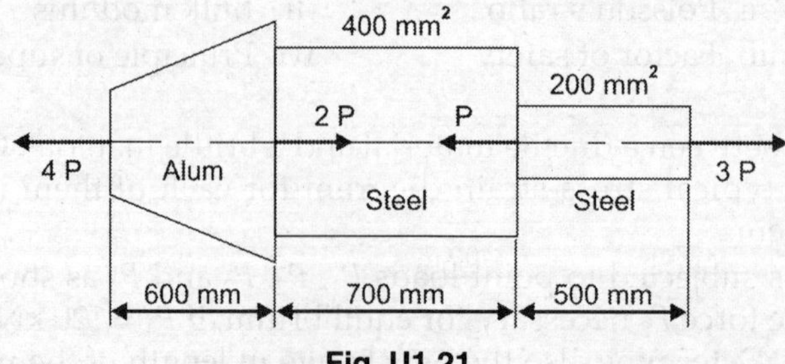

Fig. U1.21

Dec. 14/Jan. 15 (10ME34)

22. a. State Hooke's law. Sketch and explain typical stress strain curve for aluminium.
(04 Marks)

b. The tensile test was conducted on a mild steel bar. The following data was obtained from the test:

Diameter of steel bar = 16 mm, load at proportionality limit = 72 kN, load at failure = 80 kN, diameter of rod at failure = 12 mm, gauge length of the bar = 80 mm, extension at a load of 60 kN = 0.115 mm, final gauge length of the bar = 104 mm. Determine: i. Young's modulus   ii. proportionality limit   iii. true breaking stress   iv. percentage elongation
(08 Marks)

c. Determine the magnitude of load P necessary to produce zero net change in length of the straight bar shown in **Fig. U1.22**. Area of cross section = 400 mm².
(08 Marks)

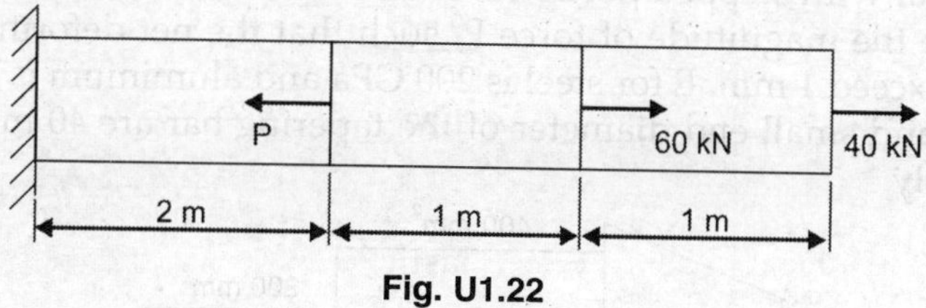

Fig. U1.22

June/July 2015 (10ME34)

23. a. State Hooke's law and define Poisson's ratio. **(03 Marks)**
    b. Explain stress – strain diagram for mild steel with salient features. **(07 Marks)**
    c. A member ABCD is subjected to points loads of P_1, P_2, P_3 and P_4 as shown in **Fig. U1.23**. Calculate the force P_2 necessary for equilibrium if P_1 = 45 kN, P_3 = 450 kN and P_4 = 130 kN. Determine the stresses in each member and also determine the total elongation of the member assuming $E = 2.1 \times 10^5 \, \text{N/mm}^2$.
(10 Marks)

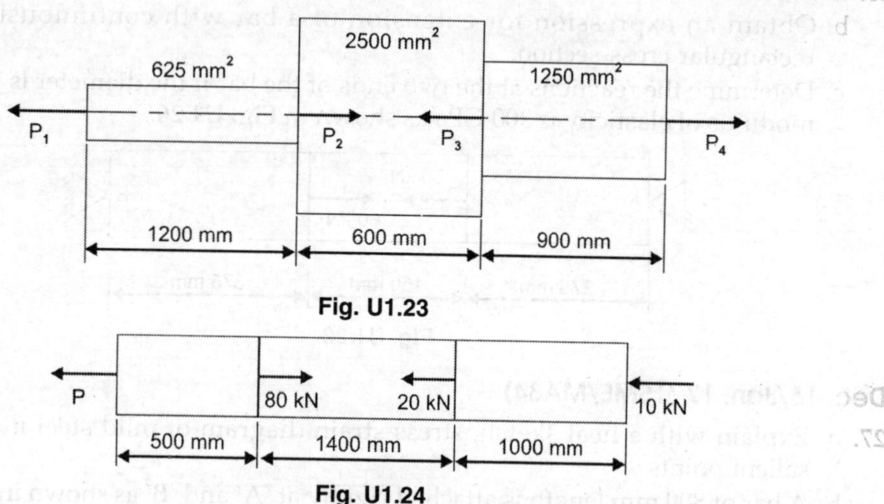

Fig. U1.23

Fig. U1.24

Dec. 15/Jan. 16 (10ME/AU34)

24. a. Define   i. Proof stress   ii. Proportionality limit
       iii. Principle of superposition   iv. Hooke's law   **(04 Marks)**

   b. Derive an expression for the total elongation of a tapered bar varying diameter from d_1 to d_2, when subjected to axial load P.   **(08 Marks)**

   c. A brass bar of uniform cross sectional area 300 mm² is subjected to a load as shown in **Fig. U1.24**. Find the total elongation of the bar and the magnitude of load P if Young's modulus is 84 GPa.   **(08 Marks)**

June/July 2016 (10ME/AU34)

25. a. State Hooke's law. Sketch the typical stress-strain diagram for mild steel indicating salient points and zones on it.   **(04 Marks)**

   b. Derive an expression for extension of a uniformly tapering circular bar subjected to axial load.   **(08 Marks)**

   c. A round bar with stepped portion is subjected to forces as shown in **Fig. U1.25**. Determine the magnitude of force P, such that the net deformation in the bar does not exceed 1 mm. E for steel is 200 GPa and aluminium is 70 GPa. Big end diameter and small end diameter of the tapering bar are 40 mm and 12.5 mm respectively.   **(10 Marks)**

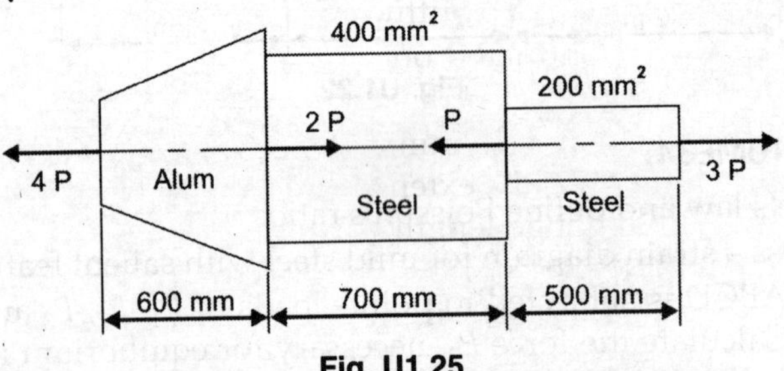

Fig. U1.25

Dec. 16/Jan. 17 (10ME/AU34)

26. a. Explain the stress-strain curve with salient points.   **(06 Marks)**

   b. Obtain an expression for extension of a bar with continuously varying rectangular cross-section.   **(08 Marks)**

   c. Determine the reactions at the two ends of the bar if the diameter is 25 mm and modulus of elasticity is 300 GPa as shown in **Fig. U1.26**.   **(06 Marks)**

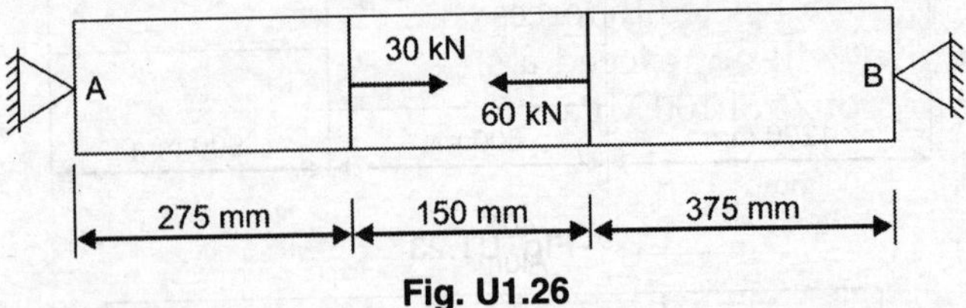

Fig. U1.26

Dec. 16/Jan. 17 (15ME/MA34)

27. a. Explain with a neat sketch, stress-strain diagram of mild steel indicating its salient points.   **(06 Marks)**

   b. A bar of 800 mm length is attached rigidly at 'A' and 'B' as shown in **Fig. U1.27**. Determine the reactions at the two ends. If the bar is of 25 mm diameter, find the stresses and change in length of each portion. Take $E = 200$ GPa.   **(10 Marks)**

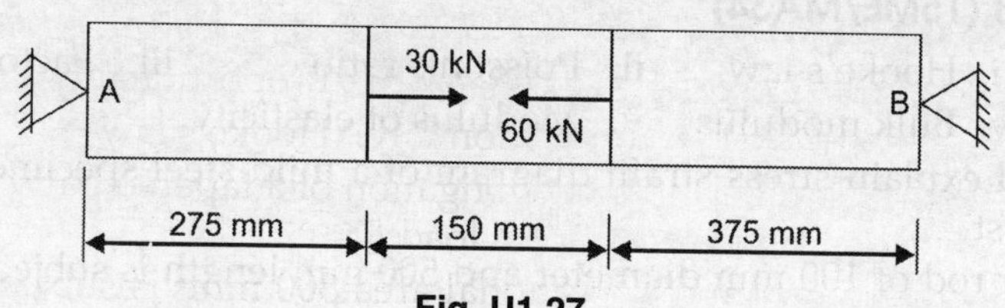

Fig. U1.27

June/July 2017 (10ME/AU34)

28. a. List and explain the mechanical properties of engineering materials.

(10 Marks)

 b. A round stepped bar is subjected to an axial load of 30 kN. Diameter and length of first portion are 40 mm and 200 mm respectively and those of the second portion are 20 mm and 100 mm respectively. Determine change in deformation when a uniform with same volume and length as that of stepped bar is subjected to 30 kN. Take $E = 200$ GPa. **(10 Marks)**

June/July 2017 (15ME/MA34)

29. a. Define the following:

  i. Elasticity   ii. Ductility   iii. Toughness

  iv. Hardness   v. Stiffness   vi. Resilience. **(06 Marks)**

 b. The tensile test was conducted on a mild steel bar. The following data was obtained from the test.

 Diameter of the steel bar = 16 mm, gauge length of the bar = 80 mm, load at proportionality limit = 72 kN, extension at a load of 72 kN = 0.115 mm, load at failure = 80 kN, final gauge length of the bar = 104 mm, dia of rod at failure = 12 mm. Determine

  i. Young's modulus   ii. Proportionality limit

  iii. True breaking stress   iv. Percentage elongation. **(10 Marks)**

Dec. 17/Jan. 18 (10ME/AU34)

30. a. Define: i. Elasticity   ii. Poisson's ratio

      iii. Hooke's law   iv. Principle of superposition. **(04 Marks)**

 b. Prove that the deformation in a bar of uniform cross-section due to self weight is equal to half the deformation due to the force equal to its self weight.

(06 Marks)

 c. A stepped bar is subjected to forces as shown in **Fig. U1.28**. Find the maximum value of P that will not exceed a stress in steel of 140 MPa in aluminium of 90 MPa or in bronze of 100 MPa. **(10 Marks)**

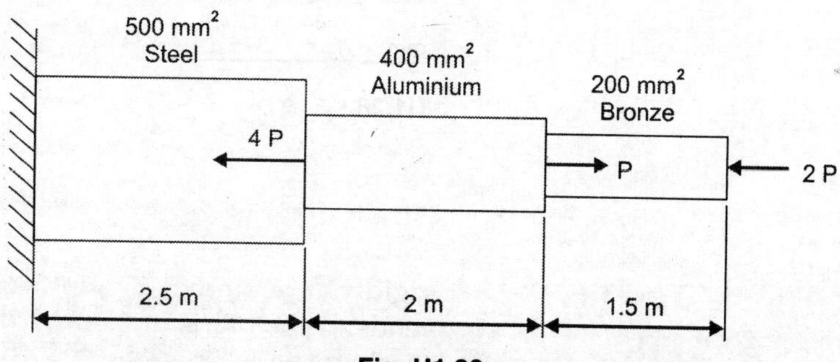

Fig. U1.28

Dec. 17/Jan. 18 (15ME/MA34)

31. a. Define: i. Hooke's law ii. Poisson's ratio iii. Factor of safety
iv. Bulk modulus v. Modulus of elasticity. **(05 Marks)**

b. Draw and explain stress-strain diagram of a mild steel specimen subjected to tension test. **(05 Marks)**

c. A circular rod of 100 mm diameter and 500 mm length is subjected to a tensile load of 1000 kN. Determine:
i. Modulus of rigidity ii. Bulk modulus iii. Change in volume.
Take Poisson's ratio as 0.30 and $E = 200$ GPa. **(06 Marks)**

Stresses in Composite Sections

Chapter Outline

2.1 COMPOSITE/COMPOUND BARS

A composite bar may be defined as a bar made of two or more different materials joined together at their ends to form a parallel arrangement and subjected to axial loading, as shown in **Fig. 2.1**. The arrangement is such that the system extends or contracts as one unit, when subjected to tensile or compressive load.

Consider a compound member made of two different materials as shown in **Fig. 2.1**.

Let, F = total load on the composite bar

        l = Length of the composite bar

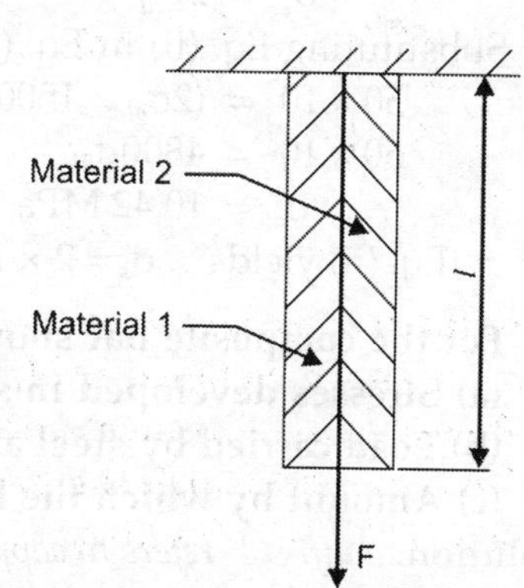

Fig. 2.1: Composite section

A_1 = Area of bar (1)

E_1 = Young's modulus of bar (1)

F_1 = Load shared by bar (1)

On similar lines let A_2, E_2 and F_2 be corresponding parameters for bar (2).

For equilibrium,
$$F = F_1 + F_2$$
$$= \sigma_1 A_1 + \sigma_2 A_2 \qquad \text{... (Eq. 2.1)}$$

For compatibility,
$$\delta l_1 = \delta l_2$$

$$\frac{F_1 l_1}{A_1 E_1} = \frac{F_2 l_2}{A_2 E_2}$$

$$\frac{\sigma_1}{E_1} = \frac{\sigma_2}{E_2} \qquad (\because l_1 = l_2) \qquad \text{... (Eq. 2.2)}$$

Or
$$\frac{\sigma_1}{\sigma_2} = \frac{E_1}{E_2} \qquad \text{... (Eq. 2.3)}$$

Note: The term $\dfrac{E_1}{E_2}$ is referred to as *modular ratio*. ... (Eq. 2.4)

1. **A compound bar rigidly joined at the ends and subjected to a load of 50 kN is shown in Fig. 2.2. Find the stresses developed and the deformation in each bar. Take E_s = 200 GPa and E_{al} = 100 GPa.**

Solution: $A_{al} = 60 \times 30 = 1800 \text{ mm}^2$, $A_s = 60 \times 25 = 1500 \text{ mm}^2$, $l = 800$ mm, $F = 50$ kN, $E_s = 200 \times 10^3$ MPa, $E_{al} = 100 \times 10^3$ MPa, $\sigma_s = ?$, $\sigma_{al} = ?$,

For a composite bar, $F = F_s + F_{al} = \sigma_s A_s + \sigma_{al} A_{al}$ ... Eq. (i)

But $\dfrac{\sigma_s}{E_s} = \dfrac{\sigma_{al}}{E_{al}}$

$$\sigma_s = \left(\frac{E_s}{Eal}\right) \sigma_{al}$$

$$= \left(\frac{200 \times 10^3}{100 \times 10^3}\right) \times \sigma_{al}$$

$$\sigma_s = 2\sigma_{al} \qquad \text{... Eq. (ii)}$$

Substituting Eq. (ii) in Eq. (i), we have,

$$50 \times 10^3 = (2\sigma_{al} \times 1500) + (\sigma_{al} \times 1800)$$
$$50 \times 10^3 = 4800\sigma_{al}$$
$$\therefore \quad \sigma_{al} = 10.42 \text{ MPa} \qquad \text{(Aluminium)}$$
$$\therefore \text{ Eq. (ii) yields... } \sigma_s = 2 \times 10.42 = 20.84 \text{ MPa} \qquad \text{(Steel)}$$

Fig. 2.2: Problem 1

2. **For the composite bar shown in Fig. 2.3, determine:**
   (a) **Stresses developed in steel and copper.**
   (b) **Load carried by steel and copper.**
   (c) **Amount by which the bar shortens.** Take E_s = 210 GPa and E_{cu} = 95 GPa.

Solution: *(suffix '1' refers to copper and '2' refers to steel)*

$d_1 = 60$ mm $\Rightarrow A_1 = (\pi \times 60^2)/4 = 2827.43$ mm^2, $(d_2)_o = 120$ mm, $(d_2)_i = 60$ mm, $\Rightarrow A_2 = \pi \times (120^2 - 60^2)/4 = 8482.30$ mm^2, $l = 2500$ mm, $F = 40$ kN, $E_{cu} = E_1 = 95 \times 10^3$ MPa, $E_s = E_2 = 210 \times 10^3$ MPa.

    (a) $\sigma_1 = ?$, $\sigma_2 = ?$ (b) $F_1 = ?$, $F_2 = ?$ (c) $\delta l = ?$

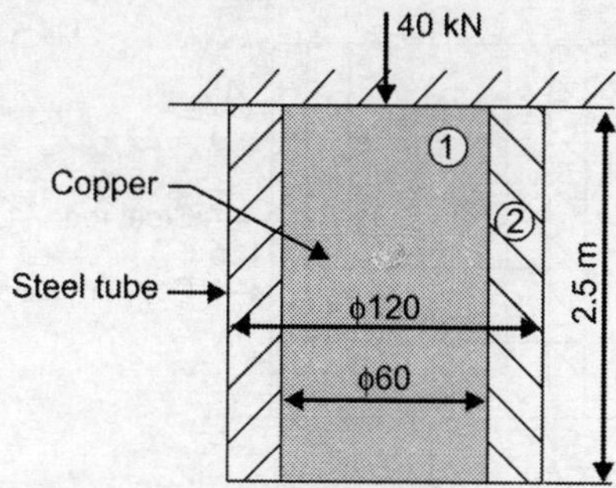

Fig. 2.3: Problem 2

a. To find stresses:

For a composite bar, $F = F_1 + F_2 = \sigma_1 A_1 + \sigma_2 A_2$ ... Eq. (i)

But
$$\frac{\sigma_1}{E_1} = \frac{\sigma_2}{E_2}$$

$$\sigma_2 = \left(\frac{E_2}{E_1}\right) \sigma_1$$

$$= \left(\frac{210 \times 10^3}{95 \times 10^3}\right) \sigma_1$$

$\therefore$ $\sigma_2 = 2.21\,\sigma_1$ ... Eq. (ii)

Substituting Eq. (ii) in Eq. (i), we have,
$$40 \times 10^3 = (2827.43\,\sigma_1) + (2.21\,\sigma_1 \times 8482.30)$$
$\therefore$ $\sigma_1 = 1.85$ MPa   (Copper)

Eq. (ii) yields... $\sigma_2 = 2.21 \times 1.85 = 4.09$ MPa   (Steel)

b. To find loads:

For copper, $\sigma_1 = \dfrac{F_1}{A_1} \Rightarrow F_1 = \sigma_1 A_1 = 1.85 \times 2827.43 = 5230.75$ N

For steel, $\sigma_2 = \dfrac{F_2}{A_2} \Rightarrow F_2 = \sigma_2 A_2 = 4.09 \times 8482.30 = 34692.61$ N

c. Amount by which the bar shortens:

Since the length of both materials is same, we have
$$\delta l_1 = \delta l_2$$

i.e. $\delta l_1 = \dfrac{\sigma_1 l}{E_1} = \dfrac{1.85 \times 2500}{95 \times 10^3} = 0.0486$ mm

3. **A steel rod of 30 mm diameter is encased by copper tube of internal diameter 35 mm and external diameter 40 mm. They are connected rigidly at the ends by rigid plates of negligible thickness. The composite bar is subjected to an axial pull of 120 kN. If the length of the composite bar is 500 mm, find the stresses in steel rod and copper tube. Take $E_s = 210$ GPa and $E_c = 105$ GPa.**

VTU – (CV) Dec 11 – 10 Marks

Solution: *(suffix '1' refers to steel and '2' refers to copper)*
$d_1 = 30$ mm $\Rightarrow A_1 = (\pi \times 30^2)/4 = 706.86$ mm^2, $(d_2)_i = 35$ mm, $(d_2)_o = 40$ mm, $\Rightarrow A_2 = \pi \times (40^2 - 35^2)/4 = 294.52$ mm^2, $F = 120$ kN, $l = 500$ mm, $E_s = E_1 = 210 \times 10^3$ MPa, $E_c = E_2 = 105 \times 10^3$ MPa, $\sigma_1 = ?$, $\sigma_2 = ?$

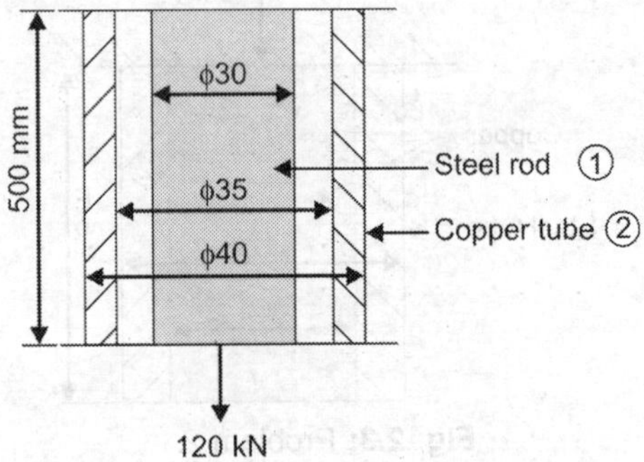

Fig. 2.4: Problem 3

For a composite bar, $F = F_1 + F_2 = \sigma_1 A_1 + \sigma_2 A_2$ ... Eq. (i)

But $\dfrac{\sigma_1}{E_1} = \dfrac{\sigma_2}{E_2}$

$$\sigma_2 = \left(\frac{E_2}{E_1}\right)\sigma_1$$

$$= \left(\frac{105 \times 10^3}{210 \times 10^3}\right)\sigma_1$$

$\therefore \qquad \sigma_2 = 0.5\,\sigma_1$ ... Eq. (ii)

Substituting Eq. (ii) in Eq. (i), we have,
$$120 \times 10^3 = (706.86\,\sigma_1) + (0.5\sigma_1 \times 294.52)$$
$\therefore \qquad \sigma_1 = 140.50$ MPa   (Steel)

Eq. (ii) yields... $\sigma_2 = 0.5 \times 140.50 = 70.25$ MPa   (Copper)

4. **A composite section comprises a steel tube 100 mm internal diameter and 120 mm external diameter fitted inside a brass tube of 140 mm internal diameter and 160 mm external diameter. The assembly is subjected to a compressive load of 500 kN. Find the load carried by the tube and the stresses generated in them. The length of the tube is 150 mm. Take $E_{steel} = 200 \times 10^3$ N/mm^2 and $E_{brass} = 100 \times 10^3$ N/mm^2. What is the change in length of the tube?**

VTU –May/ June 2010 – 10 Marks; (CV) June/ July 2008 – 10 Marks; [Similar: (CV) Dec. 15/ Jan. 16 – 10 Marks]

Solution: *(suffix '1' refers to steel and '2' refers to brass tube)*
$(d_1)_i = 100$ mm, $(d_1)_o = 120$ mm, $A_1 = \pi \times (120^2 - 100^2)/4 = 3455.75$ mm^2, $F = 500$ kN, $l_1 = l_2 = 150$ mm, $(d_2)_i = 140$ mm, $(d_2)_o = 160$ mm, $A_2 = \pi \times (160^2 - 140^2)/4 = 4712.39$ mm^2, $E_{steel} = E_1 = 200 \times 10^3$ N/mm^2, $E_{brass} = E_2 = 100 \times 10^3$ N/mm^2, $\sigma_1 = ?$, $\sigma_2 = ?$, $\delta l = ?$

a. To find stresses:

For a composite bar, $F = \sigma_1 A_1 + \sigma_2 A_2$ ... Eq. (i)

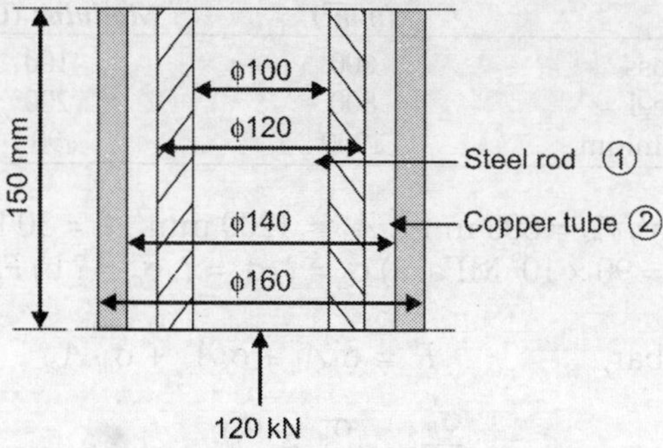

Fig. 2.5: Problem 4

$$\text{But} \qquad \frac{\sigma_1}{E_1} = \frac{\sigma_2}{E_2}$$

$$\sigma_2 = \left(\frac{E_2}{E_1}\right)\sigma_1$$

$$= \left(\frac{100 \times 10^3}{210 \times 10^3}\right)\sigma_1$$

$$\therefore \qquad \sigma_2 = 0.5\,\sigma_1 \qquad\qquad \dots \text{Eq. (ii)}$$

Substituting Eq. (ii) in Eq. (i), we have,

$$500 \times 10^3 = (3455.75\,\sigma_1) + (0.5\sigma_1 \times 4712.39)$$

$$\therefore \qquad \sigma_1 = 86.03 \text{ MPa} \qquad\qquad\qquad \text{(Steel)}$$

Eq. (ii) yields... $\sigma_2 = 0.5 \times 86.03 = 43.01$ MPa $\qquad$ (Brass tube)

b. *Change in length of the tube:*

Since the length of both materials is same, we have

$$\delta l_1 = \delta l_2$$

i.e. $\qquad \delta l_1 = \dfrac{\sigma_1 l}{E_1} = \dfrac{86.03 \times 150}{200 \times 10^3} = 0.0645 \text{ mm}$

5. Fig. 2.6 shows three bars of equal length rigidly connected at their ends. Find the stresses induced in each member and the load shared by each member.

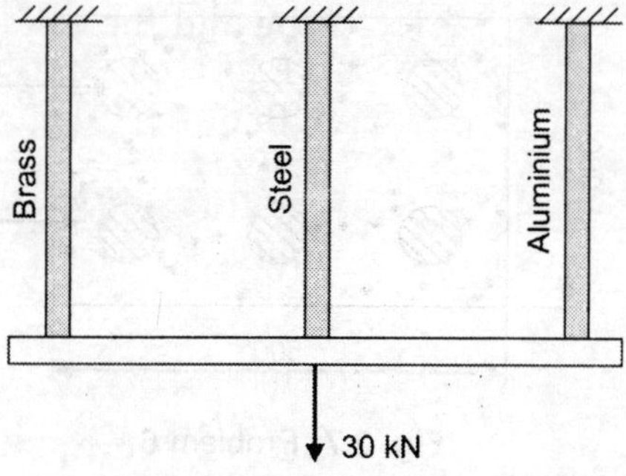

Fig. 2.6: Problem 5

Material	Area (mm²)	Young's Modulus (GPa)
Brass	600	100
Steel	800	200
Aluminium	1200	90

Solution: $A_b = 600$ mm², $A_s = 800$ mm², $A_{al} = 1200$ mm², $F = 30$ kN, $E_b = 100 \times 10^3$ MPa, $E_s = 200 \times 10^3$ MPa, $E_{al} = 90 \times 10^3$ MPa. a) $\sigma_b = ?, \sigma_s = ?, \sigma_{al} = ?$ b) $F_b = ?, F_s = ?, F_{al} = ?$

a. To find stresses:

For a composite bar,
$$F = \sigma_b A_b + \sigma_s A_s + \sigma_{al} A_{al} \qquad \text{Eq. (i)}$$

But
$$\frac{\sigma_b}{E_b} = \frac{\sigma_s}{E_s} = \frac{\sigma_{al}}{E_{al}}$$

$$\sigma_b = \left(\frac{E_b}{E_{al}}\right)\sigma_{al} = \left(\frac{100 \times 10^3}{90 \times 10^3}\right)\sigma_1 \Rightarrow \sigma_b = 1.11.\sigma_{al}$$

and
$$\sigma_s = \left(\frac{E_s}{E_{al}}\right)\sigma_{al} = \left(\frac{200 \times 10^3}{90 \times 10^3}\right)\sigma_1 \Rightarrow \sigma_s = 2.22\,\sigma_{al}$$
$$\text{Eq. (ii)}$$

Substituting Eq. (ii) in Eq. (i), we have,
$$30 \times 10^3 = (1.11\,\sigma_{al} \times 600) + (2.22\,\sigma_{al} \times 800) + 1200\sigma_{al}$$
$$\therefore \quad \sigma_{al} = 8.24\,\text{MPa}$$

Eq. (ii) yields...
$$\sigma_b = 1.11 \times 8.24 = 9.15\,\text{MPa}$$
$$\sigma_s = 2.22 \times 8.24 = 18.30\,\text{MPa}$$

b. To find loads:

For brass,
$$\sigma_b = \frac{F_b}{A_b} \Rightarrow F_b = \sigma_b A_b = 9.15 \times 600 = 5490\,\text{N}$$

For steel,
$$\sigma_s = \frac{F_s}{A_s} \Rightarrow F_s = \sigma_s A_s = 18.30 \times 800 = 14640\,\text{N}$$

For aluminium,
$$\sigma_{al} = \frac{F_{al}}{A_{al}} \Rightarrow F_{al} = \sigma_{al} A_{al} = 8.24 \times 1200 = 9888\,\text{N}$$

6. **A load of 600 kN is applied on a reinforced concrete column of size 300 mm × 500 mm. The column is reinforced with 6 numbers of steel bars of diameter 10 mm. Find the stresses developed in steel and concrete. Take $E_s = 15E_c$.**

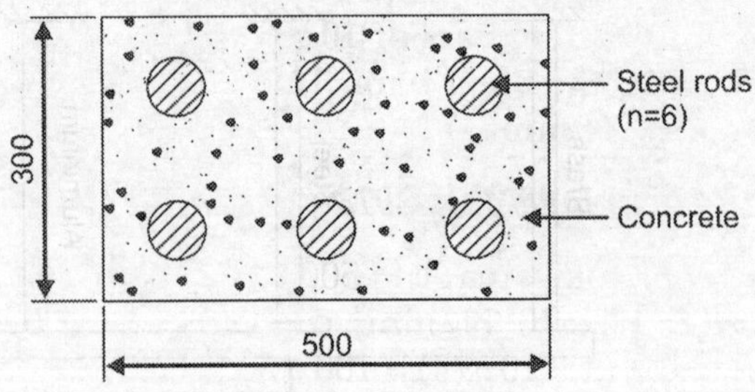

Fig. 2.7: Problem 6

Solution: $F = 600$ kN, total area $A_T = 300 \times 500 = 150000$ mm², $d_s = 10$ mm, $n = 6$, $E_s = 15E_c$, $\sigma_s = ?, \sigma_c = ?$.

Area of steel, $A_s = 6 \times (\pi \times 10^2)/4 = 150\pi$ mm^2
$\therefore$ Area of concrete, $A_c = A_T - A_s = 150000 - 150\,\pi = 149528.76$ mm^2
To find stresses:
For a composite bar, $\qquad\qquad\qquad F = F_s + F_c = \sigma_s A_s + \sigma_c A_c \qquad\qquad$ ... Eq. (i)

But $\qquad\qquad\qquad\qquad\qquad \dfrac{\sigma_s}{E_s} = \dfrac{\sigma_c}{E_c}$

$$\sigma_s = 15\,\sigma_c \qquad \textit{(using data)} \qquad ... \text{Eq. (ii)}$$

Substituting Eq. (ii) in Eq. (i), we have,
$\qquad\qquad 600 \times 10^3 = (15\sigma_c \times 150\pi) + (\sigma_c \times 149528.76)$
$\qquad \therefore \qquad\qquad \sigma_c = 3.83$ MPa
Eq. (ii) yields... $\qquad \sigma_s = 15 \times 3.83 = 57.47$ MPa

7. **A concrete column is of square section with 250 mm size and is reinforced with 8 steel bars of 16 mm diameter. The member supports an axial load of 270 kN. Evaluate the stresses in steel and concrete assuming a modular ratio as 18.**

VTU – (CV) Dec. 14/ Jan.15 – 08 Marks

Solution: Total area $A_T = 250 \times 250 = 62500$ mm^2, $d_s = 16$ mm, $n = 8$, $F = 270$ kN,

modular ratio, $\dfrac{E_s}{E_c} = 18$, $\sigma_s = ?$, $\sigma_c = ?$.

Area of steel, $A_s = 8 \times (\pi \times 16^2)/4 = 512\pi$ mm^2
$\therefore$ Area of concrete, $A_c = A_T - A_s = 62500 - 512\,\pi = 60891.50$ mm^2
To find stresses:
For a composite bar, $\quad F = F_s + F_c = \sigma_s A_s + \sigma_c A_c \qquad\qquad$ ... Eq. (i)

But $\qquad\qquad\qquad\qquad \dfrac{\sigma_s}{E_s} = \dfrac{\sigma_c}{E_c}$

$$\dfrac{\sigma_s}{\sigma_c} = \dfrac{E_s}{E_c} \Rightarrow \sigma_s = 18\,\sigma_c \quad \textit{(using data)} \qquad ... \text{Eq. (ii)}$$

Substituting Eq. (ii) in Eq. (i), we have,
$\qquad\qquad 270 \times 10^3 = (18\sigma_c \times 512\pi) + (\sigma_c \times 60891.50)$
$\qquad \therefore \qquad\qquad \sigma_c = 3.01$ MPa
Eq. (ii) yields... $\quad \sigma_s = 18 \times 3.01 = 54.18$ MPa

8. **A load of 2 MN is applied on a column 500 mm x 500 mm. The column is reinforced with four steel bars of 10 mm diameter, one in each corner. Find the stresses in concrete and steel bars. Take E for steel as 2.1 $\times$ 10^5 N/mm^2 and for concrete as 1.4 $\times$ 10^4 N/mm^2**

VTU – (CV) June/ July 2013 – 08 Marks; (CV) June/ July 2016 – 08 Marks

Solution: $F = 2 \times 10^6$ N, total area $A_T = 500 \times 500 = 250000$ mm^2, $d_s = 10$ mm, $n = 4$, $E_s = 2.1 \times 10^5$ N/mm^2, $E_c = 1.4 \times 10^4$ N/mm^2, $\sigma_s = ?$, $\sigma_c = ?$.

Area of steel, $A_s = 4 \times (\pi \times 10^2)/4 = 100\,\pi$ mm^2
$\therefore$ Area of concrete, $A_c = A_T - A_s = 250000 - 100\pi = 249685.84$ mm^2
To find stresses:
For a composite bar, $\qquad\qquad\qquad F = F_s + F_c = \sigma_s A_s + \sigma_c A_c \qquad\qquad$ ... Eq. (i)

But $\qquad\qquad\qquad\qquad\qquad \dfrac{\sigma_s}{E_s} = \dfrac{\sigma_c}{E_c}$

$$\sigma_s = \left(\frac{E_s}{E_c}\right)\sigma_c \qquad \text{... Eq. (ii)}$$

$$\therefore \quad \sigma_s = 15\,\sigma_c$$

Substituting Eq. (ii) in Eq. (i), we have,

$$2 \times 10^6 = (15\sigma_c \times 100\,\pi) + (\sigma_c \times 249685.84)$$

$$\therefore \quad \sigma_c = 7.86 \text{ MPa}$$

Eq. (ii) yields... $\quad \sigma_s = 15 \times 7.86 = 117.9 \text{ MPa}$

9. **A RCC column 300 mm × 300 mm has four reinforcement bars of steel each 20 mm in diameter placed one at each corner. Calculate the safe load on the column if the allowable stress in concrete is 4 MPa. Also calculate the shortening of the column, if the column is 3 m long. Take $E_s = 200$ GPa, and $E_s = 1.5E_c$.**

VTU – Dec. 09/ Jan. 10 – 10 Marks

Solution: Total area $A_T = 300 \times 300 = 90000 \text{ mm}^2$, $n = 4$, $d_s = 20$ mm, $\sigma_c = 4$ MPa,

$l = 3$ m, $E_s = 200 \times 10^3$ MPa, $E_s = 1.5E_c \Rightarrow \dfrac{E_s}{E_c} = 1.5$, $F = ?$, $\delta l = ?$.

a. To find load:

Area of steel, $A_s = 4 \times (\pi \times 20^2)/4 = 400\pi \text{ mm}^2$

$\therefore$ Area of concrete, $A_c = A_T - A_s = 90000 - 400\,\pi = 88743.36 \text{ mm}^2$

For a composite bar, $\qquad\qquad F = F_s + F_c = \sigma_s A_s + \sigma_c A_c \qquad\qquad \text{... Eq. (i)}$

But $\qquad\qquad\qquad\qquad \dfrac{\sigma_s}{E_s} = \dfrac{\sigma_c}{E_c}$

$$\sigma_s = \left(\frac{E_s}{E_c}\right)\sigma_c$$

$$= 1.5 \times 4 \qquad\qquad \text{... Eq. (ii)}$$

$$\therefore \quad \sigma_s = 6 \text{ MPa}$$

Substituting Eq. (ii) in Eq. (i), we have,

$$F = (6 \times 400\pi) + (4 \times 88743.36)$$

$$\therefore \quad F = 362.5 \text{ kN}$$

b. Shortening of column:

For column, $\qquad \delta l_1 = \dfrac{\sigma_c l}{E_c} = \dfrac{4 \times 3000}{(200 \times 10^3 / 1.5)} = 0.09 \text{ mm}$

10. **A square column of reinforced concrete is compressed by an axial force 'F'. What fraction of load will be carried by the concrete, if the total cross-sectional area of the steel bars is one-tenth of the cross-sectional area of concrete and modulus of elasticity of steel is ten times that of concrete?**

VTU – June 2012 – 07 Marks; [Similar: (CV) June/ July 2015 – 08 Marks]

Solution: $F_c = ?$, $F_s = ?$, $A_s = 0.1A_c$, $E_s = 10E_c$

For a composite bar, $\qquad\qquad F = F_s + F_c = \sigma_s A_s + \sigma_c A_c \qquad\qquad \text{... Eq. (i)}$

But $\qquad\qquad\qquad\qquad \dfrac{\sigma_s}{E_s} = \dfrac{\sigma_c}{E_c}$

$$\sigma_s = \left(\frac{E_s}{E_c}\right)\sigma_c$$

$$\sigma_s = 10\sigma_c \qquad\qquad \text{... Eq. (ii)}$$

Substituting Eq. (ii) in Eq. (i), we have,
$$F = (10\sigma_c) \times 0.1 A_c + \sigma_c A_c$$
$$= 2\sigma_c A_c$$
$$F = 2Fc \qquad \text{-or-}$$
$$\therefore \quad F_c = \left(\frac{1}{2}\right) F \qquad \qquad \text{... Eq. (iii)}$$

Thus load carried by concrete is half of the total load carried by column.
Substituting Eq. (iii) in Eq. (i), we have,
$$F = F_s + \left(\frac{1}{2}\right) F$$
$$\therefore \quad F_s = \left(\frac{1}{2}\right) F$$

11. **Three pillars support a rigid platform as shown in Fig. 2.8. If area of each brass rod is 1600 mm^2 and that of steel is 2000 mm^2, find the stresses developed. Take E_s = 210 GPa and E_b = 90 GPa.**

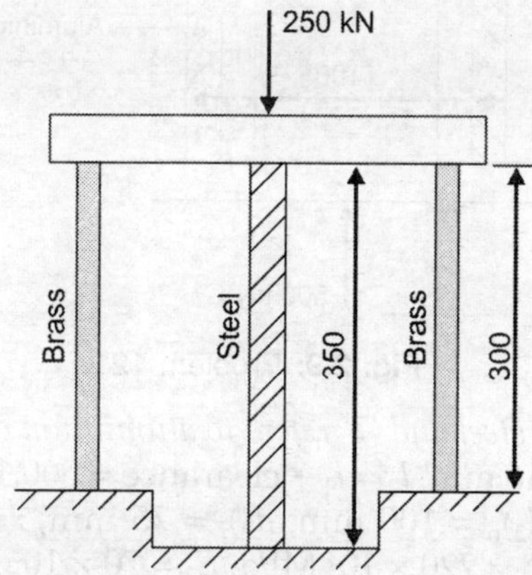

Fig. 2.8: Problem 11

Solution: A_b = 1600 mm^2, A_s = 2000 mm^2, E_s = 210 × 10^{3}MPa, E_b = 90 × 10^3 MPa, l_s = 350 mm, l_b = 300 mm, F = 250 kN, σ_s = ?, σ_b = ?.

For a composite bar,
$$F = F_s + 2F_b$$
$$F = \sigma_s A_s + 2\sigma_b A_b \qquad \qquad \text{... Eq. (i)}$$
But
$$\delta l_s = \delta l_b$$
$$\frac{\sigma_s l_s}{E_s} = \frac{\sigma_b l_b}{E_b} \qquad (\because l_s \neq l_b)$$

$$\frac{\sigma_s \times 350}{210 \times 10^3} = \frac{\sigma_b \times 300}{90 \times 10^3}$$
$$1.67 \times 10^{-3}\, \sigma_s = 3.33 \times 10^{-3}\, \sigma_b$$
$$\sigma \therefore \quad \sigma_s = 2\sigma_b \qquad \qquad \text{... Eq. (ii)}$$

Substituting Eq. (ii) in Eq. (i), we have,
$$250 \times 10^{-3} = (2\sigma_b) \times 2000 + 2\sigma_b \times 1600$$
$$\therefore \quad \sigma_b = 34.72 \text{ MPa}$$
Eq. (ii) yields... $\quad \sigma_s = 2 \times 34.72 = 69.44$ MPa

12. A solid steel cylinder 500 mm long and 70 mm in diameter is placed inside an aluminium cylinder of inside diameter 75 mm and outside diameter 100 mm. The aluminium cylinder is 0.16 mm longer than the steel cylinder. An axial load of 500 kN is applied to the bar and the cylinder through rigid cover plates as shown in Fig. 2.9. Find the stresses developed in steel and aluminium. Assume $E_s = 220$ GPa and $E_{al} = 70$ GPa.

VTU – (Similar) July 2007 – 07 Marks

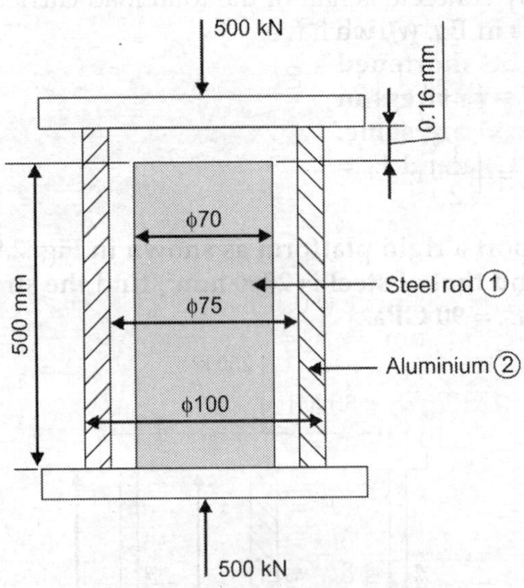

Fig. 2.9: Problem 12

Solution: *(suffix '1' refers to steel and '2' refers to aluminium cylinder)*

$l_1 = 500$ mm, clearance = 0.16 mm, $l_2 = l_1 +$ clearance = 500.16 mm, $d_1 = 70$ mm ? $A_1 = (\pi \times 70^2)/4 = 3848.45$ mm^2, $(d_2)_o = 100$ mm, $(d_2)_i = 75$ mm, $\Rightarrow A_2 = \pi \times (100^2 - 75^2)/4 = 3436.12$ mm^2, $F = 500$ kN, $E_1 = 220 \times 10^3$ MPa, $E_2 = 70 \times 10^3$ MPa, $\sigma_1 = ?$, $\sigma_2 = ?$.

For a composite bar, $\qquad F = F_1 + F_2 = \sigma_1 A_1 + \sigma_2 A_2 \qquad$ ... Eq. (i)

But $\qquad\qquad \delta l_2 = \delta l_1 +$ clearence

$$\delta l_2 = \delta l_1 + 0.16$$

$$\frac{\sigma_2 l_2}{E_2} = \left(\frac{\sigma_1 l_1}{E_1}\right) + 0.16$$

$$\left(\frac{\sigma_2 \times 500.16}{70 \times 10^3}\right) = \left(\frac{\sigma_2 \times 500}{220 \times 10^3}\right) + 0.16$$

$$7.14 \times 10^{-3}\, \sigma_2 = 2.27 \times 10^{-3}\, \sigma_1 + 0.16$$

$$\therefore \qquad \sigma_2 = 0.3183\, \sigma_1 + 22.4 \qquad\qquad \text{... Eq. (ii)}$$

Substituting Eq. (ii) in Eq. (i), we have,

$$500 \times 10^3 = \sigma_1 \times 3848.45 + (0.3183\sigma_1 + 22.41) \times 3436.12$$

$$= 3848.45\, \sigma_1 + 1093.72\, \sigma_1 + 77003.45$$

$$422995.50 = 4942.17\sigma_1$$

$$\therefore \quad \sigma_1 = 85.58\,\text{MPa} \qquad\qquad\qquad \text{(Steel)}$$

Eq. (ii) yields... $\quad \sigma_2 = (0.3183 \times 85.58) + 22.41 = 49.65$ MPa $\quad$ (Aluminium)

13. Fig. 2.10 shows a composite bar subjected to axial load F.

(a) Determine the magnitude of maximum permissible load if the compressive stress in the rod is not to exceed 110 MPa and that in tube is 80 MPa.

(b) Find the amount by which the tube will be shortened if the compressive stress in the tube and rod are same. Take E_s = 200 GPa and E_b = 100 GPa.

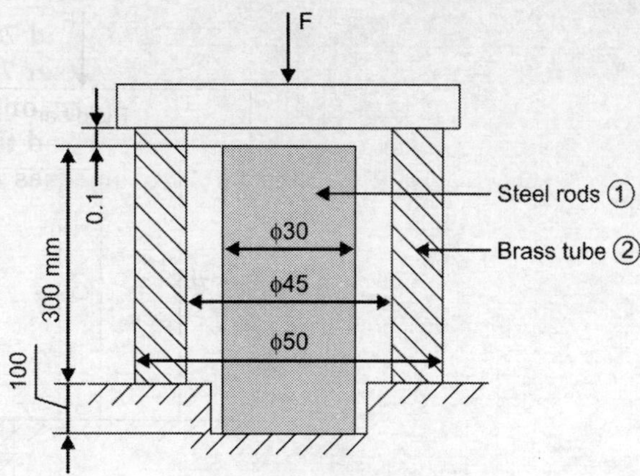

Fig. 2.10: Problem 13

Solution: *(suffix '1' refers to steel and '2' refers to brass tube)*

l_1 = 400 mm, l_2 = 300 mm, clearance = 0.1 mm, d_1 = 30 mm $\Rightarrow A_1 = (\pi \times 30^2)/4 = 706.86$ mm^2, $d_2)_o$ = 50 mm, $d_2)_i$ = 45 mm, $\Rightarrow A_2 = \pi \times (50^2 - 45^2)/4 = 373.06$ mm^2, $E_1 = 200 \times 10^3$ MPa, $E_2 = 100 \times 10^3$ MPa.

(a)　F = ?, if σ_1 = 110 MPa, σ_2 = 80 MPa

(b)　δl_2 = ?, if $\sigma_1 = \sigma_2$ = 110 MPa

a. To find load:

For a composite bar,

$$F = F_1 + F_2 = \sigma_1 A_1 + \sigma_2 A_2 \qquad \text{... Eq. (i)}$$

But

$$\delta l_2 = \delta l_1 + \text{clearence}$$

$$\delta l_2 = \delta l_1 + 0.1$$

$$\frac{\sigma_2 l_2}{E_2} = \left(\frac{\sigma_1 l_1}{E_1}\right) + 0.16$$

$$\left(\frac{\sigma_2 \times 300}{100 \times 10^3}\right) = \left(\frac{\sigma_2 \times 400}{200 \times 10^3}\right) + 0.1$$

$$3.0 \times 10^{-3}\,\sigma_2 = 2.0 \times 10^{-3}\,\sigma_1 + 0.1$$

$$\therefore \quad \sigma_2 = 0.67\sigma_1 + 33.33 \qquad \text{... Eq. (ii)}$$

Case i:　　When σ_1 = 110 MPa,

Eq. (ii) yields... $\sigma_2 = (0.67 \times 110) + 33.33 \Rightarrow \sigma_2 = 107.03$ MPa > 80 MPa (fails)

Case ii:　　When σ_2 = 80 MPa,

Eq. (ii) yields... $80 = (0.67 \times \sigma_1) + 33.33$

$$\therefore \quad \sigma_1 = 69.65 \text{ MPa} < 110 \text{ MPa (safe)}$$

Thus the safe (minimum) values are σ_1 = 69.65 MPa and σ_2 = 80 MPa

Substituting the safe values in Eq. (i), we have

Eq. (i) yields... $\quad F = (69.65 \times 706.86) + (80 \times 373.06)$

$$\therefore \quad F = 79.08 \text{ kN}$$

b. To find δl_2:

$$\delta l_2 = \frac{\sigma_2 l_2}{E_2} = \frac{110 \times 300}{100 \times 10^3} = 0.33 \text{ mm}$$

14. Determine the magnitude of 'F' that can be applied on a composite bar shown in Fig. 2.11. Allowable stress in aluminium is 130 MPa and that in copper is 65 MPa. Assume E_{al} = 70 GPa, E_{Cu} = 120 GPa, A_{al} = 1800 mm^2, A_{cu} = 1200 mm^2.

VTU – June/ July 2011 – 10 Marks

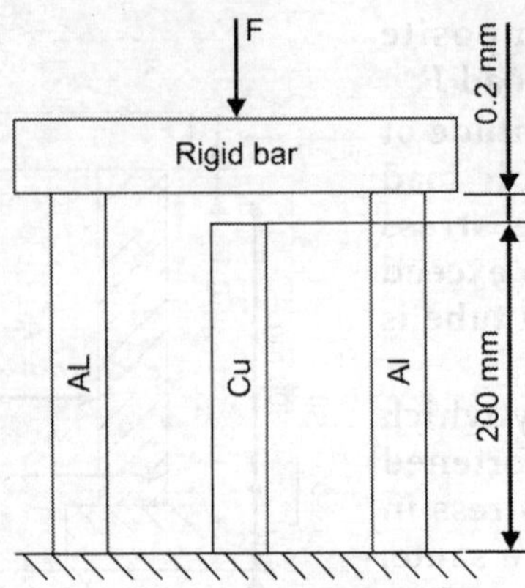

Fig. 2.11: Problem 14

Solution: *(suffix '1' refers to copper and '2' refers to aluminium)*
F = ?, l_1 = 200 mm, clearance = 0.2 mm, $l_2 = l_1$ + clearance = 200.02 mm,
A_1 = 1200 mm², A_2 = 1800 mm², $E_1 = 120 \times 10^3$ MPa, $E_2 = 70 \times 10^3$ MPa, σ_1 = 65 MPa,
σ_2 = 130 MPa.

For a composite bar, $\qquad\qquad F = F_1 + F_2 = \sigma_1 A_1 + \sigma_2 A_2 \qquad\qquad$ ... Eq. (i)

But $\qquad\qquad \delta l_2 = \delta l_1$ + clearence

$$\delta l_2 = \delta l_1 + 0.16$$

$$\frac{\sigma_2 l_2}{E_2} = \left(\frac{\sigma_1 l_1}{E_1}\right) + 0.2$$

$$\left(\frac{\sigma_2 \times 200.2}{70 \times 10^3}\right) = \left(\frac{\sigma_1 \times 200}{120 \times 10^3}\right) + 0.2$$

$$2.86 \times 10^{-3}\, \sigma_2 = 1.67 \times 10^{-3}\, \sigma_1 + 0.2$$

$$\therefore \quad \sigma_2 = 0.5839\, \sigma_1 + 69.93 \qquad\qquad\qquad \text{... Eq. (ii)}$$

Case i: When σ_1 = 65 MPa,
Eq. (ii) yields... σ_2 = (0.5839 × 65) + 69.33 $\Rightarrow \sigma_2$ = 107.28 MPa <130 MPa (safe)
Case ii: When σ_2 = 130 MPa,
Eq. (ii) yields... $\quad$ 130 = (0.5839 × σ_1) + 69.33

$$\therefore \quad \sigma_1 = 103.9 \text{ MPa} > 65 \text{ MPa (fails)}$$

Thus the safe (minimum) values are σ_1 = 65 MPa and σ_2 = 107.28 MPa
Substituting the safe values in Eq. (i), we have
Eq. (i) yields... $\quad F$ = (65 × 1200) + (107.28 × 1800)

$$\therefore \quad F = 271.10 \text{ kN}$$

15. **Determine the magnitude of 'F' that can be applied on a composite bar shown in Fig. 2.12. An allowable stress in steel is 140 MPa and that in brass is 70 MPa. Assume E_s = 200 GPa, E_{al} = 100 GPa, A_s = 1800 mm², A_{al} = 1200 mm².**

Solution: *(suffix '1' refers to steel and '2' refers to aluminium)*
F = ?, l_1 = 250 mm, , l_2 = 200 mm, A_1 = 1800 mm², A_2 = 1200 mm², $E_1 = 200 \times 10^3$ MPa,
$E_2 = E_{al} = 100 \times 10^3$ MPa, σ_1 = 140 MPa, σ_2 = 70 MPa.

For a composite bar, $\qquad\qquad F = F_s + F_{al} = F_1 + 2F_2$

$$= \sigma_1 A_1 + 2\sigma_2 A_2 \qquad\qquad \text{... Eq. (i)}$$

But $\qquad\qquad \delta l_1 = \delta l_2$

$$\frac{\sigma_1 l_1}{E_1} = \frac{\sigma_2 l_2}{E_2} \qquad (\because l_1 \neq l_2)$$

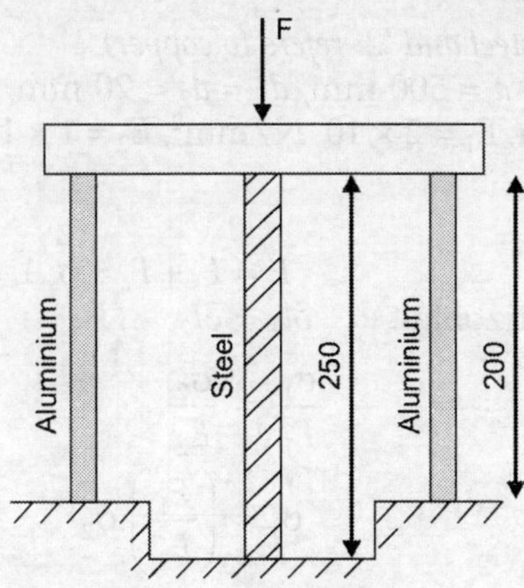

Fig. 2.12: Problem 15

$$\frac{\sigma_1 \times 250}{200 \times 10^3} = \frac{\sigma_2 \times 200}{100 \times 10^3}$$

$$1.25 \times 10^{-3}\, \sigma_1 = 2.0 \times 10^{-3}\, \sigma_2$$

$$\therefore \quad \sigma_1 = 1.6\, \sigma_2 \qquad \qquad \dots \text{Eq. (ii)}$$

Case i: When $\sigma_1 = 140$ MPa,

Eq. (ii) yields... $\sigma_2 = 140/1.6 = 87.5$ MPa > 70 MPa (fails)

Case ii: When $\sigma_2 = 70$ MPa,

Eq. (ii) yields... $\sigma_1 = 1.6 \times 70 = 112$ MPa < 140 MPa (safe)

Thus the safe (minimum) values are $\sigma_1 = 112$ MPa and $\sigma_2 = 70$ MPa

Substituting the safe values in Eq. (i), we have

Eq. (i) yields... $F = (112 \times 1800) + 2 \times (70 \times 1200)$

$$\therefore \qquad F = 369.60 \text{ kN}$$

16. **Two vertical rods one of steel and the other of copper are each rigidly fixed at the top and 500 mm apart. Diameters and lengths of each rod are 20 mm and 4 m respectively. A cross bar fixed to the rods at the lower end carries a load of 5 kN, such that the cross bar remains horizontal even after loading. Find the stresses in each rod and the position of the load on the bar. Take $E_s = 2 \times 10^5$ N/mm² and $E_c = 1 \times 10^5$ N/mm².**

VTU – Dec. 09/ Jan. 10 – 10 Marks; (CV) Dec.08/ Jan.09 – 12 Marks;
[Similar: (CV) June 2012 – 12 Marks]

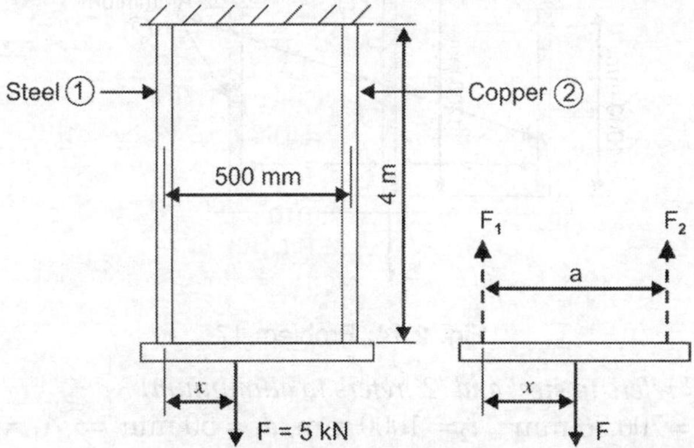

Fig. 2.13: Problem 16

Solution: *(suffix '1' refers to steel and '2' refers to copper)*
Distance between supports, $a = 500$ mm, $d_1 = d_2 = 20$ mm, $\Rightarrow A_1 = A_2 = 314.16$ mm^2, $F = 5000$ N, $l_1 = l_2 = 4000$ mm, $E_1 = 2 \times 10^5$ N/mm^2, $E_2 = 1 \times 10^5$ N/mm^2. a) $\sigma_1 = ?$, $\sigma_2 = ?$
b) $x = ?$

a. To find stresses:

For a composite bar, $\qquad\qquad\qquad F = F_s + F_c = \sigma_s A_s + \sigma_c A_c \qquad$ ... Eq. (i)

Since the bar remains horizontal, $\qquad \delta l_1 = \delta l_2 \qquad\qquad (\because l_s = l_b)$

$$\frac{\sigma_1}{E_1} = \frac{\sigma_2}{E_2}$$

$$\sigma_1 = \left(\frac{E_1}{E_2}\right)\sigma_2$$

$$\sigma_1 = \left(\frac{2 \times 10^5}{1 \times 10^5}\right)\sigma_2$$

$$\sigma_1 = 2\sigma_2 \qquad\qquad\qquad\qquad \text{... Eq. (ii)}$$

Substituting Eq. (ii) in Eq. (i), we have,
$$5000 = (2\sigma_2 \times 314.16) + (\sigma_2 \times 314.16)$$
$$\therefore \quad \sigma_2 = 5.31 \text{ N/mm}^2 \qquad\qquad\qquad\text{(Copper)}$$
Eq. (ii) yields... $\sigma = (2 \times 5.31) = 10.62$ N/mm^2 $\qquad$ (Steel)
And the corresponding loads are
$$F_2 = \sigma_2 A_2 = 5.31 \times 314.16 = 1666.67 \text{ N} \qquad \text{(Copper)}$$
$$F_1 = \sigma_1 A_1 = 10.62 \times 314.16 = 3336.34 \text{ N} \qquad \text{(Steel)}$$

b. To find x:

From **Fig. 2.13(b)**, taking moments about F_1 (steel rod), we have
$$F_2 \cdot a = F \cdot x$$
$$1666.67 \times 500 = 5000.x$$
$$\therefore \quad x = 166.67 \text{ mm}$$

17. **A rigid bar is supported by three rods in the same vertical plane and is equidistant as shown in Fig. 2.14. The outer rods are of aluminium having a diameter of 30 mm and of length 1000 mm, while the central rod is of steel having a diameter of 50 mm and length 1200 mm. Calculate the forces in the rods due to an applied force F, if the bar remains horizontal even after loading. Take $E_s = 2E_{al}$**

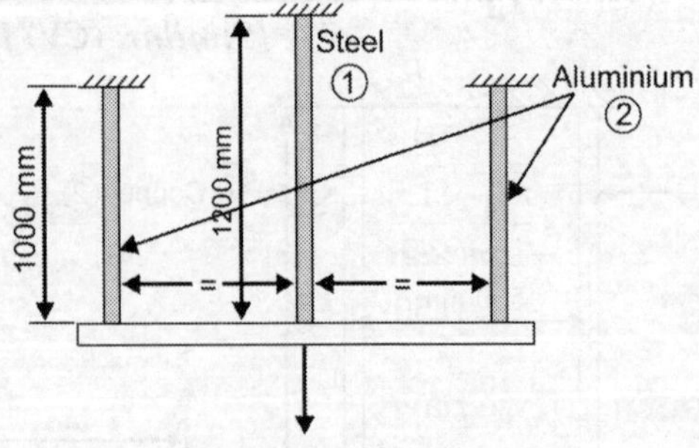

Fig. 2.14: Problem 17

Solution: *(suffix '1' refers to steel and '2' refers to aluminium)*
$d_2 = 30$ mm, $\Rightarrow A_2 = 706.86$ mm^2, $l_2 = 1000$ mm, $d_1 = 50$ mm, $\Rightarrow A_1 = 1963.50$ mm^2, $l_1 = 1200$ mm $E_s = 1.5E_{al} \Rightarrow E_1 = 1.5E_2$. $\sigma_1 = ?$, $\sigma_2 = ?$

For a composite bar, $\qquad F = F_1 + 2F_2$ ... Eq. (i)

Since the bar remains horizontal, $\qquad \delta l_1 = \delta l_2$

$$\frac{Fl_1}{A_1 E_1} = \frac{F_2 l_2}{A_2 E_2} \quad (\because l_1 \neq l_2)$$

$$\frac{F_1 \times 1200}{1963.50 \times 1.5 E_2} = \frac{F_2 \times 1000}{706.86 \times E_2}$$

$$0.407 F_1 = 1.415 \, F_2$$

$$\therefore \quad F_1 = 3.477 \, F_2 \qquad\qquad\qquad \text{... Eq. (ii)}$$

Substituting Eq. (ii) in Eq. (i), we have,

$$F = 3.477 \, F_2 + 2F_2$$
$$F = 5.477 \, F_2$$
$$F_2 = 0.1826 \, F \qquad\qquad \text{(Aluminium)}$$

Eq. (ii) yields... $F_1 = 3.477 \times (0.1826 \, F) = 0.635 \, F \qquad$ (Steel)

18. **A rigid bar is supported by three bars as shown in Fig. 2.15. Calculate the forces in the bars due to an applied force if the bar AC remains horizontal even after loading. Take $E_s = 2E_b$**

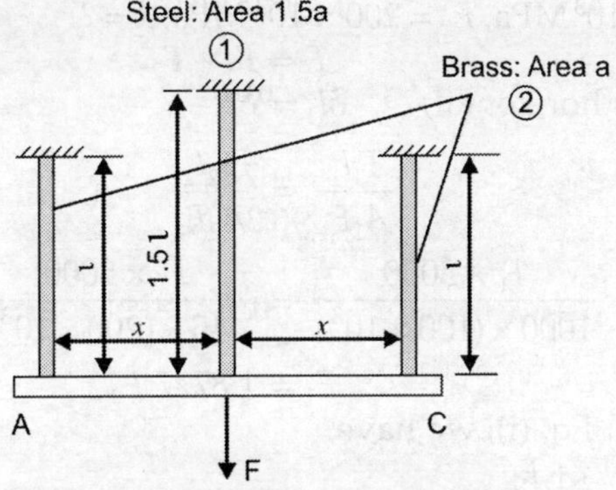

Fig. 2.15: Problem 18

Solution: (*suffix '1' refers to steel and '2' refers to brass*)

$A_2 = a$, $l_2 = l$, $A_1 = 1.5a$, $l_1 = 1.5l$, $E_s = 2E_b \Rightarrow E_1 = 2E_2$. $\sigma_1 = ?$, $\sigma_2 = ?$

For a composite bar, $\qquad F = F_1 + 2F_2$ ... Eq. (i)

Since the bar remains horizontal, $\qquad \delta l_1 = \delta l_2$

$$\frac{F_1 l_1}{A_1 E_1} = \frac{F_2 l_2}{A_2 E_2} \quad (\because l_1 \neq l_2)$$

$$\frac{F_1 \times 1.5l}{1.5a \times 2E_2} = \frac{F_2 \times l}{a \times E_2}$$

$$0.50 \, F_1 = F_2$$

$$\therefore \quad F_1 = 2 \, F_2 \qquad\qquad\qquad \text{... Eq. (ii)}$$

Substituting Eq. (ii) in Eq. (i), we have,

$$F = 2F_2 + 2F_2$$
$$F = 4 \, F_2 \Rightarrow F_2 = 0.25 \, F \qquad\qquad \text{(Brass)}$$

Eq. (ii) yields... $F_1 = 2 \times 0.25F = 0.50 \, F \qquad$ (Steel)

19. A rigid bar AB is suspended by two vertical rods A and B and as shown in Fig. 2.16. At what distance 'x' from A may a vertical load of $F = 3kN$ be applied if the bar has to remain horizontal even after the load is applied? Take $E_b = 100$ GPa, $E_s = 200$ GPa.

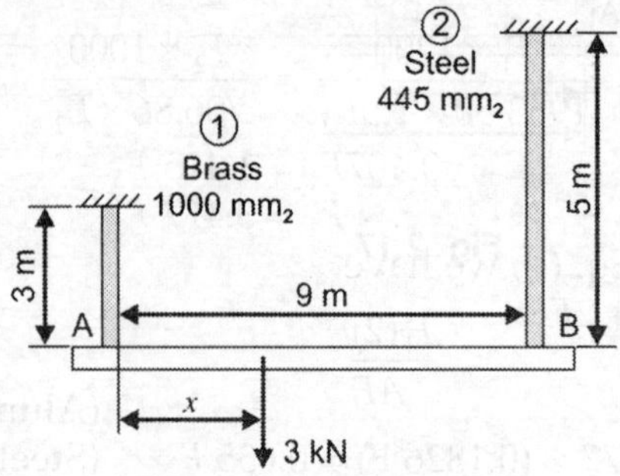

Fig. 2.16: Problem 19

Solution: *(suffix '1' refers to brass and '2' refers to steel)*
$l_1 = 3000$ mm, $A_1 = 1000$ mm^2, $l_2 = 5000$ mm, $A_2 = 445$ mm^2, distance between supports $a = 9000$ mm, $E_1 = 100 \times 10^3$ MPa, $E_2 = 200 \times 10^3$ MPa, $x = ?$

For a composite bar, $\qquad\qquad\qquad F = F_1 + F_2$ $\qquad\qquad$ ... Eq. (i)
Since the bar remains horizontal, $\qquad \delta l_1 = \delta l_2$

$$\frac{F_1 l_1}{A_1 E_1} = \frac{F_2 l_2}{A_2 E_2} \quad (\because l_1 \neq l_2)$$

$$\frac{F_1 \times 3000}{1000 \times (100 \times 10^3)} = \frac{F_2 \times 5000}{445 \times (200 \times 10^3)}$$

$$\therefore \quad F_1 = 1.8727 \, F_2 \qquad\qquad\qquad ... \text{Eq. (ii)}$$

Substituting Eq. (ii) in Eq. (i), we have,
$\qquad 3000 = 1.8727 \, F_2 + F_2$
$\qquad 3000 = 2.8727 \, F_2$
$\therefore \quad F_2 = 1044.33$ N $\qquad\qquad\qquad$ (Steel)
Eq. (ii) yields... $F_1 = 1.8727 \times 1044.33 = 1955.71$ N $\quad$ (Brass)
To find x:
Taking moments about P_1 (steel rod), we have
$\qquad\qquad F_2 \cdot a = F \cdot x$
$\qquad 1044\,33 \times 9000 = 3000 \, x$
$\qquad\qquad \therefore \quad x = 3133$ mm

20. Fig. 2.17 represents a system composed of three bars made of same material and having the same axial rigidity EA. Determine the distance x between the bars A and B in order that the rigid beam remains horizontal when a load is applied at its mid-span.

Solution: $E_1 A_1 = E_2 A_2 = E_3 A_3 = EA$, $l_1 = 2y$, $l_2 = 1.5y$, $l_3 = y$, $x = ?$

For a composite bar, $\qquad\qquad\qquad F = F_1 + F_2 + F_3$ $\qquad\qquad$ ... Eq. (i)
Since the bar remains horizontal, $\qquad \delta l_1 = \delta l_2 = \delta l_3$

$$\frac{F_1 l_1}{A_1 E_1} = \frac{F_2 l_2}{A_2 E_2} = \frac{F_3 l_3}{A_3 E_3}$$

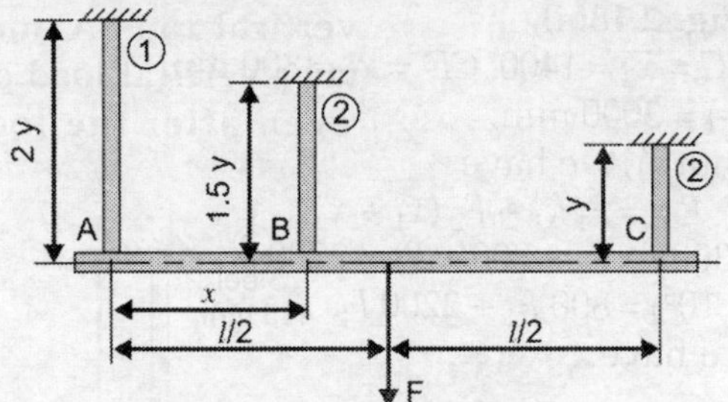

Fig. 2.17: Problem 20

$$\frac{F_1(2y)}{AE} = \frac{F_2(1.5y)}{AE} = \frac{F_3 y}{AE}$$

$$F_1 = 0.75\,F_2;\ F_3 = 1.5F_2 \qquad\qquad \text{... Eq. (ii)}$$

Substituting Eq. (ii) in Eq. (i), we have,
$$F = 0.75F_2 + F_2 + 1.5F_2 = 3.25F_2$$
$$F_2 = 0.3078\ F$$

Eq. (ii) yields... $F_1 = 0.75 \times 0.3078\ F = 0.2309\ F$
$$F_3 = 1.5 \times 0.3078\ F = 0.4617\ F \qquad\qquad \text{... Eq. (iii)}$$

To find x:

Taking moments about A, we have
$$F(l/2) = F_2 x + F_3\, l$$
$$(0.5\ F)l = (0.3078\ F)x + (0.4617\ F)l \qquad\qquad \text{... using Eq. (iii)}$$
$$(0.0383\ F)l = (0.3078\ F)\ x$$
$$\therefore\quad x = 0.124\ l$$

21. **A rigid bar AD is hinged at A and supported by a copper rod 1.5 m long and a steel rod of 0.8 m length as shown in Fig. 2.18(a). If $A_s = 400$ mm², $A_c = 600$ mm², $E_s = 210$ GPa, and $E_c = 100$ GPa, find the stresses in each rod.**

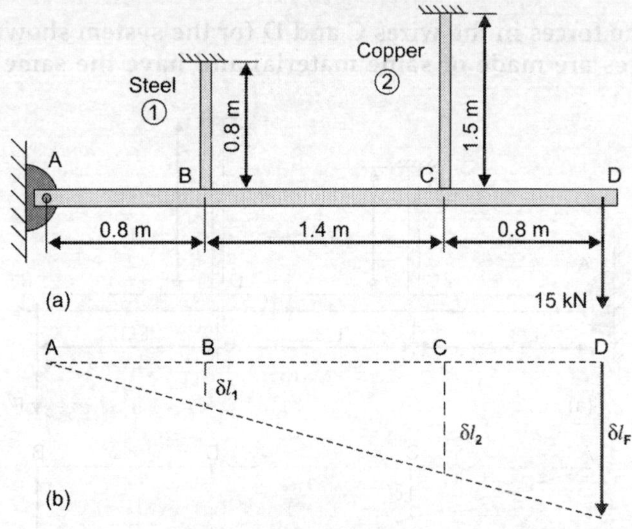

Fig. 2.18: Problem 21

Solution: *(suffix '1' refers to steel and '2' refers to copper)*
$l_1 = 800$ mm, $A_1 = A_s = 400$ mm², $l_2 = 1500$ mm, $A_2 = A_c = 600$ mm², $E_1 = 210 \times 10^3$ MPa, $E_2 = 100 \times 10^3$ MPa. $F = 15$ kN, $\sigma_1 = ?$, $\sigma_2 = ?$

Referring to given **Fig. 2.18(a)**,

$AB = x_1 = 800$ mm, $BC = x_2 = 1400$, $CD = x_3 = 800$ mm

$AD = x = (x_1 + x_2 + x_3) = 3000$ mm,

Taking moments about A, we have

$$F.x = F_1 x_1 + F_2 (x_1 + x_2)$$
$$(15 \times 10^3) \times 3000 = F_1 \times 800 + F_2 \times 2200$$
$$(45 \times 10^6) = 800\, F_1 + 2200\, F_2 \qquad \text{... Eq. (i)}$$

From **Fig. 2.18(b)**, we have

$$\frac{\delta l_1}{x_1} = \frac{\delta l_2}{x_1 + x_2}$$

$$\frac{\delta l_1}{800} = \frac{\delta l_2}{2200}$$

$$\delta l_2 = 2.75\, \delta l_1 \qquad \text{... Eq. (ii)}$$

$$\frac{F_2 l_2}{A_2 E_2} = 2.75 \left(\frac{F l_1}{A_1 E_1} \right) \qquad \text{... Eq. (ii)}$$

i.e. $\dfrac{F_2 \times 1500}{600 \times (100 \times 10^3)} = 2.75 \times \left[\dfrac{F_1 \times 800}{400 \times (210 \times 10^3)} \right]$

$$\therefore \quad F_2 = 1.0476\, F_1 \qquad \text{... Eq. (iii)}$$

Substituting Eq. (iii) in Eq. (i), we have,

$$(45 \times 10^6) = 800\, F_1 + [2200 \times (1.0476\, F_1)] = 3104.72\, F_1$$
$$\therefore \quad F_1 = 14494.06 \text{ N} \qquad \text{(Steel)}$$

Eq. (iii) yields... $F_2 = 1.0476 \times 14494.06$

$$\therefore \quad F_2 = 15184 \text{ N} \qquad \text{(Copper)}$$

Thus the stresses are:

$$\sigma_1 = F_1 / A_1 = 14494.06 / 400 = 36.24 \text{ MPa} \quad \text{(Steel)}$$
$$\sigma_2 = F_2 / A_2 = 15184 / 600 = 25.31 \text{ MPa} \quad \text{(Copper)}$$

22. **Determine the forces in the wires C and D for the system shown in Fig. 2.19(a). Both the wires are made of same material and have the same cross sectional area.**

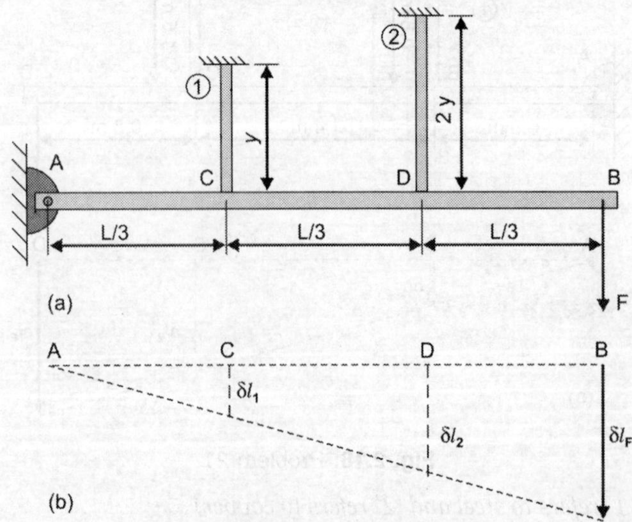

Fig. 2.19: Problem 22

Solution: $l_1 = y, l_2 = 2y, A_1 = A_2 = A, E_1 = E_2 = E, F_1 = ?, F_2 = ?$

Referring to given **Fig. 2.19(a)**,
$$AC = x_1 = L/3, CD = x_2 = L/3, DB = x_3 = L/3,$$
$$AB = x = (x_1 + x_2 + x_3) = L$$

Taking moments about A, we have
$$F.x = F_1 x_1 + F_2 (x_2 + x_1)$$
$$F.L = F_1 \times (L/3) + F_2 \times (2L/3)$$
$$\therefore \quad F = 0.334 \, F_1 + 0.667 \, F_2 \qquad \text{... Eq. (i)}$$

From **Fig. 2.19(b)**, we have

$$\frac{\delta l_1}{(L/3)} = \frac{\delta l_2}{(2L/3)}$$

$$\delta l_2 = 2\delta l_1 \qquad \text{... Eq. (ii)}$$

i.e. $\quad \dfrac{F_2 l_2}{A_2 E_2} = 2\left(\dfrac{F_1 l_1}{A_1 E_1}\right)$

$$\frac{F_2(2y)}{AE} = 2\left[\frac{F_1(y)}{AE}\right] \qquad \text{... (data)}$$

$$\therefore \quad F_2 = F_1 \qquad \text{... Eq. (iii)}$$

Substituting Eq. (iii) in Eq. (i), we have
$$F = 0.334 \, F_1 + 0.667 \, F_1$$
$$\therefore \quad F = F_1$$

Eq. (iii) yields... $F_2 = F = F_1$

23. **A rigid bar AB is hinged at A and supported by a steel rod 800 mm long and an aluminium rod of 500 m length as shown in Fig. 2.20(a). Calculate the allowable load F.**

Solution: $l_1 = 800$ mm, $d_1 = 40$ mm $\Rightarrow A_1 = 1256.64$ mm^2, $\sigma_1 = 200$ MPa, $E_1 = 200 \times 10^3$ MPa, $l_2 = 500$ mm, $d_2 = 30$ mm $\Rightarrow A_2 = 706.86$ mm^2, $\sigma_2 = 175$ MPa, $E_2 = 80 \times 10^3$ MPa. $F = ?$

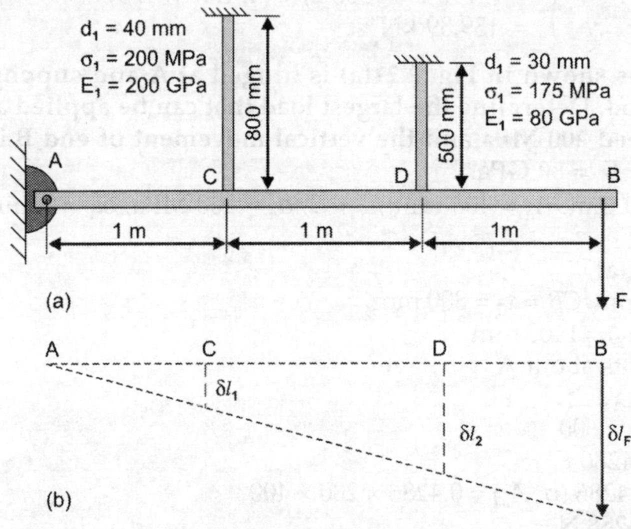

Fig. 2.20: Problem 23

Referring to given **Fig. 2.20(a)**,
$AC = x_1 = 1000$ mm, $CD = x_2 = 1000$ mm, $DB = x_3 = 1000$ mm,
$AB = x = (x_1 + x_2 + x_3) = 3000$ mm
Taking moments about A, we have

$$F.x = F_1\, x_1 + F_2\,(x_2 + x_1)$$
$$F \times 3000 = F_1 \times 1000 + F_2 \times 2000$$
$$F = 0.334\, F_1 + 0.667\, F_2$$
$$= 0.334\,(\sigma_1\, A_1) + 0.667\,(\sigma_2\, A_2)$$
$$= 0.334 \times 1256.64\,(\sigma_1) + 0.667 \times 706.86\,(\sigma_2)$$
$$\therefore \quad F = 419.72\, \sigma_1 + 471.47\, \sigma_2 \qquad \dots \text{Eq. (i)}$$

From **Fig. 2.20(b)**, we have

$$\frac{\delta l_1}{x_1} = \frac{\delta l_2}{x_1 + x_2}$$

$$\frac{\delta l_1}{1000} = \frac{\delta l_2}{2000}$$

$$\delta l_2 = 2\delta l_1 \qquad \dots \text{Eq. (ii)}$$

i.e.
$$\frac{\sigma_2 l_2}{E_2} = 2\left(\frac{\sigma_1 l_1}{E_1}\right)$$

$$\frac{\sigma_2 \times 500}{80 \times 10^3} = 2\left(\frac{\sigma_1 \times 800}{200 \times 10^3}\right)$$

$$\therefore \quad \sigma_2 = 1.28\, \sigma_1 \qquad \dots \text{Eq. (iii)}$$

Case i: When $\sigma_1 = 200$ MPa,
   Eq. (ii) yields... $\sigma_2 = 1.28 \times 200 = 256$ MPa > 175 MPa (fails)
Case ii: When $\sigma_2 = 175$ MPa,
   Eq. (ii) yields... $\sigma_1 = 175/1.28 = 136.72$ MPa < 200 MPa (safe)
Thus the safe (minimum) values are $\sigma_1 = 136.72$ MPa and $\sigma_2 = 175$ MPa
Substituting the safe values in Eq. (i), we have
   Eq. (i) yields... $\quad F = (419.72 \times 136.72) + (471.47 \times 175)$
$$\therefore \quad F = 139.89 \text{ kN}$$

24. **A rigid bar as shown in Fig. 2.21(a) is hinged at A and supported at C by an aluminium rod. Determine the largest load that can be applied at B if the stress is not to exceed 200 MPa and the vertical movement of end B is not to exceed 2.0 mm. Take $E_a = 80$ GPa.**

Solution: $l_a = 900$ mm, $A_a = 400$ mm^2, $F = ?$, $\sigma_a = 200$ MPa, $\delta l_P = 2$ mm, $E_a = 80 \times 10^3$ MPa.

From **Fig. 2.21(a)**,
$AC = x_1 = 600$ mm, $CB = x_2 = 800$ mm,
$AB = x = (x_1 + x_2) = 1400$ mm
Taking moments about A, we have

$$F.x = F_a\, x_1$$
$$F \times 1400 = F_a \times 600$$
$$F = 0.4286\, F_a \qquad \dots \text{Eq. (i)}$$
$$= 0.4286\,(\sigma_a\, A_a) = 0.4286 \times 200 \times 400$$
$$\therefore \quad F = 34288 \text{ N} \qquad \dots \text{Eq. (ii)}$$

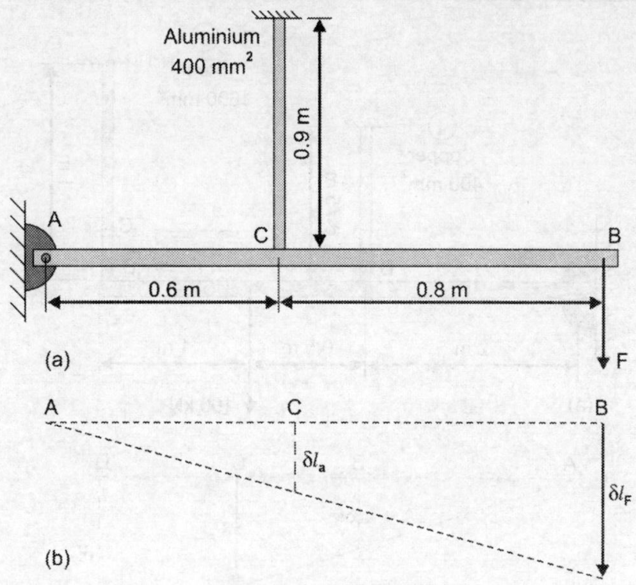

Fig. 2.21: Problem 24

From **Fig. 2.21(b)**, we have

$$\frac{\delta l_a}{x_1} = \frac{\delta l_F}{x_1 + x_2}$$

$$\frac{\delta l_a}{600} = \frac{2}{1400}$$

$$\therefore \qquad \delta l_a = 0.8571 \text{ mm}$$

But $\quad \delta l_a = \dfrac{F_a l_a}{A_a E_a}$ $\qquad\qquad\qquad\qquad$ ... Eq. (iii)

i.e. $0.8571 = \dfrac{F_a \times 900}{400 \times (80 \times 10^3)}$

$$\therefore \qquad F_a = 30474.67 \text{ N} \qquad\qquad\qquad\qquad \text{... Eq. (iv)}$$

Substituting Eq. (iv) in Eq. (i), we have

$$F = 0.4286 \times 30474.67 = 13061.44 \text{ N} \qquad\qquad \text{... Eq. (v)}$$

Thus the safe value of F is the minimum value of Eqs (ii) and (v)

i.e. $\qquad F = 13061.44$ N

25. **A rigid bar 3.5 m in length and hinged at A is as shown in Fig. 2.22(a) Determine**

   (a) Stresses in each rod

   (b) Elongation of steel rod, if 100 kN is applied on the bar at 2.5 m from hinge.
   Take E_s = 200 GPa and E_c = 120 GPa

Solution: *(suffix '1' refers to copper and '2' refers to steel)*

$l_1 = 750$ mm, $A_1 = 400$ mm², $E_1 = 120 \times 10^3$ MPa, $l_2 = 1000$ mm, $A_2 = 1600$ mm², $E_2 = 200 \times 10^3$ MPa. a) $\sigma_1 = ?$, $\sigma_2 = ?$ b) $\delta l_2 = ?$, $F = 100$ kN

   Referring to given **Fig. 2.22(a)**,

   $AB = x_1 = 2000$ mm, $BC = x_2 = 500$ mm, $CD = x_3 = 1000$ mm,

   $AD = x = (x_1 + x_2 + x_3) = 3500$ mm

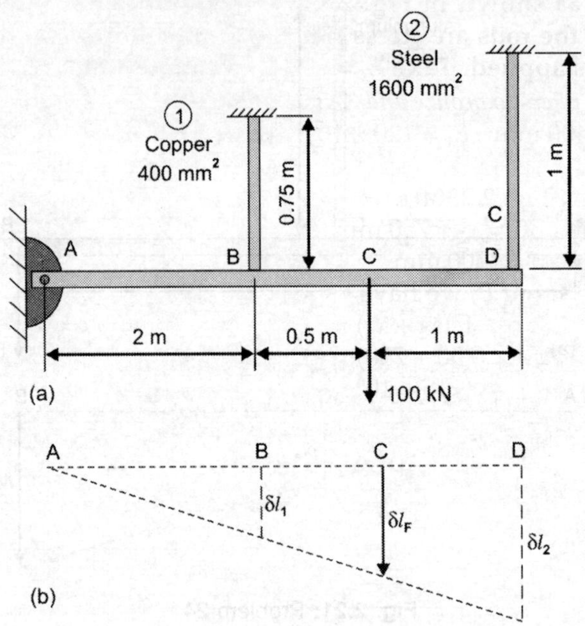

Fig. 2.22: Problem 25

a. To find stresses:

Taking moments about A, we have

$$F.(x_1 + x_2) = F_1 x_1 + F_2.x$$
$$(100 \times 10^3) \times (2000 + 500) = (F_1 \times 2000) + (F_2 \times 3500)$$
$$250 \times 10^6 = 2000 F_1 + 3500 F_2 \qquad \text{... Eq. (i)}$$

From **Fig. 2.22(b)**, we have

$$\frac{\delta l_1}{x_1} = \frac{\delta l_2}{x}$$

$$\frac{\delta l_1}{2000} = \frac{\delta l_2}{3500}$$

$$\therefore \quad \delta l_2 = 1.75 \, \delta l_1 \qquad \text{... Eq. (ii)}$$

i.e. $\dfrac{F_2 l_2}{A_2 E_2} = 1.75 \left(\dfrac{F_1 l_1}{A_2 E_2} \right)$

$$\frac{F_2 \times 1000}{1600 \times (200 \times 10^3)} = 1.75 \times \frac{F_1 \times 750}{400 \times (120 \times 10^3)}$$

$$F_2 = 8.75 \, F_1 \qquad \text{... Eq. (iii)}$$

Substituting Eq. (iii) in Eq. (i), we have,
$$250 \times 10^6 = 2000 F_1 + [3500 \times (8.75 \, F_1] = 32625 F_1$$
$$\therefore \quad F_1 = 7662.84 \text{ N} \qquad \text{(Copper)}$$

Eq. (iii) yields... $F_2 = 8.75 \times 7662.84$
$$\therefore \quad F_2 = 67049.85 \text{ N} \qquad \text{(Steel)}$$

b. To find elongation of steel rod:

We know that $\quad \delta l_2 = \dfrac{F_2 l_2}{A_2 E_2} = \dfrac{67049.85 \times 1000}{1600 \times 200 \times 10^3} = 0.2095 \text{ mm}$

26. A rigid bar is as shown in Fig. 2.23(a). Assuming that the bar was initially horizontal and the rods are stress free, determine the stress in each rod when a load of 25 kN is applied. Take E_s = 200 GPa and E_b = 120 GPa.

Solution: *(suffix '1' refers to bronze and '2' refers to steel)*

l_1 = 1500 mm, A_1 = 400 mm^2, E_1 = 120 × 10^3 MPa, l_2 = 800 mm, A_2 = 900 mm^2, E_2 = 200 × 10^3 MPa. σ_1 = ?, σ_2 = ?

Referring to given **Fig. 2.23(a)**,

AB = x_1 = 2000 mm, BC = x_2 = 750 mm, CD = x_3 = 750 mm,

AD = x = $(x_1 + x_2 + x_3)$ = 3500 mm

Taking moments about B, we have

$$F.(x_2 + x_3) = F_1 x_1 + F_2 x_2$$
$$(10 \times 10^3) \times (750 + 750) = (F_1 \times 2000) + (F_2 \times 750)$$
$$15 \times 10^6 = 2000 F_1 + 750 F_2 \qquad \text{... Eq. (i)}$$

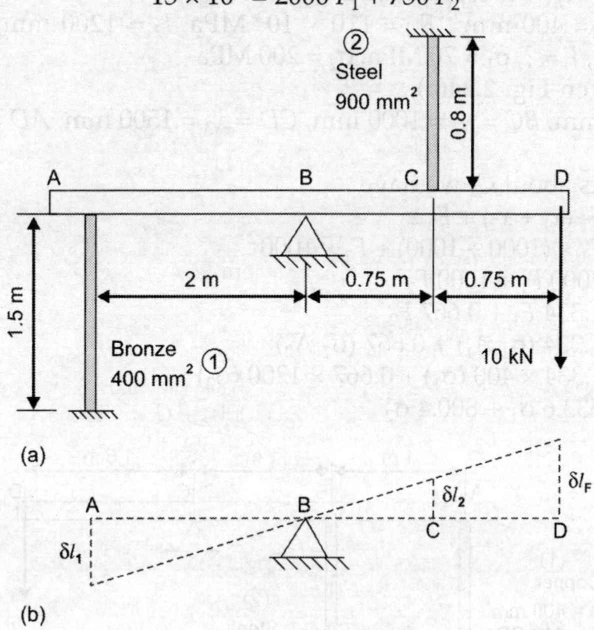

Fig. 2.23: Problem 26

From **Fig. 2.23(b)**, we have

$$\frac{\delta l_1}{x_1} = \frac{\delta l_2}{x}$$

$$\frac{\delta l_1}{2000} = \frac{\delta l_2}{750}$$

$$\therefore \quad \delta l_1 = 0.375 \, \delta l_1 \qquad \text{... Eq. (ii)}$$

$$\text{i.e.} \quad \frac{F_2 l_2}{A_2 E_2} = 0.375 \left(\frac{F_1 l_1}{A_1 E_1} \right)$$

$$\frac{F_2 \times 800}{900 \times (200 \times 10^3)} = 0.375 \times \left[\frac{F_1 \times 1500}{400 \times (120 \times 10^3)} \right]$$

$$\therefore \quad F_2 = 2.64 \, F_1 \qquad \text{... Eq. (iii)}$$

Substituting Eq. (iii) in Eq. (i), we have,
$$15 \times 10^6 = 2000\, F_1 + [750 \times (2.64\, F_1)] = 3980\, F_1$$
$$\therefore \quad F_1 = 3768.84 \text{ N} \qquad \text{(Bronze)}$$
Eq. (iii) yields… $\qquad F_2 = 2.64 \times 3768.84$
$$\therefore \quad F_2 = 9949.74 \text{ N} \qquad \text{(Steel)}$$
Thus the stresses are:
$$\sigma_1 = F_1/A_1 = 3768.84/400 = 9.42 \text{ MPa} \qquad \text{(Bronze)}$$
$$\sigma_2 = F_2/A_2 = 9949.74/900 = 11.05 \text{ MPa} \qquad \text{(Steel)}$$

27. A rigid bar is as shown in Fig. 2.24(a). Assuming that the bar were initially stress free, determine the maximum load F that can be applied at D if the stress is not to exceed 200 MPa in steel and 70 MPa in copper.

Solution: *(suffix '1' refers to copper and '2' refers to steel)*
$l_1 = 2500$ mm, $A_1 = 400$ mm^2, $E_1 = 110 \times 10^3$ MPa, $l_2 = 1200$ mm, $A_2 = 1200$ mm^2, $E_2 = 210 \times 10^3$ MPa. $F = ?$, $\sigma_1 = 70$ MPa, $\sigma_2 = 200$ MPa

Referring to given **Fig. 2.24(a)**,
$AB = x_1 = 1000$ mm, $BC = x_2 = 1000$ mm, $CD = x_3 = 1500$ mm, $AD = x = (x_1 + x_2 + x_3)$ $= 3500$ mm

Taking moments about C, we have
$$F.x_3 = F_1 (x_1 + x_2) + F_2 x_2$$
$$F \times 1500 = F_1 \times (1000 + 1000) + F_2 \times 1000$$
$$1500\, F = 2000\, F_1 + 1000\, F_2$$
$$F = 1.334\, F_1 + 0.667\, F_2$$
$$= 1.334\, (\sigma_1 A_1) + 0.667\, (\sigma_2 A_2)$$
$$= 1.334 \times 400\, (\sigma_1) + 0.667 \times 1200\, (\sigma_2)$$
$$\therefore \quad F = 533.6\, \sigma_1 + 800.4\, \sigma_2 \qquad\qquad \text{… Eq. (i)}$$

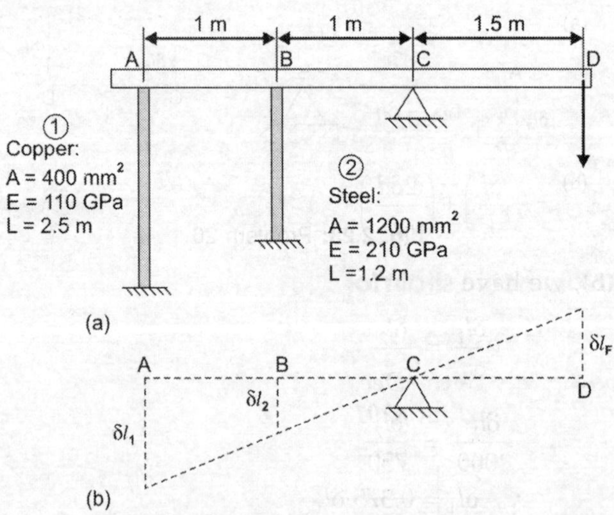

Fig. 2.24: Problem 27

From **Fig. 2.24(b)**, we have
$$\frac{\delta l_1}{x_1 + x_2} = \frac{\delta l_2}{x_2}$$

$$\frac{\delta l_1}{2000} = \frac{\delta l_2}{1000}$$

$$\therefore \qquad \delta l_1 = 2\,\delta l_2 \qquad\qquad \text{... Eq. (ii)}$$

$$\text{i.e. } \frac{\sigma_1 l_1}{E_1} = 2\left(\frac{\sigma_2 l_2}{E_2}\right)$$

$$\frac{\sigma_1 \times 2500}{110 \times 10^3} = 2\left(\frac{\sigma_2 \times 1200}{210 \times 10^3}\right)$$

$$\therefore \qquad \sigma_1 = 0.5\sigma_2 \qquad\qquad \text{... Eq. (iii)}$$

Case i: When $\qquad \sigma_1 = 70\,\text{MPa}$,

Eq. (ii) yields... $\sigma_2 = 70/0.5 = 140\,\text{MPa} < 200\,\text{MPa}$ (safe)

Case ii: When $\qquad \sigma_2 = 200\,\text{MPa}$,

Eq. (ii) yields... $\sigma_1 = 0.5 \times 200 = 100\,\text{MPa} > 70\,\text{MPa}$ (fails)

Thus the safe (minimum) values are $\sigma_1 = 70\,\text{MPa}$ and $\sigma_2 = 140\,\text{MPa}$

Substituting the safe values in Eq. (i), we have

Eq. (i) yields... $\qquad F = (533.6 \times 70) + (800.4 \times 140)$

$$\therefore \quad F = 115.81\,\text{kN}$$

2.2 VOLUMETRIC STRAIN

Volumetric strain of a deformed body is defined as the ratio of the change in volume of the body to its original volume.

$$\varepsilon_V = \frac{\delta V}{V} \qquad\qquad \text{... (Eq. 2.5a)}$$

Where $\quad V$ = original volume of the body

δV = change in volume of the body after deformation.

In general, $\quad \varepsilon_V = \dfrac{\delta V}{V} = \varepsilon_x + \varepsilon_y + \varepsilon_z$

$$\varepsilon_V = \frac{\delta l}{l} + \frac{\delta b}{b} + \frac{\delta h}{h} \qquad \text{... For a rectangular bar} \qquad \text{... (Eq. 2.5b)}$$

$$\varepsilon_V = \left(\frac{\delta l}{l}\right) + \left(\frac{2\delta d}{d}\right) \qquad \text{... For a circular rod} \qquad \text{... (Eq. 2.5c)}$$

2.2.1 Derivation of volumetric strain for a single direct stress

a. *For a rectangular bar:*

VTU – Dec.07/ Jan.08 – 05 Marks; June 2012 – 06 Marks; June/ July 2013 – 04 Marks; (CV) Dec.08/ Jan.09 – 08 Marks

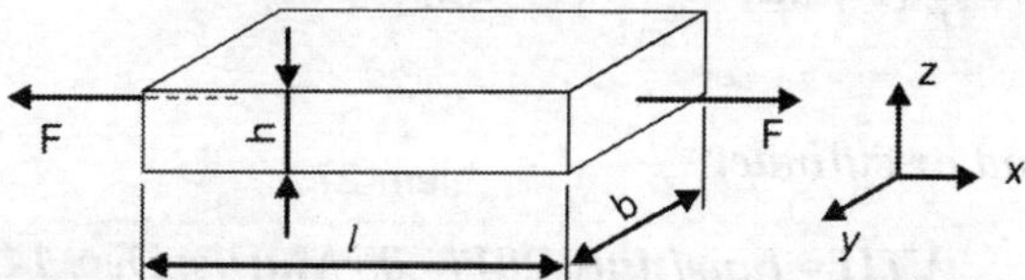

Fig. 2.25: Volumetric strain for a rectangular bar subjected to uniaxial stress

Consider a rectangular body as shown in **Fig. 2.25**, subjected to axial tensile load along the direction of length.

Let $\quad F$ = Axial tensile load

l = Length of the bar

b = Breadth of the bar

h = Depth of the bar

E = Young's modulus

μ = Poisson's ratio

For a rectangular bar, volume V = area × length = $l \times b \times h$ ... Eq. (i)

If δl, δb and δh denote the change in length, breadth and thickness of the bar in x, y and z directions respectively, then differentiating Eq. (i), we have

$$\delta V = bh.\delta l + hl.\delta b + lb.\delta h \qquad \text{... Eq. (ii)}$$

But   volumetric strain

$$\varepsilon_V = \frac{\delta V}{V}$$

$$= \frac{(bh).\delta l + (hl).\delta b + (lb).\delta h}{lbh}$$

$$\varepsilon_V = \frac{\delta l}{l} + \frac{\delta b}{b} + \frac{\delta h}{h} \qquad \text{... (Eq. 2.6)}$$

$$\varepsilon_V = \frac{\delta V}{V} = \varepsilon_x + \varepsilon_y + \varepsilon_z$$

(in respective directions) ... (Eq. 2.7)

We know that change in length, $\delta l = \dfrac{Fl}{AE} = \dfrac{\sigma l}{E}$

and linear strain $\varepsilon_x = \dfrac{\delta l}{l} = \dfrac{\sigma l / E}{l} = \dfrac{\sigma}{E}$ ... (Eq. 2.8)

also Poisson's ratio, $\mu = \dfrac{\text{lateral strain}}{\text{linear strain}}$

lateral strain = μ × linear strain   ... (Eq. 2.9)

i.e. $\varepsilon_y = \dfrac{\delta b}{b} = -\mu \dfrac{\delta l}{l} = -\mu\varepsilon_x = -\mu\left(\dfrac{\sigma}{E}\right)$

(negative sign due to decrease in width)   ... (Eq. 2.10)

$$\varepsilon_z = \dfrac{\delta h}{h} = -\mu \dfrac{\delta l}{l} = -\mu\varepsilon_x = -\mu\left(\dfrac{\sigma}{E}\right)$$

(negative sign due to decrease in thickness) ... (Eq. 2.11)

Substituting Eqs (2.8), (2.10) and (2.11) in (Eq. 2.7), we have

$$\varepsilon_V = \left(\dfrac{\sigma}{E}\right) - \mu\left(\dfrac{\sigma}{E}\right) - \mu\left(\dfrac{\sigma}{E}\right)$$

$\therefore$ $\varepsilon_V = \dfrac{\delta v}{v} = \dfrac{\sigma}{E}(1 - 2\mu) = \dfrac{F}{AE}(1 - 2\mu)$ ... (Eq. 2.12)

b.   *For a circular rod or cylinder:*

VTU – June/ July 2011– 05 Marks; Dec. 14/ Jan. 15 – 05 Marks

Consider a circular rod as shown in **Fig. 2.26**, subjected to axial tensile load along the direction of length.

Let F = Axial tensile load

l = Length of the bar

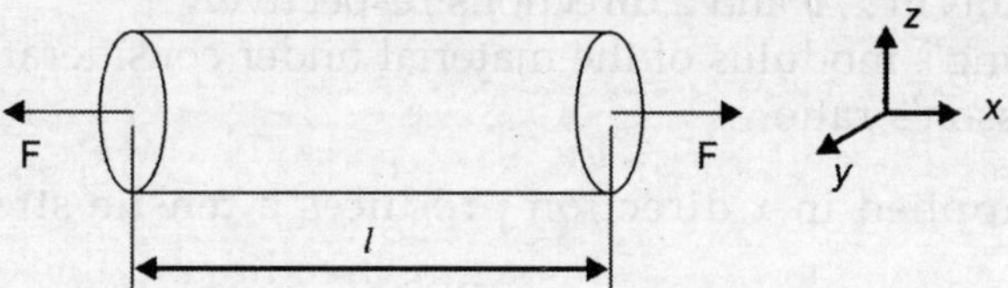

Fig. 2.26: Volumetric strain for a circular rod subjected uniaxial stress

d = diameter of the bar
E = Young's modulus
μ = Poisson's ratio

We know that volumetric strain $\varepsilon_V = \dfrac{\delta V}{V}$

For a circular rod, volume V = area × length = $A \times l = \left(\dfrac{\pi d^2}{4}\right) \times l$ ... (Eq. 2.13)

Differentiating the above equation on either side, we have

$$\delta V = \left[\left(\frac{\pi d^2}{4}\right) \times \delta l\right] + \left[l \times \left(\frac{\pi}{4}\right) 2d.\delta d\right]$$

Dividing throughout by V, we have

$$\frac{\delta V}{V} = \left(\frac{\delta l}{l}\right) + \left(\frac{2\delta d}{d}\right)$$ ... (Eq. 2.14)

But lateral strain = μ × linear strain

$$\frac{\delta d}{d} = -\mu\left(\frac{\delta l}{l}\right)$$ *– ve sign due to reduction in diameter*

Therefore (Eq. 2.14) yields... $\dfrac{\delta V}{V} = \left(\dfrac{\delta l}{l}\right) - 2\mu\left(\dfrac{\delta l}{l}\right)$

$$\therefore \frac{\delta V}{V} = \left(\frac{\delta l}{l}\right)[1 - 2\mu] = \varepsilon[1 - 2\mu] = \left(\frac{\sigma}{E}\right)[1 - 2\mu] \quad ... \text{(Eq. 2.15)}$$

2.2.2 Derivation of volumetric strain for 3 direct stresses

VTU – Dec. 13/ Jan. 14 – 09 Marks

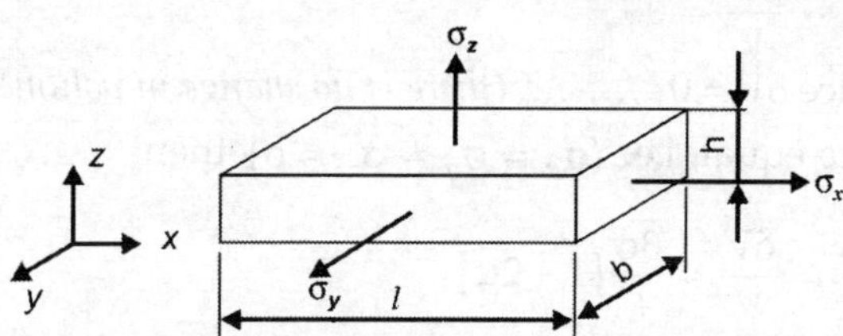

Fig. 2.27: Volumetric strain for a rectangular bar subjected to triaxial stress

Consider a rectangular body, subjected to direct tensile stresses along three mutually perpendicular directions as shown in **Fig. 2.27**.

Let σ_x = Stress in x direction.
      σ_y = Stress in y direction.
      σ_z = Stress in z direction.

$\varepsilon_x, \varepsilon_y, \varepsilon_z$ = Strains in x, y and z directions respectively.

E = Young's modulus of the material under consideration,

μ = Poisson's ratio

The stress σ_x applied in x direction produces a tensile strain of $\left(\dfrac{\sigma_x}{E}\right)$ in the direction of x and a compressive strain of $\mu\left(\dfrac{\sigma_y}{E}\right)$ in y and $\mu\left(\dfrac{\sigma_z}{E}\right)$ in z directions.

Thus the total strain in x direction due to σ_x is

$$\varepsilon_x = \left(\frac{\sigma_x}{E}\right) - \mu\left(\frac{\sigma_y}{E}\right) - \mu\left(\frac{\sigma_z}{E}\right) = \frac{1}{E}\left[\sigma_x - \mu(\sigma_y + \sigma_z)\right] \qquad \text{... (Eq. 2.16a)}$$

On similar lines in y and z directions, we have

Total strain in y direction due to σ_y is

$$\varepsilon_y = \left(\frac{\sigma_y}{E}\right) - \mu\left(\frac{\sigma_z}{E}\right) - \mu\left(\frac{\sigma_x}{E}\right) = \frac{1}{E}\left[\sigma_y - \mu(\sigma_z + \sigma_x)\right] \qquad \text{... (Eq. 2.16b)}$$

Total strain in z direction due to σ_z is

$$\varepsilon_z = \left(\frac{\sigma_z}{E}\right) - \mu\left(\frac{\sigma_x}{E}\right) - \mu\left(\frac{\sigma_y}{E}\right) = \frac{1}{E}\left[\sigma_z - \mu(\sigma_x + \sigma_y)\right] \qquad \text{... (Eq. 2.16c)}$$

Adding ε_x, ε_y and ε_z in Eq. (2.16), we have

$$\varepsilon_x + \varepsilon_y + \varepsilon_z = \frac{1}{E}\left\{\left(\sigma_x + \sigma_y + \sigma_z\right) - \mu\left[\left(\sigma_y + \sigma_z\right) + \left(\sigma_z + \sigma_x\right) + \left(\sigma_x + \sigma_y\right)\right]\right\}$$

$$= \frac{1}{E}\left\{\left(\sigma_x + \sigma_y + \sigma_z\right) - 2\mu\left(\sigma_x + \sigma_y + \sigma_z\right)\right\}$$

$$\varepsilon_x + \varepsilon_y + \varepsilon_z = \frac{\left(\varepsilon_x + \varepsilon_y + \varepsilon_z\right)}{E}\left[1 - 2\mu\right]$$

$$\therefore \left(\varepsilon_x + \varepsilon_y + \varepsilon_z\right) = \varepsilon_V = \frac{\delta v}{v} = \frac{\left(\sigma_x + \sigma_y + \sigma_z\right)}{E}\left[1 - 2\mu\right] \qquad \text{... (Eq. 2.17)}$$

Note:

- If the sum of stresses is equal to zero, i.e. $\left(\sigma_x + \sigma_y + \sigma_z\right) = 0$ then

  (Eq. 2.17) yields... $\dfrac{\delta V}{V} = 0$

  Since $V \neq 0$, hence $\delta V = 0$ .... *(there is no change in volume)* ... (Eq. 2.18)

- If the stresses are equal, i.e. $(\sigma_x = \sigma_y = \sigma_z = \sigma)$ then

  (Eq. 2.17) yields... $\dfrac{\delta V}{V} = \dfrac{3\sigma}{E}\left[1 - 2\mu\right]$ ... (Eq. 2.19)

2.3 UPPER LIMIT OF POISSON'S RATIO

OR   Show that the Poisson's ratio (μ) cannot be more than 0.5.

VTU – (CV) Dec. 10 – 04 Marks

We know that $(\varepsilon_x + \varepsilon_y + \varepsilon_z) = \dfrac{\left(\sigma_x + \sigma_y + \sigma_z\right)}{E}\left[1 - 2\mu\right]$ ... using (Eq. 2.17)

For hydrostatic state of stress, $\varepsilon_x = \varepsilon_y = \varepsilon_z = \varepsilon$ and $\sigma_x = \sigma_y = \sigma_z = \sigma$

i.e. $\qquad 3\varepsilon = \dfrac{3\sigma}{E}[1 - 2\mu]$

$\qquad\qquad \varepsilon E = \sigma[1 - 2\mu]$

Since ε, E, σ are positive values (constants), hence $[1 - 2\mu]$ should also be positive.

i.e. $[1 - 2\mu] \geq 0$

$\qquad\qquad 1 \geq 2\mu$

$\qquad \therefore \quad \mu \leq 0.5$

Note: **For most metals the value of μ varies from 0.2 to 0.45, but rubber approaches a value of 0.5.**

28. **A bar having a length of 300 mm, 40 mm wide and 25 mm thick is subjected a tensile load of 25 kN. Take Poisson's ratio of 0.25 and Young's modulus of bar material as 210 GPa. Find:**
    (a) The change in length, breadth and thickness of the bar.
    (b) Strains in length, breadth and thickness of the bar.
    (c) The change in volume of the bar.

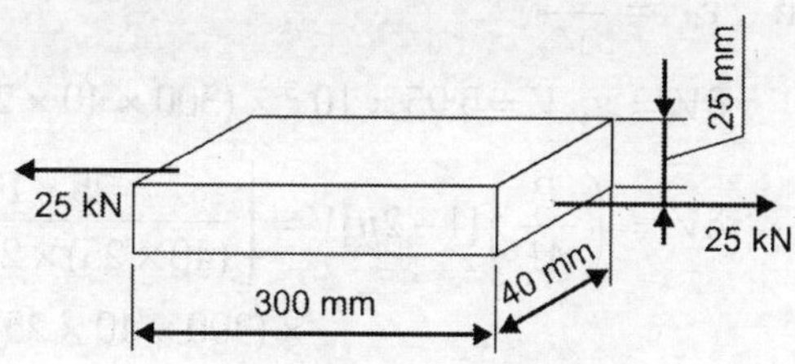

Fig. 2.28: Problem 28

Solution: $l = 300$ mm, $b = 40$ mm, $h = 25$ mm, $F = 25$ kN, $E = 210 \times 10^3$ MPa, $\mu = 0.25$.
a) δl, δb, $\delta h = ?$, b) ε_l, ε_b, $\varepsilon_h = ?$, c) $\delta V = ?$

 a. To find δl, δb, δh:

  i) To find δl:

$$\delta l = \frac{Fl}{AE} = \frac{25 \times 10^3 \times 300}{(40 \times 25) \times 210 \times 10^3} = 0.0357 \text{ mm}$$

  ii) To find δb:

$$\mu = \frac{\text{lateral strain}}{\text{linear strain}} = \frac{\text{lateral strain}}{\delta l / l}$$

$$\textit{lateral strain} = \mu\left(\frac{\delta l}{l}\right) = 0.25 \times (0.0357 / 300) = 2.975 \times 10^{-5} \text{ mm}$$

$$\text{Also lateral strain} = \left(\frac{\delta b}{b}\right)$$

$$\therefore \ \delta b = 2.975 \times 10^{-5} \times 40 = 1.19 \times 10^{-3} \text{ mm}$$

  iii) To find δh:

$$\text{Lateral strain} = \left(\frac{\delta h}{h}\right)$$

$$\therefore \ \delta h = 2.975 \times 10^{-5} \times 25 = 7.438 \times 10^{-4} \text{ mm}$$

b. To find $\varepsilon_l, \varepsilon_b, \varepsilon_h$:

$$\varepsilon_l = \frac{\delta l}{l} = \frac{0.0357}{300} = 1.19 \times 10^{-4}$$

$$\varepsilon_b = \frac{\delta b}{b} = \frac{1.19 \times 10^{-3}}{40} = -2.975 \times 10^{-5}$$

(– ve because, breadth reduces due to tensile load)

$$\varepsilon_h = \frac{\delta h}{h} = \frac{7.438 \times 10^{-4}}{25} = -2.975 \times 10^{-5}$$

(–ve because, depth reduces due to tensile load)

And volumetric strain, $\varepsilon_V = \dfrac{\delta V}{V} = \dfrac{\delta l}{l} + \dfrac{\delta b}{b} + \dfrac{\delta h}{h}$

$$= 1.19 \times 10^{-4} - 2.975 \times 10^{-5} - 2.975 \times 10^{-5}$$

$$\therefore \quad \varepsilon_V = 5.95 \times 10^{-5}$$

c. To find δV:

Volumetric strain $\quad \varepsilon_V = \dfrac{\delta V}{V}$

$$\delta V = \varepsilon_V . V = 5.95 \times 10^{-5} \times (300 \times 40 \times 25) = 17.86 \text{ mm}^3$$

or $\quad \delta V = \left(\dfrac{P}{AE}\right)[1 - 2\mu]V = \left[\dfrac{25 \times 10^3}{(40 \times 25) \times 210 \times 10^3}\right][1 - (2 \times 0.25)]$

$$\times (300 \times 40 \times 25) = 17.86 \text{ mm}^3$$

29. **A mild steel bar, 250 mm long and 80 mm × 40 mm in cross-section is subjected to axial compression of 600 kN. If E = 200 GPa, μ = 0.4, find:**
    (a) The change in length, breadth and thickness of the bar.
    (b) The change in volume of the bar

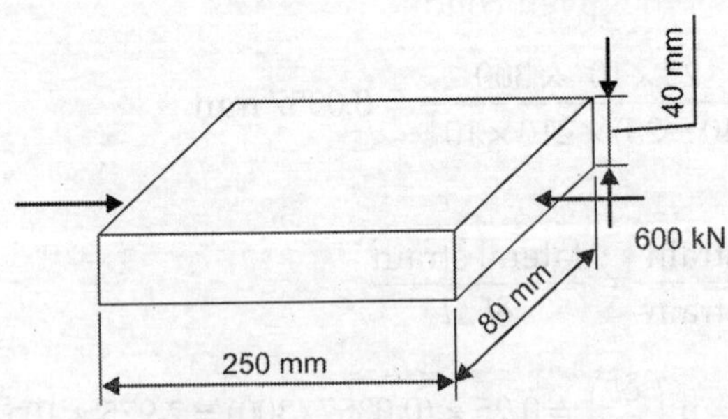

Fig. 2.29: Problem 29

Solution: l = 250 mm, b = 80 mm, h = 40 mm, F = –600 kN, E = 200 × 10³ MPa, μ = 0.4. a) $\delta l, \delta b, \delta h$ = ? b) δV = ?

a. To find $\delta l, \delta b, \delta h$:
  i) To find δl:

$$\delta l = \frac{Fl}{AE} = \frac{-600 \times 10^3 \times 250}{(80 \times 40) \times 200 \times 10^3} = -0.234 \text{ mm}$$

ii) To find δb:

$$\mu = \frac{\text{lateral strain}}{\text{linear strain}} = \frac{\text{lateral strain}}{\delta l / l}$$

Lateral strain $= \mu \left(\dfrac{\delta l}{l}\right) = 0.4 \times (-0.234/250) = -3.744 \times 10^{-4}$ mm

Also lateral strain $= \left(\dfrac{\delta b}{b}\right)$

$\therefore \quad \delta b = -3.744 \times 10^{-4} \times 80 = -0.03$ mm

iii) To find δh:

Lateral strain $= \left(\dfrac{\delta h}{h}\right)$

$\delta h = -3.744 \times 10^{-4} \times 40 = -0.015$ mm

b. To find δV:

Change in volume, $\delta V = \left(\dfrac{P}{AE}\right)[1 - 2\mu]V$

$$\delta V = \frac{-600 \times 10^3}{80 \times 40 \times 200 \times 10^3}[1 - (2 \times 0.4)] \times (250 \times 80 \times 40) = -150 \text{ mm}^3$$

30. A cube of 100 mm side is subjected to 10 N/mm² (tensile), 8 N/mm² (compressive) and 6 N/mm² (tensile) acting along X, Y and Z planes respectively. Determine the strains along the three directions and the change in volume. Take Poisson's ratio = 0.25 and $E = 2 \times 10^5$ N/mm².

VTU – Dec.07/ Jan.08 – 05 Marks

Solution: $l = b = h = 100$ mm, $\sigma_x = 10$ N/mm², $\sigma_y = -8$ N/mm², $\sigma_z = 6$ N/mm², $E = 2 \times 10^5$ MPa, $\mu = 0.25$ a) $\varepsilon_x, \varepsilon_y, \varepsilon_z = ?$, b) $\delta V = ?$

Fig. 2.30 represents the given condition of the problem.

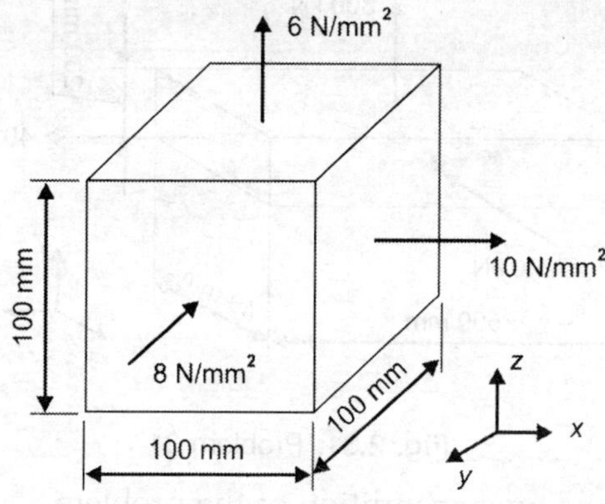

Fig. 2.30: Problem 30

a. To find $\varepsilon_x, \varepsilon_y, \varepsilon_z$:

$$\varepsilon_x = \frac{1}{E}\left[\sigma_x - \mu(\sigma_y + \sigma_z)\right]$$

$$= \frac{1}{2 \times 10^5} [10 - 0.25 \times (-8 + 6)] = 5.25 \times 10^{-5}$$

$$\varepsilon_y = \frac{1}{E} \left[\sigma_y - \mu(\sigma_z + \sigma_x) \right]$$

$$= \frac{1}{2 \times 10^5} [-8 - 0.25 \times (6 + 10)] = -6.0 \times 10^{-5}$$

$$\varepsilon_z = \frac{1}{E} \left[\sigma_z - \mu(\sigma_x + \sigma_y) \right]$$

$$= \frac{1}{2 \times 10^5} [6 - 0.25 \times (10 - 8)] = 2.75 \times 10^{-5}$$

b. To find δV:

Volumetric strain $\dfrac{\delta V}{V}$

$$\delta V = \varepsilon_V . V = (\varepsilon_x + \varepsilon_y + \varepsilon_z)V$$
$$= [(5.25 \times 10^{-5}) + (-6.0 \times 10^{-5}) + (2.75 \times 10^{-5})] \times (100 \times 100 \times 100)$$
$$\delta V = 20 \text{ mm}^3$$

31. A 500 mm long bar has a rectangular cross section 20 mm × 40 mm. This bar is subjected to:
   i. 40 kN tensile load on (20 × 40) mm faces.
   ii. 200 kN compressive load on (20 × 500) mm faces and
   iii. 300 kN tensile force on (40 × 500) mm faces.
   Find the change in volume of the bar if $E = 2 \times 10^5$ N/mm^2 and Poisson's ratio $1/m = 0.3$

VTU – Jan. 2013 – 10 Marks

Solution: $l = 500$ mm, $b = 40$ mm, $h = 20$ mm, $F_x = 40$ kN, $F_z = 300$ kN, $F_y = -200$ kN, $E = 2 \times 10^5$ MPa, $\mu = 1/m, = 0.3$, $\delta V = ?$

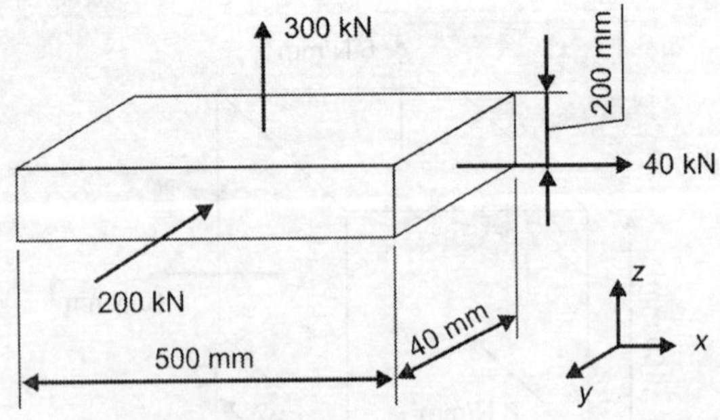

Fig. 2.31: Problem 31

Fig. 2.31 represents the given condition of the problem

Volumetric strain $\varepsilon_V = \dfrac{\delta V}{V} = \dfrac{(\sigma_x + \sigma_y + \sigma_z)}{E} [1 - 2\mu]$

$$\delta V = \frac{(\sigma_x + \sigma_y + \sigma_z)}{E} [1 - 2\mu] V \qquad \text{... Eq. (i)}$$

Here $\quad \sigma_x = \dfrac{F_x}{A_x} = \dfrac{40 \times 10^3}{40 \times 20} = 50\,\text{N/mm}^2$

$$\sigma_y = \dfrac{F_y}{A_y} = \dfrac{-200 \times 10^3}{500 \times 20} = -20\,\text{N/mm}^2$$

$$\sigma_z = \dfrac{F_z}{A_z} = \dfrac{300 \times 10^3}{500 \times 40} = 15\,\text{N/mm}^2$$

Also $\quad V = lbh = 500 \times 40 \times 20 = 4 \times 10^5\,\text{mm}^3$

Eq. (i) yields... $\delta V = \dfrac{(50 - 20 + 15)}{2 \times 10^5}\,[1 - (2 \times 0.3)] \times (4 \times 10^5) = 36\,\text{mm}^3$

32. A rectangular block 250 mm × 100 mm × 80 mm is subjected to axial loads as shown in Fig. 2.32. Assuming Poisson's ratio as 0.25 and $E = 2 \times 10^5$ MPa, calculate the change in volume of the block.

Also find the change that should be made to 1000 kN load in order that there is no change in volume of the bar.

Solution: $l = 250$ mm, $b = 100$ mm, $h = 80$ mm, $F_x = 480$ kN, $F_y = 900$ kN, $F_z = -1000$ kN, $E = 2 \times 10^5$ MPa, $\mu = 0.25$ a) $\delta V = ?$ b) $F_z = ?$, if $\delta V = 0$

a. To find δV:

Volumetric strain $\varepsilon_V = \dfrac{\delta V}{V} = \dfrac{(\sigma_x + \sigma_y + \sigma_z)}{E}[1 - 2\mu]$

$$\delta V = \dfrac{(\sigma_x + \sigma_y + \sigma_z)}{E}[1 - 2\mu]\,V \qquad\qquad \text{... Eq. (i)}$$

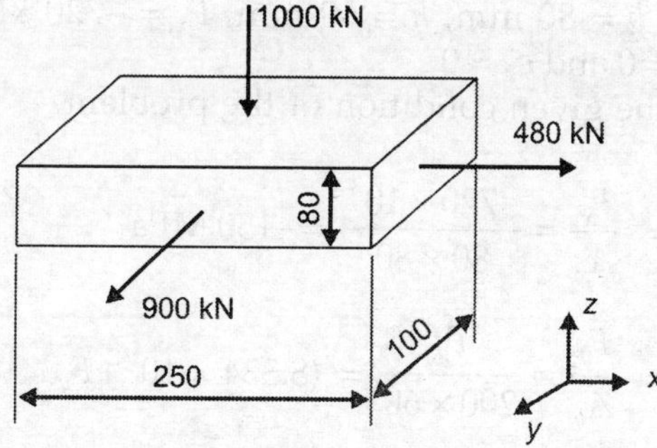

Fig. 2.32: Problem 32

Here $\quad \sigma_x = \dfrac{F_x}{A_x} = \dfrac{480 \times 10^3}{100 \times 80} = 60\,\text{MPa}$

$$\sigma_y = \dfrac{F_y}{A_y} = \dfrac{900 \times 10^3}{250 \times 80} = 45\,\text{MPa}$$

$$\sigma_z = \dfrac{F_z}{A_z} = \dfrac{-1000 \times 10^3}{250 \times 100} = -40\,\text{MPa}$$

Also $\quad V = lbh = 250 \times 100 \times 80 = 2 \times 10^6$ mm^3

Eq. (i) yields... $\delta V = \dfrac{(60 + 45 - 40)}{2 \times 10^5}\,[1 - (2 \times 0.25)] \times (2 \times 10^6)$

$$\therefore \quad \delta V = 325 \text{ mm}^3$$

b. To find $F_z = ?$, if $\delta V = 0$:

Since $\delta V = 0$, the condition is $(\sigma_x + \sigma_y + \sigma_z) = 0$ $\qquad$ *... using (Eq. 2.19)*

$$(60 + 45 + \sigma_z) = 0$$

$$\therefore \quad \sigma_z = -105 \text{ MPa}$$

But $\qquad F_z = \sigma_z\, A_z = -105 \times (250 \times 100) = -2625$ kN

Thus the net change in load for $F_z = -2625 - (-1000) = -1625$ kN

33. **A mild steel bar, 200 mm long and 80 mm × 60 mm in cross-section is subjected to axial compression of 720 kN. Determine the values of lateral forces necessary to prevent any lateral deformation. E = 200 GPa, μ = 0.25.**

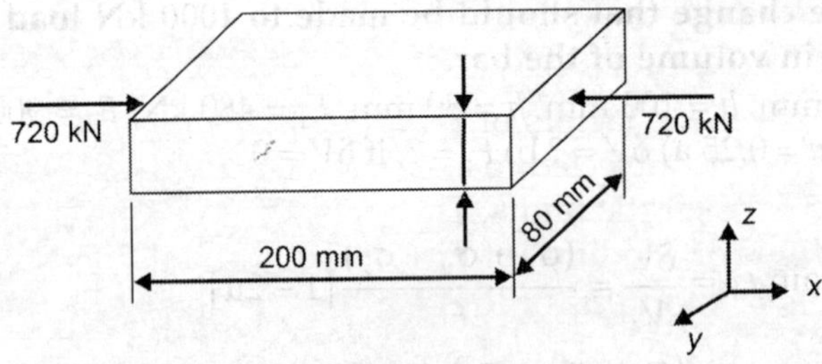

Fig. 2.33: Problem 33

Solution: l = 200 mm, b = 80 mm, h = 60 mm, F_x = –720 kN, E = 200 × 10^3 MPa, μ = 0.25, F_y, F_Z = ?, if ε_y = 0 and ε_z = 0

Fig. 2.33 represents the given condition of the problem

We know that $\quad \sigma_x = \dfrac{F_x}{A_x} = \dfrac{-720 \times 10^3}{80 \times 80} = -150$ MPa

$$\sigma_y = \dfrac{F_y}{A_y} = \dfrac{F_y}{200 \times 60} = (8.334 \times 10^{-5})\, F_y$$

$$\sigma_z = \dfrac{F_z}{A_z} = \dfrac{F_z}{200 \times 80} = (6.25 \times 10^{-5})\, F_z$$

$$V = lbh = 200 \times 80 \times 60 = 960 \times 10^3 \text{ mm}^3$$

Since lateral deformation is prevented, we have ε_y = 0 and ε_z = 0

i.e. $\qquad \varepsilon_y = \dfrac{1}{E}\,[\sigma_y - \mu(\sigma_z + \sigma_x)] = 0$

$$0 = [\sigma_y - \mu(\sigma_z + \sigma_x)]$$

$$\dfrac{\sigma_y}{\mu} = (\sigma_z + \sigma_x)$$

$$\frac{(8.334\times10^{-5})F_y}{0.25} = (6.25\times10^{-5})\,F_z - 150$$

$$(3.334\times10^{-4})\,F_y - (6.25\times10^{-5})\,F_z = -150 \qquad\qquad \text{... Eq. (i)}$$

Similarly
$$\varepsilon_z = \frac{1}{E}\,[\sigma_z - \mu(\sigma_x + \sigma_y)] = 0$$

$$0 = [\sigma_z - \mu(\sigma_x + \sigma_y)]$$

$$\frac{\sigma_z}{\mu} = (\sigma_x + \sigma_y)$$

$$\frac{(6.25\times10^{-5})F_z}{0.25} = -150 + (8.334\times10^{-5})\,F_y$$

$$(8.334\times10^{-5})F_y - (2.5\times10^{-4})\,F_z = 150 \qquad\qquad \text{... Eq. (ii)}$$

Solving Eqs (i) and (ii), we get
$$F_y = -600 \text{ kN and } F_z = -800 \text{ kN}$$

2.4 ELASTIC CONSTANTS

VTU – (CV) June/ July 2011 – 04 Marks

Elastic constants are those factors or parameters that determine the deformations of a body/ material, when subjected to a system of stresses. These factors obey Hooke's law and are within the elastic limits. These are of four types:
- Young's modulus or Modulus of Elasticity (E)
- Shear modulus or Modulus of Rigidity or Modulus of transverse elasticity (G or C or N)
- Bulk modulus (K)
- Poisson' s ratio (μ)
- *Young's modulus or Modulus of Elasticity (E):*

$$E = \frac{\text{Direct stress}}{\text{linear or longitudunal strain}} = \left(\frac{\sigma}{\varepsilon_l}\right) \qquad \text{... (Eq. 2.20)}$$

- *Bulk modulus (K):*

$$K = \frac{\text{Direct stress}}{\text{Volumetric or compressive strain}} = \left(\frac{\sigma}{\varepsilon_V}\right) \qquad \text{... (Eq. 2.21)}$$

- *Shear modulus or Modulus of rigidity (G):*

$$G = \frac{\text{Shear stress}}{\text{shear strain}} = \frac{\tau}{\gamma} \qquad \text{... (Eq. 2.22)}$$

- *Poisson's Ratio (μ):* When a bar is subject to a simple tensile loading there is an increase in length of the bar in the direction of the load, but a decrease in the lateral dimensions perpendicular to the load. The ratio of the strain in the lateral direction to that in the axial direction is defined as Poisson's ratio.

$$\mu = \frac{\text{Lateral strain}}{\text{Linear strain}} \qquad \text{... (Eq. 2.23)}$$

2.5 RELATION AMONG ELASTIC CONSTANTS

2.5.1 Relation between Young's modulus (E) and modulus of rigidity (G)

VTU (Mech) – Dec.08/ Jan.09 – 10 Marks; June/ July 2009 – 10 Marks; June/ July 2011 – 07 Marks; Dec. 2011 – 08 Marks; June/ July 2014 – 06 Marks; Dec. 14/ Jan. 15 – 07 Marks.
VTU (CV) – Dec.07/ Jan.08 – 08 Marks; Dec. 10 – 06 Marks; June/ July 2011 – 06 Marks; Dec. 2011 – 06 Marks; Dec. 2012 – 06 Marks; Jan. 2013 – 08 Marks; June/ July 2013 – 05 Marks

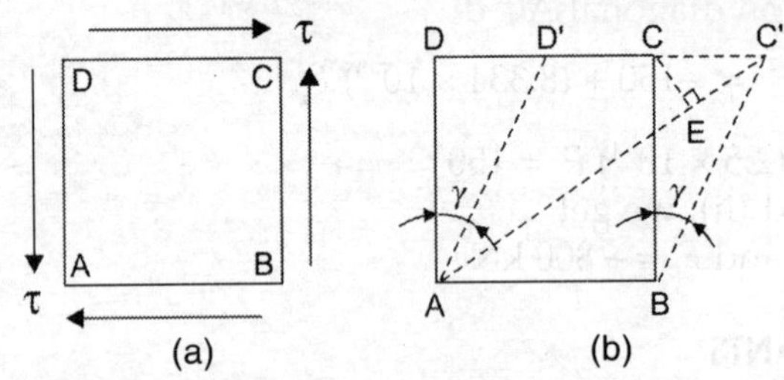

Fig. 2.34: Relation between E and G

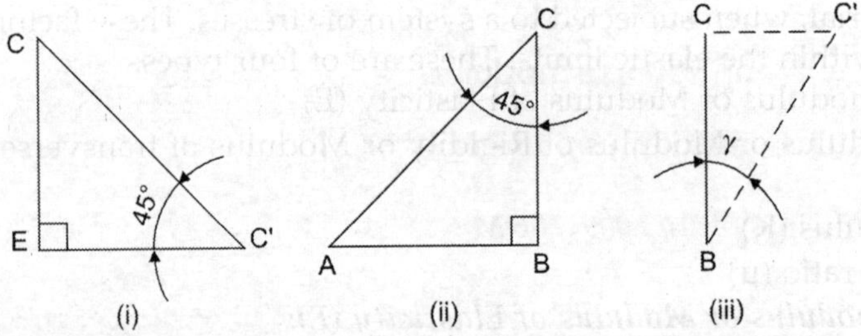

Fig. 2.34: (c)

Consider a square block *ABCD* of unit thickness subjected to pure shear (τ) as shown in **Fig. 2.34(a)**. Due to these stresses, the block undergoes deformation such that the diagonal *AC* is elongated while the diagonal *BD* is shortened. Draw a perpendicular *CE* to diagonal *AC'*.

Let G = modulus of rigidity $\qquad \gamma$ = shear strain

From **Fig. 2.34(b)** strain in diagonal $AC = \dfrac{AC' - AE}{AE} = \dfrac{EC'}{AE} = \dfrac{EC'}{AC}$ ($\because AE = AC$)

$$\ldots \text{Eq. (i)}$$

From $\triangle\, C'CE$, $\cos(45) = \dfrac{EC'}{CC'}$

$$EC' = CC' \times \cos(45)$$

$$EC' = CC'/\sqrt{2} \qquad\qquad \ldots \text{Eq. (ii)}$$

From $\triangle\, ABC$, $\cos(45) = \dfrac{BC}{AC}$

$$AC = BC/\cos(45)$$

$$AC = \sqrt{2}\ BC \qquad\qquad \ldots \text{Eq. (iii)}$$

Substituting Eqs (ii) and (iii) in Eq. (i), we have

$$\text{Strain in diagonal } AC = \frac{CC'/\sqrt{2}}{\sqrt{2}\ BC} = \frac{CC'}{2BC} = \frac{\tan\gamma}{2} \simeq \frac{\gamma}{2},$$

(since γ is very small) ... Eq. (iv)

But shear modulus, $G = \dfrac{\tau}{\gamma}$

Therefore strain in diagonal $AC = \dfrac{\tau}{2G}$ ... Eq. (v)

Now, tensile strain on diagonal AC due to tensile stress on $AC = \dfrac{\tau}{E}$

and tensile strain on diagonal AC due to compressive stress on $BD = \mu\left(\dfrac{\tau}{E}\right)$

Thus the combined strain on diagonal $AC = \dfrac{\tau}{E} + \mu\left(\dfrac{\tau}{E}\right) = \dfrac{\tau}{E}(1+\mu)$ ... Eq. (vi)

Equating Eqs (v) and (vi), we have

$$\frac{\tau}{2G} = \frac{\tau}{E}(1+\mu)$$

$$\therefore \quad E = 2G[1+\mu] \qquad \text{... (Eq. 2.24)}$$

2.5.2 Relation between Young's modulus (E) and bulk modulus (K)

VTU (Mech.) – Dec. 09/ Jan. 10 – 08 Marks; Dec. 10 – 06 Marks; Dec. 2011 – 05 Marks; Dec. 13/ Jan. 14 – 12 Marks.
VTU (CV) – June/ July 2009 – 06 Marks; Dec. 09/ Jan. 10 – 10 Marks; May/ June 2010 – 06 Marks; Dec. 14/ Jan. 15 – 05 Marks

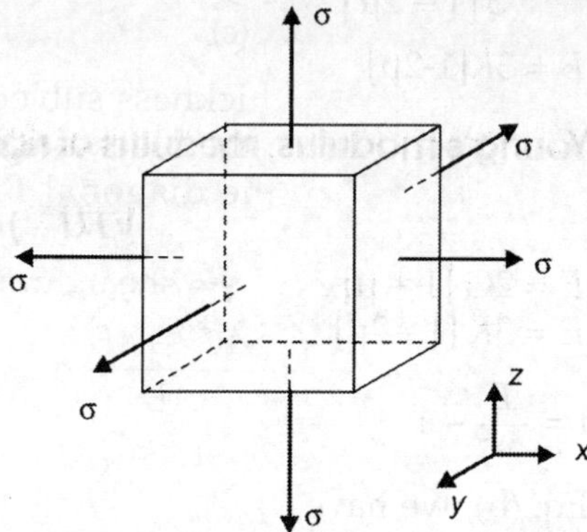

Fig. 2.35: Relation between E and K

Consider a cube of unit length subjected to three mutually perpendicular tensile stresses of equal intensity as shown in **Fig. 2.35**.

The stress σ applied in x direction produces a tensile strain of $\left(\dfrac{\sigma}{E}\right)$ in the direction of x and a compressive strain of $\mu\left(\dfrac{\sigma}{E}\right)$ in y and z directions.

Thus the total strain in x direction due to σ_x is

$$\varepsilon_x = \left(\frac{\sigma}{E}\right) - \mu\left(\frac{\sigma}{E}\right) - \mu\left(\frac{\sigma}{E}\right) = \left(\frac{\sigma}{E}\right)[1 - 2\mu] \qquad \ldots \text{(Eq. 2.25a)}$$

On similar lines in y and z directions, we have

$$\varepsilon_y = \left(\frac{\sigma}{E}\right) - \mu\left(\frac{\sigma}{E}\right) - \mu\left(\frac{\sigma}{E}\right) = \left(\frac{\sigma}{E}\right)[1 - 2\mu] \qquad \ldots \text{(Eq. 2.25b)}$$

$$\varepsilon_z = \left(\frac{\sigma}{E}\right) - \mu\left(\frac{\sigma}{E}\right) - \mu\left(\frac{\sigma}{E}\right) = \left(\frac{\sigma}{E}\right)[1 - 2\mu] \qquad \ldots \text{(Eq. 2.25c)}$$

Adding ε_x, ε_y and ε_z in (Eq. 2.25), we have

$$\varepsilon_x + \varepsilon_y + \varepsilon_z = \left(\frac{\sigma}{E}\right)[3(1 - 2\mu)]$$

$$= \left(\frac{3\sigma}{E}\right)[1 - 2\mu]$$

Thus $(\varepsilon_x + \varepsilon_y + \varepsilon_z) = \varepsilon_V = \dfrac{\delta V}{V} = \left(\dfrac{3\sigma}{E}\right)[1 - 2\mu]$ $\qquad \ldots \text{(Eq. 2.26)}$

But Bulk modulus, $K = \dfrac{\text{Direct stress}}{\text{Volumetric or compressive strain}} = \left(\dfrac{\sigma}{\varepsilon_V}\right)$

$$K = \sigma \Big/ \left(\frac{3\sigma}{E}\right)[1 - 2\mu]$$

$$K = \frac{E}{3[1 - 2\mu]}$$

$$\therefore \quad E = 3K[1\text{-}2\mu] \qquad \ldots \text{(Eq. 2.27)}$$

2.5.3 Relation between Young's modulus, modulus of rigidity and bulk modulus

VTU – June/ July 2008 – 06 Marks

We know that $\qquad E = 2G\,[1 + \mu]$ $\qquad\qquad\qquad\qquad \ldots$ Eq. (a)
and $\qquad\qquad\quad E = 3K\,[1 - 2\mu]$ $\qquad\qquad\qquad\qquad \ldots$ Eq. (b)

From Eq. (a) we have $\mu = \dfrac{E}{2G} - 1$ $\qquad\qquad\qquad\qquad\qquad \ldots$ Eq. (c)

Substituting Eq. (c) in Eq. (b), we have

$$E = 3K\left[1 - 2\left(\frac{E}{2G} - 1\right)\right]$$

$$= 3K\left[1 - \frac{E}{G} + 2\right] = 3K\left[3 - \frac{E}{G}\right]$$

$$= \frac{3K}{G}[3G - E]$$

$$E = \left(\frac{1}{G}\right)[9KG - 3KE]$$

$$EG + 3KE = 9KG$$

$$E(3K + G) = 9KG$$

$$\therefore \quad E = \left(\frac{9KG}{3K + G}\right) \qquad \qquad \dots \text{(Eq. 2.28)}$$

34. A C.I flat 300 mm long, 50 mm wide and 30 mm thick is acted upon by the following forces: 25 kN tensile in the direction of length; 350 kN compressive in the direction width; and 200 kN in the direction of thickness. Determine: (i) Change in volume of the flat (ii) Modulus of rigidity (iii) Bulk modulus Take E = 140 GN/m², and 1/m = 0.25

VTU – Dec. 2012 – 10 Marks

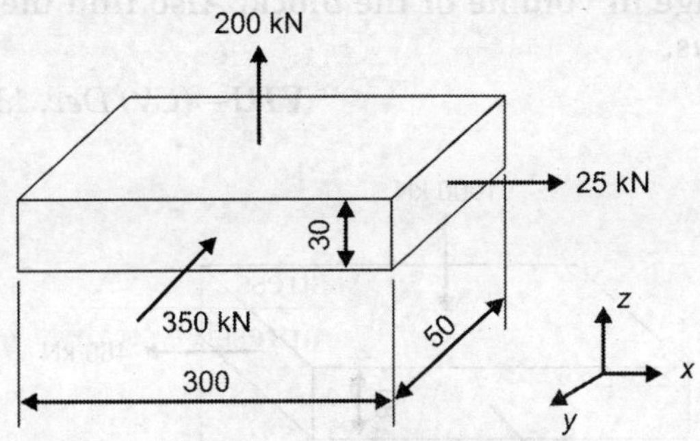

Fig. 2.36: Problem 34

Solution: l = 300 mm, b = 50 mm, h = 30 mm, F_x = 25 kN, F_y = – 350 kN, F_z = 200 kN, μ = 0.25, E = 140 × 10³ MPa. a) δV = ?, b) G = ?, c) K = ?

Fig. 2.36 represents the given condition of the problem

a. To find δV:

Volumetric strain $\varepsilon_V = \dfrac{\delta V}{V} = \dfrac{(\sigma_x + \sigma_y + \sigma_z)}{E}[1 - 2\mu]$

$$\delta V = \frac{(\sigma_x + \sigma_y + \sigma_z)}{E}[1 - 2\mu]V \qquad \qquad \dots \text{Eq. (i)}$$

Here $\quad \sigma_x = \dfrac{F_x}{A_x} = \dfrac{25 \times 10^3}{50 \times 30} = 16.67$ MPa

$$\sigma_y = \frac{F_y}{A_y} = \frac{-350 \times 10^3}{500 \times 30} = -38.89 \text{ MPa}$$

$$\sigma_z = \frac{F_z}{A_z} = \frac{200 \times 10^3}{300 \times 30} = 13.34 \text{ MPa}$$

Also $\quad V = lbh = 300 \times 50 \times 30 = 450000$ mm³

Eq. (i) yields... $\delta V = \dfrac{16.67 - 38.89 + 13.33}{140 \times 10^3}\,[1 - (2 \times 0.25)] \times (450000)$

$$\therefore \quad \delta V = -14.27 \text{ mm}^3$$

b. To find G:

We know that $\quad E = 2G[1 + \mu]$

$$140 \times 10^3 = 2G[1 + 0.25]$$

$$\therefore \quad G = 56000 \text{ MPa} = 56 \text{ GPa}$$

c. To find K:

We know that $\quad E = 3K[1-2\mu]$

$$140 \times 10^3 = 3K[1 - (2 \times 0.25)]$$

$$\therefore \quad K = 93333.34 \text{ MPa} = 93.34 \text{ GPa}$$

35. A rectangular block 250 mm × 100 mm × 80 mm is subjected to axial loads as shown in Fig. 2.37. Assuming Poisson's ratio as 0.25 and $E = 2 \times 10^5$ N/mm², calculate the change in volume of the block. Also find the modulus of rigidity and bulk modulus.

VTU – (CV) Dec. 13/ Jan. 14 – 08 Marks

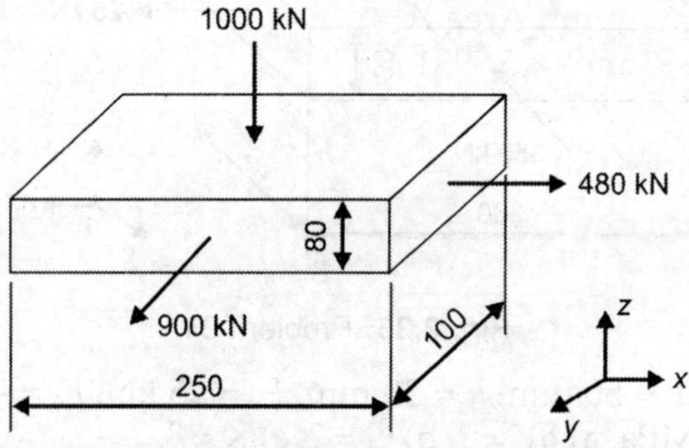

Fig. 2.37: Problem 35

Solution: $l = 250$ mm, $b = 100$ mm, $h = 80$ mm, $F_x = 480$ kN, $F_y = 900$ kN, $F_z = -1000$ kN, $\mu = 0.25$, $E = 2 \times 10^5$ MPa.

a) $\delta V = ?$,   b) $G = ?$,   c) $K = ?$

a. To find δV:

Volumetric strain $\varepsilon_V = \dfrac{\delta V}{V} = \dfrac{(\sigma_x + \sigma_y + \sigma_z)}{E}\,[1 - 2\mu]$

$$\delta V = \dfrac{(\sigma_x + \sigma_y + \sigma_z)}{E}\,[1 - 2\mu]V \qquad \ldots \text{Eq. (i)}$$

Here $\quad \sigma_x = \dfrac{F_x}{A_x} = \dfrac{480 \times 10^3}{100 \times 80} = 60 \text{ MPa}$

$$\sigma_y = \dfrac{F_y}{A_y} = \dfrac{900 \times 10^3}{250 \times 80} = 45 \text{ MPa}$$

$$\sigma_z = \dfrac{F_z}{A_z} = \dfrac{-1000 \times 10^3}{250 \times 100} = -40 \text{ MPa}$$

Also $\quad V = lbh = 250 \times 100 \times 80 = 2 \times 10^6 \text{ mm}^3$

Eq. (i) yields... $\delta V = \dfrac{(60 + 45 - 40)}{2 \times 10^5}\,[1 - (2 \times 0.25)] \times (2 \times 10^6)$

$\qquad\qquad\therefore\quad \delta V = 325\ \text{mm}^3$

b. To find G:

We know that $\quad E = 2G[1 + \mu]$

$\qquad\qquad 2 \times 10^5 = 2G[1 + 0.25]$

$\qquad\qquad\therefore\quad G = 80000\ \text{MPa} = 80\ \text{GPa}$

c. To find K:

We know that $\quad E = 3K[1 - 2\mu]$

$\qquad\qquad 2 \times 10^5 = 3K[1 - (2 \times 0.25)]$

$\qquad\qquad\therefore\quad K = 133333.34\ \text{MPa} = 133.34\ \text{GPa}$

36. **The modulus of rigidity of a member is 0.8×10^5 N/mm². When a 6 mm × 6 mm rod of this material was subjected to an axial pull of 3600 N, it was found that the lateral dimension of the rod changed to 5.9991 mm × 5.9991 mm. Find the Poisson's ratio and the modulus of elasticity.**

VTU – June 2012 – 04 Marks; [Similar: June/ July 2015 – 08 Marks]

Solution: $G = 0.8 \times 10^5$ N/mm², Area $A = bh = 6 \times 6 = 36$ mm², $F = 3600$ N, change in lateral dimension = 5.9991 mm × 5.9991 mm. a) $\mu = ?$, b) $E = ?$

To find μ:

Poisson's ratio $\mu = \dfrac{\text{lateral strain}}{\text{linear strain}}$ ... Eq. (i)

But $\quad$ lateral strain $= \dfrac{\text{Change in lateral strain}}{\text{original dimension}}$

$\qquad\qquad\qquad = \dfrac{b - \delta b}{b} = \dfrac{6 - 5.9991}{6}$

lateral strain $= 0.00015$

Also Linear strain, $\varepsilon_1 = \dfrac{F}{AE} = \dfrac{3600}{(6 \times 6)E} = \dfrac{100}{E}$

Eq. (i) yields... $\quad \mu = \dfrac{0.00015}{(100/E)}$

$\qquad\qquad\therefore\quad \mu = 1.5 \times 10^{-6}\,E$ ... Eq. (ii)

Now $\qquad\qquad E = 2G[1 + \mu]$

$\qquad\qquad E = 2 \times (0.8 \times 10^5) \times [1 + (1.5 \times 10^{-6}\,E)]$

$\qquad 6.25 \times 10^{-6}\,E = [1 + (1.5 \times 10^{-6}\,E)]$

$\qquad 4.75 \times 10^{-6}\,E = 1$

$\qquad\qquad\therefore\quad E = 210.53 \times 10^3\ \text{N/mm}^2$

37. **A bar of 20 mm diameter is tested in tension. It is observed that when a load of 37.7 kN is applied, the extension measured over a gauge length of 200 mm is 0.12 mm and contraction in diameter is 0.0036 mm. Find Poisson's ratio and elastic constants E, G and K.**

VTU – (Mech.): June/ July 2013 – 08 Marks; (Similar) Dec. 2011 – 08 Marks; (similar) June/ July 2016 – 10 Marks VTU – [Similar: (CV) Dec.07/ Jan.08 – 12 Marks; June/ July 2009 – 06 Marks; Dec. 2011 – 06 Marks; Dec. 2012 – 08 Marks

Solution: $d = 20$ mm $\Rightarrow A = 314.16$ mm^2, $F = 37.7$ kN, $l = 200$ mm, $\delta l = 0.12$ mm, $\delta d = 0.0036$ mm, a) $\mu = ?$, b) $E, K, G = ?$

a. To find μ:

Poisson's ratio $\quad \mu = \dfrac{\text{lateral strain}}{\text{linear strain}} = \dfrac{\delta d / d}{\delta l / l} = \dfrac{(0.0036 / 20)}{(0.12 / 200)} = 0.3$

b. To find E, K, G:

We know that $\quad \delta l = \dfrac{Fl}{AE}$

$$0.12 = \frac{(37.7 \times 10^3) \times 200}{314.16 \times E}$$

$$\therefore \quad E = 200 \times 10^3 \text{ MPa}$$

To find K:

We know that $\quad E = 3K[1 - 2\mu]$

$$200 \times 10^3 = 3K[1 - (2 \times 0.3)]$$

$$\therefore \quad K = 166.67 \times 10^3 \text{ MPa}$$

To find G:

We know that $\quad E = 2G[1 + \mu]$

$$200 \times 10^3 = 2G[1 + 0.3]$$

$$\therefore \quad G = 76.92 \times 10^3 \text{ MPa}$$

38. The longitudinal strain of a cylindrical bar of diameter 3 cm and length 1.5 m is four times the lateral strain during a tensile test. Determine the modulus of rigidity and bulk modulus. Also determine the change in volume when the bar is subjected to a hydrostatic pressure of 100 MPa. Take $E = 100$ GPa.

> *VTU – May/ June 2010 – 10 Marks; [Similar: (CV) June/ July 2013 – 10 Marks]*

Solution: $d = 30$ mm $\Rightarrow A = 706.86$ mm^2, $l = 1500$ mm, $\delta l = 4(\delta d) \Rightarrow \mu = 1/4 = 0.25$, $E = 100 \times 10^3$ MPa, $p = 100$ MPa. a) $K, G = ?$ b) $\delta V = ?$

a. To find K,G:

We know that $\quad E = 3K[1 - 2\mu]$

$$100 \times 10^3 = 3K[1 - (2 \times 0.25)]$$

$$\therefore \quad K = 66.67 \times 10^3 \text{ MPa}$$

Also $\quad\quad\quad\quad E = 2G[1 + \mu]$

$$100 \times 10^3 = 2G[1 + 0.25]$$

$$\therefore \quad G = 26.67 \times 10^3 \text{ MPa}$$

b. To find δV:

Change iv volume, $\quad \delta V = \varepsilon . V$ $\quad\quad\quad\quad\quad\quad\quad\quad$ ... Eq. (i)

But $\quad\quad\quad\quad \varepsilon = \dfrac{p}{K} = \dfrac{100}{66.67 \times 10^3} = 1.5 \times 10^{-3}$

Eq. (i) yields... $\quad \delta V = (1.5 \times 10^{-3}) \times 706.86 \times 1500 = 1590.36 \text{ mm}^3$

2.6 SHEAR STRESS AND SHEAR STRAIN

Shear stress (τ) is the stress state caused by a pair of opposing forces acting along parallel lines of action through the material, i.e. the stress caused by faces of the material sliding relative to one another

An example is cutting paper with scissors or stresses due to torsional loading, or a rivet subjected to tensile loading, as shown in **Fig. 2.38**.

OR

If the applied load consists of two equal and opposite parallel forces which do not share the same line of action, then there will be a tendency for one part of the body to slide over or shear from the other part.

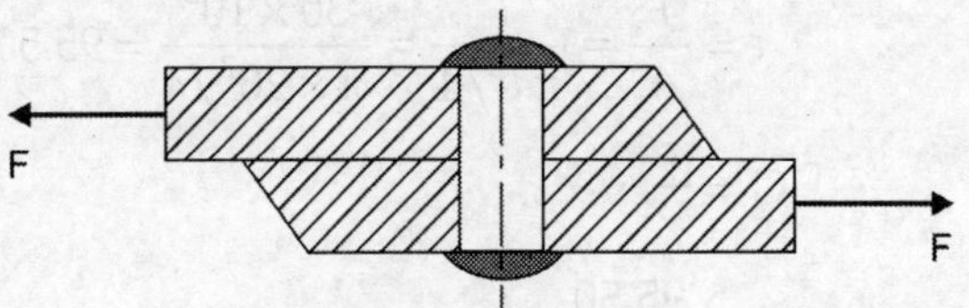

Fig. 2.38: Shear stress

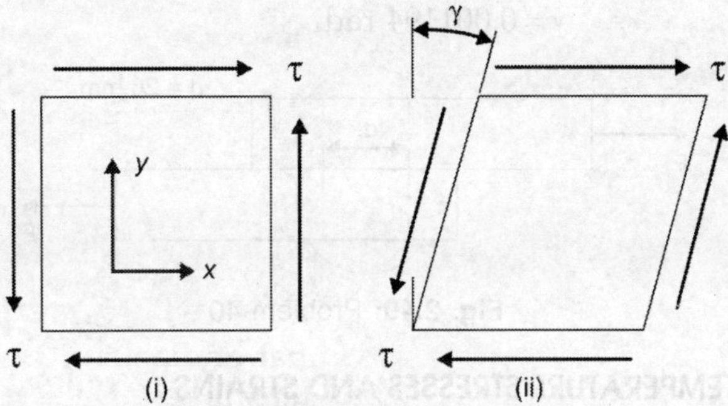

Fig. 2.39: Shear stress

$$\text{Shear stress, } \tau = \frac{F}{A} \qquad \qquad \text{... (Eq. 2.29a)}$$

where τ = the shear stress, F = the force applied,

A = Cross-sectional area of material perpendicular to the applied force.

Shear Strain (γ)

The change in angle that occurs between two line segments that were originally perpendicular to each other is referred to as shear strain, denoted by γ. It is measured in radians and is dimensionless.

$$G = \frac{\text{Shear stress}}{\text{Shear strain}} = \frac{\tau}{\gamma} \qquad \qquad \text{... (Eq. 2.29b)}$$

39. Calculate the force needed to punch a hole of 25 mm diameter in a sheet of 5 mm thick if the ultimate shear stress is 80 MPa.

Solution: $d = 25$ mm, $t = 5$ mm, $\tau = 80$ MPa, $F = ?$

$$\text{Shear stress} \qquad \tau = \frac{F}{A_s} = \frac{F}{\pi d t}$$

$$80 = \frac{F}{\pi \times 25 \times 5}$$

$$\therefore \quad F = 31.42 \text{ kN}$$

40. A riveted joint is shown in Fig. 2.40. If the diameter of the rivet is 20 mm and the load F is 30 kN, determine the shear stress and the shear strain in the rivet. Take G = 80 GPa.

VTU – June/ July 2013 – 04 Marks

Solution: d = 20 mm, F = 30 kN, τ = ?, γ = ?, G = 80 × 10³ MPa,

Shear stress
$$\tau = \frac{F}{A_s} = \frac{F}{\pi d^2/4} = \frac{30 \times 10^3}{\pi \times 20^2/4} = 95.50 \text{ MPa}$$

Shear modulus,
$$G = \frac{\tau}{\gamma}$$

$$80 \times 10^3 = \frac{95.50}{\gamma}$$

$$\therefore \quad \gamma = 0.001194 \text{ rad}$$

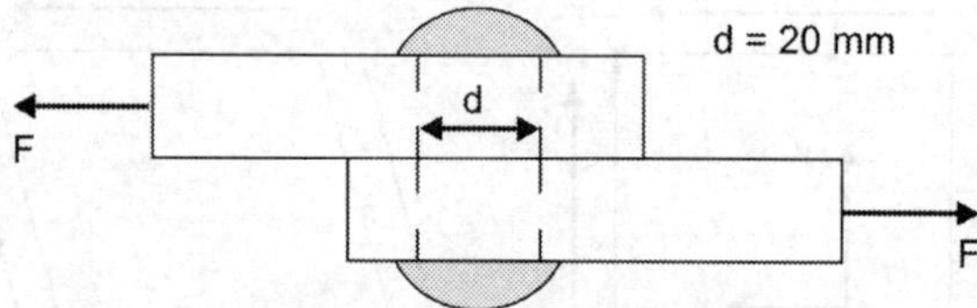

Fig. 2.40: Problem 40

2.7 THERMAL OR TEMPERATURE STRESSES AND STRAINS

Whenever a body is subjected to change in temperature, the body undergoes deformation (expansion or contraction) i.e. if there is increase in temperature the body will expand and if the temperature decreases, the body will contract. If the body is allowed to deform freely then no stresses are induced in it. On the other hand if the deformation is prevented, then some stresses are induced in the body and these stresses are referred to as thermal or temperature stresses.

This deformation is isotropic (i.e. same in every direction) and proportional to the temperature change.

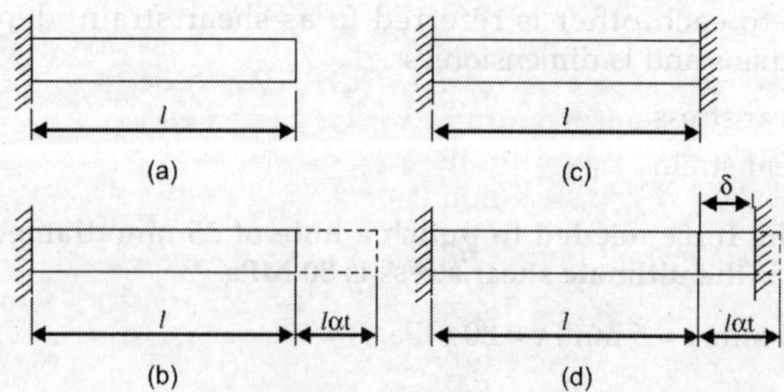

Fig. 2.41: Thermal stresses

Consider a bar as shown in **Fig. 2.41(a)** subjected to increase in temperature. Due to increase in temperature, the bar undergoes deformation as shown in **Fig. 2.41(b)**.

Let $\quad l$ = Length of the bar

$\quad t$ = Increase in temperature

$\quad \alpha$ = Coefficient of thermal or linear expansion

Thus the increase in length of the bar due to increase in temperature, $\delta l = l\alpha t$
$$\ldots \text{(Eq. 2.30)}$$
Now if the deformation is prevented (supports do not yield) as shown in **Fig. 2.40(c)** then

Compressive strain $\qquad \varepsilon = \dfrac{\delta l}{l} = \dfrac{l\alpha t}{l}$

$$\varepsilon = \alpha t \qquad\qquad\qquad\qquad \ldots \text{(Eq. 2.31a)}$$
and Compressive stress, $\sigma = \varepsilon E = \alpha t E \qquad\qquad\qquad\qquad \ldots \text{(Eq. 2.31b)}$
If the supports yield by an amount δ, as shown in **Fig. 2.41(d)**, we have
$$\delta l = (l\alpha t - \delta)$$

Compressive strain, $\qquad \varepsilon = \dfrac{\delta l}{l} = \dfrac{(l\alpha t - \delta)}{l}$

$$\varepsilon = \left(\alpha t - \frac{\delta}{l} \right) \qquad\qquad \ldots \text{(Eq. 2.32a)}$$

Compressive stress, $\qquad \sigma = \left(\alpha t - \frac{\delta}{l} \right) E \qquad\qquad \ldots \text{(Eq. 2.32b)}$

Note: The value of α is the same in both cases because a change in temperature is numerically the same in both Kelvin and degrees Celsius.

41. A rod is 10 m long at 10°C. Find the expansion of the bar, when the temperature rises to 80°C. If the expansion is prevented, determine the temperature stresses developed. Take E = 100 GPa, α = 12 × 10⁻⁶/°C

VTU – (CV) Dec. 2012 – 06 Marks

Solution: l = 10 m, t_1 = 10°C, t_2 = 80°C, E = 100 × 10³ MPa, α = 12 × 10⁻⁶/°C.
a) δl = ?, b) σ = ?, if δ = 0
  a. To find δl:
  Free expansion, $\delta l = l\alpha t$
  $\qquad\qquad\qquad = (10 \times 10^3) \times (12 \times 10^{-6}) \times 70 \qquad (t = t_2 - t_1 = 80 - 10 = 70)°C$
  $\qquad \therefore \quad \delta l = 8.4 \text{ mm}$
  b. To find σ, if δ = 0:
  Thermal stress, $\sigma = \alpha t E = (12 \times 10^{-6}) \times 70 \times (100 \times 10^3) = 84 \text{ MPa}.$

42. Calculate the nature and magnitude of stress induced in the rod of 2 m length and 20 mm diameter, when its temperature rises by 70°C, with both ends constrained. Take E = 1 × 10⁵ N/mm², and a = 1.2 × 10⁻⁵)/°C.

VTU – May/ June 2010 – 06 Marks; (CV) June/ July 2008 – 06 Marks

Solution: σ = ?, l = 2 m, d = 20 mm, t = 70°C, E = 1 × 10⁵ N/mm², α = 1.2 × 10⁻⁶/°C.
  We know that $\quad \sigma = \alpha t E = (1.2 \times 10^{-5}) \times 70 \times (1 \times 10^5) = 84 \text{ N/mm}^2 \text{ (Compressive)}$

43. A steel rod is 20 m long at a temperature of 20°C. Find the free expansion of the bar, when the temperature is raised to 65°C. Also calculate the temperature stress produced for the following cases:
  i. When the expansion of the rod is prevented
  ii. When the rod is permitted to expand by 5.8 mm. Take α = 12 × 10⁻⁶/°C and E = 200 GPa.

VTU – (CV) Dec. 2011– 06 Marks; June/ July 2016 – 06 Marks;
[Similar: (CV) June/ July 14 – 06 Marks]

Solution: $l = 20$ m, $t_1 = 20°C$, $t_2 = 65°C$, $E = 200 \times 10^3$ MPa, $d = 5.8$ mm, $\alpha = 12 \times 10^{-6}/°C$. a) $\delta l = ?$, b) $\sigma = ?$, if (i) $\delta = 0$; (ii) $\delta = 5.8$ mm

a. To find δl:

Free expansion, $\quad \delta l = l\alpha t$

$$= (20 \times 10^3) \times (12 \times 10^{-6}) \times 45 \qquad (t = t_2 - t_1 = 65 - 20 = 45)°C$$

$$\delta l = 10.8 \text{ mm}$$

b. To find σ:

i) If $\delta = 0$: $\qquad\qquad \sigma = \alpha t E = (12 \times 10^{-6}) \times 45 \times (200 \times 10^3) = 108$ MPa.

ii) If $\delta = 5.8$ mm: $\quad \sigma = \left(\alpha t - \dfrac{\delta}{l}\right) E$

$$= [(12 \times 10^{-6}) \times 45 - (5.8/(20 \times 10^3))] \times (200 \times 10^3)$$

$$\therefore \qquad \sigma = 50 \text{ MPa}$$

44. **A steel rod of diameter 25 mm is 10 m long at a temperature of 100°C. Find the pull exerted when the temperature falls to 50°C if:**
    (a) the ends do not yield
    (b) the ends yield by 1.2 mm. Take $\alpha = 12 \times 10^{-6}/°C$ and $E = 210$ GPa.

Solution: $d = 25$ mm $\Rightarrow A = 490.87$ mm^2, $l = 10$ m, $t_1 = 100°C$, $t_2 = 50°C$, $E = 210 \times 10^3$ MPa, $\alpha = 12 \times 10^{-6}/°C$. a) $F = ?$, if (i) $\delta = 0$, (ii) $\delta = 1.2$ mm

a. To find F:

i) If $\delta = 0$: $\qquad\qquad \sigma = \dfrac{F}{A}$

$$F = (\alpha t E)A \qquad\quad (\because \sigma = \alpha t E); \ \& \ (t = t_2 - t_1 = 100 - 50 = 50)°C$$

$$= (12 \times 10^{-6}) \times 50 \times (210 \times 10^3) \times 490.87$$

$$\therefore \quad F = 61.85 \text{ kN}$$

ii) If $\delta = 1.2$ mm: $\qquad F = \left(\alpha t - \dfrac{\delta}{l}\right) AE$

$$= \left[(12 \times 10^{-6}) \times 50 - \left(\frac{1.2}{10 \times 10^3}\right) \times (210 \times 10^3) \times 490.87\right]$$

$$\therefore \quad F = 49.48 \text{ kN}$$

45. **Rails are laid such that there is no stress in them at 24°C. If the rails are 32 m long, determine:**
    (a) The stress in rails at 80°C, when there is no allowance for expansion.
    (b) The stress in rails at 80°C, when there is an expansion allowance of 8 mm per rail
    (c) The expansion allowance for no stress in the rails at 80°C
    Coefficient of linear expansion $\alpha = 11 \times 10^{-6}/°C$ and Young's modulus $E = 205$ GPa.

VTU – Dec. 13/ Jan. 14 – 09 Marks

Solution: $t_1 = 24°C$, $l = 32$ m, $t_2 = 80°C$, $E = 205 \times 10^3$ MPa, $\alpha = 11 \times 10^{-6}/°C$. a) $\sigma = ?$, if $\delta = 0$, b) $\sigma = ?$, if $\delta = 8$ mm, c) $\delta = ?$, if $\sigma = 0$

a. To find σ, if $\delta = 0$:

We know that $\quad \sigma = \alpha t E$

$$= (11 \times 10^{-6}) \times 56 \times (205 \times 10^3)$$

$$\text{here } (t = t_2 - t_1 = 80 - 24 = 56)°C$$

$$\therefore \quad \sigma = 126.28 \text{ MPa}$$

b. To find σ, if δ = 8 mm

We know that $\sigma = \left(\alpha t - \dfrac{\delta}{l}\right)E$

$$= \left[(11\times10^{-6})\times 56 - \left(\dfrac{8}{32\times10^{3}}\right)\right]\times(205\times10^{3})$$

$$\therefore \quad \sigma = 75.03 \text{ MPa}$$

c. To find δ, if σ = 0

We know that $\sigma = \left(\alpha t - \dfrac{\delta}{l}\right)E$

$$0 = \left[(11\times10^{-6})\times 56 - \left(\dfrac{8}{32\times10^{3}}\right)\right]\times(205\times10^{3})$$

$$\therefore \quad \delta = 19.72 \text{ mm}$$

46. **A steel rail 12.6 m long is laid at a temperature of 24°C. The maximum temperature expected is 44°C.**
    (a) **Estimate the minimum gap between two rails to be left so that temperature stresses do not develop.**
    (b) **Calculate the thermal stresses developed in the rails if the gap of 2 mm is provided for expansion.**
    (c) **If the stress developed is 20 MN/m², what is the gap left between the rails? Take $E = 2 \times 10^5$ N/mm² and $\alpha = 12 \times 10^{-6}$/°C**

VTU – Dec. 2011 – 10 Marks

Solution: $l = 12.6$ m, $t_1 = 24°C$, $t_2 = 44°C$, $E = 2 \times 10^5$ N/mm², $\alpha = 12 \times 10^{-6}$/°C.
a) $\delta l = ?$ b) $\sigma = ?$, if $\delta = 2$ mm, c) $\delta = ?$, if $\sigma = 20$ MN/m²

a. To find δl:
Free expansion, $\delta l = l\alpha t = (12.6 \times 10^3) \times (12 \times 10^{-6}) \times 20$

here $(t = t_2 - t_1 = 44 - 24 = 20)°C$

$$\therefore \quad \delta l = 3.024 \text{ mm}$$

b. To find σ, if δ = 2 mm

We know that $\sigma = \left(\alpha t - \dfrac{\delta}{l}\right)E$

$$= \left[(12\times10^{-6})\times 20 - \left(\dfrac{2}{12.6\times10^{3}}\right)\right]\times(2\times10^{5})$$

$$\therefore \quad \sigma = 16.25 \text{ MPa}$$

c. To find δ, if σ = 20 MPa

We know that $\sigma = \left(\alpha t - \dfrac{\delta}{l}\right)E$

$$20 = \left[(12\times10^{-6})\times 20 - \left(\dfrac{\delta}{12.6\times10^{3}}\right)\right]\times(2\times10^{5})$$

$$\therefore \quad \sigma = 1.764 \text{ mm}$$

2.8 THERMAL STRESSES IN COMPOUND BARS

When a composite bar made of two different materials is subjected to change in temperature, the compound bar experiences different free expansions based on coefficient of thermal expansion (α). Hence opposite kinds of stresses are developed in the material.

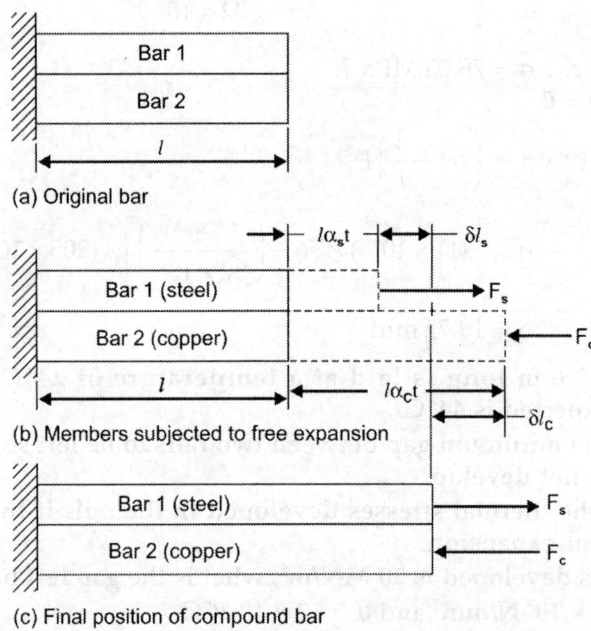

Fig. 2.42: Thermal stresses in compound bars

Consider a composite bar made of two materials [say steel (s) and copper (c)] as shown in **Fig. 2.42(a)**.

Let $\quad l$ = Length of compound bar ($l_s = l_c$)

$\quad\quad\quad t$ = Change in temperature of compound bar

$\quad\quad\quad \alpha_s$ = Coefficient of thermal expansion for steel

$\quad\quad\quad \alpha_c$ = Coefficient of thermal expansion for copper

$\quad\quad\quad F_s$ = Force in steel

$\quad\quad\quad F_c$ = Force in copper

Fig. 2.42(b) indicates bars undergoing different free expansions. This is due to the fact that coefficient of thermal expansion of copper is more than that of steel. Thus the expansion of the composite bar (Δ) as a whole would be less than that of copper and more than steel as shown in **Fig. 2.42(c)**. In order that to have common expansion, tensile stresses would be developed in steel and compressive stress in copper.

For equilibrium, tensile force in steel = compressive force in copper

$\quad\quad$ i.e. $\quad\quad\quad F_s = F_c = F$ $\qquad\qquad$ ... Eq. (i)

also for compatibility, expansion of steel = Expansion of copper

$\quad\quad$ i.e. $\quad\quad\quad \Delta_s = \Delta_c = \Delta$ $\qquad\qquad$ ... Eq. (ii)

From **Fig. 2.42(b)**, we have

$$\alpha_s lt + \delta l_s = \alpha_c lt - \delta l_c$$

$$\delta l_s + \delta l_c = lt(\alpha_c - \alpha_s) \qquad\qquad \text{... (Eq. 2.33)}$$

$$\frac{Fl}{A_s E_s} + \frac{Fl}{A_c E_c} = lt(\alpha_c - \alpha_s)$$

$$\frac{F}{A_s E_s} + \frac{F}{A_c E_c} = t(\alpha_c - \alpha_s) \qquad \text{... Eq. (iii)}$$

$$F\left[\frac{A_c E_c + A_s E_s}{A_s E_s \times A_c E_c}\right] = t(\alpha_c - \alpha_s)$$

$$F = \left[\frac{A_s E_s \times A_c E_c}{A_c E_c + A_s E_s}\right] t(\alpha_c - \alpha_s) \qquad \text{... (Eq. 2.34)}$$

By knowing the value of F, the stresses in respective materials can be calculated as

$$\sigma_s = \frac{F_s}{A_s} \text{ and } \sigma_c = \frac{F_c}{A_c} \qquad \text{... Eq. (iv)}$$

Substituting Eq. (iv) in Eq. (i), we have
$$\sigma_s A_s = \sigma_c A_c \qquad \text{... Eq. (v)}$$
Eq. (iii) can also be written as

$$\frac{\sigma_s}{E_s} + \frac{\sigma_c}{E_c} = t(\alpha_c - \alpha_s) \qquad \text{... (Eq. 2.35)}$$

$$\varepsilon_s + \varepsilon_c = t(\alpha_c - \alpha_s) \qquad \text{... (Eq. 2.36)}$$
Thus the final elongation is
$$\Delta_s = \alpha_s \, lt + \delta l_s$$
or $$\Delta_c = \alpha_c \, lt - \delta l_c$$

$$\Delta_s = \alpha_s \, lt + \frac{Fl}{A_s E_s} = \alpha_s \, lt + \frac{\sigma_s l}{E_s} \qquad \text{... (Eq. 2.37)}$$

Substituting **(Eq. 2.34)** in **(Eq. 2.37)**, and simplifying we have

$$\Delta = \frac{\left[\alpha_s A_s E_s + \alpha_c A_c E_c\right] lt}{A_c E_c + A_s E_s} \qquad \text{... (Eq. 2.38)}$$

(Eq. 2.38) gives the total deformation of the composite bar.
Where $\qquad \sigma_s$ = Tensile stress on steel
$\qquad\qquad\quad \sigma_c$ = Compressive stress on copper

47. A steel tube of 25 mm external diameter and 18 mm internal diameter encloses a copper rod of 15 mm diameter. The ends are rigidly fastened to each other. Calculate the stress in the rod and the tube when the temperature is raised from 15°C to 200°C. Take $\alpha_s = 11 \times 10^{-6}/°C$, $\alpha_c = 18 \times 10^{-6}/°C$, $E_s = 200$ GPa, $E_c = 100$ GPa.

VTU – Dec.07/ Jan.08 – 07 Marks; [Similar: (CV) Dec. 13/ Jan. 14 – 14 Marks]

Solution: Fig. 2.43 represents the given condition of the problem
$d_s)_o = 25$ mm, $d_s)_i = 18$ mm, $\Rightarrow A_s = \pi \times (25^2 - 18^2)/4 = 236.40$ mm^2, $d_c = 15$ mm, $A_c = (\pi \times 15^2)/4 = 176.71$ mm^2, $t_1 = 15°C$, $t_2 = 200°C$, $\Rightarrow t = (t_2 \sim t_1) = 185°C$, $E_s = 200 \times 10^3$ MPa, $E_c = 100 \times 10^3$ MPa, $\alpha_s = 11 \times 10^{-6}/°C$, $\alpha_c = 18 \times 10^{-6}/°C$, $\sigma_s = ?$, $\sigma_c = ?$
To find stresses:

Since $\alpha_c > \alpha_s$, we have $\dfrac{\sigma_c}{E_c} + \dfrac{\sigma_s}{E_s} = t(\alpha_c - \alpha_s)$ $\qquad \text{... Eq. (i)}$

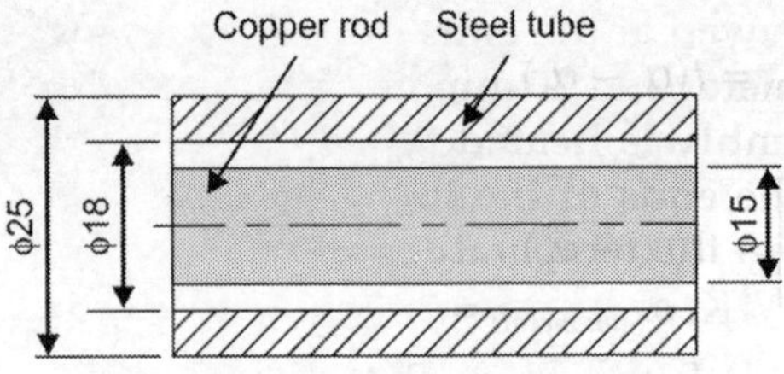

Fig. 2.43: Problem 47

But for equilibrium, tensile force in steel = compressive force in copper

i.e.
$$F_s = F_c$$
$$\sigma_s A_s = \sigma_c A_c$$
$$\sigma_s \times (236.40) = \sigma_c \times (176.71)$$
$$\therefore \quad \sigma_s = 0.748 \, \sigma_c \qquad \qquad \text{... Eq. (ii)}$$

Eq. (i) yields... $\dfrac{\sigma_c}{100 \times 10^3} + \dfrac{0.748 \, \sigma_c}{200 \times 10^3} = 185 \times (18 \times 10^{-6} - 11 \times 10^{-6})$

$$(1.374 \times 10^{-5}) \, \sigma_c = 1.295 \times 10^{-3}$$
$$\therefore \quad \sigma_c = 94.25 \, \text{MPa}$$

Eq. (ii) yields... $\sigma_s = 0.748 \times 94.25 = 70.50 \, \text{MPa}$

48. A M.S. bar 20 mm diameter and 300 mm long is encased in a brass tube whose external diameter is 30 mm and internal diameter is 25 mm. The composite bar is heated through 60°C. Calculate the stresses in each metal. Take α_s = 0.0000112/°C, α_b = 0.0000165/°C, E_s = 2 × 10⁵ N/mm², E_b = 1 × 10⁵ N/mm².

VTU – Dec. 13/ Jan. 14 – 08 Marks; [Similar: June/ July 2011 – 08 Marks; (CV) June/ July 2013 – 08 Marks;(CV) June 2012 – 10 Marks]

Solution: d_s = 20 mm $\Rightarrow A_s$ = 314.16 mm², l = 300 mm, $(d_b)_o$ = 30 mm, $(d_b)_i$ = 25 mm, $\Rightarrow A_b$ = 215.98 mm², t = 60°C, σ_s = ?, σ_b = ?, α_s = 0.0000112/°C, α_b = 0.0000165/°C, E_s = 2 × 10⁵ N/mm², E_b = 1 × 10⁵ N/mm²

To find stresses:

Since $\alpha_b > \alpha_s$, we have $\dfrac{\sigma_b}{E_b} + \dfrac{\sigma_s}{E_s} = t(\alpha_b - \alpha_s)$ $\qquad$ ... Eq. (i)

But for equilibrium, tensile force in steel = compressive force in brass

i.e.
$$F_s = F_b$$
$$\sigma_s A_s = \sigma_b A_b$$
$$\sigma_s \times (314.16) = \sigma_b \times (215.98)$$
$$\therefore \quad \sigma_s = 0.688 \, \sigma_b \qquad \qquad \text{... Eq. (ii)}$$

Eq. (i) yields... $\dfrac{\sigma_b}{100 \times 10^3} + \dfrac{0.688 \, \sigma_b}{200 \times 10^3} = 60 \times (0.0000165 - 0.0000112)$

$$(1.344 \times 10^{-5}) \, \sigma_b = 3.18 \times 10^{-4}$$
$$\therefore \quad \sigma_b = 23.66 \, \text{N/mm}^2$$

Eq. (ii) yields... $\qquad \qquad \sigma_s = 0.688 \times 23.66 = 16.28 \, \text{N/mm}^2$

49. A gun metal rod screwed at the ends passes through a steel tube. The tube has 25 mm external diameter and 20 mm internal diameter. The diameter of the rod is 16 mm. The assembly is heated to 400 K and the nuts on the rod are then screwed tightly at the ends of the tube. Find the intensity of stress in the rod and in the tube, when the temperature of the assembly falls to 300 K.
Take $\alpha_{steel} = 12 \times 10^{-6}/°K$, $\alpha_{(gun\ metal)} = 20 \times 10^{-6}/°K$, $E_{steel} = 2 \times 10^5$ N/mm^2, $E_{(gun\ metal)}$ = 0.91×10^5 N/mm^2.

VTU – (CV) Dec. 2011 – 08 Marks

Solution: Fig. 2.44 represents the given condition of the problem
$d_s)_o = 25$ mm, $d_s)_i = 20$ mm $\Rightarrow A_s = 176.71$ mm^2, $d_g = 16$ mm $\Rightarrow A_g = 201.06$ mm^2,
$t_1 = 400$ K, $t_2 = 300$ K, $t = (t_1 \sim t_2) = 100$ K, $E_s = 2 \times 10^5$ N/mm^2, $E_g = 0.91 \times 10^5$ N/mm^2,
$\alpha_s = 12 \times 10^{-6}/°K$, $\alpha_b = 20 \times 10^{-6}/°K$, $\sigma_s = ?$, $\sigma_g = ?$

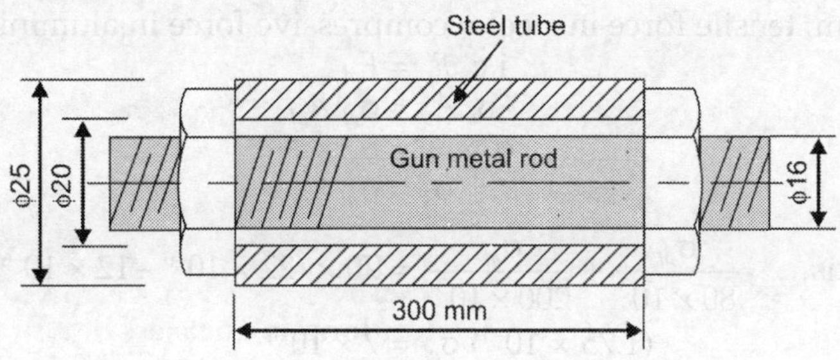

Fig. 2.44: Problem 49

To find stresses:

Since $\alpha_b > \alpha_s$, we have $\dfrac{\sigma_g}{E_g} + \dfrac{\sigma_s}{E_s} = t(\alpha_g - \alpha_s)$ ... Eq. (i)

But for equilibrium, tensile force in steel = compressive force in gun metal
     i.e. $$F_s = F_g$$
$$\sigma_s\, A_s = \sigma_g\, A_g$$
$$\sigma_s \times (176.71) = \sigma_g \times (201.06)$$
$$\therefore \quad \sigma_s = 1.138\, \sigma_g \qquad \text{... Eq. (ii)}$$

Eq. (i) yields... $\dfrac{\sigma_g}{0.91 \times 10^5} + \dfrac{1.138\, \sigma_g}{2 \times 10^5} = 100 \times (20 \times 10^{-6} - 12 \times 10^{-6})$

$$(1.668 \times 10^{-5})\, \sigma_g = 8 \times 10^{-4}$$
$$\therefore \quad \sigma_g = 47.96 \text{ N/mm}^2 \quad \text{(Tensile)}$$

Eq. (ii) yields... $\quad \sigma_s = 1.138 \times 47.96 = 54.46$ N/mm^2 (Compression)

50. A composite bar is made up of steel and aluminium plates rigidly bonded together. The bar is subjected to a temperature change of 70°C. Determine the stresses induced in both the materials and also the net deformation. Take $E_{al} = 80$ GPa, $E_s = 200$ GPa, $\alpha_{al} = 22 \times 10^{-6}/°C$, $\alpha_s = 12 \times 10^{-6}/°C$. Assume both plates have same cross sectional areas and same lengths.

VTU – (CV) June/ July 2011 – 10 Marks

Solution: Fig. 2.45 represents the given condition of the problem
$t = 70°C$, $\sigma_s = ?$, $\sigma_{al} = ?$, $E_{al} = 80 \times 10^3$ MPa, $E_s = 200 \times 10^3$ MPa, $\alpha_{al} = 22 \times 10^{-6}/°C$, $\alpha_s = 12 \times 10^{-6}/°C$, $A_s = A_{al} = A$, $l_s = l_{al} = l$

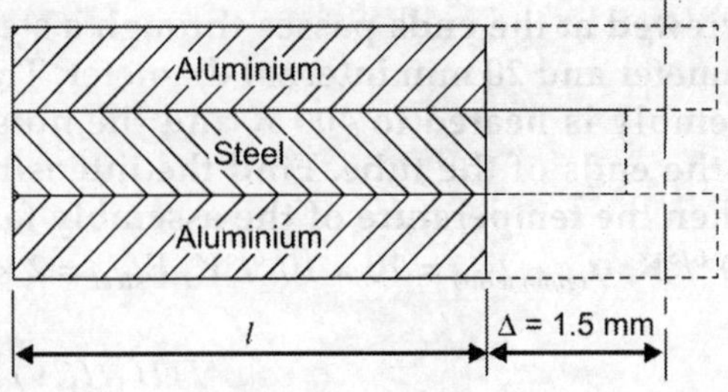

Fig. 2.45: Problem 51

To find stresses:

Since $\alpha_{al} > \alpha_s$, we have $\dfrac{\sigma_{al}}{E_{al}} + \dfrac{\sigma_s}{E_s} = t(\alpha_{al} - \alpha_s)$ ... Eq. (i)

for equilibrium, tensile force in steel = compressive force in aluminium

$$\text{i.e. } F_s = F_{al}$$
$$\sigma_s A_s = \sigma_{al} A_{al}$$
$$\sigma_s \times A = \sigma_{al} \times A$$
$$\therefore \quad \sigma_s = \sigma_{al} \qquad \qquad \text{... Eq. (ii)}$$

Eq. (i) yields... $\dfrac{\sigma_{al}}{80 \times 10^3} + \dfrac{\sigma_{al}}{200 \times 10^3} = 70 \times (22 \times 10^{-6} - 12 \times 10^{-6})$

$$(1.75 \times 10^{-5})\,\sigma_{al} = 7 \times 10^{-4}$$
$$\therefore \quad \sigma_{al} = 40 \text{ MPa}$$

Eq. (ii) yields... $\sigma_s = \sigma_{al} = 40 \text{ MPa}$

b. To find net deformation:

We know that $\Delta = \dfrac{[\alpha_s A_s E_s + \alpha_{al} A_{al} E_{al}]}{A_{al} E_{al} + A_s E_s}$

$$= \frac{\left[(12 \times 10^{-6} \times 1 \times 200 \times 10^3) + (22 \times 10^{-6} \times 1 \times 80 \times 10^3) \right] \times 1 \times 70}{1 \times 80 \times 10^3 + 1 \times 200 \times 10^3} = 1.04 \times 10^{-3} \text{ mm}$$

51. **A steel bar is placed between two copper bars, each having the same area and of length L as the steel bar at 15°C. At this stage they are rigidly connected together at both ends. The length of the composite bar is also l. When the temperature is raised to 315°C, the length of the bar increases by 1.5 mm. Determine the original length and find the stresses in the bar. Take $E_s = 2.1 \times 10^5$ MPa, $E_c = 1 \times 10^5$ MPa, $\alpha_s = 0.000012/°C$, and $\alpha_c = 0.0000175/°C$.**

VTU – Dec. 2012 – 10 Marks

Solution: $A_s = A = 2A_c,\ l_s = l_{al} = L,\, ,\ t_1 = 15°C,\ t_2 = 315°C,\ t = (t_2 \sim t_1) = 300°C,\ \Delta_s = 1.5$ mm, $E_c = 1 \times 10^5$ MPa, $E_s = 2.1 \times 10^5$ MPa, $\alpha_s = 0.000012/°C$, $\alpha_c = 0.0000175/°C$,
a) $\sigma_s = ?,\ \sigma_c = ?,$ b) $L = ?,$

  a. To find stresses:

Since $\alpha_c > \alpha_s$, we have $\dfrac{\sigma_c}{E_e} + \dfrac{\sigma_s}{E_s} = t(\alpha_c - \alpha_s)$ ... Eq. (i)

But for equilibrium, tensile force in steel = compressive force in copper

i.e.
$$F_s = F_c$$
$$\sigma_s A_s = \sigma_c A_c$$
$$\sigma_s \times A = \sigma_c \times 2A$$
$$\therefore \quad \sigma_s = 2\,\sigma_c \qquad \text{... Eq. (ii)}$$

Eq. (i) yields...
$$\frac{\sigma_c}{1 \times 10^5} + \frac{2\sigma_c}{2.1 \times 10^5} = 300 \times (0.0000175 - 0.000012)$$
$$(1.95 \times 10^{-5})\,\sigma_c = 1.65 \times 10^{-3}$$
$$\therefore \quad \sigma_c = 84.62 \text{ MPa}$$

Eq. (ii) yields...
$$\sigma_s = 2 \times 84.62 = 169.24 \text{ MPa}$$

b. To find L:

For compatibility, expansion of steel = Expansion of copper

i.e.
$$\Delta_s = \alpha_s l t + \delta l_s$$

$$\Delta_s = \alpha_s \, lt + \frac{\sigma_s L}{E_s} \qquad \text{... using (Eq. 2.37)}$$

$$1.5 = (0.000012 \times L \times 300) + \frac{(169.42)L}{2.1 \times 10^5}$$

$$1.5 = 4.405 \times 10^{-3}\,L$$

$$\therefore \quad L = 340.50 \text{ mm}$$

52. A compound bar made of central steel plate 60 mm wide and 10 mm thick to which copper plates 40 mm wide and 5 mm thick are connected rigidly on each side. The length of the bar at normal temperature is 1 meter. If the temperature is raised by 80°C, determine the stresses in each metal and change in length. Take E_s = 200 GPa, E_c = 100 GPa, α_s = 12 × 10⁻⁶/°C, and α_c = 17 × 10⁻⁶/°C.

VTU – Dec.08/ Jan.09 – 10 Marks; June 2012 – 07 Marks; Dec. 14/ Jan. 15 – 08 Marks

Solution: Fig. 2.46 represents the given condition of the problem
A_s = 60 × 10 = 600 mm², A_c = (40 × 5) = 200 mm², $l_s = l_c$ = 1000 mm, t = 80°C, E_s = 200 GPa = 200 × 10³ MPa, E_c = 100 GPa = 100 × 10³ MPa, α_s = 12 × 10⁻⁶/°C, α_c = 17 × 10⁻⁶/°C, a) σ_s = ?, σ_c = ?, b) Δ_s = ?

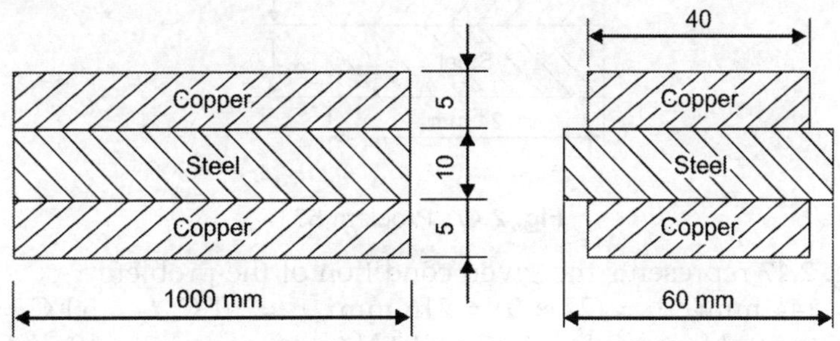

Fig. 2.46: Problem 52

a. To find stresses:

Since $\alpha_c > \alpha_s$, we have $\dfrac{\sigma_c}{E_c} + \dfrac{\sigma_s}{E_s} = t(\alpha_c - \alpha_s)$ ... Eq. (i)

But for equilibrium, tensile force in steel = compressive force in copper

i.e.
$$F_s = F_c$$
$$\sigma_s A_s = \sigma_c.(2A_c)$$
$$\sigma_s \times 600 = \sigma_c \times (2 \times 200)$$
$$\therefore \quad \sigma_s = 0.67\sigma_c \qquad \text{... Eq. (ii)}$$

Eq. (i) yields...
$$\frac{\sigma_c}{100 \times 10^3} + \frac{0.67\sigma_c}{200 \times 10^3} = 80 \times (17 \times 10^{-6} - 12 \times 10^{-6})$$
$$(1.335 \times 10^{-5})\,\sigma_c = 4 \times 10^{-4}$$
$$\therefore \quad \sigma_c = 30\,\text{MPa}$$

Eq. (ii) yields...
$$\sigma_s = 0.67 \times 30 = 20.1\,\text{MPa}$$

b. To find L:

For compatibility, expansion of steel = Expansion of copper

i.e. $\Delta_s = \alpha_s\,lt + \delta l_s = \alpha_s\,lt + \dfrac{\sigma_s l}{E_s}$ $\qquad$ ... using (Eq. 2.37)

$$= (12 \times 10^{-6} \times 1000 \times 80) + \frac{20.1 \times 1000}{200 \times 10^3}$$
$$\therefore \quad \Delta_s = 1.06\,\text{mm}$$

53. A flat bar of aluminium alloy 24 mm wide and 6 mm thick is placed between steel bars each 24 mm wide and 9 mm thick to form a composite bar (24 × 24) mm as shown in Fig. 2.47. The three bars are fastened together at their ends when the temperature is 10°C. Find the stresses in each of the material when the temperature of the whole assembly is raise to 50°C.

If at the new temperature a compressive load of 20 kN is applied to the composite bar, what are the final stresses in steel and aluminium? Take $E_s = 2 \times 10^5$ N/mm², $E_a = 2/3 \times 10^5$ N/mm², $\alpha_s = 1.2 \times 10^{-5}/°C$, $\alpha_a = 2.3 \times 10^{-5}/°C$.

VTU – (CV) Dec. 14/ Jan. 15 – 12 Marks; [Similar: (CV) Dec. 13/ Jan. 14 – 12 Marks]

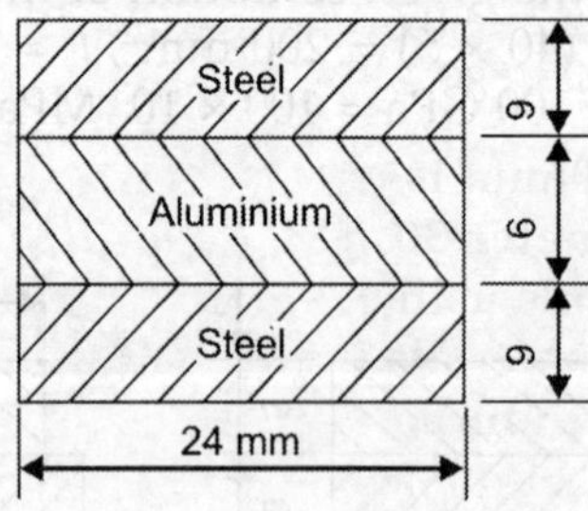

Fig. 2.47: Problem 53

Solution: Fig. 2.47 represents the given condition of the problem

$A_a = 24 \times 6 = 144$ mm², $A_s = (24 \times 9) = 216$ mm², $t_1 = 10°C$, $t_2 = 50°C$, $\Rightarrow t = (t_2 \sim t_1) = 40°C$, $E_s = 2 \times 10^5$ N/mm², $E_a = 2/3 \times 10^5$ N/mm², $\alpha_s = 1.2 \times 10^{-5}/°C$, $\alpha_a = 2.3 \times 10^{-5}/°C$. a) $\sigma_s = ?$, $\sigma_a = ?$, b) $F = 20$ kN, $\sigma_s = ?$, $\sigma_a = ?$,

a. To find stresses:

Since $\alpha_a > \alpha_s$, we have $\dfrac{\sigma_a}{E_a} + \dfrac{\sigma_s}{E_s} = t(\alpha_a - \alpha_s)$ $\qquad$ ... Eq. (i)

But for equilibrium, tensile force in steel = compressive force in aluminium

i.e.
$$F_s = F_a$$
$$\sigma_s (2A_s) = \sigma_a A_a$$
$$\sigma_s \times (2 \times 216) = \sigma_a \times 144$$
$$\therefore \quad \sigma_s = 0.34\sigma_a \qquad \text{... Eq. (ii)}$$

Eq. (i) yields...
$$\frac{\sigma_a}{(2/3)\times 10^5} + \frac{0.34\sigma_a}{2\times 10^5} = 40 \times (2.3 \times 10^{-5} - 1.2 \times 10^{-5})$$
$$(1.67 \times 10^{-5})\,\sigma_a = 4.4 \times 10^{-4}$$
$$\sigma_a = 26.38 \text{ MPa}$$

Eq. (ii) yields...
$$\sigma_s = 0.34 \times 26.38 = 9 \text{ MPa}$$

b. To find stresses, if F = 20 kN:

We know that
$$F = F_s + F_a$$
$$20 \times 10^3 = \sigma_s'(2A_s) + \sigma_a'A_a \qquad \text{... Eq. (iii)}$$

But
$$\frac{\sigma_a'}{E_a} = \frac{\sigma_s'}{E_s}$$
$$\sigma_s' = \left(\frac{E_s}{E_a}\right)\sigma_a'$$
$$= \left[\frac{2\times 10^5}{(2/3)\times 10^5}\right]\sigma_a'$$
$$\therefore \quad \sigma_s' = 3\sigma_a' \qquad \text{... Eq. (iv)}$$

Substituting Eq. (iv) in Eq. (iii), we have,
$$20 \times 10^3 = 3\sigma_a' \times (2 \times 216) + (\sigma_a' \times 144)$$
$$\therefore \quad \sigma_a' = 13.89 \text{ MPa}$$

Eq. (iii) yields... $\sigma_s' = 3 \times 13.89 = 41.67$ MPa

Thus the final (resultant) stresses are:
$$(\sigma_s)_R = \sigma_s + \sigma_s' = 9 + 41.67 = 50.67 \text{ MPa}$$
$$(\sigma_a)_R = \sigma_a + \sigma_a' = 26.38 + 13.89 = 40.27 \text{ MPa}$$

54. A brass rod of diameter 30 mm is enclosed in a steel tube of external diameter 50 mm and internal diameter 30 mm. The bar and the tube are 2 long and rigidly fastened at both ends using 20 mm diameter pins.

Find the stresses in both materials when the temperature is raised to 60°C.

Also find the shear stress induced in the pins.

Take $E_b = 1 \times 10^5$ MPa, $E_s = 2 \times 10^5$ MPa, $\alpha_b = 18 \times 10^{-6}$ per °C, $\alpha_s = 12 \times 10^{-6}$ per °C

VTU –[Similar: (CV) Dec. 13/ Jan. 2014 – 14 Marks]

Solution: Fig. 2.48 represents the given condition of the problem

$d_b = 30$ mm, $\Rightarrow A_b = (\pi \times 30^2)/4 = 706.85$ mm^2 $(d_s)_o = 50$ mm, $(d_s)_i = 30$ mm, $\Rightarrow A_s = \pi \times (50^2 - 30^2)/4 = 1256.64$ mm^2, $l = 2000$ mm, $d_p = 20$ mm, $\Rightarrow A_p = (\pi \times 20^2)/4 = 314.16$ mm^2, $t = 60°$C, $E_s = 200 \times 10^3$ MPa, $E_c = 100 \times 10^3$ MPa, $\alpha_s = 12 \times 10^{-6}/°$C, $\alpha_b = 18 \times 10^{-6}/°$C. a) $\sigma_s = ?$, $\sigma_b = ?$ b) $\tau = ?$

a. To find stresses:

Since $\alpha_b > \alpha_s$, we have $\dfrac{\sigma_b}{E_b} + \dfrac{\sigma_s}{E_s} = t(\alpha_b - \alpha_s)$ $\qquad$ ... Eq. (i)

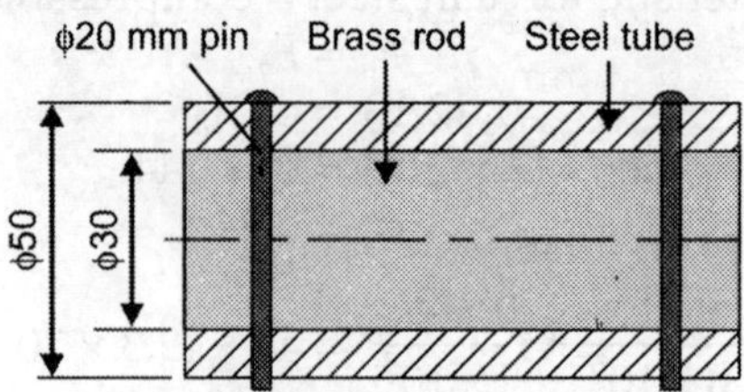

Fig. 2.48: Problem 54

But for equilibrium, tensile force in steel = compressive force in brass

i.e.
$$F_s = F_b$$
$$\sigma_s A_s = \sigma_b A_b$$
$$\sigma_s \times (1256.64) = \sigma_b \times (706.85)$$
$$\therefore \quad \sigma_s = 0.562 \, \sigma_b \qquad \qquad \text{... Eq. (ii)}$$

Eq. (i) yields...
$$\frac{\sigma_c}{100 \times 10^3} + \frac{0.562 \, \sigma_b}{200 \times 10^3} = 60 \times (18 \times 10^{-6} - 12 \times 10^{-6})$$
$$(1.281 \times 10^{-5}) \, \sigma_b = 3.6 \times 10^{-4}$$
$$\therefore \quad \sigma_b = 28.10 \, \text{MPa}$$

Eq. (ii) yields... $\quad \sigma_s = 0.562 \times 28.10 = 15.80 \, \text{MPa}$

b. To find shear stress:

We know that $\quad \tau = \dfrac{F_s}{2 A_p}$

Bur $\qquad$ shear force $\qquad F_s = F_s$ or F_b
$$= \sigma_b A_b = 28.10 \times (706.85)$$
$$\therefore \quad F_s = 19862.49 \, \text{N}$$

and $\qquad \tau = \dfrac{19862.49}{2 \times 314.16} = 31.61 \, \text{MPa}$

55. **A steel rod of 10 mm diameter passes centrally through a copper tube of 40 mm external diameter and 30 mm internal diameter and 2.0 m long. The tube is closed at each end by 20 mm thick steel plates which are secured by nuts. The nuts are tightened until the copper tube is reduced in length of 1.9996 mm. Find the stresses in the rod and tube.**

If the whole assembly is heated through 60°C, what are the corresponding stresses, assuming that the thickness of the plates remains unchanged? Take $\alpha_s = 12 \times 10^{-6}$ per °C, $\alpha_c = 17.5 \times 10^{-6}$ per °C, $E_s = 200$ GPa, $E_c = 100$ GPa.

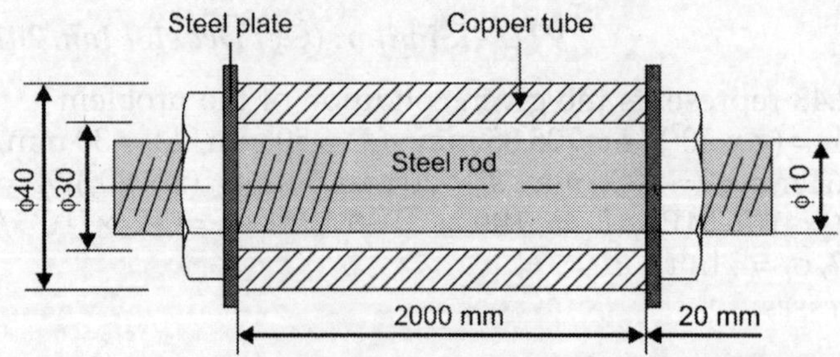

Fig. 2.49: Problem 55

Solution: Fig. 2.49 represents the given condition of the problem

$d_s = 10$ mm, $\Rightarrow A_s = (\pi \times 10^2)/4 = 78.54$ mm^2 $d_c)_o = 40$ mm, $d_c)_i = 30$ mm, $\Rightarrow A_c = \pi \times (40^2 - 30^2)/4 = 549.78$ mm^2, $l_s = 2000$ mm, $t_p = 20$ mm, $\delta_c = 1.9996$ mm, $t = 60$ °C, $E_s = 200 \times 10^3$ MPa, $E_c = 100 \times 10^3$ MPa, $\alpha_s = 12 \times 10^{-6}/$°C, $\alpha_c = 17.5 \times 10^{-6}/$°C. a) $\sigma_s = ?$, $\sigma_b = ?$ due to tightening of nuts. b) $\sigma_s = ?$, $\sigma_b = ?$ for whole assembly

a. To find stresses due to tightening of nuts:

For equilibrium, tensile force in steel = compressive force in copper

i.e.
$$F_s = F_c$$
$$\sigma_s A_s = \sigma_c A_c$$
$$\sigma_s \times (78.54) = \sigma_c \times (549.78)$$
$$\therefore \quad \sigma_s = 7\sigma_c \qquad \text{... Eq. (i)}$$

But
$$\delta l_c = l - \delta_c = 2000 - 1999.6 = 0.4 \text{ mm}$$

Also
$$\sigma_c = E_c \, \varepsilon_c = E_c \left(\frac{\delta l_c}{l_c} \right)$$

$$= (100 \times 10^3) \times \left(\frac{0.4}{2000} \right)$$

$$\therefore \quad \sigma_c = 20 \text{ MPa} \qquad \text{(Compression)}$$

Eq. (i) yields... $\qquad\qquad \sigma_s = 7 \times 20 = 140 \text{ MPa} \qquad$ (Tensile)

b. To find stresses due to change in temperature:

Let σ_c' and σ_s' be the stresses due to change in temperature then Eq. (i) yields... $\sigma_s' = 7\sigma_c'$ $\qquad\qquad\qquad$ ... Eq. (ii)

Since $\alpha_c > \alpha_s$, we have $\quad \dfrac{\sigma_c' l_c}{E_c} + \dfrac{\sigma_s' l_s}{E_s} = t(\alpha_c \, l_c - \alpha_s \, l_s)$ $\qquad$ ... Eq. (iii)

$$\text{Here} \qquad l_c = l = 2000 \text{ mm}$$
$$l_s = l + 2t_p = 2000 + (2 \times 20) = 2040 \text{ mm}$$

Eq. (iii) yields... $\dfrac{\sigma_c' \times 2000}{100 \times 10^3} + \dfrac{7\sigma_c' \times 2040}{200 \times 10^3} = 60 \times [(17.5 \times 10^{-6} \times 2000) - (12 \times 10^{-6} \times 2040)]$

$$0.0914 \, \sigma_c' = 0.6312$$
$$\therefore \quad \sigma_c' = 6.91 \text{ MPa} \qquad \text{(Compression)}$$

Eq. (ii) yields... $\qquad\qquad \sigma_s' = 7 \times 6.91 = 48.37 \text{ MPa} \qquad$ (Tensile)

Thus the final (resultant) stresses for the whole assembly are:

$$\sigma_s)_R = \sigma_s + \sigma_s' = 140 + 48.37 = 188.37 \text{ MPa} \qquad \text{(Tensile)}$$
$$\sigma_c)_R = \sigma_c + \sigma_c' = 20 + 6.91 = 26.91 \text{ MPa} \qquad \text{(Compression)}$$

56. A 12 mm steel rod passes centrally through a copper tube 48 mm external diameter and 36 mm internal diameter and 2.50 m long. The tube is closed at each end by 24 mm thick steel plates which are secured by nuts. The nuts are tightened until the copper tube is reduced in length by 0.508 mm. The whole assembly is then raised in temperature by 60°C. Calculate the stresses in copper and steel before and after raising the temperature, assuming the thickness of the plates remains to be unchanged.

Take $\qquad \alpha_s = 1.2 \times 10^{-5}$ per °C, $\qquad\qquad \alpha_c = 1.75 \times 10^{-5}$ per °C
$\qquad\qquad E_s = 2.1 \times 10^5$ N/mm^2 $\qquad\qquad E_c = 1.05 \times 10^5$ N/mm^2

VTU – June/ July 2008 – 10 Marks

Solution: Fig. 2.50 represents the given condition of the problem

$d_s = 12$ mm, $\Rightarrow A_s = (\pi \times 12^2)/4 = 113.10$ mm^2 $(d_c)_o = 48$ mm, $(d_c)_i = 36$ mm, $\Rightarrow A_c = \pi \times (48^2 - 36^2)/4 = 791.68$ mm^2, $l_s = 2500$ mm, $t_p = 24$ mm, $\delta l_c = 0.508$ mm, $t = 60°C$, $E_s = 2.1 \times 10^5$ N/mm^2, $E_c = 1.05 \times 10^5$ N/mm^2, $\alpha_s = 1.2 \times 10^{-5}/°C$, $\alpha_c = 1.75 \times 10^{-5}/°C$.

a) $\sigma_s = ?$, $\sigma_b = ?$ due to tightening of nuts;   b) $\sigma_s = ?$, $\sigma_b = ?$ for whole assembly

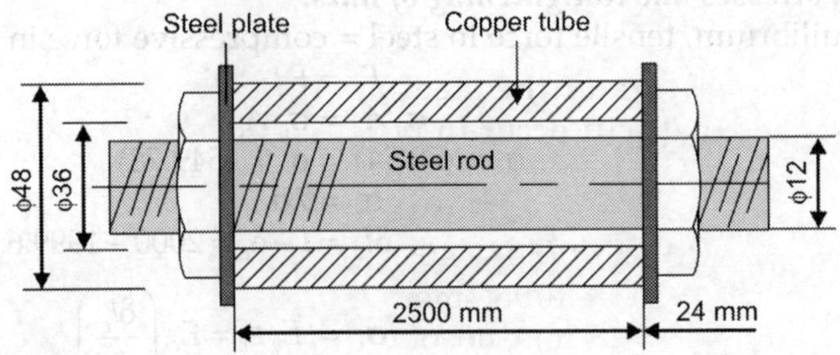

Fig. 2.50: Problem 56

a. To find stresses due to tightening of nuts:

For equilibrium, tensile force in steel = compressive force in copper

i.e. $$F_s = F_c$$
$$\sigma_s A_s = \sigma_c A_c$$
$$\sigma_s \times (113.10) = \sigma_c \times (791.68)$$
$$\therefore \quad \sigma_s = 7\sigma_c \qquad \qquad \text{... Eq. (i)}$$

Also $$\sigma_c = E_c \varepsilon_c = E_c \left(\frac{\delta l_c}{l_c} \right)$$

$$= (1.05 \times 10^5) \times \left(\frac{0.508}{2500} \right)$$

$$\therefore \quad \sigma_c = 21.34 \text{ MPa} \qquad \qquad \text{(Compression)}$$

Eq. (i) yields... $$\sigma_s = 7 \times 21.34 = 149.38 \text{ MPa} \qquad \qquad \text{(Tensile)}$$

b. To find stresses due to change in temperature:

Let σ_c' and σ_s' be the stresses due to change in temperature then Eq. (i) yields...
$$\sigma_s' = 7\sigma_c' \qquad \qquad \text{... Eq. (ii)}$$

Since $\alpha_c > \alpha_s$, we have $$\dfrac{\sigma_c' l_c}{E_c} + \dfrac{\sigma_s' l_s}{E_s} = t(\alpha_c l_c - \alpha_s l_s) \qquad \qquad \text{... Eq. (iii)}$$

Here $$l_c = 1 = 2500 \text{ mm}$$
$$l_s = 1 + 2t_p = 2500 + (2 \times 24) = 2548 \text{ mm}$$

Eq. (iii) yields... $$\frac{\sigma_c' l_c \times 2500}{1.05 \times 10^5} + \frac{7\sigma_c' l_s \times 2548}{2.1 \times 10^5} = 60 \times [(1.75 \times 10^{-5}) \times 2500 - (1.2 \times 10^{-5}) \times 2548]$$

$$0.1087 \, \sigma_c' = 0.7904$$

$$\therefore \quad \sigma_c' = 7.27 \text{ MPa} \qquad \qquad \text{(Compression)}$$

(ii) yields... $$\sigma_s' = 7 \times 7.27 = 50.89 \text{ MPa} \qquad \text{(Tensile)}$$

Thus the final (resultant) stresses for the whole assembly are:
$$\sigma_s)_R = \sigma_s + \sigma_s' = 149.38 + 50.89 = 200.27 \text{ MPa} \qquad \text{(Tensile)}$$
$$\sigma_c)_R = \sigma_c + \sigma_c' = 21.34 + 7.27 = 28.61 \text{ MPa} \qquad \qquad \text{(Compression)}$$

57. A 25 mm diameter steel rod passes concentrically through a bronze tube 400 mm long., 50 mm external diameter and 40 mm internal diameter. The end of the steel rod are threaded and provided with nuts and washers which are adjusted initially so that there is no end play at 20°C.

(a) Assuming that there is no change in thickness of the washers, find the stress produced in the steel and bronze when one of the nuts is tightened by giving one-tenth of a turn, the pitch of the thread being 2.5 mm. Take E for steel = 200 kN/mm^2, and for bronze = 100 kN/mm^2.

VTU – June/ July 2014 – 07 Marks

(b) If the temperature of the steel and bronze is then raised to 50°C find the changes that will occur in both the materials. Take α_s = 1.1 × 10^{-5}/°C, α_b = 1.8 × 10^{-5}/°C

Solution: d_s = 25 mm $\Rightarrow A_s = (\pi \times 25^2))/4$ = 490.87 mm^2, $l_b = l_s$ = 400 mm, $(d_b)_o$ = 50 mm, $(d_b)i$ = 40 mm, $\Rightarrow A_b = \pi \times (50 - 40^2)/4$ = 706.86 mm^2, t_1 = 20°C, t_2 = 50°C, $t = (t_2 \sim t_1)$ = 30°C, E_s = 200 × 10^3 N/mm^2, E_b = 100 × 10^3 N/mm^2, α_s = 1.1 × 10^{-5}/°C, α_b = 1.8 × 10^{-5}/°C, pitch = 2.5 mm, no. of turns = 1/10.

(a) σ_s = ?, σ_b = ? due to tightening of nuts;

(b) σ_s = ?, σ_b = ? due to change in temperature

a. To find stresses due to tightening of nuts:

For equilibrium, tensile force in steel = compressive force in bronz

i.e.
$$F_s = F_b$$
$$\sigma_s A_s = \sigma_b A_b$$
$$\sigma_s \times (490.87) = \sigma_b \times (706.86)$$
$$\therefore \quad \sigma_s = 1.44\, \sigma_b \qquad \qquad \text{... Eq. (i)}$$

Now axial displacement of nut = compression of bronze tube + extension of the steel rod

i.e.
$$\text{pitch} \times \text{no.of turns} = \frac{\sigma_b l_b}{E_b} + \frac{\sigma_s l_s}{E_s} \qquad (\because l_s = l_b)$$

$$2.5 \times (1/10) = \frac{\sigma_b \times 400}{100 \times 10^3} + \frac{\sigma_s \times 400}{200 \times 10^3}$$

$$0.25 = 0.004\,\sigma_b + (1.44\,\sigma_b) \times 0.002$$
$$0.25 = 0.00688\,\sigma_b$$
$$\therefore \quad \sigma_b = 36.34\,\text{MPa}$$

Eq. (i) yields... $\qquad \sigma_s = 1.44 \times 36.34 = 52.33\,\text{MPa}$ $\qquad$ (Tensile)

b. To find stresses due to change in temperature:

Let σ_b' and σ_s' be the stresses due to change in temperature then

Eq. (i) yields... $\qquad\qquad\qquad \sigma_s' = 1.44\sigma_b'$ $\qquad\qquad$ ... Eq. (ii)

Since $\alpha_b > \alpha_s$, we have $\qquad \dfrac{\sigma_b'}{E_b} + \dfrac{\sigma_s'}{E_s} = t(\alpha_b - \alpha_s)$

$$\frac{\sigma_b'}{100 \times 10^3} + \frac{1.44\,\sigma_b'}{200 \times 10^3} = 30 \times [1.8 \times 10^{-5} - 1.1 \times 10^{-5}]$$

$$1.72 \times 10^{-5}\,\sigma_b' = 2.1 \times 10^{-4}$$

$$\therefore \quad \sigma_b' = 12.21\,\text{MPa} \qquad \text{(Compression)}$$

Eq. (ii) yields... $\qquad \sigma_s' = 1.44 \times 12.21 = 17.58\,\text{MPa}$ $\qquad$ (Tensile)

Thus the final (resultant) stresses for the whole assembly are:

$$(\sigma_s)_R = \sigma_s + \sigma_s' = 52.33 + 17.58 = 69.91\,\text{MPa} \qquad \text{(Tensile)}$$
$$(\sigma_b)_R = \sigma_b + \sigma_b' = 36.34 + 12.21 = 48.55\,\text{MPa} \qquad \text{(Compression)}$$

58. Determine the stresses in the bars of system shown in Fig. 2.51, if the sectional area of each wire is 60 mm^2. The load is 25 kN and the temperature of the system raised by 15°C. The bar remains horizontal. Take E_s = 2 × 10^5 MPa, E_c = 1.2 × 10^5 MPa, α_s = 12 × 10^{-6}/°C, α_c = 16 × 10^{-6}/°C.

VTU – June/ July 2014 – 10 Marks; (CV) June/ July 2014 – 15 Marks

Solution: $A_c = A_s = 60$ mm^2, $F = 25$ kN, $t = 15°C$, $E_s = 2 \times 10^5$ MPa, $E_c = 1.2 \times 10^5$ MPa, $\alpha_s = 12 \times 10^{-6}/°C$, $\alpha_c = 16 \times 10^{-6}/°C$ a) Stresses due to 25 kN = ?; b) Stresses due to change in temperature = ?

   a. To find stresses due to 25kN:

For a composite bar, $\quad F = F_s + 2F_c = \sigma_s A_s + 2\sigma_c A_c$ ... Eq. (i)

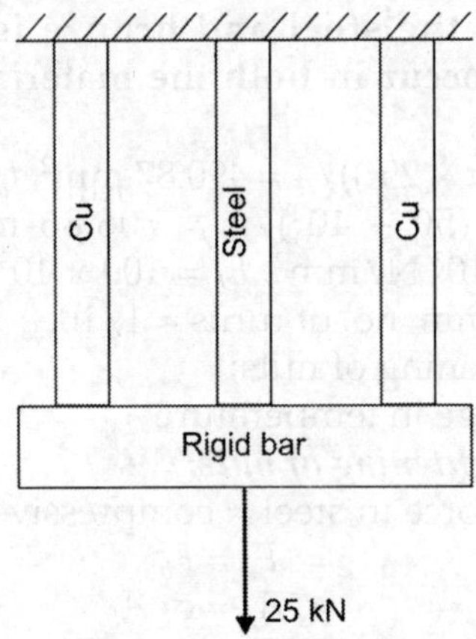

Fig. 2.51: Problem 58

Since the bar remains horizontal,

$$\delta l_s = \delta l_c$$

$$\frac{\sigma_s}{E_s} = \frac{\sigma_c}{E_c} \qquad (\because l_s = l_c)$$

$$\sigma_s = \left(\frac{E_s}{E_c}\right)\sigma_c$$

$$= \left(\frac{2 \times 10^5}{1.2 \times 10^5}\right)\sigma_c$$

$$\therefore \quad \sigma_s = 1.67\sigma_c \qquad \text{... Eq. (ii)}$$

Substituting Eq. (ii) in Eq. (i), we have,

$$25 \times 10^3 = (1.67\sigma_c) \times 60 + (2\sigma_c) \times 60$$

$$\therefore \quad \sigma_c = 113.53 \text{ MPa}$$

Eq. (ii) yields... $\qquad \sigma_s = 1.67 \times 113.53 = 189.60$ MPa

   b. To find loads due to change in temperature:

Let σ_c' and σ_s' be the stresses due to change in temperature then

Eq. (ii) yields... $\qquad\qquad \sigma_s' = 2\sigma_c' \qquad\qquad$ ... Eq. (iii)

Since $\alpha_c > \alpha_s$, we have $\qquad \dfrac{\sigma_c'}{E_c} + \dfrac{\sigma_s'}{E_s} = t(\alpha_c - \alpha_s) \qquad (\because l_s = l_c)$

$$\frac{\sigma_c'}{1.2 \times 10^5} + \frac{1.67\sigma_c'}{2 \times 10^5} = 15 \times [16 \times 10^{-6} - 12 \times 10^{-6}]$$

$$1.67 \times 10^{-5}\,\sigma_c' = 6 \times 10^{-5}$$

$$\therefore \quad \sigma_c' = 3.59 \text{ MPa}$$

Eq. (iii) yields... $\qquad \sigma_s' = 1.67 \times 3.59 = 6$ MPa

59. A horizontal rigid bar AB weighing 200 kN is hung by three vertical rods, each of 1m length and 500 mm² in cross section as shown in Fig. 2.52. The central rod is of steel and outer rods are copper. If the temperature rise is 40°C, estimate the load carried by each rod and how much the load will descend. Take E_s = 200 GN/m², E_c = 100 GN/m², α_s = 1.2 × 10⁻⁵/°C, α_c = 1.8 × 10⁻⁵/°C.

VTU – June 2012 – 10 Marks; June/ July 2014 – 10 Marks

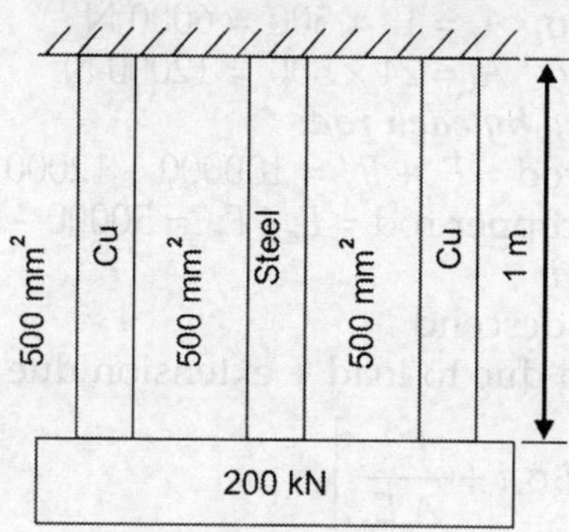

Fig. 2.52: Problem 59

Solution: $A_c = A_s = 500$ mm², $l_c = l_s = 1000$ mm, $F = 200$ kN, $t = 40$ °C, $E_s = 200 \times 10^3$ N/mm², $E_c = 100 \times 10^3$ N/mm², $\alpha_s = 1.2 \times 10^{-5}/°C$, $\alpha_c = 1.8 \times 10^{-5}/°C$. a) Loads due to 200 kN = ?; b) Loads due to change in temperature = ?; c) Amount of load carried by each rod = ?; d) Amount of bar descend = ?

Method 1:

a. To find loads due to 200 kN:

For a composite bar, $F = F_s + 2F_c = \sigma_s A_s + 2\sigma_c A_c$ ... Eq. (i)

Since the bar remains horizontal,

$$\delta l_s = \delta l_c$$

$$\frac{\sigma_s}{E_s} = \frac{\sigma_c}{E_c} \qquad (\because l_s = l_c)$$

$$\sigma_s = \left(\frac{E_s}{E_c}\right) \sigma_c$$

$$= \left(\frac{200 \times 10^3}{100 \times 10^3}\right) \sigma_c$$

$$\therefore \quad \sigma_s = 2\sigma_c \qquad \qquad ... \text{Eq. (ii)}$$

Substituting Eq. (ii) in Eq. (i), we have,

$$200 \times 10^3 = (2\sigma_c) \times 500 + (2\sigma_c) \times 500$$

$$\therefore \quad \sigma_c = 100 \, \text{MPa}$$

Eq. (ii) yields...

$$\sigma_s = 2 \times 100 = 200 \, \text{MPa}$$

Thus the loads are:

$$F_c = \sigma_c A_c = 100 \times 500 = 50000 \, \text{N}$$

$$F_s = \sigma_s A_s = 200 \times 500 = 100000 \, \text{N}$$

b. To find loads due to change in temperature:

Let $\sigma_c{}'$ and $\sigma_s{}'$ be the stresses due to change in temperature then

Eq. (ii) yields...

$$\sigma_s{}' = 2\sigma_c{}' \qquad \qquad ... \text{Eq. (iii)}$$

Since $\alpha_c > \alpha_s$, we have

$$\frac{\sigma_c{}'}{E_c} + \frac{\sigma_s{}'}{E_s} = t(\alpha_c - \alpha_s) \qquad (\because l_s = l_c)$$

$$\frac{\sigma_c'}{100 \times 10^3} + \frac{2\sigma_c'}{200 \times 10^3} = 40 \times [1.8 \times 10^{-5} - 1.2 \times 10^{-5}]$$

$$2 \times 10^{-5}\,\sigma_c' = 2.4 \times 10^{-4}$$

$$\therefore \quad \sigma_c' = 12\,\text{MPa}$$

Eq. (iii) yields…

$$\sigma_s' = 2 \times 12 = 24\,\text{MPa}$$

Thus the loads are:

$$F_c' = \sigma_c'\,A_c = 12 \times 500 = 6000\,\text{N}$$

$$F_s' = \sigma_s'\,A_s = 24 \times 500 = 12000\,\text{N}$$

c. Amount of load carried by each rod:

Load carried by steel rod $= F_s + F_s' = 100000 + 12000 = 112000\,\text{N} = 112\,\text{kN}$

Load carried by each copper rod $= F_c - F_c' = 50000 - 6000 = 44000\,\text{N} = 44\,\text{kN}$

d. Amount of bar descend:

The amount of bar descend,

$$\Delta = \text{Extension due to load} + \text{extension due to temperature}$$

$$\Delta = \frac{F_c l_c}{A_c E_c} + \left[l_s \sigma_s t + \frac{F_s' l_s}{A_s E_s} \right]$$

$$= \frac{50000 \times 1000}{500 \times (100 \times 10^3)} + \left\{ 1000 \times (1.2 \times 10^{-5}) \times 40 + \left[\frac{12000 \times 1000}{500 \times (200 \times 10^3)} \right] \right\}$$

$$= 1 + (0.48 + 0.12)$$

$\therefore$ Amount of bar descent $\Delta = 1.6\,\text{mm}$

Method 2:

a. To find loads due to 200 kN:

For a composite bar, $\qquad F = F_s + 2F_c$ $\qquad\qquad$ … Eq. (i)

Since the bar remains horizontal, $\quad \delta l_s = \delta l_c$

$$\frac{F_s}{A_s E_s} = \frac{F_c}{A_c E_c} \qquad (\because l_s = l_c)$$

$$\frac{F_s}{500 \times (200 \times 10^3)} = \frac{F_c}{500 \times (100 \times 10^3)}$$

$$F_s = 2F_c \qquad\qquad\qquad \text{… Eq. (ii)}$$

Substituting Eq. (ii) in Eq. (i), we have,

$$200 \times 10^3 = 2F_c + 2F_c$$

$$\therefore \quad F_c = 50000\,\text{N}$$

Eq. (ii) yields…

$$F_s = 2 \times 50000 = 100000\,\text{N}$$

b. To find loads due to change in temperature

Let σ_b' and σ_s' be the stresses due to change in temperature then Eq. (ii)

yields… $F_s' = 2F_c'$ $\qquad\qquad\qquad\qquad\qquad\qquad$ … Eq. (iii)

Since $\alpha_c > \alpha_s$, we have $\quad \dfrac{F_c'}{A_c E_c} + \dfrac{F_s'}{A_s E_s} = t(\alpha_c - \alpha_s) \qquad (\because l_s = l_c)$

$$\frac{F_c'}{500 \times (100 \times 10^3)} + \frac{2F_c'}{500 \times (200 \times 10^3)} = 40 \times [1.8 \times 10^{-5} - 1.2 \times 10^{-5}]$$

$$4 \times 10^{-8}\,F_c' = 2.4 \times 10^{-4}$$

$$\therefore \quad F'_c = 6000 \text{ N}$$

Eq. (iii) yields... $\qquad F'_s = 2 \times 6000 = 12000 \text{ N}$

c. Amount of load carried by each rod: $\qquad$ ...... *same as in method 1*
d. Amount of bar descend: $\qquad$ ...... *same as in method 1*

60. A horizontal bar hinged at one of its ends is supported by two vertical bars as shown in Fig. 2.53(a). If the temperature of the vertical bars increases by 40°C, determine the force, stresses and deformations induced in them. Take $E_s = 200$ GPa, $E_c = 100$ GPa, $\alpha_s = 12 \times 10^{-6}/°C$, $\alpha_c = 18 \times 10^{-6}/°C$

VTU – Jan. 2013 – 10 Marks

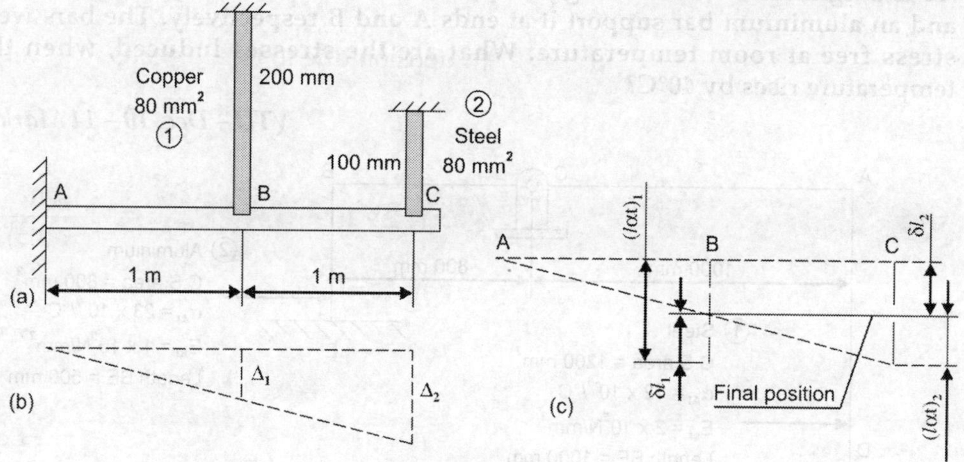

Fig. 2.53: Problem 60

Solution: *(suffix '1' refers to copper and '2' refers to steel)*
$A_1 = 80$ mm², $l_1 = 200$ mm, $A_2 = 80$ mm², $l_2 = 100$ mm, $t = 40°C$, $E_1 = 100 \times 10^3$ MPa, $E_2 = 200 \times 10^3$ MPa, $\alpha_1 = 18 \times 10^{-6}/°C$, $\alpha_2 = 12 \times 10^{-6}/°C$. a) $F_1 = ?$, $F_2 = ?$ b) $\sigma_1 = ?$, $\sigma_2 = ?$. c) $\Delta_1 = ?$, $\Delta_2 = ?$.

Referring to given **Fig. 2.53(a)**,
$\qquad AB = x_1 = 1000$ mm, $BC = x_2 = 1000$ mm.

For static equilibrium, taking moments about A, we have
$$F_1 x_1 = F_2 (x_2 + x_1)$$
$$F_1 \times 1000 = F_2 \times (1000 + 1000)$$
$$\therefore \quad F_2 = 0.5 \, F_1 \qquad \text{... Eq. (i)}$$

From **Fig. 2.53(b)**, we have
$$\frac{\Delta_1}{x_1} = \frac{\Delta_2}{x_1 + x_2}$$
$$\frac{\Delta_1}{1000} = \frac{\Delta_2}{2000}$$
$$\therefore \quad \Delta_2 = 2 \, \Delta_1 \qquad \text{... Eq. (ii)}$$
$$(l.a.t)_2 + \delta l_2 = 2 \, [(l.\alpha.t)_1 - \delta l_1] \qquad \text{... using Fig. 2.53(c)}$$
$$\delta l_2 + 2\delta l_1 = 2(l.\alpha.t)_1 - (l.\alpha.t)_2$$

i.e. $\dfrac{F_2 l_2}{A_2 E_2} + 2\left(\dfrac{F_1 l_1}{A_1 E_1}\right) = (2\alpha_1 l_1 - \alpha_2 l_2)t$

$$\frac{F_2 \times 100}{80 \times (200 \times 10^3)} + \left\{ 2 \times \left[\frac{F_1 \times 200}{80 \times (100 \times 10^3)} \right] \right\} = \{[2 \times (18 \times 10^{-6}) \times 200]$$
$$- [(12 \times 10^{-6}) \times 100]\} \times 40$$

$$(6.25 \times 10^{-6}) F_2 + (5 \times 10^{-5}) F_1 = 0.24$$
$$[(6.25 \times 10^{-6}) \times 0.5F_1] + (5 \times 10^{-5}) F_1 = 0.24 \qquad \text{... using Eq. (i)}$$
$$\therefore \quad F_1 = 4517.65 \text{ N}$$

and Eq. (i) yields...
$$F_2 = 0.5 \times 4517.65 = 2258.83 \text{ N}$$

Thus the stresses are:
$$\sigma_1 = F_1/A_1 = 4517.65/80 = 56.47 \text{ MPa} \qquad \text{(Copper)}$$
$$\sigma_2 = F_2/A_2 = 2258.83/80 = 28.24 \text{ MPa} \qquad \text{(Steel)}$$

61. **AB is a rigid bar and has a hinged support at C as shown in Fig. 2.54(a). A steel and an aluminium bar support it at ends A and B respectively. The bars were stress free at room temperature. What are the stresses induced, when the temperature rises by 40°C?**

VTU – Dec. 10 – 14 Marks

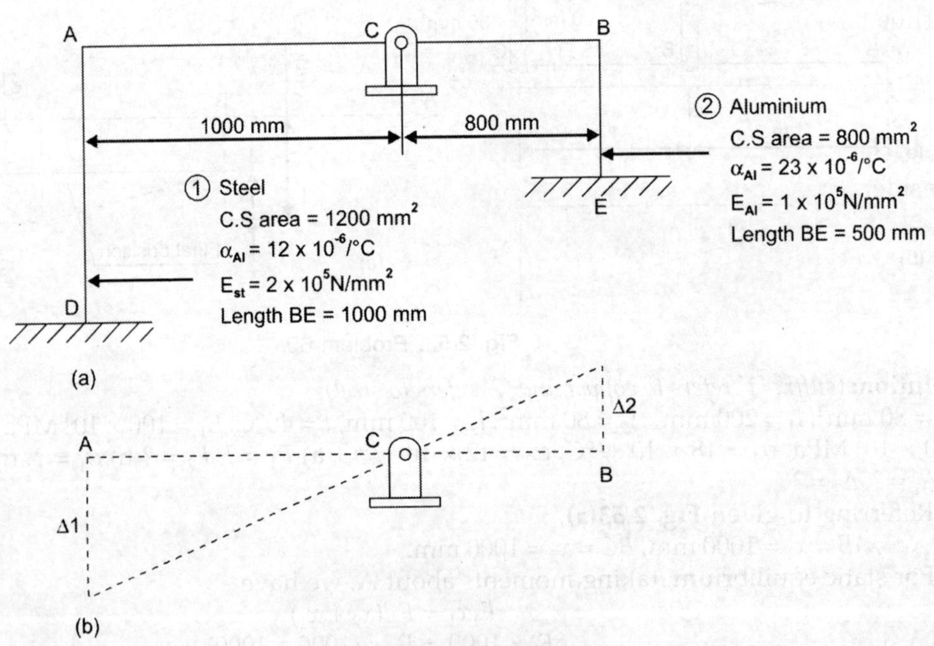

Fig. 2.54: Problem 61

Solution: *(suffix '1' refers to steel and '2' refers to Aluminium)*
$A_1 = 1200 \text{ mm}^2$, $l_1 = AD = 1000 \text{ mm}$, $\alpha_1 = 12 \times 10^{-6}/°C$, $E_1 = 2 \times 10^5 \text{ N/mm}^2$, $A_2 = 800$ mm², $l_2 = BE = 500 \text{ mm}$, $\alpha_2 = 23 \times 10^{-6}/°C$, $E_2 = 1 \times 10^5 \text{ N/mm}^2$, $t = 40°C$. $\sigma_1 = ?$, $\sigma_2 = ?$

Referring to given **Fig. 2.54(a)**,
$$A_C = x_1 = 1000 \text{ mm}, \quad CB = x_2 = 800 \text{ mm}.$$

For static equilibrium, taking moments about C, we have
$$F_1 x_1 = F_2 x_2$$
$$F_1 \times 1000 = F_2 \times 800$$
$$\therefore \quad F_2 = 1.25 F_1 \qquad \qquad \text{... Eq. (i)}$$

From **Fig. 2.54(b)**, we have
$$\frac{\Delta_1}{x_1} = \frac{\Delta_2}{x_2}$$

$$\frac{\Delta_1}{1000} = \frac{\Delta_2}{800}$$

$$\therefore \quad \Delta_2 = 0.8\,\Delta_1 \qquad\qquad \text{... Eq. (ii)}$$

$$(l.\alpha.t)_2 - \delta l_2 = 0.8\,[(\delta l_1 - (l.\alpha.t)_1]$$

$$0.8\,\delta l_1 + \delta l_2 = (l.\alpha.t)_2 + 0.8(l.\alpha.t)_1$$

$$\text{i.e. } 0.8\left(\frac{F_1 l_1}{A_1 E_1}\right) + \left(\frac{F_2 l_2}{A_2 E_2}\right) = (\alpha_2 l_2 + 0.8\alpha_1 l_1)t$$

$$\left\{0.8 \times \left[\frac{F_1 \times 1000}{1200 \times (2 \times 10^5)}\right]\right\} + \frac{F_2 \times 500}{800 \times (1 \times 10^5)} = \{[(23 \times 10^{-6}) \times 500] + [0.8 \times (12 \times 10^{-6})$$

$$\times\ 1000]\} \times 40$$

$$(3.34 \times 10^{-6})\,F_1 + (6.25 \times 10^{-6})\,F_2 = 0.844$$

$$(3.34 \times 10^{-6})\,F_1 + [(6.25 \times 10^{-6}) \times 1.25F_1] = 0.844 \qquad\qquad \text{... using Eq. (i)}$$

$$\therefore \quad F_1 = 75.67 \text{ kN} \qquad \text{(Steel)}$$

and Eq. (i) yields... $F_2 = 1.25 \times 75.67 = 94.59 \text{ kN}$ (Aluminium)

Thus the stresses are:

$$\sigma_1 = F_1/A_1 = (75.67 \times 10^3)/1200 = 63.05 \text{ MPa} \qquad \text{(Steel)}$$

$$\sigma_2 = F_2/A_2 = (94.59 \times 10^3)/800 = 118.24 \text{ MPa} \qquad \text{(Aluminium)}$$

2.9 THERMAL STRESSES IN BARS OF VARYING CROSS-SECTION

Consider a bar as shown in **Fig. 2.55** subjected to increase in temperature.

Let l_1 = length of the bar (1)

$\quad\quad\ A_1$ = Area of bar (1)

$\quad\quad\ \sigma_1$ = Stress in bar (1)

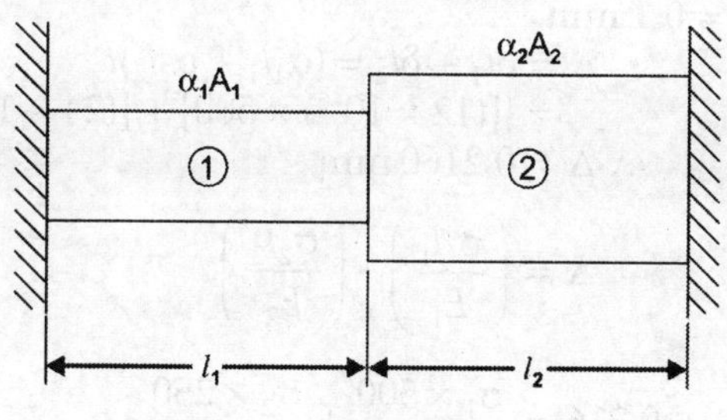

Fig. 2.55

On similar lines, let l_2, A_2, σ_2 = be the corresponding parameters of bar (2).

$\quad\quad\quad\ t$ = Increase in temperature

$\quad\quad\quad\ \alpha$ = Coefficient of thermal or linear expansion

When the bar is subjected to increase in temperature, the bar tries to expand. Since the ends are constrained, the stresses developed will be such that

$$\sigma_1 A_1 = \sigma_2 A_2$$

And the total deformation is, $\Delta = \delta l_1 + \delta l_2$

$$= \alpha t\, l_1 + \alpha t\, l_2$$

$$\Delta = t(\alpha_1 l_1 + \alpha_2 l_2) \qquad\qquad \text{... (Eq. 2.39)}$$

$$\therefore \quad \Delta = \left(\frac{\sigma_1 l_1}{E_1} + \frac{\sigma_2 l_2}{E_2}\right) \qquad\qquad \text{... (Eq. 2.40)}$$

62. **A composite bar made of aluminium and steel is held between two supports as shown in Fig. 2.56. The bars are stress free at a temperature of 42°C. What will be the stresses in the two bars when the temperature drops to 24°C, if**

(i) the supports are unyielding

(ii) the supports come nearer to each other by 0.1 mm.

The cross sectional area of the steel bar is 160 mm^2 and that of aluminium is 240 mm^2. $E_A = 0.7 \times 10^5$ MPa, $E_s = 2 \times 10^5$ MPa, $\alpha_A = 24 \times 10^{-6}$/°C, $\alpha_s = 12 \times 10^{-6}$/°C.

VTU – June/ July 2013 - 12 Marks; [Similar: June/ July 2015 – 10 Marks; (CV) June/ July 2009 – 08 Marks; (CV) Jan. 2013 – 12 Marks]

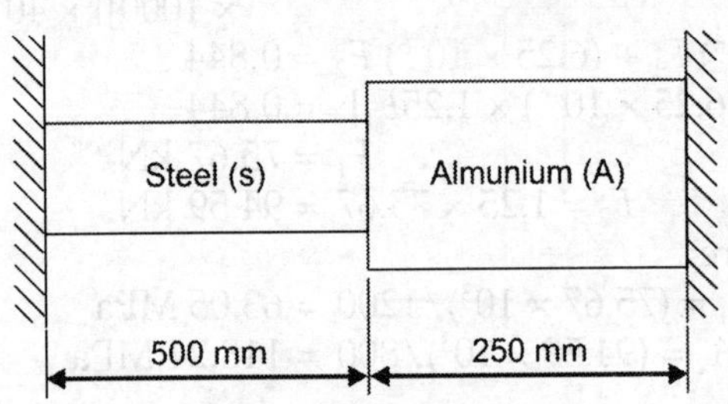

Fig. 2.56: Problem 62

Solution: *(suffix '1' refers to steel and '2' refers to Aluminium)*

$t_1 = 42$°C, $t_2 = 24$°C, $\Rightarrow t = (t_1 - t_2) = 18$°C, $A_1 = 160$ mm^2, $A_2 = 240$ mm^2, $E_s = E_1 = 2 \times 10^5$ MPa, $E_A = E_2 = 0.7 \times 10^5$ MPa, $\alpha_s = \alpha_1 = 12 \times 10^{-6}$/°C, $\alpha_A = \alpha_2 = 24 \times 10^{-6}$/°C, $l_1 = 500$ mm, $l_2 = 250$ mm. a) $\sigma_1 = ?$, $\sigma_2 = ?$, if $d = 0$, b) $\sigma_1 = ?$, $\sigma_2 = ?$, $\delta = 0.1$ mm.

a. $\sigma_1 = ?$, $\sigma_2 = ?$, if $\delta = 0.1$ mm.

We know that
$$\Delta = \delta l_1 + \delta l_2 = (\alpha_1 l_1 + \alpha_2 l_2)t$$
$$= \{[(12 \times 10^{-6}) \times 500] + [(24 \times 10^{-6}) \times 250]\} \times 18$$
$$\therefore \Delta = 0.2160 \text{ mm}$$

Also
$$\Delta = \left(\frac{\sigma_1 l_1}{E_1}\right) + \left(\frac{\sigma_2 l_2}{E_2}\right)$$

$$0.216 = \frac{\sigma_1 \times 500}{2 \times 10^5} + \frac{\sigma_2 \times 250}{0.7 \times 10^5}$$

$$0.216 = 2.5 \times 10^{-3}\, \sigma_1 + 3.571 \times 10^{-3}\, \sigma_2 \qquad \text{... Eq. (i)}$$

For equilibrium,
$$F_1 = F_2$$
$$\sigma_1 A_1 = \sigma_2 A_2$$
$$\sigma_1 \times 160 = \sigma_2 \times 240$$
$$\therefore \quad \sigma_1 = 1.5\, \sigma_2 \qquad \text{... Eq. (ii)}$$

Substituting Eq. (ii) in Eq. (i), we have,
$$0.216 = (2.5 \times 10^{-3}) \times 1.5\, \sigma_2 + (3.571 \times 10^{-3})\, \sigma_2$$
$$\sigma_2 = 29.50 \text{ MPa} \qquad \text{(Aluminium)}$$

and Eq. (ii) yields...
$$\sigma_1 = 1.5 \times 29.50 = 44.25 \text{ MPa} \qquad \text{(Steel)}$$

b. $\sigma_1 = ?$, $\sigma_2 = ?$, $\delta = 0.1$ mm:

Since d is negative,
$$\Delta' = \Delta - \delta$$
$$= 0.216 - 0.1$$
$$\therefore \quad \Delta' = 0.1160 \text{ mm} \qquad \text{... Eq. (iii)}$$

here Eq. (ii) yields... $\sigma_1' = 1.5\,\sigma_2'$ ... Eq. (iv)

Eq. (i) yields... $\sigma_2' = (2.5 \times 10^{-3})\,\sigma_1' + (3.571 \times 10^{-3})\,\sigma_2$ ... Eq. (v)

Substituting Eqs (iii) and (iv) in Eq. (v), we have,

$$0.1160 = (2.5 \times 10^{-3}) \times 1.5\,\sigma_1' + (3.571 \times 10^{-3})\,\sigma_2'$$

$$\therefore\ \sigma_2' = 15.84\ \text{MPa} \qquad \text{(Aluminium)}$$

and Eq. (iv) yields... $\sigma_1' = 1.5 \times 15.84 = 23.77\ \text{MPa}$ (Steel)

63. A composite bar is rigidly attached to the supports as shown in Fig. 2.57. Determine the stresses in the different sections of the bar when the temperature is raised by 70°C.

VTU – June/ July 2013 – 12 Marks

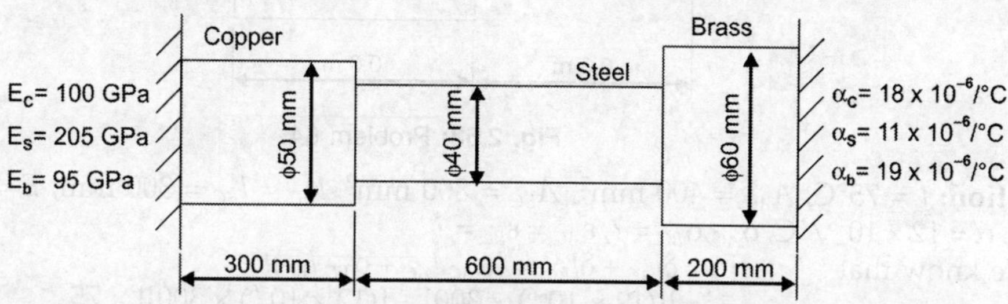

Fig. 2.57: Problem 63

Solution: *(suffix '1' refers to copper, '2' refers to steel, '3' refers to brass)*

$t = 70°C$, $d_1 = 50$ mm $\Rightarrow A_1 = (\pi \times 50^2)/4 = 1963.50$ mm², $d_2 = 40$ mm $\Rightarrow A_s = (\pi \times 40^2)/4 = 1256.64$ mm², $d_3 = 60$ mm $\Rightarrow A_3 = (\pi \times 60^2)/4 = 2827.43$ mm², $E_c = E_1 = 100 \times 10^3$ MPa, $E_s = E_2 = 205 \times 10^3$ MPa, $E_b = E_3 = 95 \times 10^3$ MPa, $\alpha_c = \alpha_1 = 18 \times 10^{-6}/°C$, $\alpha_s = \alpha_2 = 11 \times 10^{-6}/°C$, $\alpha_b = \alpha_3 = 19 \times 10^{-6}/°C$, $l_1 = 300$ mm, $l_2 = 600$ mm, $l_3 = 200$ mm. $\sigma_1 = ?$, $\sigma_2 = ?$, $\sigma_3 = ?$,

Stresses: $\sigma_1 = ?$, $\sigma_2 = ?$, $\sigma_3 = ?$ if $\delta = 0$:

We know that
$$\Delta = \delta l_1 + \delta l_2 + \delta l_3 = (\alpha_1 l_1 + \alpha_2 l_2 + \alpha^3 l_3)t$$
$$= \{[(18 \times 10^{-6}) \times 300] + [(11 \times 10^{-6}) \times 600] + [(19 \times 10^{-6}) \times 200]\} \times 70$$
$$\therefore\ \Delta = 1.106\ \text{mm}$$

Also
$$\Delta = \left(\frac{\sigma_1 l_1}{E_1}\right) + \left(\frac{\sigma_2 l_2}{E_2}\right) + \left(\frac{\sigma_3 l_3}{E_3}\right)$$

$$1.106 = \frac{\sigma_1 \times 300}{200 \times 10^3} + \frac{\sigma_2 \times 600}{205 \times 10^3} + \frac{\sigma_3 \times 200}{95 \times 10^3}$$

$$1.106 = 3 \times 10^{-3}\,\sigma_1 + 2.927 \times 10^{-3}\,\sigma_2 + 2.105 \times 10^{-3}\,\sigma_3 \qquad \text{... Eq. (i)}$$

For equilibrium, $F_1 = F_2 = F_3$

$$\sigma_1 A_1 = \sigma_2 A_2 = \sigma_3 A_3$$
$$\sigma_1 \times 1963.50 = \sigma_2 \times 1256.64 = \sigma_3 \times 2827.43$$
$$\therefore\ \sigma_2 = 1.563\,\sigma_1 \text{ and} \qquad \text{... Eq. (ii)}$$
$$\sigma_3 = 0.694\,\sigma_1 \qquad \text{... Eq. (iii)}$$

Substituting Eqs (ii) and (iii) in Eq. (i), we have,

$$1.106 = (3 \times 10^{-3})\,\sigma_1 + (2.927 \times 10^{-3}) \times 1.563\,\sigma_1 + (2.105 \times 10^{-3}) \times 0.694\,\sigma_1$$

$$\therefore\ \sigma_1 = 122.40\ \text{MPa} \qquad \text{(Copper)}$$

and Eq. (ii) yields... $\sigma_2 = 1.563 \times 122.40 = 191.31\ \text{MPa}$ (Steel)

Eq. (iii) yields... $\sigma_3 = 0.694 \times 122.40 = 84.95\ \text{MPa}$ (Brass)

64. Calculate the values of stress and strain in portion AC and CB of the steel bar shown in Fig. 2.58. A close fit exists at both the rigid supports at room temperature and the temperature is raised by 75°C. Take E = 200 GPa, α = 12 × 10^{-6}/°C for steel. Area of cross sections of AC is 400 mm² and BC is 800 mm².

VTU – Dec. 09/ Jan. 10 – 10 Marks

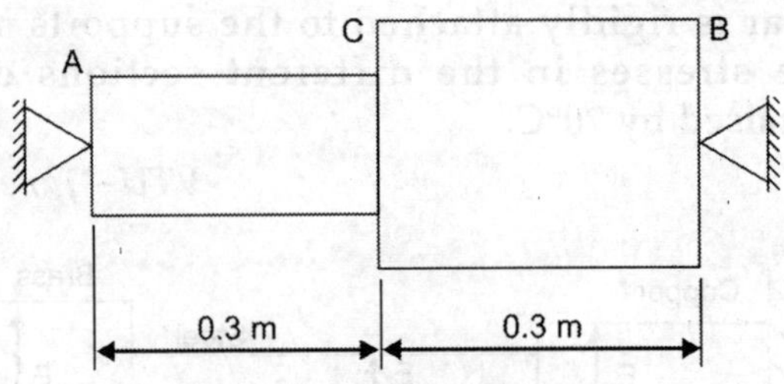

Fig. 2.58: Problem 64

Solution: t = 75°C, A_{AC} = 400 mm², A_{BC} = 800 mm², l_{AC} = l_{BC} = 300 mm, E = 2 × 10^5 MPa, α = 12 × 10^{-6}/°C, σ_{AC}, σ_{BC} = ?, ε_{AC} = ε_{BC} = ?

We know that
$$\Delta = \delta l_{AC} + \delta l_{BC} = (\alpha_{AC}\, l_{AC} + \alpha_{BC}\, l_{BC})t$$
$$= \{[(12 \times 10^{-6}) \times 300] + [(12 \times 10^{-6}) \times 300]\} \times 75$$
$$\therefore \quad \Delta = 0.540 \text{ mm}$$

Also
$$\Delta = \left(\frac{\sigma_{AC} l_{AC}}{E_{AC}}\right) + \left(\frac{\sigma_{BC} l_{BC}}{E_{BC}}\right)$$

$$0.540 = \frac{\sigma_{AC} \times 300}{200 \times 10^3} + \frac{\sigma_{BC} \times 300}{200 \times 10^3}$$

$$0.540 = (1.5 \times 10{-3})\, \sigma_{AC} + (1.5 \times 10^{-3})\, \sigma_{BC} \qquad \text{... Eq. (i)}$$

For equilibrium, $\quad F_{AC} = F_{BC}$
$$\sigma_{AC} A_{AC} = \sigma_{BC} A_{BC}$$
$$\sigma_{AC} \times 400 = \sigma_{BC} \times 800$$
$$\therefore \quad \sigma_{AC} = 2\,\sigma_{BC} \qquad \text{... Eq. (ii)}$$

Substituting Eq. (ii) in Eq. (i), we have,
$$0.540 = (1.5 \times 10^{-3}) \times 2\,\sigma_{BC} + (1.5 \times 10^{-3})\,\sigma_{BC}$$
$$\therefore \quad \sigma_{BC} = 120 \text{ MPa}$$

Eq. (ii) yields... $\quad \sigma_{AC} = 2 \times 120 = 240$ MPa

Strains:

We know that $\quad \varepsilon_{AC} = \dfrac{\sigma_{AC}}{E_{AC}} = \dfrac{240}{200 \times 10^3} = 1.2 \times 10^{-3}$

and $\quad \varepsilon_{BC} = \dfrac{\sigma_{BC}}{E_{BC}} = \dfrac{120}{200 \times 10^3} = 6 \times 10^{-4}$

65. At room temperature the gap between bar A and bar B as shown in Fig. 2.59 is 0.25 mm. what are the stresses induced in the bars, if the temperature rise is 35°C.

Given $\quad A_a$ = 1000 mm², E_a = 2 × 10^5 N/ mm², α_a = 12 × 10^{-6}/°C, l_a = 400 mm
$\quad\quad\quad A_b$ = 800 mm², E_b = 1 × 10^5 N/ mm², α_b = 23 × 10^{-6}/°C, l_b = 300 mm

VTU – June/ July 2009 – 10 Marks

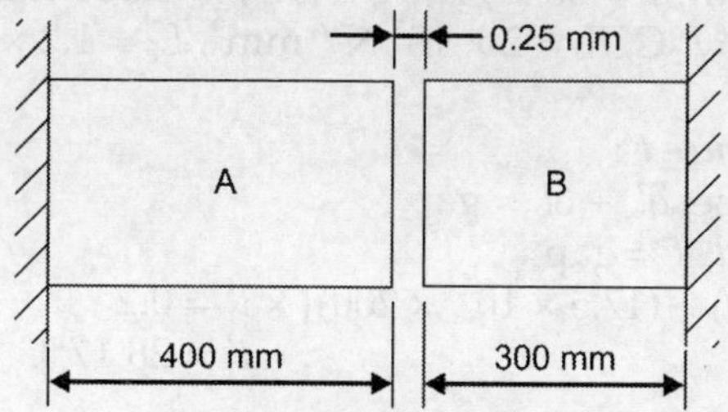

Fig. 2.59: Problem 65

Solution: gap = 0.25 mm, t = 35°C, A_a = 1000 mm², E_a = 2 × 10⁵ N/mm², α_a = 12 × 10⁻⁶/°C, l_a = 400 mm, A_b = 800 mm², E_b = 1 × 10⁵ N/mm², α_b = 23 × 10⁻⁶/°C, l_b = 300 mm, σ_a = ?, σ_b = ?

If the expansion is prevented, then total deformation is

$$\Delta = \delta l_a + \delta l_b - \text{gap}$$
$$= (\alpha_a l_a + \alpha_b l_b)t - \text{gap}$$
$$= [(12 \times 10^{-6} \times 400) + (23 \times 10^{-6} \times 300)] \times 35 - 0.25$$
$$\therefore \quad \Delta = 0.1595 \text{ mm}$$

Also
$$\Delta = \left(\frac{\sigma_a l_a}{E_a}\right) + \left(\frac{\sigma_b l_b}{E_b}\right)$$

$$0.1595 = \frac{\sigma_a \times 400}{2 \times 10^5} + \frac{\sigma_b \times 300}{1 \times 10^5}$$

$$0.1595 = 2 \times 10^{-3}\, \sigma_a + 3 \times 10^{-3}\, \sigma_b \qquad \text{... Eq. (i)}$$

For equilibrium, $\quad F_1 = F_2$
$$\sigma_a A_a = \sigma_b A_b$$
$$\sigma_a \times 1000 = \sigma_b \times 800$$
$$\therefore \quad \sigma_a = 0.8\, \sigma_b \qquad \text{... Eq. (ii)}$$

Substituting Eq. (ii) in Eq. (i), we have,
$$0.1595 = (2 \times 10^{-3}) \times 0.8\, \sigma_b + (3 \times 10^{-3})\sigma_b$$
$$\therefore \quad \sigma_b = 34.67 \text{ MPa}$$

and Eq. (ii) yields... $\sigma_a = 0.8 \times 34.67 = 27.74$ MPa

66. **The composite bar shown in Fig. 2.60 is 0.2 mm short of distance between the rigid supports at room temperature. What is the maximum temperature rise which will not produce stresses in the bar? Find the stresses induced when the temperature rise is 60°C. Take $A_s{:}A_c$ = 4:3, α_s = 12 × 10⁻⁶/°C, α_c = 17.5 × 10⁻⁶/°C, E_s = 2 × 10⁵ N/mm² and E_c = 1.2 × 10⁵ N/mm².**

VTU – Dec. 14/ Jan. 15 – 10 Marks; (similar) Dec.15/ Jan.2016 – 10 Marks

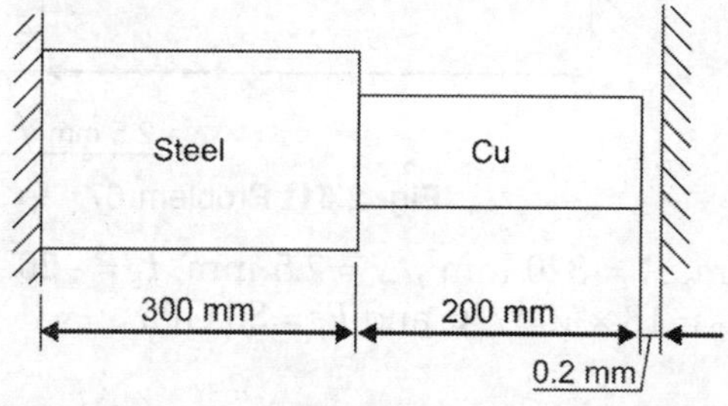

Fig. 2.60: Problem 66

Solution: gap = 0.2 mm, $t = 60°C$, $A_s:A_c = 4:3$, $l_s = 300$ mm, $l_c = 200$ mm, $\alpha_s = 12 \times 10^{-6}/°C$, $\alpha_c = 17.5 \times 10^{-6}/°C$, $E_s = 2 \times 10^5$ N/ mm^2, $E_c = 1.2 \times 10^5$ N/ mm^2, $t' = ?$ $\sigma_a = ?$, $\sigma_b = ?$

a. Raise in temperature t':

For the gap to close, $\delta l_s + \delta l_c = $ gap

$$(\alpha_s l_s + \alpha_c l_c)t' = \text{gap}$$

$$[(12 \times 10^{-6} \times 300) + (17.5 \times 10^{-6} \times 200)] \times t' = 0.2$$

$$\therefore \quad t' = 28.17°C$$

b. To find stresses:

If the expansion is prevented, then total deformation is

$$\Delta = \delta l_s + \delta l_c - \text{gap}$$
$$= (\alpha_s l_s + \alpha_c l_c)t - \text{gap}$$
$$= [(12 \times 10^{-6} \times 300) + (17.5 \times 10^{-6} \times 200)] \times 60 - 0.2$$
$$\therefore \quad \Delta = 0.226 \text{ mm}$$

Also

$$\Delta = \left(\frac{\sigma_s l_s}{E_s}\right) + \left(\frac{\sigma_c l_c}{E_c}\right)$$

$$0.226 = \frac{\sigma_s \times 300}{2 \times 10^5} + \frac{\sigma_c \times 200}{1.2 \times 10^5}$$

$$0.226 = 1.5 \times 10^{-3}\,\sigma_s + 1.67 \times 10^{-3}\,\sigma_c \qquad \text{... Eq. (i)}$$

For equilibrium, $\quad F_s = F_c$

$$\sigma_s A_s = \sigma_c A_c$$
$$\sigma_s \times (4/3) = \sigma_c$$
$$\therefore \sigma_s = 0.75\,\sigma_c \qquad \text{... Eq. (ii)}$$

Substituting Eq. (ii) in Eq. (i), we have,

$$0.226 = (1.5 \times 10^{-3}) \times 0.75\,\sigma_c + (1.67 \times 10^{-3})\,\sigma_c$$
$$\therefore \quad \sigma_c = 80.86 \text{ MPa}$$

and Eq. (ii) yields... $\sigma_s = 0.75 \times 80.86 = 60.65$ MPa

67. **The bronze bar 3m long with 320 mm^2 cross sectional area is placed between two rigid walls. At –20°C there is gap $\Delta = 2.5$ mm, as shown in Fig. 2.61. Find the magnitude and the type of stress induced in the bar when it is heated to a temperature of 50.6°C. For bronze take $\alpha_B = 18 \times 10^{-6}/°C$ and $E = 80$ GPa.**

VTU – Dec. 2011 – 07 Marks

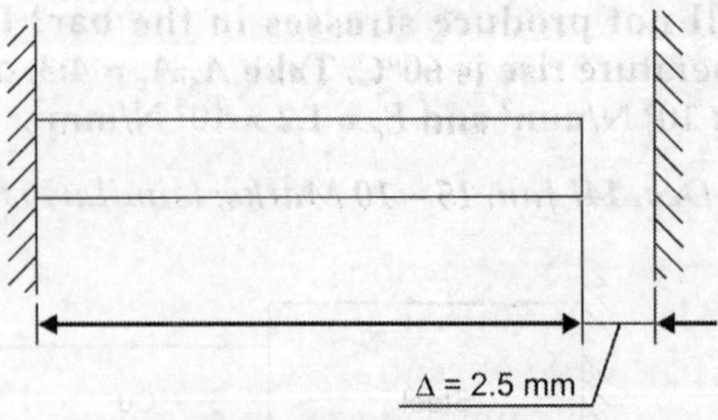

Fig. 2.61: Problem 67

Solution: $l = 3000$ mm, $A = 320$ mm^2, $\Delta = 2.5$ mm, $t_1 = -20°C$, $\sigma_b = ?$, $t_2 = 50.6°C$, $\Rightarrow$ $t = (t_2 - t_1) = 70.6°C$, $\alpha_B = 18 \times 10^{-6}/°C$ and $E_b = 80$ GPa

Total deformation, $\delta_T = \delta_{lb} + \text{gap}$

$$\alpha l t = \left(\frac{\sigma_b l_b}{E_b}\right) + 2.5$$

$$(18 \times 10^{-6} \times 3000 \times 70.6) - 2.5 = \left(\frac{\sigma_b \times 3000}{80 \times 10^3}\right)$$

$$\therefore \quad \sigma_b = 35 \, \text{MPa}$$

VTU QUESTION PAPERS

Dec. 07/Jan. 08 (06ME34)

1. a. Prove that the volumetric strain is equal to the sum of three principal strains, $\varepsilon_v = \varepsilon_x + \varepsilon_y + \varepsilon_z$. **(05 Marks)**

b. A cube of 100 mm side is subjected to 10 N/mm² (tensile), 8 N/mm² (compressive) and 6 N/mm² (tensile) acting along X, Y and Z planes respectively. Determine the strains along the three directions and the change in volume. Take Poisson's ratio = 0.25 and $E = 2 \times 10^5$ N/mm². **(05 Marks)**

c. A steel tube of 25 mm external diameter and 18 mm internal diameter encloses a copper rod of 15 mm diameter. The ends are rigidly fastened to each other. Calculate the stress in the rod and the tube when the temperature is raised from 15° to 200°C. Take $\alpha_{st} = 11 \times 10^{-6}/°C$, $\alpha_{cu} = 18 \times 10^{-6}/°C$, $E_{st} = 200$ GPa, $E_{cu} = 100$ GPa. **(07 Marks)**

June/July 2008 (06ME34)

2. a. Derive the relationship between Young's modulus and modulus of rigidity in the form of $\dfrac{9GK}{3K + G}$ **(06 Marks)**

b. A 12 mm steel rod passes centrally through a copper tube 78 mm external diameter and 36 mm internal diameter and 2.50 m long. The tube is closed at each end by 24 mm thick steel plates which are secured by nuts. The nuts are tightened until the copper tube is reduced in length by 0.508 mm. The whole assembly is then raised in temperature by 60°C. Calculate the stresses in copper and steel before and after raising the temperature, assuming the thickness of the plates remains to be unchanged.

Take $\alpha_s = 1.2 \times 10^{-5}$ per °C, $\alpha_C = 1.75 \times 10^{-5}$ per °C

$E_s = 2.1 \times 10^5$ N/mm² $E_C = 1.05 \times 10^5$ N/mm² **(10 Marks)**

Dec. 08/Jan. 09 (06ME34)

3. a. Derive an expression for relationship between Young's modulus, modulus of rigidity and Poisson's ratio. **(10 Marks)**

b. A compound bar made of central steel plate 60 mm wide and 10 mm thick to which copper plates 40 mm wide and 5 mm thick are connected rigidly on each side. The length of the bar at normal temperature is 1 meter. If the temperature is raised by 80°C, determine the stresses in each metal and change in length. Take $E_s = 200$ GPa, $E_c = 100$ GPa, $\alpha_s = 12 \times 10^{-6}/°C$, and $\alpha_c = 17 \times 10^{-6}/°C$. **(10 Marks)**

June/July 2009 (06ME34)

4. a. Establish a relationship between the modulus of elasticity and modulus of rigidity. **(10 Marks)**

   b. At room temperature the gap between bar A and bar B as shown in **Fig. U2.1** is 0.25 mm. What are the stresses induced in the bars, if the temperature rise is 35/°C.

   Given $A_a = 1000\,mm^2$ $A_b = 800\,mm^2$

           $E_a = 2 \times 10^5\,N/mm^2$ $E_b = 1 \times 10^5\,N/mm^2$

           $\alpha_a = 12 \times 10^{-6}/°C$ $\alpha_b = 23 \times 10^{-6}/°C$

           $L_a = 400\,mm$ $L_b = 300\,mm$ **(10 Marks)**

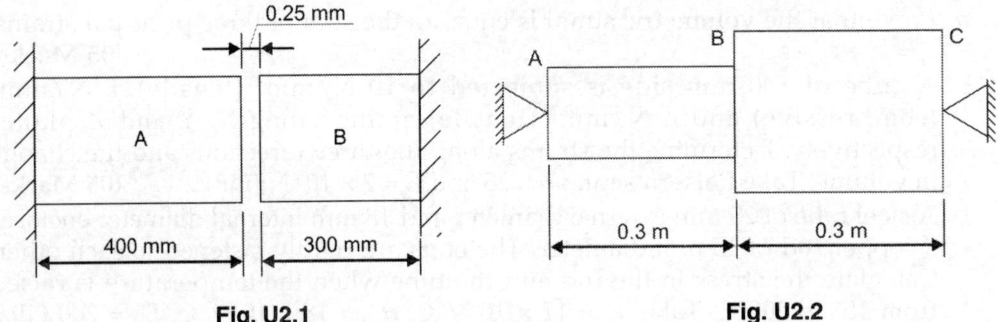

Fig. U2.1   **Fig. U2.2**

Dec. 09/Jan. 10 (06ME34)

5. Two vertical rods one of steel and the other of copper are each rigidly fixed at the top and 500 mm apart. Diameters and lengths of each rod are 20 mm and 4 m respectively. A cross bar fixed to the rods at the lower end carries a load of 5 kN, such that the cross bar remains horizontal even after loading. Find the stresses in each rod and the position of the load on the bar. Take $E_s = 2 \times 10^5\,N/mm^2$ and $E_c = 1 \times 10^5\,N/mm^2$ **(10 Marks)**

6. a. Define Bulk modulus. Derive an expression for Young's modulus in terms of Bulk modulus and Poisson's ratio. **(08 Marks)**

   b. i. Define thermal stress. **(02 Marks)**

   ii. Calculate the values of stress and strain in portion AC and CB of the steel bar shown in **Fig. U2.2**. A close fit exists at both the rigid supports at room temperature and the temperature is raised by 75°C. Take $E = 200$ GPa, $\alpha = 12 \times 10^{-6}/°C$ for steel. Area of cross sections of AC is 400 mm² and BC is 800 mm². **(10 Marks)**

May/June 2010 (06ME34)

7. a. Define: i. Modulus of rigidity   ii. Volumetric strain   **(04 Marks)**

   b. Explain the reason for development of stress in bars, when their temperature rises or falls. Accordingly calculate the nature and magnitude of stress induced in the rod of 2 m length and 20 mm diameter, when its temperature rises by 70°C, with both ends constrained. Take $E = 1 \times 10^5\,N/mm^2$, and $\alpha = 1.2 \times 10^{-5}/°C$ **(06 Marks)**

   c. A composite section comprises of a steel tube of 10 cm internal diameter and 12 cm external diameter, fitted inside a brass tube of 14 cm internal diameter and 16 cm external diameter. The assembly is subjected to a compressive load of 500 kN. Find the load carried by the tube and the stresses induced in them. The length of the tube is 150 cm. Take E_{steel} = 200 GPa and E_{brass} = 100 GPa. What is the change in length of the tubes? **(10 Marks)**

8. The longitudinal strain of a cylindrical bar of diameter 3 cm and length 1.5 m is four times the lateral strain during a tensile test. Determine the modulus of elasticity and bulk modulus. Also determine the change in volume when the bar is subjected to a hydrostatic pressure of 100 MPa. Take E = 100 GPa. **(10 Marks)**

Dec. 2010 (06ME34)

9. a. Define Poisson's ratio. Using the relationship between Young's modulus of elasticity and bulk modulus, prove that the maximum value of Poisson's ratio is 0.5. **(06 Marks)**

   b. AB is a rigid bar and has a hinged support at C as shown in **Fig. U2.3**. A steel and an aluminium bar support it at ends A and B respectively. The bars were stress free at room temperature. What are the stresses induced, when the temperature rises by 40°C? **(14 Marks)**

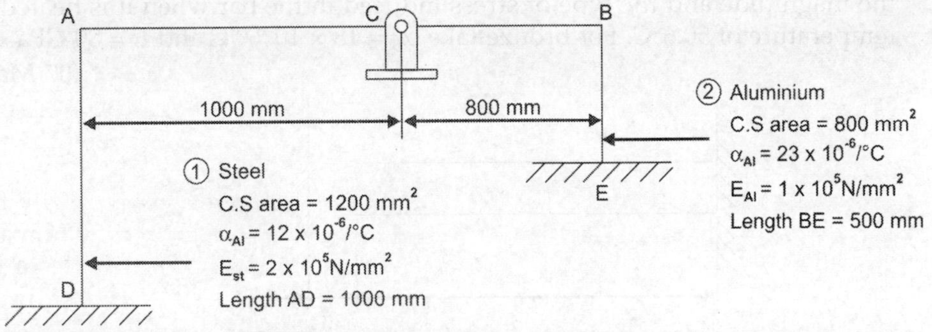

Fig. U2.3

June/July 2011 (06ME34)

10. a. Explain volumetric strain and obtain the expression for volumetric strain for a circular bar. **(05 Marks)**

    b. Establish a relationship between the modulus of elasticity and modulus of rigidity. **(07 Marks)**

    c. A steel rod of 20 mm diameter passes centrally through a copper tube of 50 mm external diameter and 40 mm internal diameter. The tube is enclosed at each end by rigid plates of negligible thickness. The nuts are tightened lightly on the projecting parts of the rod. If the temperature of the assembly is raised by 50°C, calculate the stress developed in the copper and steel members. Take E for steel as 200 GPa and for copper as 100 GPa respectively. Coefficient of expansion for steel and copper are 12×10^{-6}/°C and 18×10^{-6}/°C respectively. **(08 Marks)**

Dec. 2011 (06ME34)

11. a. Define: i. Volumetric strain   ii. Bulk modulus   **(02 Marks)**

    b. Establish the relationship between Young's modulus (E), modulus of rigidity (G) and Poisson's ratio (μ). **(08 Marks)**

   c. A steel rail 12.6 m long is laid at a temperature of 24°C. The maximum temperature expected is 44°C.

      i. Estimate the minimum gap between two rails to be left so that temperature stresses do not develop.

      ii. Calculate the thermal stresses developed in the rails if the gap of 2 mm is provided for expansion.

      iii. If the stress developed is 20 MN/m², what is the gap left between the rails?
Take $E = 2 \times 10^5$ N/mm² and $\alpha = 12 \times 10^{-6}/°C$ **(10 Marks)**

Dec. 2011 (10ME34)

12. a. With standard notations, derive an expression to relate the Modulus of elasticity (E), Bulk modulus (K) and Poisson's ratio (μ).   **(05 Marks)**

   b. When a bar of 25 mm diameter is subjected to a pull of 61 kN, the extension on a 50 mm gauge length is 0.1 mm and decrease in diameter is 0.013 mm. Calculate the value of elastic constants E, K and G.   **(08 Marks)**

   c. The bronze bar 3 m long with 320 mm² cross sectional area is placed between two rigid walls. At –20°C there is gap $\Delta = 2.5$ mm, as shown in **Fig. U2.4**. Find the magnitude and the type of stress induced in the bar when it is heated to a temperature of 50.6°C. For bronze take $\alpha_B = 18 \times 10^{-6}/°C$ and $E = 80$ GPa.

            (07 Marks)

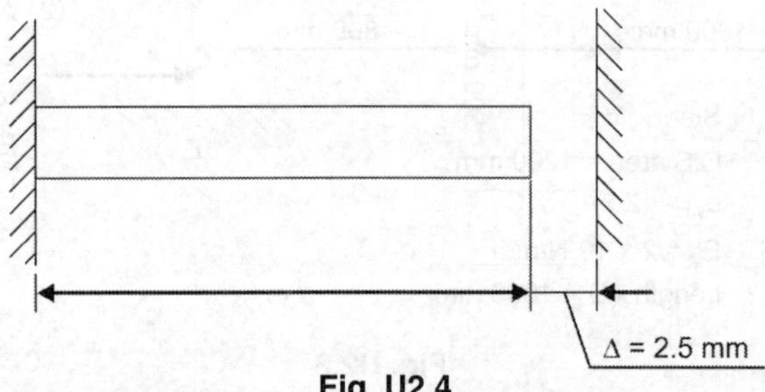

Fig. U2.4

June 2012 (06ME34)

13. a. Prove that in case of a composite section, stress in one material is modular ratio times the stress in other material.   **(05 Marks)**

   b. A square column of reinforced concrete is compressed by an axial force P. What fraction of load will be carried by the concrete, if the total cross sectional area of the steel bars is one-tenth of the cross sectional area of concrete and modulus of elasticity of steel is ten times that of concrete?   **(07 Marks)**

   c. A compound bar is made up of a central steel plate 60 mm wide and 10 mm thick to which copper plates 40 mm wide and 5 mm thick are connected rigidly on each side. The length of the bar at normal temperature is 1m. if the temperature is raised by 80°C, determine the stress in each metal and change in length. Take $E_s = 200$ GPa and $E_c = 100$ GPa; $\alpha_s = 12 \times 10^{-6}/°C$, and $\alpha_c = 17 \times 10^{-6}/°C$ **(07 Marks)**

June 2012 (10ME34)

14. Define: i. Poisson's ratio   ii. Modulus of rigidity
         iii. Bulk modulus   iv. Factor of safety.   **(04 Marks)**

15. a. Define volumetric strain. *A* bar of uniform rectangular section of area *A* is subjected to an axial load *P*. Show that the volumetric strain is given by

$$\epsilon_v = \frac{p}{AE}\left(1 - \frac{2}{m}\right)$$ where $1/m$ = Poisson's ratio, E = Young's modulus.

(06 Marks)

b. The modulus of rigidity of a member is 0.8×10^5 N/mm². When a 6 mm × 6 mm rod of this material was subjected to an axial pull of 3600 N, it was found that the lateral dimension of the rod changed to 5.9991 mm × 5.9991 mm. Find the Poisson's ratio and the modulus of elasticity. **(04 Marks)**

c. A horizontal rigid bar AB weighing 200 kN is hung by three vertical rods, each of 1m length and 500 mm² in cross section as shown in **Fig. U2.5**. The central rod is of steel and outer rods are copper. If the temperature rise is 40°C, estimate the load carried by each rod and how much the load will descend.

Take E_s = 200 GN/m², E_c = 100 GN/m², α_s = 1.2 × 10⁻⁵/°C, α_c = 1.8 × 10⁻⁵/°C

(10 Marks)

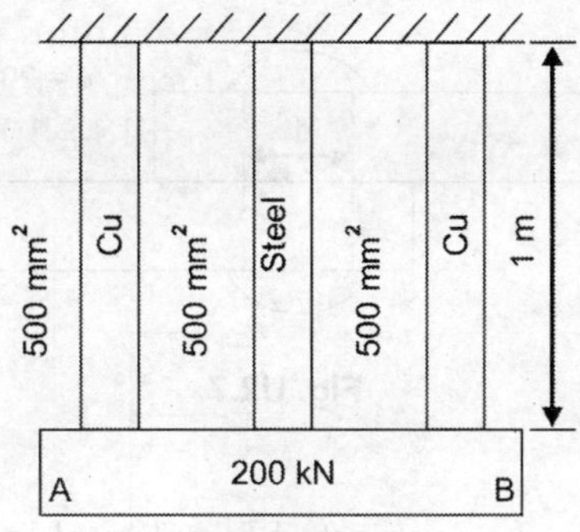

Fig. U2.5

Dec. 2012 (10ME34)

16. a. A C.I flat 300 mm long, 50 mm wide and 30 mm thick is acted upon by the following forces. 25 kN tensile in the direction of length; 350 kN compressive in the direction width; and 200 kN in the direction of thickness. Determine:

   i. Change in volume of the flat   ii. Modulus of rigidity   iii. Bulk modulus

Take E = 140 GN/m², and $1/m$ = 0.25 **(10 Marks)**

b. A steel bar is placed between two copper bars, each having the same area and of length L as the steel bar at 15°C. At this stage they are rigidly connected together at both ends. The length of the composite bar is also L. When the temperature is raised to 315°C, the length of the bar increases by 1.5 mm. Determine the original length and find the stresses in the bar.

Take E_s = 2.1 × 10⁵ N/mm², E_c = 1 × 10⁵ N/mm², α_s = 0.000012/°C, and α_c = 0.0000175/°C. **(10 Marks)**

Jan. 2013 (06ME34)

17. a. A 500 mm long bar has a rectangular cross section 20 mm × 40 mm. This bar is subjected to

   i. 40 kN tensile load on (20 × 40) mm faces.

  ii. 200 kN compressive load on (20 × 500) mm faces and

  iii. 300 kN tensile force on (40 × 500) mm faces.

Find the change in volume of the bar if $E = 2 \times 10^5$ N/mm² and Poisson's ratio $1/m = 0.3$. **(10 Marks)**

b. A horizontal bar hinged at one of its ends is supported by two vertical bars as shown in **Fig. U2.6**. If the temperature of the vertical bars increases by 40°C, determine the force, stresses and deformations induced in them. **(10 Marks)**

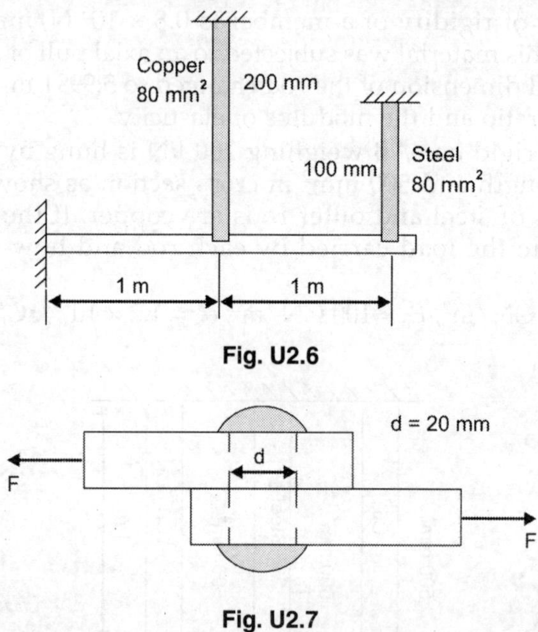

Fig. U2.6

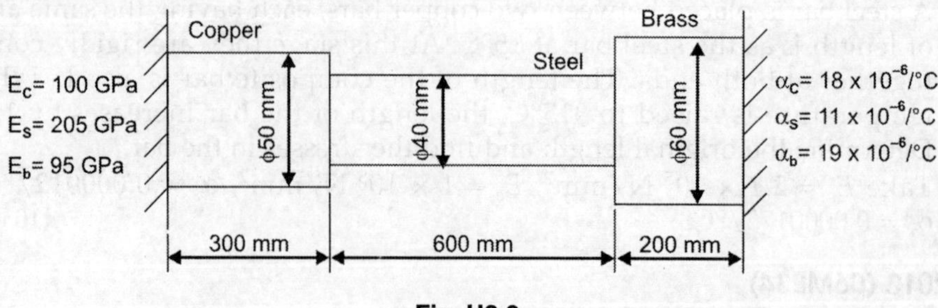

Fig. U2.7

June/July 2013 (06ME34)

18. a. Consider a rectangular bar subjected to external loads in x, y and z directions. Show that the volumetric strain is $\epsilon_v = \epsilon_x + \epsilon_y + \epsilon_z$ **(04 Marks)**

b. A riveted joint is shown in **Fig. U2.7**. if the diameter of the rivet is 20 mm and the load P is 30 kN, determine the shear stress and the shear strain in the rivet. Take $G = 80$ GPa. **(04 Marks)**

c. A composite bar is rigidly attached to the supports as shown in **Fig. U2.8**. Determine the stresses in the different sections of the bar when the temperature is raised by 70°C. **(12 Marks)**

Fig. U2.8

June/July 2013 (10ME34)

19. a. A bar of 20 mm diameter is tested in tension. It is observed that when a load of 37.7 kN is applied, the extension measured over a gauge length of 200 mm

is 0.12 mm and contraction in diameter is 0.0036 mm. Find Poisson's ratio and elastic constants E, G and K. **(08 Marks)**

b. A composite bar made of aluminium and steel is held between two supports as shown in **Fig. U2.9**. The bars are stress free at a temperature of 42°C. What will be the stresses in the two bars when the temperature drops to 24°C, if

   i. the supports are unyielding

   ii. the supports come nearer to each other by 0.1 mm.

The cross sectional area of the steel bar is 160 mm² and that of aluminium is 240 mm². $E_A = 0.7 \times 10^5$ MPa, $E_s = 2 \times 10^5$ MPa, $\alpha_A = 24 \times 10^{-6}/°C$, $\alpha_s = 12 \times 10^{-6}/°C$. **(12 Marks)**

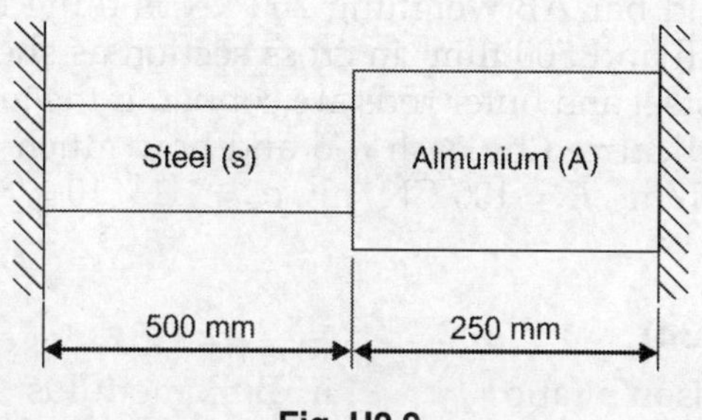

Fig. U2.9

Dec. 13/Jan. 14 (06ME34)

20. a. Define Bulk modulus. Derive an expression for Young's modulus in terms of Bulk modulus and Poisson's ratio. **(12 Marks)**

b. A M.S. bar 20 mm diameter and 300 mm long is encased in a brass tube whose external diameter is 30 mm and internal diameter is 25 mm. The composite bar is heated through 60°C. Calculate the stresses in each metal.

$\alpha_{steel} = 0.0000112/°C$ $\alpha_{brass} = 0.0000165/°C$

$E_{steel} = 2 \times 10^5$ N/mm² $E_{brass} = 1 \times 10^5$ N/mm² **(08 Marks)**

Dec. 13/Jan. 14 (10ME34)

21. a. Define: i. Volumetric strain   ii. Bulk modulus **(02 Marks)**

b. A bar of rectangular cross section shown in **Fig. U2.10** is subjected to stress, σ_x, σ_y and σ_z in x, y and z directions respectively. Show that if sum of these stresses is zero, there is no change in volume. **(09 Marks)**

c. Rails are laid such that there is no stress in them at 24°C. If the rails are 32 m long, determine:

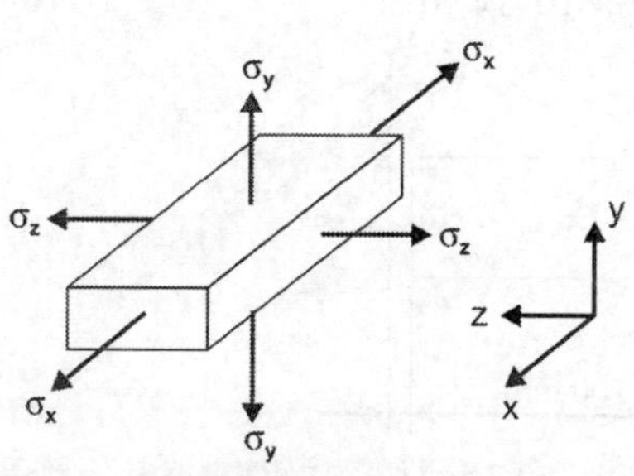

Fig. U2.10

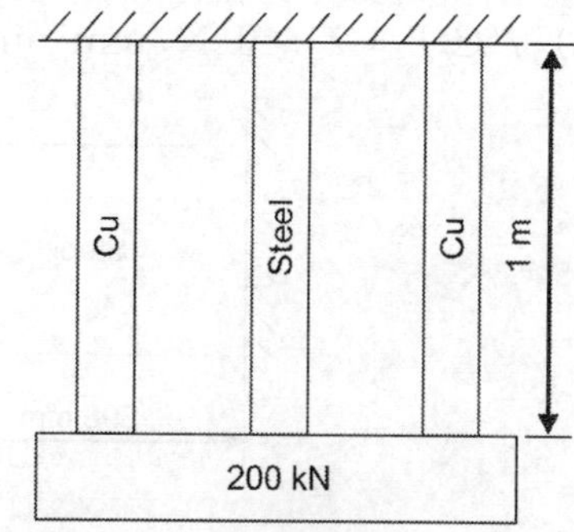

Fig. U2.11

    i. The stress in rails at 80°C, when there is no allowance for expansion.

    ii. The stress in rails at 80°C, when there is an expansion allowance of 8 mm per rail

    iii. The expansion allowance for no stress in the rails at 80°C

Coefficient of linear expansion $\alpha = 11 \times 10^{-6}/°C$ and Young's modulus $E = 205$ GPa. **(09 Marks)**

June/July 2014 (06ME34)

22. a. Establish a relationship between the modulus of elasticity and modulus of rigidity. **(10 Marks)**

   b. A horizontal rigid bar AB weighing 200 kN is hung by three vertical rods, each of 1m length and 500 mm² in cross section as shown in **Fig. U2.11**. The central rod is of steel and outer rods are copper. If the temperature rise is 40°C, estimate the load carried by each rod and how much the load will descend. Take $E_s = 200$ GN/m², $E_c = 100$ GN/m², $\alpha_s = 1.2 \times 10^{-5}/°C$, $\alpha_c = 1.8 \times 10^{-5}/°C$ **(10 Marks)**

June/July 2014 (10ME34)

23. a. Define: i. Poisson's ratio   ii. Bulk modulus   **(02 Marks)**

   b. Derive an expression for establishing the relationship between Young's modulus and modulus of rigidity **(06 Marks)**

   c. A 25 mm diameter steel rod passes concentrically through a bronze tube 400 mm long., 50 mm external diameter and 40 mm internal diameter. The end of the steel rod are threaded and provided with nuts and washers which are adjusted initially so that there is no end play at 20°C. Assuming that there is no change in thickness of the washers, find the stress produced in the steel and bronze when one of the nuts is tightened by giving one-tenth of a turn, the pitch of the thread being 2.5 mm. Take E for steel $= 200$ kN/mm², and for bronze $= 100$ kN/mm². **(07 Marks)**

Dec. 14/Jan. 15 (06ME34)

24. a. Define Bulk modulus and Poisson's ratio. **(02 Marks)**

   b. Derive an expression for the relationship between Young's Modulus, modulus of rigidity and Poisson's ratio. **(08 Marks)**

   c. The composite bar shown in **Fig. U2.12** is 0.2 mm short of distance between the rigid supports at room temperature. What is the maximum temperature rise which will not produce stresses in the bar? Find the stresses induced when the temperature rise is 60/°C. Take $A_s{:}A_c = 4{:}3$, $\alpha_s = 12 \times 10^{-6}/°C$, $\alpha_c = 17.5 \times 10^{-6}/°C$, $E_s = 2 \times 10^5$ N/mm² and $E_c = 1.2 \times 10^5$ N/mm². **(10 Marks)**

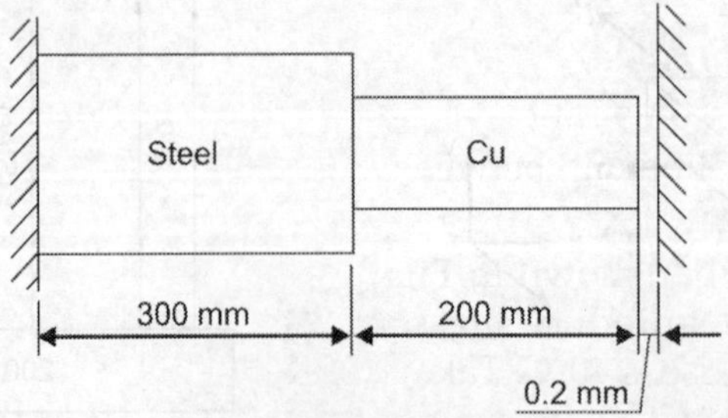

Fig. U2.12

Dec. 14/Jan. 15 (10ME34)

25. a. Explain volumetric strain and obtain the expression for volumetric strain for a circular bar. **(05 Marks)**

b. Establish a relationship between the modulus of elasticity and modulus of rigidity. **(07 Marks)**

c. A compound bar is made of a central steel plate 50 mm wide and 10 mm thick to which copper plate 50 mm wide and 5 mm thick are connected rigidly on each side. The length of the compound bar at room temperature is 1000 mm. If the temperature is raised by 100°C, determine the stress in each material and change in length of the compound bar. Assume E_s = 200 GPa, E_c = 100 GPa, α_s = 12 × 10^{-6}/°C and α_c = 18 × 10^{-6}/°C. **(08 Marks)**

June/July 15 (10ME34)

26. a. Derive an expression for volumetric strain of a rectangular bar subjected to normal stress σ along its axis. **(06 Marks)**

b. Define 3 modulli of elasticity and the write the relationship between them. **(04 Marks)**

c. A composite bar consisting of steel and aluminium components shown in **Fig. U2.13** is held firmly between two grips at the ends at a temperature of 60°C. Find the stresses in the two rods, when temperature falls to 20°C, if :
   i. The ends don't yield
   ii. The ends yield by 0.25 mm **(10 Marks)**

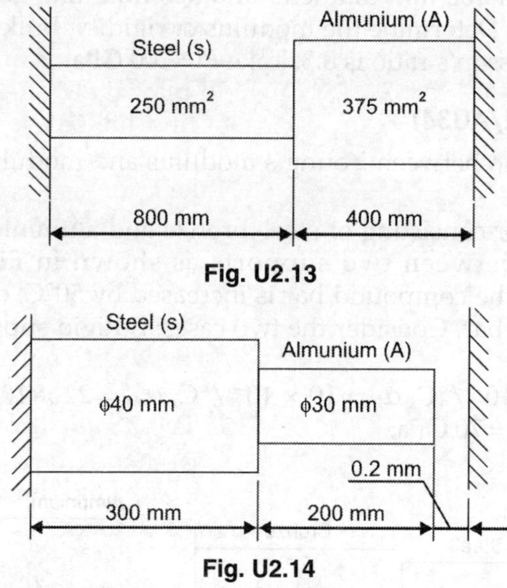

Fig. U2.13

Fig. U2.14

Dec. 15/Jan. 16 (10ME/AU34)

27. a. Define   i. Poisson's ratio   ii. Modular ratio. **(02 Marks)**

b. Establish the relationship between Young's modulus and rigidity modulus. **(08 Marks)**

c. For the stepped bar shown in **Fig. U2.14**, what is the maximum temperature rise which will not produce stress in the bar. Also find the stress induced when the temperature rise is 40°C. Take E_s = 200 GPa, E_A = 100 GPa, α_s = 12 × 10^{-6}/°C and α_A = 18 × 10^{-6}/°C. **(10 Marks)**

June/July 2016 (10ME/AU34)

28. a. Define Poisson's ratio. Determine an expression for volumetric strain of a rectangular bar, subjected to normal stress along the axis. **(10 Marks)**

 b. When a bar of 25 mm diameter is subjected to a pull of 61 kN, the extension on a 50 mm gauge length is 0.1 mm and decrease in diameter is 0.013 mm. Calculate the values of elastic constants E, G, K and μ. **(10 Marks)**

Dec. 16/Jan. 17 (10ME/AU34)

29. a. Derive an equation for volumetric strain for tri-axial stress system. **(06 Marks)**

 b. A compound bar is made of a central steel plate 60 mm wide and 10 mm thick to which copper plates 40 mm wide by 5 mm thick are connected rigidly on each side. The length of the bar at normal temperature is one meter. If the temperature is raised by 80°C, determine the stresses in each metal and change in length. Take $E_s = 200$ GPa, $E_c = 100$ GPa, $\alpha_s = 12 \times 10^{-6}/°C$ and $\alpha_c = 17 \times 10^{-6}/°C$. **(14 Marks)**

Dec. 16/Jan. 17 (15ME/MA34)

30. A bar of brass 25 mm diameter is enclosed in a steel tube of 50 mm external diameter and 25 mm internal diameter. The bar and the tube are rigidly fastened at the ends and are 1.5 m long. Find the stresses in the two materials when the temperature raises from 30°C to 100°C. Take $E_{steel} = 200$ kN/mm², $E_{brass} = 100$ kN/mm², $\alpha_{steel} = 11.6 \times 10^{-6}/°C$, $\alpha_{brass} = 18.7 \times 10^{-6}/°C$ **(08 Marks)**

 b. A circular rod of 100 mm diameter and 500 mm long is subjected to a tensile load of 1000 kN. Determine the modulus of rigidity, Bulk modulus and change in volume if Poisson's ratio is 0.3. Take $E = 200$ GPa. **(08 Marks)**

June/July 2017 (10ME/AU34)

31. a. Show the relation between Young's modulus and modulus of rigidity. **(10 Marks)**

 b. A compound bar consisting of steel, bronze and aluminium bars connected in series is held between two supports as shown in **Fig. U2.15**. When the temperature of the compound bar is increased by 50°C, determine the stresses induced in each bar. Consider the two cases: i) Rigid supports and ii) supports yield by 0.5 mm.
 Take $\alpha_s = 12 \times 10^{-6}/°C$, $\alpha_B = 19 \times 10^{-6}/°C$, $\alpha_{Al} = 22 \times 10^{?-6}/°C$, $E_s = 200$ GPa, $E_B = 83$ GPa, $E_{Al} = 70$ GPa. **(10 Marks)**

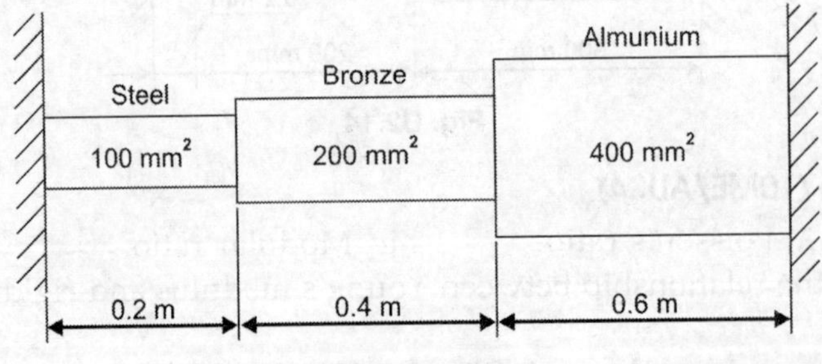

Fig. U2.15

June/July 2017 (15ME/MA34)

32. a. Derive a relation between modulus of elasticity and bulk modulus.**(06 Marks)**

b. At room temperature, the gap between bars A and B shown in **Fig. U2.16** is 0.25 mm. What are the stresses induced in the bars, if the temperature rise is 35/°C. Given A_A = 1000 mm^2, A_B = 800 mm^2, E_A = 200 GPa, E_B = 100 GPa, α_A = 12 × 10^{-6}/°C, α_B = 23 × 10^{-6}/°C, L_A = 400 mm, L_B = 300 mm. **(10 Marks)**

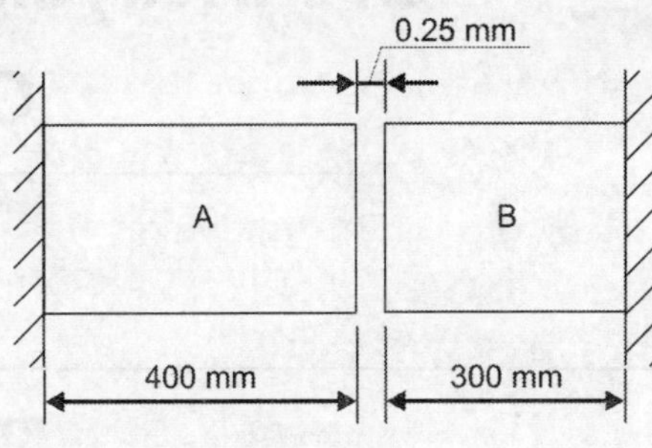

Fig. U2.16

Dec. 17/Jan. 18 (10ME/AU34)

33. a. Define: i. Volumetric strain ii. Modulus of rigidity **(02 Marks)**

b. Derive relation $E = 3K(1 - 2\mu)$ between Young's modulus(E), bulk modulus (K) and Poisson's ratio(μ). **(08 Marks)**

c. A steel tube of 30 mm external diameter and 20 mm internal diameter encloses a copper rod of 15 mm diameter to which it is rigidly joined at each end. If at a temperature of 10°C there is no longitudinal stress, calculate stresses in rod and tube when the temperature is raised to 200°C. Take E for steel and copper as 2.1 × 10^5 MPa and 1 × 10^5 MPa respectively. The value of α for steel and copper as 11 × 10^{-6}/°C and 18 × 10^{-6}/°C respectively. **(10 Marks)**

Dec. 17/Jan. 18 (15ME/MA34)

34. a. Derive a relation between modulus of elasticity and bulk modulus.**(05 Marks)**

b. A bar of brass 25 mm diameter is enclosed in a steel tube of 50 mm external diameter and 25 mm internal diameter. The bar and the tube is fastened at the ends and are 1.5 m long. Find the stresses in the two materials, when the temperature raises from 30°C to 80°C.

Take E_{steel} = 200 GPa, E_{brass} = 100 GPa, α_{steel} = 11.6 × 10^{-6}/°C, α_{brass} = 18.7 × 10^{-6}/°C **(06 Marks)**

Compound Stresses or Analysis of Stress and Strain

Chapter Outline

3.1 INTRODUCTION

In **chapters 1 and 2,** we have dealt with problems relating to simple direct stress and shear stress. But in most practical applications or problems we have to deal with combinations of these stresses.

For example, we have considered a bar subjected to only one loading at a time. But frequently such bars are subjected to several kinds of loadings simultaneously and it is required to determine the state of stress under these conditions. Since normal and shearing stresses are tensor quantities, care should be taken in combining the stresses given by the expressions for single loadings. In this chapter, we investigate the state of stress on an arbitrary plane through an element in a body subjected to both normal and shearing stresses.

In general, simple stresses mean only tensile stress or compressive stress or only shear stress. Tensile and compressive stresses act on a plane normal to the line of action of these stresses, and shear stress acts on a plane parallel to the line of action of this stress. But when a plane in a strained body is *oblique (inclined)* to the applied external force, this plane may be subjected to tensile or compressive stress and shear stress. i.e. a system or a plane in which direct or normal stresses and shear stresses act simultaneously are called *compound stresses or complex stresses*.

3.2 PLANE STRESS

A basic concept of stress analysis is the state of stress at a point. *The state of stress at a point is defined by the stress components acting on the sides of a differential volume element that encloses the point.* Knowing the state of stress at a point enables us to calculate the stress components that act on any plane passing through that point, which in turn enables us to compute the maximum stresses in a body.

A plane state of stress is a 2-dimensional (2D) state of stress in a sense that the stress components in one direction are all zero.

i.e. $$\sigma_z = \tau_{yz} = \tau_{zx} = 0$$

Examples: Plane state of stress includes – bars in tension and compression, shafts in torsion, and beams in bending, plates and shells.

3.2.1 Stress Tensor or Components of Stress

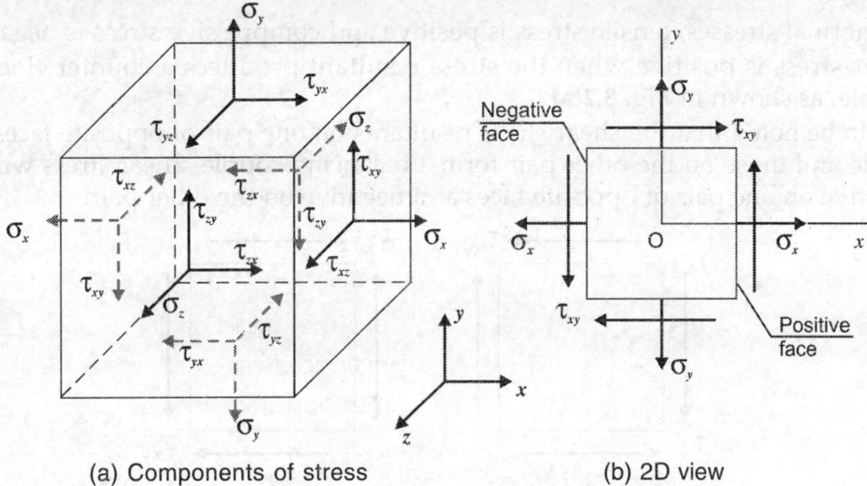

Fig. 3.1: Elements of plane stress

Consider the stress element shown in **Fig. 3.1(a)**. This element is infinitesimal in size and can be sketched either as a cube or as a rectangular parallelepiped. The x, y, z axes are parallel to the edges of the element, and the faces of the element are designated by the directions of their outward normals. For convenience in sketching plane-stress elements, we usually draw only a two-dimensional view of the element, as shown in **Fig. 3.1(b)**.

The state of stress at any point of a continuous body is determined entirely by the components of stress in three mutually perpendicular planes which pass through the chosen point. These planes are usually taken perpendicular to the orthogonal coordinate system.

To define the stresses acting on six faces of the cubical element, we need 3 normal stresses: σ_x, σ_y, and σ_z and 6 shear stresses are τ_{xy}, τ_{yx}, τ_{yz}, τ_{zy}, τ_{zx} and τ_{xz}. Thus the state of stress at a point using three mutually perpendicular (orthogonal) planes can be described by the nine distinct values of stress represented in the matrix form shown below.

$$\tau_{ij} = \begin{bmatrix} \tau_{xx} & \tau_{xy} & \tau_{xz} \\ \tau_{yx} & \tau_{yy} & \tau_{yz} \\ \tau_{zx} & \tau_{zy} & \tau_{zz} \end{bmatrix} = \begin{bmatrix} \sigma_x & \tau_{xy} & \tau_{xz} \\ \tau_{yx} & \sigma_y & \tau_{yz} \\ \tau_{zx} & \tau_{zy} & \sigma_z \end{bmatrix} \qquad \text{... (Eq. 3.1)}$$

To ensure the static equilibrium, the following equations must hold:

$$\tau_{xy} = \tau_{yx}, \tau_{yz} = \tau_{zy}, \text{ and } \tau_{zx} = \tau_{xz} \qquad \text{... (Eq. 3.2)}$$

$\therefore$ (Eq. 3.1) yields...
$$\tau_{ij} = \begin{bmatrix} \sigma_x & \tau_{xy} & \tau_{xz} \\ \tau_{xy} & \sigma_y & \tau_{yz} \\ \tau_{xz} & \tau_{yz} & \sigma_z \end{bmatrix} \qquad \text{... (Eq. 3.3)}$$

These components together form a *stress tensor* or *stress matrix*. A tensor matrix describes the property of a system which is invariant with respect to coordinate system.

3.2.2 Sign convention

- For normal stresses, tensile stress is positive and compressive stress is negative.
- Shear stress is positive when the stress resultant produces a counter clockwise couple, as shown in **Fig. 3.2(a)**.

It is to be noted that the shear stress resultants on one pair of opposite faces form a couple and those on the other pair form a balancing couple. Shear stress will thus be positive on one pair of opposite faces and negative on the other pair.

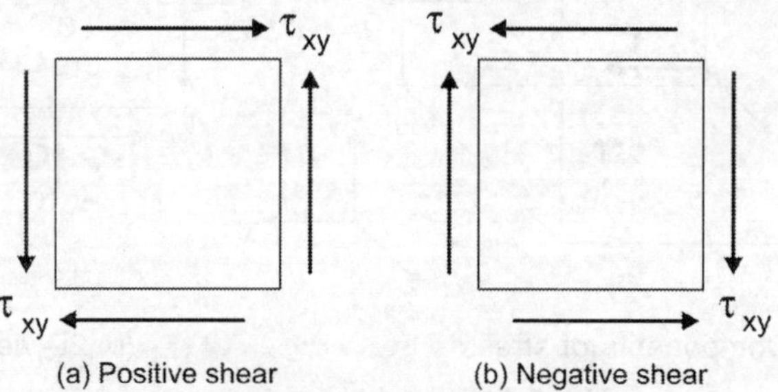

(a) Positive shear   (b) Negative shear

Fig. 3.2: Sign convention for shear force

3.2.3 Notation of stress

The normal stress is represented as σ_n and the tangential (shear) stress is represented as τ. Subscripts are used to indicate the direction of the plane on which the stress is acting. For example σ_x indicates that the stress is acting on a plane normal to the x-axis.

The shear stress is further resolved into two components parallel to the coordinate axis. Two subscripts are used in this case;

- The first indicating the direction of normal to the plane (face) and
- The second indicates the direction of component of stress as shown:

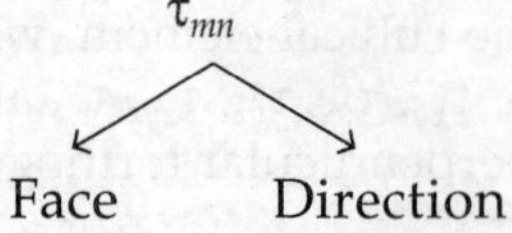

i.e. The first is the plane in which the stress acts and the second is the direction in which the stress acts.

Examples: τ_{yz} is the shear stress in a plane perpendicular to y axis in z direction. Each component represents a magnitude for that particular plane and direction.

3.3 METHODS OF STRESS DETERMINATION

The stresses on an oblique or inclined plane can be determined by following methods:
1. Analytical method
2. Graphical method

The above methods are applied for the following cases:
a. Uniaxial stress system
b. Biaxial stress system
c. General two-dimensional stress system

3.4 STRESSES ON AN INCLINED PLANE SUBJECTED TO UNIAXIAL STRESSES

Consider a body subjected to uniaxial stress as shown in **Fig. 3.3(a)**. The thickness is assumed to be unity as shown in **Fig. 3.3(b)**. **Fig. 3.3(c)** represents the two-dimensional view of the element. Consider an oblique/inclined plane AB at an angle ϕ with plane AC in counter-clockwise direction. **Fig. 3.3(d)** represents the stresses acting on the wedge shaped element.

Let $\sigma_x = \sigma$ = tensile stress acting along x axis

ϕ = angle made by AB with vertical AC in CCW direction

σ_n = normal stress

τ = tangential stress.

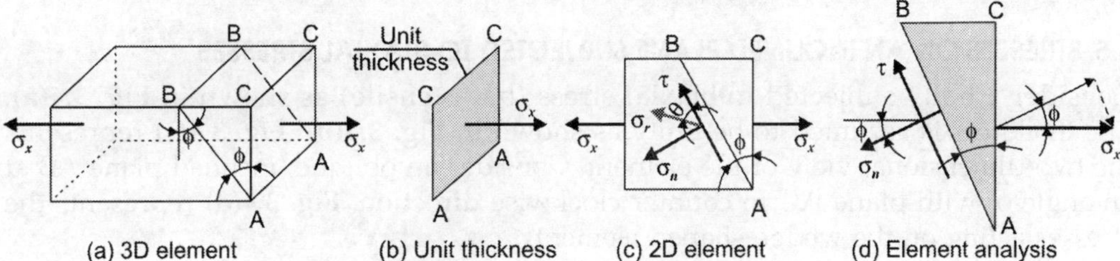

Fig. 3.3: Uniaxial stress system

- Resolving forces normal to plane AB,

$\sigma_n.AB - (\sigma_x.AC)\cos\phi = 0$

$\sigma_n.AB = (\sigma_x.AC)\cos\phi$

$$\text{From \textbf{Fig. 3.3(d)} } \cos\phi = \frac{AC}{AB} \Rightarrow AC = AB.\cos\phi$$

$$\text{and } \sin\phi = \frac{BC}{AB} \Rightarrow BC = AB.\sin\phi$$

$\sigma_n.AB = (\sigma_x\cos\phi)(AB.\cos\phi)$

$\qquad = (\sigma_x\cos^2\phi)AB$

$\therefore \quad \sigma_n = \sigma_x\cos^2\phi$ $\qquad\qquad\qquad$ ... (Eq. 3.4)

- Resolving forces parallel to plane AB,

$\tau.AB - (\sigma_x.AC)\sin\phi = 0$

$$\tau.AB = (\sigma_x.AC)\sin\phi$$
$$= (\sigma_x \sin\phi)(AB.\cos\phi)$$
$$\tau.AB = (\sigma_x \sin\phi.\cos\phi)AB$$

$$\therefore \quad \tau = (\sigma_x \sin\phi.\cos\phi) = \left(\frac{\sigma_x}{2}\right)\sin 2\phi \qquad \text{... (Eq. 3.5)}$$

- The resultant stress is calculated as $\sigma_r = \sqrt{\sigma_n^2 + \tau^2}$ ... (Eq. 3.6)

- Angle of obliquity, $\tan\theta = \left(\dfrac{\sigma_n}{\tau}\right)$ ... (Eq. 3.7)

Angle of obliquity refers to the angle made by the resultant stress with normal stress.

Note:

→ Maximum normal stress occurs when $\phi = 0$: $\sigma_n)_{max} = \sigma_1 = \sigma_x \cos^2(0) = \sigma_x$

     ... (Eq. 3.8a)

→ Minimum normal stress occurs when $\phi = 90°$: $\sigma_n)_{min} = \sigma_x \cos^2(90) = 0$

     ... (Eq. 3.8b)

→ Maximum shear stress (or maximum in-plane shear stress) occurs when $\phi = 45°$ or $2\phi = 90°$:

$$\tau_{max} = \left(\frac{\sigma_x}{2}\right)\sin 2\phi = \left(\frac{\sigma_x}{2}\right)\sin(90)$$

$$\tau_{max} = \left(\frac{\sigma_x}{2}\right) \qquad \text{... (Eq. 3.8c)}$$

Thus any material whose yield stress in shear is less than half that in tension or compression will yield initially in shear under the action of direct tensile or compressive forces

3.5 STRESSES ON AN INCLINED PLANE SUBJECTED TO BIAXIAL STRESSES

Consider a body subjected to biaxial stress (both tensile) as shown in **Fig. 3.4(a)**. The thickness is assumed to be unity as shown in **Fig. 3.4(b)**. **Fig. 3.4(c)** represents the two-dimensional view of the element. Consider an oblique/inclined plane AB at an angle ϕ with plane AC in counter clockwise direction. **Fig. 3.4(d)** represents the stresses acting on the wedge shaped element.

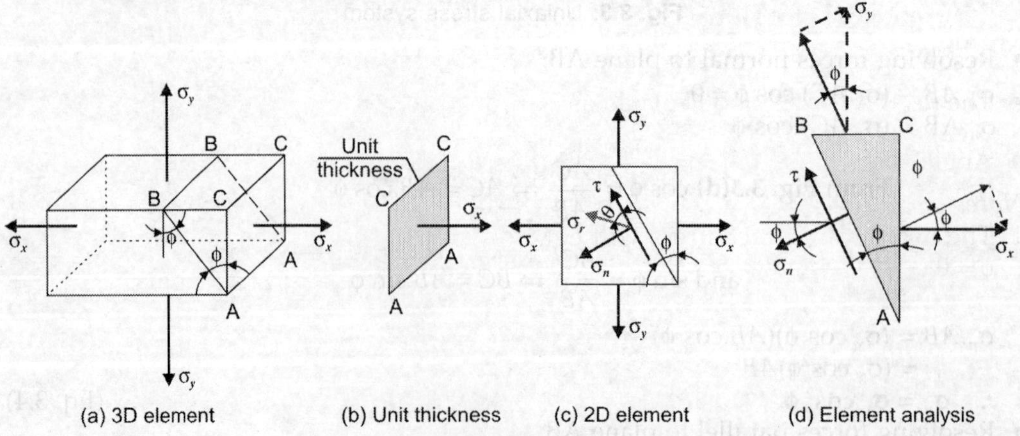

Fig. 3.4: Uniaxial stress system

Let $\quad \sigma_x$ = tensile stress acting along x axis

$\quad\quad \sigma_y$ = tensile stress acting along y axis

$\quad\quad \phi$ = angle made by AB with vertical AC in CCW direction

$\quad\quad \sigma_n$ = normal stress

$\quad\quad \tau$ = tangential stress.

- Resolving forces normal to plane AB,

$$\sigma_n.AB - (\sigma_x.AC) \cos \phi - (\sigma_y.BC) \sin \phi = 0$$
$$\sigma_n.AB = (\sigma_x.AC) \cos \phi + (\sigma_y.BC) \sin \phi$$

From **Fig. 3.4(d)**, $\cos \phi = \dfrac{AC}{AB} \Rightarrow AC = AB.\cos \phi$

and $\quad \sin \phi = \dfrac{BC}{AB} \Rightarrow BC = AB.\sin \phi$

$$\sigma_n.AB = (\sigma_x \cos \phi)(AB.\cos \phi) + (\sigma_y \sin \phi)(AB.\sin \phi)$$
$$= (\sigma_x \cos^2 \phi + \sigma_y \sin^2 \phi)AB$$
$$\therefore \ \sigma_n = (\sigma_x \cos^2 \phi + \sigma_y \sin^2 \phi) \quad\quad\quad\quad \text{... (Eq. 3.9a)}$$

But $\cos^2 \phi = \left(\dfrac{1 + \cos 2\phi}{2}\right)$ and $\sin^2 \phi = \left(\dfrac{1 - \cos 2\phi}{2}\right)$

i.e. $\sigma_n = \sigma_x \left(\dfrac{1 + \cos 2\phi}{2}\right) + \sigma_y \left(\dfrac{1 - \cos 2\phi}{2}\right)$

$$= \dfrac{\sigma_x}{2}\left(\dfrac{\sigma_x \cos 2\phi}{2}\right) + \dfrac{\sigma_y}{2} - \left(\dfrac{\sigma_y \cos 2\phi}{2}\right)$$

$$\therefore \ \sigma_n = \left(\dfrac{\sigma_x + \sigma_y}{2}\right) + \left(\dfrac{\sigma_x - \sigma_y}{2}\right) \cos 2\phi \quad\quad\quad \text{... (Eq. 3.9b)}$$

- Resolving forces parallel to plane AB,

$$\tau.AB - (\sigma_x.AC) \sin \phi + (\sigma_y.BC) \cos \phi = 0$$
$$\tau.AB = (\sigma_x.AC) \sin \phi - (\sigma_y.BC) \cos \phi$$
$$= (\sigma_x \sin \phi)(AB.\cos \phi) - (\sigma_y \cos \phi)(AB.\sin \phi)$$
$$= (\sigma_x \sin \phi.\cos \phi - \sigma_y \sin \phi.\cos \phi)AB$$
$$\tau.AB = [(\sigma_x - \sigma_y) \sin \phi.\cos \phi]AB$$
$$\therefore \ \tau = (\sigma_x - \sigma_y) \sin \phi.\cos \phi \quad\quad\quad\quad \text{... (Eq. 3.10a)}$$

or $\quad \therefore \ \tau = \left(\dfrac{\sigma_x - \sigma_y}{2}\right) \sin 2\phi \quad\quad\quad\quad \text{... (Eq. 3.10b)}$

- The resultant stress is calculated as $\sqrt{\sigma_n^2 + \tau^2}$ $\quad\quad\quad\quad \text{... (Eq. 3.11)}$

- Angle of obliquity, $\tan \theta = \left(\dfrac{\sigma_n}{\tau}\right)$ $\quad\quad\quad\quad \text{... (Eq. 3.12)}$

Note:

1. The maximum direct stress will equal σ_x or σ_y, whichever is the greater, when $\phi = 0$ or $90°$.

- @ $\phi = 0$: Maximum normal stress, $\sigma_n)_{max} = \sigma_1 = \left(\dfrac{\sigma_x + \sigma_y}{2}\right) + \left(\dfrac{\sigma_x - \sigma_y}{2}\right) \cos(0)$

$$= \left(\dfrac{\sigma_x + \sigma_y}{2}\right) + \left(\dfrac{\sigma_x - \sigma_y}{2}\right)$$

$$\sigma_n)_{max} = \sigma_1 = \sigma_x \quad\quad\quad\quad \text{... (Eq. 3.13a)}$$

- @ $\phi = 90°$: Minimum normal stress, $\sigma_n)_{min} = \sigma_2 = \left(\dfrac{\sigma_x + \sigma_y}{2}\right) + \left(\dfrac{\sigma_x - \sigma_y}{2}\right) \cos(180)$

$$= \left(\dfrac{\sigma_x + \sigma_y}{2}\right) + \left(\dfrac{\sigma_x - \sigma_y}{2}\right)$$

$$\sigma_n)_{max} = \sigma_2 = \sigma_y \qquad \text{... (Eq. 3.13b)}$$

2. Maximum shear stress (or maximum in-plane shear stress) occurs when $\phi = 45°$ or $2\phi = 90°$:

$$\tau_{max} = \left(\dfrac{\sigma_x - \sigma_y}{2}\right) \sin 2\phi = \left(\dfrac{\sigma_x - \sigma_y}{2}\right) \sin(90)$$

$$\tau_{max} = \left(\dfrac{\sigma_x - \sigma_y}{2}\right) \qquad \text{... (Eq. 3.13c)}$$

Using Eqs (3.13a) and (3.13b), we have $\tau_{max} = \left(\dfrac{\sigma_1 - \sigma_2}{2}\right) \qquad \text{... (Eq. 3.13d)}$

3.6 STRESSES DUE TO PURE SHEARING

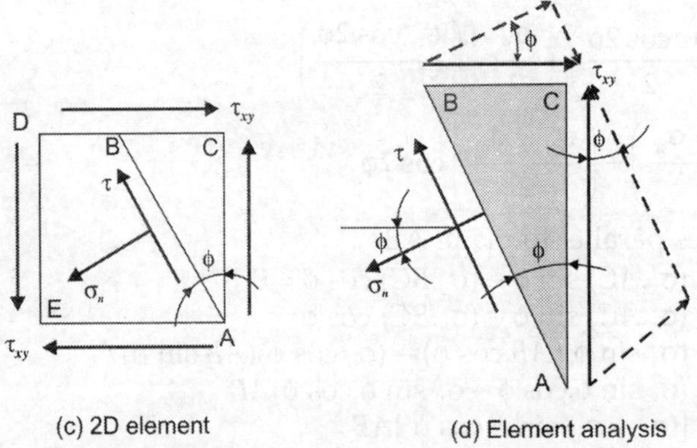

(c) 2D element   (d) Element analysis

Fig. 3.5: Material subjected to pure shear stress

Consider the element of unit thickness shown in **Fig. 3.5(a)** subjected to shear stresses on faces DC and AE. *Complementary shear stresses* of equal value but of opposite effect are then set up on sides DE and AC so as to prevent rotation of the element. **Fig. 3.5(b)** represents the stresses acting on the wedge shaped element.

- Resolving forces normal to plane AB,

$\sigma_n.AB - (\tau_{xy}.AC) \sin \phi - (\tau_{xy}.BC) \cos \phi = 0$

$\sigma_n.AB = (\tau_{xy}.AC) \sin \phi + (\tau_{xy}.BC) \cos \phi$

From **Fig. 3.5(b)**, $\cos \phi = \dfrac{AC}{AB} \Rightarrow AC = AB.\cos \phi$

and $\quad \sin \phi = \dfrac{BC}{AB} \Rightarrow BC = AB.\sin \phi$

$\sigma_n.AB = (\tau_{xy} \sin \phi)(AB.\cos \phi) + (\tau_{xy} \cos \phi)(AB.\sin \phi)$

$\qquad = (\tau_{xy} \sin \phi.\cos \phi + \tau_{xy} \sin \phi.\cos \phi)AB$

$$\sigma_n.AB = (2\tau_{xy} \sin \phi.\cos \phi)AB$$
$$\therefore \ \boldsymbol{\sigma_n = (\tau_{xy} \sin 2\phi)} \qquad \qquad \dots \text{(Eq. 3.14)}$$

- Resolving forces tangential to plane AB

$$\tau.AB + (\tau_{xy}.AC) \cos \phi - (\tau_{xy}.BC) \sin \phi = 0$$
$$\tau.AB = - (\tau_{xy}.AC) \cos \phi + (\tau_{xy}.BC) \sin \phi$$
$$= - (\tau_{xy} \cos \phi)(AB.\cos \phi) + (\tau_{xy} \sin \phi)(AB.\sin \phi)$$
$$= (- \tau_{xy} \cos^2 \phi + \tau_{xy} \sin^2 \phi)AB$$
$$\tau.AB = [- \tau_{xy} (\cos^2 \phi - \sin^2 \phi)]AB$$
$$\therefore \ \tau = - \tau_{xy} (\cos^2 \phi - \sin^2 \phi)$$

$$\text{But } \cos^2 \phi = \left(\frac{1 + \cos 2\phi}{2} \right) \text{ and } \sin^2 \phi = \left(\frac{1 - \cos 2\phi}{2} \right)$$

$$\text{i.e. } \tau = - \tau_{xy} \left(\frac{1 + \cos 2\phi}{2} \right) - \left(\frac{1 - \cos 2\phi}{2} \right)$$

$$= - \left(\frac{\tau_{xy}}{2} \right) 2 \cos 2\phi$$

$$\therefore \ \boldsymbol{\tau = - \tau_{xy} \cos 2\phi} \qquad \qquad \dots \text{(Eq. 3.15)}$$

Negative sign indicates that τ will be acting downwards on the plane AB

The maximum value of τ, is τ_{xy} when $\phi = 0°$ or $90°$ and it has a value of zero when $\phi = 45°$, i.e. on the planes of maximum direct stress.

*Applications:*This has great significance in the measurement of shear stresses or torques on shafts using strain gauges where the gauges are arranged to record the direct strains at 45° to the shaft axis.

3.7 GENERAL TWO-DIMENSIONAL STRESS SYSTEM OR PLANE STRESS SYSTEM

Consider a body subjected to biaxial stress (both tensile) as shown in **Fig. 3.6(a)**. The thickness is assumed to be unity as shown in **Fig. 3.6(b)**. **Fig. 3.6(c)** represents the two-dimensional view of the element. Consider an oblique/inclined plane AB at an angle ϕ with plane AC in counter clockwise direction. **Fig. 3.6(d)** represents the stresses acting on the wedge shaped element.

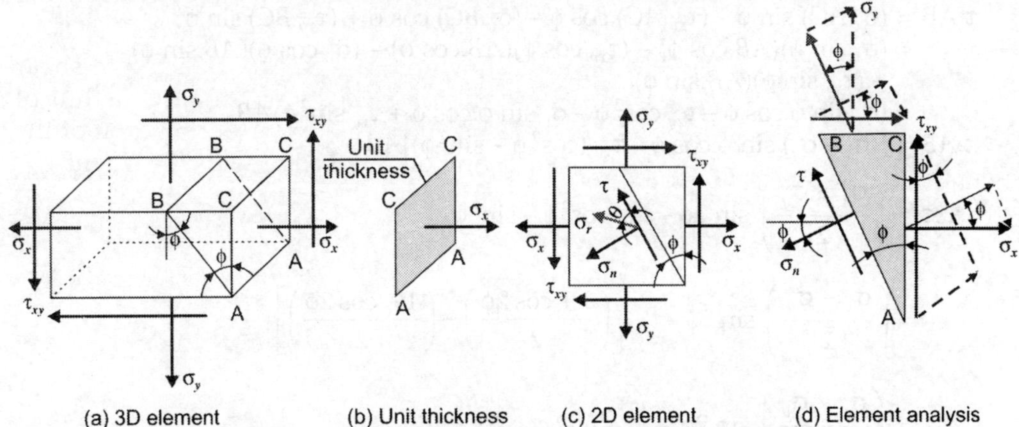

(a) 3D element   (b) Unit thickness   (c) 2D element   (d) Element analysis

Fig. 3.6: Plane stress system or 2D generalized system

Let σ_x = tensile stress acting along x axis

σ_y = tensile stress acting along y axis

τ_{xy} = shear stress

ϕ = angle made by AB with vertical AC in CCW direction

σ_n = normal stress

τ = tangential stress.

Resolving forces normal to plane AB,

$$\sigma_n.AB - (\sigma_x.AC)\cos\phi - (\tau_{xy}.AC)\sin\phi - (\sigma_y.BC)\sin\phi - (\tau_{xy}.BC)\cos\phi = 0$$

$$\sigma_n.AB = (\sigma_x.AC)\cos\phi + (\tau_{xy}.AC)\sin\phi + (\sigma_y.BC)\sin\phi + (\tau_{xy}.BC)\cos\phi$$

From **Fig. 3.6(d)**, $\cos\phi = \dfrac{AC}{AB} \Rightarrow AC = AB.\cos\phi$

and $\sin\phi = \dfrac{BC}{AB} \Rightarrow BC = AB.\sin\phi$

$$\sigma_n.AB = (\sigma_x\cos\phi)(AB.\cos\phi) + (\tau_{xy}\sin\phi)(AB.\cos\phi) + (\sigma_y\sin\phi)(AB.\sin\phi)$$
$$+ (\tau_{xy}\cos\phi)(AB.\sin\phi)$$
$$= (\sigma_x\cos^2\phi + \tau_{xy}\sin\phi.\cos\phi + \sigma_y\sin^2\phi + \tau_{xy}\sin\phi.\cos\phi)AB$$
$$\sigma_n.AB = (\sigma_x\cos^2\phi + \sigma_y\sin^2\phi + 2\tau_{xy}\sin\phi.\cos\phi)AB$$
$$\therefore\ \sigma_n = (\sigma_x\cos^2\phi + \sigma_y\sin^2\phi + \tau_{xy}\sin 2\phi) \qquad\qquad \dots \text{(Eq. 3.16a)}$$

But $\cos^2\phi = \left(\dfrac{1+\cos 2\phi}{2}\right)$ and $\sin^2\phi = \left(\dfrac{1-\cos 2\phi}{2}\right)$

$$= \sigma_x\left(\frac{1+\cos 2\phi}{2}\right) + \sigma_y\left(\frac{1-\cos 2\phi}{2}\right) + \tau_{xy}\sin 2\phi$$

$$= \frac{\sigma_x}{2} + \left(\frac{\sigma_x\cos 2\phi}{2}\right) + \frac{\sigma_y}{2} - \left(\frac{\sigma_y\cos 2\phi}{2}\right) + \tau_{xy}\sin 2\phi$$

$$\therefore\ \sigma_n = \left(\frac{\sigma_x+\sigma_y}{2}\right) + \left(\frac{\sigma_x-\sigma_y}{2}\right)\cos 2\phi + \tau_{xy}\sin 2\phi \qquad\qquad \dots \text{(Eq. 3.16b)}$$

- Resolving forces tangential to plane AB

$$\tau.AB - (\sigma_x.AC)\sin\phi + (\tau_{xy}.AC)\cos\phi + (\sigma_y.BC)\cos\phi - (\tau_{xy}.BC)\sin\phi = 0$$
$$\tau.AB = (\sigma_x.AC)\sin\phi - (\tau_{xy}.AC)\cos\phi - (\sigma_y.BC)\cos\phi + (\tau_{xy}.BC)\sin\phi$$
$$= (\sigma_x\sin\phi)(AB.\cos\phi) - (\tau_{xy}\cos\phi)(AB.\cos\phi) - (\sigma_y\cos\phi)(AB.\sin\phi)$$
$$+ (\tau_{xy}\sin\phi)(AB.\sin\phi)$$
$$= (\sigma_x\sin\phi.\cos\phi - \tau_{xy}\cos^2\phi - \sigma_y\sin\phi.\cos\phi + \tau_{xy}\sin^2\phi)AB$$
$$\tau.AB = [(\sigma_x-\sigma_y)\sin\phi.\cos\phi - \tau_{xy}(\cos^2\phi - \sin^2\phi)]AB$$

$$\therefore\ \tau = \left(\frac{\sigma_x-\sigma_y}{2}\right)\sin 2\phi - \tau_{xy}(\cos^2\phi - \sin^2\phi)$$

$$= \left(\frac{\sigma_x-\sigma_y}{2}\right)\sin 2\phi - \tau_{xy}\left[\left(\frac{1+\cos 2\phi}{2}\right) - \left(\frac{1-\cos 2\phi}{2}\right)\right]$$

$$= \left(\frac{\sigma_x-\sigma_y}{2}\right)\sin 2\phi - \left(\frac{\tau_{xy}}{2}\right)2\cos 2\phi$$

$$\therefore \quad \tau = \left(\frac{\sigma_x - \sigma_y}{2}\right) \sin 2\phi - \tau_{xy} \cos 2\phi \qquad \text{... (Eq. 3.17)}$$

- The resultant stress is calculated as $\sigma_r = \sqrt{\sigma_n^2 + r^2}$ $\qquad$ ... (Eq. 3.18)

- Angle of obliquity, $\tan \theta = \dfrac{\tau}{\sigma_n}$ $\qquad$ ... (Eq. 3.19)

Principal Stresses

To determine maximum normal stress induced at a given point, there can be infinite number of planes passing through a point, and normal stress on each plane will be different from one another.

But there will be one plane on which normal stress value is *maximum*, known as *principal plane or maximum principal plane* and normal stress on this plane is known as *principal stress or maximum principal stress*.

Similarly there will be one more plane on which normal stress value is *minimum*, this is also a principal plane or minimum principal plane and normal stress on this plane is known as *principal stress or minimum principal stress*.

Thus to find the principal stresses, the maximum and minimum values of s_n must be obtained by equating t to zero

$$\text{i.e.} \quad \left(\frac{\sigma_x - \sigma_y}{2}\right) \sin 2\phi - \tau_{xy} \cos 2\phi = 0$$

$$\left(\frac{\sigma_x - \sigma_y}{2}\right) \sin 2\phi = \tau_{xy} \cos 2\phi$$

$$\tan 2\phi = \frac{\tau_{xy}}{(\sigma_x - \sigma_y)/2} \qquad \text{... (Eq. 3.20a)}$$

$$\text{or} \quad \tan 2\phi = \left(\frac{2\tau_{xy}}{\sigma_x - \sigma_y}\right) \qquad \text{... (Eq. 3.20b)}$$

Equation (3.20a) can be represented as shown in **Fig. 3.7**. From this equation we have two values of 2ϕ which differ by 180° [i.e. ϕ_1 and ϕ_2 differ by 90°].

If $2\phi_1$ and $2\phi_2$ be the solutions, then

$$\sin 2\phi_1 = \frac{\tau_{xy}}{\sqrt{\left(\dfrac{\sigma_x - \sigma_y}{2}\right)^2 + \tau_{xy}^2}} \quad \text{and} \quad \cos 2\phi_1 = \frac{(\sigma_x - \sigma_y)/2}{\sqrt{\left(\dfrac{\sigma_x - \sigma_y}{2}\right)^2 + \tau_{xy}^2}} \qquad \text{... Eq. (3.21)}$$

Fig. 3.7: Direction or principal stress

Similarly, $\sin 2\phi_2 = \dfrac{-\tau_{xy}}{\sqrt{\left(\dfrac{\sigma_x - \sigma_y}{2}\right)^2 + \tau_{xy}^2}}$ and $\cos 2\phi_2 = \dfrac{-(\sigma_x - \sigma_y)/2}{\sqrt{\left(\dfrac{\sigma_x - \sigma_y}{2}\right)^2 + \tau_{xy}^2}}$ ... Eq. (3.22)

Substituting Eqs (3.21) and (3.22) in Eq. (3.16), we get two principal stresses. i.e. substituting Eq. (3.21) in Eq. (3.16b) for major principal stress, we have

maximum or major principal stress $\sigma_1 = \left(\dfrac{\sigma_x + \sigma_y}{2}\right) + \left(\dfrac{\sigma_x - \sigma_y}{2}\right) \cos 2\phi_1 + \tau_{xy} \sin 2\phi_1$

$$= \left(\frac{\sigma_x + \sigma_y}{2}\right) + \left(\frac{\sigma_x - \sigma_y}{2}\right)\left[\frac{(\sigma_x - \sigma_y)/2}{\sqrt{\left(\dfrac{\sigma_x - \sigma_y}{2}\right)^2 + \tau_{xy}^2}}\right] + \tau_{xy}\left[\frac{\tau_{xy}}{\sqrt{\left(\dfrac{\sigma_x - \sigma_y}{2}\right)^2 + \tau_{xy}^2}}\right]$$

$$= \left(\frac{\sigma_x + \sigma_y}{2}\right) + \left(\frac{\sigma_x - \sigma_y}{2}\right)\left[\frac{(\sigma_x - \sigma_y)/2}{\dfrac{1}{2}\sqrt{(\sigma_x - \sigma_y)^2 + 4\tau_{xy}^2}}\right] + \tau_{xy}\left[\frac{\tau_{xy}}{\dfrac{1}{2}\sqrt{(\sigma_x - \sigma_y)^2 + 4\tau_{xy}^2}}\right]$$

$$= \left(\frac{\sigma_x + \sigma_y}{2}\right) + \left[\frac{(\sigma_x - \sigma_y)^2}{2\sqrt{(\sigma_x - \sigma_y)^2 + 4\tau_{xy}^2}}\right] + \left[\frac{2\tau_{xy}^2}{\sqrt{(\sigma_x - \sigma_y)^2 + 4\tau_{xy}^2}}\right]$$

$$= \left(\frac{\sigma_x + \sigma_y}{2}\right) + \frac{(\sigma_x - \sigma_y)^2 + 4\tau_{xy}^2}{2\sqrt{(\sigma_x - \sigma_y)^2 + 4\tau_{xy}^2}}$$

$$= \left(\frac{\sigma_x + \sigma_y}{2}\right) + \frac{\sqrt{(\sigma_x - \sigma_y)^2 + 4\tau_{xy}^2}}{2}$$

$$\therefore \sigma_1 = \left(\frac{\sigma_x + \sigma_y}{2}\right) - \sqrt{\left(\frac{\sigma_x - \sigma_y}{2}\right)^2 + \tau_{xy}^2} \qquad \text{... (Eq. 3.23)}$$

Similarly substituting Eq. (3.22) in Eq. (3.16b) for minor principal stress, we have

minimum or minor principal stress $\sigma_2 = \left(\dfrac{\sigma_x + \sigma_y}{2}\right) + \left(\dfrac{\sigma_x - \sigma_y}{2}\right) \cos 2\phi_2 + \tau_{xy} \sin 2\phi_2$

$$= \left(\frac{\sigma_x + \sigma_y}{2}\right) + \left(\frac{\sigma_x - \sigma_y}{2}\right)\left[\frac{-(\sigma_x - \sigma_y)/2}{\sqrt{\left(\dfrac{\sigma_x - \sigma_y}{2}\right)^2 + \tau_{xy}^2}}\right] + \tau_{xy}\left[\frac{-\tau_{xy}}{\sqrt{\left(\dfrac{\sigma_x - \sigma_y}{2}\right)^2 + \tau_{xy}^2}}\right]$$

$$= \left(\frac{\sigma_x + \sigma_y}{2}\right) - \left(\frac{\sigma_x - \sigma_y}{2}\right)\left[\frac{(\sigma_x - \sigma_y)/2}{\frac{1}{2}\sqrt{(\sigma_x - \sigma_y)^2 + 4\tau_{xy}^2}}\right] - \tau_{xy}\left[\frac{\tau_{xy}}{\frac{1}{2}\sqrt{(\sigma_x - \sigma_y)^2 + 4\tau_{xy}^2}}\right]$$

$$= \left(\frac{\sigma_x + \sigma_y}{2}\right) - \left[\frac{(\sigma_x - \sigma_y)^2}{2\sqrt{(\sigma_x - \sigma_y)^2 + 4\tau_{xy}^2}}\right] - \left[\frac{2\tau_{xy}^2}{\sqrt{(\sigma_x - \sigma_y)^2 + 4\tau_{xy}^2}}\right]$$

$$= \left(\frac{\sigma_x + \sigma_y}{2}\right) - \frac{(\sigma_x - \sigma_y)^2 + 4\tau_{xy}^2}{2.\sqrt{(\sigma_x - \sigma_y)^2 + 4\tau_{xy}^2}}$$

$$= \left(\frac{\sigma_x + \sigma_y}{2}\right) + \frac{\sqrt{(\sigma_x - \sigma_y)^2 + 4\tau_{xy}^2}}{2}$$

$$\therefore \; \sigma_2 = \left(\frac{\sigma_x + \sigma_y}{2}\right) - \sqrt{\left(\frac{\sigma_x - \sigma_y}{2}\right)^2 + \tau_{xy}^2} \qquad \ldots \text{(Eq. 3.24)}$$

For maximum value of τ, differentiating (Eq. 3.17) with respect to ϕ and equating to zero, we have

$$\left(\frac{d\tau}{d\phi}\right)_{\phi = \phi_s} = 0$$

i.e. $$\left(\frac{\sigma_x - \sigma_y}{2}\right)2\cos 2\phi_s + \tau_{xy}2\sin 2\phi_s = 0$$

$$(\sigma_x - \sigma_y)\cos 2\phi_s = -\tau_{xy}2\sin 2\phi_s$$

i.e. Direction of shear stress $$\tan 2\phi_s = -\left(\frac{\sigma_x - \sigma_y}{2\tau_{xy}}\right) \qquad \ldots \text{Eq. (3.25)}$$

Eq. (3.25) can be represented as shown in **Fig. 3.8.**

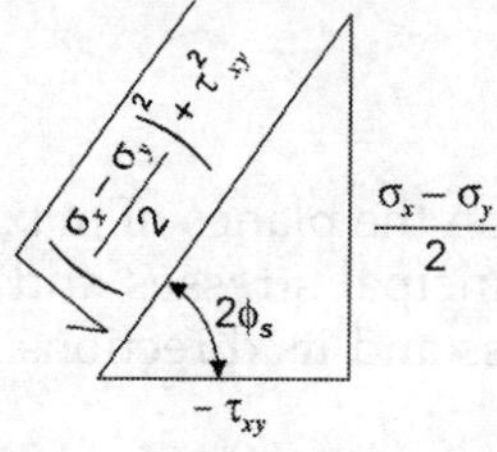

Fig. 3.8: Direction of shear stress

From **Fig. 3.8**, we have

$$\sin 2\phi_s = \frac{(\sigma_x - \sigma_y)/2}{\sqrt{\left(\frac{\sigma_x - \sigma_y}{2}\right)^2 + \tau_{xy}^2}} \quad \text{and} \quad \cos 2\phi_s = \frac{-\tau_{xy}}{\sqrt{\left(\frac{\sigma_x - \sigma_y}{2}\right)^2 + \tau_{xy}^2}} \qquad \ldots \text{(Eq. 3.26)}$$

Substituting (Eq. 3.26) in (Eq. 3.17), we have

$$\tau_{max} = \left(\frac{\sigma_x - \sigma_y}{2}\right)\sin 2\phi_s - \tau_{xy}\cos 2\phi_s$$

$$= \left(\frac{\sigma_x - \sigma_y}{2}\right)\left[\frac{(\sigma_x - \sigma_y)/2}{\sqrt{\left(\frac{\sigma_x - \sigma_y}{2}\right)^2 + \tau_{xy}^2}}\right] - \tau_{xy}\left[\frac{-\tau_{xy}}{\sqrt{\left(\frac{\sigma_x - \sigma_y}{2}\right)^2 + \tau_{xy}^2}}\right]$$

$$= \left(\frac{\sigma_x - \sigma_y}{2}\right)\left[\frac{(\sigma_x - \sigma_y)/2}{\frac{1}{2}\sqrt{\left(\sigma_x - \sigma_y\right)^2 + 4\tau_{xy}^2}}\right] + \tau_{xy}\left[\frac{\tau_{xy}}{\frac{1}{2}\sqrt{\left(\sigma_x - \sigma_y\right)^2 + 4\tau_{xy}^2}}\right]$$

$$= \left[\frac{(\sigma_x - \sigma_y)^2}{2\sqrt{\left(\sigma_x - \sigma_y\right)^2 + 4\tau_{xy}^2}}\right] + \left[\frac{2\tau_{xy}^2}{\sqrt{\left(\sigma_x - \sigma_y\right)^2 + 4\tau_{xy}^2}}\right]$$

$$= \frac{(\sigma_x - \sigma_y)^2 + 4\tau_{xy}^2}{2.\sqrt{\left(\sigma_x - \sigma_y\right)^2 + 4\tau_{xy}^2}}$$

$$= \frac{1}{2}\sqrt{\left(\sigma_x - \sigma_y\right)^2 + 4\tau_{xy}^2}$$

$$\therefore \quad \tau_{max} = \sqrt{\left(\frac{\sigma_x - \sigma_y}{2}\right)^2 + \tau_{xy}^2} \qquad \ldots \text{(Eq. 3.27a)}$$

$$\text{or} \quad \tau_{max} = \left(\frac{\sigma_1 - \sigma_2}{2}\right) \qquad \ldots \text{(Eq. 3.27b)}$$

- Further there is an average (normal) stress on the planes of maximum shear stress, given as

$$\sigma_{avg} = \left(\frac{\sigma_x + \sigma_y}{2}\right) \qquad \ldots \text{(Eq. 3.27c)}$$

This same normal stress acts on the planes of maximum negative shear stress.

Fig. 3.9(a) represents the principal stresses and its directions, while **Fig. 3.9(b)** represents maximum shear stress and its directions.

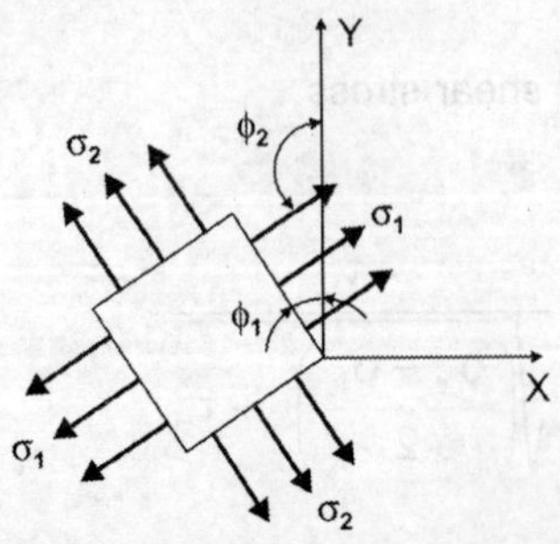

Fig. 3.9(a): Principal stresses and directions

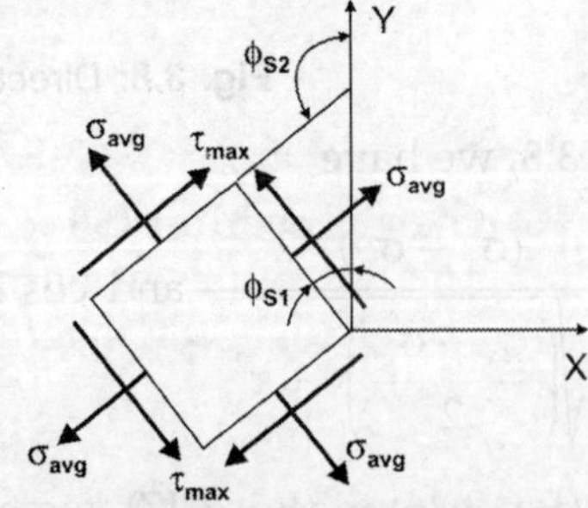

Fig. 3.9(b): Maximum shear and directions

Note:

→ Direction of principal stresses: $\phi_1 = \dfrac{1}{2} \tan^{-1}\left(\dfrac{2\tau_{xy}}{\sigma_x - \sigma_y}\right)$ ... using (Eq. 3.20b)

and $\phi_2 = \phi_1 + 90°$

→ Direction of shear stresses: $\phi_{s\,max} = \phi_{s1} = \dfrac{1}{2}\tan^{-1}\left[-\left(\dfrac{\sigma_x - \sigma_y}{2\tau_{xy}}\right)\right]$

... using (Eq. 3.25)

and $\phi_{s\,min} = \phi_{s2} = \phi_{s1} + 90°$

or $\phi_{s\,max} = \phi_{s1} = \phi_1 + 45°$

and $\phi_{s\,min} = \phi_{s2} = \phi_1 + 135°$

Fig. 3.9(c) gives information regarding planes and axes.

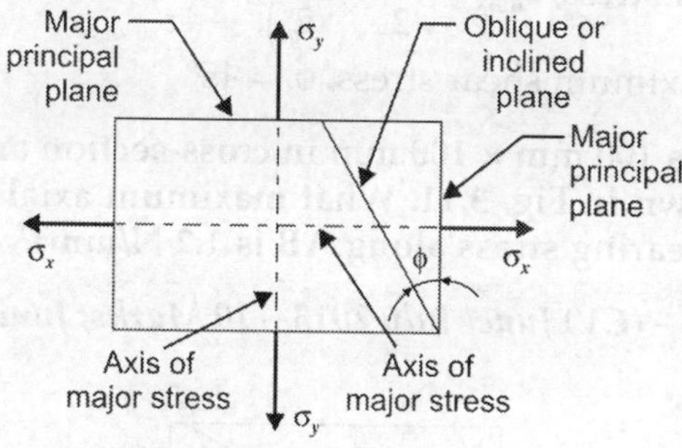

Fig. 3.9(c): Planes and axes

Application of Principal Stresses

- Plane stress is a common stress condition that exists in all ordinary structures, including buildings, machines, vehicles, and aircrafts, thin – walled spherical and cylindrical vessels, such as storage tanks containing compressed gases or liquids and in a wide variety of structures subjected to the combined effects of axial, shear, and bending loads, as well as internal pressure.
- Values of principal stresses at a given point are important in design of components. Material failure theories extensively use this data to predict whether the design would withstand the given load at a specified location.
- Fatigue failures of structures such as machines and aircraft are often associated with the maximum stresses, and hence their magnitudes and orientations should be determined as part of the design process.

Problems on uniaxial stress

1. **A rectangular bar of section (50 × 25) mm is subjected to a tensile load of 25 kN. Determine the values of normal and shear stresses on a plane 30° with the vertical. Also calculate the magnitude and direction of the maximum shear stress.**

Solution: $A = 50 \times 25 = 1250$ mm^2, $F = 25$ kN, $\sigma_n = ?$, $\tau = ?$, $\tau_{max} = ?$, $\phi = 30°$.

(a) Normal stress, $\sigma_n = \sigma_x \cos^2 \phi$

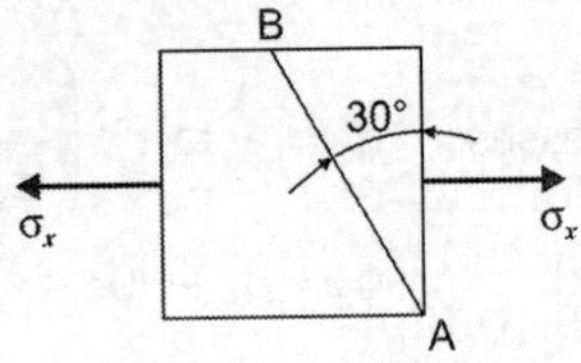

Fig. 3.10: Problem 1

$$\text{But} \quad \sigma_x = \frac{F}{A} = \frac{25000}{1250} = 20 \text{ MPa}$$

$$\sigma_n = 20 \times \cos^2(30) = 15 \text{ MPa}$$

(b) Shear stress, $\quad \tau = \dfrac{\sigma_x}{2} \sin 2\phi = \left(\dfrac{20}{2}\right) \sin (2 \times 30) = 8.66 \text{ MPa}$

(c) Maximum shear stress, $\tau_{\max} = \dfrac{\sigma_x}{2} = \dfrac{20}{2} = 10 \text{ MPa}$

(d) Direction of maximum shear stress, $\phi_s = 45°$

2. **Two wooden pieces 100 mm × 100 mm in cross-section are glued together along the line AB as shown in Fig. 3.11. What maximum axial force F can be applied if the allowable shearing stress along AB is 1.2 N/mm²?**

VTU – (CV) June/ July 2013 – 10 Marks; June/ July 2016 – 10 Marks

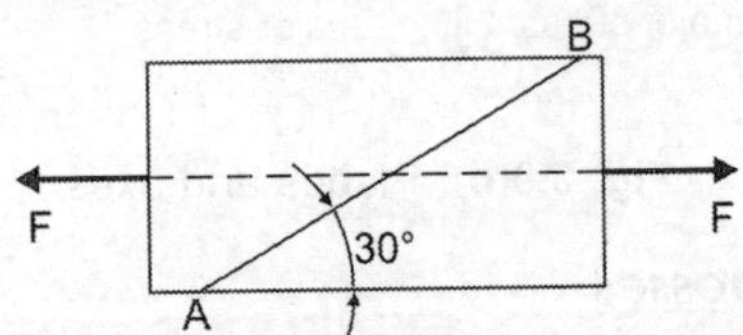

Fig. 3.11: Problem 2

Solution: $A = 100 \times 100 = 10000 \text{ mm}^2$, $F = ?$, $\tau_n = 1.2 \text{ MPa}$, $\phi' = 30°$ (with horizontal), $\phi = 60°$ (with vertical)

$$\text{We know that} \quad \tau = \frac{\sigma_x}{2} \sin 2\phi$$

$$1.2 = \left(\frac{\sigma_x}{2}\right) \sin(2 \times 60)$$

$$\sigma_x = 2.771 \text{ MPa}$$

$$\text{Also} \quad \sigma_x = F/A$$

$$2.771 = F/10000$$

$$F = 27.71 \times 10^3 \text{ N}$$

2A. **A circular bar of 20 mm diameter is subjected to compression. If the permissible stresses in compression and shear are 90 MPa and 25 MPa respectively, determine the failure load and plane.**

VTU – June/ July 2013 – 06 Marks

Solution: $d = 20$ mm $\Rightarrow A = \pi \times 20^2/4 = 314.16$ mm^2, $\sigma_c = 90$ MPa, $\tau = 25$ MPa.

We know that $\qquad \tau = \dfrac{\sigma_c}{2} = \dfrac{90}{2} = 45$ MPa

Since 45 MPa > 25 MPa, failure of the specimen occurs in shear. The failure surface is at 45° to the plane of axial stress.

Thus the corresponding safe compressive stress, $\sigma_c = 2 \times 25 = 50$ MPa
and the corresponding failure load, $F_c = \sigma_c.A = 50 \times 314.16 = 15708$ N $= 15.71$ kN

Problems on biaxial stress

3. **For the system shown in Fig. 3.12, determine:**
   (a) The normal and tangential stress intensities.
   (b) Magnitude and direction of resultant stress.
   (c) Maximum shear stress

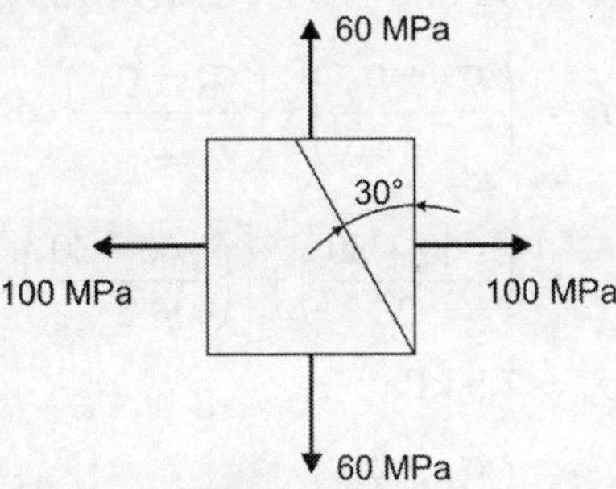

Fig. 3.12: Problem 3

Solution: $\sigma_x = 100$ MPa, $\sigma_y = 60$ MPa, $\phi = 30°$

  a. Normal and tangential stress intensities:

$$\text{Normal stress,} \quad \sigma_n = \left(\frac{\sigma_x + \sigma_y}{2}\right) + \left(\frac{\sigma_x - \sigma_y}{2}\right)\cos 2\phi$$

$$= \left(\frac{100 + 60}{2}\right) + \left[\left(\frac{100 - 60}{2}\right)\cos(2 \times 30)\right]$$

$$\sigma_n = 90\ \text{MPa}$$

$$\text{Tangential stress,}\ \tau = \left(\frac{\sigma_x - \sigma_y}{2}\right)\sin 2\phi = \left(\frac{100 - 60}{2}\right)\sin(2 \times 30) = 17.32\ \text{MPa}$$

  b. Magnitude and direction of resultant stress:

$$\text{Magnitude,} \quad \sigma_r = \sqrt{\sigma_n^2 + r^2} = \sqrt{90^2 + 17.32^2} = 91.65\ \text{MPa}$$

$$\text{Direction, } \tan\theta = \left(\frac{\sigma_n}{\tau}\right) = \left(\frac{90}{17.32}\right)$$

$$\theta = 79.11°$$

  c. Maximum shear stress, $\tau_{\max} = \dfrac{\sigma_x - \sigma_y}{2} = \dfrac{100 - 60}{2} = 20$ MPa

4. **The stresses acting in a strained material is as shown in Fig. 3.13. Find the normal and tangential stress acting on a plane AB.**

VTU – Dec. 14/ Jan. 15 – 05 Marks

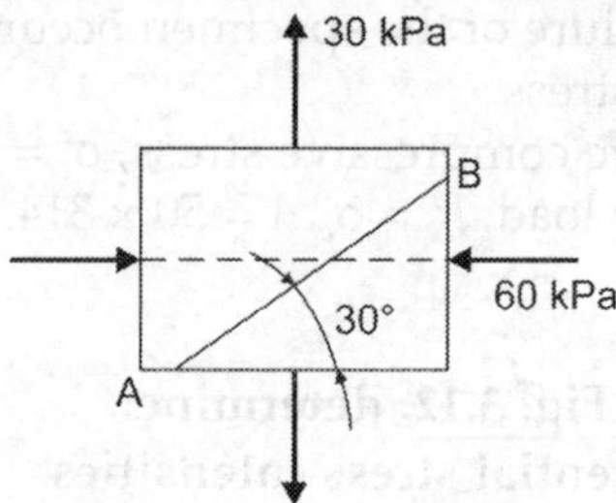

Fig. 3.13: Problem 4

Solution: $\sigma_x = -60$ kPa, $\sigma_y = 30$ kPa, $\phi' = 30°$ (with horizontal), $\phi = 60°$ (with vertical)

- Normal stress, $\quad \sigma_n = \left(\dfrac{\sigma_x + \sigma_y}{2}\right) + \left(\dfrac{\sigma_x - \sigma_y}{2}\right)\cos 2\phi$

$$= \left(\dfrac{-60 + 30}{2}\right) + \left[\left(\dfrac{-60 - 30}{2}\right)\cos(2 \times 60)\right]$$

$$\sigma_n = 7.5 \text{ kPa}$$

- Tangential stress, $\quad \tau = \left(\dfrac{\sigma_x - \sigma_y}{2}\right)\sin 2\phi$

$$= \left(\dfrac{-60 - 30}{2}\right)\sin(2 \times 60)$$

$$\tau = -38.97 \text{ kPa}$$

5. **Determine the magnitude and direction of resultant stresses on a plane inclined at an angle of 60° to major principal stress plane, when the bar is subjected to principal stresses at a point 200 MPa tensile and 100 MPa compressive. Also determine the resultant stress and its obliquity.**

VTU – (CV) June/ July 2016 – 06 Marks

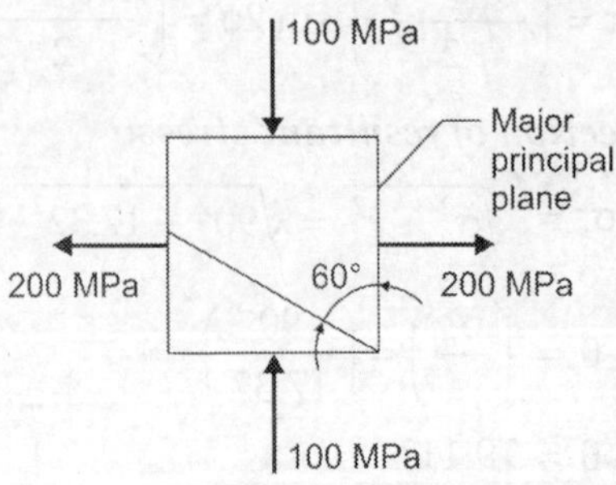

Fig. 3.14: Problem 5

Solution: $\sigma_x = 200$ MPa, $\sigma_y = -100$ MPa, $\phi = 60°$, $\sigma_r = ?$, $\theta = ?$, *a.* ***Resultant stress,*** $\sigma_r = \sqrt{\sigma_n^2 + \tau}$ ... Eq. (i)

But Normal stress, $\sigma_n = \left(\dfrac{\sigma_x + \sigma_y}{2}\right) + \left(\dfrac{\sigma_x - \sigma_y}{2}\right)\cos 2\phi$

$$= \left(\dfrac{200 - 100}{2}\right) + \left[\left(\dfrac{200 + 100}{2}\right)\cos(2 \times 60)\right]$$

$$\sigma_n = -2.5\,\text{MPa}$$

and tangential stress, $\tau = \left(\dfrac{\sigma_x - \sigma_y}{2}\right)\sin 2\phi$

$$= \left(\dfrac{200 + 100}{2}\right)\sin(2 \times 60) = 129.90\,\text{MPa}$$

$\therefore$ Eq. (i) yields... $\sigma_r = \sqrt{(-25)^2 + 129.90^2} = 132.28\,\text{MPa}$

b. ***Direction of resultant stress,*** $\tan\theta = \left(\dfrac{\sigma_n}{\tau}\right) = \left(\dfrac{-25}{129.90}\right)$

$$\theta = -10.81°$$

Problems on pure shear stress

6. **A rectangular block of material is subjected to a shear stress of 30 MPa together with its associated complementary shear stress. Determine the magnitude of the stresses on a plane inclined at 30° to the directions of the applied stresses, which may be taken as horizontal.**

Solution: $\tau_{xy} = 30$ MPa, $\phi' = 30°$ (with horizontal), $\tau = 60°$ (with vertical)

Normal stress, $\sigma_n = (\tau_{xy}\sin 2\phi) = 30 \times \sin(2 \times 60) = 25.98$ MPa

Tangential stress, $\tau = -\tau_{xy}\cos 2\phi = -30 \times \cos(2 \times 60) = 15$ MPa

Problems on generalized stress system

7. **Prove that the sum of normal stresses on any two mutually perpendicular planes is a constant in a general two-dimensional stress system.**

VTU – Dec.08/ Jan.09 – 07 Marks; Dec. 2011 – 06 Marks; June/ July 2013 – 08 Marks; Dec. 13/ Jan. 14 – 08 Marks; June/ July 2014 – 05 Marks; Dec. 14/ Jan. 15 – 08 Marks; (CV) May/ June 2010 – 06 Marks

Solution:

For a generalized system, Normal stress, $\sigma_n = \left(\dfrac{\sigma_x + \sigma_y}{2}\right) + \left(\dfrac{\sigma_x - \sigma_y}{2}\right)\cos 2\phi + \tau_{xy}\sin 2\phi,$

     ... Eq. (i)

where ϕ = inclination with the major principal plane

Let $(\phi + 90°)$ = inclination with the major principal plane and $\sigma_n{'}$ = Normal stress on the plane $(\phi + 90°)$

Then
$$\sigma_n' = \left(\frac{\sigma_x + \sigma_y}{2}\right) + \left(\frac{\sigma_x - \sigma_y}{2}\right)\cos(2\phi + 180°) + \tau_{xy}\sin(2 + 180°)$$

$$= \left(\frac{\sigma_x + \sigma_y}{2}\right) - \left(\frac{\sigma_x - \sigma_y}{2}\right)\cos 2\phi - \tau_{xy}\sin 2\phi \qquad \text{... Eq. (ii)}$$

Adding Eqs (i) and (ii), we have

$$\sigma_n + \sigma_n' = \left[\left(\frac{\sigma_x + \sigma_y}{2}\right) + \left(\frac{\sigma_x - \sigma_y}{2}\right)\cos 2\phi + \tau_{xy}\sin 2\phi\right]$$

$$+ \left[\left(\frac{\sigma_x + \sigma_y}{2}\right) - \left(\frac{\sigma_x - \sigma_y}{2}\right)\cos 2\phi - \tau_{xy}\sin 2\phi\right]$$

$$\sigma_n + \sigma_n' = 2\left(\frac{\sigma_x + \sigma_y}{2}\right)$$

$$\therefore \quad \sigma_n + \sigma_n' = \sigma_x + \sigma_y$$

Thus the sum of normal stresses on any two mutually perpendicular planes is a constant.

8. **Show that the principal planes are planes of maximum normal stress also. VTU**

June/ July 2014 – 05 Marks

Solution:

For a biaxial system, normal stress, $\sigma_n = \left(\frac{\sigma_x + \sigma_y}{2}\right) + \left(\frac{\sigma_x - \sigma_y}{2}\right)\cos 2\phi + \tau_{xy}\sin 2\phi$

$$\text{... Eq. (i)}$$

For maximum value of σ_n, differentiating Eq. (i) with respect to ϕ and equating to zero, we have

$$\left(\frac{d\sigma_n}{d\phi}\right) = 0$$

i.e. $\left(\frac{\sigma_x - \sigma_y}{2}\right)2(-\sin 2\phi) + \tau_{xy}2\cos 2\phi = 0$

i.e. $\left(\frac{\sigma_x - \sigma_y}{2}\right)\sin 2\phi - \tau_{xy}\cos 2\phi = 0$

Thus principal planes are planes of maximum normal stress

9. **The principal stresses at a point in a strained material are σ_x and σ_y. Show that the resultant stress σ_r on the plane carrying the maximum shear stress is**

$$\sigma_r = \sqrt{\frac{\sigma_x^2 + \sigma_y^2}{2}}$$

Solution:

We know that the resultant stress, $\sigma = \sqrt{\sigma_n^2 + \tau^2}$ $\qquad$ ... Eq. (i)

But normal stress, $\sigma_n = \left(\frac{\sigma_x + \sigma_y}{2}\right) + \left(\frac{\sigma_x - \sigma_y}{2}\right)\cos 2\phi + \tau_{xy}\sin 2\phi$

i.e.
$$\sigma_n = \left(\frac{\sigma_x + \sigma_y}{2}\right) + \left(\frac{\sigma_x - \sigma_y}{2}\right)\cos 2\phi \ \ (\text{since } \tau_{xy} = 0) \quad \dots \text{Eq. (ii)}$$

and shear stress,
$$\tau = \left(\frac{\sigma_x - \sigma_y}{2}\right)\sin 2\phi - \tau_{xy}\cos 2\phi$$

i.e.
$$\tau = \left(\frac{\sigma_x - \sigma_y}{2}\right)\sin 2\phi \qquad \dots \text{Eq. (iii)}$$

For maximum shear stress, $\phi = 45°$

$\therefore$ Eq. (i) yields…

$$\sigma_r = \sqrt{\left[\left(\frac{\sigma_x + \sigma_y}{2}\right) + \left(\frac{\sigma_x - \sigma_y}{2}\right)\cos(2 \times 45)\right]^2 + \left[\left(\frac{\sigma_x - \sigma_y}{2}\right)\sin(2 \times 45)\right]^2}$$

$$= \sqrt{\left(\frac{\sigma_x + \sigma_y}{2}\right)^2 + \left(\frac{\sigma_x - \sigma_y}{2}\right)^2}$$

i.e.
$$\sigma_r^2 = \frac{1}{4}\left(\sigma_x^2 + \sigma_y^2 + 2\sigma_x\sigma_y\right) + \frac{1}{4}\left(\sigma_x^2 + \sigma_y^2 - 2\sigma_x\sigma_y\right)$$

$$= \frac{1}{4}\left(2\sigma_x^2 + 2\sigma_y^2\right)$$

$$= \frac{1}{2}\left(\sigma_x^2 + \sigma_y^2\right)$$

$\therefore$
$$\sigma_r = \sqrt{\frac{\sigma_x^2 + \sigma_y^2}{2}}$$

10. At a point in a 2D stress system, the normal stresses on two mutually perpendicular planes are σ_x and σ_y (both alike) and the shear stress is τ_{xy}. If $\tau_{xy}^2 = \sigma_x \cdot \sigma_y$, show that one of the principal stresses is zero.

Solution:

We know that
$$\sigma_{1,2} = \left(\frac{\sigma_x + \sigma_y}{2}\right) \pm \sqrt{\left(\frac{\sigma_x + \sigma_y}{2}\right)^2 + \tau_{xy}^2}$$

$$= \left(\frac{\sigma_x + \sigma_y}{2}\right) \pm \sqrt{\frac{\sigma_x^2 + \sigma_y^2 - 2\sigma_x\sigma_y}{4} + \sigma_x\sigma_y}$$

$$= \left(\frac{\sigma_x + \sigma_y}{2}\right) \pm \sqrt{\frac{\sigma_x^2 + \sigma_y^2 - 2\sigma_x\sigma_y + 4\sigma_x\sigma_y}{4}}$$

$$= \left(\frac{\sigma_x + \sigma_y}{2}\right) \pm \sqrt{\frac{\sigma_x^2 + \sigma_y^2 + 2\sigma_x\sigma_y}{4}}$$

$$= \left(\frac{\sigma_x + \sigma_y}{2}\right) \pm \sqrt{\left(\frac{\sigma_x + \sigma_y}{2}\right)^2}$$

$$\sigma_{1,2} = \left(\frac{\sigma_x + \sigma_y}{2}\right) \pm \left(\frac{\sigma_x + \sigma_y}{2}\right)$$

$$\therefore \quad \sigma_1 = (\sigma_x + \sigma_y) \quad \text{and} \quad \sigma_2 = 0$$

11. A point in a plate girder is subjected to a horizontal tensile stress of 100 N/mm^2 and a vertical shear stress of 60 N/mm^2. Find the magnitude of principal stresses and its location.

VTU – Dec. 14/ Jan. 15 – 05 Marks

Solution: $\sigma_x = 100 \text{ N/mm}^2$, $\tau_{xy} = 60 \text{ N/mm}^2$, $\sigma_1 = ?$, $\sigma_2 = ?$, $\phi_1 = ?$, $\phi_2 = ?$,

- Maximum principal stress,

$$\sigma_1 = \left(\frac{\sigma_x + \sigma_y}{2}\right) + \sqrt{\left(\frac{\sigma_x - \sigma_y}{2}\right)^2 + \tau_{xy}^2}$$

$$= \left(\frac{100 + 0}{2}\right) + \sqrt{\left(\frac{100 - 0}{2}\right)^2 + 60^2}$$

$$\sigma_1 = 128.10 \text{ N/mm}^2$$

Minimum principal stress,

$$\sigma_1 = \left(\frac{\sigma_x + \sigma_y}{2}\right) - \sqrt{\left(\frac{\sigma_x - \sigma_y}{2}\right)^2 + \tau_{xy}^2}$$

$$= \left(\frac{100 + 0}{2}\right) - \sqrt{\left(\frac{100 - 0}{2}\right)^2 + 60^2}$$

$$\sigma_1 = -28.10 \text{ N/mm}^2$$

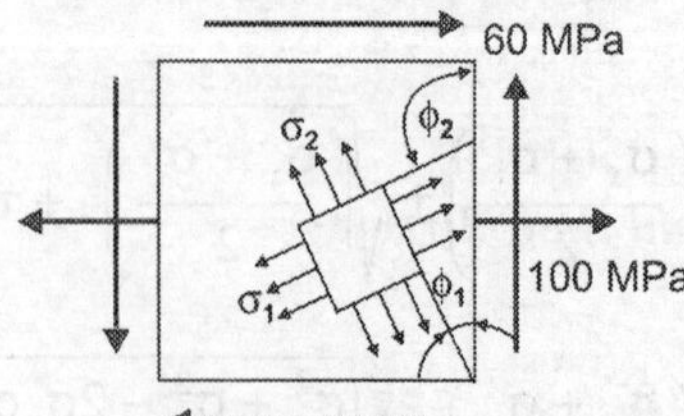

Fig. 3.15: Problem 11

Directions:

We know that
$$\tan 2\phi_1 = \left(\frac{2\tau_{xy}}{\sigma_x - \sigma_y}\right) = \left(\frac{2 \times 60}{100 - 0}\right) = 1.2$$

$$2\phi_1 = 50.19°$$
$$\therefore \quad \phi_1 = 25.09° \text{ and}$$
$$\phi_2 = \phi_1 + 90° = 25.09° + 90° = 115.09°$$

12. **An element is subjected to stresses as shown in Fig. 3.16. Determine**
    (a) Stress acting on the plane PP
    (b) Principal stresses and principal planes
    (c) Maximum shear stress and its plane

VTU – (CV) May/ June 2010 – 14 Marks

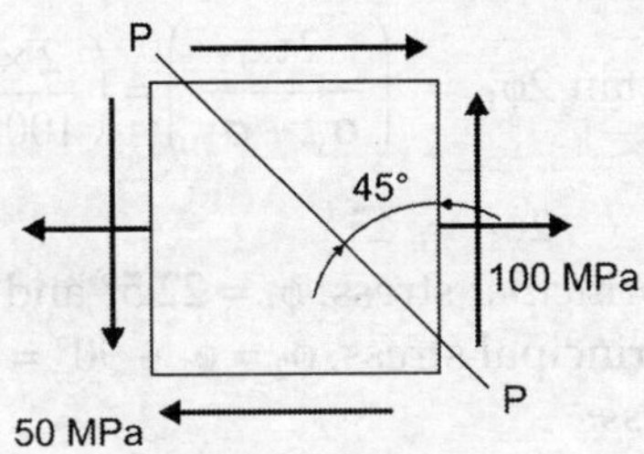

Fig. 3.16: Problem 12

Solution: $\sigma_x = 100$ MPa, $\tau_{xy} = 50$ MPa. a) $\sigma_n = ?$, $\tau = ?$ b) $\sigma_1 = ?$, $\sigma_2 = ?$, $\phi_1 = ?$, $\phi_2 = ?$
b) $\tau_{max} = ?$, $\phi_{s1} = ?$, $\phi_{s2} = ?$

  a. **Normal and tangential stress intensities:**

$$\text{Normal stress, } \sigma_n = \left(\frac{\sigma_x + \sigma_y}{2}\right) + \left(\frac{\sigma_x - \sigma_y}{2}\right)\cos 2\phi + \tau_{xy}\sin 2\phi$$

$$= \left(\frac{100 + 0}{2}\right) + \left[\left(\frac{100 - 0}{2}\right)\cos(2 \times 45)\right] + 50 \times \sin(2 \times 45)$$

$$\sigma_n = 100 \text{ MPa}$$

$$\text{Tangential stress, } \tau = \left(\frac{\sigma_x - \sigma_y}{2}\right)\sin 2\phi - \tau_{xy}\cos 2\phi$$

$$= \left[\left(\frac{100 - 0}{2}\right)\sin(2 \times 45)\right] - 50 \times \cos(2 \times 45)$$

$$\tau = 50 \text{ MPa}$$

  b. **Principal stresses and their directions:**

$$\text{Maximum principal stress, } \sigma_1 = \left(\frac{\sigma_x + \sigma_y}{2}\right) + \sqrt{\left(\frac{\sigma_x - \sigma_y}{2}\right)^2 + \tau_{xy}^2}$$

$$= \left(\frac{100 + 0}{2}\right) + \sqrt{\left(\frac{100 - 0}{2}\right)^2 + 50^2}$$

$$\sigma_1 = 120.71 \text{ MPa}$$

Minimum principal stress, $\sigma_2 = \left(\dfrac{\sigma_x + \sigma_y}{2}\right) - \sqrt{\left(\dfrac{\sigma_x - \sigma_y}{2}\right)^2 + \tau_{xy}^2}$

$$= \left(\dfrac{100 + 0}{2}\right) - \sqrt{\left(\dfrac{100 - 0}{2}\right)^2 + 50^2}$$

$$\sigma_2 = -20.71 \text{ MPa}$$

Directions:

We know that $\quad \tan 2\phi_1 = \left(\dfrac{2\tau_{xy}}{\sigma_x - \sigma_y}\right) = \left(\dfrac{2 \times 50}{100 - 0}\right) = 1$

$$2\phi_1 = 45°$$

Direction of maximum principal stress, $\phi_1 = 22.5°$ and
Direction of minimum principal stress, $\phi_2 = \phi_1 + 90° = 22.5° + 90° = 112.5°$

c. ***Maximum shear stress:***

Maximum shear stress,

$$\tau_{max} = \pm \sqrt{\left(\dfrac{\sigma_x - \sigma_y}{2}\right)^2 + \tau_{xy}^2} = \sqrt{\left(\dfrac{100 - 0}{2}\right)^2 + 50^2} = \pm 70.71 \text{ MPa}$$

Directions:

We know that $\quad \tan 2\phi_s = -\left(\dfrac{\sigma_x - \sigma_y}{2\tau_{xy}}\right) = -\left(\dfrac{100 - 0}{2 \times 50}\right) = -1$

$$2\phi_s = -45°$$

Direction of maximum shear stress, $\phi_{s1} = -22.5°$ and
Direction of minimum shear stress, $\phi_{s2} = \phi_1 + 90° = -22.5° + 90° = 67.5°$

13. The state of stress at a point in a structural member is as shown in Fig. 3.17. The tensile principal stress is known to be 84 MPa. Determine:
(a) The maximum shear stress at the point and orientation of its plane.
(b) The shearing stress τ_{xy}.

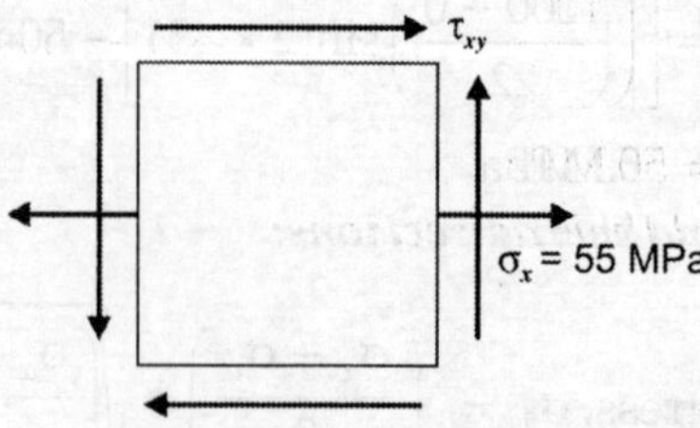

Fig. 3.17: Problem 13

Solution: $\sigma_x = 55$ MPa, $\sigma_1 = 84$ MPa $\quad$ a) $\tau_{max} = ?$, $\phi_s = ?$ b) $\tau_{xy} = ?$

b. ***Shear stress τ_{xy}:***

Maximum principal stress, $\sigma_1 = \left(\dfrac{\sigma_x + \sigma_y}{2}\right) + \sqrt{\left(\dfrac{\sigma_x - \sigma_y}{2}\right)^2 + \tau_{xy}^2}$

$$84 = \left(\frac{55 + 0}{2}\right) + \sqrt{\left(\frac{55 - 0}{2}\right)^2 + \tau_{xy}^2}$$

$$\therefore \quad \tau_{xy} = 49.36 \text{ MPa}$$

a. Maximum shear stress and orientation of its plane:

Maximum shear stress, $\tau_{max} = \pm \sqrt{\left(\dfrac{\sigma_x - \sigma_y}{2}\right)^2 + \tau_{xy}^2} = \sqrt{\left(\dfrac{55 - 0}{2}\right)^2 + (49.36)^2}$

$$= \pm 56.50 \text{ MPa}$$

Shear stress directions:

We know that $\quad \tan 2\phi_s = -\left(\dfrac{\sigma_x - \sigma_y}{2\tau_{xy}}\right) = -\left(\dfrac{55 - 0}{2 \times 49.36}\right) = -0.56$

$$2\phi_s = -29.13°$$

$$\therefore \quad \phi_{s1} = -14.56° \text{ and } \phi_{s2} = \phi_1 + 90° = -14.56° + 90° = 75.44°$$

14. **A direct stresses of 120 MPa in tension and 90 MPa in compression are applied to an elastic material at a certain point on the planes at right angles. The maximum principal stress is 150 MPa. What is the corresponding shear stress on the given planes and what will be the maximum shearing stress at that point?**

VTU – (CV) Dec.07/ Jan.08 – 12 Marks

Solution: $\sigma_x = 120$ MPa, $\sigma_y = -90$ MPa, $\sigma_1 = 150$ N/mm^2 a) $\tau_{xy} = ?$, b) $\tau_{max} = ?$

b. Shear stress τ_{xy}:

Maximum principal stress, $\sigma_1 = \left(\dfrac{\sigma_x + \sigma_y}{2}\right) + \sqrt{\left(\dfrac{\sigma_x - \sigma_y}{2}\right)^2 + \tau_{xy}^2}$

$$150 = \left(\frac{120 - 90}{2}\right) + \sqrt{\left(\frac{120 + 90}{2}\right)^2 + \tau_{xy}^2}$$

$$\therefore \quad \tau_{xy} = 84.85 \text{ MPa}$$

a. Maximum shear stress:

Maximum shear stress,

$$\tau_{max} = \sqrt{\left(\frac{\sigma_x - \sigma_y}{2}\right)^2 + \tau_{xy}^2} = \pm \sqrt{\left(\frac{120 + 90}{2}\right)^2 + (84.85)^2} = \pm 135 \text{ MPa}$$

15. **The state of stress at a point in a strained material is as shown in Fig. 3.18. Determine:**
    (a) The direction of principal planes.
    (b) The magnitude of principal stresses
    (c) The magnitude of maximum shear stress and its direction. Indicate all the above planes by a sketch.

VTU – Dec. 2011 – 10 Marks; (CV) Dec. 2012 – 10 Marks

Solution: $\sigma_x = 180$ MPa, $\sigma_y = 120$ MPa, $\tau_{xy} = 80$ MPa. a) $\phi_1 = ?$, $\phi_2 = ?$, b) $\sigma_1 = ?$, $\sigma_2 = ?$, c) $\tau_{max} = ?$, $\phi_{s1} = ?$, $\phi_{s2} = ?$

a. Direction of principal planes:

We know that $\quad \tan 2\phi_1 = \left(\dfrac{2\tau_{xy}}{\sigma_x - \sigma_y}\right) = \left(\dfrac{2 \times 30}{180 - 120}\right) = 2.67$

$$2\phi_1 = 69.44°$$
$$\therefore \quad \phi_1 = 34.72° \text{ and}$$
$$\phi_2 = \phi_1 + 90° = 34.72° + 90° = 124.72°$$

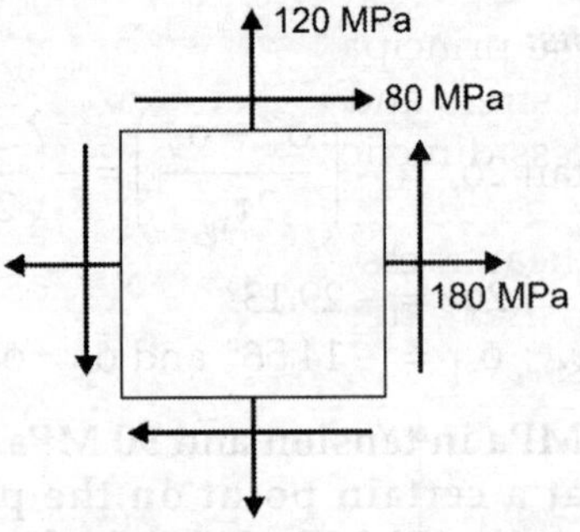

Fig. 3.18(a): Problem 15

b. Principal stresses:

Maximum principal stress, $\quad \sigma_1 = \left(\dfrac{\sigma_x + \sigma_y}{2}\right) + \sqrt{\left(\dfrac{\sigma_x - \sigma_y}{2}\right)^2 + \tau_{xy}^2}$

$$= \left(\dfrac{180 + 120}{2}\right) + \sqrt{\left(\dfrac{180 - 120}{2}\right)^2 + 80^2}$$

$$\therefore \quad \sigma_1 = 235.44 \text{ MPa}$$

Minimum principal stress, $\quad \sigma_2 = \left(\dfrac{\sigma_x + \sigma_y}{2}\right) - \sqrt{\left(\dfrac{\sigma_x - \sigma_y}{2}\right)^2 + \tau_{xy}^2}$

$$= \left(\dfrac{180 + 120}{2}\right) + \sqrt{\left(\dfrac{180 - 120}{2}\right)^2 + 80^2}$$

$$\therefore \quad \sigma_2 = 64.56 \text{ MPa}$$

c. Maximum shear stress and orientation of its plane:

Maximum shear stress, $\quad \tau_{max} = \pm\sqrt{\left(\dfrac{\sigma_x - \sigma_y}{2}\right)^2 + \tau_{xy}^2}$

$$= \pm\sqrt{\left(\dfrac{180 - 120}{2}\right)^2 + 80^2}$$

$$\tau_{max} = \pm 85.44 \text{ MPa}$$

Average (normal) stress on the planes of maximum shear stress is,

$$\sigma_{avg} = \left(\frac{\sigma_x + \sigma_y}{2}\right) = \frac{180 + 120}{2} = 150 \, MPa$$

Shear stress directions:

$$We \ know \ that \quad \tan 2\phi_s = -\left(\frac{\sigma_x - \sigma_y}{2\tau_{xy}}\right) = -\left(\frac{180 - 120}{2 \times 80}\right) = -0.375$$

$$2\phi_s = -20.56°$$

$$\therefore \quad \phi_{s1} = -10.28° \ and \ \phi_{s2} = \phi_{s1} + 90 = -10.28° + 90° = 79.72°$$

Fig. 3.18(b) represents the principal stresses and its directions, while **Fig. 3.18(c)** represents maximum shear stress and its directions.

The maximum shear stress directions shown in **Fig. 3.18(d)** can also be found as follows:

Direction of maximum shear stress, $\phi_{s1} = \phi_1 + 45° = 34.72° + 45° = 79.72°$

Direction of minimum shear stress, $\phi_{s2} = \phi_1 + 135° = 34.72° + 135° = 169.72°$ [or $\phi_{s1} + 90°$]

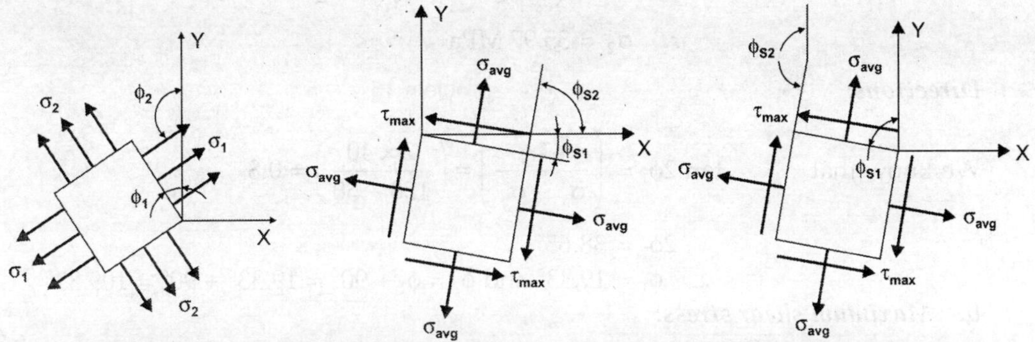

Fig. 3.18(b): Problem 15　　**Fig. 3.18(c): Problem 15**　or　**Fig. 3.18(d): Problem 15**

Principal stresses and direction　　**Principal stresses and direction**

16. **An element is subjected to stresses as shown in Fig. 3.19. Determine a) Principal stresses and principal planes b) maximum shear stress and its plane.**

VTU – (CV) June/ July 2013 – 10 Marks; [Similar (CV): June/ July 2014 – 12 Marks; Jan. 2013 – 10 Marks]

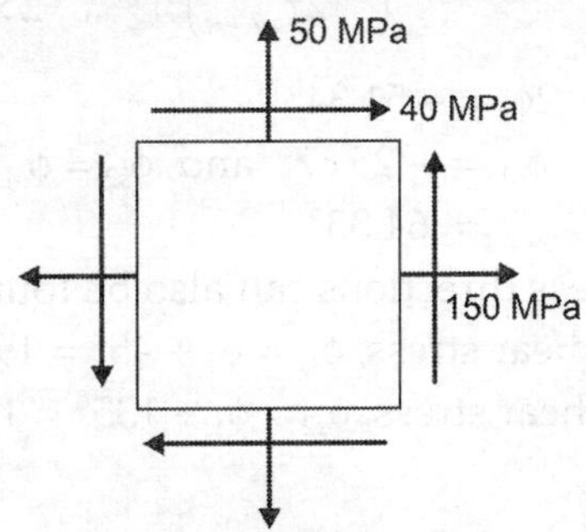

Fig. 3.19: Problem 16

Solution: $\sigma_x = 150$ MPa, $\sigma_y = 50$ MPa, $\tau_{xy} = 40$ MPa. a) $\sigma_1 = ?$, $\sigma_2 = ?$, $\phi_1 = ?$, $\phi_2 = ?$, b) $\sigma_{max} = ?$, $\phi_{s1} = ?$, $\phi_{s2} = ?$

a. Principal stresses and their directions:

Maximum principal stress, $\quad \sigma_1 = \left(\dfrac{\sigma_x + \sigma_y}{2}\right) + \sqrt{\left(\dfrac{\sigma_x - \sigma_y}{2}\right)^2 + \tau_{xy}^2}$

$$= \left(\frac{150 + 50}{2}\right) + \sqrt{\left(\frac{150 - 50}{2}\right)^2 + 40^2}$$

$$\therefore \quad \sigma_1 = 164.03 \text{ MPa}$$

Minimum principal stress, $\quad \sigma_2 = \left(\dfrac{\sigma_x + \sigma_y}{2}\right) - \sqrt{\left(\dfrac{\sigma_x - \sigma_y}{2}\right)^2 + \tau_{xy}^2}$

$$= \left(\frac{150 + 50}{2}\right) - \sqrt{\left(\frac{150 - 50}{2}\right)^2 + 40^2}$$

$$\therefore \quad \sigma_2 = 35.97 \text{ MPa}$$

Directions:

We know that $\qquad \tan 2\phi_1 = \left(\dfrac{2\tau_{xy}}{\sigma_x - \sigma_y}\right) = \left(\dfrac{2 \times 40}{150 - 50}\right) = 0.8$

$$2\phi_1 = 38.65°$$
$$\therefore \quad \phi_1 = 19.33° \text{ and } \phi_2 = \phi_1 + 90° = 19.33° + 90° = 109.33°$$

b. Maximum shear stress:

Maximum shear stress, $\quad \tau_{max} = \sqrt{\left(\dfrac{\sigma_x - \sigma_y}{2}\right)^2 + \tau_{xy}^2} = \pm\sqrt{\left(\dfrac{150 - 50}{2}\right)^2 + 40^2}$

$$= \pm 64.03 \text{ MPa}$$

Directions:

We know that $\qquad \tan 2\phi_s = -\left(\dfrac{\sigma_x - \sigma_y}{2\tau_{xy}}\right) = -\left(\dfrac{150 - 50}{2 \times 40}\right) = -1.25$

$$2\phi_s = -51.34°$$
$$\therefore \quad \phi_{s1} = -25.67° \text{ and } \phi_{s2} = \phi_{s1} + 90° = -25.67° + 90°$$
$$= 64.33°$$

The maximum shear stress directions can also be found as:

Direction of maximum shear stress, $\phi_{s1} = \phi_1 + 45° = 19.33° + 45° = 64.33°$

Direction of minimum shear stress, $\phi_{s2} = \phi_1 + 135° = 19.33° + 135° = 154.33°$
[or $\phi_{s1} + 90°$]

17. A rectangular block of material is subjected to a tensile stress of 100 N/mm² on one plane and tensile stress of 47 N/mm² on the plane at right angle to the first as shown in Fig. 3.20(a). Each of the above stresses is accompanied by a shear stress of 63 N/mm². Determine the magnitude and direction of each principal stress and magnitude of maximum shear stress. Sketch the planes and mark the stresses on the planes.

VTU – June 2012 – 06 Marks

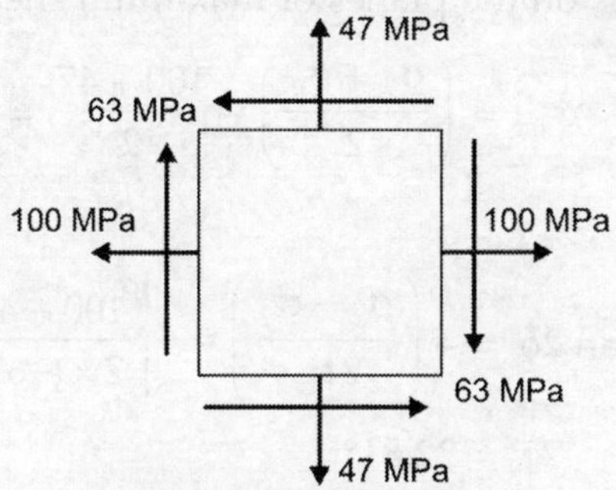

Fig. 3.20(a): Problem 17

Solution: $\sigma_x = 100$ MPa, $\sigma_y = 47$ MPa, $\tau_{xy} = -63$ MPa. a) $\sigma_1 = ?$, $\sigma_2 = ?$, $\phi_1 = ?$, $\phi_2 = ?$, b) $\tau_{max} = ?$, $\phi_{s1} = ?$, $\phi_{s2} = ?$

a. Principal stresses and their directions:

Maximum principal stress,

$$\sigma_1 = \left(\frac{\sigma_x + \sigma_y}{2}\right) + \sqrt{\left(\frac{\sigma_x - \sigma_y}{2}\right)^2 + \tau_{xy}^2}$$

$$= \left(\frac{100 + 47}{2}\right) + \sqrt{\left(\frac{100 - 47}{2}\right)^2 + (-63)^2}$$

$$\therefore \quad \sigma_1 = 141.85 \text{ MPa}$$

Minimum principal stress,

$$\sigma_2 = \left(\frac{\sigma_x + \sigma_y}{2}\right) - \sqrt{\left(\frac{\sigma_x - \sigma_y}{2}\right)^2 + \tau_{xy}^2}$$

$$= \left(\frac{100 + 47}{2}\right) - \sqrt{\left(\frac{100 - 47}{2}\right)^2 + (-63)^2}$$

$$\therefore \quad \sigma_2 = 5.15 \text{ MPa}$$

Directions:

We know that

$$\tan 2\phi_1 = \left(\frac{2\tau_{xy}}{\sigma_x - \sigma_y}\right) = \left[\frac{2 \times (-63)}{100 - 47}\right] = -2.38$$

$$2\phi_1 = -67.21°$$

$$\therefore \quad \phi_1 = -33.60° \text{ and } \phi_2 = \phi_1 + 90° = -33.60° + 90° = 56.40°$$

b. Maximum shear stress:

$$2\phi_s = 22.81°$$

Maximum shear stress, $\tau_{max} = \pm\sqrt{\left(\dfrac{\sigma_x - \sigma_y}{2}\right)^2 + \tau_{xy}^2} = \pm\sqrt{\left(\dfrac{100 - 47}{2}\right)^2 + (-63)^2}$

$$= \pm 68.35 \text{ MPa}$$

Average (normal) stress on the planes of maximum shear stress is,

$$\sigma_{avg} = \left(\frac{\sigma_x + \sigma_y}{2}\right) = \frac{100 + 47}{2} = 73.5 \text{ MPa}$$

Directions:

We know that $\qquad \tan 2\phi_s = -\left(\dfrac{\sigma_x - \sigma_y}{2\tau_{xy}}\right) = -\left[\dfrac{100 - 47}{2\times(-63)}\right] = 0.42$

$$2\phi_s = 22.81°$$
$$\therefore \quad \phi_{s1} = 11.41° \text{ and}$$
$$\phi_{s2} = \phi_{s1} + 90° = 11.41° + 90° = 101.41°$$

Fig. 3.20(b) represents the principal stresses and its directions and **Fig. 3.20(c)** represents the maximum shear stress and its directions

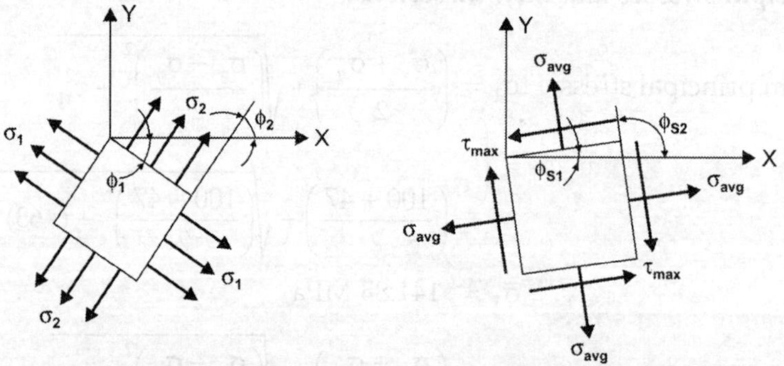

Fig. 3.20(b): Problem 17 **Fig. 3.20(c): Problem 17**
Principal stresses and directions **Maximum shear stress and directions**

18. At a certain point in a strained material the value of normal stresses across two planes at right angles to each other are 80 MPa and 32 MPa, both tensile and there is a shear stress of 32 MPa clockwise on the plane carrying 80 MPa stresses across the planes as shown in Fig. 3.21(a). Determine:
    (a) Maximum and minimum normal stresses and locate their planes.
    (b) Maximum shear stress and specify its plane.

VTU – Dec. 15/ Jan. 16 – 10 Marks; June/ July 2013 – 12 Marks

Solution: $\sigma_x = 80$ MPa, $\sigma_y = 32$ MPa, $\tau_{xy} = -32$ MPa. a) $\sigma_1 = ?$, $\sigma_2 = ?$, $\phi_1 = ?$, $\phi_2 = ?$,
b) $\tau_{max} = ?$, $\phi_{s1} = ?$, $\phi_{s2} = ?$

a. Maximum principal stress, $\sigma_1 = \left(\dfrac{\sigma_x + \sigma_y}{2}\right) + \sqrt{\left(\dfrac{\sigma_x - \sigma_y}{2}\right)^2 + \tau_{xy}^2}$

Fig. 3.21(a): Problem 18

$$= \left(\frac{80 + 32}{2} \right) + \sqrt{\left(\frac{80 - 32}{2} \right)^2 + (-32)^2}$$

$$\therefore \quad \sigma_1 = 96 \, \text{MPa}$$

Minimum principal stress, $\quad \sigma_2 = \left(\frac{\sigma_x + \sigma_y}{2} \right) - \sqrt{\left(\frac{\sigma_x - \sigma_y}{2} \right)^2 + \tau_{xy}^2}$

$$= \left(\frac{80 + 32}{2} \right) - \sqrt{\left(\frac{80 - 32}{2} \right)^2 + (-32)^2}$$

$$\therefore \quad \sigma_2 = 16 \, \text{MPa}$$

Directions:

We know that $\quad \tan 2\phi_1 = \left(\frac{2\tau_{xy}}{\sigma_x - \sigma_y} \right) = \left[\frac{2 \times (-32)}{80 - 32} \right] = -1.34$

$$2\phi_1 = -53.13°$$
$$\therefore \quad \phi_1 = -26.57° \quad \text{and} \quad \phi_2 = \phi_1 + 90° = -26.57° + 90° = 63.43°$$

b. *Maximum shear stress:*

Maximum shear stress, $\tau_{\max} = \pm \sqrt{\left(\frac{\sigma_x - \sigma_y}{2} \right)^2 + \tau_{xy}^2} = \pm \sqrt{\left(\frac{80 - 32}{2} \right)^2 + (-32)^2}$

$$= \pm 40 \, \text{MPa}$$

Average (normal) stress on the planes of maximum shear stress is,

$$\sigma_{avg} = \left(\frac{\sigma_x + \sigma_y}{2} \right) = \frac{80 + 32}{2} = 56 \, \text{MPa}$$

Directions:

We know that $\quad \tan 2\phi_s = -\left(\frac{\sigma_x - \sigma_y}{2\tau_{xy}} \right) = -\left[\frac{80 - 32}{2 \times (-32)} \right] = 0.75$

$$2\phi_s = 36.86°$$
$$\therefore \quad \phi_{s1} = 18.43° \quad \text{and}$$
$$\phi_{s2} = \phi_{s1} + 90° = 18.43° + 90° = 108.43°$$

Fig. 3.21(b) represents the principal stresses and its directions and **Fig. 3.21(c)** represents the maximum shear stress and its directions

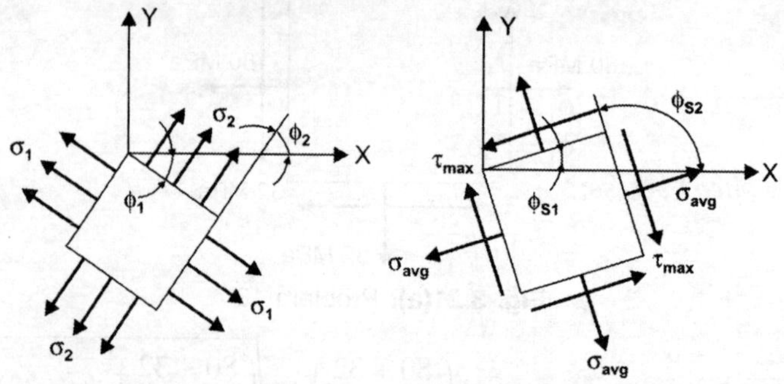

Fig. 3.21(b): Problem 18   **Fig. 3.21(c): Problem 18**

Principal stresses and directions   **Maximum shear stress and directions**

19. **A plane element is subjected to stresses as shown in Fig. 3.22(a). Determine principal stresses, maximum shear stress and their planes. Sketch the planes determined.**

VTU – Dec.08/ Jan.09 – 07 Marks

Solution: $\sigma_x = 60$ MPa, $\sigma_y = -40$ MPa, $\tau_{xy} = 10$ MPa. a) $\sigma_1 = ?$, $\sigma_2 = ?$, $\phi_1 = ?$, $\phi_2 = ?$, b) $\tau_{max} = ?$, $\phi_{s1} = ?$, $\phi_{s2} = ?$

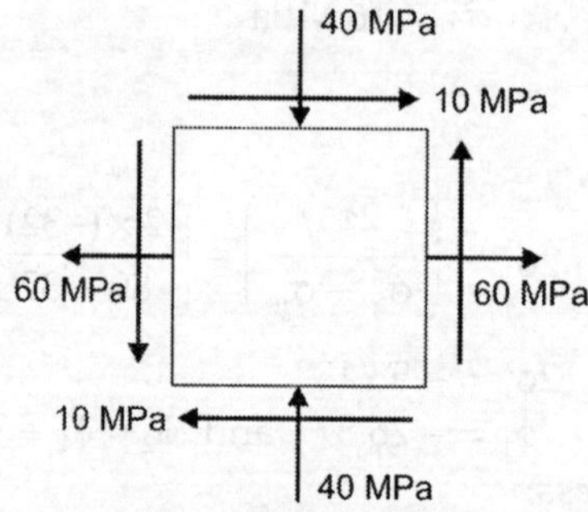

Fig. 3.22(a): Problem 19

a. Principal stresses and their directions:

Maximum principal stress, $\sigma_1 = \left(\dfrac{\sigma_x + \sigma_y}{2}\right) + \sqrt{\left(\dfrac{\sigma_x - \sigma_y}{2}\right)^2 + \tau_{xy}^2}$

$$= \left(\frac{60 - 40}{2}\right) + \sqrt{\left(\frac{60 + 40}{2}\right)^2 + 10^2}$$

$$\therefore \quad \sigma_1 = 61 \text{ MPa}$$

Minimum principal stress, $\sigma_2 = \left(\dfrac{\sigma_x + \sigma_y}{2}\right) - \sqrt{\left(\dfrac{\sigma_x - \sigma_y}{2}\right)^2 + \tau_{xy}^2}$

$$= \left(\frac{60 - 40}{2}\right) - \sqrt{\left(\frac{60 + 40}{2}\right)^2 + 10^2}$$

$$\therefore \quad \sigma_2 = -41 \text{ MPa}$$

Directions:

We know that $\tan 2\phi_1 = \left(\dfrac{2\tau_{xy}}{\sigma_x - \sigma_y}\right) = \left(\dfrac{2 \times 10}{60 + 40}\right) = 0.20$

$$2\phi_1 = 11.31°$$
$$\therefore \quad \phi_1 = 5.65° \text{ and } \phi_2 = \phi_1 + 90° = 5.65° + 90° = 95.65°$$

b. *Maximum shear stress:*

Maximum shear stress, $\tau_{max} = \pm\sqrt{\left(\dfrac{\sigma_x - \sigma_y}{2}\right)^2 + \tau_{xy}^2} = \pm\sqrt{\left(\dfrac{60 + 40}{2}\right)^2 + 10^2}$

$$= \pm\, 51 \text{ MPa}$$

Average (normal) stress on the planes of maximum shear stress is,

$$\sigma_{avg} = \left(\dfrac{\sigma_x + \sigma_y}{2}\right) = \dfrac{60 - 40}{2} = 10 \text{ MPa}$$

Directions:

We know that $\tan 2\phi_s = -\left(\dfrac{\sigma_x - \sigma_y}{2\tau_{xy}}\right) = -\left[\dfrac{60 - (-40)}{2 \times 10}\right] = -5$

$$2\phi_s = -78.69°$$
$$\therefore \quad \phi_{s1} = -39.35° \text{ and}$$
$$\phi_{s2} = \phi_{s1} + 90° = -39.35° + 90° = 50.65°$$

Fig. 3.22(b) represents the principal stresses and its directions and **Fig. 3.22(c)** represents the maximum shear stress and its directions

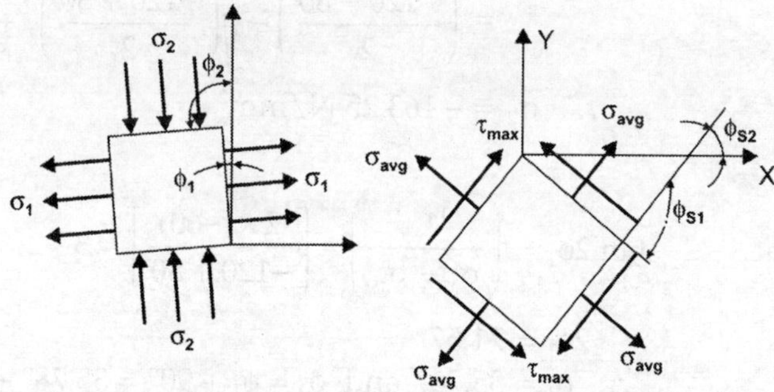

Fig. 3.22(b): Problem 19   **Fig. 3.22(c): Problem 19**

Principal stresses and directions   **Maximum shear stress and directions**

20. **The state of stress in two-dimensional stressed body is as shown in Fig. 3.23. Determine the principal planes, principal stresses, maximum shear stress and their planes.**

> *VTU – June/ July 2008 – 12 Marks; May/ June 2010 – 15 Marks; Dec. 2012 – 20 Marks; June/ July 2014 – 10 Marks; (CV) Dec. 2011 – 14 Marks; [Similar: (CV) Dec.08/ Jan.09 – 10 Marks; (CV) June 2012 – 10 Marks]*

Solution: $\sigma_x = -120 \text{ N/mm}^2$, $\sigma_y = -80 \text{ N/mm}^2$, $\tau_{xy} = -60 \text{ N/mm}^2$. a) $\sigma_1 = ?$, $\sigma_2 = ?$, $\phi_1 = ?$, $\phi_2 = ?$, b) $\tau_{max} = ?$, $\phi_{s1} = ?$, $\phi_{s2} = ?$

a. Principal stresses and their directions:

Maximum principal stress, $\sigma_1 = \left(\dfrac{\sigma_x + \sigma_y}{2}\right) + \sqrt{\left(\dfrac{\sigma_x - \sigma_y}{2}\right)^2 + \tau_{xy}^2}$

$$= \left(\dfrac{-120 - 80}{2}\right) + \sqrt{\left(\dfrac{-120 + 80}{2}\right)^2 + (-60)^2}$$

$$\therefore \quad \sigma_1 = -36.75 \text{ N/mm}^2$$

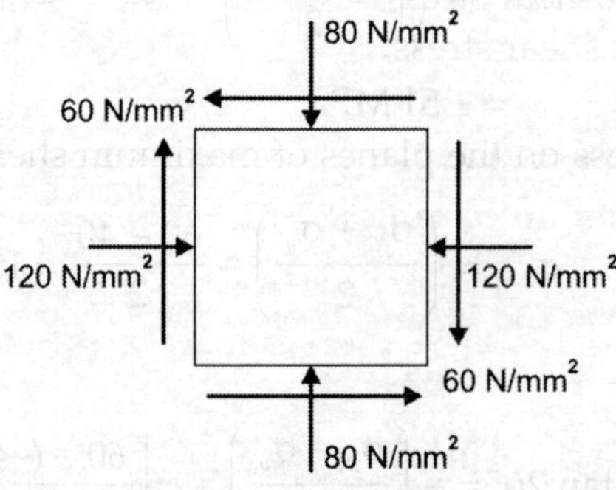

Fig. 3.23: Problem 20

Minimum principal stress, $\sigma_2 = \left(\dfrac{\sigma_x + \sigma_y}{2}\right) - \sqrt{\left(\dfrac{\sigma_x - \sigma_y}{2}\right)^2 + \tau_{xy}^2}$

$$= \left(\dfrac{-120 - 80}{2}\right) - \sqrt{\left(\dfrac{-120 + 80}{2}\right)^2 + (-60)^2}$$

$$\therefore \quad \sigma_2 = -163.25 \text{ N/mm}^2$$

Directions:

We know that $\qquad \tan 2\phi_1 = \left(\dfrac{2\tau_{xy}}{\sigma_x - \sigma_y}\right) = \left[\dfrac{2 \times (-60)}{-120 + 80}\right] = 3$

$$2\phi_1 = 71.57°$$
$$\therefore \quad \phi_1 = 35.78° \text{ and } \phi_2 = \phi_1 + 90° = 35.78° + 90° = 125.78°$$

b. Maximum shear stress:

Maximum shear stress, $\tau_{max} = \pm \sqrt{\left(\dfrac{\sigma_x - \sigma_y}{2}\right)^2 + \tau_{xy}^2} = \pm \sqrt{\left(\dfrac{-120 + 80}{2}\right)^2 + (-60)^2}$

$$= \pm 63.25 \text{ N/mm}^2$$

Average (normal) stress on the planes of maximum shear stress is,

$$\sigma_{avg} = \left(\dfrac{\sigma_x + \sigma_y}{2}\right) = \dfrac{-120 - 80}{2} = -100 \text{ N/mm}^2$$

Directions:

We know that
$$\tan 2\phi_s = -\left(\frac{\sigma_x - \sigma_y}{2\tau_{xy}}\right) = -\left[\frac{-120 + 80}{2 \times (-60)}\right] = -0.33$$

$$2\phi_s = -18.43°$$
$$\therefore \phi_{s1} = -9.22° \text{ and}$$
$$\phi_{s2} = \phi_{s1} + 90° = -9.22° + 90° = 80.78°$$

The maximum shear stress directions can also be found as:

Direction of maximum shear stress, $\phi_{s1} = \phi_1 + 45° = 35.78° + 45° = 80.78°$

Direction of minimum shear stress, $\phi_{s2} = \phi_1 + 135° = 35.78° + 135° = 170.78°$
[or $\phi_{s1} + 90°$]

21. **A point in a structural member is subjected to plane state of stress as shown in Fig. 3.24. Determine the following:**
    (a) Normal and tangential stress intensities.
    (b) Principal stresses σ_1 and σ_2 and their directions.
    (c) Maximum shear stress and its plane.

Solution: $\sigma_x = 40$ MPa, $\sigma_y = -30$ MPa, $\tau_{xy} = 25$ MPa, $\phi = 45°$, a) $\sigma_n = ?$, $\tau = ?$ b) $\sigma_1 = ?$, $\sigma_2 = ?$, $\phi_1 = ?$, $\phi_2 = ?$ b) $\tau_{max} = ?$, $\phi_{s1} = ?$, $\phi_{s2} = ?$

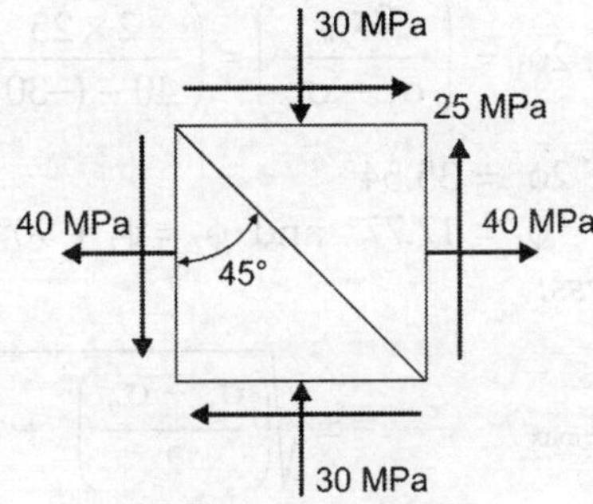

Fig. 3.24: Problem 21

a. Normal and tangential stress intensities:

Normal stress,
$$\sigma_n = \left(\frac{\sigma_x + \sigma_y}{2}\right) + \left(\frac{\sigma_x - \sigma_y}{2}\right)\cos 2\phi + \tau_{xy}\sin 2\phi$$

$$= \left(\frac{40 - 30}{2}\right) + \left[\left(\frac{40 + 30}{2}\right)\cos(2 \times 45)\right] + 25 \times \sin(2 \times 45)$$

$$\sigma_n = 30 \text{ MPa}$$

Tangential stress,
$$\tau = \left(\frac{\sigma_x - \sigma_y}{2}\right)\sin 2\phi - \tau_{xy}\cos 2\phi$$

$$= \left[\left(\frac{40 + 30}{2}\right)\sin(2 \times 45)\right] - 25 \times \cos(2 \times 45)$$

$$\tau = 35 \text{ MPa}$$

b. *Principal stresses and their directions:*

Maximum principal stress, $\quad \sigma_1 = \left(\dfrac{\sigma_x + \sigma_y}{2}\right) + \sqrt{\left(\dfrac{\sigma_x - \sigma_y}{2}\right)^2 + \tau_{xy}^2}$

$$= \left(\dfrac{40 - 30}{2}\right) + \sqrt{\left(\dfrac{40 + 30}{2}\right)^2 + 25^2}$$

$$\therefore \quad \sigma_1 = 48.01 \text{ MPa}$$

Minimum principal stress, $\quad \sigma_2 = \left(\dfrac{\sigma_x + \sigma_y}{2}\right) - \sqrt{\left(\dfrac{\sigma_x - \sigma_y}{2}\right)^2 + \tau_{xy}^2}$

$$= \left(\dfrac{40 - 30}{2}\right) - \sqrt{\left(\dfrac{40 + 30}{2}\right)^2 + 25^2}$$

$$\therefore \quad \sigma_2 = -38.01 \text{ MPa}$$

Directions:

We know that $\quad \tan 2\phi_1 = \left(\dfrac{2\tau_{xy}}{\sigma_x - \sigma_y}\right) = \left(\dfrac{2 \times 25}{40 - (-30)}\right) = 0.714$

$$2\phi_1 = 35.54°$$
$$\therefore \quad \phi_1 = 17.77° \text{ and } \phi_2 = \phi_1 + 90° = 17.77° + 90° = 107.77°$$

c. *Maximum shear stress:*

Maximum shear stress, $\tau_{max} \quad = \pm \sqrt{\left(\dfrac{\sigma_x - \sigma_y}{2}\right)^2 + \tau_{xy}^2} = \pm \sqrt{\left(\dfrac{40 + 30}{2}\right)^2 + 25^2}$

$$= \pm 43.01 \text{ MPa}$$

Directions:

We know that $\quad \tan 2\phi_s = -\left(\dfrac{\sigma_x - \sigma_y}{2\tau_{xy}}\right) = -\left[\dfrac{40 - (-30)}{2 \times 25}\right] = -1.4$

$$2\phi_s = -54.46°$$
$$\therefore \quad \phi_{s1} = -27.23° \text{ and}$$
$$\phi_{s2} = \phi_{s1} + 90° = -27.23° + 90° = 62.77°$$

22. **For the state of stress shown in Fig. 3.25, determine:**
    (a) Principal planes
    (b) Principal stresses
    (c) Maximum shear stress and their planes
    (d) Normal and shear stress acting on plane DE.

VTU – June/ July 2013 – 14 Marks [Similar: (CV) June/ July 2014 – 10 Marks]

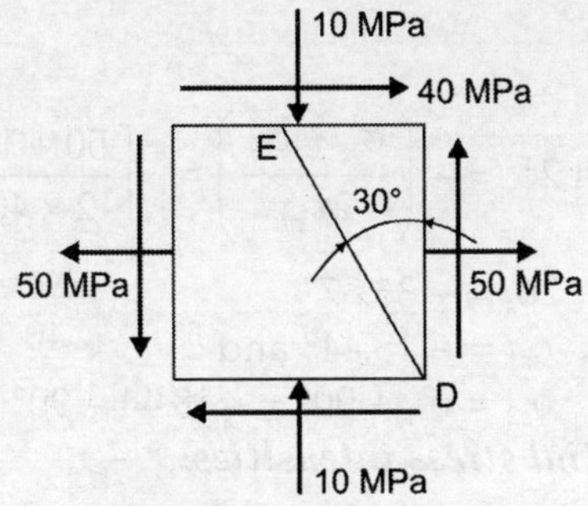

Fig. 3.25: Problem 22

Solution: $\sigma_x = 50$ MPa, $\sigma_y = -10$ MPa, $\tau_{xy} = 40$ MPa, $\phi = 30°$. a) $\phi_1 = ?$, $\phi_2 = ?$, b) $\sigma_1 = ?$, $\sigma_2 = ?$, c) $\tau_{max} = ?$, $\phi_{s1} = ?$, $\phi_{s2} = ?$, d) $\sigma_n = ?$, $\tau = ?$,

a. Principal directions:

We know that

$$\tan 2\phi_1 = \left(\frac{2\tau_{xy}}{\sigma_x - \sigma_y}\right) = \left[\frac{2 \times 40}{50 \times 10}\right] = 1.33$$

$$2\phi_1 = 53.13°$$

$$\therefore \quad \phi_1 = 26.57° \text{ and}$$

$$\phi_2 = \phi_1 + 90° = 26.57° + 90° = 116.57°$$

b. Principal stresses and their directions:

Maximum principal stress, $\quad \sigma_1 = \left(\frac{\sigma_x + \sigma_y}{2}\right) + \sqrt{\left(\frac{\sigma_x - \sigma_y}{2}\right)^2 + \tau_{xy}^2}$

$$= \left(\frac{50 - 10}{2}\right) + \sqrt{\left(\frac{50 + 10}{2}\right)^2 + 40^2}$$

$$\therefore \quad \sigma_1 = 70 \text{ MPa}$$

Minimum principal stress, $\quad \sigma_2 = \left(\frac{\sigma_x + \sigma_y}{2}\right) - \sqrt{\left(\frac{\sigma_x - \sigma_y}{2}\right)^2 + \tau_{xy}^2}$

$$= \left(\frac{50 - 10}{2}\right) - \sqrt{\left(\frac{50 + 10}{2}\right)^2 + 40^2}$$

$$\therefore \quad \sigma_2 = -30 \text{ MPa}$$

c. Maximum shear stress:

Maximum shear stress, $\quad \tau_{max} = \pm \sqrt{\left(\frac{\sigma_x - \sigma_y}{2}\right)^2 + \tau_{xy}^2} = \pm \sqrt{\left(\frac{50 + 10}{2}\right)^2 + 40^2}$

$$= \pm 50 \text{ MPa}$$

Directions:

We know that
$$\tan 2\phi_s = -\left(\frac{\sigma_x - \sigma_y}{2\tau_{xy}}\right) = -\left[\frac{50 + 10}{2 \times 40}\right] = -0.75$$

$$2\phi_s = -36.87°$$
$$\therefore \; \phi_{s1} = -18.44° \text{ and}$$
$$\phi_{s2} = \phi_{s1} + 90° = -18.44 + 90° = 71.56°$$

d. *Normal and tangential stress intensities:*

Normal stress,
$$\sigma_n = \left(\frac{\sigma_x + \sigma_y}{2}\right) + \left(\frac{\sigma_x - \sigma_y}{2}\right)\cos 2\phi + \tau_{xy} \sin 2\phi$$

$$= \left(\frac{50 - 10}{2}\right) + \left[\left(\frac{50 + 10}{2}\right)\cos(2 \times 30)\right] + 40 \times \sin(2 \times 30)$$

$$\sigma_n = 69.64 \text{ MPa}$$

Tangential stress,
$$\tau = \left(\frac{\sigma_x - \sigma_y}{2}\right)\sin 2\phi - \tau_{xy} \cos 2\phi$$

$$= \left[\left(\frac{50 + 10}{2}\right)\sin(2 \times 30)\right] - 40 \times \cos(2 \times 30)$$

$$\tau = 35 \text{ MPa}$$

23. **At a point in a strained material, the state of stress is as shown in Fig. 3.26. Calculate the normal and shearing stresses on the plane AC. Also find the principal stresses and their planes. Determine the maximum shear stress and their planes.**

> *VTU – (CV) June – July 2015 – 12 Marks; [Similar: (CV) Dec. 2011 – 10 Marks; (CV) June/ July 2009 – 10 Marks; (CV) Dec. 15/ Jan. 16 – 14 Marks; June/ July 2014 – 10 Marks]*

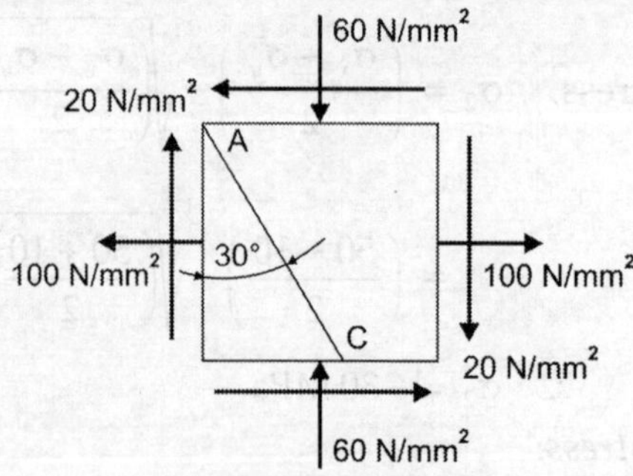

Fig. 3.26: Problem 23

Solution: $\sigma_x = 100$ MPa, $\sigma_y = -60$ MPa, $\tau_{xy} = -20$ MPa. a) $\sigma_n = ?, \tau = ?$, b) $\sigma_1 = ?, \sigma_2 = ?$, $\phi_1 = ?, \phi_2 = ?$, c) $\tau_{max} = ?, \phi_{s1} = ?, \phi_{s2} = ?$

a. *Normal and tangential stress intensities:*

Normal stress,
$$\sigma_n = \left(\frac{\sigma_x + \sigma_y}{2}\right) + \left(\frac{\sigma_x - \sigma_y}{2}\right)\cos 2\phi + \tau_{xy} \sin 2\phi$$

$$= \left(\frac{100 - 60}{2}\right) + \left[\left(\frac{100 + 60}{2}\right)\cos(2 \times 30)\right] + \left[(-20) \times \sin(2 \times 30)\right]$$

$$\sigma_n = 42.68 \text{ MPa}$$

Tangential stress, $\tau = \left(\dfrac{\sigma_x - \sigma_y}{2}\right)\sin 2\phi - \tau_{xy}\cos 2\phi$

$$= \left[\left(\frac{100 + 60}{2}\right)\sin(2 \times 30)\right] - \left[(-20) \times \cos(2 \times 30)\right]$$

$$\tau = 79.28 \text{ MPa}$$

b. Principal stresses and their directions:

Maximum principal stress, $\quad \sigma_1 = \left(\dfrac{\sigma_x + \sigma_y}{2}\right) + \sqrt{\left(\dfrac{\sigma_x - \sigma_y}{2}\right)^2 + \tau_{xy}^2}$

$$= \left(\frac{100 - 60}{2}\right) + \sqrt{\left(\frac{100 + 60}{2}\right)^2 + (-20)^2}$$

$$\therefore \quad \sigma_1 = 102.46 \text{ MPa}$$

Minimum principal stress, $\quad \sigma_2 = \left(\dfrac{\sigma_x + \sigma_y}{2}\right) - \sqrt{\left(\dfrac{\sigma_x - \sigma_y}{2}\right)^2 + \tau_{xy}^2}$

$$= \left(\frac{100 - 60}{2}\right) - \sqrt{\left(\frac{100 + 60}{2}\right)^2 + (-20)^2}$$

$$\therefore \quad \sigma_2 = -62.46 \text{ MPa}$$

Directions:

We know that $\quad \tan 2\phi_1 = \left(\dfrac{2\tau_{xy}}{\sigma_x - \sigma_y}\right) = \left[\dfrac{2 \times (-20)}{100 + 60}\right] = -0.25$

$$2\phi_1 = -14.04°$$
$$\therefore \quad \phi_1 = -7.02° \text{ and}$$
$$\phi_2 = \phi_1 + 90° = -7.02° + 90° = 82.98°$$

c. Maximum shear stress:

Maximum shear stress, $\tau_{max} = \pm\sqrt{\left(\dfrac{\sigma_x - \sigma_y}{2}\right)^2 + \tau_{xy}^2} = \pm\sqrt{\left(\dfrac{100 + 60}{2}\right)^2 + (-20)^2}$

$$= \pm 82.46 \text{ MPa}$$

Directions:

We know that $\quad \tan 2\phi_s = -\left(\dfrac{\sigma_x - \sigma_y}{2\tau_{xy}}\right) = -\left[\dfrac{100 + 60}{2 \times (-20)}\right] = 4$

$$2\phi_s = 75.96°$$
$$\therefore \phi_{s1} = 37.98° \text{ and}$$
$$\phi_{s2} = \phi_{s1} + 90° = 37.98° + 90° = 127.98°$$

24. At a certain point in a strained material the stress condition shown in Fig. 3.27 exists. Find

(a) The normal and shear stresses on the inclined plane AB

(b) Principal stresses and principal planes

(c) Maximum shear stress.

VTU – June/ July – 10 Marks; Dec. 13! Jan. 14 – 10 Marks;
[Similar: Dec. 14/ Jan. 15 – 12 Marks]

Solution: $\sigma_x = -30$ MPa, $\sigma_y = 120$ MPa, $\tau_{xy} = -40$ MPa, $\phi' = 30°$ (CCW with horizontal), $\phi = 90° - 30° = 60°$ (CW with vertical). $\therefore \phi = -60°$ (opposite) a) $\sigma_n = ?$, $\tau = ?$, b) $\sigma_1 = ?$, $\sigma_2 = ?$, $\phi_1 = ?$, $\phi_2 = ?$, c) $\tau_{max} = ?$, $\phi_{s1} = ?$, $\phi_{s2} = ?$

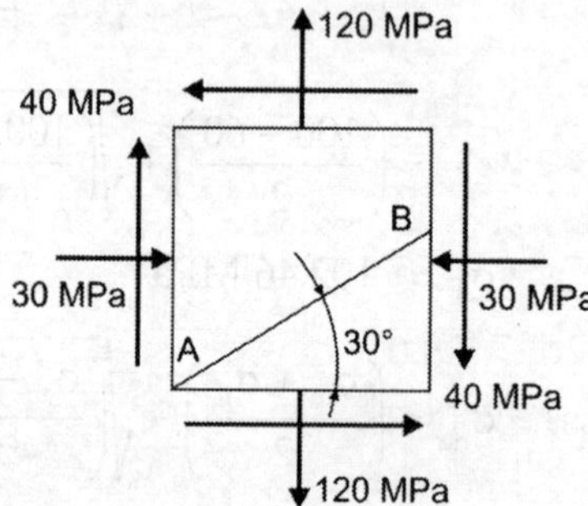

Fig. 3.27: Problem 24

a.   Normal and shear stresses:

Normal stress, $\quad \sigma_n = \left(\dfrac{\sigma_x + \sigma_y}{2}\right) + \left(\dfrac{\sigma_x - \sigma_y}{2}\right)\cos 2\phi + \tau_{xy}\sin 2\phi$

$$= \left(\dfrac{-30 + 120}{2}\right) + \left[\left(\dfrac{-30 - 120}{2}\right)\cos(2 \times -60)\right]$$

$$+ \left[(-40) \times \sin(2 \times -60)\right]$$

$$\sigma_n = 117.14 \text{ MPa}$$

Tangential stress, $\tau = \left(\dfrac{\sigma_x - \sigma_y}{2}\right)\sin 2\phi - \tau_{xy}\cos 2\phi$

$$= \left[\left(\dfrac{-30 - 120}{2}\right)\sin(2 \times -60)\right] - \left[(-40) \times \cos(2 \times -60)\right]$$

$$\tau = 44.95 \text{ MPa}$$

b.   Principal stresses and their directions:

Maximum principal stress, $\quad \sigma_1 = \left(\dfrac{\sigma_x + \sigma_y}{2}\right) + \sqrt{\left(\dfrac{\sigma_x - \sigma_y}{2}\right)^2 + \tau_{xy}^2}$

$$= \left(\frac{-30 + 120}{2}\right) + \sqrt{\left(\frac{-30 - 120}{2}\right)^2 + (-40)^2}$$

$$= 130 \, \text{MPa}$$

Minimum principal stress, $\quad \sigma_2 = \left(\frac{\sigma_x + \sigma_y}{2}\right) - \sqrt{\left(\frac{\sigma_x - \sigma_y}{2}\right)^2 + \tau_{xy}^2}$

$$= \left(\frac{-30 + 120}{2}\right) - \sqrt{\left(\frac{-30 - 120}{2}\right)^2 + (-40)^2}$$

$$= -40 \, \text{MPa}$$

Directions:

We know that $\quad \tan 2\phi_1 = \left(\frac{2\tau_{xy}}{\sigma_x - \sigma_y}\right)$

$$\tan 2\phi_1 = \left[\frac{2 \times (-40)}{-30 - 120}\right] = 0.53$$

$$\therefore \quad 2\phi_1 = 28.07°$$
$$\phi_1 = 14.04°$$
$$\phi_2 = \phi_1 + 90° = 14.04° + 90° = 104.04°$$

c.   *Maximum shear stress:*

Maximum shear stress, $\quad \tau_{max} = \pm \sqrt{\left(\frac{\sigma_x - \sigma_y}{2}\right)^2 + \tau_{xy}^2} = \pm\sqrt{\left(\frac{-30 - 120}{2}\right)^2 + (-40)^2}$

$$= \pm 85 \, \text{MPa}$$

Directions:

We know that $\quad \tan 2\phi_s = -\left(\frac{\sigma_x - \sigma_y}{2\tau_{xy}}\right) = -\left[\frac{-30 - 120}{2 \times (-40)}\right] = -1.88$

$$2\phi_s = -61.93°$$
$$\therefore \quad \phi_{s1} = -30.97° \text{ and}$$
$$\phi_{s2} = \phi_{s1} + 90° = -30.97° + 90° = 59.03°$$

25. **In an elastic material, the stresses acting on an elementary block are as shown in Fig. 3.28. Compute:**
(a) Normal and tangential (shear) stresses on plane AC
(b) Principal stresses and principal planes
(c) Maximum shear stress.

VTU – (CV) Dec. 10 – 10 Marks; [Similar: CV) June/ July 2011 – 12 Marks]

Solution: $\sigma_x = -100$ MPa, $\sigma_y = 60$ MPa, $\tau_{xy} = 40$ MPa, $\phi' = 60°$ (CCW with horizontal), $\phi = 90° - 60° = 30°$ (CW with vertical). $\therefore \phi = -30\phi$ (opposite). a) σ_n = ?, τ = ?, b) σ_1 = ?, σ_2 = ?, ϕ_1 = ?, ϕ_2 = ?, c) τ_{max} = ?, ϕ_{s1} = ?, ϕ_{s2} = ?

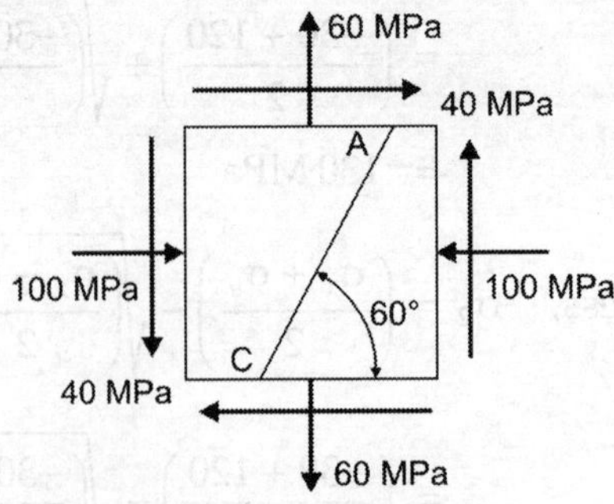

Fig. 3.28: Problem 25

a. *Normal and shear stresses:*

Normal stress, $\sigma_n = \left(\dfrac{\sigma_x + \sigma_y}{2}\right) + \left(\dfrac{\sigma_x - \sigma_y}{2}\right)\cos 2\phi + \tau_{xy}\sin 2\phi$

$$= \left(\dfrac{-100 + 60}{2}\right) + \left[\left(\dfrac{-100 - 60}{2}\right)\cos(2\times -30)\right]$$

$$+ \, 40 \times \sin(2 \times -30)$$

$$\sigma_n = -94.64 \text{ MPa}$$

Tangential stress, $\tau = \left(\dfrac{\sigma_x - \sigma_y}{2}\right)\sin 2\phi - \tau_{xy}\cos 2\phi$

$$= \left[\left(\dfrac{-100 - 60}{2}\right)\sin(2\times -30)\right] - 40 \times \cos(2\times -30)$$

$$= 49.28 \text{ MPa}$$

b. *Principal stresses and their directions:*

Maximum principal stress, $\sigma_1 = \left(\dfrac{\sigma_x + \sigma_y}{2}\right) + \sqrt{\left(\dfrac{\sigma_x - \sigma_y}{2}\right)^2 + \tau_{xy}^2}$

$$= \left(\dfrac{-100 + 60}{2}\right) + \sqrt{\left(\dfrac{-100 - 60}{2}\right)^2 + 40^2}$$

$$= 69.44 \text{ MPa}$$

Minimum principal stress, $\sigma_2 = \left(\dfrac{\sigma_x + \sigma_y}{2}\right) - \sqrt{\left(\dfrac{\sigma_x - \sigma_y}{2}\right)^2 + \tau_{xy}^2}$

$$= \left(\dfrac{-100 + 60}{2}\right) - \sqrt{\left(\dfrac{-100 - 60}{2}\right)^2 + 40^2}$$

$$= -109.44 \text{ MPa}$$

Directions:

We know that
$$\tan 2\phi_1 = \left(\dfrac{2\tau_{xy}}{\sigma_x - \sigma_y}\right)$$

$$\tan 2\phi_1 = \left(\dfrac{2 \times 40}{-100 - 60}\right) = -0.5$$

$$2\phi_1 = -26.57°$$
$$\therefore \ \phi_1 = -13.28° \text{ and}$$
$$\phi_2 = \phi_1 + 90° = -13.28° + 90° = 76.72°$$

c. *Maximum shear stress:*

Maximum shear stress, $\tau_{max} = \pm \sqrt{\left(\dfrac{\sigma_x - \sigma_y}{2}\right)^2 + \tau_{xy}^2} = \pm \sqrt{\left(\dfrac{-100 - 60}{2}\right)^2 + 40^2}$

$$= \pm \, 89.44 \text{ MPa}$$

Directions:

We know that
$$\tan 2\phi_s = -\left(\dfrac{\sigma_x - \sigma_y}{2\tau_{xy}}\right) = -\left[\dfrac{-100 - 60}{2 \times 40}\right] = 2$$

$$2\phi_s = 63.43°$$
$$\therefore \ \phi_{s1} = 31.72° \text{ and}$$
$$\phi_{s2} = \phi_{s1} + 90° = 31.72° + 90° = 121.72°$$

26. **The state of stress at a point is shown in Fig. 3.29(a). If the plane EF cuts the element, determine the normal and shear stresses on the plane and show them clearly on the portion of the element ABFE.**

VTU – Dec. 10 – 08 Marks

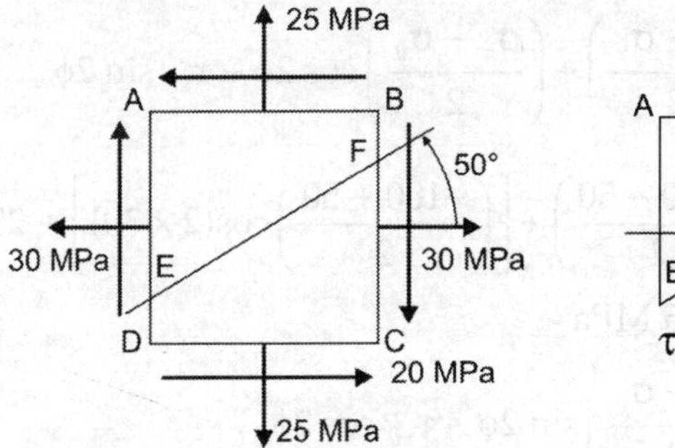

Fig. 3.29(a): Problem 26   **Fig. 3.29(b):** Problem 26

Solution: $\sigma_x = 30$ MPa, $\sigma_y = 25$ MPa, $\tau_{xy} = -20$ MPa, $\phi' = 50°$ (CCW with horizontal), $\phi = 90° - 50° = 40°$ (CW with vertical). $\therefore \phi = -40°$ (opposite). $\sigma_n = ?$, $\tau = ?$,

Normal and shear stresses:

Normal stress, $\sigma_n = \left(\dfrac{\sigma_x + \sigma_y}{2}\right) + \left(\dfrac{\sigma_x - \sigma_y}{2}\right)\cos 2\phi + \tau_{xy} \sin 2\phi$

$$= \left(\dfrac{30 + 25}{2}\right) + \left[\left(\dfrac{30 - 25}{2}\right)\cos(2 \times -40)\right]$$

$$+\left[(-20)\times\sin(2\times-40)\right]$$

$$\sigma_n = 47.63\ \text{MPa}$$

Tangential stress, $\tau = \left(\dfrac{\sigma_x - \sigma_y}{2}\right)\sin 2\phi - \tau_{xy}\cos 2\phi$

$$= \left[\left(\dfrac{30-25}{2}\right)\sin(2\times-40)\right] - \left[(-20)\times\cos(2\times-40)\right]$$

$$\tau = 1.01\ \text{MPa}$$

Fig 3.29(b) represents the normal and shear stresses on the element ABFE.

27. **A machine component is subjected to stresses as shown in Fig. 3.30. Determine:**
    (a) Normal, shear and resultant stresses
    (b) Principal stresses and their directions

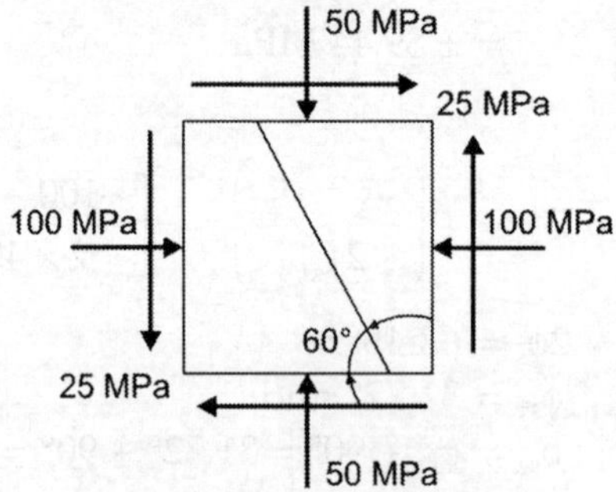

Fig. 3.30: Problem 27

Solution: $\sigma_x = -100$ MPa, $\sigma_y = -50$ MPa, $\tau_{xy} = 25$ MPa, $\phi' = 60°$ (CW with horizontal), $\phi = 30°$ (CCW with vertical). a) $\sigma_n = ?$, $\tau = ?$, $\sigma_r = ?$, b) $\sigma_1 = ?$, $\sigma_2 = ?$, $\phi_1 = ?$, $\phi_2 = ?$,

a. *Normal, shear and resultant stresses:*

Normal stress, $\sigma_n = \left(\dfrac{\sigma_x + \sigma_y}{2}\right) + \left(\dfrac{\sigma_x - \sigma_y}{2}\right)\cos 2\phi + \tau_{xy}\sin 2\phi$

$$= \left(\dfrac{-100-50}{2}\right) + \left[\left(\dfrac{-100+50}{2}\right)\cos(2\times 30)\right] + 25\times\sin(2\times 30)$$

$$= -65.85\ \text{MPa}$$

Tangential stress, $\tau = \left(\dfrac{\sigma_x - \sigma_y}{2}\right)\sin 2\phi - \tau_{xy}\cos 2\phi$

$$= \left[\left(\dfrac{-100+50}{2}\right)\sin(2\times 30)\right] - 25\times\cos(2\times 30)$$

$$= -34.15\ \text{MPa}$$

Resultant stress, $\sigma_r = \sqrt{\sigma_n^2 + \tau^2}$

$$= \sqrt{(-65.85)^2 + (-34.15)^2}$$

$$\sigma_r = 74.18\ \text{MPa}$$

b. *Principal stresses and their directions:*

Maximum principal stress, $\sigma_1 = \left(\dfrac{\sigma_x + \sigma_y}{2}\right) + \sqrt{\left(\dfrac{\sigma_x - \sigma_y}{2}\right)^2 + \tau_{xy}^2}$

$$= \left(\dfrac{-100 - 50}{2}\right) + \sqrt{\left(\dfrac{-100 + 50}{2}\right)^2 + 25^2}$$

$$= -39.64 \text{ MPa}$$

Minimum principal stress, $\sigma_2 = \left(\dfrac{\sigma_x + \sigma_y}{2}\right) - \sqrt{\left(\dfrac{\sigma_x - \sigma_y}{2}\right)^2 + \tau_{xy}^2}$

$$= \left(\dfrac{-100 - 50}{2}\right) - \sqrt{\left(\dfrac{-100 + 50}{2}\right)^2 + 25^2}$$

$$= -110.36 \text{ MPa}$$

Directions:

We know that $\quad \tan 2\phi_1 = \left(\dfrac{2\tau_{xy}}{\sigma_x - \sigma_y}\right)$

$$\tan 2\phi_1 = \left[\dfrac{2 \times 25}{-100 - (-50)}\right] = -1$$

$$2\phi_1 = -45°$$
$$\therefore \ \phi_1 = -22.5° \text{ and}$$
$$\phi_2 = \phi_1 + 90° = -22.5° + 90° = 67.5°$$

28. **At a certain point in a material under stress, the intensity of resultant stress on a vertical plane is 10 MPa inclined at 30° to the normal plane and the stress on the horizontal plane has a normal tensile stress of 6 MPa, as shown in Fig. 3.31. Find the principal stresses and the location of the planes on which they act.**

VTU – Jan. 2013 – 08 Marks

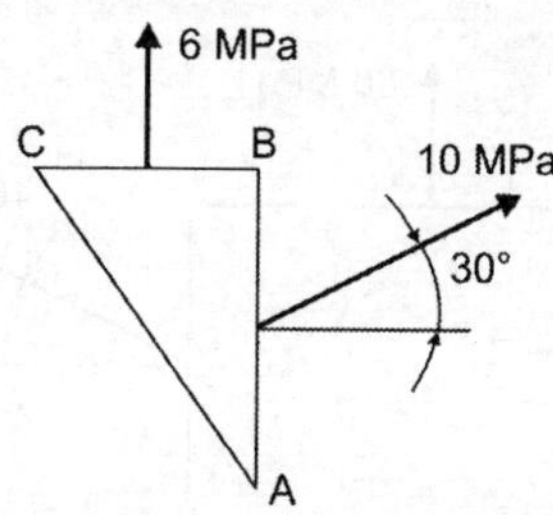

Fig. 3.31: Problem 28

Solution: $\sigma_r = 10$ MPa, $\sigma_y = 6$ MPa, $\phi = 30°$. $\sigma_1 = ?$, $\sigma_2 = ?$, $\phi_1 = ?$, $\phi_2 = ?$,
Horizontal component of stress, $\sigma_x = \sigma_r \cos\phi = 10 \cos(30) = 8.66$ MPa
Vertical component of stress, $\tau_{xy} = \sigma_r \sin\phi = 10 \sin(30) = 5$ MPa

Principal stresses and their directions:

Maximum principal stress, $\sigma_1 = \left(\dfrac{\sigma_x + \sigma_y}{2}\right) + \sqrt{\left(\dfrac{\sigma_x - \sigma_y}{2}\right)^2 + \tau_{xy}^2}$

$$= \left(\dfrac{8.66 + 6}{2}\right) + \sqrt{\left(\dfrac{8.66 - 6}{2}\right)^2 + 25^2}$$

$$= 12.50 \text{ MPa}$$

Minimum principal stress, $\sigma_2 = \left(\dfrac{\sigma_x + \sigma_y}{2}\right) - \sqrt{\left(\dfrac{\sigma_x - \sigma_y}{2}\right)^2 + \tau_{xy}^2}$

$$= \left(\dfrac{8.66 + 6}{2}\right) - \sqrt{\left(\dfrac{8.66 - 6}{2}\right)^2 + 25^2}$$

$$= 2.16 \text{ MPa}$$

Directions:

We know that $\qquad \tan 2\phi_1 = \left(\dfrac{2\tau_{xy}}{\sigma_x - \sigma_y}\right)$

$$\tan 2\phi_1 = \left(\dfrac{2 \times 5}{8.66 - 6}\right) = 3.76$$

$$2\phi_1 = 75.10°$$
$$\therefore \ \phi_1 = 37.55° \text{ and}$$
$$\phi_2 = \phi_1 + 90° = 37.55° + 90° = 127.55°$$

29. At a point in a strained material, the state of stress is shown in Fig. 3.32(a). Determine:
   (a) Principal planes and stresses,
   (b) Critical shear planes and sketches.
   Sketch the orientation of the planes and mark the principal stresses on the planes.

VTU – (CV) Dec. 13/ Jan. 14 – 10 Marks

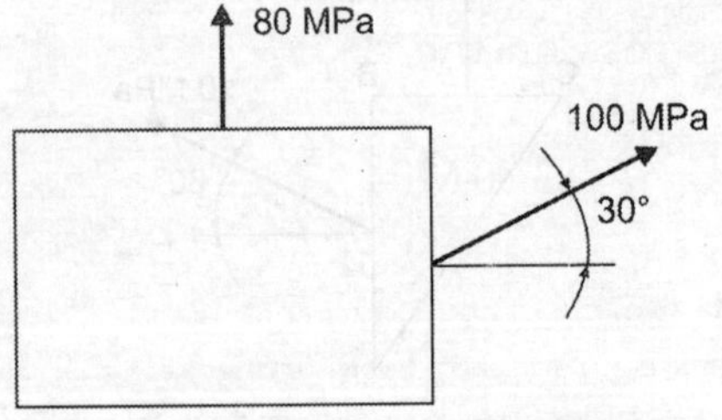

Fig. 3.32(a): Problem 29

Solution: $\sigma_r = 100$ MPa, $\sigma_y = 80$ MPa, $\phi = 30°$. a) $\sigma_1 = ?$, $\sigma_2 = ?$, $\phi_1 = ?$, $\phi_2 = ?$, b) $\tau_{max} = ?$, $\phi_{s1} = ?$, $\phi_{s2} = ?$

Horizontal component of stress, $\quad \sigma_x = \sigma_r \cos\phi = 100\cos(30) = 86.60$ MPa

Vertical component of stress, $\quad \tau_{xy} = \sigma_r \sin\phi = 100\sin(30) = 50$ MPa

a. Principal stresses and their directions:

Maximum principal stress, $\quad \sigma_1 = \left(\dfrac{\sigma_x + \sigma_y}{2}\right) + \sqrt{\left(\dfrac{\sigma_x - \sigma_y}{2}\right)^2 + \tau_{xy}^2}$

$$= \left(\frac{86.60 + 80}{2}\right) + \sqrt{\left(\frac{86.60 - 80}{2}\right)^2 + 50^2}$$

$$= 133.41 \text{ MPa}$$

Minimum principal stress, $\quad \sigma_2 = \left(\dfrac{\sigma_x + \sigma_y}{2}\right) - \sqrt{\left(\dfrac{\sigma_x - \sigma_y}{2}\right)^2 + \tau_{xy}^2}$

$$= \left(\frac{86.60 + 80}{2}\right) - \sqrt{\left(\frac{86.60 - 80}{2}\right)^2 + 50^2}$$

$$= 33.20 \text{ MPa}$$

Directions:

We know that $\quad \tan 2\phi_1 = \left(\dfrac{2\tau_{xy}}{\sigma_x - \sigma_y}\right)$

$$\tan 2\phi_1 = \left(\frac{2 \times 25}{86.60 - 80}\right) = 15.15$$

$$2\phi_1 = 86.22°$$

$$\therefore\ \phi_1 = 43.11° \text{ and}$$

$$\phi_2 = \phi_1 + 90° = 43.11° + 90° = 133.11°$$

b. Maximum shear stress:

Maximum shear stress, $\quad \tau_{max} = \pm\sqrt{\left(\dfrac{\sigma_x - \sigma_y}{2}\right)^2 + \tau_{xy}^2} = \pm\sqrt{\left(\dfrac{86.60 - 80}{2}\right)^2 + 50^2}$

$$= \pm 50.11 \text{ MPa}$$

Average (normal) stress on the planes of maximum shear stress is, $\sigma_{avg} = \left(\dfrac{\sigma_x + \sigma_y}{2}\right) = \dfrac{86.60 + 80}{2} = 83.30$ MPa

Directions:

We know that $\quad \tan 2\phi_s = -\left(\dfrac{\sigma_x - \sigma_y}{2\tau_{xy}}\right) = -\left[\dfrac{86.60 - 80}{2 \times 50}\right] = -0.066$

$$2\phi_s = -3.77°$$

$$\therefore\ \phi_{s1} = -1.88° \text{ and}$$

$$\phi_{s2} = \phi_{s1} + 90° = -1.88° + 90° = 88.11°$$

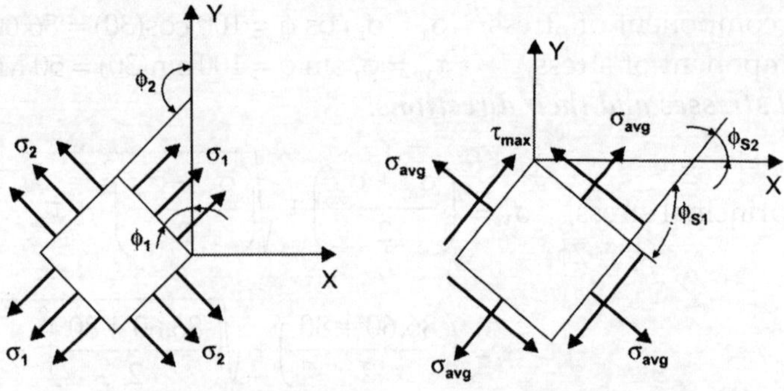

Fig. 3.32(b): Problem 29   **Fig. 3.32(c):** Problem 29

Principal stresses and directions   **Maximum shear stress and directions**

30. **A point in a machine member is subjected to stresses as shown in Fig. 3.33. A circle of diameter 200 mm on the member is converted into ellipse after the application of stresses. Determine the major and minor axes of the ellipse and their orientations. Take $E = 2 \times 105$ MPa and the Poisson's ratio as 0.3.**

VTU – June/ July 2009 – 15 Marks

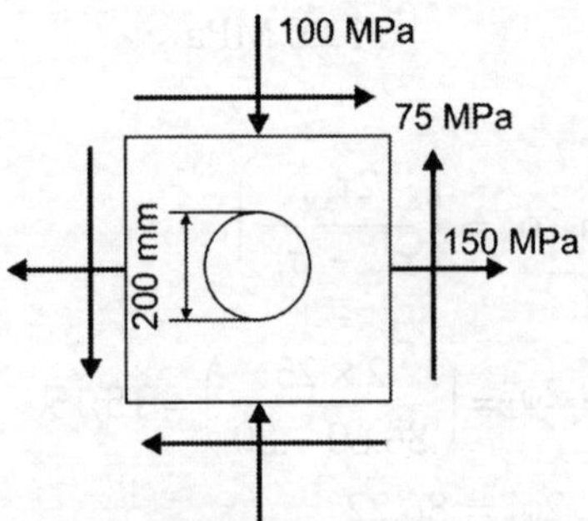

Fig. 3.33: Problem 30

Solution: $\sigma_x = 150$ MPa, $\sigma_y = -100$ MPa, $\tau_{xy} = 75$ MPa, $\mu = 0.3$, $E = 2 \times 10^5$ MPa, $d = 200$ mm, $2a = ?$, $2b = ?$.

Principal stresses and their directions:

Maximum principal stress,
$$\sigma_1 = \left(\frac{\sigma_x + \sigma_y}{2}\right) + \sqrt{\left(\frac{\sigma_x - \sigma_y}{2}\right)^2 + \tau_{xy}^2}$$

$$= \left(\frac{150 - 100}{2}\right) + \sqrt{\left(\frac{150 + 100}{2}\right)^2 + 75^2}$$

$$\sigma_1 = 170.77 \text{ MPa}$$

Minimum principal stress,
$$\sigma_2 = \left(\frac{\sigma_x + \sigma_y}{2}\right) - \sqrt{\left(\frac{\sigma_x - \sigma_y}{2}\right)^2 + \tau_{xy}^2}$$

$$= \left(\frac{150 - 100}{2}\right) - \sqrt{\left(\frac{150 + 100}{2}\right)^2 + 75^2}$$

$$= -120.77 \text{ MPa}$$

Directions:

We know that
$$\tan 2\phi_1 = \left(\frac{2\tau_{xy}}{\sigma_x - \sigma_y}\right)$$

$$\tan 2\phi_1 = \left(\frac{2 \times 75}{150 + 100}\right) = 0.6$$

$$2\phi_1 = 30.96°$$
$$\therefore \quad \phi_1 = 15.48° \text{ and}$$
$$\phi_2 = \phi_1 + 90° = 15.48° + 90° = 105.48°$$

Principal strains:

Major Principal strain, $\in_1 = \dfrac{\sigma_1}{E} - \mu\dfrac{\sigma_2}{E} = \dfrac{1}{E}(\sigma_1 - \mu\sigma_2) = \dfrac{1}{2 \times 10^5}(170.77 + 0.3$
$$\times 120.77) = 1.035 \times 10^{-3}$$

Minor Principal strain, $\in_2 = \dfrac{\sigma_2}{E} - \mu\dfrac{\sigma_1}{E} = \dfrac{1}{E}(\sigma_2 - \mu\sigma_1) = \dfrac{1}{2 \times 10^5}(-120.77 - 0.3$
$$\times 170.77) = -8.6 \times 10^{-4}$$

Thus Major axis, $2a = d(1 + \in_1) = 200 \times (1 + 1.035 \times 10^{-3}) = 200.21$ mm

Minor axis, $2b = d(1 + \in_2) = 200 \times (1 - 8.6 \times 10^{-4}) = 199.83$ mm

3.8 GRAPHICAL SOLUTION: MOHR'S CIRCLE METHOD

The transformation equations for plane stress can be represented in a graphical form known as Mohr's circle. In this method, normal stresses are plotted along the horizontal axis (abscissa) and shearing stresses along the vertical axis (ordinate).

Sign convention:

- *Direct stresses:* Tensile stresses are considered to be positive and compressive stresses negative. Thus tensile stresses are plotted to the right of the origin while compressive stresses are plotted to the left of the origin.
- *Shear stresses:* clockwise rotation is considered positive and is plotted above the axis; while counter clockwise rotation is considered negative and is plotted below the axis.
- *Angle* ϕ is considered positive when measured in CCW direction.

Mohr's circle is drawn for the following cases:

(a) Two mutually perpendicular like stresses (both tensile or both compressive).

(b) Two mutually perpendicular unlike stresses (one tensile and other compressive).

(c) Two mutually perpendicular like or unlike stresses accompanied by shear stress.

3.8.1 Mohr's circle for two Mutually perpendicular like stresses

1. Let σ_x and σ_y be the two like stresses (both tensile), as shown in **Fig. 3.34(a)**.
2. Using suitable scale, cut-off OA equal to σ_x and OB equal to σ_y on the same side of the O (right side of origin).
3. Bisect AB at M. With M as center and radius equal to MA or MB, draw a circle. This circle is known as Mohr's circle.
4. From M draw a line MP at an angle 2ϕ in the same direction as the normal to the plane makes with the direction of σ_x to get P.
5. From P, drop a perpendicular PQ on OX axis. Join OP.

From **Fig. 3.34(b)**, we have:

- $OM = \left(\dfrac{\sigma_x + \sigma_y}{2}\right)$ $MP = MA = \left(\dfrac{\sigma_x - \sigma_y}{2}\right)$

- Normal stress, $\sigma_n = OQ$
- Tangential stress, $\tau = PQ$
- Resultant stress, $\sigma_r = OP$
- Angle of obliquity, $\theta = \angle POQ$
- Maximum principal stress, $\sigma_1 = \sigma_x = OA$
- Minimum principal stress, $\sigma_2 = \sigma_y = OB$
- Maximum shear stress = Radius of Mohr's circle, $MN = MA = MB = \tau_{max}$

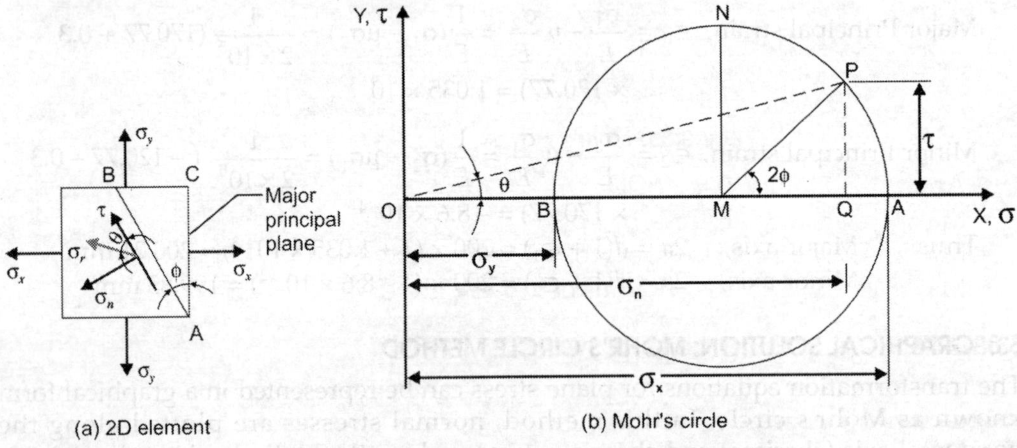

Fig. 3.34: Mohr's circle for two like stresses

Note: If σ_x and σ_y are two like stresses (both compressive), the entire diagram shown in **Fig 3.34** has to be constructed towards the left side of origin O.

3.8.2 Mohr's circle for two mutually perpendicular unlike stresses

1. Let σ_x and σ_y be the two unlike stresses (one tensile and other compressive), as shown in **Fig. 3.35(a)**.
2. Using suitable scale, cut – off OA equal to σ_x (tensile) on the right side of O and OB equal to σ_y (compressive) on left side of O.
3. Bisect AB at M. With M as center and radius equal to MA or MB, draw a circle. This circle is known as Mohr's circle.
4. From M draw a line MP at an angle 2ϕ in the same direction as the normal to the plane makes with the direction of σ_x to get P.
5. From P, drop a perpendicular PQ on OX axis. Join OP.

From **Fig. 3.35(b)**, we have:

- $OM = \left(\dfrac{\sigma_x + \sigma_y}{2}\right)$ $MP = MA = \left(\dfrac{\sigma_x - \sigma_y}{2}\right)$

- Normal stress, $\sigma_n = OQ$
- Tangential stress, $\tau = PQ$
- Resultant stress, $\sigma_r = OP$

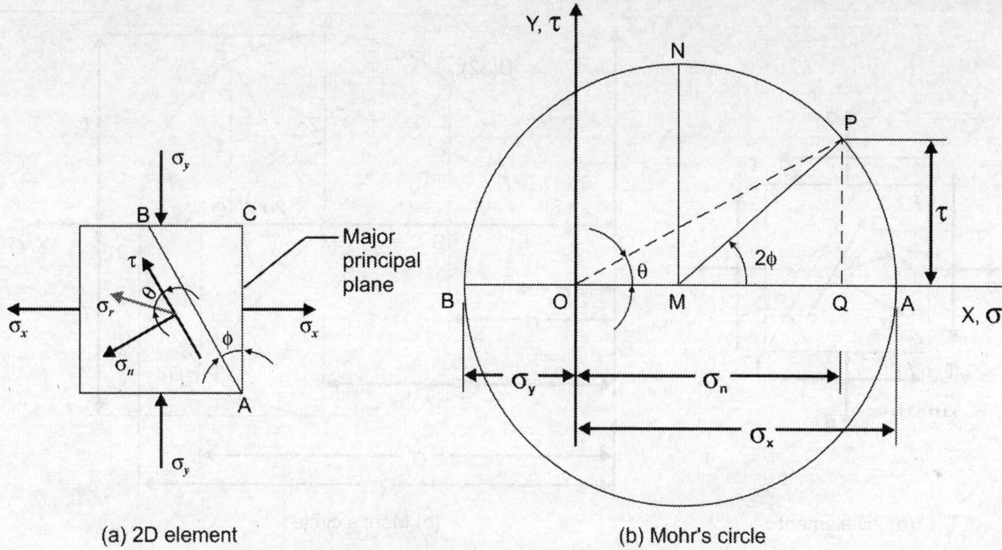

(a) 2D element   (b) Mohr's circle

Fig. 3.35: Mohr's circle for two unlike stresses

- Angle of obliquity, $\theta = \angle POQ$
- Maximum principal stress, $\sigma_1 = \sigma_x = OA$
- Minimum principal stress, $\sigma_2 = \sigma_y = OB$
- Maximum shear stress = Radius of Mohr's circle, $MN = MA = MB = \tau_{max}$

3.8.3 Mohr's circle for general two-dimensional stress system or plane stress system

Sign convention:

- *Direct stresses:* Tensile stresses are considered to be positive and compressive stresses negative. Thus tensile stresses are plotted to the right of the origin while compressive stresses are plotted to the left of the origin.
- *Shear stresses:* clockwise rotation is considered positive ($\overline{32}$) and is plotted above x-axis; while counter clockwise rotation is considered negative ($\overline{12}$) and is plotted below x-axis.
- *Angle* ϕ is considered positive when measured in CCW direction.

1. Let σ_x and σ_y be the two like stresses (both tensile), accompanied by a positive shear stress τ_{xy}, as shown in **Fig. 3.36(a)**.
2. Using suitable scale, cut-off OA equal to σ_x and OB equal to σ_y on the same side of the O (right side of origin).
3. Bisect AB at M.
4. Erect perpendiculars at A and B and cut-off AC and BD each equal to τ_{xy}
5. With M as center and radius equal to MC or MD, draw a circle to get points E and F on OX axis. This circle is known as *Mohr's circle.*
6. On the line MC, draw a line MP at an angle 2ϕ in CCW direction.
7. From P, drop a perpendicular PQ on OX axis. Join OP.
8. Now OQ and PQ will give the required normal and tangential stresses, while OP gives the resultant stress.
9. Also OE and OF gives the maximum and minimum values of normal stress, while MN gives the maximum value of shear stress.

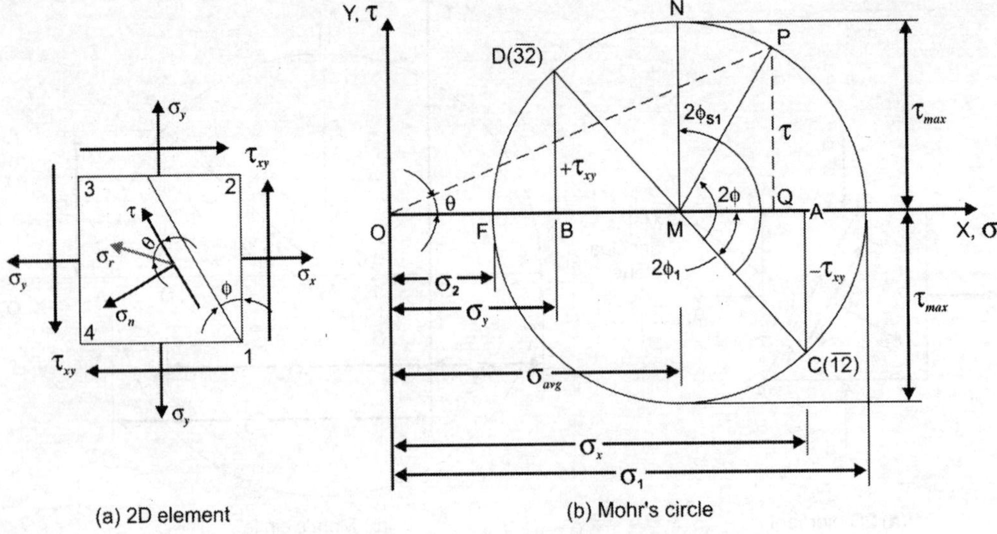

(a) 2D element   (b) Mohr's circle

Fig. 3.36: Mohr's circle for plane stress system

From **Fig. 3.36(b)**, we have:

$$\bullet \ \sigma_{avg} = OM = \left(\frac{\sigma_x + \sigma_y}{2}\right) \qquad MA = \left(\frac{\sigma_x - \sigma_y}{2}\right)$$

- Normal stress, $\sigma_n = OQ$
- Tangential stress, $\tau = PQ$
- Resultant stress, $\sigma_r = OP$
- Angle of obliquity, $\theta = \angle POQ$
- $\tau_{xy} = AC = BD$
- Maximum principal stress, $\sigma_1 = OE$
- Minimum principal stress, $\sigma_2 = OF$
- Maximum shear stress = Radius of Mohr's circle, $\tau_{max} = MN = ME = MF$

- Direction of principal stresses: $\quad 2\phi_1 = \angle CME \Rightarrow \phi_1 = \dfrac{\angle CME}{2}$ and $\phi_2 = \phi_1 + 90°$

- Direction of shear stresses: $\quad 2\phi_{S1} = \angle CMN \Rightarrow \phi_{S1} = \dfrac{\angle CMN}{2}$ and $\phi_{s2} = \phi_{s1} + 90°$

31. **Construct the Mohr's circle for a point in the machine member subjected to pure shear of 50 MPa. Determine the maximum and minimum stresses induced and orientation of their planes.**

VTU – June/ July 2009 – 08 Marks

Solution: $\tau_{xy} = 50$ MPa. Since the normal stresses are absent, the radius of Mohr's circle is equal to 50 MPa, as shown in **Fig. 3.37**.

- Maximum principal stress, $\sigma_1 = OA \times scale = 5 \times 10 = 50$ MPa (Tensile)
- Minimum principal stress, $\sigma_2 = OB \times scale = 5 \times 10 = 50$ MPa (Compressive)
- Maximum principal stress plane/direction, $2\phi_1 = 90° \Rightarrow \phi_1 = 45°$
- Minimum principal stress plane/direction, $\phi_2 = \phi_1 + 90° = 45° + 90° = 135°$
- Maximum shear stress = Radius of Mohr's circle, $\tau_{max} = OA = OB = 50$ MPa
- Maximum shear stress plane/direction, $2\phi_{s1} = 180° \Rightarrow \phi_{s1} = 90°$
- Minimum shear stress plane/direction, $\phi_{s2} = \phi_{s1} + 90° = 90° + 90° = 180°$

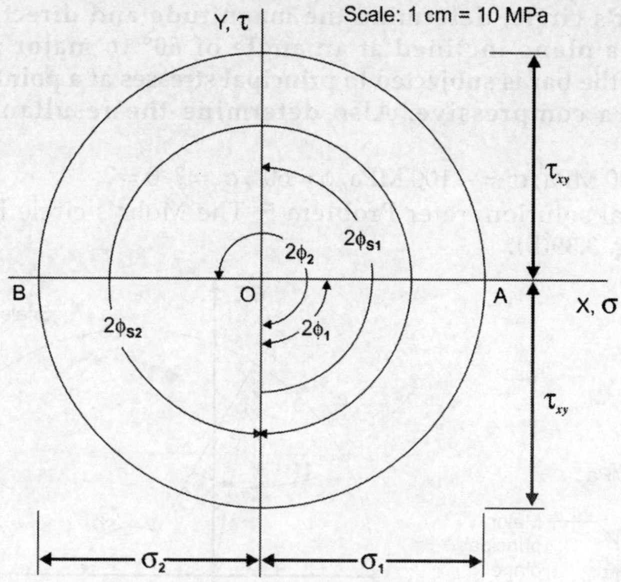

Fig. 3.37: Problem 31

32. Construct the Mohr's circle for the system shown in Fig. 3.38(a) and determine:
   (a) The normal and tangential stress intensities.
   (b) Magnitude and direction of resultant stress.
   (c) Maximum shear stress

Solution: $\sigma_x = 100$ MPa, $\sigma_y = 60$ MPa, $\phi = 30°$

For analytical solution, *refer Problem 3*. The Mohr's circle is constructed as shown in **Fig. 3.38(b)**.

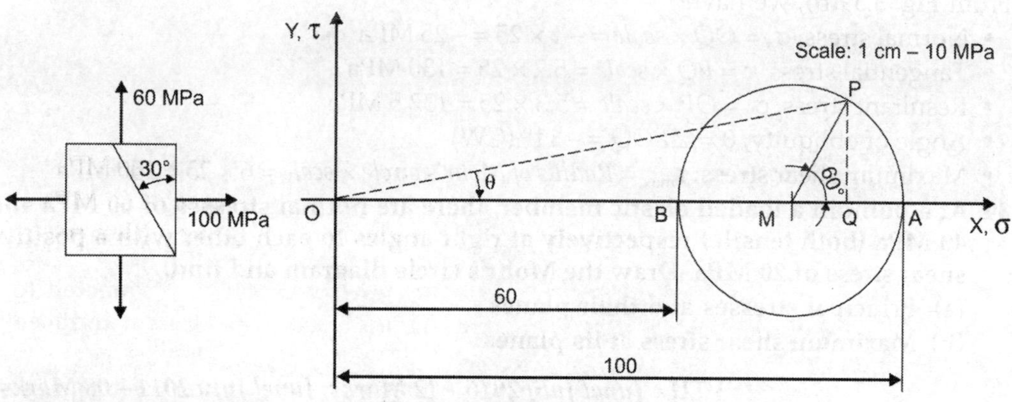

Fig. 3.38(a): Problem 32   **Fig. 3.38(b):** Problem 32

Fig. 3.38(b), we have
   - Normal stress, $\sigma_n = OQ \times scale = 9 \times 10 = 90$ MPa
   - Tangential stress, $\tau = PQ \times scale = 1.7 \times 10 = 17$ MPa
   - Resultant stress, $\sigma_r = OP \times scale = 9.2 \times 10 = 92$ MPa
   - Angle of obliquity, $\theta = \angle POQ = -11°$ (CW)
   c. **Maximum shear stress,** $\tau_{max} = Radius\ of\ Mohr's\ circle \times scale = 2 \times 10 = 20$ MPa

33. **Using Mohr's circle, determine the magnitude and direction of resultant stresses on a plane inclined at an angle of 60° to major principal stress plane, when the bar is subjected to principal stresses at a point 200 MPa tensile and 100 MPa compressive. Also determine the resultant stress and its obliquity.**

Solution: $\sigma_x = 200$ MPa, $\sigma_y = -100$ MPa, $\phi = 60°$, $\sigma_r = ?$, $\theta = ?$

For analytical solution, refer **Problem 5**. The Mohr's circle is constructed as shown in **Fig. 3.39(b)**.

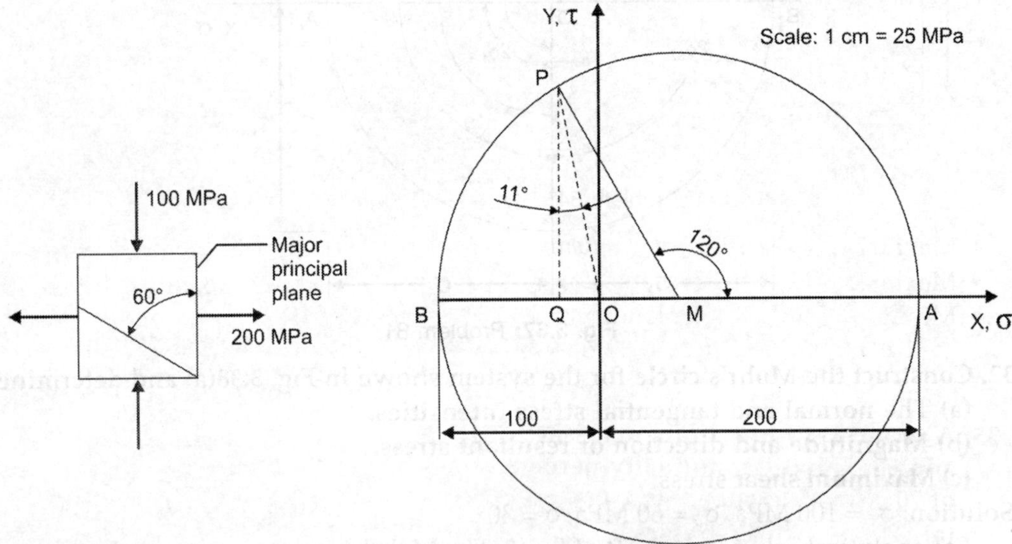

Fig. 3.39(a): Problem 33   **Fig. 3.39(b):** Problem 33

From **Fig. 3.39(b)**, we have
- Normal stress, $\sigma_n = OQ \times scale = -1 \times 25 = -25$ MPa
- Tangential stress, $\tau = PQ \times scale = 5.2 \times 25 = 130$ MPa
- Resultant stress, $\sigma_r = OP \times scale = 5.3 \times 25 = 132.5$ MPa
- Angle of obliquity, $\theta = \angle POQ = -11°$ (CW)
- Maximum shear stress, $\tau_{max} = Radius\ of\ Mohr's\ circle \times scale = 6 \times 25 = 150$ MPa

34. **At a point in a loaded elastic member, there are normal stresses of 60 MPa and 40 MPa (both tensile) respectively at right angles to each other with a positive shear stress of 20 MPa. Draw the Mohr's circle diagram and find:**
    (a) Principal stresses and their planes
    (b) Maximum shear stress at its plane.

VTU – June/ July 2016 – 12 Marks; June/ July 2011 – 08 Marks

Solution: Fig. 3.40(a) represents the stresses acting on the member. The Mohr's circle is constructed as shown in **Fig. 3.40(b)**.

From **Fig. 3.40(b)**, we have
- Maximum principal stress, $\sigma_1 = OE \times scale = 7.2 \times 10 = 72$ MPa
- Minimum principal stress, $\sigma_2 = OF \times scale = 2.8 \times 10 = 28$ MPa
- Maximum principal stress plane, $2\phi_1 = \angle CME = 63.5° \Rightarrow \phi_1 = 31.75°$
- Minimum principal stress plane, $\phi_2 = \phi_1 + 90° = 31.5° + 90° = 121.75°$

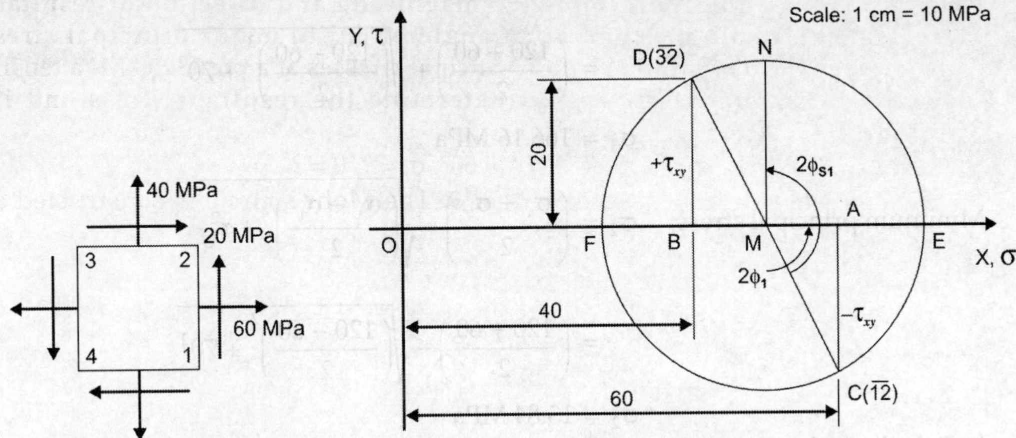

Fig. 3.40(a): Problem 34   **Fig. 3.40(b):** Problem 34

- Maximum shear stress, τ_{max} = *Radius of Mohr's circle* × *scale* = 2.3 × 10 = 23 MPa
- Maximum shear stress plane, $2\phi_{s1} = \angle CMN = 153° \Rightarrow \phi_{s1} = 76.5°$
- Minimum shear stress plane, $\phi_{s2} = \phi_{s1} + 90° = 76.5° + 90° = 166.5°$

$$\text{Or} \quad \phi_{s1} = \phi_1 + 45° = 31.75° + 45° = 76.75°$$
$$\phi_{s2} = \phi_1 + 135° = 31.75° + 135° = 166.75°$$

35. **A rectangular block of a material is subjected to tensile stresses of 120 N/mm²
and 60 N/mm² on mutually perpendicular planes together with a shear stress
of 70 N/mm². Find:**
    (a) The principal stresses
    (b) The principal planes
    (c) The maximum shear stress. Verify the results by constructing the Mohr's circle.

VTU – (CV) Dec. 14/ Jan. 15 – 12 Marks

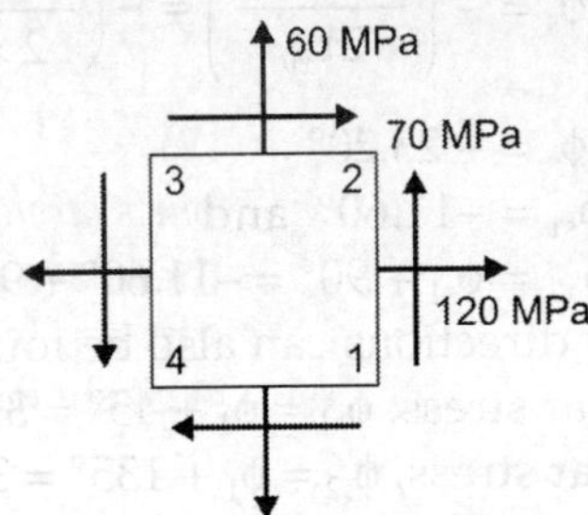

Fig. 3.41(a): Problem 35

Solution: σ_x = 120 MPa, σ_y = 60 MPa, τ_{xy} = 70 MPa. a) σ_1 = ?, σ_2 = ?, b) ϕ_1 = ?, ϕ_2 = ?,
c) τ_{max} = ?.

Fig. 3.41(a) represents the stresses acting on the member.

I. Analytical method

a. Principal stresses and their directions:

Maximum principal stress, $\quad \sigma_1 = \left(\dfrac{\sigma_x + \sigma_y}{2}\right) + \sqrt{\left(\dfrac{\sigma_x - \sigma_y}{2}\right)^2 + \tau_{xy}^2}$

$$= \left(\frac{120 + 60}{2}\right) + \sqrt{\left(\frac{120 - 60}{2}\right)^2 + 70^2}$$

$$\sigma_1 = 166.16 \text{ MPa}$$

Minimum principal stress, $\sigma_2 = \left(\frac{\sigma_x + \sigma_y}{2}\right) - \sqrt{\left(\frac{\sigma_x - \sigma_y}{2}\right)^2 + \tau_{xy}^2}$

$$= \left(\frac{120 + 60}{2}\right) - \sqrt{\left(\frac{120 - 60}{2}\right)^2 + 70^2}$$

$$\sigma_2 = 13.84 \text{ MPa}$$

b. Principal planes:

We know that $\tan 2\phi_1 = \left(\dfrac{2\tau_{xy}}{\sigma_x - \sigma_y}\right) = \left(\dfrac{2 \times 70}{120 - 60}\right) = 2.33$

$$2\phi_1 = 66.8°$$

$$\therefore \phi_1 = 33.40° \quad \text{and} \quad \phi_2 = \phi_1 + 90° = 33.40° + 90° = 123.40°$$

c. Maximum shear stress:

Maximum shear stress, $\tau_{max} = \pm \sqrt{\left(\dfrac{\sigma_x - \sigma_y}{2}\right)^2 + \tau_{xy}^2} = \pm \sqrt{\left(\dfrac{120 - 60}{2}\right)^2 + 70^2}$

$$= \pm 76.15 \text{ MPa}$$

Directions:

We know that $\tan 2\phi_s = -\left(\dfrac{\sigma_x - \sigma_y}{2\tau_{xy}}\right) = -\left(\dfrac{120 - 60}{2 \times 70}\right) = -0.43$

$$2\phi_s = -23.20°$$

$$\therefore \phi_{s1} = -11.60° \quad \text{and}$$

$$\phi_{s2} = \phi_{s1} + 90° = -11.60° + 90° = 78.40°$$

The maximum shear stress directions can also be found as:

Direction of maximum shear stress, $\phi_{s1} = \phi_1 + 45° = 33.40° + 45° = 78.40°$

Direction of minimum shear stress, $\phi_{s2} = \phi_1 + 135° = 33.40° + 135° = 168.40°$
[or $\phi_{s1} + 90°$]

II. Graphical method – Mohr's circle: The Mohr's circle is constructed as shown in Fig. 3.41(b)

From **Fig. 3.41(b)**, we have

- Maximum principal stress, $\sigma_1 = OE \times scale = 8.3 \times 20 = 166$ MPa
- Minimum principal stress, $\sigma_2 = OF \times scale = 0.69 \times 20 = 13.8$ MPa
- Maximum principal stress plane, $2\phi_1 = \angle CME = 67° \Rightarrow \phi_1 = 33.5°$
- Minimum principal stress plane, $\phi_2 = \phi_1 + 90° = 33.5° + 90° = 123.5°$
- Maximum shear stress, $\tau_{max} = Radius \ of \ Mohr's \ circle \times scale = 3.8 \times 20 = 76$ MPa
- Maximum shear stress plane, $2\phi_{s1} = \angle CMN = 157° \Rightarrow \phi_{s1} = 78.5°$
- Maximum shear stress plane, $\phi_{s2} = \phi_{s1} + 90° = 78.5° + 90° = 168.5°$

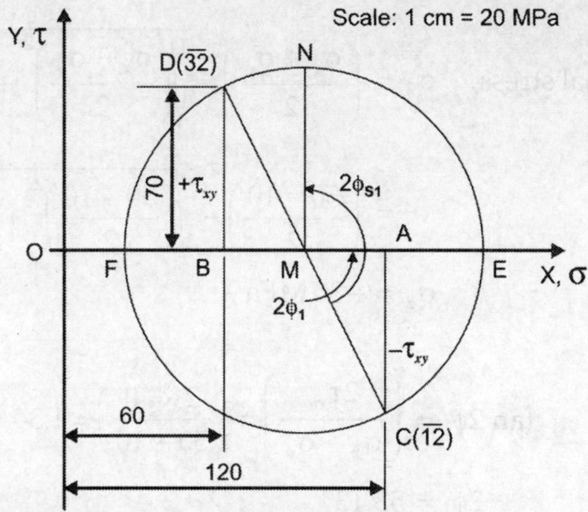

Fig. 3.41(b): Problem 35

36. For the state of stress shown in Fig. 3.42(a), determine:
   (a) The principal stresses and principal planes
   (b) Maximum in – plane shear stress and plane on which it is acting. Also find the normal stress on the maximum shear plane
   (c) Sketch the element aligned with planes of principal stresses and planes of maximum shear.

   Also draw the Mohr's circle for the above stress state.

VTU – Dec. 2011 – 20 Marks

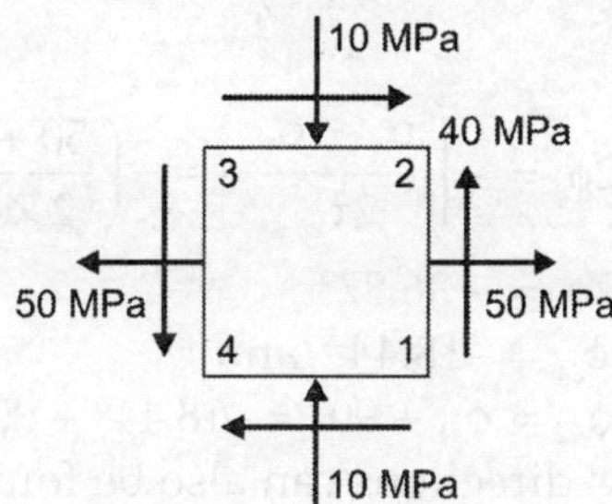

Fig. 3.42(a): Problem 36

Solution: $\sigma_x = 50$ MPa, $\sigma_y = -10$ MPa, $\tau_{xy} = 40$ MPa. a) $\sigma_1 = ?$, $\sigma_2 = ?$, $\phi_1 = ?$, $\phi_2 = ?$, b) $\tau_{max} = ?$, $\phi_{s1} = ?$, $\phi_{s2} = ?$

I. Analytical method

a. Principal stresses and their directions:

Maximum principal stress,

$$\sigma_1 = \left(\frac{\sigma_x + \sigma_y}{2}\right) + \sqrt{\left(\frac{\sigma_x - \sigma_y}{2}\right)^2 + \tau_{xy}^2}$$

$$= \left(\frac{50 - 10}{2}\right) + \sqrt{\left(\frac{50 + 10}{2}\right)^2 + 40^2}$$

$$\sigma_1 = 70 \text{ MPa}$$

Minimum principal stress, $\quad \sigma_2 = \left(\dfrac{\sigma_x + \sigma_y}{2}\right) - \sqrt{\left(\dfrac{\sigma_x - \sigma_y}{2}\right)^2 + \tau_{xy}^2}$

$$= \left(\dfrac{50 - 10}{2}\right) - \sqrt{\left(\dfrac{50 + 10}{2}\right)^2 + 40^2}$$

$$\sigma_2 = -30\,\text{MPa}$$

Directions:

We know that $\quad \tan 2\phi_1 = \left(\dfrac{2\tau_{xy}}{\sigma_x - \sigma_y}\right) = \left(\dfrac{2 \times 40}{50 + 10}\right) = 1.34$

$$2\phi_1 = 53.13°$$
$$\therefore \ \phi_1 = 26.56° \ \text{ and } \ \phi_2 = \phi_1 + 90° = 26.56° + 90° = 116.56°$$

b. Maximum shear stress and planes:

Maximum shear stress, $\quad \tau_{max} = \pm \sqrt{\left(\dfrac{\sigma_x - \sigma_y}{2}\right)^2 + \tau_{xy}^2} = \pm \sqrt{\left(\dfrac{50 + 10}{2}\right)^2 + 40^2}$

$$= \pm 50\,\text{MPa}$$

Average (normal) stress on the planes of maximum shear stress is,

$$\sigma_{avg} = \left(\dfrac{\sigma_x + \sigma_y}{2}\right) = \dfrac{50 - 10}{2} = 20\,\text{MPa}$$

Directions:

$$\tan 2\phi_s = -\left(\dfrac{\sigma_x - \sigma_y}{2\tau_{xy}}\right) = -\left(\dfrac{50 + 10}{2 \times 40}\right) = -0.75$$

$$2\phi_s = -36.87°$$
$$\therefore \ \phi_{s1} = -18.44° \ \text{ and}$$
$$\phi_{s2} = \phi_{s1} + 90° = -18.44° + 90° = 71.56°$$

The maximum shear stress directions can also be found as:

Direction of maximum shear stress, $\phi_{s1} = \phi_1 + 45° = 26.56° + 45° = 71.56°$

Direction of minimum shear stress, $\phi_{s2} = \phi_1 + 135° = 26.56° + 135° = 161.56°$

[or $\phi_{s1} + 90°$]

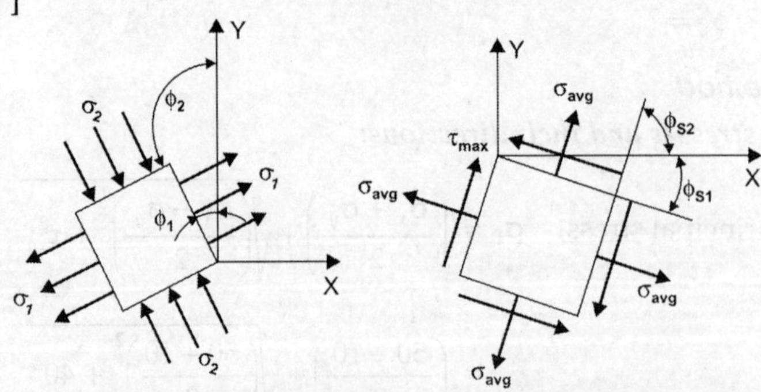

Fig. 3.42(b): Problem 36   **Fig. 3.42(c): Problem 36**

Principal stresses and directions   **Maximum shear stress and directions**

II. Graphical method – Mohr's circle: The Mohr's circle is constructed as shown in Fig. 3.42(d)

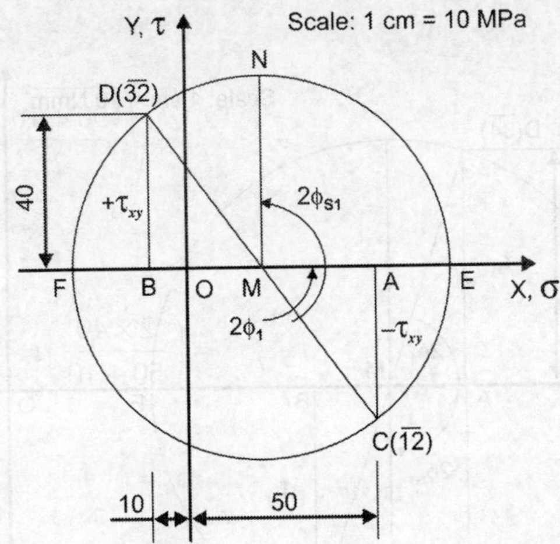

Fig. 3.42(d): Problem 36

From **Fig. 3.42(d)**, we have

- Maximum principal stress, $\sigma_1 = OE \times scale = 7 \times 10 = 70$ MPa
- Minimum principal stress, $\sigma_2 = OF \times scale = -3 \times 10 = -30$ MPa
- Maximum principal stress plane, $2\phi_1 = \angle CME = 53° \Rightarrow \phi_1 = 26.5°$
- Minimum principal stress plane, $\phi_2 = \phi_1 + 90° = 26.5° + 90° = 116.5°$
- Maximum shear stress, $\tau_{max} = Radius\ of\ Mohr's\ circle \times scale = 5 \times 10 = 50$ MPa
- Maximum shear stress plane, , $2\phi_{s1} = \angle CMN = 143° \Rightarrow \phi_{s1} = 71.5°$ (CCW)
- Maximum shear stress plane, $\phi_{s2} = \phi_{s1} + 90° = 71.5° + 90° = 161.5°$
- Average (normal) stress on the planes of maximum shear stress is, $\sigma_{avg} = OM \times scale = 2 \times 10 = 20$ MPa

37. The state of stress in a two-dimensionally stressed body is shown in Fig. 3.43(a). Determine the principal planes, principal stresses, maximum shear stress and their planes. Also draw the Mohr's circle to verify the results obtained analytically. Indicate all the above planes by a sketch.

VTU – Dec. 2012 – 20 Marks; Dec. 13/ Jan. 14 – 08 Marks; (CV) Dec. 2011 – 14 Marks

Solution: $\sigma_x = -120$ N/mm^2, $\sigma_y = -80$ N/mm^2, $\tau_{xy} = -60$ N/mm^2. a) $\sigma_1 = ?$, $\sigma_2 = ?$, $\phi_1 = ?$, $\phi_2 = ?$, b) $\tau_{max} = ?$, $\sigma_{s1} = ?$, $\phi_{s2} = ?$

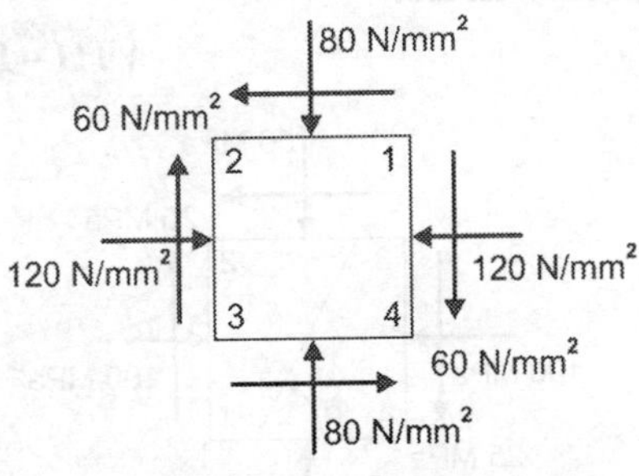

Fig. 3.43(a): Problem 37

I. Analytical method: For analytical solution, refer to Problem 20

II. Graphical method – Mohr's circle: The Mohr's circle is constructed as shown in Fig. 3.43(b)

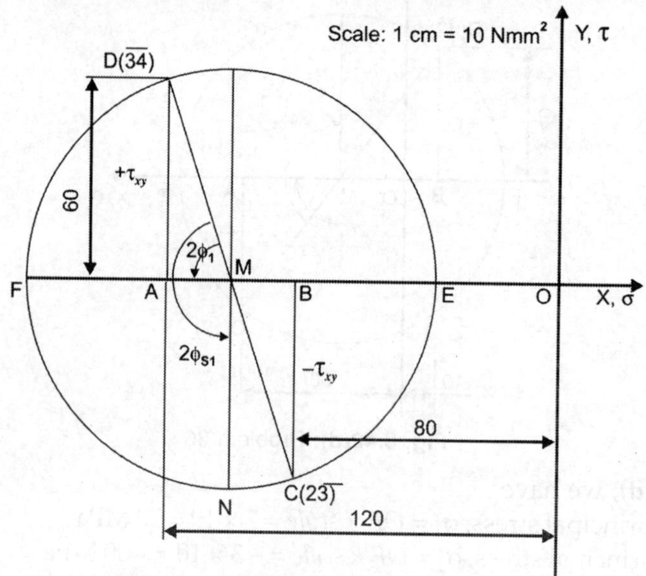

Fig. 3.43(b): Problem 37

From **Fig. 3.43(b)**, we have

- Maximum principal stress, $\sigma_1 = OE \times scale = -3.7 \times 10 = -37$ MPa
- Minimum principal stress, $\sigma_2 = OF \times scale = -16.3 \times 10 = -163$ MPa
- Maximum principal stress plane, $2\phi_1 = \angle DMF = 71.6° \Rightarrow \phi_1 = 35.8°$
- Minimum principal stress plane, $\phi_2 = \phi_1 + 90° = 35.8° + 90° = 125.8°$
- Maximum shear stress, $\tau_{max} = Radius\ of\ Mohr's\ circle \times scale = 6.3 \times 10 = 63$ MPa
- Maximum shear stress plane, , $2\phi_{s1} = \angle DMN = 161.6° \Rightarrow \phi_{s1} = 80.8°$ (CCW)
- Maximum shear stress plane, $\phi_{s2} = \phi_{s1} + 90° = 80.8° + 90° = 170.8°$
- Average (normal) stress on the planes of maximum shear stress is, $\sigma_{avg} = OM \times scale = 10 \times 10 = 100$ MPa

38. **A machine component is subjected to stresses as shown in Fig. 3.44(a). Find the normal and shearing stresses on the section AB inclined at an angle of 600° with x-axis. Also find the resultant stress on the section. Verify the above results by drawing Mohr's circle.**

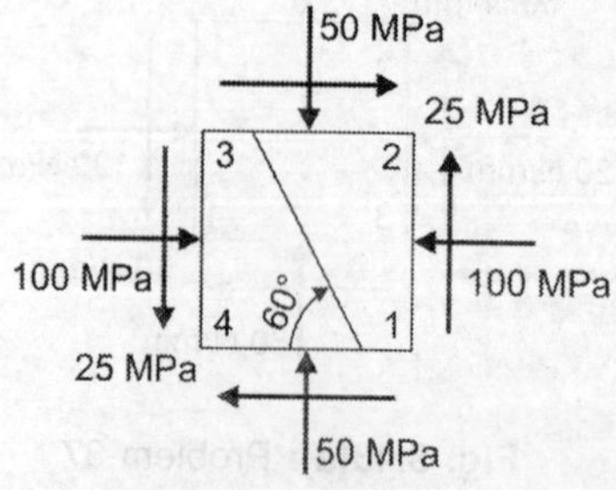

Fig. 3.44(a): Problem 38

Solution: $\sigma_x = -100$ MPa, $\sigma_y = -50$ MPa, $\tau_{xy} = 25$ MPa, $\phi' = 60°$ (with horizontal), $\phi = 30°$ (with vertical). $\sigma_n = ?, \sigma_r = ?, \tau = ?$.

I.. Analytical method: For analytical solution, refer to Problem 27

II. Graphical method – Mohr's circle

The Mohr's circle is constructed as shown in **Fig. 3.44(b)**

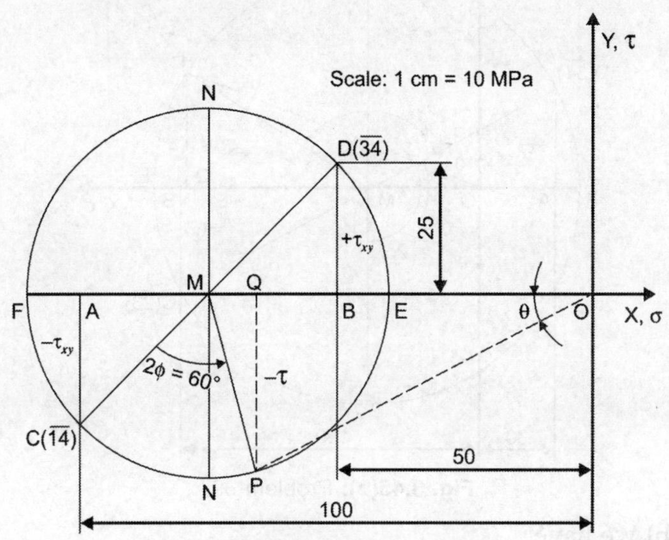

Fig. 3.44(b): Problem 38

From **Fig. 3.44(b)** we have:

- Normal stress, $\sigma_n = OQ \times scale = -6.6 \times 10 = -66$ MPa
- Tangential stress, $\tau = PQ \times scale = -3.4 \times 10 = -34$ MPa
- Resultant stress, $\sigma_r = OP \times scale = 7.4 \times 10 = 74$ MPa
- Angle of obliquity, $\theta = \angle POQ = -27.4°$ (CW)

39. At a certain point in a strained material the stress condition shown in Fig. 3.45(a) exists. Find

    a. The normal and shear stress on the inclined plane AB

    b. Principal stresses and principal planes

    c. Maximum shear stress.

VTU – June/ July 15 – 10 Marks

Solution: $\sigma_x = -30$ MPa, $\sigma_y = 120$ MPa, $\tau_{xy} = -40$ MPa, $\phi' = 30°$ (CCW with horizontal), $\phi = 90 - 30° = 60°$ (CW with vertical). $\therefore \ \phi = -60°$ (opposite) a) $\sigma_n = ?$, $\tau = ?$, b) $\sigma_1 = ?, \sigma_2 = ?, \phi_1 = ?, \phi_2 = ?$, c) $\tau_{max} = ?, \phi_{s1} = ?, \phi_{s2} = ?$

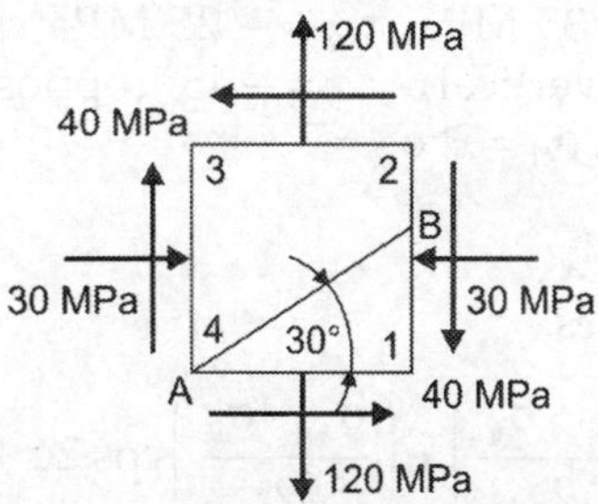

Fig. 3.45(a): Problem 39

For analytical solution, refer **Problem 24**.

Graphical method – Mohr's circle: The Mohr's circle is constructed as shown in Fig. 3.45(b)

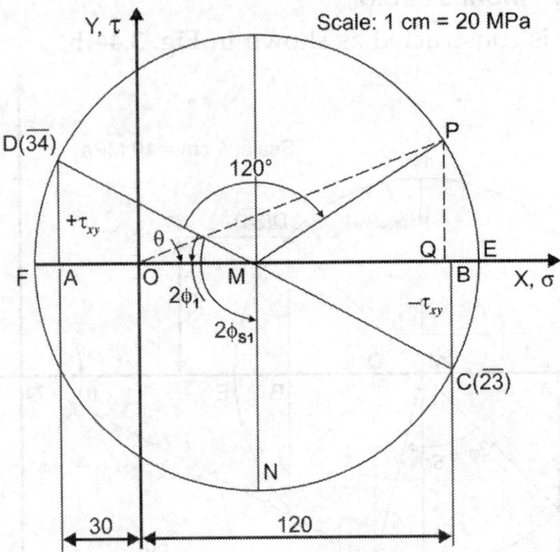

Fig. 3.45(b): Problem 39

From **Fig. 3.45(b)** we have:
- Normal stress, $\sigma_n = OQ \times scale = 5.8 \times 20 = 116$ MPa
- Tangential stress, $\tau = PQ \times scale = 2.3 \times 20 = 46$ MPa
- Resultant stress, $\sigma_r = OP \times scale = 6.3 \times 20 = 126$ MPa
- Angle of obliquity, $\theta = \angle POQ = -21°$ (CW)
- Maximum principal stress, $\sigma_1 = OE \times scale = 6.5 \times 20 = 130$ MPa
- Minimum principal stress, $\sigma_2 = OF \times scale = -2 \times 20 = -40$ MPa
- Maximum principal stress plane, $2\phi_1 = \angle DMF = 28° \Rightarrow \phi_1 = 14°$
- Minimum principal stress plane, $\phi_2 = \phi_1 + 90° = 14° + 90° = 104°$
- Maximum shear stress, $\tau_{max} = Radius\ of\ Mohr's\ circle \times scale = 4.3 \times 20 = 86$ MPa
- Maximum shear stress plane, , $2\phi_{s1} = \angle DMN = 118° \Rightarrow \phi_{s1} = 59°$
- Maximum shear stress plane, $\phi_{s2} = \phi_{s1} + 90° = 59° + 90° = 149°$

40. **A point in a strained material is subjected to stresses shown in Fig. 3.46(a). Using Mohr's circle, determine the normal and tangential stresses across the oblique plane. Check the answer analytically.**

VTU – June 2012 – 12 Marks

Solution: $\sigma_x = 65$ MPa, $\sigma_y = 35$ MPa, $\tau_{xy} = -25$ MPa, $\phi' = 45°$ (CW with vertical), $\phi = 90° - 45° = 45°$ (CW with vertical). $\therefore \tau = -45°$ (opposite) a) $\sigma_n = ?, \tau = ?,$ b) $\sigma_1 = ?,$ $\sigma_2 = ?, \phi_1 = ?, \phi_2 = ?,$ c) $\tau_{max} = ?, \phi_{s1} = ?, \phi_{s2} = ?$

Analytical method

Normal and tangential stresses:

$$\text{Normal stress,} \quad \sigma_n = \left(\frac{\sigma_x + \sigma_y}{2}\right) + \left(\frac{\sigma_x - \sigma_y}{2}\right)\cos 2\phi + \tau_{xy}\sin 2\phi$$

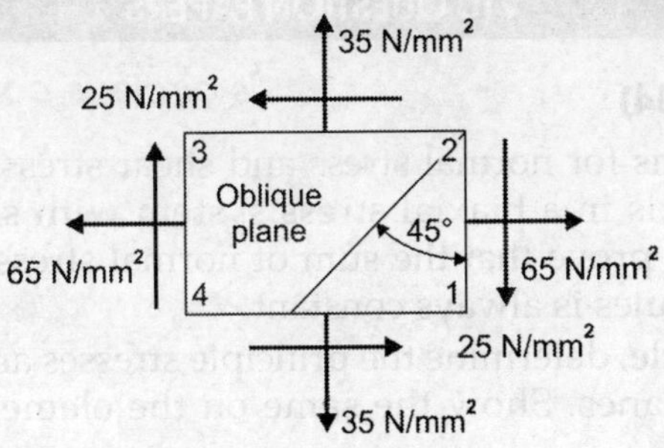

Fig. 3.46(a): Problem 40

$$= \left(\frac{65+35}{2}\right) + \left[\left(\frac{65-35}{2}\right)\cos(2\times-45)\right] + (-25)\times\sin(2\times-45)$$

$$\sigma_n = 75\,\text{MPa}$$

Tangential stress, $\tau = \left(\dfrac{\sigma_x - \sigma_y}{2}\right)\sin 2\phi - \tau_{xy}\cos 2\phi$

$$= \left[\left(\frac{65-35}{2}\right)\cos(2\times-45)\right] - (-25)\times\sin(2\times-45)$$

$$\tau = -15\,\text{MPa}$$

Graphical method – Mohr's circle: The Mohr's circle is constructed as shown in Fig. 3.46(b).

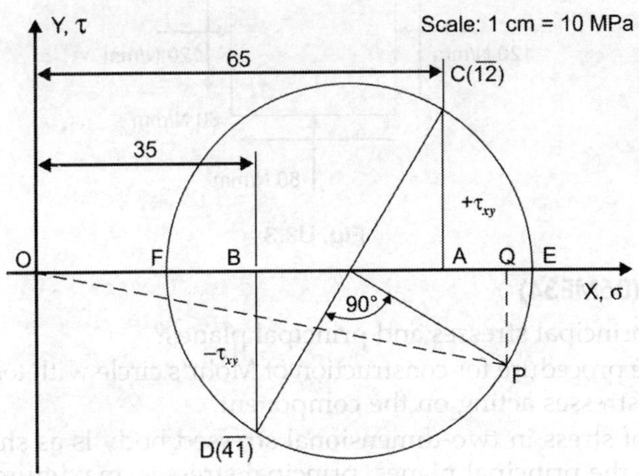

Fig. 3.46(b): Problem 40

From **Fig. 3.46(b)** we have:
- Normal stress, $\sigma_n = OQ \times scale = 7.5 \times 10 = 75\,\text{MPa}$
- Tangential stress, $\tau = PQ \times scale = -1.51 \times 10 = -15.1\,\text{MPa}$

Dec.07/Jan.08 (06ME34)

1. a. Derive expressions for normal stress and shear stress on a plane inclined at θ to the vertical axis in a biaxial stress system with shear stress as shown in **Fig. U3.1**. Hence, prove that the sum of normal stresses on any two mutually perpendicular planes is always constant. **(10 Marks)**

b. Using Mohr's circle, determine the principle stresses and the planes, max. shear stress and the planes. Show the same on the elements separately. Refer to **Fig. U3.2**. **(10 Marks)**

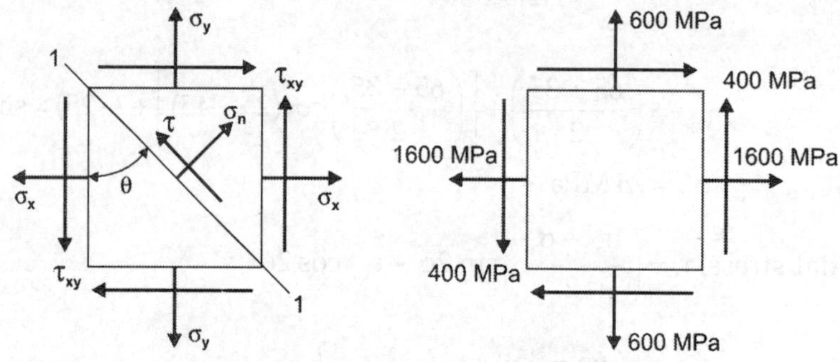

Fig. U3.1   **Fig. U3.2**

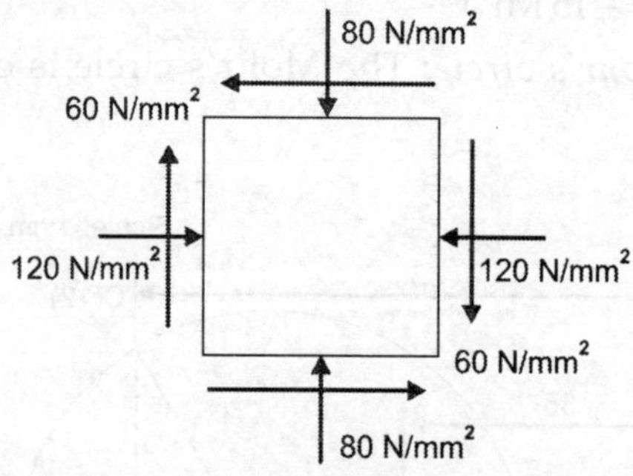

Fig. U3.3

June/July 2008 (06ME34)

2. a. What are principal stresses and principal planes? **(02 Marks)**

b. Explain the procedure for construction of Mohr's circle with tensile, compressive and shear stresses acting on the component. **(06 Marks)**

c. The state of stress in two-dimensional stressed body is as shown in **Fig. U3.3**. Determine the principal planes, principal stresses, maximum shear stress and their planes. **(12 Marks)**

Dec.08/Jan.09 (06ME34)

3. a. Define principal stresses and principal planes. **(03 Marks)**

b. Prove that the sum of normal stresses on any two mutually perpendicular planes is a constant in a general two-dimensional stress system. **(07 Marks)**

c. A plane element is subjected to stresses as shown in **Fig. U3.4**. Determine principal stresses, maximum shear stress and their planes. Sketch the planes determined. **(07 Marks)**

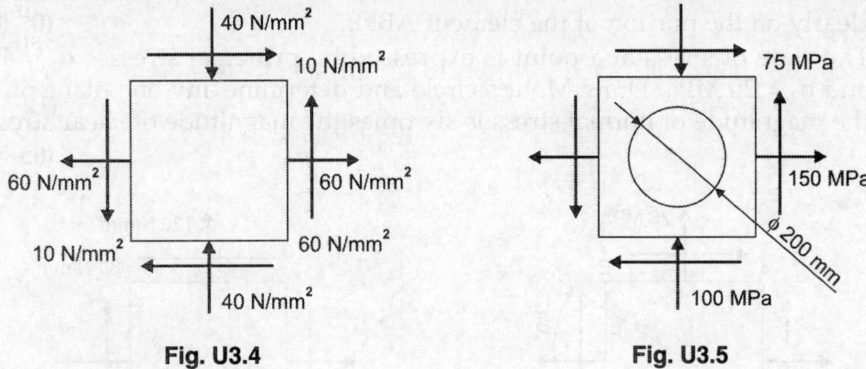

Fig. U3.4   **Fig. U3.5**

June/July 2009 (06ME34)

4. a. Construct the Mohr's circle for a point in the machine member subjected to pure shear of 50 MPa. Determine the maximum and minimum stresses induced and orientation of their planes. **(08 Marks)**

   b. A point in a machine member is subjected to stresses as shown in **Fig. U3.5**. A circle of diameter 200 mm on the member is converted into ellipse after the application of stresses. Determine the major and minor axes of the ellipse and their orientations. Take $E = 210$ GPPa and the Poisson's ratio as 0.3. **(15 Marks)**

Dec. 09/Jan. 10 (06ME34)

5. a. Define   i. Principal stress   ii. Principal strain. **(04 Marks)**

   b. A machine component is subjected to stresses as shown in **Fig. U3.6**. Find the normal and shearing stresses on the section AB inclined at an angle of 60° with x-axis. Also find the resultant stress on the section. Verify the above results by drawing Mohr's circle. **(16 Marks)**

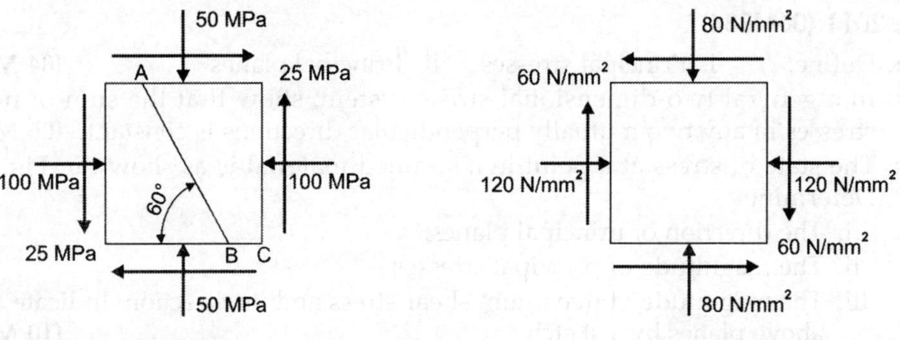

Fig. U3.6   **Fig. U3.7**

May/June 2010 (06ME34)

6. The state of stress in a two-dimensional stressed body is shown in **Fig. U3.7**. Determine the principal planes, principal stress, maximum shear stress and their planes. Schematically represent these planes on $x - y$ coordinates. **(15 Marks)**

Dec. 10 (06ME34)

7. a. Explain in brief 'plane stress'. **(04 Marks)**

   b. The state of stress at a point is shown in **Fig. U3.8**. If the plane EF cuts the element, determine the normal and shear stresses on the plane and show them clearly on the portion of the element ABFE. **(08 Marks)**

   c. The state of stress at a point is expressed by principal stresses σ_1 = 40 MPa and σ_2 = 20 MPa. Draw Mohr's circle and determine any one plane on which the magnitude of normal stress is six times the magnitude of shear stress. **(08 Marks)**

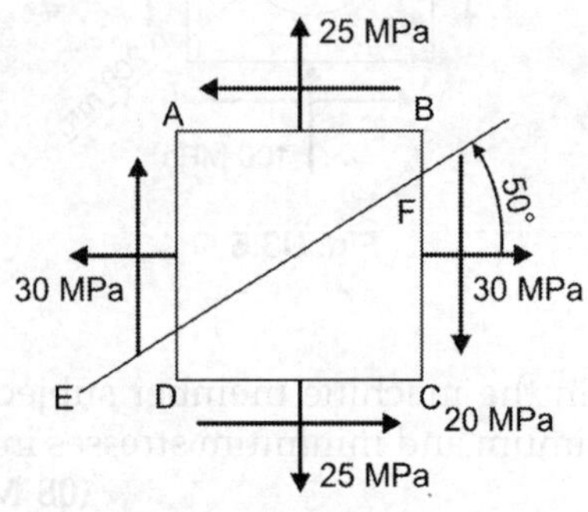

Fig. U3.8

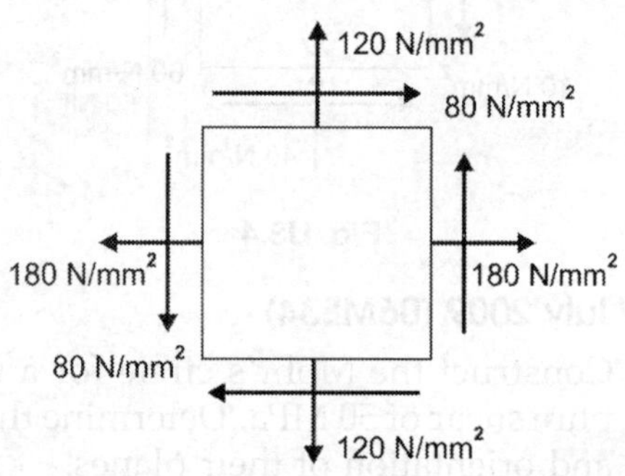

Fig. U3.9

June/July 2011 (06ME34)

8. a. Derive an expression for the normal stress and shear stress on a plane inclined at θ to the vertical axis in an biaxial stress system with shear. Also prove that the sum of normal stresses on any two mutually perpendicular planes is always a constant. **(12 Marks)**

   b. At a point in a loaded elastic member, there are normal stresses of 60 MPa and 40 MPa (both tensile) respectively at right angles to each other with positive shear stress of 20 MPa. Draw the Mohr's circle diagram and find:

   i. Principal stresses and their planes

   ii. Maximum shear stress and its plane. **(08 Marks)**

Dec. 2011 (06ME34)

9. a. Define: i. Principal stresses   ii. Principal planes   **(04 Marks)**

   b. In a general two-dimensional stress system, show that the sum of normal stresses in any two mutually perpendicular directions is constant. **(06 Marks)**

   c. The state of stress at a point in a strained material is as shown in **Fig. U3.9**. Determine:

   i. The direction of principal planes.

   ii. The magnitude of principal stresses

   iii. The magnitude of maximum shear stress and its direction. Indicate all the above planes by a sketch. **(10 Marks)**

Dec. 2011 (10ME34)

10. a. For the state of stress shown in **Fig. U3.10**, determine:

   i. The principal stresses and principal planes.

ii. Maximum in – plane shear stress and plane on which it is acting. Also find the normal stress on the maximum shear plane.

iii. Sketch the element aligned with planes of principal stresses and planes of maximum shear.

Also draw the Mohr's circle for the above stress state. **(20 Marks)**

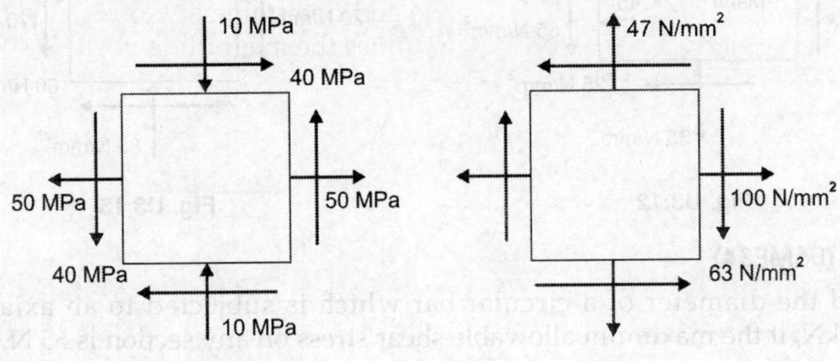

Fig. U3.10   Fig. U3.11

June 2012 (06ME34)

11. **a.** What are the principal stresses and principal planes? Explain their uses.

(04 Marks)

b. Explain the procedure for construction of Mohr's circle with tensile, compressive and shear stresses acting in the component. **(06 Marks)**

c. A rectangular block of material is subjected to a tensile stress of 100 N/mm^2 on one plane and tensile stress of 47 N/mm^2 on the plane at right angle to the forms as shown in **Fig. U3.11**. Each of the above stresses is accompanied by a shear stress of 63 N/mm^2. Determine the magnitude and direction of each principal stress and magnitude of maximum shear stress. Sketch the planes and mark the stresses on the planes. **(06 Marks)**

June 2012 (10ME34)

12. **a.** A rectangular bar is subjected to two direct stresses σ_x and σ_y in two mutually perpendicular directions. Prove that the normal stress σ_n and shear stress τ on an oblique plane which is inclined at θ with the axis of minor stress are given by

$$\sigma_n = \left(\frac{\sigma_x + \sigma_y}{2}\right) + \left(\frac{\sigma_x - \sigma_y}{2}\right)\cos 2\theta \text{ and } \tau = \left(\frac{\sigma_x - \sigma_y}{2}\right)\sin 2\theta \qquad \textbf{(08 Marks)}$$

b. A point in a strained material is subjected to stresses shown in **Fig. U3.12**. Using Mohr's circle, determine the normal and tangential stresses across the oblique plane. Check the answer analytically. **(12 Marks)**

Dec. 2012 (10ME34)

13. **a.** The state of stress in a two-dimensionally stressed body is shown in **Fig. U3.13**. Determine the principal planes, principal stresses, maximum shear stress and their planes. Also draw the Mohr's circle to verify the results obtained analytically. Indicate all the above planes by a sketch. **(20 Marks)**

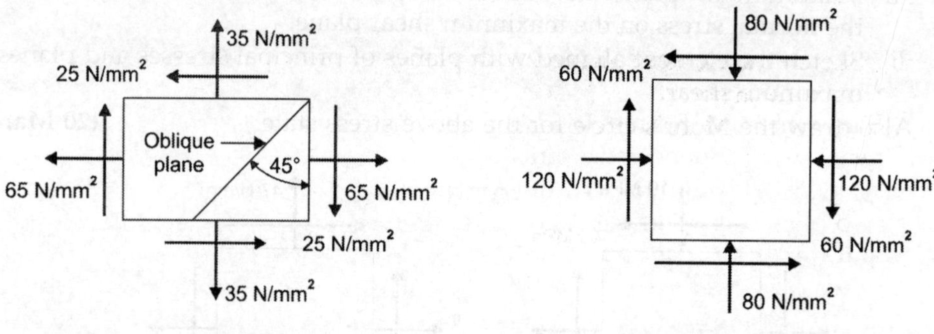

Fig. U3.12

Fig. U3.13

Jan. 2013 (06ME34)

14. a. Find the diameter of a circular bar which is subjected to an axial pull of 160 kN, if the maximum allowable shear stress on any section is 65 N/mm².

(05 Marks)

b. A rectangular bar is subjected to two direct stresses σ_x and σ_y in two mutually perpendicular directions. Prove that the normal stress on an oblique plane which is inclined at θ with the axis of minor stress are given by

$$\sigma_n = \left(\frac{\sigma_x + \sigma_y}{2}\right) + \left(\frac{\sigma_x - \sigma_y}{2}\right) \cos 2\theta$$

(07 Marks)

c. At a certain point in a material under stress, the intensity of resultant stress on a vertical plane is 10 N/mm² inclined to 30° to the normal to that plane and the stress on the horizontal plane has a normal tensile stress of 6 N/mm², as shown in **Fig. U3.14**. Find the principal stresses and the location of the planes on which they act.

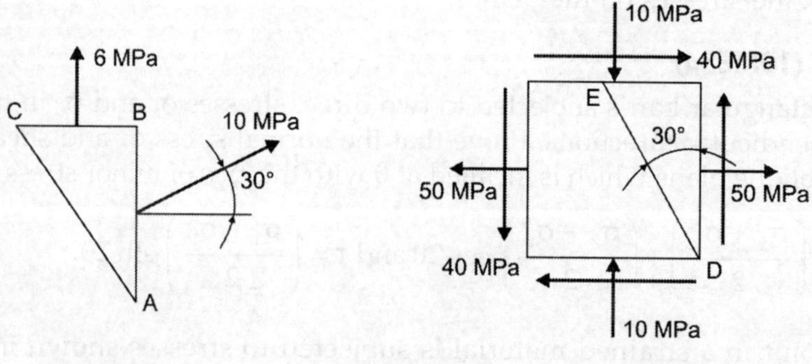

Fig. U3.14

Fig. U3.15

June/July 2013 (06ME34)

15. a. A circular bar of 20 mm diameter is subjected to compression. If the permissible stresses in compression and shear are 90 MPa and 25 MPa respectively, determine the failure load and plane. **(06 Marks)**

b. For the state of stress shown in **Fig. U3.15**, determine:
   i. Principal planes
   ii. Principal stresses

iii. Maximum shear stress and their planes

iv. Normal and shear stress acting on plane DE. **(14 Marks)**

June/July 2013 (10ME34)

16. a. Show that the sum of normal stresses on any two planes at right angles in a general two-dimensional stress system is constant. **(08 Marks)**

b. At a certain point in a strained material the value of normal stresses across two planes at right angles to each other are 80 MPa and 32 MPa, both tensile and there is a shear stress of 32 MPa clockwise on the plane carrying 80 MPa stresses across the planes as shown in **Fig. U3.16**. Determine:

i. Maximum and minimum normal stresses and locate their planes.

ii. Maximum shear stress and specify its plane. **(12 Marks)**

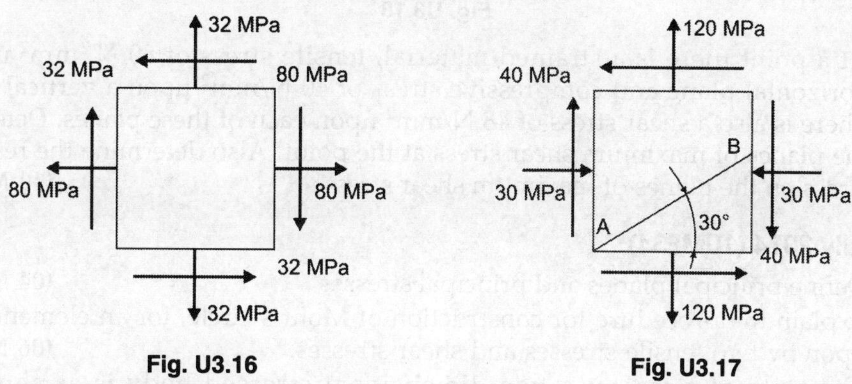

<table>
<tr><td align="center">**Fig. U3.16**</td><td align="center">**Fig. U3.17**</td></tr>
</table>

Dec. 13/Jan. 14 (06ME34)

17. a. Define Principal stress and principal strain. **(02 Marks)**

b. Prove that sum of normal stresses in any two mutually perpendicular directions is a constant. **(08 Marks)**

c. At a certain point in a strained material the stress condition is obtained as shown in **Fig. U3.17**.

Find: i. Normal and shear stresses on the inclined plane AB

ii. Major and minor principal stresses. **(10 Marks)**

Dec. 13/Jan. 14 (10ME34)

18. a. Determine the expressions for normal and tangential stress on a plane inclined at θ to the plane of stress in x-direction in a general two-dimensional stress system and show that the sum of normal stress in any two mutually perpendicular directions is constant. **(12 Marks)**

b. The state of stress in a two-dimensional stressed body is shown in **Fig. U3.18**. Determine graphically (by drawing Mohr's circle), the principal stresses, principal planes, maximum shear stress and its planes. **(08 Marks)**

June/July 2014 (10ME34)

19. a. Show that:

i. Sum of normal stresses in any two mutually perpendicular directions is constant.

ii. Principal planes are planes of maximum normal stress also. **(10 Marks)**

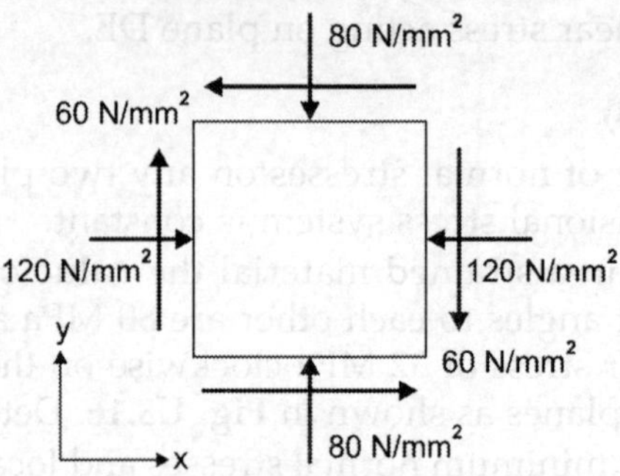

Fig. U3.18

b. At a point there is a strained material, tensile stress of 80 N/mm^2 upon a horizontal plane and compressive stress of 40 N/mm^2 upon a vertical plane. There is also a shear stress of 48 N/mm^2 upon each of these planes. Determine the planes of maximum shear stress at the point. Also determine the resultant stress on the planes of maximum shear stress. **(10 Marks)**

June/July 2014 (10ME34)

20. a. Define principal planes and principal stresses **(04 Marks)**
   b. Explain the procedure for construction of Mohr's circle, for an element acted upon by two tensile stresses and shear stresses. **(06 Marks)**
   c. The state of stress in a two-dimensional stressed body is as shown in **Fig. U3.19**. Determine the principal planes, principal stresses, maximum shear stress and their planes. **(10 Marks)**

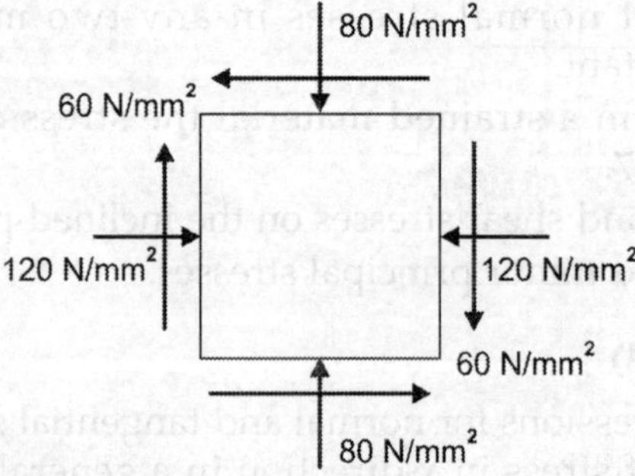

Fig. U3.19

Dec. 14/Jan. 15 (06ME34)

21. a. Define principal planes. Prove that the sum of normal stresses on any two mutually perpendicular planes is constant in a general two-dimensional stress system. **(08 Marks)**
   b. The state of stress in a two-dimensionally stressed body is as shown in **Fig. U3.20**. Determine principal stresses, principal planes and maximum shear stress. Also determine the normal and tangential stresses on plane AC. **(12 Marks)**

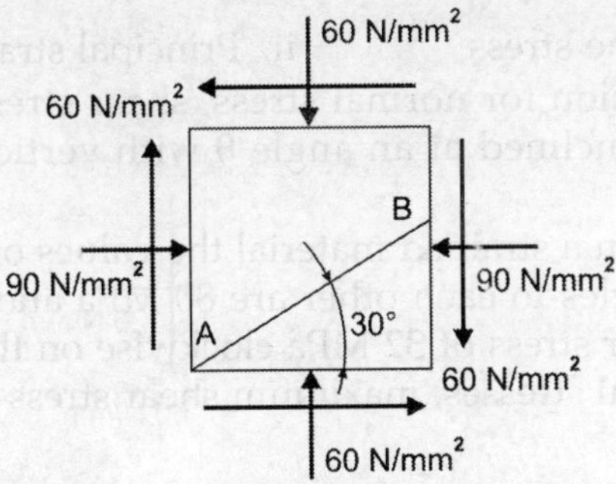

Fig. U3.20

Dec. 14/Jan. 15 (10ME34)

22. a. A point in a plate girder is subjected to a horizontal tensile stress of 100 N/mm^2 and a vertical shear stress of 60 N/mm^2. Find the magnitude of principal stresses and its location. **(05 Marks)**

b. An element with the stresses acting on it is as shown in **Fig. U3.21**. By Mohr's circle method, determine:

   i. Normal and shear stress acting on a plane whose normal is at an angle of 110° with respect to x-axis.

   ii. Principal stresses and its locations

   iii. Maximum shear stresses and its location. **(15 Marks)**

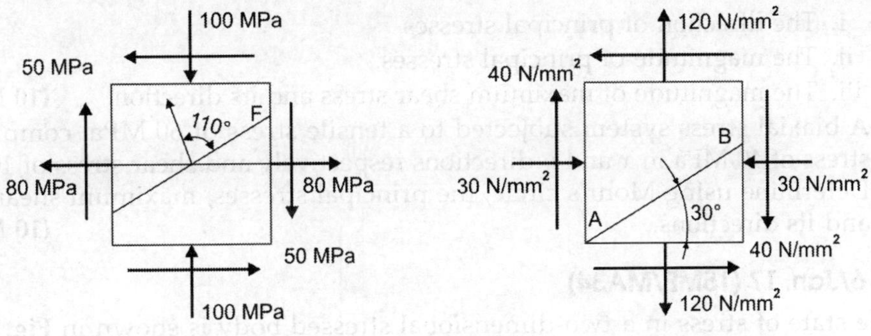

Fig. U3.21   **Fig. U3.22**

June/July 15 (10ME34)

23. a. Define principal stresses and principal planes. **(03 Marks)**

b. Explain the construction of Mohr's circle and represent principal stress. **(07 Marks)**

c. At a certain point in a strained material the stress condition shown in **Fig. U3.22** exists. Find

   i. The normal and shear stress on the inclined plane AB

   ii. Principal stresses and principal planes

   iii. Maximum shear stress. **(10 Marks)**

Dec. 15/Jan. 16 (10ME/AU34)

24. a. Define   i. Plane stress   ii. Principal strain   **(02 Marks)**

b. Derive the expression for normal stress, shear stress and resultant stress on an oblique plane inclined at an angle θ with vertical axis in a biaxial direct stress system.   **(08 Marks)**

c. At a certain point in a strained material the values of normal stress across two planes at right angles to each other are 80 MPa and 32 MPa, both are tensile and there is a shear stress of 32 MPa clockwise on the plane carrying 80 MPa. Determine principal stresses, maximum shear stress and their planes.

    (10 Marks)

June/July 2016 (10ME/AU34)

25. a. Derive an expression for the normal stress and shear stress on a plane inclined at θ to the vertical axis in a biaxial stress system.   **(08 Marks)**

b. At a point in a loaded elastic member, there are normal stresses of 60 MPa and 40 MPa (both tensile) respectively at right angles to each other with a positive shear stress of 20 MPa. Draw the Mohr's circle diagram and find:

    i. Principal stresses and their planes

    ii. Maximum shear stress at its plane.   **(12 Marks)**

Dec. 16/Jan. 17 (10ME/AU34)

26. a. State of stress at a point is a strained material with tensile stress of 180 MPa in x-direction, tensile stress of 120 MPa in y-direction and shear stress of 80 MPa. Determine:

    i. The direction of principal stresses

    ii. The magnitude of principal stresses.

    iii. The magnitude of maximum shear stress and its direction.   **(10 Marks)**

b. A biaxial stress system subjected to a tensile stress of 60 MPa, compressive stress of 40 MPa in x and y-directions respectively and shear stress of 10 MPa. Determine using Mohr's circle, the principal stresses, maximum shear stress and its directions.   **(10 Marks)**

Dec. 16/Jan. 17 (15ME/MA34)

27. The state of stress in a two-dimensional stressed body is shown in **Fig. U3.23**. Determine the principal plane, principal stresses and maximum shear stresses. Sketch the results. Construct the Mohr's circle and verify the answer graphically.

    (20 Marks)

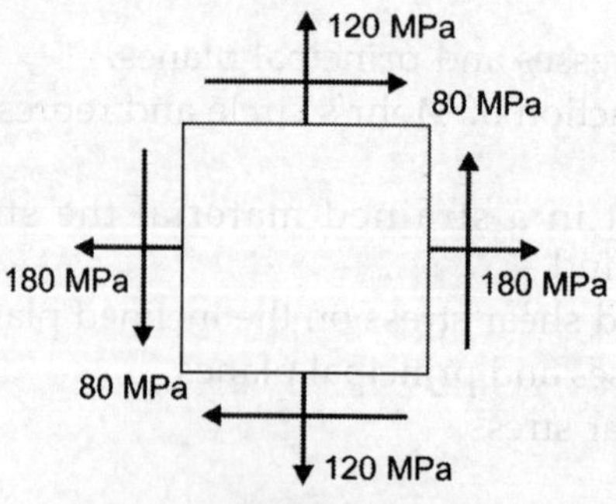

Fig. U3.23

June/July 2017 (10ME/AU34)

28. a. Explain:
    i. Principal planes and principal stresses
    ii. Maximum and minimum shear stresses with respect to compound stress.
    (06 Marks)
   b. Describe the construction of Mohr's circle for plane stress. **(06 Marks)**
   c. A point in a beam is subjected to maximum tensile stress of 110 MPa and shear stress 30 MPa. Find the magnitudes and direction of principal stresses. If the point in the beam is in the compression zone under the same magnitude of bending stress and shear stress, find magnitudes of principal stresses and their directions. **(08 Marks)**

June/July 2017 (15ME/MA34)

29. A point in a strained material is subjected to tensile stress of 500 MPa and 300 MPa in two mutually perpendicular planes. Calculate the normal, tangential, resultant stresses and its obliquity on a plane making an angle of 30° with the axis of second stress. Also find the maximum stress. **(10 Marks)**

30. An elemental cube is subjected to tensile stress of 30 MPa and 10 MPa acting on two mutually perpendicular planes and a shear stress of 10 MPa on these planes. Draw the Mohr's circle of stresses and hence determine the magnitudes and directions of principal stresses and also the greatest shear stress. **(08 Marks)**

Dec. 17/Jan. 18 (10ME/AU34)

31. a. Show that the sum of the normal stresses on any two planes at right angles in a general two-dimensional stress system is constant. **(06 Marks)**
   b. Sketch the Mohr's circle for the following cases (**Fig. U3.24**): **(04 Marks)**

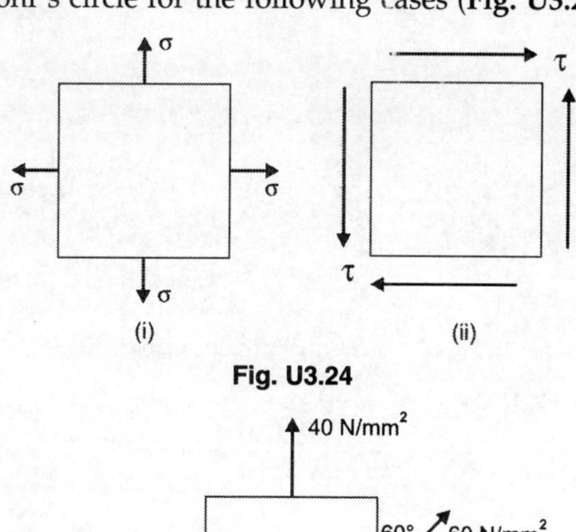

Fig. U3.24

Fig. U3.25

c. A point in a strained material is subjected to the stresses as shown in **Fig. U3.25**. Evaluate principal stresses and locate principal planes. Sketch the planes. **(10 Marks)**

Dec. 17/Jan. 18 (15ME/MA34)

32. Derive an expression for normal stress, shear stress and resultant stress on an oblique plane inclined at an angle θ with vertical axis (x-plane) in a biaxial stress system subjected to σ_x, σ_y and τ_{xy}. Also find the obliquity ϕ. **(10 Marks)**

33. A point in a strained material is subjected to a tensile stress of 500 MPa and 300 MPa in two mutually perpendicular planes and also these planes carries a shear stress of 100 MPa. Calculate the normal, tangential, resultant stresses on a plane making an angle of 30° with the vertical axis (x-plane). Also find the principal stresses. **(10 Marks)**

Thick and Thin Cylinders

Chapter Outline

4.1 INTRODUCTION

Cylinders and spheres are most commonly used in engineering works to hold liquid or gases under internal pressure. Examples include air compressors, boilers, tanks, engine cylinders, gas cylinders, roof domes, airplane wings, submarine hulls, etc. Failure occurs when the internal pressure causes a high tensile stress across the walls of the cylinder.

When gas is used, pressure is constant in all parts of the vessel. In case of liquids, the pressure is lowest at the top and increases with depth. On the other hand, if the vessels are empty, they are subjected to atmospheric pressure both internally and externally and hence the resultant effect of atmospheric pressure is zero (nil).

The shells are classified into two types based on the ratio of wall thickness to that of the diameter of the shell as:

- **Thin shells:** A cylinder is regarded as thin if the thickness is less than 1/20 of diameter

$$t < \frac{d}{20} \text{ or } t < \frac{r}{10} \qquad (t = \text{thickness of shell}) \qquad \text{... (Eq. 4.1)}$$

Here the normal stresses (tensile/compressive) are assumed to be uniformly distributed through the thickness of the wall. The operating pressure is around 30 MPa and more.

Examples: Boilers, tanks, steam pipes, water pipes, submarine hulls, etc.
- *Thick shells:* A cylinder is regarded as thick if the thickness is more than 1/20 of diameter

$$t > \frac{d}{20} \text{ or } t > \frac{r}{10} \qquad \text{... (Eq. 4.2)}$$

Here the normal stresses (tensile/compressive) vary along the thickness of the wall. The analysis of thick shells is more complex than that of thin shells. The operating pressure is more than 250 MPa.

4.2 THIN CYLINDRICAL SHELLS SUBJECTED TO INTERNAL PRESSURE

When a cylinder is subjected to internal pressure which may be due to a fluid or gas enclosed within the cylinder, the following types of stresses are developed:

1. *Circumferential or hoop or tangential stress:* This acts in a tangential direction to the circumference of the shell.
2. *Longitudinal or axial stress:* This acts parallel to the longitudinal axis of the shell.
3. *Radial stress:* This acts radially which are too small and hence can be neglected.

In the analysis of a thin-walled vessel, following assumptions are made:

1. The stress distribution over the thickness is assumed to be uniform.
2. The radial stress is too small and hence can be neglected.

4.2.1 Circumferential or hoop or tangential stress

Consider the cross section of a cylinder as shown in **Fig. 4.1** subjected to internal pressure.

Let, $\quad$ d = diameter of the cylinder

$\qquad$ t = thickness of the cylinder

$\qquad$ p = internal pressure in the cylinder

$\qquad$ σ_c or σ_1 = circumferential stress

$\qquad$ L = length of the cylinder

The internal pressure acting on the long sides of the cylinder gives rise to a circumferential stress in the wall of the cylinder (σ_c or σ_1). The bursting force is equal to the product of pressure and the projected area (pdL). Due to this bursting force, the cylinder has a tendency to get split into two parts along the horizontal diameter. The resistance to this action is offered by the development of hoop stress (σ_1) as shown in **Fig. 4.1**.

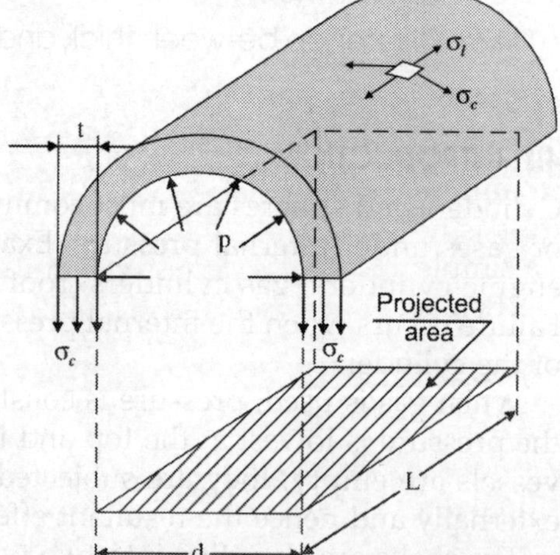

Fig. 4.1: Circumferential or hoop or tangential stress

For equilibrium, $\quad$ bursting force = resisting strength

pressure × projected area = circumferential stress × resisting area

$$p(dL) = \sigma_c \,(2tL)$$

$$\sigma_c = \frac{pd}{2t} \qquad \text{... (Eq. 4.3a)}$$

If η is the efficiency of the riveted joint then, $\sigma_c = \dfrac{pd}{2t\eta} \qquad \text{... (Eq. 4.3b)}$

4.2.2 Longitudinal or axial stress

Consider the cross section of a cylinder as shown in **Fig. 4.2** subjected to internal pressure.

Let,

d = diameter of the cylinder

t = thickness of the cylinder

p = internal pressure in the cylinder

σ_l or σ_2 = longitudinal stress

L = length of the cylinder

Since the ends of the cylinder are closed at its ends, the bursting force is equal to $p \times \left(\dfrac{\pi d^2}{4} \right)$. Due to this bursting force, the cylinder has a tendency to be split into two smaller cylinders, longitudinally.

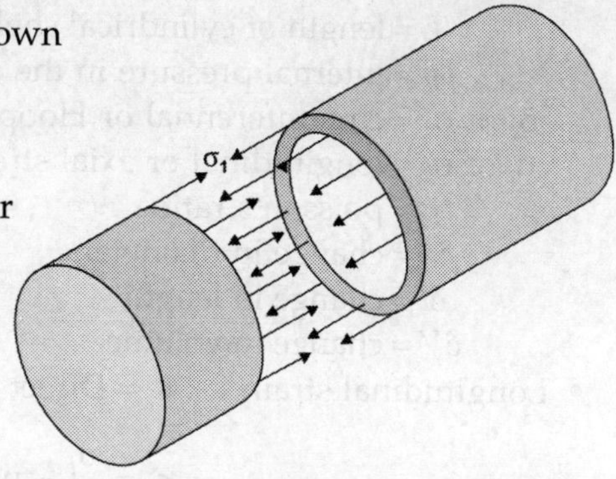

Fig. 4.2: Longitudinal stress

For equilibrium,   bursting force = resisting strength

pressure × projected area = longitudinal stress × resisting area

$$p \left(\frac{\pi}{4} d^2 \right) = \sigma_l (\pi d t)$$

$$\sigma_l = \frac{pd}{4t} \qquad \text{... (Eq. 4.4a)}$$

If η is the efficiency of the riveted joint then, $\sigma_l = \dfrac{pd}{4t\eta}$ ... (Eq. 4.4b)

Thus the longitudinal stress is half that of circumferential stress or circumferential stress is twice that of longitudinal stress.

4.2.3 Maximum shear stress

The stresses acting on an element of the wall of the cylinder consist of a circumferential stress(σ_c), a longitudinal stress (σ_l), and a radial stress. If radial stress is neglected, the state of stress in the wall of the cylinder approximates then to a simple two-dimensional system with principal stresses σ_c and σ_l.

Therefore the maximum shear stress,

$$\tau_{max} = \frac{\sigma_c - \sigma_l}{2} = \frac{\sigma_1 - \sigma_2}{2} \qquad \text{... (Eq. 4.5a)}$$

$$= \left(\frac{pd}{2t} - \frac{pd}{4t} \right) / 2$$

$$\tau_{max} = \frac{pd}{8t} \qquad \text{... (Eq. 4.5b)}$$

4.3 CHANGE IN DIMENSION OF A THIN CYLINDRICAL SHELL SUBJECTED TO INTERNAL PRESSURE

VTU – June/ July 2014– 07 Marks; June 2012 – 05 Marks; June/ July 2011 – 08 Marks; June/ July 2009 – 08 Marks; Dec.07/ Jan.08 – 10 Marks; Jan. 2013 – 10 Marks

Consider a thin cylindrical shell subjected to internal pressure.

Let, d = diameter of cylindrical shell

$$t = \text{thickness of cylindrical shell}$$
$$L = \text{length of cylindrical shell}$$
$$p = \text{internal pressure in the cylinder}$$
$$\sigma_c \text{ or } \sigma_1 = \text{circumferential or Hoop stress}$$
$$\sigma_l \text{ or } \sigma_2 = \text{longitudinal or axial stress}$$
$$\mu = \text{poisson's ratio}$$
$$\delta d = \text{change in diameter}$$
$$\delta l = \text{change in length}$$
$$\delta V = \text{change in volume}$$

- Longitudinal strain $\quad \epsilon_l = \text{Direct strain} - \text{laterial strain due to direct strain}$

$$\epsilon_l = \frac{\sigma_l}{E} - \mu\left(\frac{\sigma_c}{E}\right)$$

$$= \frac{1}{E}\left(\sigma_l - \mu\sigma_c\right)$$

$$= \frac{1}{E}\left[\frac{pd}{4t} - \frac{\mu pd}{2t}\right]$$

$$\therefore \quad \epsilon_l = \frac{pd}{2tE}\left[\frac{1}{2} - \mu\right] = \frac{pd}{4tE}(1 - 2\mu) \qquad \ldots \text{(Eq. 4.6)}$$

- Circumferential strain $\quad \epsilon_c = \text{Direct strain} - \text{laterial strain due to direct strain}$

$$\epsilon_c = \frac{\sigma_c}{E} - \mu\left(\frac{\sigma_l}{E}\right)$$

$$= \frac{1}{E}\left(\sigma_c - \mu\sigma_l\right)$$

$$= \frac{1}{E}\left[\frac{pd}{2t} - \frac{\mu pd}{4t}\right]$$

$$\therefore \quad \epsilon_c = \frac{pd}{2tE}\left[1 - \frac{\mu}{2}\right] = \frac{pd}{4tE}(2 - \mu) \qquad \ldots \text{(Eq. 4.7)}$$

- Change in length:

We know that $\quad \epsilon_l = \dfrac{\text{Change in length}}{\text{Original length}} = \dfrac{\delta L}{L}$

$$\delta L = \epsilon_l . L$$

$$\therefore \quad \delta L = \frac{pdL}{4tE}(1 - 2\mu) \qquad \ldots \text{(Eq. 4.8)}$$

- Change in diameter:

We know that $\quad \epsilon_c = \dfrac{\text{Change in diameter}}{\text{Original diameter}} = \dfrac{\delta d}{d}$

$$\delta d = \epsilon_c . d$$

$$\therefore \quad \delta d = \frac{pd^2}{4tE}(2 - \mu) \qquad \qquad \text{... (Eq. 4.9)}$$

- **Change in volume:**

We know that $\qquad \epsilon_v = \dfrac{\text{Change in volume}}{\text{Original volume}} = \dfrac{\delta V}{V}$

But volume, $\qquad V = \left(\dfrac{\pi d^2}{4}\right) L$

Since V is a function of d and L, we have

$$\delta V = \frac{\pi}{4}\left[L.2d.\delta d + d^2.\delta L \right]$$

$$\therefore \quad \frac{\delta V}{V} = \frac{\pi\left[L.2d.\delta d + d^2.\delta L \right]/4}{\pi d^2 L / 4}$$

$$\frac{\delta V}{V} = 2\left(\frac{\delta d}{d}\right) + \frac{\delta l}{L} \qquad \qquad \text{... (Eq. 4.10a)}$$

$$\therefore \quad \frac{\delta V}{V} = \epsilon_v = 2\epsilon_c + \epsilon_l \qquad \qquad \text{... (Eq. 4.10b)}$$

Thus the volumetric strain is the sum of twice the hoop strain and the longitudinal strain.

$$\frac{\delta V}{V} = \epsilon_v = 2\left[\frac{pd}{4tE}(2 - \mu) \right] + \left[\frac{pd}{4tE}(1 - 2\mu) \right]$$

$$= \frac{pd}{4tE}\left[(4 - 2\mu) + (1 - 2\mu)\right]$$

$$\therefore \quad \frac{\delta V}{V} = \epsilon_v = \frac{pd}{4tE}(5 - 4\mu) \qquad \qquad \text{... (Eq. 4.11a)}$$

$$\text{or} \qquad \delta V = \frac{pdV}{4tE}(5 - 4\mu) \qquad \qquad \text{... (Eq. 4.11b)}$$

Note: **All the above relations holds good for seamless shells; i.e. shells without joints**

1. **Calculate the a) change in diameter b) change in length and c) change in volume of a thin cylindrical shell 1000 mm diameter, 10 mm thick and 5 m long when subjected to internal pressure of 3 N/mm². Take the value of $E = 2 \times 10^5$ N/mm² and $1/m = 0.3$**

VTU – June 2012 – 06 Marks; [Similar: June/ July 2008 – 10 Marks]

Solution: $d = 1000$ mm, $t = 10$ mm, $L = 5000$ mm, $p = 3$ N/mm², $E = 2 \times 10^5$ N/mm², $\dfrac{1}{m} = \mu = 0.3$. a) $\delta d = ?$, b) $\delta L = ?$, c) $\delta V = ?$

- Circumferential stress $\qquad \sigma_c = \dfrac{pd}{2t} = \dfrac{3 \times 1000}{2 \times 10} = 150 \text{ N/mm}^2$

- Longitudinal stress $\qquad \sigma_l = \dfrac{pd}{4t} = \dfrac{3 \times 1000}{4 \times 10} = 75 \text{ N/mm}^2$

a. Change in diameter:

$$\epsilon_c = \frac{\delta d}{d} = \frac{1}{E}(\sigma_c - \mu\sigma_l) = \frac{1}{2 \times 10^5}(150 - 0.3 \times 75) = 6.375 \times 10^{-4}$$

$$\therefore \quad \delta d = (6.375 \times 10^{-4}) \times 1000 = 0.6375 \text{ mm}$$

$$\text{or} \quad \delta d = \frac{pd^2}{4tE}(2 - \mu) = \frac{3 \times 1000^2}{4 \times 10 \times 2 \times 10^5}(2 - 0.3) = 0.6375 \text{ mm}$$

b. Change in Length:

$$\epsilon_l = \frac{\delta L}{L} = \frac{1}{E}(\sigma_l - \mu\sigma_c) = \frac{1}{2 \times 10^5}(75 - 0.3 \times 150) = 1.5 \times 10^{-4}$$

$$\therefore \quad \delta L = (1.5 \times 10^{-4}) \times 5000 = 0.75 \text{ mm}$$

$$\text{or} \quad \delta L = \frac{pdL}{4tE}(1 - 2\mu) = \frac{3 \times 1000 \times 5000}{4 \times 10 \times 2 \times 10^5}(1 - 2 \times 0.3) = 0.75 \text{ mm}$$

c. Change in volume:

$$\epsilon_v = \frac{\delta V}{V} = 2\epsilon_c + \epsilon_l = 2 \times (6.375 \times 10^{-4}) + 1.5 \times 10^{-4} = 1.425 \times 10^{-3}$$

$$\therefore \quad \delta V = (1.425 \times 10^{-3}) \times \left(\frac{\pi \times 1000^2}{4}\right) \times 5000 = 5.60 \times 10^6 \text{ mm}^3$$

$$\text{or} \quad \delta V = \frac{pdV}{4tE}(5 - 4\mu) = \left(\frac{3 \times 1000}{4 \times 10 \times 2 \times 10^5}\right) \times \left(\frac{\pi \times 1000^2}{4}\right) \times 5000 \times (5 - 4 \times 0.3)$$

$$= 5.60 \times 10^6 \text{ mm}^3$$

2. **A cylindrical shell is 3 m long and is having 1m internal diameter and 15 mm thickness. Calculate the maximum intensity of shear stress induced and also the changes in dimensions of the shell, if it is subjected to an internal pressure of 1.5 N/mm². Take $E = 2 \times 10^5$ N/mm² and $\mu = 0.3$**

Solution: $L = 3000$ mm, $d = 1000$ mm, $t = 15$ mm, $p = 1.5$ N/mm², $E = 2 \times 10^5$ N/mm², $\mu = 0.3$. a) $\tau_{max} = ?$, b) $\delta d = ?$, $\delta L = ?$, $\delta V = ?$

a. Maximum shear stress:

$$\text{Maximum shear stress,} \quad \tau_{max} = \frac{\sigma_c - \sigma_l}{2} \qquad \dots \text{Eq. (i)}$$

$$\text{But circumferential stress} \quad \sigma_c = \frac{pd}{2t} = \frac{1.5 \times 1000}{2 \times 15} = 50 \text{ N/mm}^2$$

$$\text{Longitudinal stress} \quad \sigma_l = \frac{pd}{4t} = \frac{1.5 \times 1000}{4 \times 15} = 25\,\text{N/mm}^2$$

$$\therefore \quad \text{Eq. (i) yields...} \qquad \tau_{max} = \frac{50 - 25}{2} = 12.5\,\text{N/mm}^2$$

b. Change in diameter:

$$\epsilon_c = \frac{\delta d}{d} = \frac{1}{E}(\sigma_c - \mu\sigma_l) = \frac{1}{2 \times 10^5}(50 - 0.3 \times 25) = 2.125 \times 10^{-4}$$

$$\therefore \quad \delta d = (2.125 \times 10^{-4}) \times 1000 = 0.2125\,\text{mm}$$

c. Change in Length:

$$\epsilon_l = \frac{\delta L}{L} = \frac{1}{E}(\sigma_l - \mu\sigma_c) = \frac{1}{2 \times 10^5}(25 - 0.3 \times 50) = 5 \times 10^{-5}$$

$$\therefore \quad \delta L = (5 \times 10^{-5}) \times 3000 = 0.15\,\text{mm}$$

d. Change in volume:

$$\epsilon_v = \frac{\delta V}{V} = 2\epsilon_c + \epsilon_l = 2 \times (2.125 \times 10^{-4}) + 5 \times 10^{-5}$$

$$= 4.75 \times 10^{-4}$$

$$\therefore \quad \delta V = (4.75 \times 10^{-4}) \times \left(\frac{\pi \times 1000^2}{4}\right) \times 3000 = 1.12 \times 10^6\,\text{mm}^3$$

3. A thin cylinder, 2 m long and 200 mm in diameter with 10 mm thickness is filled completely with a fluid, at atmospheric pressure. If an additional 25000 mm³ of fluid is pumped in, find the longitudinal and hoop stress developed. Also determine the changes in diameter and length if $E = 2 \times 10^5$ N/mm² and Poisson's ratio = 0.3.

VTU – Dec. 10 – 10 Marks

Solution: $L = 2000$ mm, $d = 200$ mm, $t = 10$ mm, $\delta V = 25000$ mm³, $E = 2 \times 10^5$ N/mm², $\mu = 0.3$. a) $\sigma_c = ?$, $\sigma_l = ?$, b) $\delta d = ?$, $\delta L = ?$

a. To find Circumferential and Longitudinal:

$$\text{Circumferential stress} \qquad \sigma_c = \frac{pd}{2t} = \frac{200\,p}{2 \times 10} = 10\,p \qquad \text{... (i)}$$

$$\text{Longitudinal stress} \qquad \sigma_l = \frac{pd}{4t} = \frac{200\,p}{4 \times 10} = 5\,p \qquad \text{... (ii)}$$

$$\text{Change in volume} \qquad \delta V = \epsilon_v \cdot V = (2\epsilon_c + \epsilon_l)V \qquad \text{... (iii)}$$

$$\text{But } \epsilon_c = \frac{\delta d}{d} = \frac{1}{E}(\sigma_c - \mu\sigma_l) = \frac{1}{2 \times 10^5}(10p - 0.3 \times 5p) = (4.25 \times 10^{-5})p$$

$$\therefore \quad \epsilon_l = \frac{\delta d}{d} = \frac{1}{E}(\sigma_l - \mu\sigma_c) = \frac{1}{2 \times 10^5}(5p - 0.3 \times 10p) = (1 \times 10^{-5})p$$

$$\therefore \text{ Eq. (iii) yields... } 25000 = [2 \times (4.25 \times 10^{-5})p + (1 \times 10^{-5})p] \times \left(\frac{\pi \times 200^2}{4}\right) \times 2000$$

$$\therefore \quad p = 4.19\,\text{N/mm}^2$$

$\therefore$ Eq. (ii) yields... $\qquad \sigma_l = 5 \times 4.19 = 20.95 \text{ N/mm}^2$

$\therefore$ Eq. (i) yields... $\qquad \sigma_c = 10 \times 4.19 = 41.90 \text{ N/mm}^2$

   b. To find changes in diameter and length:

Change in diameter, $\qquad \delta d = \epsilon_c . d = (4.25 \times 10^{-5}) \times 4.18 \times 200 = 0.0355 \text{ mm}$

Change in length, $\qquad \delta L = \epsilon_l . L = (1 \times 10^{-5}) \times 4.18 \times 2000 = 0.0836 \text{ mm}$

4. A water main 80 cm diameter contains water at a pressure head of 100 m. If the weight density of water is 9810 N/m³, find the thickness of the metal required for the water main. Given the permissible stress as 20 N/mm².

VTU – Dec. 13/ Jan. 14 – 06 Marks

Solution: $d = 800$ mm, $h = 100$ m $= 100000$ mm, $w = 9810$ N/m³ $= 9.81 \times 10^{-6}$ N/mm³, $t = ?$, $\sigma_c = 20$ N/mm².

Circumferential stress $\sigma_c = \dfrac{pd}{2t}$ $\qquad\qquad\qquad\qquad$ ... Eq. (i)

$\qquad$ But $\qquad p = wh = (9.81 \times 10^{-6}) \times 100000 = 0.981 \text{ N/mm}^2$

$\therefore$ Eq. (i) yields... $\qquad 20 = \dfrac{0.9810 \times 800}{2t}$

$$\therefore \quad t = 19.62 \text{ mm}$$

5. For a thin cylindrical shell, the L/d ratio is 3 and its initial volume is 20 m³. The ultimate stress for the cylinder material is 200 MPa. Determine the wall thickness, if it has to convey water under a head of 200 m. Take FOS = 2.

VTU – Dec. 15/ Jan. 16 – 08 Marks

Solution: $L/d = 3$ mm, V $= 20$ m³ $= 20 \times 10^9$ mm³, $\sigma_u = 200$ MPa, $FOS = 2$, $t = ?$, $h = 200$ m $= 200000$ mm.

• Volume $\qquad\qquad V = AL$

$$20 \times 10^9 = \left(\frac{\pi \times d^2}{4} \right) \times 3d$$

$$\therefore \quad d = 2040 \text{ mm}$$

Circumferential stress $\sigma_c = \dfrac{pd}{2t}$ $\qquad\qquad\qquad\qquad$ ... Eq. (i)

$\qquad$ But $\qquad\qquad p = wh = (9.81 \times 10^{-6}) \times 200000 = 1.962 \text{ N/mm}^2$

$(w = 9.81 \text{ kN/m}^3)$

$\qquad$ Also $\qquad\qquad \sigma_c = \dfrac{\sigma_u}{FOS} = \dfrac{200}{2} = 100 \text{ MPa}$

$\therefore$ Eq. (i) yields... $\quad 100 = (1.962 \times 2040)/2t$

$$\therefore \quad t = 20.01 \text{ mm}$$

6. Determine the change in volume of a thin cylinder of original volume 65.5 $\times$ 10⁻³ m³ and length 1.3 m if its wall thickness is 6 mm and the internal pressure 14 bar. For the cylinder material E = 210 GPa, μ = 0.3.

Solution: $\delta V = ?$, $V = 65.5 \times 10^{-3}$ m³ $= 65.5 \times 10^6$ mm³, $L = 1300$ mm, $t = 6$ mm, $p = 14$ bar $= 1.4$ MPa, $E = 210 \times 10^3$ MPa, $\mu = 0.3$

- Change in volume $dV = (2\epsilon_c + \epsilon_l)V$ ... Eq. (i)
- Volume $V = AL$

$$65.5 \times 10^6 = \left(\frac{\pi \times d^2}{4}\right) \times 1300$$

$$\therefore \quad d = 253.28 \text{ mm} \approx 254 \text{ mm}$$

- Circumferential stress $\sigma_c = \dfrac{pd}{2t} = \dfrac{1.4 \times 254}{2 \times 6} = 29.63 \text{ MPa}$

- Longitudinal stress $\sigma_l = \dfrac{pd}{4t} = \dfrac{1.4 \times 254}{4 \times 6} = 14.82 \text{ MPa}$

- $\epsilon_c = \dfrac{1}{E}(\sigma_c - \mu\sigma_l) = \dfrac{1}{210 \times 10^3}(29.63 - 0.3 \times 14.82) = 1.20 \times 10^{-4}$

- $\epsilon_l = \dfrac{1}{E}(\sigma_l - \mu\sigma_c) = \dfrac{1}{210 \times 10^3}(14.82 - 0.3 \times 29.63) = 2.82 \times 10^{-5}$

$\therefore$ Eq. (i) yields... $\delta V = [2 \times (1.20 \times 10^{-4}) + (2.82 \times 10^{-5})] \times 65.5 \times 10^6$

$$\therefore \quad \delta V = 17567.1 \text{ mm}^3$$

7. **A steel cylinder 1 m long, of 150 mm internal diameter and plate thickness 5 mm, is subjected to an internal pressure of 7 MPa, the increase in volume owing to the pressure is 16.8×10^{-6} m^3. Find the values of Poisson's ratio and the modulus of rigidity. Assume $E = 210$ GPa.**

Solution: $L = 1000$ mm, $d = 150$ mm, $t = 5$ mm, $p = 7$ MPa, $\delta V = 16.8 \times 10^{-6}$ m$^3 = 16.8 \times 10^3$ mm^3, $\mu = ?$, $G = ?$ $E = 210 \times 10^3$ MPa.

a. Change in volume:

We know that $\delta V = \dfrac{pdV}{4tE}(5 - 4\mu)$

$$16.8 \times 10^3 = \frac{7 \times 150 \times (5 - 4\mu)}{4 \times 5 \times 210 \times 10^3} \times \left(\frac{\pi \times 150^2}{4}\right) \times 1000$$

$$16.8 \times 10^3 = 4417.86 \times (5 - 4\mu)$$

$$(5 - 4\mu) = 3.80$$

$$\therefore \quad \mu = 0.299 \approx 0.3$$

b. Modulus of rigidity:

We know that $E = 2G(1 + \mu)$

$$210 \times 10^3 = 2G(1 + 0.3)$$

$$\therefore \quad G = 80769.23 \text{ MPa}$$

8. **Define bulk modulus K, and show that the decrease in volume of a fluid under pressure p is $\left(\dfrac{pV}{k}\right)$. Hence derive a formula to find the extra fluid which must be pumped into a thin cylinder to raise its pressure by an amount p.**

Solution: Bulk modulus is defined as the ratio of volumetric stress to volumetric strain i.e. $\quad K = \dfrac{\text{Volumetric stress}}{\text{Volumetric strain}}$

in this case *volumetric stress = pressure (p)*

$$K = \dfrac{p}{\epsilon_v} = \dfrac{pV}{\delta V}$$

Thus change in volume under pressure, $\delta V = \dfrac{pV}{K}$ $\qquad$ ... (Eq. 4.12)

If a fluid is used as the pressurization medium, the fluid itself will change in volume as pressure is increased and this must be taken into account when calculating the amount of fluid which must be pumped into the cylinder in order to raise the pressure by a specified amount, the cylinder being initially full of fluid at atmospheric pressure.

The extra fluid required to raise the pressure must, therefore, take up this volume together with the increase in internal volume of the cylinder itself.

Thus extra fluid required to raise the cylinder pressure $= \dfrac{pdV}{4tE}(5 - 4\mu) + \dfrac{pV}{K}$

$$\text{... (Eq. 4.13)}$$

9. **How much fluid is required to raise the pressure in a thin cylinder of length 3 m, internal diameter 700 mm and wall thickness 12 mm by 7 MPa? Take $E = 210$ GPa and $\mu = 0.3$ for the material of the cylinder and $K = 2.1$GPa for the fluid.**

Solution: $L = 3000$ mm, $d = 700$ mm, $t = 12$ mm, $p = 7$ MPa, $E = 210 \times 10^3$ MPa, $\mu = 0.3$, $K = 2.1 \times 10^3$ MPa.

Fluid required in raising the cylinder pressure $= \dfrac{pdV}{4tE}(5 - 4\mu) + \dfrac{pV}{K}$

Volume, $\quad V = \left(\dfrac{\pi \times 700^2}{4}\right) \times 3000 = 1.16 \times 10^9 \text{ mm}^3$

$$= pV\left[\dfrac{d}{4tE}(5 - 4\mu) + \dfrac{1}{K}\right]$$

$$= 7 \times (1.16 \times 10^9)\left[\dfrac{700}{4 \times 12 \times 210 \times 10^3}(5 - 4 \times 0.3) + \dfrac{1}{2.1 \times 10^3}\right]$$

Fluid required in raising the cylinder pressure $= 5.98 \times 10^6 \text{ mm}^3$

4.4 THICK CYLINDERS

A cylinder is regarded as thick if the thickness is more than 1/20 of diameter

i.e. $\quad t > \dfrac{d}{20} \quad \text{or} \quad t > \dfrac{r}{10}$ $\qquad$ ... (Eq. 4.14)

The thin cylinders are basically used for low internal pressure. Due to this the pressure was considered negligible compared to the circumferential and longitudinal stresses. On the other hand thick cylinders are subjected to high internal pressures and hence the radial stresses can't be neglected.

Radial stress varies from the inner surface where it is equal to the magnitude of the fluid pressure to the outer surface where usually it is equal to zero if exposed to atmosphere. Circumferential stress also varies with thickness of the shell.

4.5 LAME'S THEORY

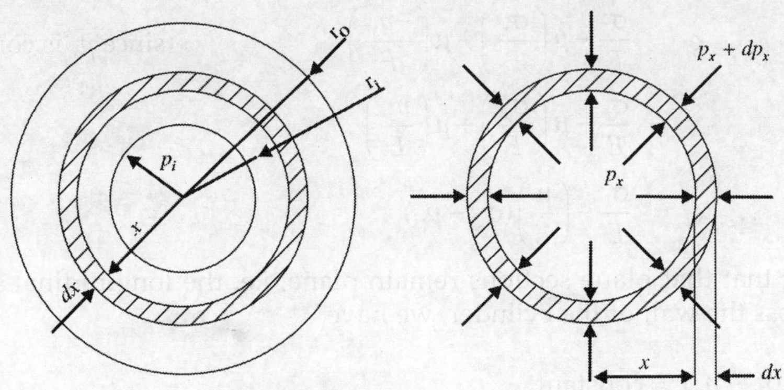

Fig. 4.3: Thick cylinder subjected to internal pressure

Assumptions:

- The material of the shell is homogeneous and isotropic.
- Plane sections of the cylinder, perpendicular to the longitudinal axis remain plane under the pressure.
- The longitudinal strain is assumed to be constant.

Let, r_o = Outer radius of the cylinder.

r_i = Inner radius of the cylinder.

L = Length of the cylinder.

p_x = Radial pressure on the inner surface of the ring.

$(p_x + dp_x)$ = Radial pressure on the outer surface of the ring

σ_x = Circumferential stress induced in the elementary ring.

Fig 4.3 shows a thick cylinder subjected to internal pressure p_i, and external pressure p_o. These pressures are compressive and act radially.

Consider an elementary ring of radius 'x' and thickness 'dx' as shown.

Bursting force, $= p_x (2xL) - (p_x + dp_x)[2(x + dx)L]$ ... Eq. (i)

Resisting strength = circumferential stress × resisting area = $\sigma_x (2dx.L)$ ... Eq. (ii)

For radial equilibrium of the element, equating the above equations, we have

$$p_x.(2xL) - (p_x + dp_x)[2(x + dx)L] = \sigma_x (2dx.L)$$

Dividing the above equation with 2L, we have

$$p_x.x - (p_x + dp_x)(x + dx) = \sigma_x.dx$$

$$p_x.x - p_x (x + dx) - dp_x (x + dx) = \sigma_x.dx$$

$$p_x x - p_x.x - p_x.dx - dp_x.x - dp_x.dx = \sigma_x.dx$$

Neglecting second – order small quantities, we have

$$- p_x.dx - dp_x.x = \sigma_x.dx$$

$$\sigma_x.dx = - p_x.dx - dp_x.x$$

$$\therefore \quad \sigma_x = - p_x - x \left(\frac{dp_x}{dx} \right) \qquad \qquad \text{... Eq. (iii)}$$

As discussed in Section 4.2, at any point in a cylindrical pressure vessel, there are three stresses acting in three perpendicular directions namely:

- Circumferential stress,
- Longitudinal stress and
- Radial stress.

Longitudinal strain is given as

$$\epsilon_l = \frac{\sigma_l}{E} - \mu\left(\frac{\sigma_x}{E}\right) - \mu\left(\frac{-p_x}{E}\right) \qquad \text{(since } p_x \text{ is compressive)}$$

$$= \frac{\sigma_l}{E} - \mu\left(\frac{\sigma_x}{E}\right) + \mu\left(\frac{p_x}{E}\right)$$

$$\therefore \quad \epsilon_l = \frac{\sigma_l}{E} - \left(\frac{\mu}{E}\right)(\sigma_x - p_x) \qquad \text{... Eq. (iv)}$$

Assuming that that plane sections remain plane, i.e. the longitudinal strain ϵ_l is constant across the wall of the cylinder, we have

$$\frac{\sigma_l}{E} - \left(\frac{\mu}{E}\right)(\sigma_x - p_x) = \text{constant} \qquad \text{... Eq. (v)}$$

It is also assumed that the longitudinal stress (σ_l) is constant across the cylinder walls at points remote from the ends of the cylinder. Further μ and E are material properties which remain constant for a given material. Thus we have

$$(\sigma_x - p_x) = \text{constant}$$
$$(\sigma_x - p_x) = 2a \qquad \text{where } 2a = \text{constant}$$
$$\therefore \sigma_x = p_x + 2a \qquad \text{... Eq. (vi)}$$

Substituting Eq. (vi) in Eq. (iii), we have

$$p_x + 2a = -p_x - x\left(\frac{dp_x}{dx}\right)$$

$$2p_x + 2a = -x\left(\frac{dp_x}{dx}\right)$$

$$\left(\frac{dp_x}{dx}\right) = -\frac{2(p_x + a)}{x}$$

$$\left(\frac{dp_x}{p_x + a}\right) = -\frac{2}{x}\,dx$$

Integrating the above equation, we have

$$\log_e (p_x + a) = -2\log_e x + \log_e b \qquad \text{where } \log_e b = \text{Integration constant}$$
$$= -\log_e x^2 + \log_e b$$

$$\log_e (p_x + a) = \log_e\left(\frac{b}{x^2}\right)$$

$$\therefore \quad (p_x + a) = \left(\frac{b}{x^2}\right)$$

$$\therefore \quad p_x = \left(\frac{b}{x^2}\right) - a \qquad \text{... Eq. (vii)}$$

It is to be noted that radial stress p_x is compressive
Substituting Eq. (vii) in Eq. (vi), we have

$$\sigma_x = \left(\frac{b}{x^2}\right) - a + 2a$$

$$\therefore \quad \sigma_x = \left(\frac{b}{x^2}\right) + a \qquad \qquad \dots \text{Eq. (viii)}$$

Eqs (viii) and (vii) are referred to as Lame's equations for thick cylinders, where a and b are constants to be evaluated from boundary conditions. **Fig. 4.4** represents the hoop and radial stress distribution

Case 1: Internal pressure p_i and external pressure zero:
- at $x = r_i$, $p_x = p_i$ (internal pressure)
- at $x = r_o$, $p_x = p_o = 0$ (external pressure)

Case 2: Internal pressure zero and external pressure p_o:
- at $x = r_i$, $p_x = p_i = 0$ (internal pressure)
- at $x = r_o$, $p_x = p_o$ (external pressure)

Case 3: Internal pressure p_i and external pressure p_o:
- at $x = r_i$, $p_x = p_i$ (internal pressure)
- at $x = r_o$, $p_x = p_o$ (external pressure)

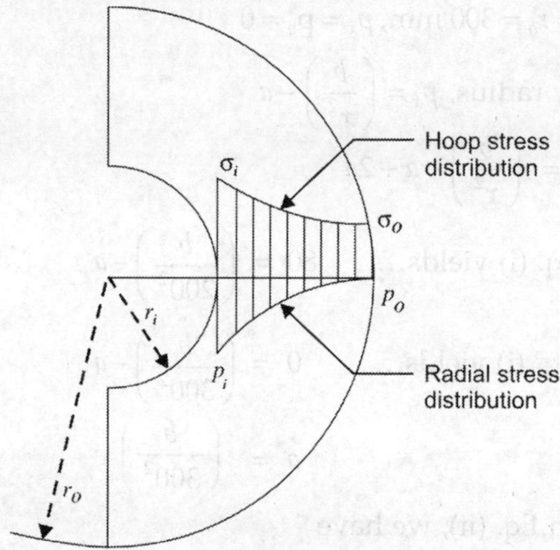

Fig. 4.4: Hoop and radial stress distribution

4.6 DIFFERENCE BETWEEN THICK AND THIN CYLINDERS

Sl No.	Thin cylinder	Thick cylinder
1.	Thickness: $t < \dfrac{d}{20}$	Thickness: $t > \dfrac{d}{20}$
2.	Stress distribution over the thickness is assumed to be uniform.	Stress distribution varies with thickness of the shell.
3.	Radial stress is too small and hence neglected.	Radial stress varies from the inner surface where it is equal to the magnitude of the fluid pressure to the outer surface where usually it is equal to zero if exposed to atmosphere.
4.	Analysis is simple.	Complex.
5.	The operating pressure is around 30 MPa and more.	The operating pressure is more than 250 MPa.

Problems on stresses

10. A pipe of 400 mm internal diameter and 100 mm thickness contains a fluid at a pressure of 80 MPa. Find the maximum and minimum hoop stresses across the section. Also sketch the radial and hoop stress distribution across the section.

VTU – Dec. 14/ Jan. 15 – 12 Marks; June/ July 2014 – 10 Marks;
Dec. 13/ Jan. 14 – 08 Marks; June/ July 2013 – 10 Marks; June 2012 – 05 Marks
Dec. 2011 – 10 Marks; May/ June 2010 – 12 Marks; Dec.08/ Jan.09 – 10 Marks

Solution: $d_i = 400$ mm, $t = 100$ mm, $p_i = 80$ MPa, $\sigma_{ri} = ?$, $\sigma_{ro} = ?$

Now $\qquad d_o = d_i + 2t = 400 + (2 \times 100) = 600$ mm

$$\therefore \quad r_i = 200 \text{ mm}, r_o = 300 \text{ mm and } r_m = \frac{200 + 300}{2} = 250 \text{ mm}$$

Boundary conditions:

- at inner radius: $x = r_i = 200$ mm, $p_x = p_i = 80$ MPa
- at outer radius: $x = r_o = 300$ mm, $p_x = p_o = 0$

Radial pressure at any radius, $p_x = \left(\dfrac{b}{x^2}\right) - a$ $\qquad\qquad$ ... Eq. (i)

$$\sigma_x = \left(\frac{b}{x^2}\right) - a + 2a$$

At inner radius, Eq. (i) yields... $\qquad 80 = \left(\dfrac{b}{200^2}\right) - a$ $\qquad$ ... Eq. (ii)

At outer radius, Eq. (i) yields... $\qquad 0 = \left(\dfrac{b}{300^2}\right) - a$

$$a = \left(\frac{b}{300^2}\right) \qquad\qquad \text{... Eq. (iii)}$$

Substituting Eq. (iii) in Eq. (ii), we have

$$80 = \left(\frac{b}{200^2}\right) - \left(\frac{b}{300^2}\right)$$

$$= b\left(\frac{1}{200^2} - \frac{1}{300^2}\right)$$

$$\therefore \quad b = 5760000$$

Eq. (iii) yields... $\qquad\qquad a = \left(\dfrac{5760000}{300^2}\right) = 64$

Circumferential stress at any radius, $\sigma_x = \left(\dfrac{b}{x^2}\right) + a$

At inner radius, $\sigma_r)_i = \left(\dfrac{5760000}{200^2}\right) + 64 = 208$ MPa

At mean radius, $\sigma_r)_m = \left(\dfrac{5760000}{250^2}\right) + 64 = 156.16$ MPa

At outer radius, $\sigma_r)_o = \left(\dfrac{5760000}{300^2}\right) + 64 = 128$ MPa

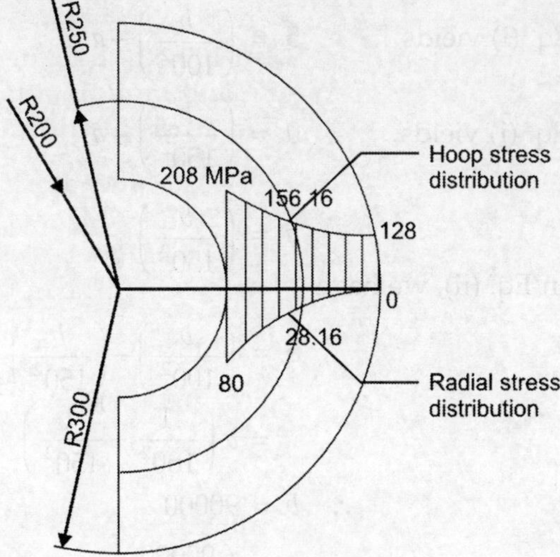

Fig. 4.5: Problem 10

Values of pressure:

At inner radius, Eq. (i) yields... $p_r)_i = \left(\dfrac{5760000}{200^2} \right) - 64 = 80$ MPa

At mean radius, Eq. (i) yields... $p_r)_m = \left(\dfrac{5760000}{250^2} \right) - 64 = 28.16$ MPa

At outer radius, Eq. (i) yields... $p_r)_o = \left(\dfrac{5760000}{300^2} \right) - 64 = 0$ MPa

The pressures and stress distribution diagrams are shown in **Fig. 4.5**.

11. **A CI pipe has 200 mm internal diameter and 50 mm metal thickness and carries water under a pressure of 5 MPa. Calculate the maximum and minimum intensities of circumferential stress and sketch the distribution of circumferential stress intensity and intensity of radial pressure across the section.**
    What is the percentage change if the maximum hoop stress is found using the relation of thin pipe?

VTU – June/ July 15 – 10 Marks; June/ July 2014 – 10 Marks

Solution: $d_i = 200$ mm, $t = 50$ mm, $p_i = 5$ MPa, $\sigma_{ri} = ?$, $\sigma_{ro} = ?$

Now $\quad d_o = d_i + 2t = 200 + (2 \times 50) = 300$ mm

$$\therefore \quad r_i = 100 \text{ mm}, r_o = 150 \text{ mm and } r_m = \frac{100+150}{2} = 125 \text{ mm}$$

Boundary conditions:
- at inner radius: $x = r_i = 100$ mm, $p_x = p_i = 5$ MPa
- at outer radius: $x = r_o = 150$ mm, $p_x = p_o = 0$

Radial pressure at any radius, $\qquad p_x = \left(\dfrac{b}{x^2} \right) - a \qquad$ ... Eq. (i)

At inner radius, Eq. (i) yields... $\quad 5 = \left(\dfrac{b}{100^2}\right) - a$ $\qquad$ ... Eq. (ii)

At outer radius, Eq. (i) yields... $\quad 0 = \left(\dfrac{b}{150^2}\right) - a$

$$a = \left(\dfrac{b}{150^2}\right) \qquad \text{... Eq. (iii)}$$

Substituting Eq. (iii) in Eq. (ii), we have

$$5 = \left(\dfrac{b}{100^2}\right) - \left(\dfrac{b}{150^2}\right)$$

$$= b\left(\dfrac{1}{100^2} - \dfrac{1}{150^2}\right)$$

$$\therefore \quad b = 90000$$

Eq. (iii) yields... $\qquad a = \left(\dfrac{90000}{150^2}\right) = 4$

Circumferential stress at any radius, $\quad \sigma_x = \left(\dfrac{b}{x^2}\right) + a$

At inner radius, $\qquad \sigma_r)_i = \left(\dfrac{90000}{100^2}\right) + 4 = 13\,\text{MPa}$

At mean radius, $\qquad \sigma_r)_m = \left(\dfrac{90000}{125^2}\right) + 4 = 9.76\,\text{MPa}$

At outer radius, $\qquad \sigma_r)_o = \left(\dfrac{90000}{150^2}\right) + 4 = 8\,\text{MPa}$

Values of pressure:

At inner radius, Eq. (i) yields... $\quad p_r)_i = \left(\dfrac{90000}{100^2}\right) - 4 = 5\,\text{MPa}$

At mean radius, Eq. (i) yields... $\quad p_r)_m = \left(\dfrac{90000}{125^2}\right) - 4 = 1.76\,\text{MPa}$

At outer radius, Eq. (i) yields... $\quad p_r)_o = \left(\dfrac{90000}{150^2}\right) - 4 = 0\,\text{MPa}$

Percentage error:

For a thin cylinder, hoop stress $\qquad \sigma_c = \dfrac{pd}{2t} = \dfrac{p_i d_i}{2t} = \dfrac{5 \times 200}{2 \times 50} = 10\,\text{MPa}$

$$\therefore \quad \% \text{ Error} = \left(\dfrac{\sigma_i - \sigma_c}{\sigma_i}\right) \times 100 = \left(\dfrac{13 - 10}{13}\right) \times 100$$

$$= 23.07\%$$

The pressures and stress distribution diagrams may be drawn similar to **Fig. 4.5** of Problem 10.

12. **A pressure vessel with outer and inner diameters of 400 mm and 320 mm respectively is subjected to an external pressure of 8 MPa. Determine the circumferential stress induced at the inner and outer surface. Prove that the longitudinal strain is constant throughout the cylinder.**

VTU – June 2012 – 08 Marks

Solution: $d_o = 400$ mm, $d_i = 320$ mm, $p_o = 8$ MPa, $\sigma_{ri} = ?$, $\sigma_{ro} = ?$

$$\therefore \quad r_o = 200 \text{ mm}, r_i = 160 \text{ mm and } r_m = \frac{200 + 160}{2} = 180 \text{ mm}$$

a. Stresses:

Boundary conditions:

- at inner radius: $x = r_i = 160$ mm, $p_x = p_i = 0$
- at outer radius: $x = r_o = 200$ mm, $p_x = p_o = 8$ MPa

Radial pressure at any radius, $\qquad p_x = \left(\dfrac{b}{x^2}\right) - a \qquad$ ... Eq. (i)

At inner radius, Eq. (i) yields... $\qquad 0 = \left(\dfrac{b}{160^2}\right) - a$

$$a = \left(\frac{b}{160^2}\right) \qquad \text{... Eq. (ii)}$$

At outer radius, Eq. (i) yields... $\qquad 8 = \left(\dfrac{b}{200^2}\right) - a \qquad$ ... Eq. (iii)

Substituting Eq. (ii) in Eq. (iii), we have

$$8 = \left(\frac{b}{200^2}\right) - \left(\frac{b}{160^2}\right)$$

$$= b\left(\frac{1}{200^2} - \frac{1}{160^2}\right)$$

$$\therefore \quad b = -568888.89$$

Eq. (iii) yields... $\qquad a = \left(\dfrac{-568888.89}{160^2}\right) = -22.22$

Circumferential stress at any radius, $\qquad \sigma_x = \left(\dfrac{b}{x^2}\right) + a$

At inner radius, $\qquad \sigma_r)_i = \left(\dfrac{-568888.89}{160^2}\right) - 22.22 = -44.44$ MPa

At mean radius, $\qquad \sigma_r)_m = \left(\dfrac{-568888.89}{180^2}\right) - 22.22 = -39.78$ MPa

At outer radius, $\qquad \sigma_r)_o = \left(\dfrac{-568888.89}{200^2}\right) - 22.22 = -36.44$ MPa

b. Longitudinal strain:

We know that $\qquad \epsilon_l = \dfrac{\sigma_l}{E} - \left(\dfrac{\mu}{E}\right)(\sigma_x - p_x)$

At inner radius: $\sigma_l = 0$, $\sigma_x = \sigma_{ri}$ and $p_x = p_i = 0$

Assume $E = 200\,\text{GPa}$ and $\mu = 0.25$

$$\epsilon_l = 0 - \left(\frac{\mu}{E}\right)(\sigma_{ri} - p_i) = 0 - \left(\frac{0.25}{2 \times 10^5}\right) \times (-44.44 - 0)$$

$$= 5.55 \times 10^{-5}$$

At outer radius: $\sigma_l = 0$, $\sigma_x = \sigma_{ro}$ and $p_x = p_0 = 8\,\text{MPa}$

$$\epsilon_l = 0 - \left(\frac{\mu}{E}\right)(\sigma_{ro} - p_o) = 0 - \left(\frac{0.25}{2 \times 10^5}\right) \times (-36.44 - 8)$$

$$= 5.55 \times 10^{-5}$$

Thus longitudinal strain is constant throughout the cylinder

13. **A thick cylinder with internal diameter 80 mm and external diameter 120 mm is subjected to an external pressure of 40 MPa, when the internal pressure is 120 MPa, calculate the circumferential stress at external and internal surfaces of the cylinder. Plot the variation of circumferential stress and radial pressure on the thickness of the cylinder.**

VTU – Dec. 14/ Jan. 15 – 10 Marks; Dec.07/ Jan.08 – 10 Marks

Solution: $d_i = 80\,\text{mm}$, $d_o = 120\,\text{mm}$, $p_o = 40\,\text{MPa}$, $p_i = 120\,\text{MPa}$, $\sigma_{ri} = ?$, $\sigma_{ro} = ?$

$$\therefore \quad r_i = 40\,\text{mm}, r_o = 60\,\text{mm} \text{ and } r_m = \frac{40 + 60}{2} = 50\,\text{mm}$$

a. Stresses:

Boundary conditions:
- at inner radius: $x = r_i = 40\,\text{mm}$, $p_x = p_i = 120\,\text{MPa}$
- at outer radius: $x = r_o = 60\,\text{mm}$, $p_x = p_o = 40\,\text{MPa}$

Radial pressure at any radius, $p_x = \left(\dfrac{b}{x^2}\right) - a$ ... Eq. (i)

At inner radius, Eq. (i) yields... $120 = \left(\dfrac{b}{40^2}\right) - a$ ... Eq. (ii)

At outer radius, Eq. (i) yields... $40 = \left(\dfrac{b}{60^2}\right) - a$ ... Eq. (iii)

Eq. (ii) – Eq. (iii) yields... $80 = \left(\dfrac{b}{40^2}\right) - \left(\dfrac{b}{60^2}\right)$

$$= b\left(\frac{1}{40^2} - \frac{1}{60^2}\right)$$

$$\therefore \quad b = 230400$$

Eq. (iii) yields... $40 = \left(\dfrac{230400}{60^2}\right) - a$

$$\therefore \quad a = 24$$

Circumferential stress at any radius, $\sigma_x = \left(\dfrac{b}{x^2}\right) + a$

At inner radius, $\qquad \sigma_r)_i = \left(\dfrac{230400}{40^2}\right) + 24 = 168\text{ MPa}$

At mean radius, $\qquad \sigma_r)_m = \left(\dfrac{230400}{50^2}\right) + 24 = 116.16\text{ MPa}$

At outer radius, $\qquad \sigma_r)_o = \left(\dfrac{230400}{60^2}\right) + 24 = 88\text{ MPa}$

Values of pressure:

At inner radius, Eq. (i) yields... $\quad p_r)_i = \left(\dfrac{230400}{40^2}\right) - 24 = 120\text{ MPa}$

At mean radius, Eq. (i) yields... $\quad p_r)_m = \left(\dfrac{230400}{50^2}\right) - 24 = 68.16\text{ MPa}$

At outer radius, Eq. (i) yields... $\quad p_r)_o = \left(\dfrac{230400}{60^2}\right) - 24 = 40\text{ MPa}$

The pressures and stress distribution diagrams are shown in **Fig. 4.6.**

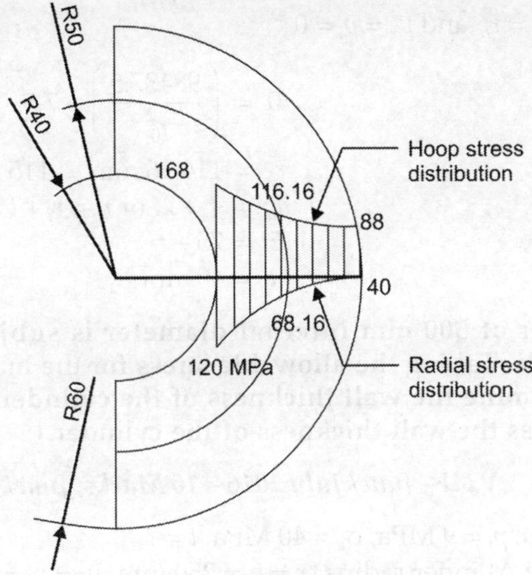

Fig. 4.6: Problem 13

Problems on thickness

14. **Find the thickness of metal necessary for a thick cylinder of internal diameter 150 mm to withstand an internal pressure of 10 MPa. The maximum hoop stress in the section is not to exceed 25 MPa.**

VTU – Dec. 13/ Jan. 14 – 10 Marks; June/ July 2009 – 08 Marks

Solution: $t = ?$, $d_i = 150$ mm, $p_i = 10$ MPa, $\sigma_c = 25$ MPa

Boundary conditions: at inner radius: $x = r_i = 75$ mm, $p_x = p_i = 10$ MPa, $\sigma_x = \sigma_c = \sigma_r)_i = 25$ MPa

Radial pressure at any radius, $\qquad p_x = \left(\dfrac{b}{x^2}\right) - a \qquad\qquad$ ... Eq. (i)

At inner radius, Eq. (i) yields ... $10 = \left(\dfrac{b}{75^2}\right) - a$ ... Eq. (ii)

Circumferential stress at any radius, $\sigma_x = \left(\dfrac{b}{x^2}\right) + a$ ... Eq. (iii)

At inner radius, Eq. (iii) yields... $25 = \left(\dfrac{b}{75^2}\right) + a$ ... Eq. (iv)

Eq. (ii) + Eq. (iv) yields... $35 = \left(\dfrac{b}{75^2}\right) + \left(\dfrac{b}{75^2}\right)$

$$= \left(\dfrac{2b}{75^2}\right)$$

$$\therefore \quad b = 98437.5$$

Eq. (iv) yields... $25 = \left(\dfrac{98437.5}{75^2}\right) + a$

$$\therefore \quad a = 7.5$$

At outer radius, $x = r_o$ and $p_x = p_i = 0$

Eq. (i) yields... $0 = \left(\dfrac{98437.5}{r_0^2}\right) - 7.5$

$$\therefore \quad r_o = 114.56 \text{ mm} \approx 115 \text{ mm}$$

But $d_o = d_i + 2t \text{ or } r_o = r_i + t$

$$115 = 75 + t$$

$$t = 40 \text{ mm}$$

15. **A thick cylinder of 500 mm internal diameter is subjected to an internal pressure of 9 MPa. Taking the allowable stress for the material of the cylinder as 40 MPa, determine the wall thickness of the cylinder. Also plot the stress distribution across the wall thickness of the cylinder.**

VTU – June/ July 2016 – 10 Marks; June/ July 2011 – 12 Marks

Solution: $d_i = 500$ mm, $p_i = 9$ MPa, $\sigma_c = 40$ MPa, $t = ?$

Boundary conditions: At inner radius: $x = r_i = 250$ mm, $p_x = p_i = 9$ MPa, $\sigma_x = \sigma_c = \sigma_r)_i = 40$ MPa

Radial pressure at any radius, $p_x = \left(\dfrac{b}{x^2}\right) - a$ ... Eq. (i)

At inner radius, Eq. (i) yields... $9 = \left(\dfrac{b}{250^2}\right) - a$ ... Eq. (ii)

Circumferential stress at any radius, $\sigma_x = \left(\dfrac{b}{x^2}\right) + a$ ... Eq. (iii)

At inner radius, Eq. (iii) yields... $40 = \left(\dfrac{b}{250^2}\right) + a$ ... Eq. (iv)

Eq. (ii) + Eq. (iv) yields... $49 = \left(\dfrac{b}{250^2}\right) + \left(\dfrac{b}{250^2}\right)$

$$= \left(\frac{2b}{250^2} \right)$$

$$\therefore \quad b = 1531250$$

Eq. (iv) yields...
$$40 = \left(\frac{1531250}{250^2} \right) + a$$

$$\therefore \quad a = 15.5$$

At outer radius, $x = r_o$ and $p_x = p_i = 0$

Eq. (i) yields...
$$0 = \left(\frac{1531250}{r_0^2} \right) - 15.5$$

$$\therefore \quad r_o = 314.31 \text{ mm}$$

But
$$d_o = d_i + 2t \text{ or } r_o = r_i + t$$
$$314.31 = 250 + t$$
$$t = 64.31 \text{ mm}$$

And
$$r_m = \frac{250 + 314.31}{2} = 282.15 \text{ mm}$$

Values of Circumferential stress:

At inner radius,
$$\sigma_r)_i = \frac{1531250}{250^2} + 15.5 = 40 \text{ MPa}$$

At mean radius,
$$\sigma_r)_m = \frac{1531250}{282.15^2} + 15.5 = 34.73 \text{ MPa}$$

At outer radius,
$$\sigma_r)_o = \frac{1531250}{314.31^2} + 15.5 = 31 \text{ MPa}$$

Values of pressure:

At inner radius, Eq. (i) yields...
$$p_r)_i = \frac{1531250}{250^2} - 15.5 = 9 \text{ MPa}$$

At mean radius, Eq. (i) yields...
$$p_r)_m = \frac{1531250}{282.15^2} - 15.5 = 3.73 \text{ MPa}$$

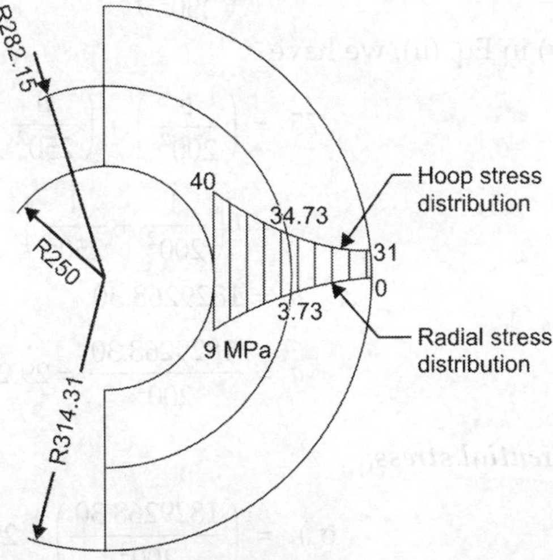

Fig. 4.7: Problem 15

At outer radius, Eq. (i) yields... $\quad p_r)_o = \dfrac{1531250}{314.31^2} - 15.5 = 0\,\text{MPa}$

The pressures and stress distribution diagrams are shown in **Fig. 4.7**.

Problems on pressure

16. **A cylindrical pressure vessel has inner and outer radii of 200 mm and 250 mm respectively. The material of the cylinder has an allowable normal stress of 75 MN/m². Determine the maximum internal pressure that can be applied and draw a sketch of radial pressure and circumferential stress distribution.**

VTU – Dec. 2012 – 10 Marks

Solution: $\quad r_i = 200\,\text{mm}, r_o = 250\,\text{mm}, \sigma_c = 75\,\text{MN/m}^2 = 75\,\text{N/mm}^2, p_i = ?$

$$r_m = \frac{200 + 250}{2} = 225\,\text{mm}$$

Boundary conditions:
- at inner radius: $x = r_i = 200\,\text{mm},\ \sigma_x = \sigma_c = \sigma_r)_i = 75\,\text{N/mm}^2$
- at outer radius: $x = r_o = 250\,\text{mm},\ p_x = p_o = 0$

Circumferential stress at any radius, $\sigma_x = \left(\dfrac{b}{x^2}\right) + a$ $\qquad$ ... Eq. (i)

Since maximum stress occurs at inner radius, we have

$$75 = \left(\frac{b}{200^2}\right) + a \qquad \text{... Eq. (ii)}$$

Radial pressure at any radius, $\qquad p_x = \left(\dfrac{b}{x^2}\right) - a$ $\qquad$ ... Eq. (iii)

At outer radius, Eq. (i) yields... $\qquad 0 = \left(\dfrac{b}{250^2}\right) - a$

$$a = \left(\frac{b}{250^2}\right) \qquad \text{... Eq. (iv)}$$

Substituting Eq. (iv) in Eq. (ii), we have

$$75 = \left(\frac{b}{200^2}\right) + \left(\frac{b}{250^2}\right)$$

$$= b\left(\frac{1}{200^2} + \frac{1}{250^2}\right)$$

$$\therefore \quad b = 1829268.30$$

Eq. (iv) yields... $\qquad a = \dfrac{1829268.30}{200^2} = 29.27$

Values of Circumferential stress:

At inner radius, $\qquad \sigma_r)_i = \left(\dfrac{1829268.30}{200^2}\right) + 29.27 = 75\,\text{N/mm}^2$

At mean radius, $\qquad \sigma_r)_m = \left(\dfrac{1829268.30}{225^2}\right) + 29.27 = 65.40 \text{ N/mm}^2$

At outer radius, $\qquad \sigma_r)_o = \left(\dfrac{1829268.30}{250^2}\right) + 29.27 = 58.54 \text{ N/mm}^2$

Values of pressure:

At inner radius, Eq. (i) yields... $\quad p_r)_i = \left(\dfrac{1829268.30}{200^2}\right) - 29.27 = 16.46 \text{ N/mm}^2$

At mean radius, Eq. (i) yields... $\quad p_r)_m = \left(\dfrac{1829268.30}{225^2}\right) - 29.27 = 6.86 \text{ N/mm}^2$

At outer radius, Eq. (i) yields... $\quad p_r)_o = \left(\dfrac{1829268.30}{250^2}\right) - 29.27 = 0 \text{ N/mm}^2$

The pressures and stress distribution diagrams are shown in **Fig. 4.8**.

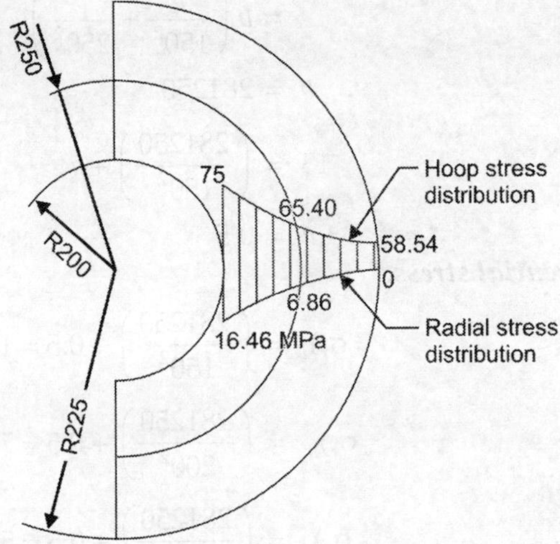

Fig. 4.8: Problem 16

17. **The internal and external diameters of a thick cylinder are 300 mm and 500 mm respectively. It is subjected to an external pressure of 4 N/mm². Find the internal pressure that can be applied if the permissible stress in the cylinder is limited to 13 N/mm². Sketch the variation of hoop stress and radial stress across the thickness of the cylinder.**

VTU – Jan. 2013 – 10 Marks

Solution: $\quad d_i = 300 \text{ mm},\ d_o = 500 \text{ mm},\ p_o = 4 \text{ N/mm}^2\ \sigma_c = 13 \text{ MN/m}^2 = 13 \text{ N/mm}^2,$
$\qquad p_i = ?$

$$\therefore\quad r_i = 150 \text{ mm},\ r_o = 250 \text{ mm and } r_m = \frac{150 + 250}{2} = 200 \text{ mm}$$

Boundary conditions:
- at inner radius: $x = r_i = 150 \text{ mm},\ \sigma_x = \sigma_c = \sigma_r)_i = 13 \text{ N/mm}^2$
- at outer radius: $x = r_o = 250 \text{ mm},\ p_x = p_o = 4 \text{ N/mm}^2$

Circumferential stress at any radius, $\sigma_x = \left(\dfrac{b}{x^2}\right) + a$ ... Eq. (i)

Since maximum stress occurs at inner radius, we have

$$13 = \left(\dfrac{b}{150^2}\right) + a \qquad \text{... Eq. (ii)}$$

Radial pressure at any radius, $\qquad p_x = \left(\dfrac{b}{x^2}\right) - a$ ... Eq. (iii)

At inner radius, Eq. (i) yields... $\qquad 4 = \left(\dfrac{b}{250^2}\right) - a$ ... Eq. (iv)

Eq. (ii) + Eq. (iv) yields... $\qquad 17 = \left(\dfrac{b}{150^2}\right) + \left(\dfrac{b}{250^2}\right)$

$$= b\left(\dfrac{b}{150^2} + \dfrac{b}{250^2}\right)$$

$$\therefore \quad b = 281250$$

Eq. (ii) yields... $\qquad 13 = \left(\dfrac{281250}{150^2}\right) + a$

$$\therefore \quad a = 0.5$$

Values of circumferential stress:

At inner radius, $\qquad \sigma_r)_i = \left(\dfrac{281250}{150^2}\right) + 0.5 = 13\,\text{N/mm}^2$

At mean radius, $\qquad \sigma_r)_m = \left(\dfrac{281250}{200^2}\right) + 0.5 = 7.53\,\text{N/mm}^2$

At outer radius, $\qquad \sigma_r)_o = \left(\dfrac{281250}{250^2}\right) + 0.5 = 5\,\text{N/mm}^2$

Values of pressure:

At inner radius, Eq. (i) yields... $\quad p_r)_i = \left(\dfrac{281250}{150^2}\right) - 0.5 = 12\,\text{N/mm}^2$

At mean radius, Eq. (i) yields... $\quad p_r)_m = \left(\dfrac{281250}{200^2}\right) - 0.5 = 6.53\,\text{N/mm}^2$

At outer radius, Eq. (i) yields... $\quad p_r)_o = \left(\dfrac{281250}{250^2}\right) - 0.5 = 4\,\text{N/mm}^2$

The pressures and stress distribution diagrams may be drawn similar to **Fig. 4.8**.

18. Find the ratio of maximum circumferential stress to the internal pressure for a tube subjected to internal pressure if the external pressure is zero.

Solution: Radial pressure at any radius, $p_x = \left(\dfrac{b}{x^2}\right) - a$ ... Eq. (i)

Boundary conditions:

- at inner radius: $x = r_i$, $\sigma_x = \sigma_c = \sigma_r)_i$
- at outer radius: $x = r_o$, $p_x = p_o$

At inner radius, Eq. (i) yields...

$$p_i = \left(\frac{b}{r_i^2}\right) - a \qquad \text{... Eq. (ii)}$$

At outer radius, Eq. (i) yields...

$$0 = \left(\frac{b}{r_o^2}\right) - a$$

$$a = \left(\frac{b}{r_o^2}\right) \qquad \text{... Eq. (iii)}$$

Substituting Eq. (iii) in Eq. (ii), we have

$$p_i = \left(\frac{b}{r_i^2}\right) - \left(\frac{b}{r_o^2}\right)$$

$$= b\left(\frac{r_o^2 - r_i^2}{r_o^2 \cdot r_i^2}\right)$$

$$b = p_i\left(\frac{r_o^2 \cdot r_i^2}{r_o^2 - r_i^2}\right) \qquad \text{... Eq. (iv)}$$

Substituting Eq. (iv) in Eq. (iii), we have

$$a = \left(\frac{p_i}{r_o^2}\right)\left(\frac{r_o^2 \cdot r_i^2}{r_o^2 - r_i^2}\right)$$

$$a = \left(\frac{p_i \cdot r_i^2}{r_o^2 - r_i^2}\right) \qquad \text{... Eq. (v)}$$

Circumferential stress at any radius, $\sigma_x = \left(\dfrac{b}{x^2}\right) + a$

Substituting a and b in the above equation, we have

$$\sigma_x = \left(\frac{p_i}{x^2}\right)\left(\frac{r_o^2 \cdot r_i^2}{r_o^2 - r_i^2}\right) + \left(\frac{p_i \cdot r_i^2}{r_o^2 - r_i^2}\right)$$

$$= \left(\frac{p_i \cdot r_i^2}{r_o^2 - r_i^2}\right)\left(\frac{r_o^2}{x^2} + 1\right)$$

$$\therefore \quad \sigma_x = \left(\frac{p_i \cdot r_i^2}{x^2}\right)\left(\frac{r_o^2 + x^2}{r_o^2 - r_i^2}\right) \qquad \text{... Eq. (vi)}$$

Since maximum stress occurs at inner radius, we have

$$\sigma_r)_i = \left(\frac{p_i \cdot r_i^2}{r_i^2}\right)\left(\frac{r_o^2 + r_i^2}{r_o^2 - r_i^2}\right)$$

$$(\sigma_r)_i = p_i \left(\frac{r_o^2 + r_i^2}{r_o^2 - r_i^2} \right)$$

or

$$\frac{(\sigma_r)_i}{p_i} = \left(\frac{r_o^2 + r_i^2}{r_o^2 - r_i^2} \right) = \left(\frac{K^2 + 1}{K^2 - 1} \right)$$

$$(\text{where } K = r_o/r_i) \qquad \ldots \text{Eq. (vii)}$$

On similar lines it can be proved that $\dfrac{p_x}{p_i} = \left(\dfrac{r_o^2 - r_i^2}{r_o^2 + r_i^2} \right) = \left(\dfrac{K^2 - 1}{K^2 + 1} \right)$ $\qquad \ldots$ Eq. (viii)

19. Find the ratio of thickness to internal diameter for a tube subjected to internal pressure, when the ratio of internal pressure to maximum circumferential stress is 5/8.

Solution: $\dfrac{t}{d_i} = ?, \ \dfrac{p_i}{(\sigma_r)_i} = \dfrac{5}{8}$

Circumferential stress at any radius $\dfrac{(\sigma_r)_i}{p_i} = \left(\dfrac{r_o^2 + r_i^2}{r_o^2 - r_i^2} \right) = \left(\dfrac{K^2 + 1}{K^2 - 1} \right)$

$$(\text{where } K = r_o/r_i) \qquad \ldots \text{using Eq. (vii)}$$

$$\frac{8}{5} = \left(\frac{K^2 + 1}{K^2 - 1} \right)$$

$$8(K^2 - 1) = 5(K^2 + 1)$$
$$3K^2 = 13$$
$$K = 2.08$$

i.e.
$$2.08\, r_i = r_o$$
$$2.08\, r_i = r_i + t$$
$$t = 1.08\, r_i$$
$$t/r_i = 1.08 \text{ or } t/d_i = 0.54$$

20. Calculate the maximum external to internal radius ratio for a thick cylinder with internal fluid pressure of 15 MPa and maximum hoop stress is 60 MPa.

VTU – Dec. 15/ Jan. 16 – 08 Marks

Solution: $\dfrac{d_o}{d_i} = ?, \ p_i = 15 \text{ MPa}, \ (\sigma_r)_i = 60 \text{ MPa}$

Circumferential stress at any radius $\dfrac{(\sigma_r)_i}{p_i} = \left(\dfrac{r_o^2 + r_i^2}{r_o^2 - r_i^2} \right) = \left(\dfrac{K^2 + 1}{K^2 - 1} \right)$

$$(\text{where } K = r_o/r_i) \qquad \ldots \text{using Eq. (vii)}$$

$$\frac{60}{15} = \left(\frac{K^2 + 1}{K^2 - 1} \right)$$

$$4(K^2 - 1) = (K^2 + 1)$$
$$3K^2 = 5$$
$$K = 2.29 = r_o/r_i$$

Dec.07/ Jan.08 (06ME34)

1. a. Prove that the volumetric strain in a thin cylinder is given by $\varepsilon_V = (2\varepsilon_C + \varepsilon_L)$, where ε_C = hoop strain, ε_L = longitudinal strain and express the same in terms of diameter of the cylinder (D), thickness (t), Young's Modulus (E), internal pressure (p), and Poisson's ratio (μ). **(10 Marks)**

   b. A thick cylinder with internal diameter 80 mm and external diameter 120 mm is subjected to an external pressure of 40 kN/m^2, when the internal pressure is 120 kN/m^2. Calculate the circumferential stress at external and internal surfaces of the cylinder. Plot the variation of circumferential stress and radial pressure on the thickness of the cylinder. **(10 Marks)**

June/July 2008 (06ME34)

2. a. What are the differences between thin and thick cylinder? **(02 Marks)**

   b. Derive Lame's equation for thick cylinder. **(08 Marks)**

   c. A thin cylindrical shell 1.2 m in diameter and 3 m long has a metal wall thickness of 12 mm. It is subjected to an internal fluid pressure of 3.2 MPa. Find the circumferential and longitudinal stress in the wall. Determine the change in length, diameter and volume of the cylinder. Assume E = 210 GPa and μ = 0.3. **(10 Marks)**

Dec.08/Jan.09 (06ME34)

3. a. Derive an expression of circumferential and longitudinal stress for thin cylinder. **(10 Marks)**

   b. A pipe of 400 mm internal diameter and 100 mm thickness contains a fluid at a pressure of 80 N/mm^2. Find the maximum and minimum hoop stresses across the section. Also sketch the radial and hoop stress distribution across the section. **(10 Marks)**

June/July 2009 (06ME34)

4. a. Briefly discuss the stresses developed and their distribution along the thickness of the walls of pressure vessels. **(04 Marks)**

   b. A thin cylinder of diameter d, thickness t is subjected to an internal pressure p. Prove that the change in volume is $dV = \dfrac{pd}{4tE}(5 - 4\mu)V$, where E = Young's modulus , μ = Poisson's ratio and V = volume of the pressure vessel. **(08 Marks)**

   c. A thick cylinder of internal diameter 160 mm is subjected to an internal pressure of 40 N/mm^2. If the allowable stress in the material is 120 N/mm^2, find the required wall thickness of the cylinder. **(08 Marks)**

Dec. 09/Jan. 10 (06ME34)

5. a. Derive an expression for circumferential stress and longitudinal stress for a thin shell subjected to an internal pressure. **(06 Marks)**

   b. Derive an expression for the radial pressure and hoop stress for a thick spherical shell. **(06 Marks)**

   c. A thick spherical shell of 200 mm internal diameter is subjected to an internal fluid pressure of 7 N/mm². If the permissible tensile stress in the shell material is 8 N/mm², find the thickness of the shell. **(08 Marks)**

May/June 2010 (06ME34)

6. a. Obtain an expression for the volumetric strain of a thin cylinder, subjected to internal fluid pressure. **(08 Marks)**

   b. Determine the hoop stress and radial pressure across the section of a thick cylinder of internal diameter 40 cm and thickness 10 cm, when it contains a fluid at a pressure of 8 N/mm². Also sketch the distribution of hoop stress and radial pressure. **(12 Marks)**

Dec. 10 (06ME34)

7. a. A thin cylinder, 2 m long and 200 mm in diameter with 10 mm thickness is filled completely with a fluid, at atmospheric pressure. If an additional 25000 mm³ of fluid is pumped in, find the longitudinal and hoop stress developed. Also determine the changes in diameter and length if $E = 2 \times 10^5$ N/mm² and Poisson's ratio = 0.3. **(10 Marks)**

   b. Derive the expression for radial and hoop stresses (Lame's equation) for a thick cylinder. **(12 Marks)**

June/July 2011 (06ME34)

8. a. A thin cylinder of diameter d, thickness t, is subjected to an internal pressure of p. Prove that the change in volume is $dV = \dfrac{pd}{4tE}\,(5-4\mu)V$. Where E = Young's modulus, μ = Poisson's ratio and V = volume of the cylinder. **08 Marks)**

   b. A thick cylinder of 500 internal diameter is subjected to an internal pressure of 9 MPa. Taking the allowable stress for the material of the cylinder as 40 MPa, determine the wall thickness of the cylinder. Also plot the stress distribution across the wall thickness of the cylinder. **(12 Marks)**

Dec. 2011 (06ME34)

9. a. A cylindrical shell is 3 m long and is having 1m internal diameter and 15 mm thickness. Calculate the maximum intensity of shear stress induced and also the changes in dimensions of the shell, if it is subjected to an internal pressure of 1.5 N/mm². Take $E = 2 \times 10^5$ N/mm² and $\mu = 0.3$. **(10 Marks)**

   b. A pipe of 400 mm internal diameter and 100 mm thickness contains a fluid at a pressure of 80 N/mm². Find the maximum and minimum hoop stress across the section. Also sketch the radial and hoop stress distribution across the section. **(10 Marks)**

Dec. 2011 (10ME34)

10. A thin cylinder of 75 mm internal diameter and 250 mm long has 2.5 mm thick walls. The cylinder is subjected to an internal pressure of 7 MN/m². Determine the change in internal diameter and change in length of the cylinder. Also compute the hoop stress and longitudinal stress in the cylinder. Take $E = 2 \times 10^5$ N/mm² and $\mu = 0.3$. **(06 Marks)**

June 2012 (06ME34)

11. a. Show that the volumetric strain in a thin cylinder is given by $\epsilon_v = \dfrac{pd}{2tE}\left(\dfrac{5}{2} - \dfrac{2}{m}\right)$,

where ϵ_v = volumetric strain, $1/m$ = Poisson's ratio, E = Young's modulus

(05 Marks)

b. A cylindrical shell has an external diameter of 500 mm and wall thickness 10 mm and length of the cylinder is 1.7 m. Determine the increase in its internal diameter and length when inside pressure is 1 N/mm^2. Take E = 210 GPa and $\mu = 0.3$. **(05 Marks)**

c. A cast iron pipe of 400 mm internal diameter and 10 mm wall thickness carries water under pressure of 10 MPa. Determine the maximum and minimum intensities of hoop stress across the section. Also sketch the radial and hoop stress distribution diagram across the section. **(05 Marks)**

June 2012 (10ME34)

12. a. Calculate the i) change in diameter ii) change in length and iii) change in volume of a thin cylindrical shell 1000 mm diameter, 10 mm thick and 5 m long when subjected to internal pressure of 3 N/mm^2. Take the value of $E = 2 \times 10^5$ N/mm^2 and $1/m = 0.3$. **(06 Marks)**

b. A pressure vessel with outer and inner diameters of 400 mm and 320 mm respectively is subjected to an external pressure of 8 MPa. Determine the circumferential stress induced at the inner and outer surface. Prove that the longitudinal strain is constant throughout the cylinder. **(08 Marks)**

Dec. 2012 (10ME34)

13. a. Derive an expression for the circumferential stress of a thin cylinder.

(05 Marks)

b. A cylindrical pressure vessel has inner and outer radii of 200 mm and 250 mm respectively. The material of the cylinder has an allowable normal stress of 75 MN/m^2. Determine the maximum internal pressure that can be applied and draw a sketch of radial pressure and circumferential stress distribution.

(10 Marks)

Jan. 2013 (06ME34)

14. a. Derive expressions for circumferential and longitudinal stresses in a thin cylinder subjected to internal fluid pressure. Show that the circumferential stress is twice the longitudinal stress. **(10 Marks)**

b. The internal and external diameters of a thick cylinder are 300 mm and 500 mm respectively. It is subjected to an external pressure of 4 N/mm^2. Find the internal pressure that can be applied if the permissible stress in the cylinder is limited to 13 N/mm^2. Sketch the variation of hoop stress and radial stress across the thickness of the cylinder. **(10 Marks)**

June/July 2013 (06ME34)

15. a. For a thin cylinder, if hoop stress $\sigma_1 = pd/2t$ and longitudinal stress $\sigma_2 = pd/4t$, derive the expression for volumetric strain. **(10 Marks)**

   b. A pipe of 400 mm internal diameter and 100 mm thickness contains a fluid at a pressure of 80 MPa. Sketch the radial and hoop stress distribution across the section. **(10 Marks)**

June/July 2013 (10ME34)

16. A thin cylindrical shell 1m in diameter and 3 m long has a metal thickness of 10 mm. It is subjected to an internal fluid pressure of 3 MPa. Determine the change in length, diameter and volume. Also find the maximum shearing stress in the shell. Assume Poisson's ratio as 0.3 and $E = 210$ GPa. **(10 Marks)**

Dec. 13/Jan. 14 (06ME34)

17. a. Derive an expression for the circumferential and longitudinal stress of a thin cylinder subjected to an internal pressure. **(10 Marks)**
   b. Find the thickness of metal necessary for a thick cylinder of internal diameter 150 mm to withstand an internal pressure of 10 N/mm². The maximum hoop stress in the section is not to exceed 25 N/mm². **(10 Marks)**

Dec. 13/Jan. 14 (10ME34)

18. a. A water main 80 cm diameter contains water at a pressure head of 100 m. If the weight density of water is 9810 N/m³, find the thickness of the metal required for the water main. Given the permissible stress as 20 N/mm². **(06 Marks)**
   b. A pipe of 400 mm internal diameter and 100 mm thickness contains a fluid at a pressure of 8 N/mm². Find the maximum and minimum hoop stress across the section. Also sketch the variation of radial pressure distribution and hoop stress distribution across the section. **(08 Marks)**

June/July 2014 (06ME34)

19. a. Derive the expression for circumferential and radial stresses in the wall of thick cylinder (Lame's equation). **(10 Marks)**
   b. Determine the maximum and minimum hoop stress across the section of 400 mm internal diameter and 100 thick when the pipe contains a fluid at a pressure of 8 N/mm². Also sketch the radial pressure distribution and hoop stress distribution across the section. **(10 Marks)**

June/July 2014 (10ME34)

20. a. Prove that the volumetric strain in a thin cylinder is given by $\dfrac{pd}{4tE}$ $(5 - 4\mu)$ **(07 Marks)**
   b. A C.I. pipe has 200 mm internal diameter and 50 mm metal thickness and carries water under a pressure of 5 N/mm². Calculate the maximum and minimum intensities of circumferential stress and sketch the distribution of circumferential stress and radial pressure across the section. **(10 Marks)**

Dec. 14/Jan. 15(06ME34)

21. a. Derive an expression for circumferential and longitudinal stress for thin cylinder. **(08 Marks)**

b. A pipe of 400 mm internal diameter and 100 mm thickness contains a fluid at a pressure of 80 N/mm². Find the maximum and minimum hoop stresses across the section. Also sketch the radial and hoop stress distribution across the section. **(12 Marks)**

Dec. 14/Jan. 15(10ME34)

22. A thick cylinder with internal diameter 80 mm and external diameter 120 mm is subjected to an external pressure of 40 N/mm², when the internal pressure is 120 N/mm², calculate the circumferential stress at external and internal surfaces of the cylinder. Plot the variation of circumferential stress and radial pressure on the thickness of the cylinder. **(10 Marks)**

June/July 15(10ME34)

23. a. Derive an expression for circumferential stress of a thin cylinder. **(04 Marks)**
    b. A C.I pipe has 200 mm internal diameter and 50 mm metal thickness and carries water under a pressure of 5 N/mm². Calculate the maximum and minimum intensities of circumferential stress and sketch the distribution of circumferential stress intensity and intensity of radial pressure across the section.   **(10 Marks)**

Dec. 15/Jan. 16 (10ME/AU34)

24. a. For a thin cylindrical shell, the L/d ratio is 3 and its initial volume is 20 m³. The ultimate stress for the cylinder material is 200 MPa. Determine the wall thickness, if it has to convey water under a head of 200 m. Take FOS = 2.
    (08 Marks)
    b. Calculate the maximum external to internal radius ratio for a thick cylinder with internal fluid pressure of 15 MPa and maximum hoop stress of 60 MPa.
    (08 Marks)

June/July 2016 (10ME/AU34

25. a. Derive an expression for circumferential stress of a thin cylinder. **(05 Marks)**
    b. A thick cylinder of 500 mm inner diameter is subjected to an internal pressure of 9 MPa. Taking the allowable stress for the material of the cylinder as 40 MPa, determine the wall thickness of the cylinder.   **(10 Marks)**

Dec. 16/Jan. 17 (10ME/AU34)

26. a. A cylindrical shell is 3m long and is having 1m internal diameter and 15 mm thickness. Calculate the maximum intensity of shear stress induced and also the changes in the dimensions of the shell if is subjected to an internal fluid pressure of 1.5 MPa. Take E = 200 GPa and Poisson's ratio as 0.3.   **(10 Marks)**
    b. A thick cylindrical pipe of outside diameter 300 mm and internal diameter 200 mm is subjected to an internal fluid pressure of 14 MPa. Determine the maximum hoop stress developed in the cross-section. What is the percentage of error if the maximum hoop stress is found from the equation for thin pipes?
    (10 Marks)

Dec. 16/Jan. 17 (15ME/MA34)

27. a. A thin cylinder 3 m long is having 1m internal diameter and 15 mm thickness. Calculate the maximum intensity of shear stress induced and also the changes in the dimensions of the cylinder if it is subjected to an internal pressure of 1.5 N/mm². **(08 Marks)**

b. A thick cylindrical vessel is 250 mm internal diameter and has 50 mm thick wall. It is subjected to an internal pressure of 10 MPa due to movement of the fluid. Find the maximum hoop stress developed in the cylinder. Also calculate the radial and hoop stresses at a point 20 mm from the inner surface. Sketch the stresses. **(08 Marks)**

June/July 2017 (10ME/AU34)

28. a. Explain the concept of circumferential stress and longitudinal stress corresponding to thin cylinders. **(10 Marks)**
    b. A cylindrical pressure vessel of 1m inner diameter and 1.5 m long is subjected to an internal pressure p, thickness of the cylinder wall is 15 mm. Taking allowable stress for cylinder material as 90 MPa, determine:
       i. Magnitude of maximum internal pressure p that the pressure vessel can withstand and
       ii. Change in dimensions. Take $E = 200$ GPa and $\mu = 0.3$. **(10 Marks)**

June/July 2017 (15ME/MA34)

29. A thick cylindrical shell of 160 mm internal diameter is subjected to an internal pressure of 8 MPa. Find the thickness of the shell if the permissible or hoop stress in the section is not to exceed 35 MPa. **(06 Marks)**
30. A thin cylindrical shell with following dimensions is filled with a liquid at atmospheric pressure:
    Length = 1.2 m, external diameter = 200 mm, thickness of metal = 8 mm. Find the value of pressure exerted by the liquid on the walls of the cylinder and the hoop stress induced if an additional volume of 25000 mm^3 of liquid is pumped into the cylinder. Take $E = 2.1$ GPa and $\mu = 0.33$. **(08 Marks)**

Dec. 17/Jan. 18 (10ME/AU34)

31. Derive expressions for circumferential and radial stresses in the wall of thick cylinder (Lame's equation). **(10 Marks)**

Dec. 17/Jan. 18 (15ME/MA34)

32. Derive expressions for hoop stress and longitudinal stress for a thin cylinder subjected to internal fluid pressure. **(06 Marks)**
33. A thin cylindrical shell 1.3 m in diameter and 3 m long has a metal wall thickness of 12 mm. It is subjected to an internal pressure of 3.2 MPa. Find the circumferential and longitudinal stresses in the wall. Also determine the change in volume of the cylinder. Assume $E = 210$ GPa and $\mu = 0.30$. **(10 Marks)**

Shear Forces and Bending Moments

Chapter Outline

5.1 INTRODUCTION

A beam is a structural member that is designed to support transverse loads, i.e. loads act perpendicular to the longitudinal axis of the beam. A beam resists the applied loads by a combination of internal transverse shear force and bending moment which usually vary from point to point along the axis of the beam. On the other hand, axial and torsional loads often result in internal forces that are constant along the axis of the beam.

The beams shown in **Fig. 5.1** are planar structures because all loads act in the plane of the figure and all deflections occur in that same plane, which is called the plane of bending.

5.2 TYPES OF BEAMS

Based on the type of support, beams are classified as:
- Cantilever beam
- Simply supported beam
- Overhanging beam
- Continuous beam
- Fixed beam
- Beam fixed at one end and supported at the other end or Propped cantilever beam

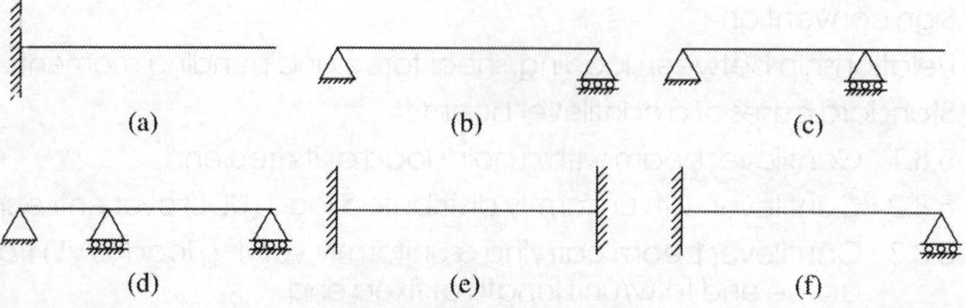

Fig. 5.1: Types of beams

- *Cantilever beam:* A beam whose one end is fixed while the other end is free as shown in **Fig. 5.1(a)** is a cantilever beam.
- *Simply supported beam:* A beam with a pin support at one end and a roller support at the other end as shown in **Fig. 5.1(b)** is a simply supported beam.
  Here at least one of the supports should undergo horizontal movement so that no force exists in the direction of the axis of the beam. Thus, a roller is shown as one of the supports.
- *Overhanging beam:* A beam that extends beyond the support at one end or at both ends as shown in **Fig. 5.1(c)** is an overhanging beam.
- *Continuous Beam:* A beam with a pin support at one end, a roller support at the other end, and one or more intermediate roller supports, as shown in **Fig. 5.1(d)** is a continuous beam.
- *Fixed beam:* A beam whose both ends are fixed as shown in **Fig. 5.1(e)** is a continuous beam.
- *Propped cantilever beam:* A beam with a cantilever support (i.e. fixed end) at one end and a roller at the other end as shown in **Fig. 5.1(f)** is a propped cantilever beam.

- **Fig's 5.1 (a) to (c)** are known as *statically determinate beams* since the support reactions of these beams can be determined by using the equations of static equilibrium [$\Sigma H = 0$, $\Sigma V = 0$ and $\Sigma M = 0$] and the reactions are independent of the deformation of beams. While **Fig's 5.1 (d) to (f)** are referred to as *statically indeterminate beams* as their support reactions cannot be determined by the equations of static equilibrium alone and requires consideration of the deflections caused by bending.

  Further the beams may be straight or curved and/or horizontal, vertical and inclined.

5.3 TYPES OF SUPPORTS

Three types of support are shown in **Fig. 5.1**.

- *Cantilever support (or fixed end):* prevents displacement in the axial direction and in the transverse direction, and also prevents z-rotation; the reaction consists of a force with both axial and transverse components.
- *Pin support:* prevents displacement in the axial direction and in the transverse direction, but permits z-rotation; the reaction is a force with both axial and transverse components.
- *Roller support:* prevents displacement in the transverse (i.e., y) direction, but permits z-rotation and displacement in the axial direction; the reaction is a force in the $+ y$ or $- y$ direction.

5.4 TYPES OF LOADING

Irrespective of the type of beam, a beam may be subjected to either of the loads or a combination of these loads:

- Concentrated or point load
- Uniformly distributed load (UDL)
- Uniformly varying load (UVL) and
- A couple.

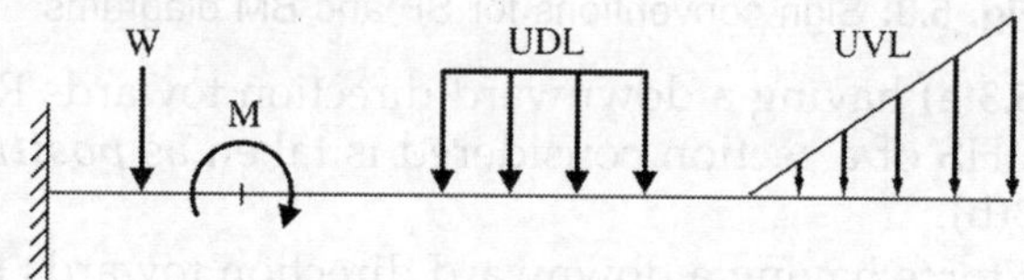

Fig. 5.2: Types of loads

- *Point load (W)* is one which is considered to act at a point. In actual practice, the load has to be distributed over a small area because such knife-edge contacts are generally neither possible nor desirable.
- *Distributed load* is one which is distributed or spread over some area along the length of the beam. Such loads are measured by their intensity and are expressed as force per unit distance along the axis of the beam.

  If the spread is uniform, the beam is called *uniformly distributed load (UDL)*, and if the spread is not uniform, the beam is called as *uniformly varying load (UVL)*. The intensity of UVL may vary from 0 to w or from w_1 to w_2.
- Another kind of load is a couple, represented as M in **Fig. 5.2**.

5.5 DEFINITIONS

- *Bending:* It indicates the deformation of a bar produced by loads perpendicular to its axis as well as force-couples acting in a plane passing through the axis of the bar.
- *Plane bending:* If the plane of the loading passes through one of the principal centroidal axes of the cross section of the beam, the bending is said to be plane/direct bending.
- *Oblique bending:* If the plane of loading does not pass through one of the principal centroidal axes of the cross section of the beam, the bending is said to be oblique.
- *Shear force* may be defined as the algebraic sum of all the vertical forces, either to the left or right side of the section.
- *Bending moment* may be defined as the algebraic sum of moments of all the forces either to the left or right of the section.
- *Maximum bending moment* is defined as the point at which shear force is zero or changes its sign.
- *Point of contraflexure* is defined as the point at which bending moment changes its sign. It is also called as **point of inflection**.

5.6 SIGN CONVENTION

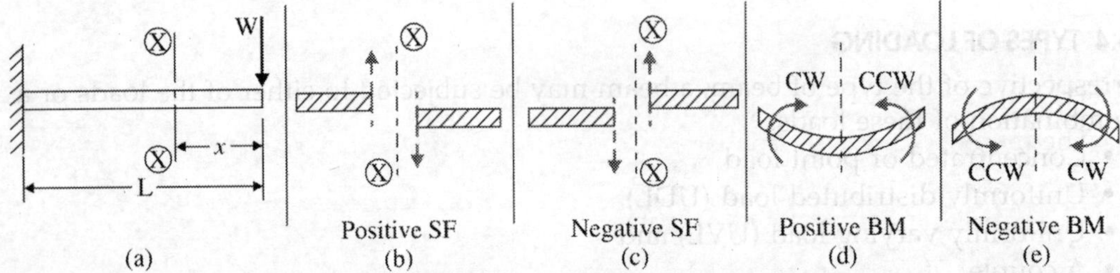

Fig. 5.3: Sign conventions for SF and BM diagrams

- Shear force **Fig. 5.3(a)** having a downward direction towards RHS or an upward direction to the LHS of a section considered is taken as *positive shear force*, as shown in **Fig. 5.3(b)**.

  Similarly shear force having a downward direction towards LHS of the section or an upward direction to RHS of the section considered is taken as *negative shear force*, as shown in **Fig. 5.3(c)**.

  In other words, clockwise shear is taken as positive, while counter clockwise shear is taken as negative.

- The force that tends to bend the beam so as to produce a concave surface is taken as *positive bending moment* (sagging bending moment); while that producing a convex surface is taken as *negative bending moment* (hogging bending moment) as shown in **Figs 5.3 (d) and (e)** respectively.

  In other words upward forces always cause positive bending moments (sagging) while downward forces cause negative bending moment (hogging), regardless of whether they act to the left or to the right of the section considered

5.7 RELATIONSHIP BETWEEN LOADING, SHEAR FORCE AND BENDING MOMENTS

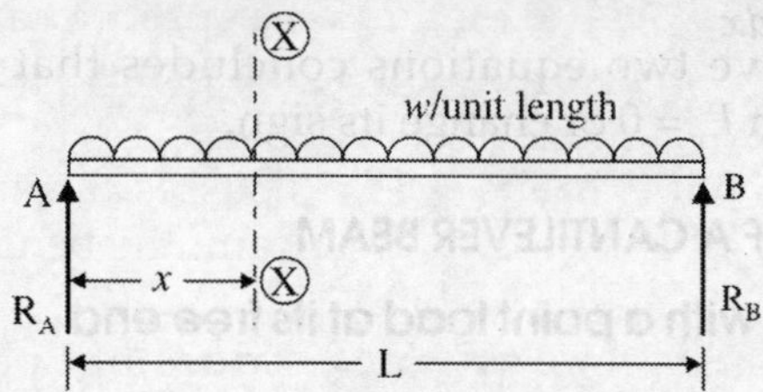

Fig. 5.4: Relation between load, SF and BM

Consider a beam subjected to a uniformly distributed load of w/unit length as shown in **Fig. 5.4**. Due to symmetry, the reaction at each support will be

$$R_A = R_B = \frac{wL}{2}$$

Consider a section X-X at a distance x from the left support. The shear force at this section is

$$F_x = R_A - wx = \frac{wL}{2} - wx \qquad \text{... (Eq. 5.1)}$$

Differentiating Eq. (5.1), we have

$$\frac{dF_x}{dx} = -w \qquad \text{... (Eq. 5.2)}$$

Thus the rate of change of shear force is $-w$ at any location x.

The moment at this section is

$$M_x = R_A.x - wx\left(\frac{x}{2}\right)$$

$$M_x = \left(\frac{wL}{2}\right)x - \frac{wx^2}{2} \qquad \text{... (Eq. 5.3)}$$

Differentiating the above equation, we have

$$\frac{dM_x}{dx} = \left(\frac{wL}{2}\right) - wx = F_x \qquad \text{... (Eq. 5.4)}$$

Thus the rate of change of bending moment is equal to shear force at any location x.

The terms $w.dx$ and $F.dx$ from Eqs (5.2) and (5.4) represent the differential areas under the distributed load and shear force diagrams respectively.

(Eq. 5.2) can be integrated between two locations x_1 and x_2 on the beam as

$$\int_{x_1}^{x_2} dF_x = \int_{x_1}^{x_2} - w.dx \qquad \text{... (Eq. 5.5)}$$

On similar lines, Eq. (5.4) can be written as

$$\int_{x_1}^{x_2} dM_x = \int_{x_1}^{x_2} F_x.dx \qquad \text{... (Eq. 5.6)}$$

The maximum bending moment occurs when $\dfrac{dM_x}{dx} = 0$.

But from (Eq. 5.4), $\dfrac{dM_x}{dx} = F_x$

Combining the above two equations concludes that the maximum bending moment occurs when $F_x = 0$ or change its sign.

5.8 STANDARD CASES OF A CANTILEVER BEAM

5.8.1 Cantilever beam with a point load at its free end

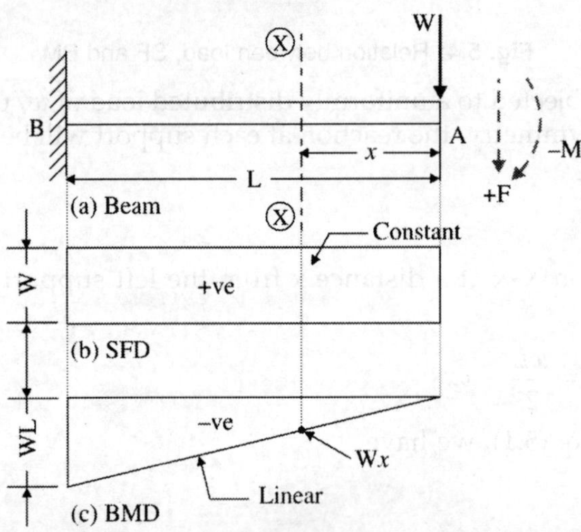

Fig. 5.5: Cantilever beam with point load at fee end

Fig. 5.5(a) indicates a cantilever beam subjected to point load at free end.

Let $\quad$ W = Point load at free end

$\quad\quad$ L = Length of the beam

$\quad\quad$ F_n = Shear force at salient points

$\quad\quad$ M_n = Bending moment at salient points

Consider a section X - X at a distance x from free end A.

Shear force at X - X is $\quad\quad\quad\quad F_x = W$

Boundary conditions:

$\quad\quad$ At A, $x = 0$, $\quad\quad\quad\quad F_A = W$

$\quad\quad$ At B, $x = L$, $\quad\quad\quad\quad F_B = W$

Bending moment at X-X is $\quad\quad M_x = -W.x \quad\quad$ (Negative because of hogging)

Applying the boundary conditions, we have

$\quad\quad$ At A, $x = 0$, $\quad\quad\quad\quad M_A = 0$

$\quad\quad$ At B, $x = L$, $\quad\quad\quad\quad M_B = -WL$

The SFD and BMD diagrams are shown in **Figs 5.5(b) & (c)** respectively.

5.8.2 Cantilever with uniformly distributed load over entire span

Fig. 5.6(a) indicates a cantilever beam subjected to uniformly distributed load over entire span.

Let $\quad$ w = Uniformly distributed load per unit length

$\quad\quad$ L = Length of the beam

$\quad\quad$ F_n = Shear force at salient points

$\quad\quad$ M_n = Bending moment at salient points

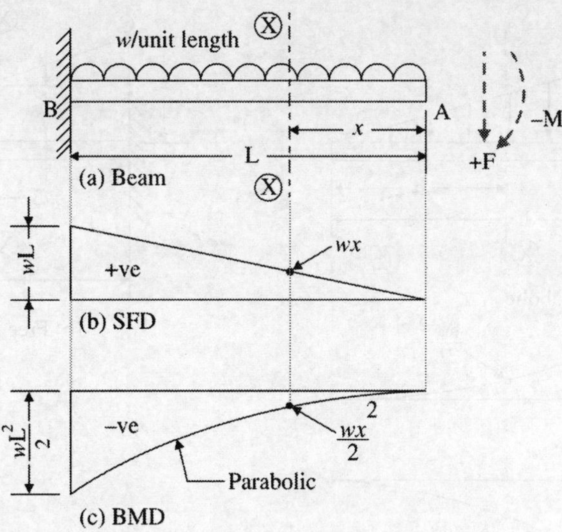

Fig. 5.6: Cantilever beam with UDL over entire span

Consider a section X-X at a distance x from free end A.

Shear force at X-X is $\qquad\qquad F_x = wx$

Boundary conditions:

At A, $x = 0$, $\qquad\qquad F_A = 0$

At B, $x = L$, $\qquad\qquad F_B = wL$

Bending moment at X - X is $\qquad M_x = -wx\left(\dfrac{x}{2}\right) = -\left(\dfrac{wx^2}{2}\right)$

(Negative because of hogging)

Applying the boundary conditions, we have

At A, $x = 0$, $\qquad\qquad M_A = 0$

At B, $x = L$, $\qquad\qquad M_B = -\left(\dfrac{wL^2}{2}\right)$

The SFD and BMD diagrams are shown in **Figs 5.6(b) & (c)** respectively.

5.8.3 Cantilever beam carrying a uniformly varying load from zero at free end to w/unit length at fixed end

Fig. 5.7(a) indicates a cantilever beam subjected to uniformly varying load of intensity 0 at free end and w/unit length at fixed end. **Fig. 5.7(b)** represents the free body diagram of the beam.

Let $\qquad w$ = Uniformly varying load per unit length

$\qquad\qquad L$ = Length of the beam

$\qquad\qquad F_n$ = Shear force at salient points

$\qquad\qquad M_n$ = Bending moment at salient points

To find rate of loading or load intensity:

Consider a section X-X at a distance x from free end A. From similar triangles ABC and AXD

$$\frac{y}{w} = \frac{x}{L}$$

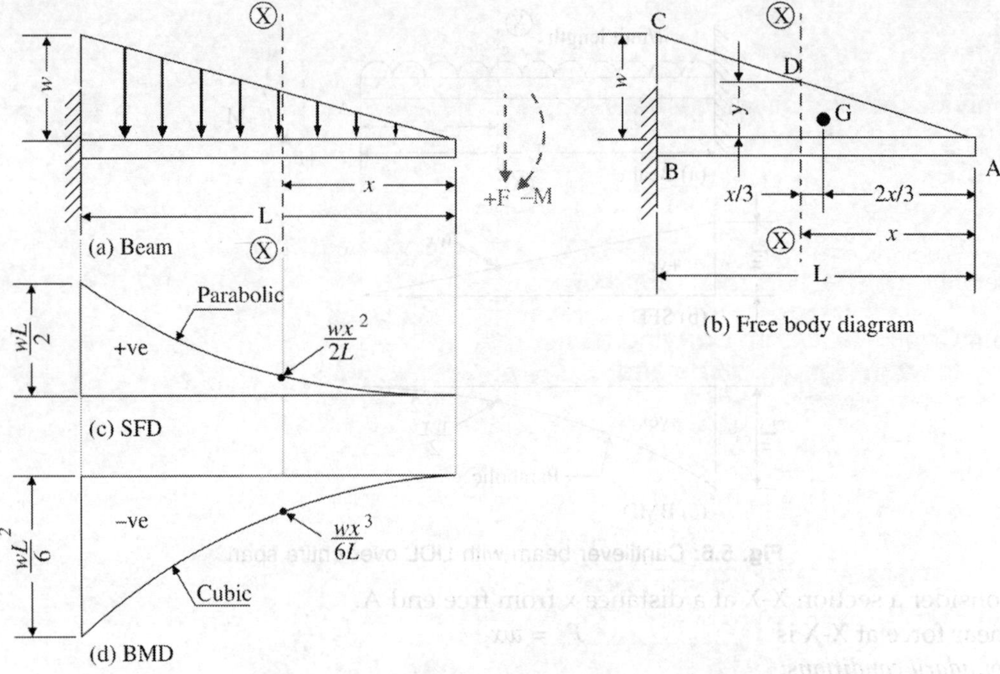

Fig. 5.7: Cantilever beam with UVL over entire span
(Zero at free end to w/unit length at fixed end)

$$y = \frac{wx}{L} \qquad\qquad \dots \text{Eq. (i)}$$

Eq. (i) gives the load intensity at a distance x from the free end.

i.e. $$y = w_x = \frac{wx}{L}$$

With the load intensity known, the resultant of the distributed loading is determined from the area under the diagram.

Shear force at X - X is $\qquad F_x$ = area of load diagram between A and X

$$= \frac{1}{2}\, y.x = \frac{1}{2}\, w_x.x = \frac{1}{2}\left(\frac{wx}{L}\right).x$$

$$F_x = \left(\frac{wx^2}{2L}\right)$$

Boundary conditions:

At A, $x = 0$, $\qquad\qquad F_A = 0$

At B, $x = L$, $\qquad\qquad F_B = \left(\frac{wL^2}{2L}\right) = \left(\frac{wL}{2}\right)$

Bending moment at X - X is $\qquad M_x$ = Moment of load acting on XA about X

$$= - F_x \times \text{distance of G from XX}$$

(Negative because of hogging)

$$= -\left(\frac{wx^2}{2L}\right)\left(\frac{x}{3}\right)$$

$$M_x = -\left(\frac{wx^3}{6L}\right)$$

Applying the boundary conditions, we have

      At A, $x = 0$, $M_A = 0$

      At B, $x = L$, $M_B = -\left(\frac{wL^3}{6L}\right) = -\left(\frac{wL^2}{6}\right)$

The SFD and BMD diagrams are shown in **Fig's 5.7(c) & (d)** respectively.

5.8.4 Cantilever beam carrying a uniformly varying load from zero at fixed end to w/unit length at free end

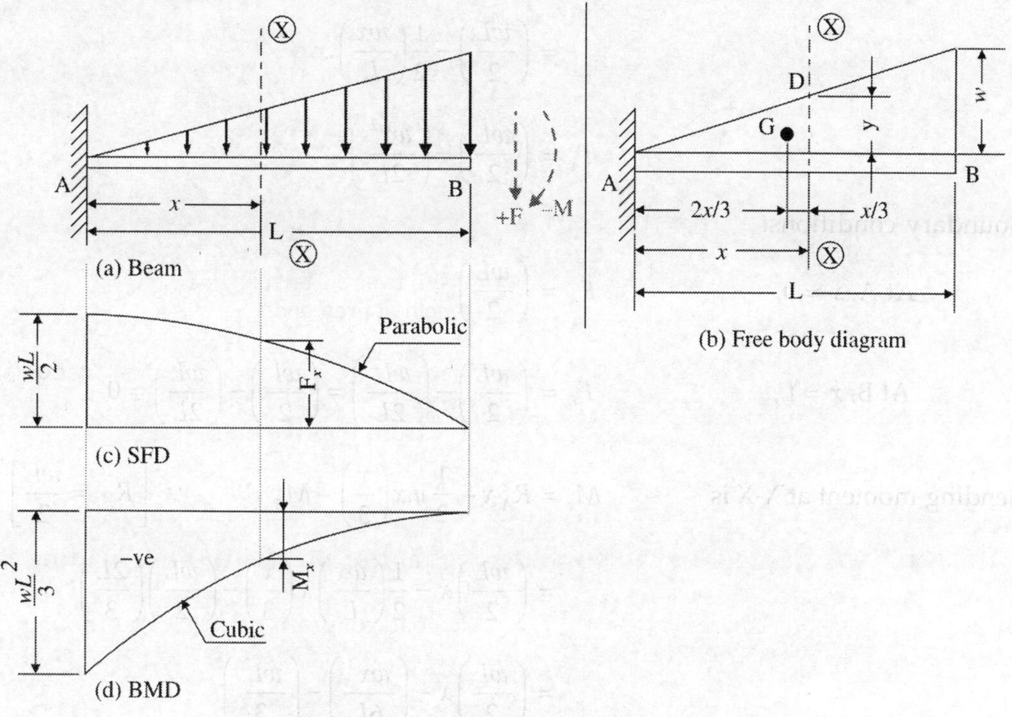

Fig. 5.8: Cantilever beam with UVL over entire span
(Zero at fixed end to w/unit length at free end)

Fig. 5.8(a) indicates a cantilever beam subjected to uniformly varying load of intensity 0 at fixed end and w/unit length at free end. **Fig. 5.8(b)** represents the free body diagram of the beam.

    Let w = Uniformly varying load per unit length

                L = Length of the beam

                F_n = Shear force at salient points

                M_n = Bending moment at salient points

To find rate of loading or load intensity:

Consider a section X-X at a distance x from fixed end A. From similar triangles ABC and AXD

$$\frac{y}{w} = \frac{x}{L}$$

$$y = \frac{wx}{L} \qquad\qquad \ldots \text{Eq. (i)}$$

Eq. (i) gives the load intensity at a distance x from the free end.

i.e. $\qquad y = w_x = \dfrac{wx}{L}$

With the load intensity known, the resultant of the distributed loading is determined from the area under the diagram.

Shear force at X-X is $\qquad\qquad F_x$ = area of load diagram between A and X

$$= \frac{1}{2}\,w.L - \frac{1}{2}\,y.x$$

$$= \left(\frac{wL}{2}\right) - \frac{1}{2}\left(\frac{wx}{L}\right).x$$

$$F_x = \left(\frac{wL}{2}\right) - \left(\frac{wx^2}{2L}\right)$$

Boundary conditions:

At A, $x = 0$, $\qquad\qquad F_A = \left(\dfrac{wL}{2}\right)$

At B, $x = L$, $\qquad\qquad F_B = \left(\dfrac{wL}{2}\right) - \left(\dfrac{wL^2}{2L}\right) = \left(\dfrac{wL}{2}\right) - \left(\dfrac{wL}{2L}\right) = 0$

Bending moment at X-X is $\qquad M_x = R_A x - \dfrac{1}{2}\,y.x\left(\dfrac{x}{3}\right) - M_A \qquad \because \left[R_A = \dfrac{wL}{2}\right]$

$$= \left(\frac{wL}{2}\right)x - \frac{1}{2}\left(\frac{wx}{L}\right)x\left(\frac{x}{3}\right) - \left(\frac{wL}{2}\right)\left(\frac{2L}{3}\right)$$

$$= \left(\frac{wL}{2}\right)x - \left(\frac{wx^3}{6L}\right) - \left(\frac{wL^2}{3}\right)$$

Applying the boundary conditions, we have

At A, $x = 0$, $\qquad\qquad M_A = -\left(\dfrac{wL^2}{3}\right)$

At B, $x = L$, $\qquad\qquad M_B = 0$

The SFD and BMD diagrams are shown in **Fig's 5.8(c) & (d)** respectively.

5.8.5 Cantilever beam subjected to couple

Fig. 5.9(a) indicates a cantilever beam subjected to a CW couple at free end.

Let $\qquad M$ = couple

$\qquad\qquad L$ = Length of the beam

Since no force is acting on the beam, shear force is zero as shown in **Fig. 5.9(b)**.

At every section in the beam the bending moment will be $-M$ which remains constant throughout as shown in **Fig. 5.9(c)**.

Note: In case of cantilever beams, moments at the free end is always zero, unless the beam is subjected to a moment at the free end.

1. **Draw the shear force and bending moment diagrams for the cantilever beam shown in Fig. 5.10(a).**

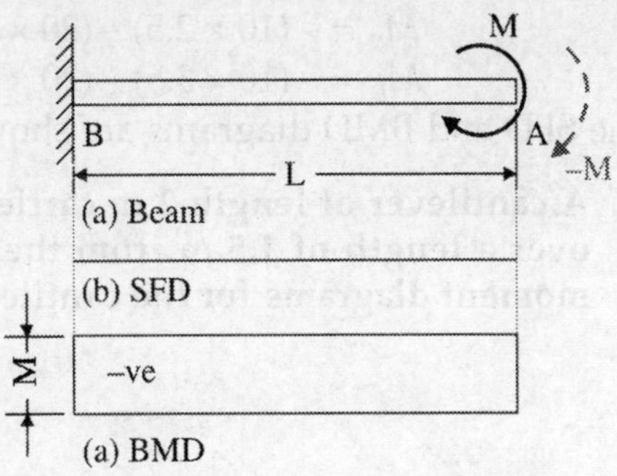

Fig. 5.9: Cantilever beam with a couple

VTU – Dec. 16/ Jan. 17 – 08 Marks; [similar: (CV) June/ July 2011– 06 Marks]

Solution:

Let F_n = Shear force at salient points

M_n = Bending moment at salient points

Shear force calculations:

$$F_A = 10 \text{ kN}$$
$$F_B = F_A + 20 = 10 + 20 = 30 \text{ kN}$$
$$F_C = F_B + 30 = 30 + 20 = 50 \text{ kN}$$
$$F_D = F_C + 0 = 50 \text{ kN}$$

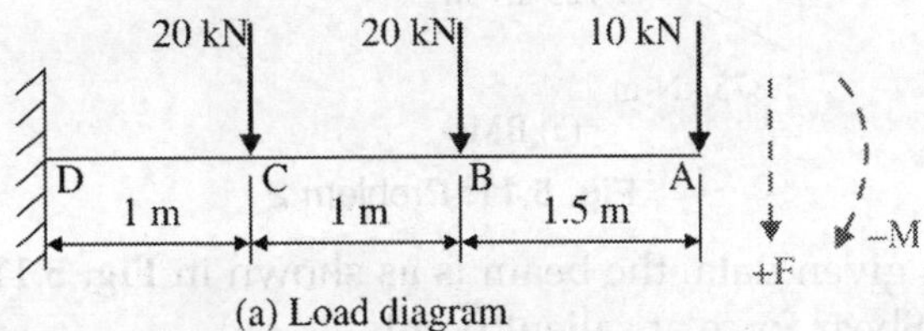

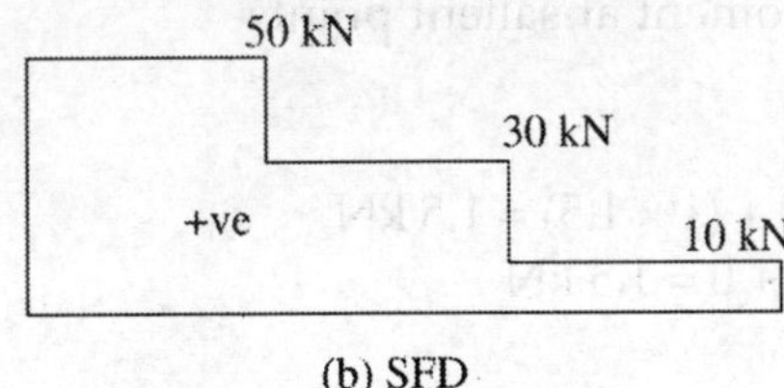

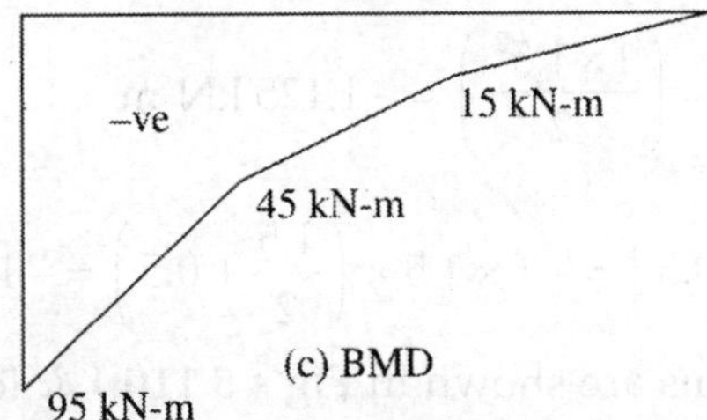

Fig. 5.10: Problem 1

Bending moment calculations:

$$M_A = 0$$
$$M_B = -10 \times 1.5 = 15 \text{ kN-m or kJ}$$

$$M_C = -(10 \times 2.5) - (20 \times 1) = -45 \text{ kN-m or kJ}$$
$$M_D = -(10 \times 3.5) - (20 \times 2) - (20 \times 1) = -95 \text{ kN-m or kJ}$$

The SFD and BMD diagrams are shown in **Fig's 5.10(b) & (c)** respectively.

2. **A cantilever of length 2 m carries a uniformly distributed load of 1 kN/m run over a length of 1.5 m from the free end. Draw the shear force and bending moment diagrams for the cantilever.**

VTU – Dec. 2012 – 06 Marks

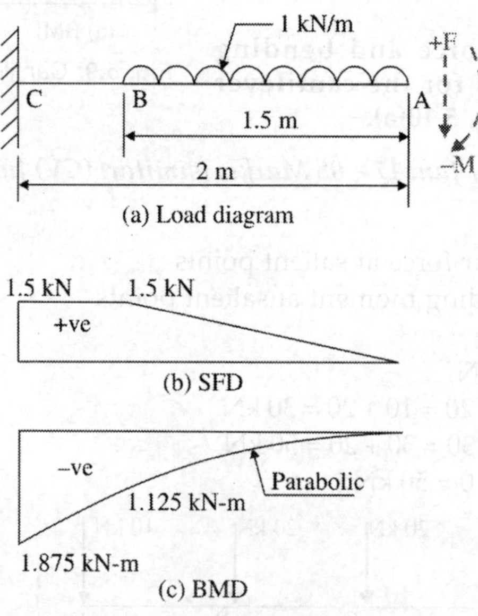

Fig. 5.11: Problem 2

Solution: Based on given data, the beam is as shown in **Fig. 5.11(a)**.

Let F_n = Shear force at salient points

M_n = Bending moment at salient points

Shear force calculations:

$$F_A = 0$$
$$F_B = F_A + wL = 0 + (1 \times 1.5) = 1.5 \text{ kN}$$
$$F_C = F_B + 0 = 1.5 + 0 = 1.5 \text{ kN}$$

Bending moment calculations:

$$M_A = 0$$

$$M_B = -\left(\frac{wL^2}{2}\right) = -\left(\frac{1 \times 1.5^2}{2}\right) = -1.125 \text{ kN-m}$$

$$M_C = -wL\left(\frac{L}{2} + 0.5\right) = -1 \times 1.5 \times \left(\frac{1.5}{2} + 0.5\right) = -1.875 \text{ kN-m}$$

The SFD and BMD diagrams are shown in **Fig's 5.11(b) & (c)** respectively.

3. **For the cantilever beam shown in Fig. 5.12(a), obtain the shear force and bending moment diagrams.**

VTU – (CV) June/ July 2016 – 06 Marks; (CV) Dec. 2012 – 05 Marks

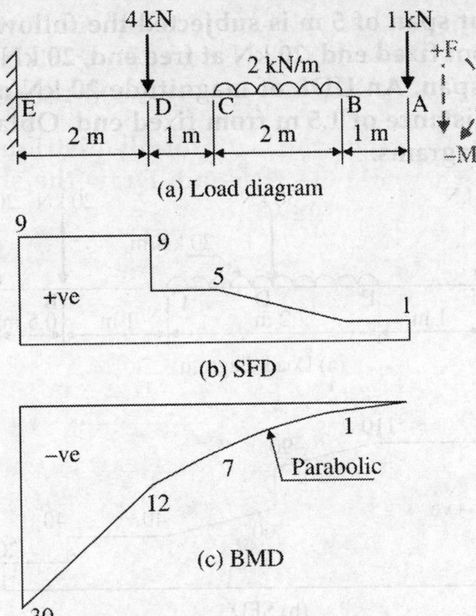

Fig. 5.12: Problem 3

Solution: Based on given data, the beam is as shown in **Fig. 5.12(a)**.

Let $\quad F_n$ = Shear force at salient points

$\quad\quad\quad M_n$ = Bending moment at salient points

Shear force calculations:

$$F_A = 1$$

$$F_B = F_A + 0 = 1 \text{ kN}$$

SF changes between B to C as

$$F_{B-C} = F_B + wL = 1 + (2 \times 2) = 5 \text{ kN}$$

$$F_C = F_{B-C} + 0 = 5 \text{ kN}$$

SF changes between C to D as

$$F_{C-D} = F_C + 0 = 5 \text{ kN}$$

$$F_D = F_{C-D} + 4 = 9 \text{ kN}$$

$$F_E = F_D + 0 = 9 \text{ kN}$$

Bending moment calculations:

$$M_A = 0$$

$$M_B = -1 \times 1 = 1 \text{ kN-m}$$

$$M_C = -(1 \times 3) - \left(\frac{2 \times 2^2}{2}\right) = -7 \text{ kN-m}$$

$$M_D = -(1 \times 4) - \left[2 \times 2 \times \left(\frac{2}{2} + 1\right)\right] = -12 \text{ kN-m}$$

$$M_E = -(1 \times 6) - \left[2 \times 2 \times \left(\frac{2}{2} + 3\right)\right] - (4 \times 2) = -30 \text{ kN-m}$$

The SFD and BMD diagrams are shown in **Fig's 5.12(b) & (c)** respectively.

4. **A cantilever beam of span of 5 m is subjected the following loads. Point loads of 10 kN at 0.5 m from fixed end, 20 kN at free end, 20 kN at 0.5 m from free end and 30 kN an mid span. An UDL of magnitude 20 kN/m run over a length of 2 m is located at a distance of 1.5 m from fixed end. Obtain the shear force and bending moment diagrams.**

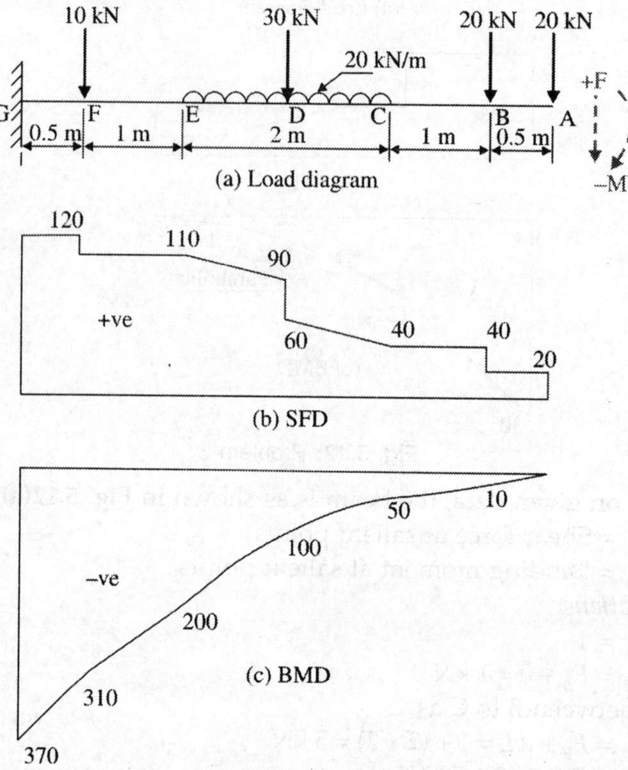

Fig. 5.13: Problem 4

Solution: Based on given data, the beam is as shown in **Fig. 5.13(a)**.

Let $\quad F_n$ = Shear force at salient points

$\qquad M_n$ = Bending moment at salient points

Shear force calculations:

$$F_A = 20 \text{ kN}$$

$$F_B = F_A + 20 = 20 + 20 = 40 \text{ kN}$$

$$F_C = F_B + 0 = 40 \text{ kN}$$

SF changes between C to D as

$$F_{C-D} = F_C + wL = 40 + (20 \times 1) = 60 \text{ kN}$$

$$F_D = F_{C-D} + 30 = 60 + 30 = 90 \text{ kN}$$

SF changes between D to E as

$$F_{D-E} = F_D + wL = 90 + (20 \times 1) = 110 \text{ kN}$$

$$F_E = F_{D-E} + 0 = 110 \text{ kN}$$

$$F_F = F_E + 10 = 110 + 10 = 120 \text{ kN}$$

$$F_G = F_F + 0 = 120 \text{ kN}$$

Bending moment calculations:

$$M_A = 0$$

$$M_B = -20 \times 0.5 = 10 \text{ kN-m or kJ}$$

$$M_C = -(20 \times 1.5) - (20 \times 1) = -50 \text{ kN-m}$$

$$M_D = -(20 \times 2.5) - (20 \times 2) - \left(\frac{20 \times 1^2}{2}\right) = -100 \text{ kN-m}$$

$$M_E = -(20 \times 3.5) - (20 \times 3) - (30 \times 1) - \left(\frac{20 \times 2^2}{2}\right) = -200 \text{ kN-m}$$

$$M_F = -(20 \times 4.5) - (20 \times 4) - (30 \times 2) - \left[20 \times 2 \times \left(\frac{2}{2} + 1\right)\right] = -310 \text{ kN-m}$$

$$M_G = -(20 \times 5) - (20 \times 4.5) - (30 \times 2.5) - (10 \times 0.5) - \left[20 \times 2 \times \left(\frac{2}{2} + 1.5\right)\right]$$

$$= -370 \text{ kN-m}$$

The SFD and BMD diagrams are shown in **Fig's 5.13(b) & (c)** respectively.

5. **For the cantilever beam shown in Fig. 5.14(a), obtain SFD and BMD.**

VTU – Dec. 15/ Jan. 16 – 06 Marks

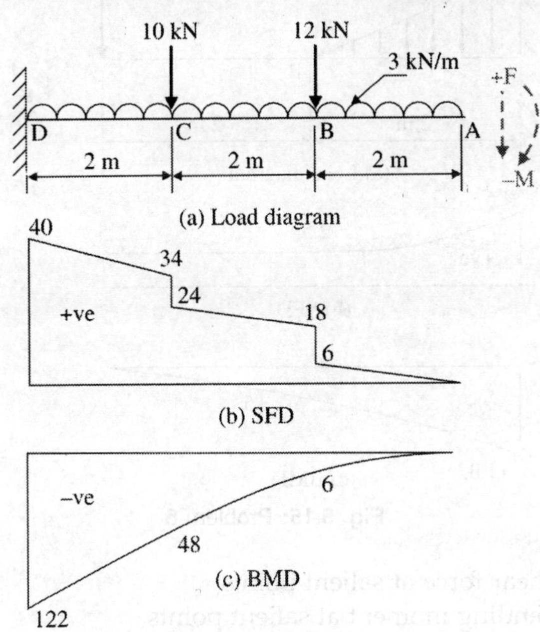

Fig. 5.14: Problem 5

Solution:

Let $\quad F_n$ = Shear force at salient points

$\qquad M_n$ = Bending moment at salient points

Shear force calculations:

$$F_A = 0 \text{ kN}$$

SF changes between A to B as

$$F_{A-B} = F_A + wL = 0 + (3 \times 2) = 6 \text{ kN}$$

$$F_B = F_{A-B} + 12 = 6 + 12 = 18 \text{ kN}$$

SF changes between B to C as

$$F_{B-C} = F_B + wL = 18 + (3 \times 2) = 24 \text{ kN}$$
$$F_C = F_{B-C} + 10 = 24 + 10 = 34 \text{ kN}$$
$$F_D = F_C + wL = 34 + (3 \times 2) = 40 \text{ kN}$$

Bending moment calculations:

$$M_A = 0$$

$$M_B = -\left(\frac{3 \times 2^2}{2}\right) = -6 \text{ kN-m}$$

$$M_C = -\left(\frac{3 \times 4^2}{2}\right) - (12 \times 2) = -48 \text{ kN-m}$$

$$M_D = -\left(\frac{3 \times 6^2}{2}\right) - (12 \times 4) - (10 \times 2) = -122 \text{ kN-m}$$

The SFD and BMD diagrams are shown in **Fig's 5.14(b) & (c)** respectively.

6. **Draw the shear-force and bending-moment diagrams for the beam shown in Fig. 5.15(a).**

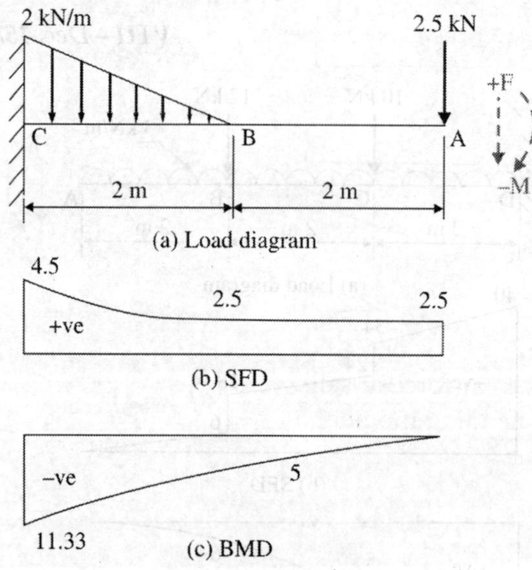

Fig. 5.15: Problem 6

Solution:

Let $\quad F_n$ = Shear force at salient points

$\qquad M_n$ = Bending moment at salient points

Shear force calculations:

$$F_A = 2.5 \text{ kN}$$
$$F_B = F_A + 0 = 2.5 \text{ kN}$$

$$F_C = F_B + \left(\frac{wL}{2}\right) = 2.5 + \left(\frac{1}{2} \times 2 \times 2\right) = 4.5 \text{ kN}$$

Bending moment calculations:

$$M_A = 0$$
$$M_B = -2.5 \times 2 = -5 \text{ kN-m}$$

$$M_C = -2.5 \times 4 - \left[\frac{1}{2} \times 2 \times 2 \times \left(\frac{2}{3}\right)\right] = -11.33 \text{ kN-m}$$

The SFD and BMD diagrams are shown in **Fig's 5.15(b) & (c)** respectively.

7. **Draw the shear-force and bending-moment diagrams for the beam shown in Fig. 5.16(a).**

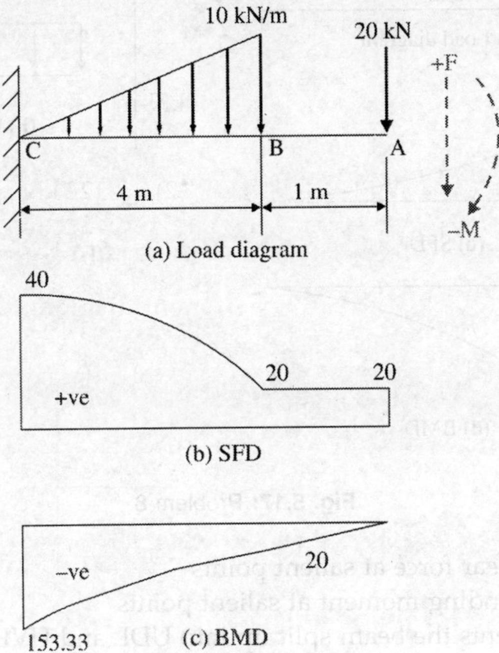

Fig. 5.16: Problem 7

Solution:

Let F_n = Shear force at salient points

M_n = Bending moment at salient points

Shear force calculations:

$$F_A = 20 \text{ kN}$$
$$F_B = F_A + 0 = 20 \text{ kN}$$
$$F_C = F_B + \left(\frac{wL}{2}\right) = 20 + \left(\frac{1}{2} \times 10 \times 4\right) = 40 \text{ kN}$$

Bending moment calculations:

$$M_A = 0$$
$$M_B = -20 \times 1 = -20 \text{ kN-m}$$
$$M_C = -20 \times 5 - \left[\frac{1}{2} \times 10 \times 4 \left(\frac{2 \times 4}{3}\right)\right] = -153.33 \text{ kN-m}$$

The SFD and BMD diagrams are shown in **Fig's 5.16(b) & (c)** respectively.

8. **Draw the shear force and bending moment diagram for the cantilever beam Fig. 5.17(a) with varying load of 5 kN/m at free end and 15 kN/m at fixed end.**

VTU – (CV) Dec. 10 – 08 Marks

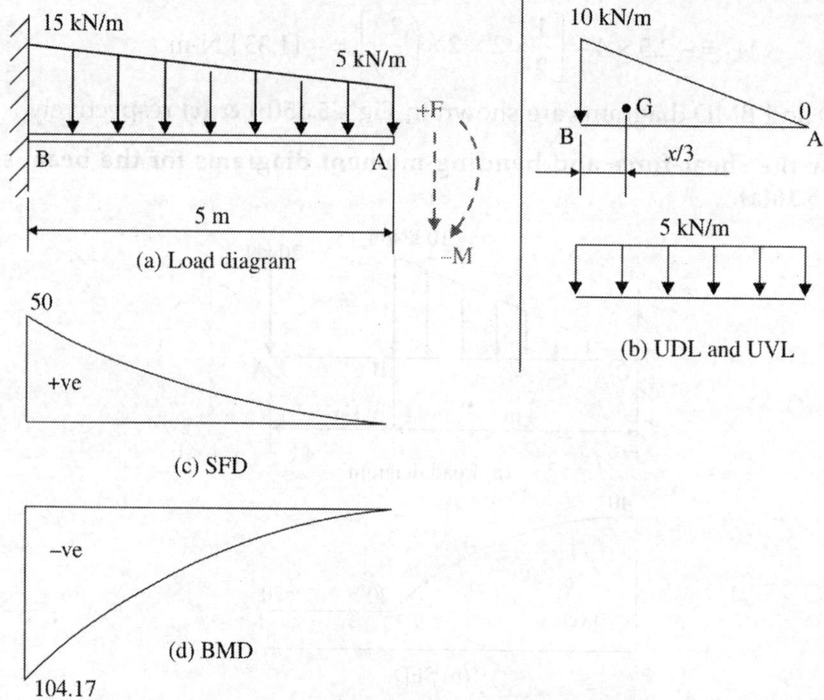

Fig. 5.17: Problem 8

Solution:

Let F_n = Shear force at salient points

M_n = Bending moment at salient points

Fig. 5.17(b) represents the beam split up into UDL and UVL. Thus the shear force and bending moments at salient points are the summation of the above two loads.

Shear force calculations:

$$F_A = 0 \text{ kN}$$

$$F_B = F_A + [UDL + UVL] = 0 + \left[(5 \times 5) + \left(\frac{1}{2} \times 10 \times 5 \right) \right] = 50 \text{ kN}$$

Bending moment calculations:

$$M_A = 0$$

$$M_B = -\left(\frac{5 \times 5^2}{2} \right) - \left[\frac{1}{2} \times 10 \times 5 \times \left(\frac{5}{3} \right) \right] = -104.17 \text{ kN-m}$$

The SFD and BMD diagrams are shown in **Fig's 5.17(b) & (c)** respectively.

9. Draw the shear force and bending moment diagram for the cantilever beam shown in Fig. 5.18(a).

Solution:

Let F_n = Shear force at salient points

M_n = Bending moment at salient points

Fig. 5.18(b) represents the beam split up into UDL and UVL. Thus the shear force and bending moments at salient points are the summation of the above two loads.

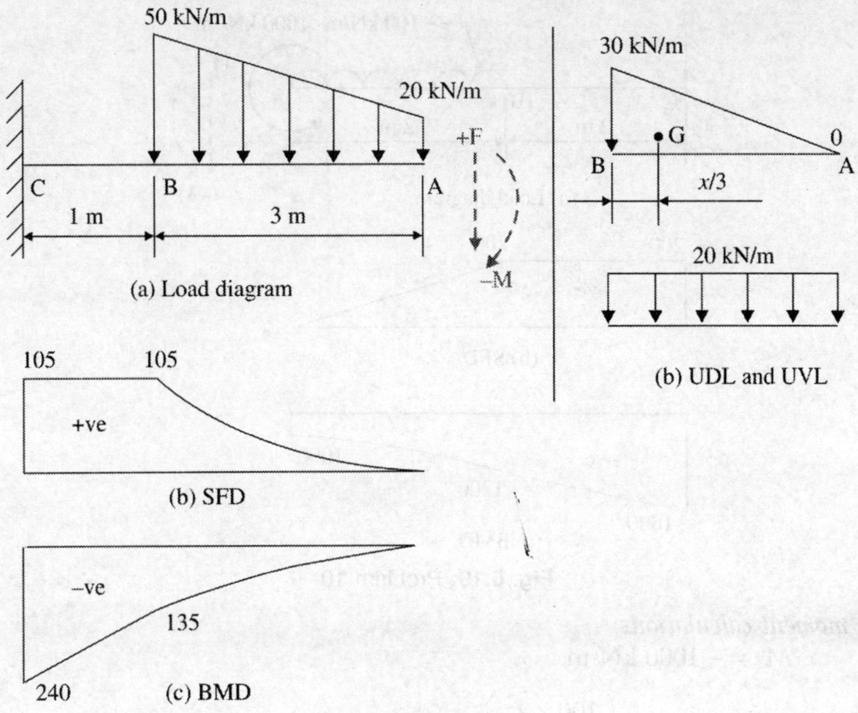

Fig. 5.18: Problem 9

Shear force calculations:

$$F_A = 0 \text{ kN}$$

$$F_B = F_A + [UDL + UVL] = 0 + \left[(20 \times 3) + \left(\frac{1}{2} \times 30 \times 3 \right) \right] = 105 \text{ kN}$$

$$F_C = F_B + 0 = 105 \text{ kN}$$

Bending moment calculations:

$$M_A = 0$$

$$M_B = -\left(\frac{20 \times 3^2}{2} \right) - \left[\frac{1}{2} \times 30 \times \left(\frac{3}{3} \right) \right] = -135 \text{ kN-m}$$

$$M_C = -\left[20 \times 3 \times \left(\frac{3}{2} + 1 \right) \right] - \left[\frac{1}{2} \times 30 \times 3 \times \left(\frac{3}{3} + 1 \right) \right] = -240 \text{ kN-m}$$

The SFD and BMD diagrams are shown in **Fig's 5.18(b) & (c)** respectively.

10. Draw the shear force and bending moment diagram for the cantilever beam shown in Fig. 5.19(a).

Solution:

Let $\quad F_n$ = Shear force at salient points

$\qquad M_n$ = Bending moment at salient points

Shear force calculations:

$$F_A = 0 \text{ kN}$$
$$F_B = (100 \times 2) = 200 \text{ kN}$$
$$F_C = F_B + 0 = 200 \text{ kN}$$

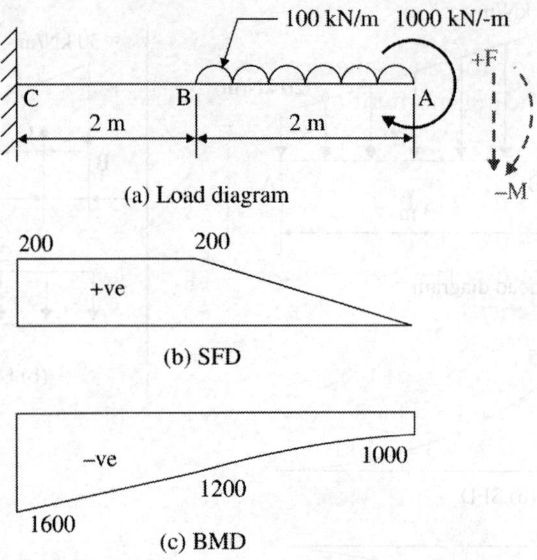

Fig. 5.19: Problem 10

Bending moment calculations:

$$M_A = -1000 \text{ kN-m}$$

$$M_B = -1000 - \left(\frac{100 \times 2^2}{2}\right) = -1200 \text{ kN-m}$$

$$M_C = -1000 - \left[100 \times 2 \times \left(\frac{2}{2} + 2\right)\right] = -1600 \text{ kN-m}$$

The SFD and BMD diagrams are shown in **Fig's 5.19(b) & (c)** respectively.

11. Draw the shear force and bending moment diagrams for the beam shown in Fig. 5.20(a), locating the point of contraflexure.

VTU – (CV) May/ June 2010 – 10 Marks

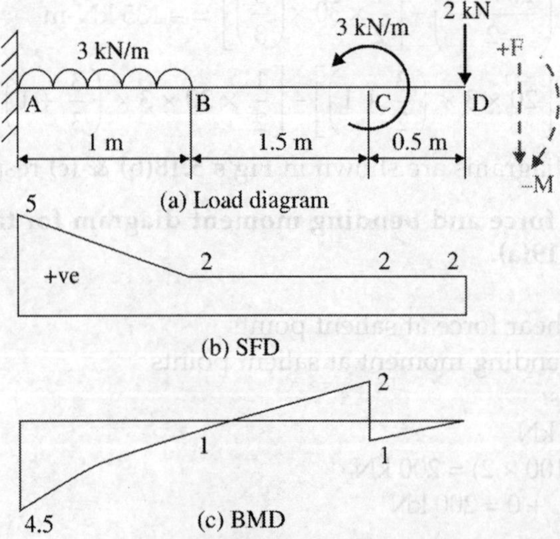

Fig. 5.20: Problem 11

Solution:

Let $\qquad F_n$ = Shear force at salient points

$\qquad\qquad M_n$ = Bending moment at salient points

Shear force calculations:

$$F_D = 2 \text{ kN}$$
$$F_C = F_D + 0 = 2 \text{ kN}$$
$$F_B = F_C + 0 = 2 \text{ kN}$$
$$F_A = F_B + (3 \times 1) = 2 + 3 = 5 \text{ kN}$$

Bending moment calculations:

$$M_D = 0$$
$$M_{D-C} = -(2 \times 0.5) = -1 \text{ kN-m}$$
$$M_C = M_{D-C} + 3 = -1 + 3 = 2 \text{ kN-m}$$
$$M_B = -(2 \times 2) + 3 = -1 \text{ kN-m}$$

$$M_A = -(2 \times 3) + 3 - \left(\frac{3 \times 1^2}{2}\right) = -4.5 \text{ kN-m}$$

The SFD and BMD diagrams are shown in **Fig's 5.20(b) & (c)** respectively.

12. Draw the shear force and bending moment diagrams for the cantilever shown in Fig. 5.21(a).

VTU – Jan. 2013 – 08 Marks

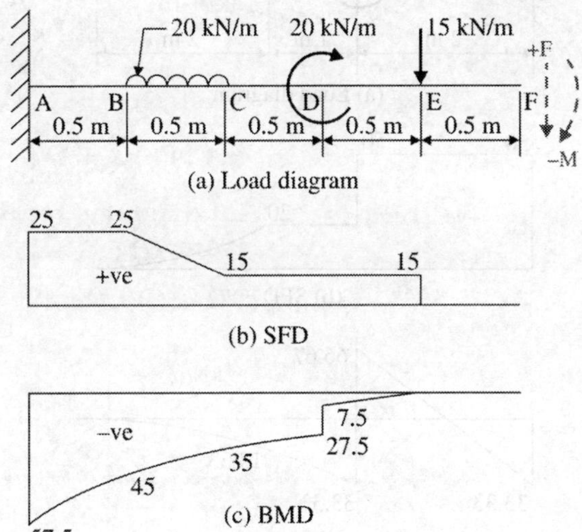

Fig. 5.21: Problem 12

Solution:

Let $\qquad F_n$ = Shear force at salient points

$\qquad\qquad M_n$ = Bending moment at salient points

Shear force calculations:

$$F_F = 0 \text{ kN}$$
$$F_E = 15 \text{ kN}$$
$$F_D = F_E + 0 = 15 \text{ kN}$$
$$F_C = F_D + 0 = 15 \text{ kN}$$
$$F_B = F_D + (20 \times 0.5) = 15 + 10 = 25 \text{ kN}$$
$$F_A = F_B + 0 = 25 \text{ kN}$$

Bending moment calculations:

$$M_F = 0$$
$$M_E = 0$$
$$M_{E-D} = -(15 \times 0.5) = -7.5 \text{ kN-m}$$
$$M_D = M_{D-C} - 20 = -7.5 - 20 = -27.5 \text{ kN-m}$$
$$M_C = -(15 \times 1) - 20 = -35 \text{ kN-m}$$

$$M_B = -(15 \times 1.5) - 20 - \left(\frac{20 \times 0.5^2}{2}\right) = -45 \text{ kN-m}$$

$$M_A = -(15 \times 2) - 20 - \left[20 \times 0.5 \times \left(\frac{0.5}{2} + 0.5\right)\right] = -57.5 \text{ kN-m}$$

The SFD and BMD diagrams are shown in **Fig's 5.21(b) & (c)** respectively.

13. A cantilever is loaded as shown in Fig. 5.22(a). Draw the shear force and bending moment diagrams for the beam.

VTU – June 2012 – 12 Marks

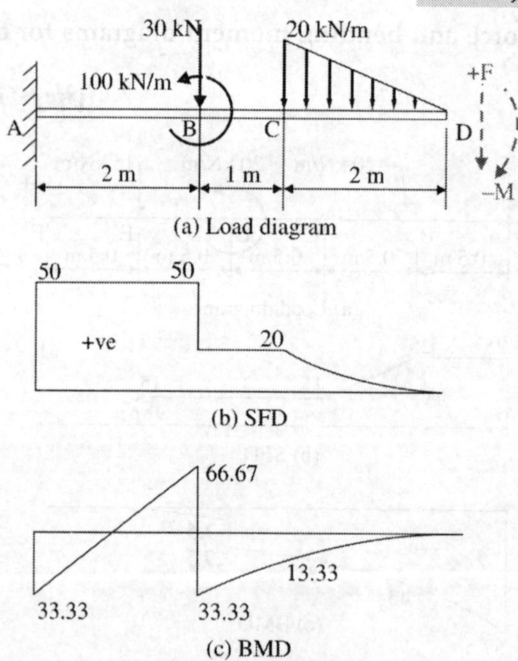

Fig. 5.22: Problem 13

Solution:

Let F_n = Shear force at salient points

M_n = Bending moment at salient points

Shear force calculations:

$$F_D = 0 \text{ kN}$$

$$F_C = F_D + \left(\frac{wL}{2}\right) = 0 + \left(\frac{1}{2} \times 20 \times 2\right) = 20 \text{ kN}$$

$$F_B = F_C + 30 = 20 + 30 = 50 \text{ kN}$$
$$F_A = F_B + 0 = 50 \text{ kN}$$

Bending moment calculations:

$$M_D = 0$$

$$M_C = -\left[\frac{1}{2} \times 20 \times 2 \times \left(\frac{2}{3}\right)\right] = -13.33 \text{ kN-m}$$

$$M_{C-B} = -\left[\frac{1}{2} \times 20 \times 2 \times \left(\frac{2}{3} + 1\right)\right] = -33.33 \text{ kN-m}$$

$$M_B = M_{C-B} + 20 = -33.33 + 100 = 66.67 \text{ kN-m}$$

$$M_A = -\left[\frac{1}{2} \times 20 \times 2 \times \left(\frac{2}{3} + 3\right)\right] + 100 - (30 \times 2)$$

$$= -33.33 \text{ kN-m}$$

The SFD and BMD diagrams are shown in **Fig's 5.22(b) & (c)** respectively.

14. Obtain the shear force and bending moment diagrams for the beam shown in Fig. 5.23(a).

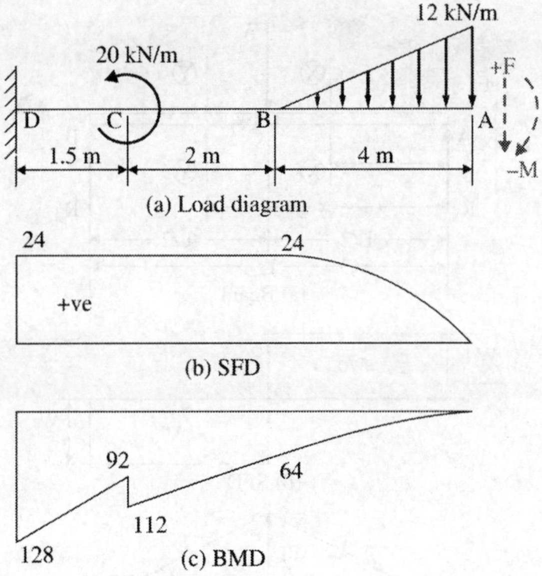

Fig. 5.23: Problem 14

Solution:

Let F_n = Shear force at salient points

M_n = Bending moment at salient points

Shear force calculations:

$$F_A = 0 \text{ kN}$$

$$F_B = F_A + \left(\frac{wL}{2}\right) = 0 + \left(\frac{1}{2} \times 12 \times 4\right) = 24 \text{ kN}$$

$$F_C = F_B + 0 = 24 \text{ kN}$$

$$F_D = F_C + 0 = 24 \text{ kN}$$

Bending moment calculations:

$$M_A = 0$$

$$M_B = -\left[\frac{1}{2} \times 12 \times 4 \times \left(\frac{2 \times 4}{3}\right)\right] = -64 \text{ kN-m}$$

$$M_{B-C} = -\left[\frac{1}{2} \times 12 \times 4 \times \left(\frac{2 \times 4}{3} + 2\right)\right] = -112 \text{ kN-m}$$

$$M_C = M_{B-C} + 20 = -112 + 20 = -92 \text{ kN-m}$$

$$M_D = -\left[\frac{1}{2} \times 12 \times 4 \times \left(\frac{2 \times 4}{3} + 3.5\right)\right] + 20 = -128 \text{ kN-m}$$

The SFD and BMD diagrams are shown in **Fig's 5.23(b) & (c)** respectively.

5.9 STANDARD CASES OF A SIMPLY SUPPORTED BEAM (SSB)

5.9.1 Simply supported beam with a point load at mid-span

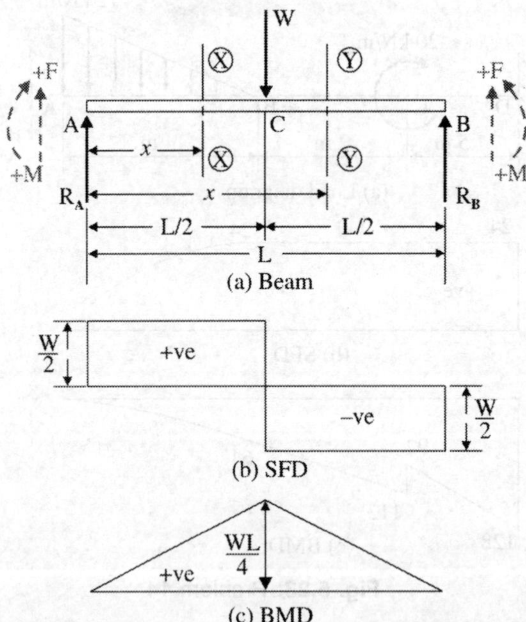

Fig. 5.24: Simply supported beam with point load at mid span

Fig. 5.24(a) indicates a simply supported beam subjected to point load at mid-span.

Let W = Point load

L = Length of the beam

F_n = Shear force at salient points

M_n = Bending moment at salient points

R_A = Reaction at support A

R_B = Reaction at support B

Reactions at supports:

$$R_A + R_B = W \qquad \qquad \dots \text{Eq. (i)}$$

Taking moments about A and equating to zero, we have

$$R_B L = W(L/2)$$

$$R_B = \frac{W}{2} \qquad \qquad \text{... Eq. (ii)}$$

Substituting Eq. (ii) in Eq. (i), we have

$$R_A + (W/2) = W$$

$$R_A = \frac{W}{2} \qquad \qquad \text{... Eq. (iii)}$$

Here the reactions are equal as the beam is symmetrically loaded.

Region AC: $\quad 0 < x < L/2$

Consider a section X-X at a distance x from left support A.

Shear force at X-X is $\qquad \qquad F_x = R_A = \dfrac{W}{2}$

Bending moment at X-X is $\qquad M_x = R_A.x = \left(\dfrac{W}{2}\right) x$

(Positive because, sagging)

Boundary conditions:

At A, $x = 0$, $\qquad \qquad F_A = R_A = \dfrac{W}{2} \qquad$ remains constant up to C

$$M_A = 0$$

At C, $x = L/2$, $\qquad \qquad F_C = R_A - W = \dfrac{W}{2} - W = -\dfrac{W}{2}$

remains constant from C to B

$$M_C = \left(\frac{W}{2}\right)\left(\frac{L}{2}\right) = \left(\frac{WL}{4}\right)$$

Region CB: $\quad L/2 < x < L$

Consider a section Y-Y at a distance x from left support A.

Shear force at Y-Y is $\qquad \qquad F_x = R_A - W = \dfrac{W}{2} - W = -\dfrac{W}{2}$

Bending moment at Y-Y is $\qquad M_x = R_A.x - W\left(x - \dfrac{L}{2}\right)$

Applying the boundary conditions, we have

At C, $x = L/2$ $\qquad \qquad M_C = R_A (L/2) = \left(\dfrac{W}{2}\right)\left(\dfrac{L}{2}\right) = \left(\dfrac{WL}{4}\right)$

At B, $x = L$, $\qquad \qquad M_B = 0$

The SFD and BMD diagrams are shown in **Fig's 5.24(b) & (c)** respectively.

5.9.2 Simply supported beam with an eccentric point load

Fig. 5.25(a) indicates a simply supported beam subjected to an eccentric point load.

Let $\qquad W$ = Point load

$\qquad \qquad L$ = Length of the beam

$\qquad \qquad F_n$ = Shear force at salient points

M_n = Bending moment at salient points
R_A = Reaction at support A
R_B = Reaction at support B

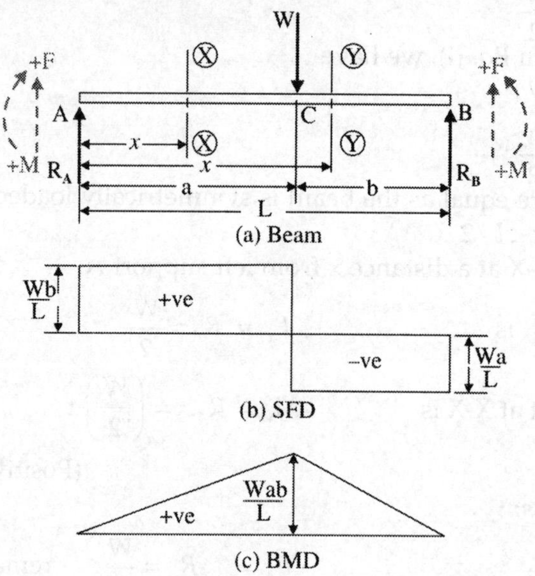

Fig. 5.25: Simply supported beam with eccentric point load

Reactions at supports:

$$R_A + R_B = W \qquad\qquad \text{... Eq. (i)}$$

Taking moments about A and equating to zero, we have

$$R_B L = Wa$$

$$R_B = \frac{Wa}{L} \qquad\qquad \text{... Eq. (ii)}$$

Substituting Eq. (ii) in Eq. (i), we have

$$R_A + \frac{Wa}{L} = W$$

$$R_A = W - \frac{Wa}{L} = \frac{WL - Wa}{L} = \frac{W(L-a)}{L}$$

$$R_A = \frac{Wb}{L} \qquad (\because L - a = b) \qquad \text{... Eq. (iii)}$$

Region AC: $\quad 0 < x < a$

Consider a section X-X at a distance x from end A.

Shear force at X-X is
$$F_x = R_A = \frac{Wb}{L}$$

Bending moment at X-X is
$$M_x = R_A.x = \left(\frac{Wb}{L}\right)x$$

(Positive because of sagging)

Boundary conditions:

At A, $x = 0$, $\qquad F_A = R_A = \dfrac{Wb}{L}$ remains constant up to C

$$M_A = 0$$

At C, $x = a$, $\qquad F_C = R_A - W = \dfrac{Wb}{L} - W = \dfrac{Wb - WL}{L}$

$$(\because b - L = -a)$$

$$F_C = -Wa/L \quad \text{remains constant from C to B}$$

$$M_C = R_A\, a = \left(\dfrac{Wb}{L}\right) a = \left(\dfrac{Wab}{L}\right)$$

Region CB: $\qquad a < x < L$

Consider a section Y-Y at a distance x from left support A.

Shear force at Y-Y is $\qquad F_x = R_A - W = \dfrac{Wb}{L} - W = \dfrac{Wb - WL}{L} = -\dfrac{Wa}{L}$

Bending moment at Y-Y is $\qquad M_x = R_A.x - W(x - a)$

Applying the boundary conditions, we have

At C, $x = a$ $\qquad M_C = R_A\, a = -\left(\dfrac{Wb}{L}\right) a = \left(\dfrac{Wab}{L}\right)$

At B, $x = L$ $\qquad M_B = R_A.L - W(L - a)$

$$M_B = R_A L - Wb = \left(\dfrac{Wb}{L}\right) L - Wb = 0$$

$$(\because L - a = b)$$

The SFD and BMD diagrams are shown in **Fig's 5.25(b) & (c)** respectively.

5.9.3 Simply Supported beam with a uniformly distributed load over entire span

Fig. 5.26(a) indicates a simply supported beam subjected to UDL over entire span.

Let $\qquad w = $ Uniformly distributed load per unit length

$\qquad L = $ Length of the beam

$\qquad F_n = $ Shear force at salient points

$\qquad M_n = $ Bending moment at salient points

$\qquad R_A = $ Reaction at support A

$\qquad R_B = $ Reaction at support B

Reactions at supports:

$$R_A + R_B = wL \qquad\qquad\qquad\qquad \text{... Eq. (i)}$$

Taking moments about A and equating to zero, we have

$$R_B L = wL \left(\dfrac{L}{2}\right)$$

$$R_B = \dfrac{wL}{2} \qquad\qquad\qquad\qquad \text{... Eq. (ii)}$$

Substituting Eq. (ii) in Eq. (i), we have

$$R_A + \dfrac{wL}{2} = wL$$

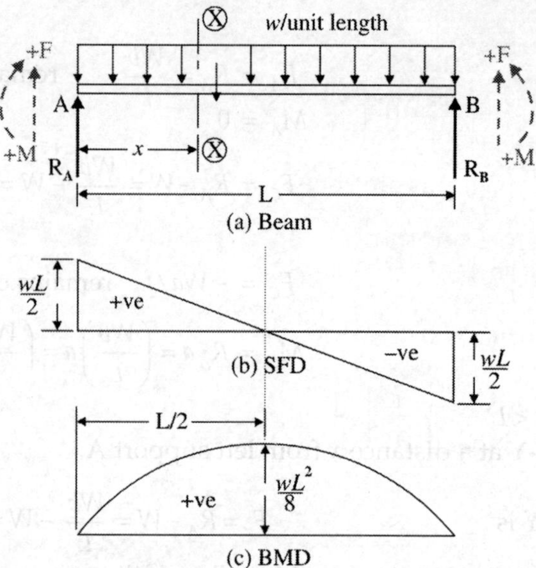

Fig. 5.26: Simply supported beam with UDL over entire span

$$R_A = \frac{wL}{2} \qquad\qquad \dots \text{Eq. (iii)}$$

Here the reactions are equal as the beam is symmetrically loaded.
Consider a section X-X at a distance x from end A.

Shear force at X-X is
$$F_x = R_A - wx = \frac{wL}{2} - wx \qquad\qquad \dots \text{Eq. (iv)}$$

Boundary conditions:

$$\text{At A, } x = 0, \qquad F_A = \frac{wL}{2}$$

$$\text{At B, } x = L, \qquad F_B = \frac{wL}{2} - wL = -\frac{wL}{2}$$

Bending moment at X-X is
$$M_x = R_A.x - wx\left(\frac{x}{2}\right) = \left(\frac{wL}{2}\right)x - \left(\frac{wx^2}{2}\right)$$

$$\dots \text{Eq. (v)}$$

Applying the boundary conditions, we have

$$\text{At A, } x = 0, \qquad M_A = 0$$
$$\text{At B, } x = L, \qquad M_B = 0$$

Maximum bending moment: It is defined as the point at which shear force is zero or changes its sign.

i.e. $\qquad F_x = 0$

$$\frac{wL}{2} - wx = 0 \qquad\qquad \dots \text{using Eq. (iv)}$$

$$\frac{wL}{2} = wx$$

$$x = \frac{L}{2}$$

Thus the maximum bending moment occurs at a distance of $L/2$ from either of the supports and its value is

$$M_C = M_{max} = \left(\frac{wL^2}{4}\right) - \left(\frac{wL^2}{8}\right) = \left(\frac{wL^2}{8}\right) \qquad \text{... using Eq. (v)}$$

The SFD and BMD diagrams are shown in **Fig's 5.26(b) & (c)** respectively.

5.9.4 Simply supported beam carrying a UVL from zero at one end to w/unit length at other end

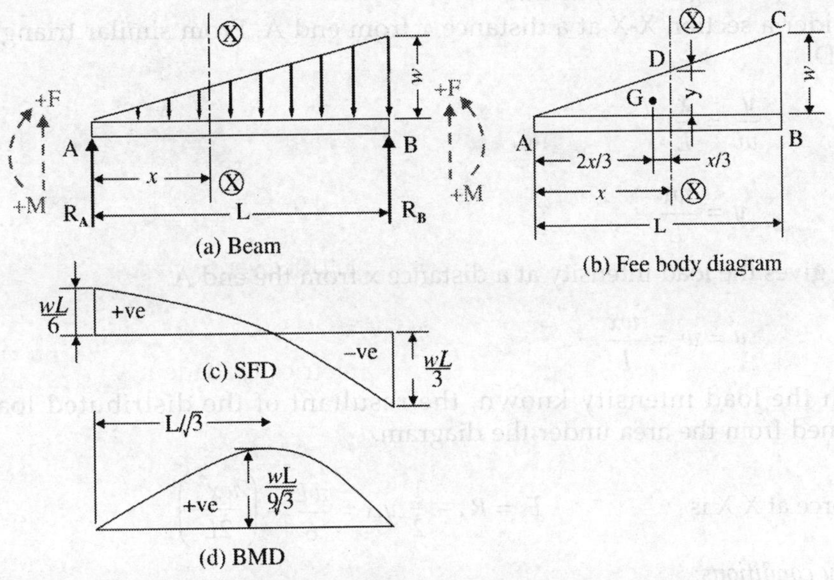

Fig. 5.27: Simply supported beam with UVL over entire span
(Zero at one end to w/ unit length at other end)

Fig. 5.27(a) indicates a simply supported beam subjected to uniformly varying load of intensity 0 at one end to w/unit length at other end. **Fig. 5.27(b)** represents the free body diagram of the beam.

Let w = Uniformly varying load per unit length

            L = Length of the beam

            F_n = Shear force at salient points

            M_n = Bending moment at salient points

Reactions at supports:

$$R_A + R_B = \frac{wL}{2} \qquad \text{... Eq. (i)}$$

Taking moments about A and equating to zero, we have

$$R_B L = \frac{1}{2} wL \left(\frac{2L}{3}\right)$$

$$R_B = \frac{wL}{3} \qquad \text{... Eq. (ii)}$$

Substituting Eq. (ii) in Eq. (i), we have

$$R_A + \frac{wL}{3} = \frac{wL}{2}$$

$$R_A = \frac{wL}{2} - \frac{wL}{3}$$

$$R_A = \frac{wL}{6} \qquad \ldots \text{Eq. (iii)}$$

To find rate of loading or load intensity:

Consider a section X-X at a distance x from end A. From similar triangles ABC and AXD

$$\frac{y}{w} = \frac{x}{L}$$

$$y = \frac{wx}{L} \qquad \ldots \text{Eq. (iv)}$$

Eq. (iv) gives the load intensity at a distance x from the end A.

i.e. $$y = w_x = \frac{wx}{L} \qquad \ldots \text{Eq. (v)}$$

With the load intensity known, the resultant of the distributed loading is determined from the area under the diagram.

Shear force at X-X is $$F_x = R_A - \frac{1}{2}\, y.x = \frac{wL}{6} - \left(\frac{wx^2}{2L}\right) \qquad \ldots \text{Eq. (vi)}$$

Boundary conditions:

At A, $x = 0$, $$F_A = \frac{wL}{6}$$

At B, $x = L$, $$F_B = \frac{wL}{6} - \left(\frac{wL^2}{2L}\right) = -\frac{wL}{3}$$

Bending moment at X-X is $$M_x = R_A.x - \frac{1}{2}\, y.x \left(\frac{x}{3}\right) = \left(\frac{wL}{6}\right).x - \left(\frac{wx^3}{6L}\right) \qquad \ldots \text{Eq. (vii)}$$

Applying the boundary conditions, we have

At A, $x = 0$, $\qquad\qquad\qquad M_A = 0$

At B, $x = L$, $\qquad\qquad\qquad M_B = 0$

Maximum bending moment: It is defined as the point at which shear force is zero or changes its sign.

i.e. $$F_x = 0$$

$$\frac{wL}{6} - \left(\frac{wx^2}{2L}\right) = 0 \qquad \ldots \text{using Eq. (vi)}$$

$$\frac{wL}{6} = \left(\frac{wx^2}{2L}\right)$$

$$x^2 = \frac{L^2}{3}$$

$$x = \frac{L}{\sqrt{3}}$$

Thus the maximum bending moment occurs at a distance of $L/\sqrt{3}$ from support A and its value is

$$M_{max} = \left(\frac{wL}{6}\right)\frac{L}{\sqrt{3}} - \left(\frac{w}{6L}\right)\left(\frac{L}{\sqrt{3}}\right)^3 \qquad \text{... using Eq. (vii)}$$

$$= \left(\frac{wL^2}{6\sqrt{3}}\right) - \left(\frac{wL^2}{18\sqrt{3}}\right) = \left(\frac{wL^2}{\sqrt{3}}\right) - \left(\frac{1}{6} - \frac{1}{18}\right)$$

$$M_{max} = \left(\frac{wL^2}{9\sqrt{3}}\right)$$

The SFD and BMD diagrams are shown in **Fig's 5.27(c) & (d)** respectively.

5.9.5 Simply supported beam carrying a uniformly varying load from zero at both ends to w/unit length at the centre

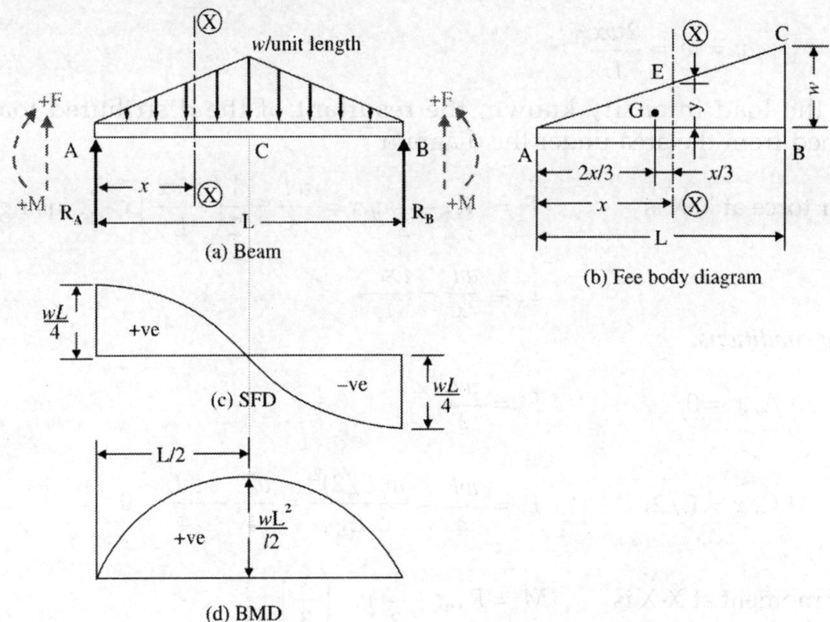

Fig. 5.28: Simply supported beam with UVL over entire span
(Zero at one end to w/ unit length at other end)

Fig. 5.28(a) indicates a simply supported beam subjected to uniformly varying load of intensity zero at each end to w/unit length at mid-span. **Fig. 5.28(b)** represents the free body diagram of the beam.

Let w = Uniformly varying load per unit length

     L = Length of the beam

F_n = Shear force at salient points

M_n = Bending moment at salient points

Reactions at supports:

$$R_A + R_B = \frac{wL}{2} \qquad \text{... Eq. (i)}$$

Due to symmetry of loading, the reactions at A and B are equal

$$R_A = R_B = \frac{wL/2}{2}$$

$$R_A = R_B = \frac{wL}{4} \qquad \text{... Eq. (ii)}$$

To find rate of loading or load intensity:

Consider a section X-X at a distance x from end A. From similar triangles ACD and AXE

$$\frac{y}{w} = \frac{x}{L/2}$$

$$y = \frac{2wx}{L} \qquad \text{... Eq. (iii)}$$

Eq. (iv) gives the load intensity at a distance x from the free end.

i.e. $$y = w_x = \frac{2wx}{L} \qquad \text{... Eq. (iv)}$$

With the load intensity known, the resultant of the distributed loading is determined from the area under the diagram

Shear force at X-X is $$F_x = R_A - \frac{1}{2}\,y.x = \frac{wL}{4} - \frac{1}{2}\left(\frac{2wx}{L}\right)x \quad \text{... using Eq. (iv)}$$

$$F_x = \frac{wL}{4} - \frac{wx^2}{L} \qquad \text{... Eq. (v)}$$

Boundary conditions:

At A, $x = 0$, $$F_A = \frac{wL}{4}$$

At C, $x = L/2$, $$F_C = \frac{wL}{4} - \frac{w(L/2)^2}{L} = \frac{wL}{4} - \frac{wL}{4} = 0$$

Bending moment at X-X is $$M_x = R_A.x - \frac{1}{2}\,y.x\left(\frac{x}{3}\right)$$

$$= \left(\frac{wL}{4}\right)x - \frac{1}{2}\left(\frac{2wx}{L}\right)x\left(\frac{x}{3}\right)$$

$$M_x = \left(\frac{wL}{4}\right)x - \frac{wx^3}{3L} \qquad \text{... Eq. (vi)}$$

Applying the boundary conditions, we have

$$\text{At A, } x = 0, \qquad\qquad M_B = 0$$
$$\text{At B, } x = L, \qquad\qquad M_B = 0$$

Maximum bending moment: It is defined as the point at which shear force is zero or changes its sign.

$$\text{i.e.} \qquad\qquad F_x = 0$$

$$\frac{wL}{4} - \frac{wx^2}{L} = 0 \qquad\qquad\qquad\qquad \text{... using Eq. (v)}$$

$$\frac{wL}{4} = \frac{wx^2}{L}$$

$$x^2 = \frac{L^2}{4}$$

$$x = \frac{L}{2}$$

Thus the maximum bending moment occurs at a distance of $L/2$ from support A and its value is

$$M_{\max} = \left(\frac{wL}{4}\right)\frac{L}{2} - \left(\frac{w}{3L}\right)\left(\frac{L}{2}\right)^3 \qquad\qquad \text{... using Eq. (vi)}$$

$$= \left(\frac{wL^2}{8}\right) - \left(\frac{wL^2}{24}\right) = wL^2\left(\frac{3-1}{24}\right)$$

$$M_{\max} = \left(\frac{wL^2}{12}\right)$$

The SFD and BMD diagrams are shown in **Fig's 5.28(c) & (d)** respectively.

5.9.6 Simply supported beam subjected to couple at mid-span

Fig. 5.29(a) indicates a simply supported beam subjected to a CCW couple at mid-span.

$$\text{Let} \qquad\qquad M = \text{couple}$$
$$L = \text{Length of the beam}$$

Reactions at supports:

Taking moments about A and equating to zero, we have

$$R_B L + M = 0$$

$$R_B = -\frac{M}{L}$$

Since no other load is acting on the beam, reaction at the other support would be in the opposite sense to keep the system in equilibrium as shown in **Fig. 5.29(b)**.

$$R_A = \frac{M}{L}$$

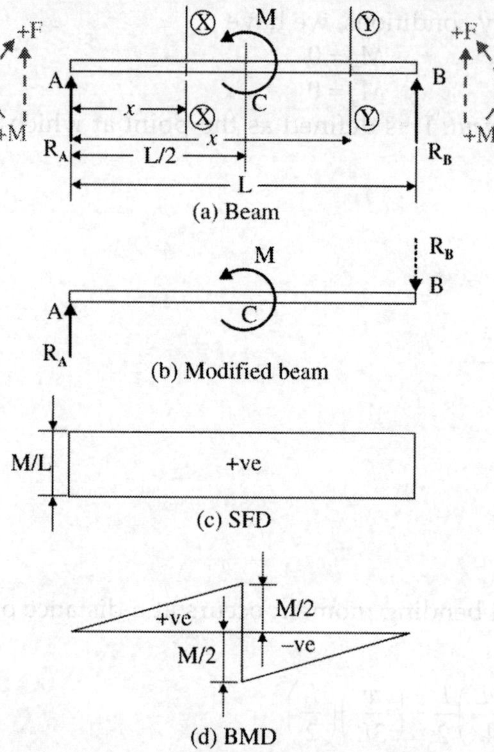

Fig. 5.29: Simply supported beam subjected to couple

Region AC: $0 < x < L/2$

Consider a section X-X at a distance x from left support A.

Shear force at X-X is
$$F_x = R_A = \frac{M}{L}$$

Since no force is acting on the beam, shear force remains constant at $\dfrac{M}{L}$ as shown in **Fig. 5.29(c)**.

Bending moment at X-X is $M_x = R_A.x = \dfrac{M}{L}x$

Boundary conditions:

At A, $x = 0$, $\qquad M_A = 0$

At C, $x = L/2$, $\qquad M_x = \dfrac{M}{L}\left(\dfrac{L}{2}\right) = \dfrac{M}{2}$

Region CB: $L/2 < x < L$

Consider a section Y-Y at a distance x from left support A.

Shear force at Y-Y remains constant at $\dfrac{M}{L}$

Bending moment at Y-Y is $M_x = R_A.x - M = \dfrac{M}{L}x - M$

Applying the boundary conditions, we have

At C, $x = L/2$, $\qquad\qquad M_C = \dfrac{M}{L}\left(\dfrac{L}{2}\right) - M = -\dfrac{M}{2}$

At B, $x = L$, $\qquad\qquad M_B = 0$

The SFD and BMD diagrams are shown in **Fig's 5.29(c) & (d)** respectively.

Note:

1. If the moment is applied at a distance a from left support, then the values are

$$F_x = R_A = \dfrac{M}{L} \qquad\qquad M_A = 0 \qquad\qquad M_B = 0$$

$$M_x = \dfrac{Ma}{L}, \text{ in region AC} \qquad M_x = -\dfrac{M(L-a)}{L}, \text{ in region CB}$$

2. In case of SS beams, moments at the supports are always zero, unless the beam is subjected to a moment at the support.

15. Draw SFD and BMD for the beam shown in Fig. 5.30(a).

Solution:

Reactions at supports:

$$R_A + R_B = 20 + 40 = 60 \text{ kN} \qquad\qquad\qquad \text{... Eq. (i)}$$

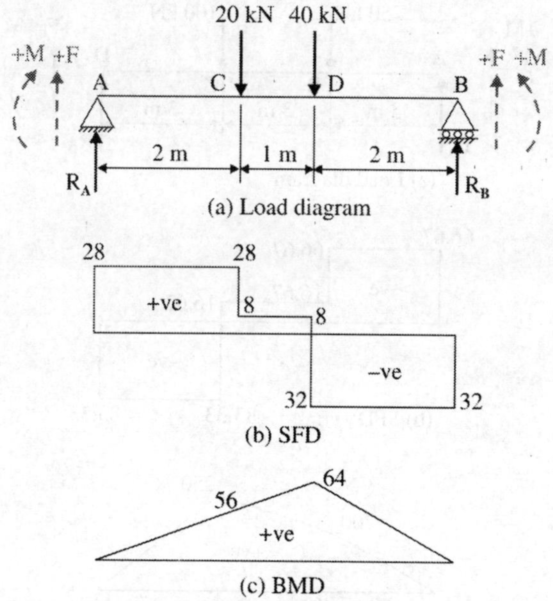

Fig. 5.30: Problem 15

Taking moments about A and equating to zero, we have

$$R_B \times 5 = (20 \times 2) + (40 \times 3)$$
$$R_B = 32 \text{ kN} \qquad\qquad\qquad\qquad\qquad \text{... Eq. (ii)}$$

Substituting Eq. (ii) in Eq. (i), we have

$$R_A + 32 = 60$$
$$R_A = 28 \text{ kN} \qquad\qquad\qquad\qquad\qquad \text{... Eq. (iii)}$$

Shear force calculations:

$$F_A = R_A = 28 \text{ kN}$$
$$F_C = F_A - 20 = 28 - 20 = 8 \text{ kN}$$
$$F_D = F_C - 40 = 8 - 40 = -32 \text{ kN} \qquad \text{remains constant up to B}$$
$$F_B = F_D = -32 \text{ kN} = R_B$$

Bending moment calculations:

$$M_A = 0$$
$$M_C = R_A \times 2 = 28 \times 2 = 56 \text{ kN-m}$$
$$M_D = R_A \times 3 - (20 \times 1) = (28 \times 3) - 20 = 64 \text{ kN-m}$$

Or $\quad M_D = R_B \times 2 = 32 \times 2 = 64 \text{ kN-m} \qquad$ (from RHS)

$$M_B = R_A \times 5 - (20 \times 3) - (40 \times 2)$$
$$= (28 \times 5) - 60 - 80 = 0$$

Or $\quad M_B = 0 \qquad\qquad\qquad$ (from RHS)

The SFD and BMD diagrams are shown in **Fig's 5.30(b) & (c)** respectively.

16. Draw SFD and BMD for the beam shown in Fig. 5.31(a).

Solution:

Reactions at supports:

$$R_A + R_D = 50 + 100 = 150 \text{ kN} \qquad\qquad\qquad \text{... Eq. (i)}$$

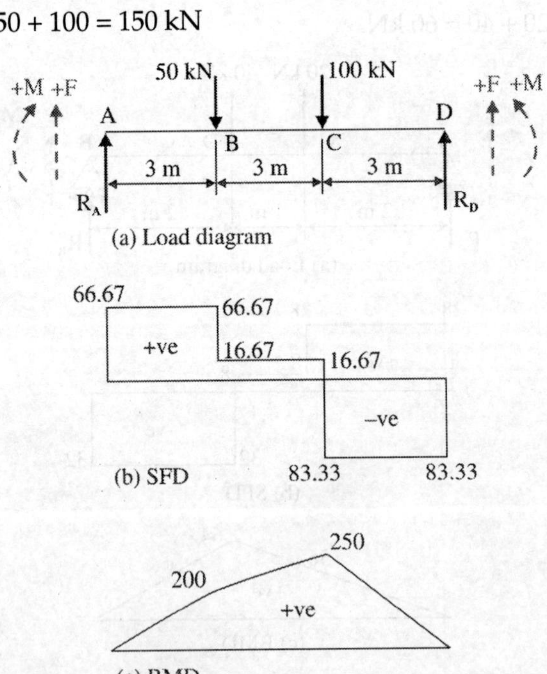

Fig. 5.31: Problem 16

Taking moments about A and equating to zero, we have

$$R_D \times 9 = (50 \times 3) + (100 \times 6)$$
$$R_D = 83.33 \text{ kN} \qquad\qquad\qquad \text{... Eq. (ii)}$$

Substituting Eq. (ii) in Eq. (i), we have

$$R_A + 83.33 = 150$$
$$R_A = 66.67 \text{ kN} \qquad\qquad\qquad \text{... Eq. (iii)}$$

Shear force calculations:

$$F_A = R_A = 66.67 \text{kN}$$
$$F_B = R_A - 50 = 66.67 - 50 = 16.67 \text{ kN}$$
$$F_C = F_B - 100 = 16.67 - 100 = -83.33 \text{ kN} \qquad \text{remains constant up to D}$$
$$F_D = F_C = -83.33 \text{ kN} = R_D$$

Bending moment calculations:

$$M_A = 0$$
$$M_B = R_A \times 3 = 66.67 \times 3 = 200 \text{ kN-m}$$
$$M_C = R_A \times 6 - (50 \times 3) = (66.67 \times 6) - 150$$
$$= 250 \text{ kN-m}$$
$$M_D = R_A \times 9 - (50 \times 6) - (100 \times 3)$$
$$= (66.67 \times 9) - 300 - 300 = 0$$

Or $\qquad M_D = 0 \qquad\qquad$ (from RHS)

The SFD and BMD diagrams are shown in **Fig's 5.31(b) & (c)** respectively.

17. A beam is simply supported at its ends and carries uniformly distributed load of 20 N per m length over its entire length. Derive expression for shear force and bending moment at an section at a distance 'X' from the left support. Draw the shear force and bending moment diagrams.

VTU – Jan. 2013 – 08 Marks

Solution: Based on the given data, the beam is as shown in **Fig. 5.32(a)** having a lengh of 1 m.

Reactions at supports:

$$R_A + R_B = 20 \times 1 = 20 \text{ N} \qquad\qquad \text{... Eq. (i)}$$

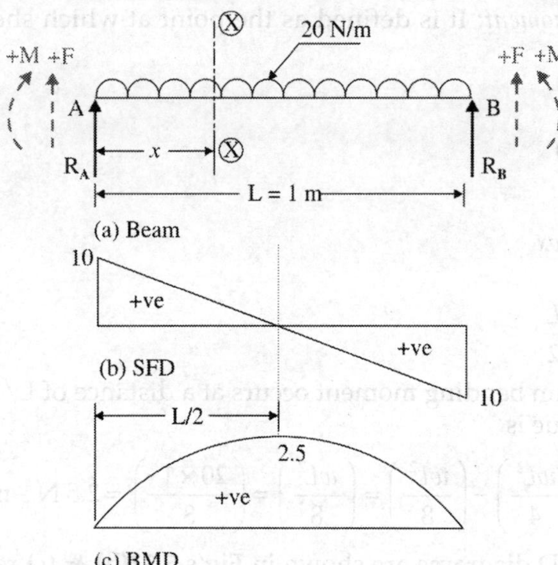

Fig. 5.32: Problem 17

Taking moments about A and equating to zero, we have

$$R_B \times 1 = 20 \times 1 \left(\frac{1}{2} \right)$$
$$R_B = 10 \text{ N} \qquad\qquad \text{... Eq. (ii)}$$

Substituting Eq. (ii) in Eq. (i), we have

$$R_A + 10 = 20$$
$$R_A = 10\,N \qquad \text{... Eq. (iii)}$$

Here the reactions are equal since the beam is symmetrically loaded.

Shear force calculations:

Consider a section X-X at a distance x from free end A.

Shear force at X-X is
$$F_x = R_A - wx = \frac{wL}{2} - wx \qquad \text{... Eq. (iv)}$$

Applying the boundary conditions, we have

At A, $x = 0$,
$$F_A = \frac{wL}{2} = \frac{20 \times 1}{2} = 10\,N$$

At B, $x = L$,
$$F_B = \frac{wL}{2} - wL = -\frac{wL}{2} = -\frac{20 \times 1}{2}$$
$$F_B = -10\,N = R_B \qquad \text{(downward)}$$

BM at X-X is
$$M_x = R_A \cdot x - wx\left(\frac{x}{2}\right)$$
$$= \left(\frac{wL}{2}\right)x - \left(\frac{wx^2}{2}\right) \qquad \text{... Eq. (v)}$$

Applying the boundary conditions, we have

At A, $x = 0$, $M_A = 0$

At B, $x = L$, $M_B = 0$

Maximum bending moment: It is defined as the point at which shear force is zero or changes its sign.

i.e. $F_x = 0$

$$\frac{wL}{2} - wx = 0 \qquad \text{... using Eq. (iv)}$$

$$\frac{wL}{2} = wx$$

$$x = \frac{L}{2}$$

Thus the maximum bending moment occurs at a distance of L/2 from either of the supports and its value is

$$M_C = M_{max} = \left(\frac{wL^2}{4}\right) - \left(\frac{wL^2}{8}\right) = \left(\frac{wL^2}{8}\right) = \left(\frac{20 \times 1^2}{8}\right) = 2.5\,N-m \quad \text{... using Eq. (v)}$$

The SFD and BMD diagrams are shown in **Fig's 5.32(b) & (c)** respectively.

18. Draw SFD and BMD for the beam shown in Fig. 5.33(a). Also find the maximum bending value.

Solution:

Reactions at supports:

$$R_A + R_B = wL = 40 \times 4 = 160\,kN \qquad \text{... Eq. (i)}$$

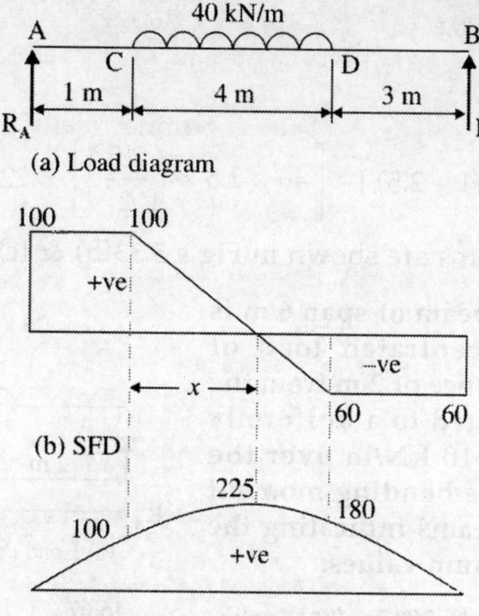

Fig. 5.33: Problem 18

Taking moments about A and equating to zero, we have

$$R_B \times 8 = \left[40 \times 4 \times \left(\frac{4}{2} + 1 \right) \right]$$

$$R_B = 60 \text{ kN} \hspace{3cm} \dots \text{Eq. (ii)}$$

Substituting Eq. (ii) in Eq. (i), we have

$$R_A + 60 = 160$$

$$R_A = 100 \text{ kN} \hspace{3cm} \dots \text{Eq. (iii)}$$

Shear force calculations:

$$F_A = R_A = 100 \text{ kN}$$
$$F_C = 100 - 0 = 100 \text{ kN}$$
$$F_{C-D} = 100 - (40 \times 4) = -60 \text{ kN}$$
$$F_D = -60 + 0 = -60 \text{ kN} \hspace{1.5cm} \text{remains constant up to B}$$
$$F_B = F_D = -60 \text{ kN} = R_B$$

Bending moment calculations:

$$M_A = 0$$
$$M_C = 100 \times 1 = 100 \text{ kN-m}$$

$$M_D = (100 \times 5) - 40 \times 4 \times \left(\frac{4}{2} \right) = 180 \text{ kN-m}$$

Or $\hspace{2cm} M_B = 60 \times 3 = 180 \text{ kN-m} \hspace{2cm}$ (from RHS)

$$M_B = (100 \times 8) - 40 \times 4 \times \left(\frac{4}{2} + 3 \right) = 0$$

Or $\hspace{2cm} M_B = 0 \hspace{4cm}$ (from RHS)

Maximum bending moment:

$$\frac{x}{100} = \frac{4 - x}{60}$$

$$60x = 400 - 100x$$
$$400 = 160x$$
$$x = 2.5 \text{ m}$$

$$M_{max} = [100 \times (1 + 2.5)] - \left[40 \times 2.5 \times \left(\frac{2.5}{2}\right)\right] = 225 \text{ kN-m}$$

The SFD and BMD diagrams are shown in **Fig's 5.33(b) & (c)** respectively.

19. **A simply supported beam of span 6 m is subjected to a concentrated load of 25 kN acting at a distance of 2 m from the left end. Also subjected to a uniformly distributed load of 10 kN/m over the entire span. Draw the bending moment and shear force diagrams indicating the maximum and minimum values.**

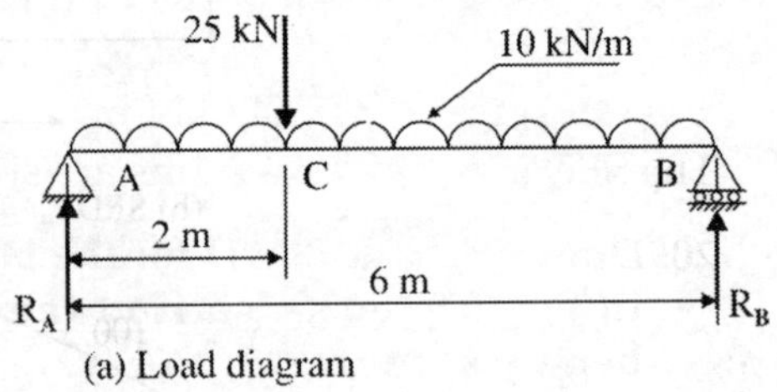

(a) Load diagram

Solution: Based on the given data, the beam is as shown in **Fig. 5.34(a)**.

Reactions at supports:

$$R_A + R_B = 25 + (10 \times 6) = 85 \text{ kN} \quad \dots \text{Eq. (i)}$$

Taking moments about A and equating to zero, we have

$$R_B \times 6 = (25 \times 2) + \left[10 \times 6 \times \left(\frac{6}{2}\right)\right]$$

$$R_B = 38.33 \text{ kN} \qquad \dots \text{Eq. (ii)}$$

Substituting Eq. (ii) in Eq. (i), we have

$$R_A + 38.33 = 85$$

$$R_A = 46.67 \text{ kN} \qquad \dots \text{Eq. (iii)}$$

Shear force calculations:

$$F_A = R_A = 46.67 \text{kN}$$
$$F_{A-C} = 46.67 - (10 \times 2) = 26.67 \text{ kN}$$
$$F_C = 26.67 - 25 = 1.67 \text{ kN}$$
$$F_{C-B} = 1.67 - (10 \times 4) = -38.33 \text{ kN}$$
$$F_B = F_{C-B} = -38.33 \text{ kN} = R_B$$

Bending moment calculations:

$$M_A = 0$$

$$M_C = (6.67 \times 2) - \left[10 \times 2 \times \left(\frac{2}{2}\right)\right] = 73.34 \text{ kN-m}$$

$$M_B = (46.67 \times 6) - (25 \times 4) - \left[10 \times 6 \times \left(\frac{6}{2}\right)\right] = 0.02 \text{ kN-m} \approx 0$$

Or $\qquad M_B = 0 \qquad$ (from RHS)

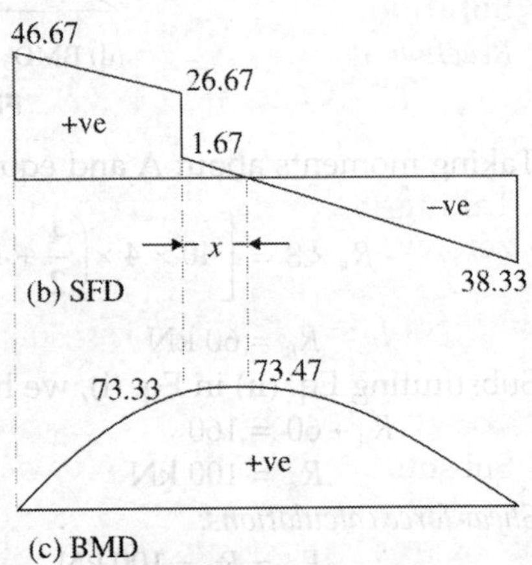

Fig. 5.34: Problem 19

Maximum bending moment:

$$\frac{x}{1.67} = \frac{4 - x}{38.33}$$

$$38.33x = 1.67(4 - x)$$

$$36.66x = 6.68$$

$$x = 0.17 \text{ m}$$

$$M_{max} = [46.67 \times (2 + 0.17)] - (25 \times 0.17) - \left[10 \times (2 + 0.17) \times \left(\frac{2 + 0.17}{2}\right)\right]$$

$$= 73.47 \text{ kN-m}$$

The SFD and BMD diagrams are shown in **Fig's 5.34(b) & (c)** respectively.

20. Draw SFD and BMD for the beam shown in Fig. 5.35(a). Also find the maximum bending value.

Solution:

Reactions at supports:

$$R_A + R_B = 50 + (50 \times 2) = 150 \text{ kN}$$

$$\dots \text{ Eq. (i)}$$

Taking moments about A and equating to zero, we have

$$R_B \times 4 = (50 \times 1) + \left[50 \times 2 \times \left(\frac{2}{2} + 2\right)\right]$$

$$R_B = 87.5 \text{ kN} \qquad \dots \text{ Eq. (ii)}$$

Substituting Eq. (ii) in Eq. (i), we have

$$R_A + 87.5 = 150$$

$$R_A = 62.5 \text{ kN} \qquad \dots \text{ Eq. (iii)}$$

Shear force calculations:

$$F_A = R_A = 62.5 \text{ kN}$$

$$F_C = 62.5 - 50 = 12.5 \text{ kN}$$

$$F_D = 12.5 + 0 = 12.5 \text{ kN}$$

$$F_{D-B} = 12.5 - (50 \times 2) - 50 = -87.5 \text{ kN}$$

$$F_B = F_{D-B} = -87.5 \text{ kN} = R_B$$

Bending moment calculations:

$$M_A = 0$$

$$M_C = (62.5 \times 1) = 62.5 \text{ kN-m}$$

$$M_D = (62.5 \times 2) - (50 \times 1) = 75 \text{ kN-m}$$

$$M_B = (62.5 \times 4) - (50 \times 3) - \left[50 \times 2 \times \left(\frac{2}{2}\right)\right] = 0 \text{ kN-m}$$

Or $M_B = 0$ (from RHS)

Maximum bending moment:

$$\frac{x}{12.5} = \frac{2 - x}{87.5}$$

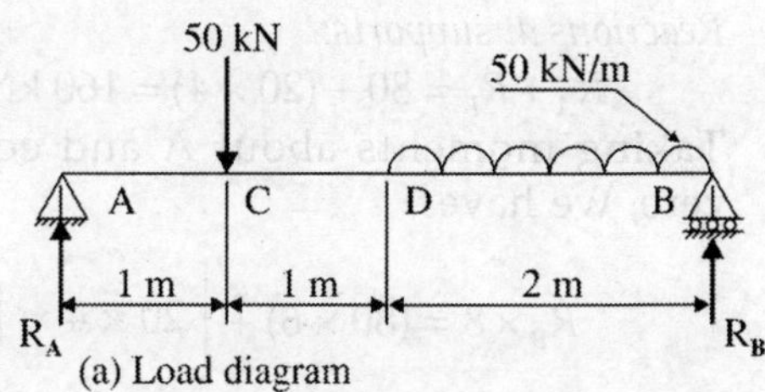

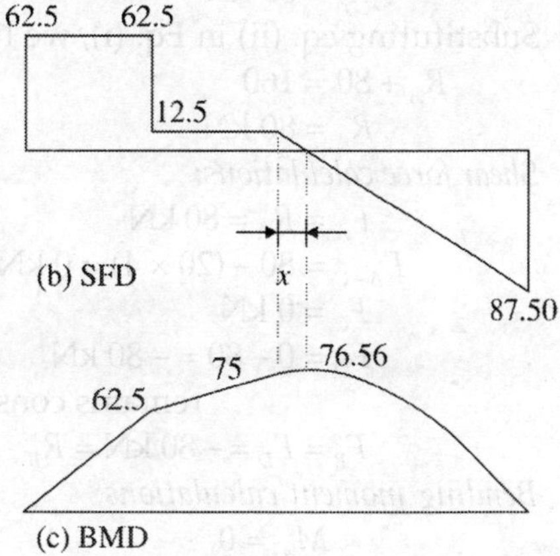

Fig. 5.35: Problem 20

$$87.5x = 12.5(2 - x)$$
$$100x = 25$$
$$x = 0.25 \text{ m}$$

$$M_{max} = [62.5 \times (2 + 0.25)] - (50 \times 1.25) - \left[50 \times 0.25 \times \left(\frac{0.25}{2}\right)\right] = 76.56 \text{ kN-m}$$

The SFD and BMD diagrams are shown in **Fig's 5.35(b) & (c)** respectively.

21. Draw SFD and BMD for the beam shown in Fig. 5.36(a).

Solution:
Reactions at supports:

$$R_A + R_B = 80 + (20 \times 4) = 160 \text{ kN} \dots \text{Eq. (i)}$$

Taking moments about A and equating to zero, we have

$$R_B \times 8 = (80 \times 6) + \left[20 \times 4 \times \left(\frac{4}{2}\right)\right]$$

$$R_B = 80 \text{ kN} \qquad \dots \text{Eq. (ii)}$$

Substituting eq. (ii) in Eq. (i), we have

$$R_A + 80 = 160$$
$$R_A = 80 \text{ kN} \qquad \dots \text{Eq. (iii)}$$

Shear force calculations:

$$F_A = R_A = 80 \text{ kN}$$
$$F_{A-C} = 80 - (20 \times 4) = 0 \text{ kN}$$
$$F_C = 0 \text{ kN}$$
$$F_D = 0 - 80 = -80 \text{ kN}$$

remains constant up to B

$$F_B = F_D = -80 \text{ kN} = R_B$$

Bending moment calculations:

$$M_A = 0$$

$$M_C = (80 \times 4) - \left[20 \times 4 \times \left(\frac{4}{2}\right)\right] = 160 \text{ kN-m}$$

$$M_D = (80 \times 2) = 160 \text{ kN-m} \qquad \text{(from RHS)}$$
$$M_B = 0 \qquad \text{(from RHS)}$$

The SFD and BMD diagrams are shown in **Fig's 5.36(b) & (c)** respectively.

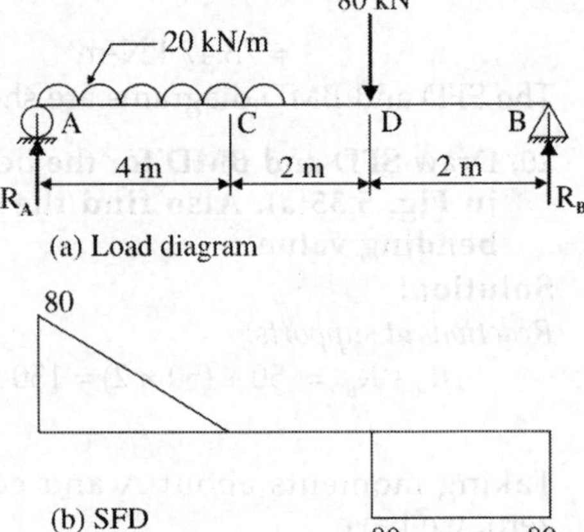

Fig. 5.36: Problem 21

22. Draw the shear force and bending moment diagrams for the beam shown in Fig. 5.37(a). Also calculate the maximum bending moment.

Solution:
Reactions at supports:

$$R_A + R_B = 50 + 40 + (10 \times 4) = 130 \text{ kN} \qquad \dots \text{Eq. (i)}$$

Taking moments about A and equating to zero, we have

$$R_B \times 10 = (40 \times 6) + \left[10 \times 4 \times \left(\frac{4}{2} + 2 \right) \right] + (50 \times 2)$$

$$R_B = 50 \text{ kN} \qquad \text{... Eq. (ii)}$$

Substituting Eq. (ii) in Eq. (i), we have

$$R_A + 50 = 130$$
$$R_A = 80 \text{ kN} \qquad \text{... Eq. (iii)}$$

Shear force calculations:

$$F_A = R_A = 80 \text{ kN}$$
$$F_C = 80 - 50 = 30 \text{ kN}$$
$$F_{C-D} = 30 - (10 \times 4) = -10 \text{ kN}$$
$$F_D = -10 - 40 = -50 \text{ kN}$$
$$\text{remains constant up to B}$$
$$F_B = F_D = -50 \text{ kN} = R_B$$

Bending moment calculations:

$$M_A = 0$$
$$M_C = (80 \times 2) = 160 \text{ kN-m}$$
$$M_D = (50 \times 4) = 200 \text{ kN-m}$$
$$\text{(from RHS)}$$
$$M_B = 0 \qquad \text{(from RHS)}$$

Maximum bending moment:

$$\frac{x}{30} = \frac{4-x}{10}$$
$$10x = 30(4-x)$$
$$40x = 120$$
$$x = 3 \text{ m}$$

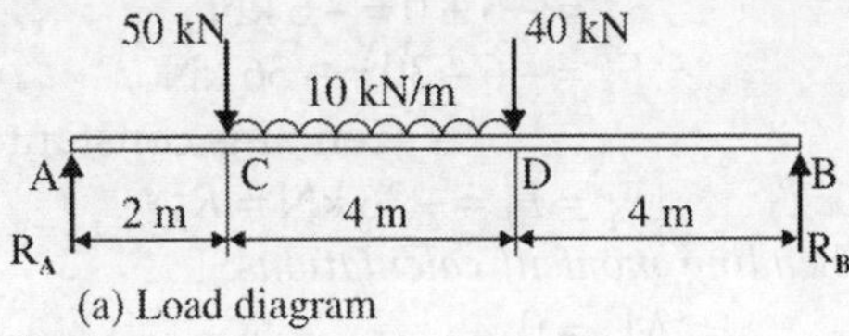

(a) Load diagram

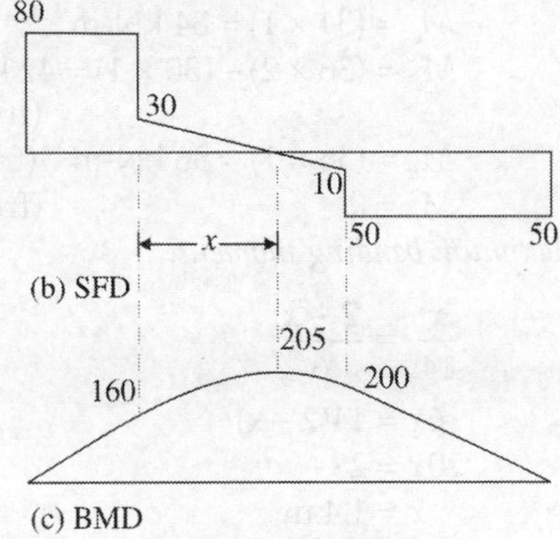

Fig. 5.37: Problem 22

$$M_{\text{max}} = [80 \times (2 + 3)] - (50 \times 3) - \left[10 \times 3 \times \left(\frac{3}{2} \right) \right] = 205 \text{ kN-m}$$

The SFD and BMD diagrams are shown in **Fig's 5.37(b) & (c)** respectively.

23. Draw the shear force and bending moment diagrams for the beam shown in Fig. 5.38(a). Also calculate the maximum bending moment.

Solution:

Reactions at supports:

$$R_A + R_B = 20 + 30 + (10 \times 2) = 70 \text{ kN} \qquad \text{... Eq. (i)}$$

Taking moments about A and equating to zero, we have

$$R_B \times 5 = (30 \times 4) + \left[10 \times 2 \times \left(\frac{2}{2} + 1 \right) \right] + (20 \times 1)$$

$$R_B = 36 \text{ kN} \qquad \text{... Eq. (ii)}$$

Substituting Eq. (ii) in Eq. (i), we have

$$R_A + 36 = 70$$
$$R_A = 34 \text{ kN} \qquad \text{... Eq. (iii)}$$

Shear force calculations:

$$F_A = R_A = 34 \text{ kN}$$
$$F_C = 34 - 20 = 14 \text{ kN}$$
$$F_{C-D} = 14 - (10 \times 2) = -6 \text{ kN}$$
$$F_D = -6 + 0 = -6 \text{ kN}$$
$$F_E = -6 - 30 = -36 \text{ kN}$$
$$\text{remains constant up to B}$$
$$F_B = F_E = -36 \text{ kN} = R_B$$

Bending moment calculations:

$$M_A = 0$$
$$M_C = (34 \times 1) = 34 \text{ kN-m}$$
$$M_D = (36 \times 2) - (30 \times 1) = 42 \text{ kN-m}$$
$$\text{(from RHS)}$$
$$M_E = (36 \times 1) = 36 \text{ kN-m} \quad \text{(from RHS)}$$
$$M_B = 0 \quad \text{(from RHS)}$$

Maximum bending moment:

$$\frac{x}{14} = \frac{2 - x}{6}$$
$$6x = 14(2 - x)$$
$$20x = 28$$
$$x = 1.4 \text{ m}$$

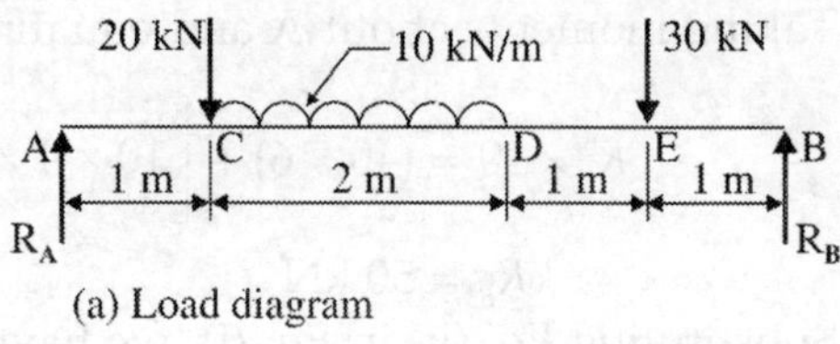

(a) Load diagram

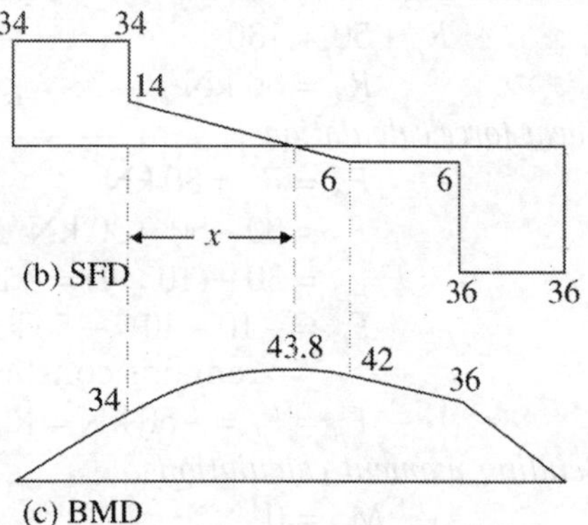

Fig. 5.38: Problem 23

$$M_{\max} = [34 \times (1 + 1.4)] - (20 \times 1.4) - \left[10 \times 1.4 \times \left(\frac{1.4}{2}\right)\right] = 43.8 \text{ kN-m}$$

Or $\quad M_{\max} = [36 \times (2 + 0.6)] - (30 \times 1.6) - \left[10 \times 0.6 \times \left(\frac{0.6}{2}\right)\right] = 43.8 \text{ kN-m}$

(from RHS)

The SFD and BMD diagrams are shown in **Fig's 5.38(b) & (c)** respectively.

24. Draw the shear force and bending moment diagrams for the beam shown in Fig. 5.38(a).

Solution:

Reactions at supports:

$$R_A + R_B = 40 + \left(\frac{1}{2} \times 20 \times 3\right) = 70 \text{ kN} \qquad \text{... Eq. (i)}$$

Taking moments about A and equating to zero, we have

$$R_B \times 8 = 40 + (40 \times 4) + \left[\left(\frac{1}{2} \times 20 \times 3\right) \times \left(\frac{2 \times 3}{3}\right)\right]$$

$$R_B = 32.5 \text{ kN} \qquad \text{... Eq. (ii)}$$

Substituting Eq. (ii) in Eq. (i), we have

$$R_A + 32.5 = 70$$
$$R_A = 37.5 \text{ kN} \qquad \text{... Eq. (iii)}$$

Shear force calculations:

$$F_A = R_A = 37.5 \text{ kN-m}$$
$$F_C = 37.5 - (1/2 \times 20 \times 3) = 7.5 \text{ kN-m}$$

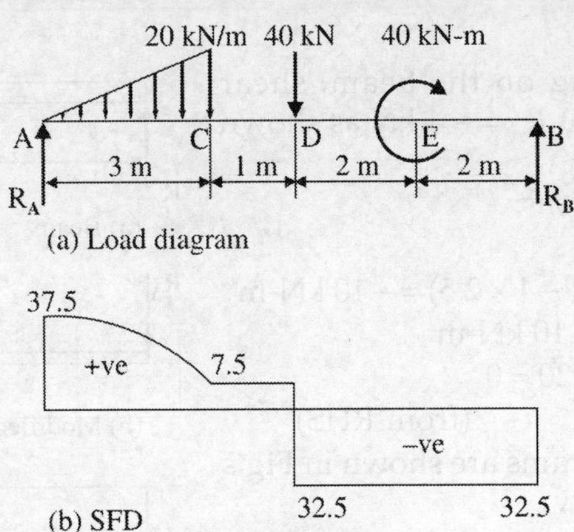

Fig. 5.39: Problem 24

$$F_D = 7.5 + 40 = -32.5 \text{ kN-m} \qquad\qquad \text{remains constant up to B}$$
$$F_E = -32.5 + 0 = -32.5 \text{ kN-m}$$
$$F_B = F_E = -32.5 \text{ kN} = R_B$$

Bending moment calculations:

$$M_A = 0$$

$$M_C = (37.5 \times 3) - \left[\left(\frac{1}{2} \times 20 \times 3\right) \times \left(\frac{3}{3}\right)\right] = 82.5 \text{ kN-m}$$

$$M_D = (37.5 \times 4) - \left[\left(\frac{1}{2} \times 20 \times 3\right) \times \left(\frac{3}{3} + 1\right)\right] = 90 \text{ kN-m}$$

$$M_{D-E} = (37.5 \times 6) - \left[\left(\frac{1}{2} \times 20 \times 3\right) \times \left(\frac{3}{3} + 3\right)\right] - (40 \times 2) = 25 \text{ kN-m}$$

$$M_E = 25 + 40 = 65 \text{ kN-m}$$
$$M_B = 0 \qquad\qquad \text{(from RHS)}$$

The SFD and BMD diagrams are shown in **Fig's 5.39(b) & (c)** respectively.

25. Draw the SFD and BMD for the beam shown in Fig. 5.40(a).

VTU – Dec. 2011– 12 Marks

Solution:

Reactions at supports:

Taking moments about A and equating to zero, we have

$$R_B \times 5 - 20 = 0$$
$$R_B = 4 \text{ kN}$$

Since no other load is acting on the beam, reaction at the other support would be in the opposite sense to keep the system in equilibrium as shown in **Fig. 5.40(b)**.

$$R_A = -4 \text{ kN}$$

Shear force calculations:

Since no force is acting on the beam, shear force remains constant at $R_A = -4$ kN as shown in **Fig. 5.40(c)**.

Bending moment calculations:

$$M_A = 0$$
$$M_{A-C} = R_A \times 2.5 = (-4 \times 2.5) = -10 \text{ kN-m}$$
$$M_C = -10 + 20 = 10 \text{ kN-m}$$
$$M_B = (-4 \times 5) + 20 = 0$$

or $\quad M_B = 0 \qquad$ (from RHS)

The SFD and BMD diagrams are shown in **Fig's 5.40(b) & (c)** respectively.

26. Draw the SFD and BMD for the beam shown in Fig. 5.41(a).

Solution:

Reactions at supports:

$$R_A + R_B = 80 \text{ kN} \qquad \text{... Eq. (i)}$$

Taking moments about A and equating to zero, we have

$$R_B \times 8 = (80 \times 5) + 120$$
$$R_B = 65 \text{ kN} \qquad \text{... Eq. (ii)}$$

Substituting Eq. (ii) in Eq. (i), we have

$$R_A + 65 = 80$$
$$R_A = 15 \text{ kN} \qquad \text{... Eq. (iii)}$$

Shear force calculations:

$$F_A = R_A = 15 \text{ kN}$$
$$F_C = 15 + 0 = 15 \text{ kN}$$
$$F_D = 15 - 80 = -65 \text{ kN}$$

$\qquad\qquad$ remains constant up to B

$$F_E = F_D = -65 \text{ kN} = R_B$$

Bending moment calculations:

$$M_A = 0$$
$$M_{A-C} = (15 \times 2) = 30 \text{ kN-m}$$
$$M_C = 30 + 120 = 150 \text{ kN-m}$$
$$M_D = (15 \times 5) + 120 = 195 \text{ kN-m}$$

or $\quad M_D = (65 \times 3) = 195 \text{ kN-m}$

$\qquad\qquad\qquad$ (from RHS)

$$M_B = 0 \qquad \text{(from RHS)}$$

The SFD and BMD diagrams are shown in **Fig's 5.41(b) & (c)** respectively

27. For the beam shown in Fig. 5.42(a), draw the shear force and bending moment diagrams. Clearly indicate the point of contra flexure.

VTU – Dec. 14/ Jan. 15 – 15 Marks

Solution:

Reactions at supports:

$$R_A + R_B = (20 \times 3) + 40 = 100 \text{ kN} \qquad\qquad \text{... Eq. (i)}$$

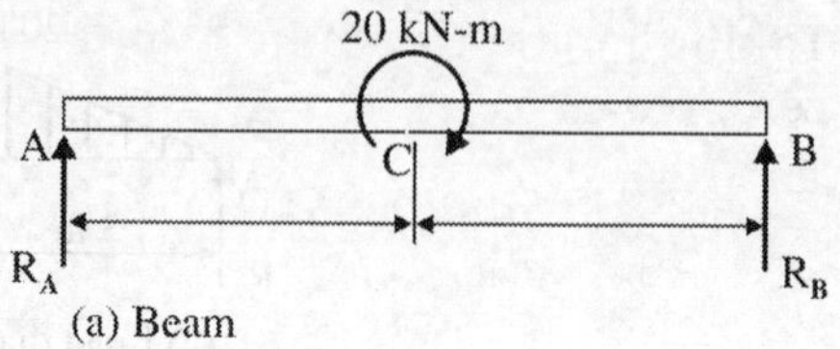

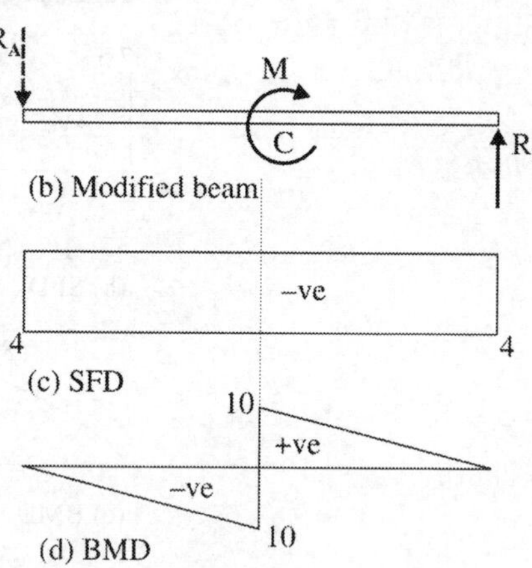

Fig. 5.40: Problem 25

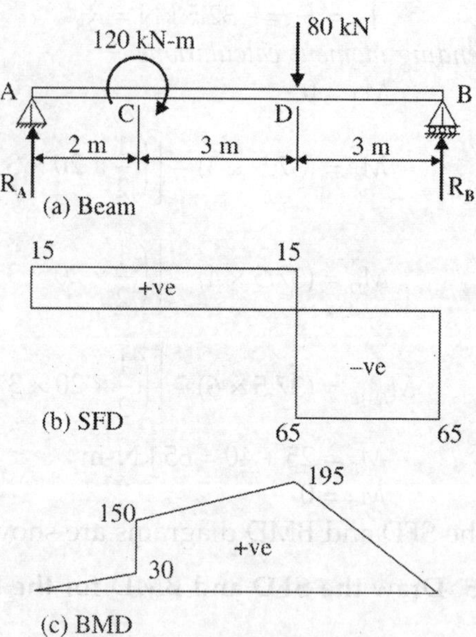

Fig. 5.41: Problem 26

Taking moments about A and equating to zero, we have

$$R_B \times 6 = 120 + (40 \times 3) + \left[(20 \times 3) \times \left(\frac{3}{2}\right) \right]$$

$$R_B = 55 \text{ kN} \qquad \text{... Eq. (ii)}$$

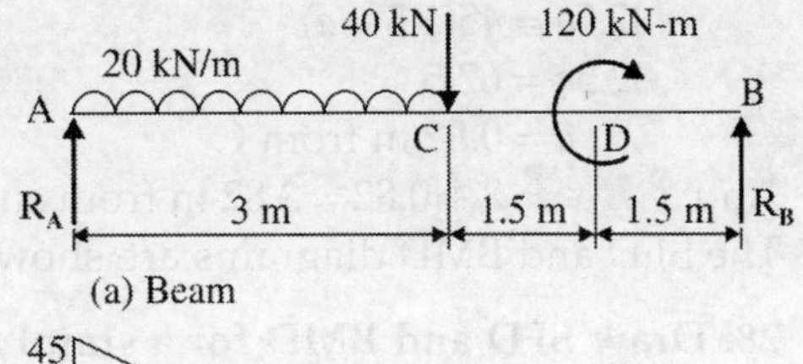

Substituting Eq. (ii) in Eq. (i), we have

$$R_A + 55 = 100$$

$$R_A = 45 \text{ kN} \qquad \text{... Eq. (iii)}$$

Shear force calculations:

$$F_A = R_A = 45 \text{ kN}$$

$$F_{A-C} = 45 - (20 \times 3) = -15 \text{ kN}$$

$$F_C = -15 - 40 = -55 \text{ kN}$$

$$\qquad\qquad \text{remains constant up to B}$$

$$F_D = -15 + 0 = -15 \text{ kN}$$

$$F_B = F_D = -65 \text{ kN} = R_B$$

Bending moment calculations:

$$M_A = 0$$

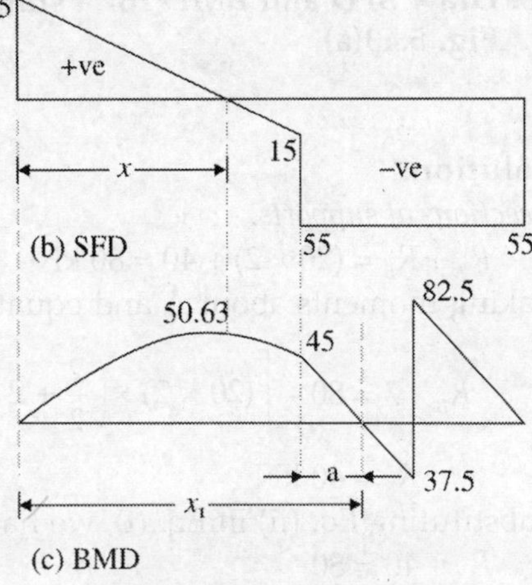

Fig. 5.42: Problem 27

$$M_C = (45 \times 3) - \left[(20 \times 3) \times \left(\frac{3}{2}\right) \right]$$

$$= 45 \text{ kN-m}$$

$$M_{C-D} = (45 \times 4.5) - \left[(20 \times 3) \times \left(\frac{3}{2} + 1.5\right) \right] - (40 \times 1.5) = -37.5 \text{ kN-m}$$

Or $\quad M_{B-D} = (55 \times 1.5) - 120 = -37.5 \text{ kN-m} \quad$ (from RHS)

$$M_D = -37.5 + 120 = 82.5 \text{ kN-m}$$

Or $\quad M_D = (55 \times 1.5) = 82.5 \text{ kN-m} \qquad$ (from RHS)

$$M_B = 0 \qquad\qquad\qquad\qquad\qquad \text{(from RHS)}$$

Maximum bending moment:

$$\frac{x}{45} = \frac{3-x}{15}$$

$$15x = 45(3 - x)$$

$$60x = 135$$

$$x = 2.25 \text{ m}$$

$$M_{max} = (45 \times 2.25) - \left[(20 \times 2.25) \times \left(\frac{2.25}{2}\right) \right] = 50.63 \text{ kN-m}$$

Point of contraflexure: Occurs when bending moment changes its sign.

$$M_{x1} = 0$$

$$45x_1 - [(20 \times 3)(x_1 - 3/2)] - 40(x_1 - 3) = 0$$

$$45x_1 - 60x_1 + 90 - 40x_1 + 120 = 0$$

$$210 = 55x_1$$

$$x_1 = 3.82 \text{ m}$$

Or $\quad \dfrac{a}{45} = \dfrac{1.5 - a}{37.5}$

$$37.5a = 45(1.5 - a)$$
$$82.5a = 67.5$$
$$a = 0.82 \text{ m from C}$$

And $\quad x_1 = 3 + 0.82 = 3.82$ m from support A

The SFD and BMD diagrams are shown in **Fig's 5.42(b) & (c)** respectively.

28. Draw SFD and BMD for a simply supported beam carrying loads as shown in Fig. 5.43(a).

VTU – (CV) Dec. 16/ Jan. 17– 10 Marks

Solution:

Reactions at supports:

$$R_A + R_B = (20 \times 2) + 40 = 80 \text{ kN} \qquad \qquad \text{... Eq. (i)}$$

Taking moments about A and equating to zero, we have

$$R_B \times 7 = 80 + \left[(20 \times 2) \times \left(\frac{2}{2} + 2 \right) \right] + (40 \times 2)$$

$$R_B = 40 \text{ kN} \qquad \text{... Eq. (ii)}$$

Substituting Eq. (ii) in Eq. (i), we have

$$R_A + 40 = 80$$
$$R_A = 40 \text{ kN} \qquad \text{... Eq. (iii)}$$

Shear force calculations:

$$F_A = R_A = 40 \text{ kN}$$
$$F_C = 40 - 40 = 0$$
$$F_{C-D} = 0 - (20 \times 2) = -40 \text{ kN}$$

$$\text{remains constant up to B}$$

$$F_D = -40 + 0 = -40 \text{ kN}$$
$$F_E = -40 + 0 = -40 \text{ kN}$$
$$F_B = F_E = -40 \text{ kN} = R_B$$

Bending moment calculations:

$$M_A = 0$$
$$M_C = 40 \times 2 = 80 \text{ kN-m}$$

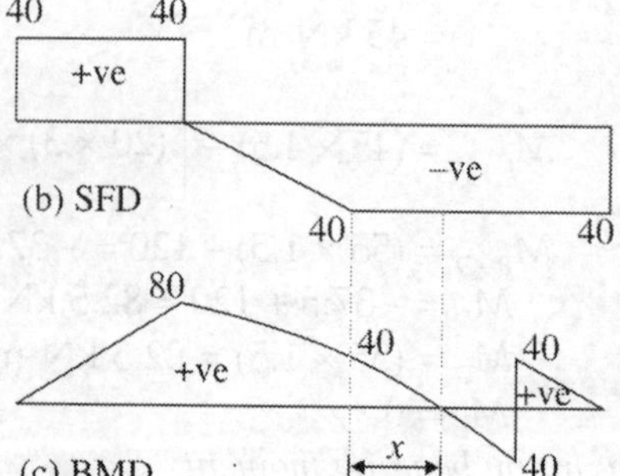

Fig. 5.43: Problem 28

$$M_D = (40 \times 4) - (40 \times 2) - \left[(20 \times 2) \times \left(\frac{2}{2} \right) \right] = -40 \text{ kN-m}$$

$$M_{D-E} = (40 \times 6) - (40 \times 4) - \left[(20 \times 2) \times \left(\frac{2}{2} + 2 \right) \right] = -40 \text{ kN-m}$$

$$M_E = -40 + 80 = 40 \text{ kN-m}$$

or $\qquad M_E = (40 \times 1) = 40$ kN-m $\qquad \qquad$ (from RHS)

$\qquad M_B = 0 \qquad \qquad$ (from RHS)

Point of contraflexure: We have two points of contraflexure as seen in **Fig. 5.43(c)**.

Case 1: The first occurs at a distance of 1m from support B

Case 2: Since the value of moments at points D and E are 40 kN-m each, the second one occurs at mid-span of DE. i.e. 1m either from D or E.

Or $\qquad \dfrac{x}{40} = \dfrac{2 - x}{40}$

$$2x = 2$$
$$x = 1 \text{ m from D or E}$$

The SFD and BMD diagrams are shown in **Fig's 5.43(b) & (c)** respectively.

29. Draw SFD and BMD for the beam shown in Fig. 5.44(a). Determine the point of maximum bending moment and also locate the point of contraflexure.

VTU – (CV) June/July 2011 – 10 Marks

Solution:

Reactions at supports:

$$R_A + R_D = (20 \times 2) + 40 = 80 \text{ kN} \quad \dots \text{ Eq. (i)}$$

Taking moments about A and equating to zero, we have

$$R_D \times 8 = -100 + (40 \times 5) + 200$$

$$+ \left[(20 \times 2) \times \left(\frac{2}{2} \right) \right]$$

$$R_D = 42.5 \text{ kN} \quad \dots \text{ Eq. (ii)}$$

Substituting Eq. (ii) in Eq. (i), we have

$$R_A + 42.5 = 80$$

$$R_A = 37.5 \text{ kN} \quad \dots \text{ Eq. (iii)}$$

Shear force calculations:

$$F_A = R_A = 37.5 \text{ kN}$$
$$F_B = 37.5 - (20 \times 2) = -2.5 \text{ kN}$$
$$F_C = -2.5 - 40 = -42.5 \text{ kN}$$
$$\text{remains constant up to B}$$
$$F_D = F_C = -42.5 \text{ kN} = R_D$$

Bending moment calculations:

$$M_A = 0$$

$$M_{A-B} = (37.5 \times 2) - \left[(20 \times 2) \times \left(\frac{2}{2} \right) \right] = 35 \text{ kN-m}$$

$$M_B = 35 + 200 = 235 \text{ kN-m}$$

$$M_{B-C} = (37.5 \times 5) + 200 - \left[(20 \times 2) \times \left(\frac{2}{2} + 3 \right) \right] = 227.5 \text{ kN-m}$$

$$M_C = 227.5 - 100 = 127.5 \text{ kN-m}$$
$$M_D = 0 \qquad \text{(from RHS)}$$

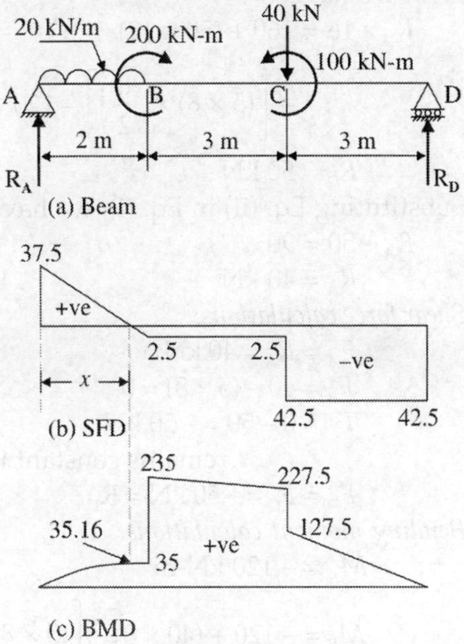

Maximum bending moment:

$$\frac{x}{37.5} = \frac{2 - x}{2.5}$$

$$2.5x = 37.5(2 - x)$$
$$40x = 75$$
$$x = 1.88 \text{ m}$$

$$M_{max} = (37.5 \times 1.88) - \left[(20 \times 1.88) \times \left(\frac{1.88}{2} \right) \right] = 35.16 \text{ kN-m}$$

The SFD and BMD diagrams are shown in **Fig's 5.44(b) & (c)** respectively.

Fig. 5.44: Problem 29

30. For the beam shown in Fig. 5.45(a), obtain SFD and BMD. Locate points of contraflexure, if any.

VTU – (CV) June/ July 2009 – 14 Marks

Solution:

Reactions at supports:

$$R_A + R_D = (5 \times 8) + 50 = 90 \text{ kN} \quad \ldots \text{Eq. (i)}$$

Taking moments about A and equating to zero, we have

$$R_D \times 16 = 160 + (50 \times 12)$$

$$+ \left[(5 \times 8) \times \left(\frac{8}{2} \right) \right] - 120$$

$$R_D = 50 \text{ kN} \quad \ldots \text{Eq. (ii)}$$

Substituting Eq. (ii) in Eq. (i), we have

$$R_A + 50 = 90$$

$$R_A = 40 \text{ kN} \quad \ldots \text{Eq. (iii)}$$

Shear force calculations:

$$F_A = R_A = 40 \text{ kN}$$

$$F_B = 40 - (5 \times 8) = 0$$

$$F_C = 0 - 50 = -50 \text{ kN}$$

$$\text{remains constant up to B}$$

$$F_D = F_C = -50 \text{ kN} = R_D$$

Bending moment calculations:

$$M_A = -120 \text{ kN-m}$$

$$M_B = -120 + (40 \times 8) - \left[(5 \times 8) \times \left(\frac{8}{2} \right) \right] = 40 \text{ kN-m}$$

$$M_C = -120 + (40 \times 12) - \left[(5 \times 8) \times \left(\frac{8}{2} + 4 \right) \right] = 40 \text{ kN-m}$$

$$M_D = -160 \quad \text{(from RHS)}$$

Point of contraflexure: We have two points of contraflexure as seen in **Fig. 5.45(c)**.

To find x_1:

$$M_{x1} = -120 + 40x_1 - \left[(5x_1) \times \left(\frac{x_1}{2} \right) \right] = 0$$

$$0 = -120 + 40x - 2.5x^2$$

$$x = 4 \text{ m from support A}$$

To find x_2:

$$M_{x2} = 50x_1 - 160 = 0$$

$$50x_1 = 160$$

$$x = 3.2 \text{ m from support D}$$

or

$$\frac{x_2}{160} = \frac{4 - x_2}{40}$$

$$40x_2 = 640 - 160x_2$$

$$x_2 = 3.2 \text{ m}$$

The SFD and BMD diagrams are shown in **Figs 5.45(b) & (c)** respectively.

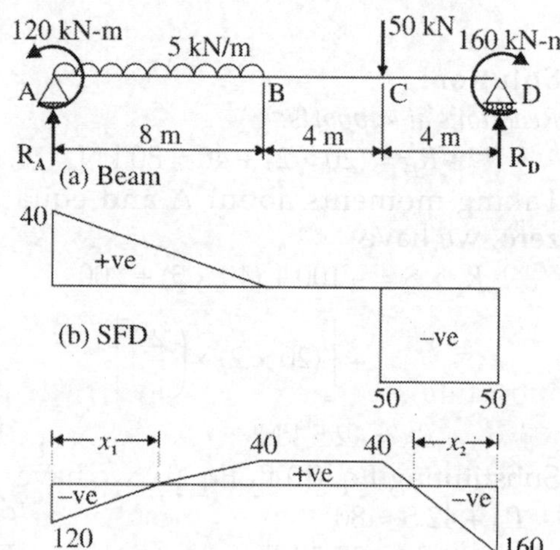

Fig. 5.45: Problem 30

5.10 STANDARD CASES OF AN OVERHANGING BEAM (OHB)

5.10.1 Overhanging beam with point load at each end

Fig. 5.46(a) indicates an overhanging beam subjected to a point load at each end.

Let W = Point load

L = Length of the beam

F_n = Shear force at salient points

M_n = Bending moment at salient points

R_A = Reaction at support A

R_B = Reaction at support B

Reactions at supports:

$$R_A + R_B = 2W \qquad \text{... Eq. (i)}$$

Taking moments about A and equating to zero, we have

$$R_B L = W(L + a) - Wa$$
$$R_B = W \qquad \text{... Eq. (ii)}$$

Substituting Eq. (ii) in Eq. (i), we have

$$R_A + W = 2W$$
$$R_A = W \qquad \text{... Eq. (iii)}$$

Here the reactions are equal as the beam is symmetrically loaded.

Shear force calculations:

$$F_D = -W$$
$$F_A = -W + W = 0$$
$$F_B = +W$$
$$F_C = +W$$

Bending moment calculations:

$$M_D = 0$$
$$M_A = -Wa$$
$$M_B = -W(a + L) + WL = -Wa$$
$$M_C = 0 \qquad \text{(from RHS)}$$

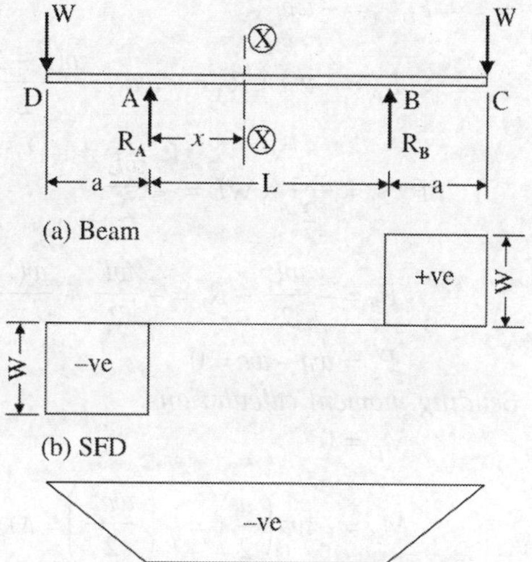

Fig. 5.46: Overhanging beam with point load at each end

Consider a section X-X at a distance x from support A.

Shear force at X-X is $\quad F_x = -W + R_A = -W + W = 0$

Bending moment at X-X is $\quad M_x = -W(a + x) + R_A x$
$$= -W(a + x) + Wx$$
$$M_x = -Wa$$

The SFD and BMD diagrams are shown in **Figs 5.46(b) & (c)** respectively.

5.10.2 Overhanging beam with UDL over entire span

Fig. 5.47(a) indicates a overhanging beam subjected to UDL over entire span.

Let w = Uniformly distributed load per unit length

L = Length of the beam

F_n = Shear force at salient points

M_n = Bending moment at salient points

R_A = Reaction at support A

R_B = Reaction at support B

Reactions at supports:

$$R_A + R_B = w(L + 2a) \qquad \text{... Eq. (i)}$$

Since the beam is symmetrically loaded,

$$R_A = R_B = \frac{w(L + 2a)}{2} \qquad \text{... Eq. (ii)}$$

Shear force calculations:

$$F_D = 0$$

$$F_{D-A} = -wa$$

$$F_A = -wa + R_A = -wa + \frac{w(L + 2a)}{2} = \frac{wL}{2}$$

$$F_{A-B} = \frac{wL}{2} - wL = -\frac{wL}{2}$$

$$F_B = -\frac{wL}{2} + R_B = -\frac{wL}{2} + \frac{w(L + 2a)}{2} = wa$$

$$F_C = wa - wa = 0$$

Bending moment calculations:

$$M_D = 0$$

$$M_A = -wa\left(\frac{a}{2}\right) = -\left(\frac{wa^2}{2}\right) = M_B$$

$$M_C = 0$$

Moment at a distance x_1 from left end D is

$$M_{x1} = -\left(\frac{wx_1^2}{2}\right) + R_A(x_1 - a)$$

$$= -\left(\frac{wx_1^2}{2}\right) + \frac{w(L + 2a)}{2}(x_1 - a)$$

$$M_{x1} = \frac{w}{2}\left[-x_1^2 + (L + 2a)(x_1 - a)\right] \qquad \text{... Eq. (iii)}$$

At $x_1 = a,$ $\qquad M_{x1} = M_A = -\left(\frac{wa^2}{2}\right)$

At $x_1 = a + L,$ $\qquad M_{x1} = M_B = \frac{w}{2}\left[-(a + L)^2 + (L + 2a)\{(a + L) - a\}\right]$

$$= \frac{w}{2}\left[-a^2 - L^2 - 2aL + (L^2 + 2aL)\right]$$

$$M_B = -\left(\frac{wa^2}{2}\right)$$

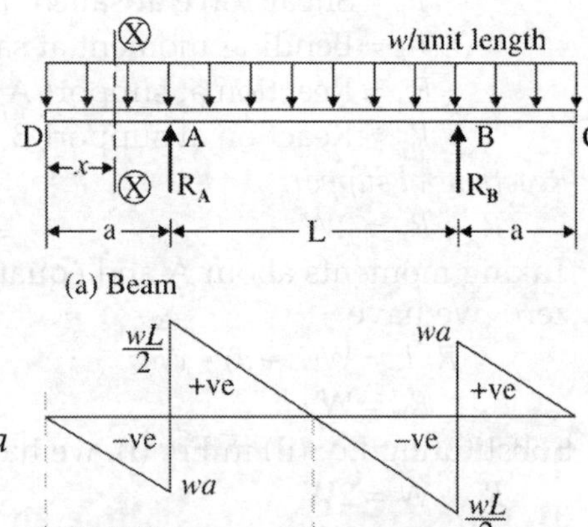

Fig. 5.47: Overhanging beam with UDL over entire span

At $x_1 = a + (L/2)$,

$$M_{x1} = M_{max} = \frac{w}{2}\left[-[a+(L/2)]^2 + (L+2a)\{[a+(L/2)]-a\}\right]$$

$$= \frac{w}{2}\left[-\left(a^2 + \frac{L^2}{4} + aL\right) + (L+2a)(L/2)\right]$$

$$= \frac{w}{2}\left[-a^2 - \frac{L^2}{4} - aL + \frac{L^2}{2} + aL\right]$$

$$= \frac{w}{2}\left[-a^2 - \frac{L^2}{4} + \frac{L^2}{2}\right] = \frac{w}{2}\left[\frac{-4a^2 - L^2 + 2L^2}{4}\right]$$

$$M_{max} = \frac{w(L^2 - 4a^2)}{8}$$

The SFD and BMD diagrams are shown in **Figs 5.47(b) & (c)** respectively.

31. Calculate the shear force and bending moments for the beam shown in Fig. 5.48(a).

Solution:

Reactions at supports:

$R_C + R_D = 40 + 20 = 60$ kN   ... Eq. (i)

Taking moments about C and equating to zero, we have

$R_D \times 4 = (20 \times 6) - (40 \times 2)$

$R_D = 10$ kN   ... Eq. (ii)

Substituting Eq. (ii) in Eq. (i), we have

$R_C + 10 = 60$

$R_C = 50$ kN   ... Eq. (iii)

Shear force calculations:

$F_A = -40$ kN

$F_C = -40 + R_C = -40 + 50 = 10$ kN

$F_D = 10 + R_D = 10 + 10 = 20$ kN

$F_B = F_D = 20$ kN

Bending moment calculations:

$M_A = 0$

$M_C = -(40 \times 2) = -80$ kN-m

$M_D = -(40 \times 6) + (50 \times 4) = -40$ kN-m

or $M_D = -(20 \times 2) = -40$ kN-m   (from RHS)

$M_B = 0$

The SFD and BMD diagrams are shown in **Figs 5.48(b) & (c)** respectively.

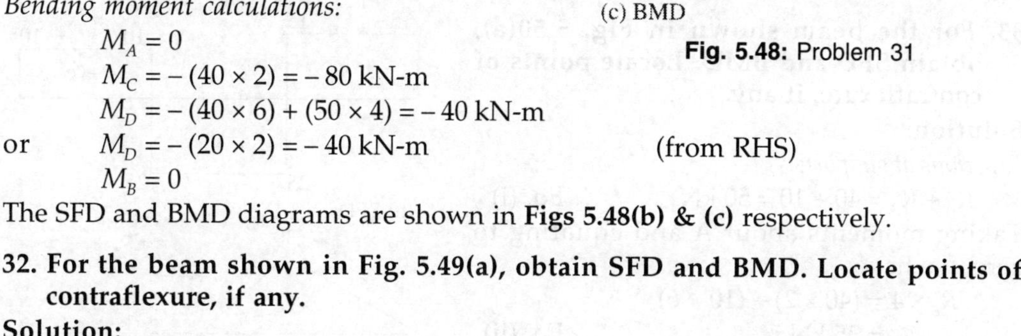

Fig. 5.48: Problem 31

32. For the beam shown in Fig. 5.49(a), obtain SFD and BMD. Locate points of contraflexure, if any.

Solution:

Reactions at supports:

$R_A + R_B = 2 + 20 + 2 = 24$ kN   ... Eq. (i)

Taking moments about A and equating to zero, we have

$$R_B \times 6 = (2 \times 8) + (20 \times 3) - (2 \times 2)$$
$$R_B = 12 \text{ kN} \qquad \text{... Eq. (ii)}$$

Substituting Eq. (ii) in Eq. (i), we have

$$R_A + 12 = 24$$
$$R_A = 12 \text{ kN} \qquad \text{... Eq. (iii)}$$

Shear force calculations:

$$F_C = -2 \text{ kN}$$
$$F_A = -2 + R_A = -2 + 12 = 10 \text{ kN}$$
$$F_D = 10 - 20 = -10 \text{ kN}$$
$$F_B = -10 + R_B = -10 + 12 = 2 \text{ kN}$$
$$F_E = F_B = 2 \text{ kN}$$

Bending moment calculations:

$$M_C = 0$$
$$M_A = -(2 \times 2) = -4 \text{ kN-m}$$
$$M_D = -(2 \times 5) + (12 \times 3) = 26 \text{ kN-m}$$
$$M_B = -(2 \times 2) = -4 \text{ kN-m} \qquad \text{(from RHS)}$$
$$M_E = 0$$

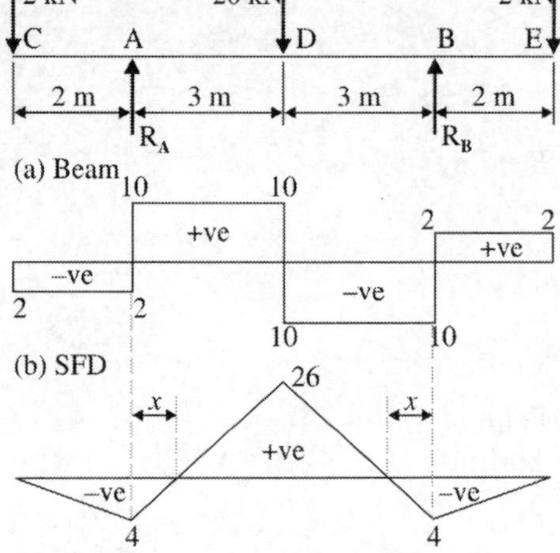

Fig. 5.49: Problem 32

Point of contraflexure: We have two points of contraflexure as seen in **Fig. 5.49(c)**. To find x:

$$M_{x1} = -2 \times (2 + x) + R_A.x = 0$$
$$0 = -4 - 2x + 12x$$
$$10x = 4$$
$$x = 2.5 \text{ m from support A}$$

Or

$$\frac{x}{4} = \frac{3 - x}{26}$$
$$26x = 12 - 4x$$
$$x = 2.5 \text{ m from support A}$$

Since the beam is symmetrically loaded, the second point of contraflexure occurs at 2.5 m from support B

The SFD and BMD diagrams are shown in **Figs 5.49(b) & (c)** respectively.

33. For the beam shown in Fig. 5.50(a), obtain SFD and BMD. Locate points of contraflexure, if any.

Solution:

Reactions at supports:

$$R_A + R_B = 40 + 10 = 50 \text{ kN} \qquad \text{... Eq. (i)}$$

Taking moments about A and equating to zero, we have

$$R_B \times 4 = (40 \times 2) + (10 \times 6)$$
$$R_B = 35 \text{ kN} \qquad \text{... Eq. (ii)}$$

Substituting Eq. (ii) in Eq. (i), we have

$$R_A + 35 = 50$$
$$R_A = 15 \text{ kN} \qquad \text{... Eq. (iii)}$$

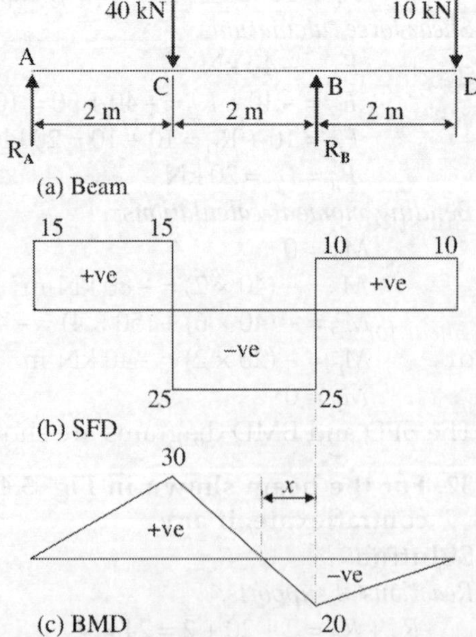

Fig. 5.50: Problem 33

Shear force calculations:
$$F_A = R_A = 15 \text{ kN}$$
$$F_C = 15 - 40 = -25 \text{ kN}$$
$$F_B = -25 + R_B = -25 + 35 = 10 \text{ kN}$$
$$F_D = F_B = 10 \text{ kN}$$

Bending moment calculations:
$$M_A = 0$$
$$M_C = (15 \times 2) = 30 \text{ kN-m}$$
$$M_B = (15 \times 4) - (40 \times 2) = -20 \text{ kN-m}$$
Or $\quad M_B = -(10 \times 2) = -20 \text{ kN-m} \qquad$ (from RHS)
$$M_D = 0$$

Point of contraflexure:

To find x:
$$M_x = -10 \times (2 + x) + R_B.x = 0$$
$$0 = -20 - 10x + 35x$$
$$25x = 20$$
$$x = 0.8 \text{ m from support B}$$

Or $\quad \dfrac{x}{20} = \dfrac{2 - x}{30}$

$$30x = 40 - 20x$$
$$x = 0.8 \text{ m from support B}$$

The SFD and BMD diagrams are shown in **Figs 5.50(b) & (c)** respectively.

34. Draw the shear force and bending moment diagram for the beam shown in Fig. 5.51(a). Locate the point of contra-flexure.

Solution:

Reactions at supports:
$$R_A + R_D = 20 + 15 + 10 = 45 \text{ kN} \quad \text{... Eq. (i)}$$
Taking moments about A and equating to zero, we have
$$R_D \times 5 = (10 \times 6) + (15 \times 4) + (20 \times 2.5)$$
$$R_D = 34 \text{ kN} \qquad \text{... Eq. (ii)}$$
Substituting Eq. (ii) in Eq. (i), we have
$$R_A + 34 = 45$$
$$R_A = 11 \text{ kN} \qquad \text{... Eq. (iii)}$$

Shear force calculations:
$$F_A = R_A = 11 \text{ kN}$$
$$F_B = 11 - 20 = -9 \text{ kN}$$
$$F_C = -9 - 15 = -24 \text{ kN}$$
$$F_D = -24 + R_D = -24 + 34 = 10 \text{ kN}$$
$$F_E = F_D = 10 \text{ kN}$$

Bending moment calculations:
$$M_A = 0$$
$$M_B = (11 \times 2.5) = 27.5 \text{ kN-m}$$

VTU – June/ July 2016 – 15 Marks

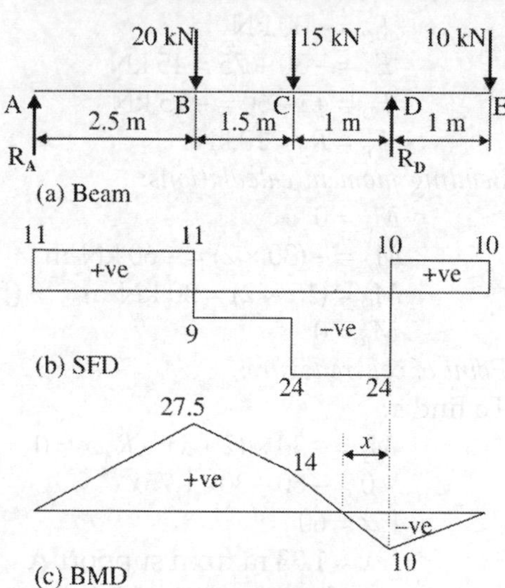

Fig. 5.51: Problem 34

$$M_C = (11 \times 4) - (20 \times 1.5) = 14 \text{ kN-m}$$

Or $\quad M_C = -(10 \times 2) + (34 \times 1) = 14 \text{ kN-m} \quad$ (from RHS)

$$M_D = -(10 \times 1) = -10 \text{ kN-m}$$

$$M_E = 0$$

Point of contraflexure:

To find x:

$$M_x = -10 \times (1 + x) + R_D.x = 0$$

$$0 = -10 - 10x + 34x$$

$$24x = 10$$

$$x = 0.416 \text{ m from support D}$$

Or $\quad \dfrac{x}{10} = \dfrac{1-x}{14}$

$$14x = 10 - 10x$$

$$x = 0.416 \text{ m from support D}$$

The SFD and BMD diagrams are shown in **Figs 5.51(b) & (c)** respectively.

35. Draw the shear force and bending moment diagram for the beam shown in Fig. 5.52(a). Also locate the point of contra-flexure.

Solution:

Reactions at supports:

$$R_A + R_B = 30 + 60 = 90 \text{ kN} \qquad \text{... Eq. (i)}$$

Taking moments about A and equating to zero, we have

$$R_B \times 4 = (60 \times 2) - (30 \times 2)$$

$$R_B = 15 \text{ kN} \qquad \text{... Eq. (ii)}$$

Substituting Eq. (ii) in Eq. (i), we have

$$R_A + 15 = 90$$

$$R_A = 75 \text{ kN} \qquad \text{... Eq. (iii)}$$

Shear force calculations:

$$F_C = -30 \text{ kN}$$

$$F_A = -30 + 75 = 45 \text{ kN}$$

$$F_D = 45 - 60 = -15 \text{ kN}$$

$$F_B = R_B = 10 \text{ kN}$$

Bending moment calculations:

$$M_C = 0$$

$$M_A = -(30 \times 2) = -60 \text{ kN-m}$$

$$M_D = (15 \times 2) = 30 \text{ kN-m} \quad \text{(from RHS)}$$

$$M_B = 0$$

Point of contraflexure:

To find x:

$$M_x = -30 \times (2 + x) + R_A.x = 0$$

$$0 = -60 - 30x + 75x$$

$$45x = 60$$

$$x = 1.33 \text{ m from support A}$$

Or $\quad \dfrac{x}{60} = \dfrac{2-x}{30}$

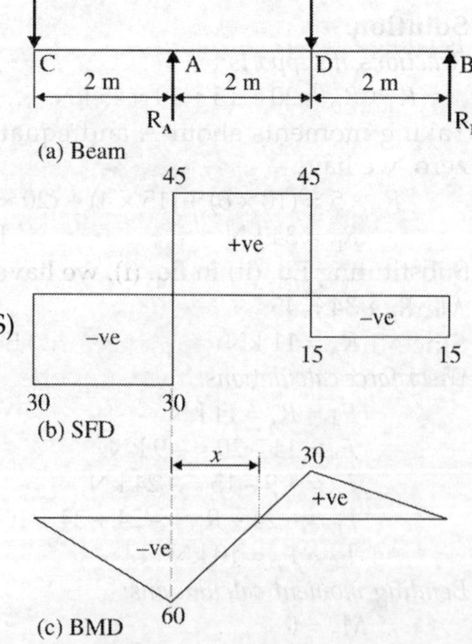

Fig. 5.52: Problem 35

$$30x = 120 - 60x$$
$$x = 1.33 \text{ m from support A}$$

The SFD and BMD diagrams are shown in **Figs 5.52(b) & (c)** respectively.

36. Draw SF and BM diagrams for the loading pattern on the beam shown in Fig. 5.53(a). Indicate where the inflexion and contraflexure points are located. Also locate the maximum BM and its magnitude.

VTU – Dec. 07/ Jan. 08 – 12 Marks; May/ June 2010 – 14 Marks; June/ July 2014 – 12 Marks

Solution:

Reactions at supports:

$$R_A + R_B = (5 \times 14) = 70 \text{ kN} \qquad \text{... Eq. (i)}$$

Taking moments about A and equating to zero, we have

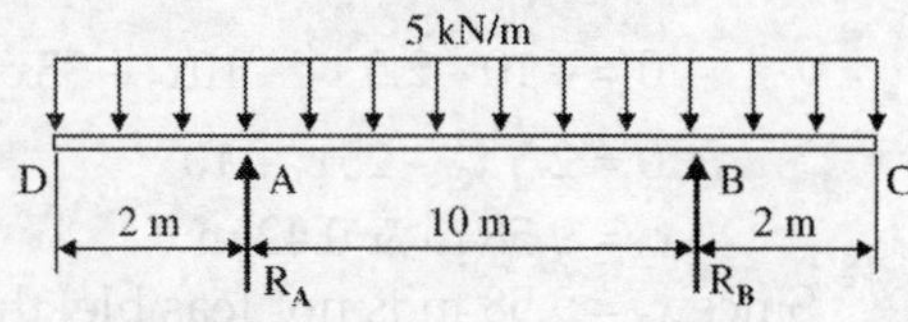

$$R_B \times 10 = (5 \times 12) \times \left(\frac{12}{2}\right) - (5 \times 2) \times \left(\frac{2}{2}\right)$$

$$R_B = 35 \text{ kN} \qquad \text{... Eq. (ii)}$$

Substituting Eq. (ii) in Eq. (i), we have

$$R_A + 35 = 70$$
$$R_A = 35 \text{ kN} \qquad \text{... Eq. (iii)}$$

Shear force calculations:

$$F_D = 0 \text{ kN}$$
$$F_{D-A} = -(5 \times 2) = -10 \text{ kN}$$
$$F_A = -10 + R_A = -10 + 35 = 25 \text{ kN}$$
$$F_{A-B} = 25 - (5 \times 10) = -25 \text{ kN}$$
$$F_B = -25 + R_B = -25 + 35 = 10 \text{ kN}$$
$$F_C = 10 - (5 \times 2) = 0 \text{ kN}$$

Bending moment calculations:

$$M_D = 0$$

$$M_A = -(5 \times 2)\left(\frac{2}{2}\right) = -10 \text{ kN-m}$$

$$M_B = -(5 \times 2)\left(\frac{2}{2}\right) = -10 \text{ kN-m} \qquad \text{(from RHS)}$$

$$M_C = 0$$

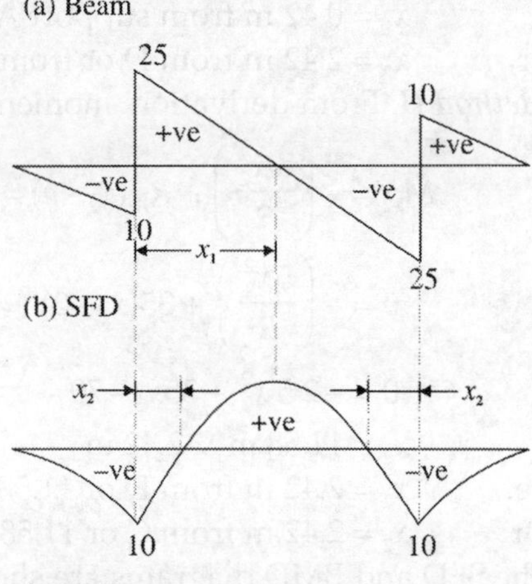

Fig. 5.53: Problem 36

Maximum bending moment:

Since the beam is symmetrically loaded, maximum bending moment occurs at a distance of 5m from either supports.

$$\frac{x_1}{25} = \frac{10 - x_1}{25}$$

$$20x_1 = 10$$
$$x_1 = 5 \text{ m from support A or support B}$$

$$M_{max1} = -(5 \times 7)\left(\frac{7}{2}\right) + (35 \times 5) = 52.5 \text{ kN-m}$$

Or from derivation,

$$M_{\max} = \frac{w(L^2 - 4a^2)}{8} = \frac{5(10^2 - 4 \times 2^2)}{8} = 52.5 \text{ kN-m}$$

Point of contraflexure: We have two points of contraflexure as seen in **Fig. 5.53(c)**.
To find x_2 :

$$M_{x2} = -5 \times (2 + x_2)\left(\frac{2 + x_2}{2}\right) + 35x_2 = 0$$

$$0 = -[2.5 \times (4 + x_2^2 + 4x_2)] + 35x_2$$
$$0 = -10 - 2.5\,x_2^2 - 10x_2 + 35x_2$$
$$0 = 2.5\,x_2^2 - 25x_2 + 10$$
$$x_2 = 9.58 \text{ m} \,\&\, 0.42 \text{ m}$$

Since $x_2 = 9.58$ m is not feasible, the correct value is

$$x_2 = 0.42 \text{ m from support A or support B}$$

or $\qquad x_2 = 2.42$ m from D or from C

Method II: From derivation, moment at a distance x_2 from left end D is

$$M_{x2} = -\left(\frac{wx_2^2}{2}\right) + R_A\,(x_2 - a) = 0$$

$$0 = -\left(\frac{5x_2^2}{2}\right) + 35(x_2 - 2)$$

$$0 = -2.5\,x_2^2 + 35x_2 - 70$$
$$x_2 = 11.58 \text{ m} \,\&\, 2.42 \text{ m}$$

i.e. $\qquad x_2 = 2.42$ m from D or 11.58 m from C

Or $\qquad x_2 = 2.42$ m from C or 11.58 m from D

The SFD and BMD diagrams are shown in **Figs 5.53(b) & (c)** respectively.

**37. Draw the shear force and bending moment diagram for the overhanging beam
carrying a uniformly distributed load of 2 kN/m over the entire length and a
point load of 2 kN as shown in Fig. 5.54(a). Locate the point of contraflexure.**

VTU – Dec. 2012 – 14 Marks, Dec. 13/ Jan. 14 – 14 Marks

Solution:

Reactions at supports:

$$R_A + R_B = 2 + (2 \times 6) = 14 \text{ kN} \qquad \text{... Eq. (i)}$$

Taking moments about A and equating to zero, we have

$$R_B \times 4 = (2 \times 6) + (2 \times 6) \times \left(\frac{6}{2}\right)$$

$$R_B = 12 \text{ kN} \qquad \text{... Eq. (ii)}$$

Substituting Eq. (ii) in Eq. (i), we have

$$R_A + 12 = 14$$
$$R_A = 2 \text{ kN} \qquad \text{... Eq. (iii)}$$

Shear force calculations:

$$F_A = R_A = 2 \text{ kN}$$
$$F_{A-B} = 2 - (2 \times 4) = -6 \text{ kN}$$

$$F_B = -6 + R_B = -6 + 12 = 6 \text{ kN}$$
$$F_{B-C} = 6 - (2 \times 2) = +2 \text{ kN}$$
$$F_C = +2 \text{ kN}$$

Bending moment calculations:
$$M_A = 0$$

$$M_B = -(2 \times 2) - (2 \times 2) \times \left(\frac{2}{2}\right) = -8 \text{ kN-m}$$

$$M_C = 0$$

Maximum bending moment:
$$\frac{x_1}{2} = \frac{4 - x_1}{6}$$
$$3x_1 = 4 - x_1$$
$$x_1 = 1 \text{ m from support A}$$

$$M_{max1} = (2 \times 1) - (2 \times 1)\left(\frac{1}{2}\right) = 1 \text{ kN-m}$$

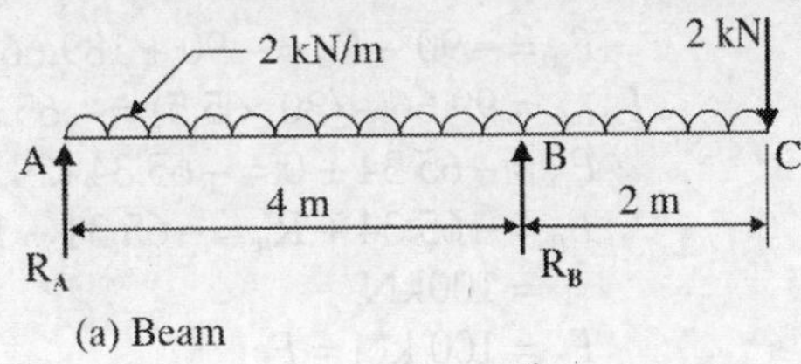

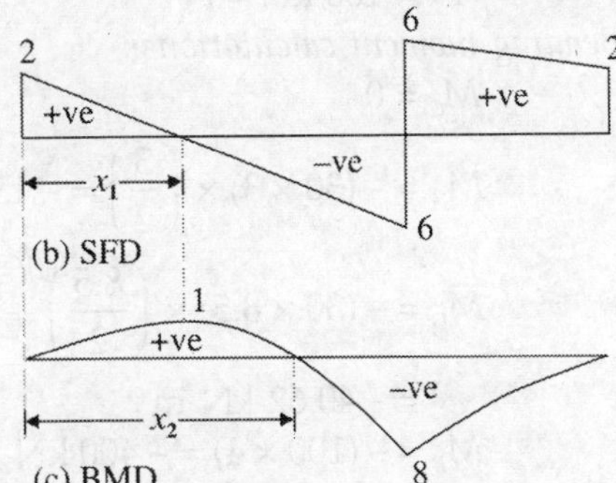

Fig. 5.54: Problem 37

Point of contraflexure: We have two points of contraflexure as seen in **Fig. 5.54(c)**.
To find x_2 :

$$M_{x2} = -\left(\frac{wx_2^2}{2}\right) + R_A x_2 = 0$$

$$0 = -\left(\frac{2x_2^2}{2}\right) + 2x_2$$

$$0 = -x_2^2 + 2x_2$$

$$x_2 = 2 \text{ m from support A}$$

The SFD and BMD diagrams are shown in **Figs 5.54(b) & (c)** respectively.

38. Draw the shear force and bending moment diagrams for the beam loaded as shown in Fig. 5.55(a).

VTU – Dec. 09/ Jan. 10 – 20 Marks

Solution:
Distance CA = 8.5 + 5.5 – 11 = 3 m
Reactions at supports:
$$R_A + R_B = 100 + (30 \times 8.5) = 355 \text{ kN} \qquad \ldots \text{Eq. (i)}$$
Taking moments about A and equating to zero, we have

$$R_B \times 11 = (100 \times 15) + (30 \times 5.5) \times \left(\frac{5.5}{2}\right) - (30 \times 3) \times \left(\frac{3}{2}\right)$$

$$R_B = 165.34 \text{ kN} \qquad \ldots \text{Eq. (ii)}$$

Substituting Eq. (ii) in Eq. (i), we have
$$R_A + 165.34 = 190$$
$$R_A = 189.66 \text{ kN} \qquad \ldots \text{Eq. (iii)}$$

Shear force calculations:
$$F_C = 0$$
$$F_{C-A} = 0 - (30 \times 3) = -90 \text{ kN}$$

$$F_A = -90 + R_A = -90 + 189.66 = 99.66 \text{ kN}$$
$$F_{A-D} = 99.66 - (30 \times 5.5) = -65.34 \text{ kN}$$
$$F_D = -65.34 + 0 = -65.34 \text{ kN}$$
$$F_B = -65.34 + R_B = -65.34 + 165.34$$
$$= 100 \text{kN}$$
$$F_E = 100 \text{ kN} = F_B$$

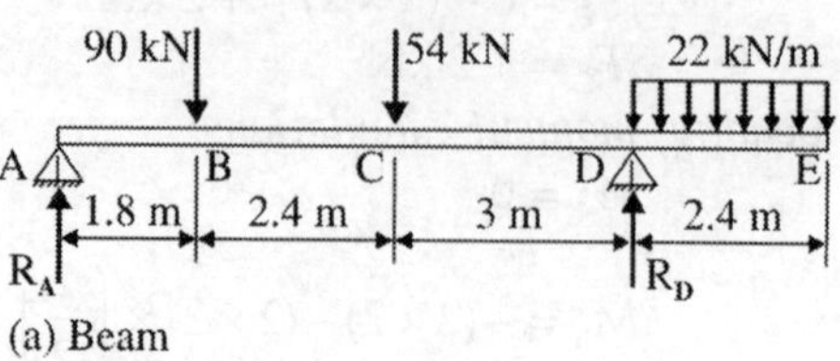

Bending moment calculations:
$$M_C = 0$$
$$M_A = -(30 \times 3) \times \left(\frac{3}{2}\right) = -135 \text{ kN-m}$$
$$M_D = -(30 \times 8.5) \times \left(\frac{8.5}{2}\right) + (189.66 \times 5.5)$$
$$= -40.62 \text{ kN-m}$$
$$M_B = -(100 \times 4) = -400 \text{ kN-m}$$
$$M_E = 0$$

Maximum bending moment:

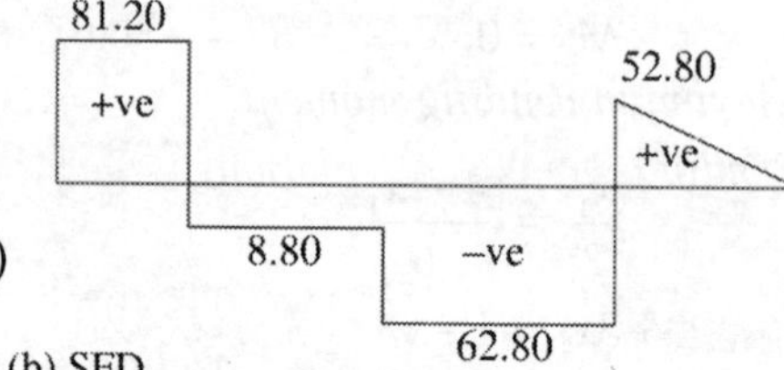

$$\frac{x_1}{99.66} = \frac{5.5 - x_1}{65.34}$$
$$65.34 x_1 = 584.13 - 99.66 x_1$$
$$1654 x_1 = 584.02$$
$$x_1 = 3.32 \text{ m from support A}$$
$$= 6.32 \text{ m from C}$$

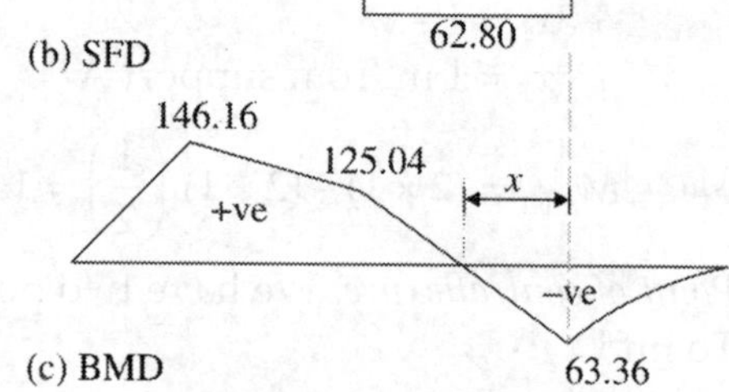

Fig. 5.55: Problem 38

$$M_{\text{max1}} = -(30 \times 6.32)\left(\frac{6.32}{2}\right) + (189.66 \times 3.32) = 30.54 \text{ kN-m}$$

Point of contraflexure: We have two points of contraflexure as seen in **Fig. 5.55(c)**.

$$M_{x2} = -30 x_2 \times \left(\frac{x_2}{2}\right) + 189.66(x_2 - 3) = 0$$
$$0 = -15 x_2^2 + 189.66 x_2 - 568.98$$
$$15 x_2^2 - 189.66 x_2 + 568.98 = 0$$
$$x_2 = 7.748 \text{ m } \& 4.895 \text{ m}$$

i.e. $\quad x_2 = 4.895$ m from C $\quad$ and $\quad x_3 = 7.748$ m from C

The SFD and BMD diagrams are shown in **Figs 5.55(b) & (c)** respectively

39. Draw the SFD and BMD for the beam shown in Fig. 5.56(a), showing the salient features. Also locate the points of contraflexure if any.

VTU – (CV)Dec. 2011– 12 Marks; [Similar: (CV) Dec. 2012 – 10 Marks]

Solution:

Reactions at supports:
$$R_A + R_B = 3 + 5 + (10 \times 6) = 68 \text{ kN} \qquad \text{... Eq. (i)}$$

Taking moments about A and equating to zero, we have

$$R_B \times 6 = (5 \times 8) + (10 \times 6) \times \left(\frac{6}{2}\right) - (3 \times 2)$$
$$R_B = 35.67 \text{ kN} \qquad \text{... Eq. (ii)}$$

Substituting Eq. (ii) in Eq. (i), we have

$$R_A + 35.67 = 68$$
$$R_A = 32.33 \text{ kN} \qquad \text{... Eq. (iii)}$$

Shear force calculations:

$$F_C = -3 \text{ kN}$$
$$F_A = -3 + R_A = -3 + 32.33 = 29.33 \text{ kN}$$
$$F_{A-B} = 29.33 - (10 \times 6) = -30.67 \text{ kN}$$
$$F_B = -30.67 + R_B = -30.67 + 35.67 = 5 \text{ kN}$$
$$F_D = 5 \text{ kN} = F_B$$

Bending moment calculations:

$$M_C = 0$$
$$M_A = -(3 \times 2) = -6 \text{ kN-m}$$
$$M_B = -(5 \times 2) = -10 \text{ kN-m} \quad \text{(from RHS)}$$
$$M_D = 0 \qquad\qquad\qquad\quad \text{(from RHS)}$$

Maximum bending moment:

$$\frac{x_1}{29.33} = \frac{6 - x_1}{30.67}$$
$$30.67x_1 = 175.98 - 29.33x_1$$
$$60x_1 = 175.98$$
$$x_1 = 2.93 \text{ m from support A}$$

$$M_{max1} = -(3 \times 4.93) + (32.33 \times 2.93) - (10 \times 2.93) \times \left(\frac{2.93}{2}\right) = 37.02 \text{ kN-m}$$

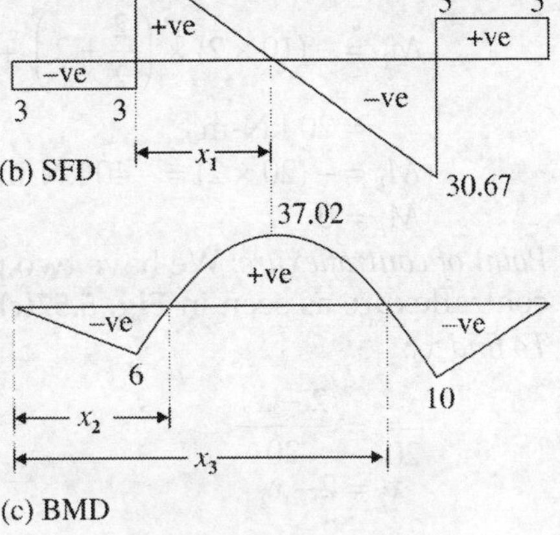

Fig. 5.56: Problem 39

Point of contraflexure: We have two points of contraflexure as seen in **Fig. 5.56(c)**. The SFD and BMD diagrams are shown in **Figs 5.56(b) & (c)** respectively

40. Draw the shear force and bending moment diagrams for the beam shown in Fig. 5.57(a).

VTU – Dec. 2011 – 14 Marks; Dec. 16/ Jan. 17 – 16 Marks

Solution:

Reactions at supports:

$$R_A + R_B = 40 + 20 + (10 \times 2) + (10 \times 2) = 100 \text{ kN} \qquad \text{... Eq. (i)}$$

Taking moments about A and equating to zero, we have

$$R_B \times 4 = (20 \times 6) + (40 \times 2) + (10 \times 2) \times \left(\frac{2}{2} + 2\right) - (10 \times 2) \times \left(\frac{2}{2}\right)$$
$$R_B = 60 \text{ kN} \qquad \text{... Eq. (ii)}$$

Substituting Eq. (ii) in Eq. (i), we have

$$R_A + 60 = 100$$
$$R_A = 40 \text{ kN} \qquad \text{... Eq. (iii)}$$

Shear force calculations:

$$F_C = 0$$
$$F_{C-A} = -(10 \times 2) = -20 \text{ kN}$$
$$F_A = -20 + R_A = -20 + 40 = 20 \text{ kN}$$
$$F_D = 20 - 40 = -20 \text{ kN}$$

$$F_{D-B} = -20 - (10 \times 2) = -40 \text{kN}$$
$$F_B = -40 + R_B = -40 + 60 = 20 \text{ kN}$$
$$F_E = 20 \text{ kN} = F_B$$

Bending moment calculations:

$$M_C = 0$$

$$M_A = -(10 \times 2) \times \left(\frac{2}{2}\right) = -20 \text{ kN-m}$$

$$M_D = -(10 \times 2) \times \left(\frac{2}{2} + 2\right) + (40 \times 2)$$

$$= 20 \text{ kN-m}$$

$$M_B = -(20 \times 2) = -40 \text{ kN-m} \quad \text{(from RHS)}$$

$$M_E = 0 \qquad\qquad\qquad \text{(from RHS)}$$

Point of contraflexure: We have two points of contraflexure as seen in **Fig. 5.57(c)**.

To find x_2:

$$\frac{x_2}{20} = \frac{2 - x_2}{20}$$
$$x_2 = 2 - x_2$$
$$2x_2 = 2$$
$$x_2 = 1 \text{ m from support A}$$

Or

$$M_{x2} = -(10 \times 2) \times \left(\frac{2}{2} + x_2\right) + 40x_2 = 0$$

$$0 = -20 - 20x_2 + 40x_2$$
$$20 = 20x_2$$
$$x_2 = 1 \text{ m from support A}$$

To find x_3:

$$M_{x3} = -20 \times (2 + x_3) + 60x_3 - 10x_3\left(\frac{x_3}{2}\right) = 0$$

$$0 = -40 - 20x_3 + 60x_3 - 5x_3^2$$
$$0 = -5x_3^2 + 40x_3 - 40$$
$$x_3 = 1.17 \text{ m \& } 6.83 \text{ m}$$
$$x_3 = 1.17 \text{ m from support B}$$

Or

$$M_{x3} = -20x_3 + 60(x_3 - 2) - 10 \times \frac{(x_3 - 2)^2}{2} = 0$$

$$0 = -20x_3 + 60x_3 - 120 - 5(x_3^2 + 4 - 4x_3)$$
$$0 = -5x_3^2 + 60x_3 - 140$$
$$x_3 = 3.17 \text{ \& } 8.83 \text{ m}$$
$$x_3 = 3.17 \text{m from End E}$$

The SFD and BMD diagrams are shown in **Figs 5.57(b) & (c)** respectively.

41. **Draw the SF and BM diagrams indicating principal values for an overhanging beam as shown in Fig. 5.58(a). Locate the point of contraflexure, if any.**

VTU – Dec. 09/ Jan. 10– 15 Marks, June/ July 2013 – 10 Marks; [Similar: (CV) Dec. 2010 – 12 Marks]

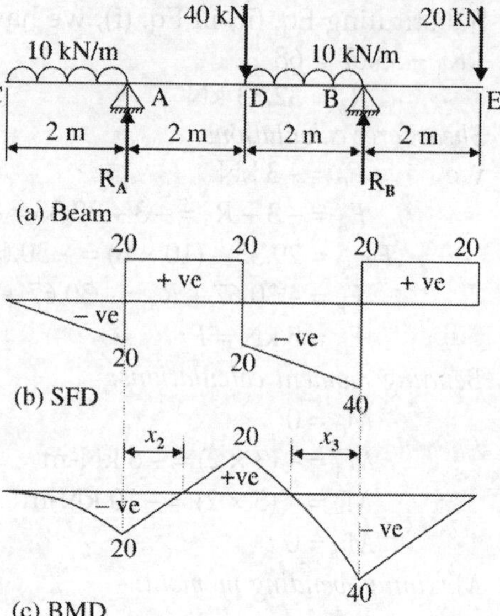

Fig. 5.57: Problem 40

Solution:

Reactions at supports:

$$R_A + R_B = 6 + (20 \times 2) = 46 \text{ kN} \qquad \text{... Eq. (i)}$$

Taking moments about A and equating to zero, we have

$$R_B \times 4 = (6 \times 6) + (20 \times 2) \times \left(\frac{2}{2}\right)$$

$$R_B = 19 \text{ kN} \qquad \text{... Eq. (ii)}$$

Substituting Eq. (ii) in Eq. (i), we have

$$R_A + 19 = 46$$

$$R_A = 27 \text{ kN} \qquad \text{... Eq. (iii)}$$

Shear force calculations:

$$F_A = 27 \text{ kN}$$

$$F_{A-C} = 27 - (20 \times 2) = -13 \text{ kN}$$

$$F_C = -13 + 0 = -13 \text{ kN}$$

$$\text{remains constant up to B}$$

$$F_B = -13 + R_B = -13 + 19 = 6 \text{ kN}$$

$$F_D = 6 \text{ kN} = F_B$$

Bending moment calculations:

$$M_A = 0$$

$$M_C = (27 \times 2) - (20 \times 2) \times \left(\frac{2}{2}\right) = 14 \text{ kN-m}$$

$$M_B = -(6 \times 2) = -12 \text{ kN-m} \qquad \text{(from RHS)}$$

$$M_D = 0 \qquad \text{(from RHS)}$$

Maximum bending moment:

$$\frac{x_2}{27} = \frac{2 - x_2}{13}$$

$$13x_1 = 54 - 27x_1$$

$$40x_1 = 54$$

$$x_1 = 1.35 \text{ m from support A}$$

$$M_{max1} = (27 \times 1.35) - (20 \times 1.35) \times \left(\frac{1.35}{2}\right) = 18.23 \text{ kN-m}$$

Point of contraflexure:

$$\frac{x_2}{12} = \frac{2 - x_2}{14}$$

$$14x_2 = 24 - 12x_2$$

$$26x_2 = 24$$

$$x_2 = 0.92 \text{ m from support B}$$

Or $\quad M_{max2} = -6 \times (2 + x_2) + 19x_2 = 0$

$$0 = -12 - 6x_2 + 19x_2$$

$$12 = 13x_2$$

$$x_2 = 0.92 \text{ m from support B}$$

The SFD and BMD diagrams are shown in **Figs 5.58(b) & (c)** respectively

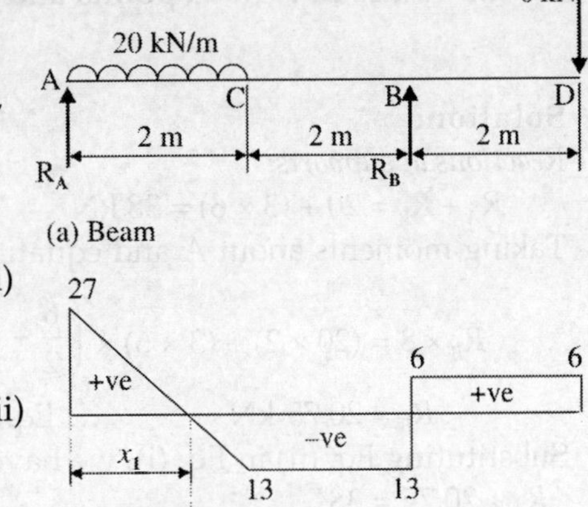

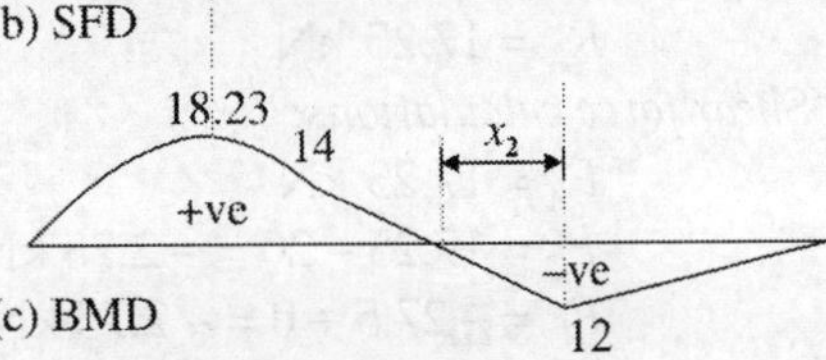

Fig. 5.58: Problem 41

42. Draw SFD and BMD for the beam loaded as shown in Fig. 5.59(a). Indicate the values at various points and locate the point of contraflexure, if any.

VTU – June/ July 2014 – 14 Marks

Solution:

Reactions at supports:

$$R_A + R_B = 20 + (3 \times 6) = 38 \text{ kN} \qquad \text{... Eq. (i)}$$

Taking moments about A and equating to zero, we have

$$R_B \times 8 = (20 \times 2) + (3 \times 6) \times \left(\frac{6}{2} + 4 \right)$$

$$R_B = 20.75 \text{ kN} \qquad \text{... Eq. (ii)}$$

Substituting Eq. (ii) in Eq. (i), we have

$$R_A + 20.75 = 38$$

$$R_A = 17.25 \text{ kN} \qquad \text{... Eq. (iii)}$$

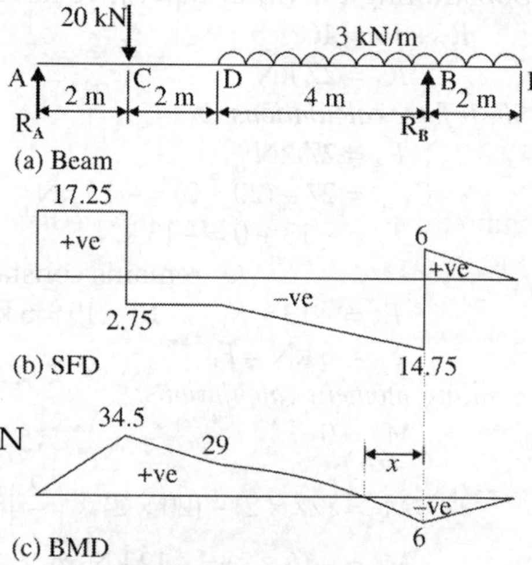

Shear force calculations:

$$F_A = 17.25 \text{ kN}$$
$$F_C = 17.25 - 20 = -2.75 \text{ kN}$$
$$F_D = -27.5 + 0 = -2.75 \text{ kN}$$
$$F_{D-B} = -2.75 - (3 \times 4) = -14.75 \text{ kN}$$
$$F_B = -14.75 + R_B = -14.75 + 20.75 = 6 \text{ kN}$$
$$F_E = -6 + (3 \times 2) = 0$$

Bending moment calculations:

$$M_A = 0$$
$$M_C = (17.25 \times 2) = 34.5 \text{ kN-m}$$
$$M_D = (17.25 \times 4) - (20 \times 2) = 29 \text{ kN-m}$$

$$M_B = -(3 \times 2) \times \left(\frac{2}{2} \right) = -6 \text{ kN-m} \qquad \text{(from RHS)}$$

$$M_E = 0 \qquad \text{(from RHS)}$$

Point of contraflexure:

$$M_{max} = -3 \times \frac{(2 + x)^2}{2} + 20.75x = 0$$

$$0 = -1.5(4 + x^2 + 4x) + 20.75x$$
$$0 = -6 - 6x - 1.5x^2 + 20.75x$$
$$1.5x^2 - 14.75x + 6 = 0$$
$$x = 9.41 \text{ m} \ \& \ 0.43 \text{ m}$$

i.e $x = 0.43$ m from support B

Or $$M_{max} = -3 \times \left(\frac{x^2}{2} \right) + 20.75(x - 2) = 0$$

$$0 = -1.5x^2 + 20.75x - 41.5$$
$$1.5x^2 - 20.75x + 41.5 = 0$$
$$x = 11.41 \text{ m} \ \& \ 2.43 \text{ m}$$

i.e $x = 2.43$ m from E

or $x = 0.43$ m from support B

The SFD and BMD diagrams are shown in **Figs 5.59(b) & (c)** respectively

20 kN
3 kN/m
A
C
D
B
E
2 m
2 m
4 m
2 m
R_A
R_B
(a) Beam
17.25
+ve
6
+ve
2.75
−ve
(b) SFD
14.75
34.5
29
+ve
x
−ve
6
(c) BMD

Fig. 5.59: Problem 42

43. Draw the shear force and bending moment diagrams for the beam shown in Fig. 5.60(a). Locate the point of contraflexure.

VTU – June/July 2013 – 20 Marks

Solution:

Reactions at supports:

$$R_A + R_D = 90 + 54 + (22 \times 2.4)$$
$$= 196.8 \text{ kN} \qquad \text{... Eq. (i)}$$

Taking moments about A and equating to zero, we have

$$R_D \times 7.2 = (90 \times 1.8) + (54 \times 4.2) + (22 \times 2.4)$$
$$\times \left(\frac{2.4}{2} + 7.2 \right)$$
$$R_D = 115.60 \text{ kN} \qquad \text{... Eq. (ii)}$$

Substituting Eq. (ii) in Eq. (i), we have

$$R_A + 115.6 = 196.80$$
$$R_A = 81.20 \text{ kN} \qquad \text{... Eq. (iii)}$$

Shear force calculations:

$$F_A = R_A = 81.20 \text{ kN}$$
$$F_B = 81.20 - 90 = -8.80 \text{ kN}$$
$$F_C = -8.80 - 54 = -62.80 \text{ kN}$$
$$F_D = -62.8 + R_B = -62.80 + 115.60$$
$$= 52.80 \text{ kN}$$
$$F_{D-E} = 52.80 - (22 \times 2.4) = 0 \text{ kN} = F_E$$

Bending moment calculations:

$$M_A = 0$$
$$M_B = (81.20 \times 1.8) = 146.16 \text{ kN-m}$$
$$M_C = (81.20 \times 4.2) - (90 \times 2.4) = 125.04 \text{ kN-m}$$

$$M_D = -(22 \times 2.4) \times \left(\frac{2.4}{2} \right) = -63.36 \text{ kN-m} \qquad \text{(from RHS)}$$

$$M_E = 0 \qquad \text{(from RHS)}$$

Point of contraflexure:

$$\frac{x}{63.36} = \frac{3 - x}{125.04}$$
$$125.04x = 190.08 - 63.36x$$
$$188.40x = 190.08$$
$$x = 1.01 \text{ m from support D}$$

$$\text{Or} \quad M_{\max} = -22 \times 2.4 \times \left(\frac{2.4}{2} + x \right) + 115.60x = 0$$

$$0 = -63.36 - 52.8x + 115.60x$$
$$0 = -63.36 + 62.8x$$
$$x = 1.01 \text{ m from support D}$$

The SFD and BMD diagrams are shown in **Figs 5.60(b) & (c)** respectively.

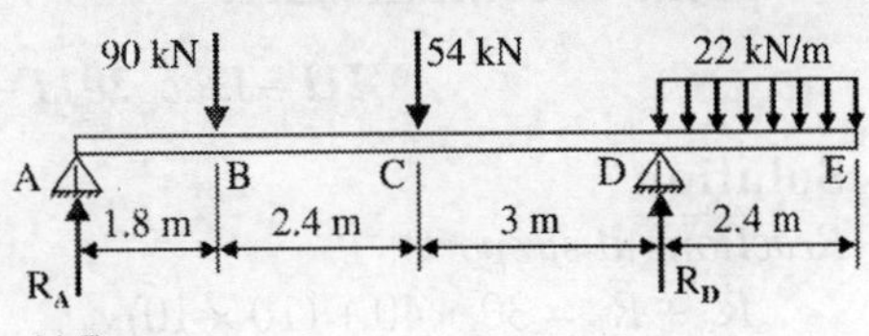

(a) Beam

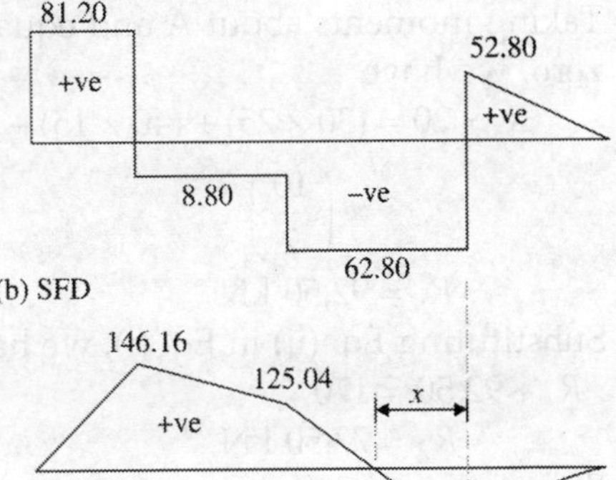

(b) SFD

(c) BMD

Fig. 5.60: Problem 43

44. A beam 25 m long is supported at A and B and is loaded as shown in Fig. 5.61(a). Draw the shear force and bending moment diagrams for the beam computing shear force and bending moments at A, E, D, B and C. Find the position and magnitude of maximum bending moment. Also determine the point of contraflexure.

VTU – Dec. 2011 – 14 Marks, [Similar: (CV) Dec. 2011– 16 Marks]

Solution:

Reactions at supports:

$$R_A + R_B = 30 + 40 + (10 \times 10)$$
$$= 170 \text{ kN} \qquad \text{... Eq. (i)}$$

Taking moments about A and equating to zero, we have

$$R_B \times 20 = (30 \times 25) + (40 \times 15) + (10 \times 10) \times \left(\frac{10}{2}\right)$$

$$R_B = 92.50 \text{ kN} \qquad \text{... Eq. (ii)}$$

Substituting Eq. (ii) in Eq. (i), we have

$$R_A + 92.50 = 170$$
$$R_A = 77.50 \text{ kN} \qquad \text{... Eq. (iii)}$$

Shear force calculations:

$$F_A = R_A = 77.50 \text{ kN}$$
$$F_{A-E} = 77.50 - (10 \times 10) = -22.50 \text{ kN}$$
$$F_E = -22.50 - 0 = -22.50 \text{ kN}$$
$$F_D = -22.50 - 40 = -62.50 \text{ kN}$$
$$F_B = -62.50 + R_B = -62.50 + 92.50$$
$$= 30 \text{ kN}$$
$$F_C = 30 \text{ kN} = F_B$$

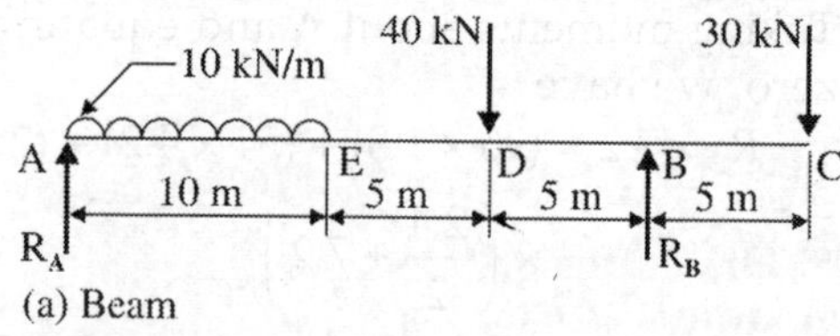

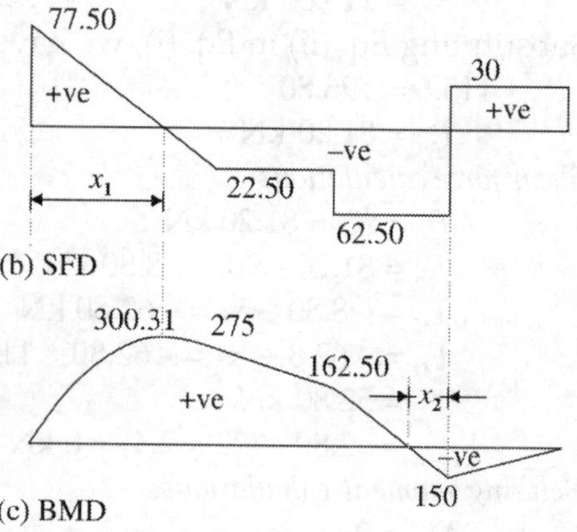

Fig. 5.61: Problem 44

Bending moment calculations:

$$M_A = 0$$

$$M_E = (77.50 \times 10) - (10 \times 10) \times \left(\frac{10}{2}\right) = 275 \text{ kN-m}$$

$$M_D = -(30 \times 10) + (92.50 \times 5) = 162.50 \text{ kN-m} \quad \text{(from RHS)}$$
$$M_B = -(30 \times 5) = -150 \text{ kN-m} \quad \text{(from RHS)}$$
$$M_C = 0 \quad \text{(from RHS)}$$

Maximum bending moment:

$$\frac{x_1}{77.50} = \frac{10 - x_1}{22.50}$$

$$22.50 x_1 = 775 - 77.50 x_1$$
$$100 x_1 = 775$$
$$x_1 = 7.75 \text{ m from support A}$$

$$M_{\text{max1}} = (77.50 \times 7.75) - (10 \times 7.75) \times \left(\frac{7.75}{2}\right) = 300.31 \text{ kN-m}$$

Point of contraflexure:

$$\frac{x_2}{150} = \frac{5 - x_2}{162.50}$$

$$162.50x_2 = 750 - 150x_2$$

$$312.50x_2 = 750$$

$$x_2 = 2.4 \text{ m from support B}$$

Or $\quad M_{max2} = -30 \times (5 + x_2) + 92.50x_2 = 0$

$$0 = -150 - 30x_2 + 92.50x_2$$

$$x_2 = 2.4 \text{ m from support B}$$

The SFD and BMD diagrams are shown in **Figs 5.61(b) & (c)** respectively

45. Draw the shear force and bending moment diagrams for the overhanging beam shown in Fig. 5.62(a). Locate the point of contraflexure, if any.

VTU – (CV) Dec. 13/ Jan. 14 – 10 Marks; (CV) Dec. 13/ Jan. 14 – 12 Marks; [similar: (CV) June – July 2015 – 14 Marks]

Solution:

Reactions at supports:

$$R_A + R_B = 20 + 40 + (20 \times 2)$$

$$= 100 \text{ kN} \qquad \text{... Eq. (i)}$$

Taking moments about A and equating to zero, we have

$$R_B \times 4 = (20 \times 5) + (40 \times 2) + (20 \times 2)$$

$$\times \left(\frac{2}{2}\right)$$

$$R_B = 55 \text{ kN} \qquad \text{... Eq. (ii)}$$

Substituting Eq. (ii) in Eq. (i), we have

$$R_A + 55 = 100$$

$$R_A = 45 \text{ kN} \qquad \text{... Eq. (iii)}$$

Shear force calculations:

$$F_A = R_A = 45 \text{ kN}$$

$$F_{A-C} = 45 - (20 \times 2) = 5 \text{ kN}$$

$$F_C = 5 - 40 = -35 \text{ kN}$$

$$F_B = -35 + + R_B = -35 + 55 = 20 \text{ kN}$$

$$F_D = 20 \text{ kN} = F_B$$

Bending moment calculations:

$$M_A = 0$$

$$M_C = (45 \times 2) - (20 \times 2) \times \left(\frac{2}{2}\right) = 50 \text{ kN-m}$$

$$M_B = -(20 \times 1) = -20 \text{ kN-m} \qquad \text{(from RHS)}$$

$$M_D = 0 \qquad \text{(from RHS)}$$

Point of contraflexure:

$$\frac{x}{20} = \frac{2 - x}{50}$$

$$50x = 40 - 20x$$

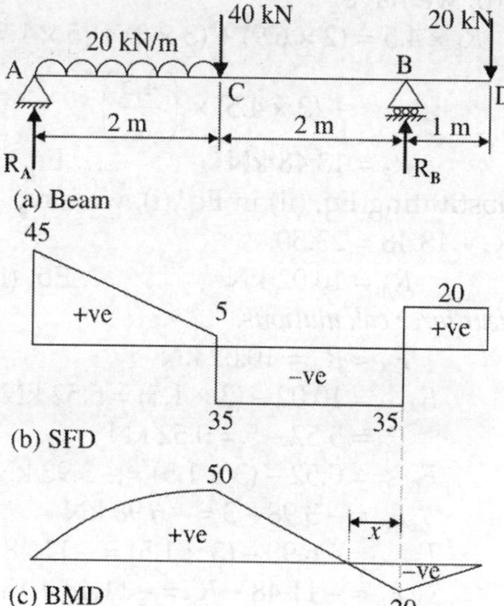

Fig. 5.62: Problem 45

$$70x = 40$$
$$x = 0.57 \text{ m from support B}$$

Or
$$M_{max} = -20 \times (1 + x) + 55x = 0$$
$$0 = -20 - 20x + 55x$$
$$20 = 35x$$
$$x = 0.57 \text{ m from support B}$$

The SFD and BMD diagrams are shown in **Figs 5.62(b) & (c)** respectively.

46. Draw the SFD and BMD for the loaded beam as shown in Fig. 5.63(a). Mark the salient values on the figure.

VTU – June 2012 – 16 Marks

Solution:

Reactions at supports:

$$R_A + R_B = 5 + 3 + 2 + (3 \times 4.5)$$
$$= 23.50 \text{ kN} \qquad \dots \text{Eq. (i)}$$

Taking moments about A and equating to zero, we have

$$R_B \times 4.5 = (2 \times 6.9) + (3 \times 3) + (5 \times 1.5)$$
$$+ (3 \times 4.5) \times \left(\frac{4.5}{2}\right)$$
$$R_B = 13.48 \text{ kN} \qquad \dots \text{Eq. (ii)}$$

Substituting Eq. (ii) in Eq. (i), we have

$$R_A + 13.48 = 23.50$$
$$R_A = 10.02 \text{ kN} \qquad \dots \text{Eq. (iii)}$$

Shear force calculations:

$$F_A = R_A = 10.02 \text{ kN}$$
$$F_{A-C} = 10.02 - (3 \times 1.5) = 5.52 \text{ kN}$$
$$F_C = 5.52 - 5 = 0.52 \text{ kN}$$
$$F_{C-D} = 0.52 - (3 \times 1.5) = -3.98 \text{ kN}$$
$$F_D = -3.98 - 3 = -6.98 \text{ kN}$$
$$F_{D-B} = -6.98 - (3 \times 1.5) = -11.48 \text{ kN}$$
$$F_B = -11.48 + R_B = -11.48 + 13.48 = 2 \text{ kN}$$
$$F_E = 2 \text{ kN} = F_B$$

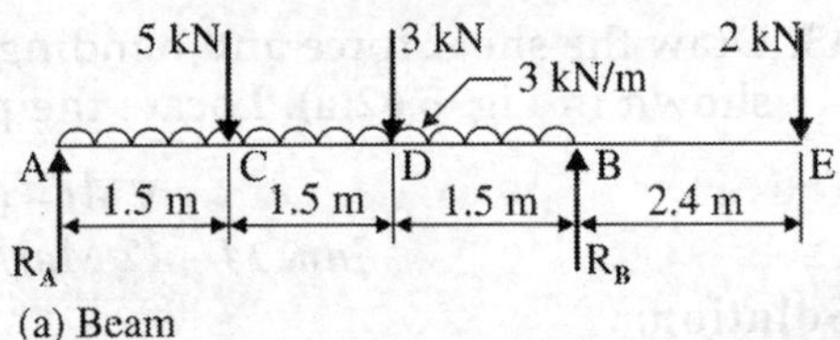

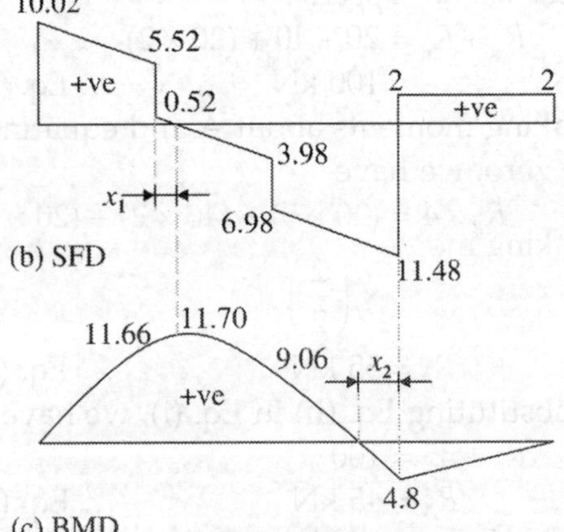

Fig. 5.63: Problem 46

Bending moment calculations:

$$M_A = 0$$
$$M_C = (10.02 \times 1.5) - (3 \times 1.5) \times \left(\frac{1.5}{2}\right) = 11.66 \text{ kN-m}$$
$$M_D = (10.02 \times 3) - (3 \times 3) \times \left(\frac{3}{2}\right) - (5 \times 1.5) = 9.06 \text{ kN-m}$$

$$M_B = -(2 \times 2.4) = -4.8 \text{ kN-m} \qquad \text{(from RHS)}$$
$$M_E = 0 \qquad \text{(from RHS)}$$

Maximum bending moment:

$$\frac{x_1}{0.52} = \frac{1.5 - x_1}{3.98}$$
$$3.98x_1 = 0.78 - 0.52x_1$$

$$4.5x_1 = 0.78$$
$$x_1 = 0.17 \text{ m from C}$$

$$M_{max1} = (10.02 \times 1.67) - (5 \times 0.17) - (3 \times 1.67) \times \left(\frac{1.67}{2}\right) = 11.70 \text{ kN-m}$$

Point of contraflexure:
$$M_{max2} = -2 \times (2.4 + x_2) + 13.48x_2 = 0$$
$$0 = -4.8 - 2x_2 + 13.48x_2$$
$$4.8 = 11.48x_2$$
$$x_2 = 0.42$$

Or $\quad M_{max2} = -2x_2 + 13.48(x_2 - 2.4) = 0$
$$0 = -2x_2 + 13.48x_2 - 32.35$$
$$4.8 = 11.48x_2$$
$$x_2 = 2.82 \text{ from E}$$

Or $\qquad x_2 = 0.42 \text{ from B}$

The SFD and BMD diagrams are shown in **Figs 5.63(b) & (c)** respectively.

47. Draw the shear force and bending moment diagrams for the beam shown in Fig. 5.64(a).

VTU – June/ July 2016 – 10 Marks

Solution:

Reactions at supports:
$$R_A + R_B = 40 + (15 \times 2) + (10 \times 2)$$
$$= 90 \text{ kN} \qquad \text{... Eq. (i)}$$

Taking moments about A and equating to zero, we have

$$R_B \times 8 = (40 \times 4) + (15 \times 2) \times \left(\frac{2}{2} + 1\right)$$
$$+ (10 \times 2) \times \left(\frac{2}{2} + 8\right)$$
$$R_B = 50 \text{ kN} \qquad \text{... Eq. (ii)}$$

Substituting Eq. (ii) in Eq. (i), we have
$$R_A + 50 = 90$$
$$R_A = 40 \text{ kN} \qquad \text{... Eq. (iii)}$$

Shear force calculations:
$$F_A = R_A = 40 \text{ kN}$$
$$F_D = 40 + 0 = 40 \text{ kN}$$
$$F_E = 40 - (15 \times 2) = 10 \text{ kN}$$
$$F_F = 10 - 40 = -30 \text{ kN}$$
$$F_B = -30 + R_B = -30 + 50 = 20 \text{ kN}$$
$$F_C = 20 - (10 \times 2) = 0 \text{ kN}$$

Bending moment calculations:
$$M_A = 0$$
$$M_D = (40 \times 1) = 40 \text{ kN-m}$$
$$M_E = (40 \times 3) - (15 \times 2) \times \left(\frac{2}{2}\right) = 90 \text{ kN-m}$$
$$M_F = -(10 \times 2) \times \left(\frac{2}{2} + 4\right) + (50 \times 4) = 100 \text{ kN-m} \qquad \text{(from RHS)}$$

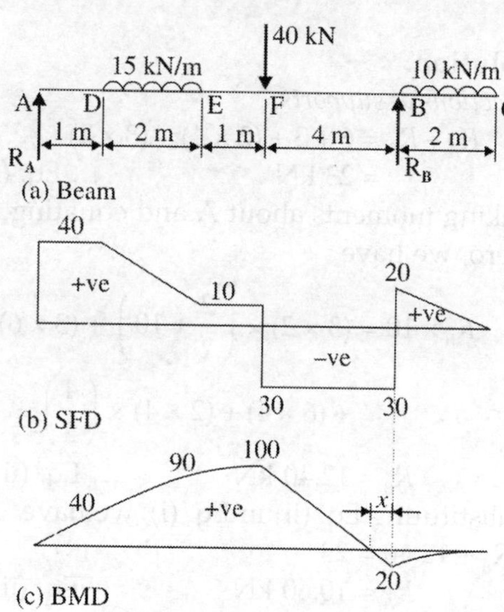

Fig. 5.64: Problem 47

$$M_B = -(10 \times 2) \times \left(\frac{2}{2}\right) = -20 \text{ kN-m} \qquad \text{(from RHS)}$$

$$M_C = 0 \qquad \text{(from RHS)}$$

Point of contraflexure:

$$\frac{x}{20} = \frac{4-x}{100}$$

$$100x = 80 - 20x$$

$$120x = 80$$

$$x = 0.67 \text{ m from B}$$

Or
$$M_{max} = -(10 \times 2) \times \left(\frac{2}{2} + x\right) + 50x = 0$$

$$0 = -20 - 20x + 50x$$

$$20 = 30x$$

$$x = 0.67 \text{ m from B}$$

The SFD and BMD diagrams are shown in **Figs 5.64(b) & (c)** respectively.

48. Draw shear force and bending moment diagram for the beam shown in Fig. 5.65(a), indicating the principal values.

VTU – June/ July 2008 – 16 Marks

Solution:

Reactions at supports:

$$R_A + R_B = 6 + 3 + (2 \times 4) + (3 \times 2)$$

$$= 23 \text{ kN} \qquad \text{... Eq. (i)}$$

Taking moments about A and equating to zero, we have

$$R_B \times 10 = (3 \times 2) \times \left(\frac{2}{2} + 10\right) + (3 \times 6)$$

$$+ (6 \times 4) + (2 \times 4) \times \left(\frac{4}{2}\right)$$

$$R_B = 12.40 \text{ kN} \qquad \text{... Eq. (ii)}$$

Substituting Eq. (ii) in Eq. (i), we have

$$R_A + 12.40 = 23$$

$$R_A = 10.60 \text{ kN} \qquad \text{... Eq. (iii)}$$

Shear force calculations:

$$F_A = R_A = 10.60 \text{ kN}$$

$$F_{A-C} = 10.60 - (2 \times 4) = 2.60 \text{ kN}$$

$$F_C = 2.60 - 6 = -3.40 \text{ kN}$$

$$F_D = -3.40 - 3 = -6.40 \text{ kN}$$

$$F_B = -6.40 + R_B = -6.40 + 12.40 = 6 \text{ kN}$$

$$F_E = 6 - (3 \times 2) = 0 \text{ kN}$$

Bending moment calculations:

$$M_A = 0$$

$$M_C = (10.60 \times 4) - (2 \times 4) \times \left(\frac{4}{2}\right) = 26.40 \text{ kN-m}$$

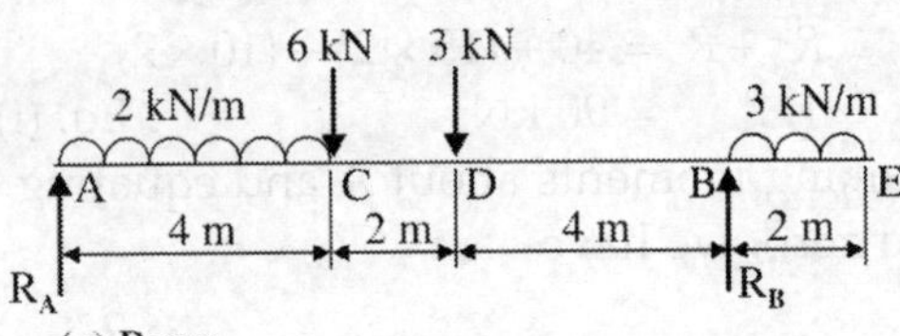

(a) Beam

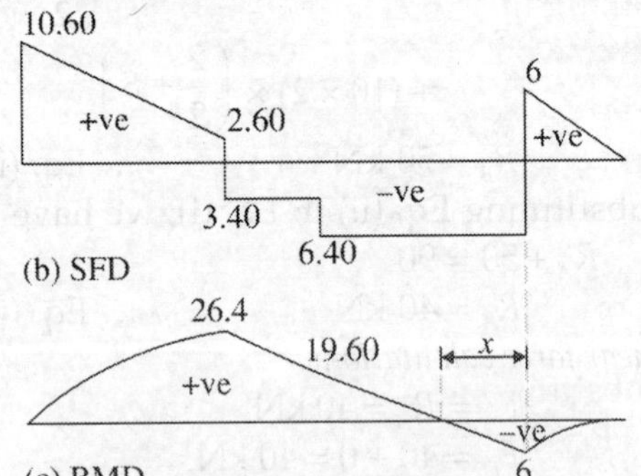

(b) SFD

(c) BMD

Fig. 5.65: Problem 48

$$M_D = (10.60 \times 6) - (2 \times 4) \times \left(\frac{4}{2} + 2\right) - (6 \times 2) = 19.60 \text{ kN-m}$$

$$M_B = -(3 \times 2) \times \left(\frac{2}{2}\right) = -6 \text{ kN-m} \qquad \text{(from RHS)}$$

$$M_E = 0 \qquad \text{(from RHS)}$$

Point of contraflexure:

$$\frac{x}{6} = \frac{4-x}{19.60}$$

$$19.60x = 24 - 6x$$

$$24.60x = 24$$

$$x = 0.94 \text{ m from B}$$

Or $\quad M_{\max} = -(3 \times 2) \times \left(\frac{2}{2} + x\right) + 12.40x = 0$

$$0 = -6 - 6x + 12.40x$$

$$6 = 6.40x$$

$$x = 0.94 \text{ m from B}$$

The SFD and BMD diagrams are shown in **Figs 5.65(b) & (c)** respectively.

49. For the beam shown in Fig. 5.66(a), draw shear force and bending moment diagrams. Locate the point of contraflexure, if any.

VTU – Dec. 08/ Jan. 09 – 15 Marks

Reactions at supports:

$$R_A + R_B = (10 \times 2) + 30 + 40 + (20 \times 4)$$
$$= 170 \text{ kN} \qquad \dots \text{Eq. (i)}$$

Taking moments about A and equating to zero, we have

$$R_B \times 6 = (20 \times 4) \times \left(\frac{4}{2} + 4\right) + (40 \times 4)$$

$$\qquad\qquad + (30 \times 2) + (10 \times 2) \times \left(\frac{2}{2}\right)$$

$$R_B = 120 \text{ kN} \qquad \dots \text{Eq. (ii)}$$

Substituting Eq. (ii) in Eq. (i), we have

$$R_A + 120 = 170$$

$$R_A = 50 \text{ kN} \qquad \dots \text{Eq. (iii)}$$

Shear force calculations:

$$F_A = R_A = 50 \text{ kN}$$

$$F_{A-C} = 50 - (10 \times 2) = 30 \text{ kN}$$

$$F_C = 30 - 30 = 0 \text{ kN}$$

$$F_D = 0 - 40 = -40 \text{ kN}$$

$$F_{D-B} = -40 - (20 \times 2) = -80 \text{kN}$$

$$F_B = -80 + R_B = -80 + 120 = 40 \text{ kN}$$

$$F_E = 40 - (20 \times 2) = 0 \text{ kN}$$

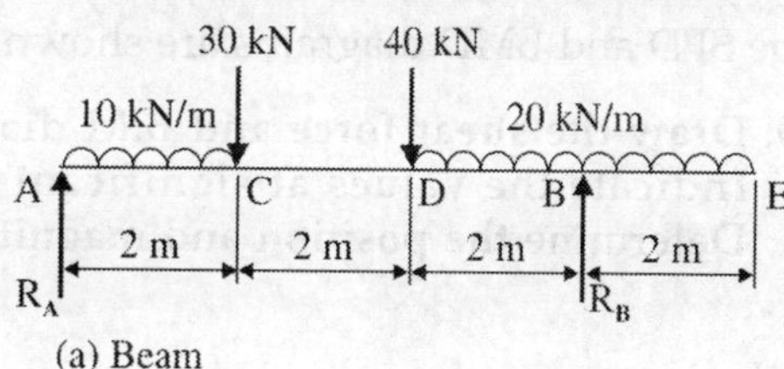

(a) Beam

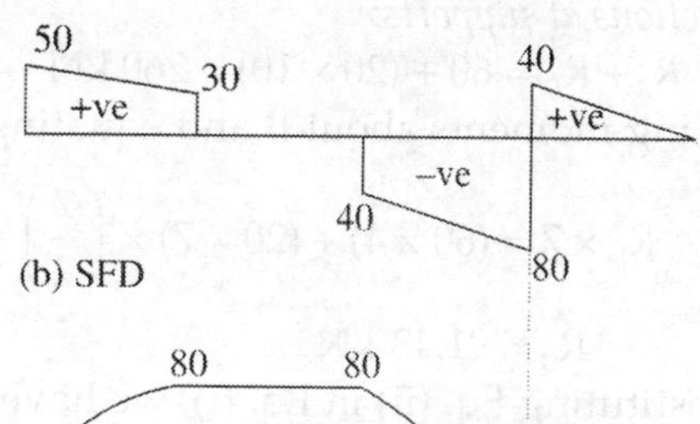

(b) SFD

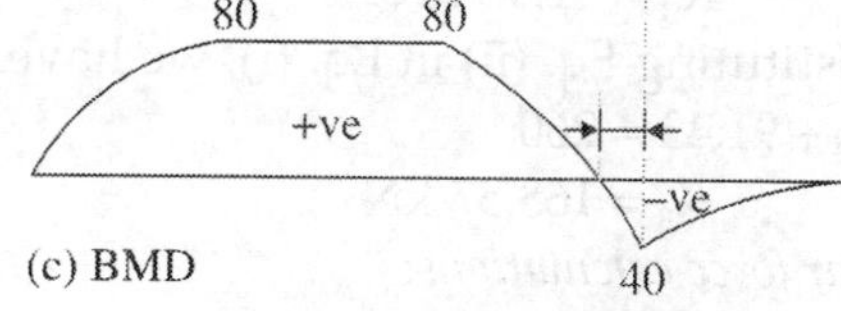

(c) BMD

Fig. 5.66: Problem 49

Bending moment calculations:

$$M_A = 0$$

$$M_C = (50 \times 2) - (10 \times 2) \times \left(\frac{2}{2}\right) = 80 \text{ kN-m}$$

$$M_D = (50 \times 4) - (10 \times 2) \times \left(\frac{2}{2} + 2\right) - (30 \times 2) = 80 \text{ kN-m}$$

$$M_B = -(20 \times 2) \times \left(\frac{2}{2}\right) = -40 \text{ kN-m} \qquad \text{(from RHS)}$$

$$M_E = 0 \qquad \text{(from RHS)}$$

Point of contraflexure:

$$M_{max} = -20 \times \left[\frac{(2+x)^2}{2}\right] + 120x = 0$$

$$0 = -10 \times (4 + x^2 + 4x) + 120x$$
$$0 = -40 - 10x^2 - 40x + 120x$$
$$0 = 10x^2 - 80x + 40$$
$$x = 0.54 \text{ m \& } 7.46 \text{ m}$$
$$x = 0.54 \text{ m from B}$$

Or $\quad M_{max} = -20x \times \left(\dfrac{x}{2}\right) + 120(x - 2) = 0$

$$0 = -10x^2 + 120x - 240$$
$$x = 2.54 \text{ m from E}$$

The SFD and BMD diagrams are shown in **Figs 5.66(b) & (c)** respectively.

50. **Draw the shear force and B.M diagrams for the beam shown in Fig. 5.67(a). Indicate the values at significant points. Locate the point of contraflexure. Determine the position and magnitude of the maximum B.M.**

VTU – June/ July 2014 – 15 Marks

Solution:

Reactions at supports:

$$R_B + R_D = 60 + (20 \times 10) = 260 \text{ kN} \qquad \text{... Eq. (i)}$$

Taking moments about B and equating to zero, we have

$$R_D \times 7 = (60 \times 4) + (20 \times 7) \times \left(\frac{7}{2}\right) - (20 \times 3) \times \left(\frac{3}{2}\right)$$

$$R_D = 91.43 \text{ kN} \qquad \text{... Eq. (ii)}$$

Substituting Eq. (ii) in Eq. (i), we have

$$R_B + 91.43 = 260$$
$$R_B = 168.57 \text{ kN} \qquad \text{... Eq. (iii)}$$

Shear force calculations:

$$F_A = 0 \text{ kN}$$
$$F_{A-B} = 0 - (20 \times 3) = -60 \text{ kN}$$
$$F_B = -60 + R_B = -60 + 168.57 = 108.57 \text{ kN}$$
$$F_{B-C} = 108.57 - (20 \times 4) = 28.50 \text{ kN}$$
$$F_C = 28.57 - 60 = -31.43 \text{ kN}$$

$$F_{C-D} = -31.43 - (20 \times 3) = -91.43 \text{ kN}$$
$$F_D = -91.43 = R_D$$

Bending moment calculations:
$$M_A = 0$$
$$M_B = -(20 \times 3) \times \left(\frac{3}{2}\right) = -90 \text{ kN-m}$$
$$M_C = (91.43 \times 3) - (20 \times 3) \times \left(\frac{3}{2}\right)$$
$$= 184.29 \text{ kN-m} \qquad \text{(from RHS)}$$
$$M_D = 0 \qquad \text{(from RHS)}$$

Point of contraflexure:

$$M_{max} = -20 \times \left[\frac{(3+x)^2}{2}\right] + 168.57x = 0$$

$$0 = -10 \times (9 + x^2 + 6x) + 168.57x$$
$$0 = -90 - 10x^2 - 60x + 168.57x$$
$$0 = 10x^2 - 108.57x + 90$$
$$x = 9.95 \text{ m} \ \& \ 0.90 \text{ m}$$
$$x = 0.90 \text{ m from B}$$

Or $\quad M_{max} = -20x \times \left(\dfrac{x}{2}\right) + 168.57(x-3) = 0$

$$0 = -10x^2 + 168.57x - 505.71$$
$$x = 3.90 \text{ m} \ \& \ 12.95 \text{ m from A}$$
$$x = 3.90 \text{ m from A}$$

The SFD and BMD diagrams are shown in **Figs 5.67(b)** & **(c)** respectively.

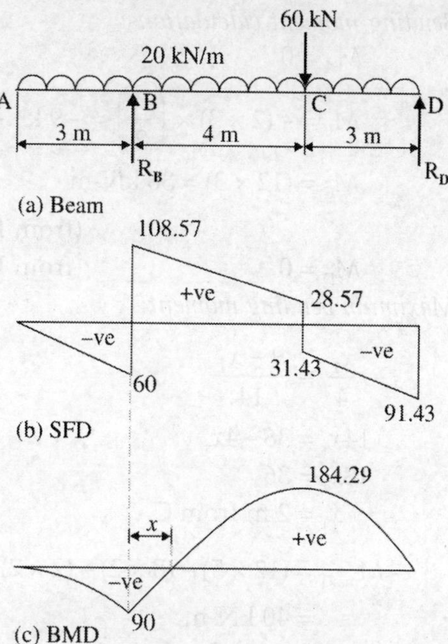

Fig. 5.67: Problem 50

51. For the beam shown in Fig. 5.68(a), draw SFD and BMD and mark the values of salient points.

Solution:

Reactions at supports:
$$R_B + R_D = 8 + (2 \times 12) = 32 \text{ kN} \qquad \dots \text{Eq. (i)}$$

Taking moments about B and equating to zero, we have

$$R_D \times 12 = (8 \times 9) + (2 \times 9) \times \left(\frac{9}{2}\right) - (2 \times 3) \times \left(\frac{3}{2}\right)$$
$$R_D = 12 \text{ kN} \qquad \dots \text{Eq. (ii)}$$

Substituting Eq. (ii) in Eq. (i), we have
$$R_B + 12 = 32$$
$$R_B = 20 \text{ kN} \qquad \dots \text{Eq. (iii)}$$

Shear force calculations:
$$F_A = 0 \text{ kN}$$
$$F_{A-B} = 0 - (2 \times 3) = -6 \text{ kN}$$
$$F_B = -6 + R_B = -6 + 20 = 14 \text{ kN}$$
$$F_{B-C} = 14 - (2 \times 9) = -4 \text{ kN}$$
$$F_C = -4 - 8 = -12 \text{ kN}$$
$$F_D = -12 \text{ kN} = R_D$$

Bending moment calculations:

$$M_A = 0$$

$$M_B = -(2 \times 3) \times \left(\frac{3}{2}\right) = -9 \text{ kN-m}$$

$$M_C = (12 \times 3) = 36 \text{ kN-m}$$

$$\text{(from RHS)}$$

$$M_D = 0 \qquad \text{(from RHS)}$$

Maximum bending moment:

$$\frac{x_1}{4} = \frac{9 - x_1}{14}$$

$$14x_1 = 36 - 4x_1$$

$$18x_1 = 36$$

$$x_1 = 2 \text{ m from C}$$

$$M_{\text{max1}} = (12 \times 5) - (8 \times 2) - (2 \times 2) \times \left(\frac{2}{2}\right)$$

$$= 40 \text{ kN-m}$$

Point of contraflexure:

$$M_{\text{max2}} = -2 \times \left[\frac{(3 + x_2)^2}{2}\right] + 20x_2 = 0$$

$$0 = -(9 + x_2^2 + 6x_2) + 20x_2$$

$$0 = -9 - x_2^2 - 6x_2 + 20x_2$$

$$0 = x_2^2 - 14x_2 + 9$$

$$x_2 = 13.32 \text{ m} \ \& \ 0.68 \text{ m}$$

$$x_2 = 0.68 \text{ m from B}$$

Or
$$M_{\text{max2}} = -2x_2 \times \left(\frac{x_2}{2}\right) + 20(x_2 - 3) = 0$$

$$0 = -x_2^2 + 20x_2 - 60$$

$$x_2 = 3.68 \text{ m} \ \& \ 16.32 \text{ m}$$

$$x_2 = 3.68 \text{ m from A}$$

The SFD and BMD diagrams are shown in **Figs 5.68(b) & (c)** respectively.

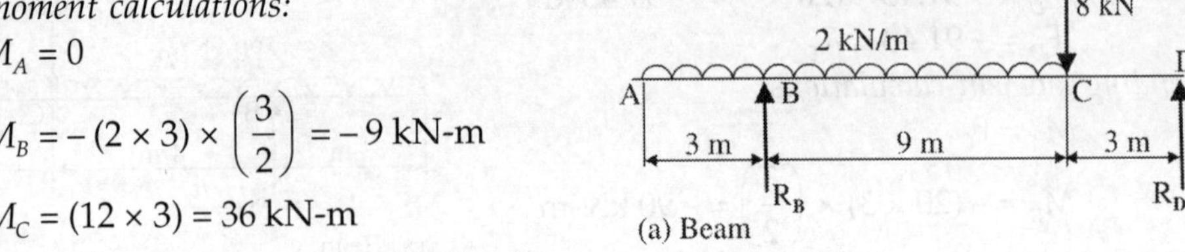

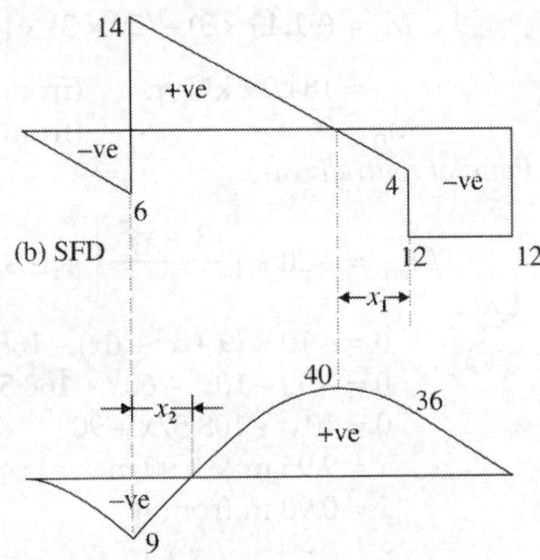

Fig. 5.68: Problem 51

52. Draw the SFD and BMD for the overhanging beam shown in Fig. 5.69(a). Indicate all the significant values including point of contraflexure.

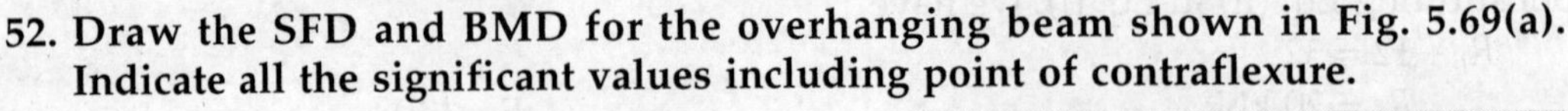

Solution:

Reactions at supports:

$$R_A + R_B = 20 + \left(\frac{1}{2} \times 60 \times 2\right) = 80 \text{ kN} \qquad \qquad \text{... Eq. (i)}$$

Taking moments about A and equating to zero, we have

$$R_B \times 4 = (20 \times 5) + \left[\left(\frac{1}{2} \times 60 \times 2\right) \times \left(\frac{2 \times 2}{3} + 1\right)\right]$$

$$R_B = 60 \text{ kN} \hspace{4cm} \dots \text{Eq. (ii)}$$

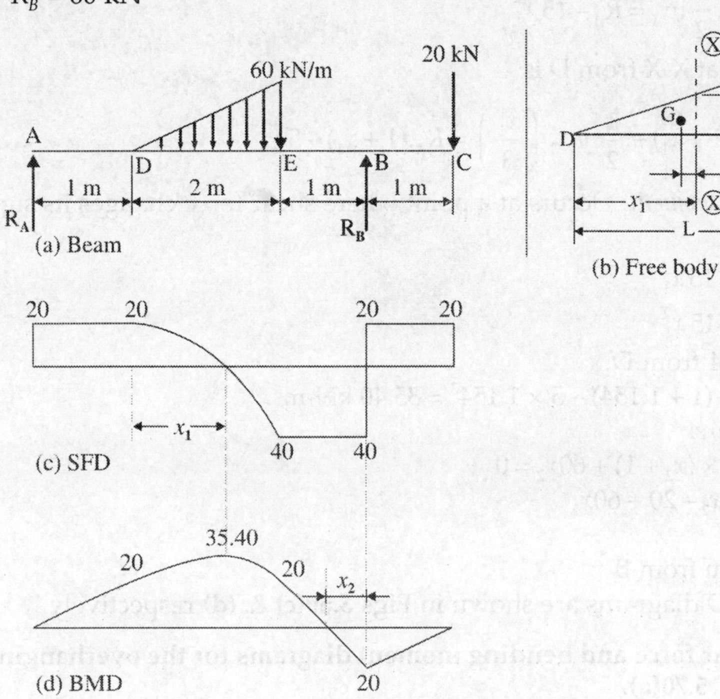

Fig. 5.69: Problem 52

Substituting Eq. (ii) in Eq. (i), we have

$$R_A + 60 = 80$$

$$R_A = 20 \text{ kN} \hspace{4cm} \dots \text{Eq. (iii)}$$

Shear force calculations:

$$F_A = 20 \text{ kN}$$

$$F_D = 20 \text{ kN}$$

$$F_E = 20 - \left(\frac{1}{2} \times 60 \times 2\right) = -40 \text{ kN}$$

$$F_B = -40 + R_B = -40 + 20 = 20 \text{ kN}$$

$$F_C = 20 \text{ kN} = F_B$$

Bending moment calculations:

$$M_A = 0$$

$$M_D = (20 \times 1) = 20 \text{ kN-m}$$

$$M_E = (60 \times 1) - (20 \times 2) = 20 \text{ kN-m} \hspace{1cm} \text{(from RHS)}$$

$$M_B = (-20 \times 1) = -20 \text{ kN-m}$$

$$M_C = 0 \hspace{4cm} \text{(from RHS)}$$

To find rate of loading or load intensity **(Refer to sec 5.9.4):**

Consider a section X-X at a distance x_1 from end D as shown in **Fig. 5.69 (b)**. From similar triangles

$$\frac{y}{w} = \frac{x_1}{L} \Rightarrow y = \frac{wx_1}{L} = \frac{60x_1}{2} = 30x_1 \qquad \text{... Eq. (iv)}$$

Shear force at X-X between D and E is

$$F_{x1} = R_A - \frac{1}{2} yx_1 = R_A - 15\,x_1^2 \qquad \text{... Eq. (v)}$$

Bending moment at X-X from D is

$$M_{x1} = R_A \cdot (1 + x_1) - \frac{1}{2}\, y.x_1 \left(\frac{x_1}{3} \right) = R_A \cdot (1 + x_1) - 5\,x_1^3 \qquad \text{... Eq. (vi)}$$

Maximum bending moment: Occurs at a point where shear force changes its sign.

i.e. $\qquad F_{x1} = 0$

$$0 = R_A - 15\,x_1^2$$
$$0 = 20 - 15\,x_1^2$$
$$x_1 = 1.154 \text{ from D}$$
$$M_{x1} = 20 \times (1 + 1.154) - 5 \times 1.154^3 = 35.40 \text{ kN-m}$$

Point of contraflexure:
$$M_{\max} = -20 \times (x_2 + 1) + 60x_2 = 0$$
$$0 = -20x_2 - 20 + 60x_2$$
$$20 = 40x_2$$
$$x_2 = 0.5 \text{ m from B}$$

The SFD and BMD diagrams are shown in **Figs 5.69(c) & (d)** respectively.

53. Draw the shear force and bending moment diagrams for the overhanging beam shown in Fig. 5.70(a).

VTU – June/ July 2009 – 20 Marks

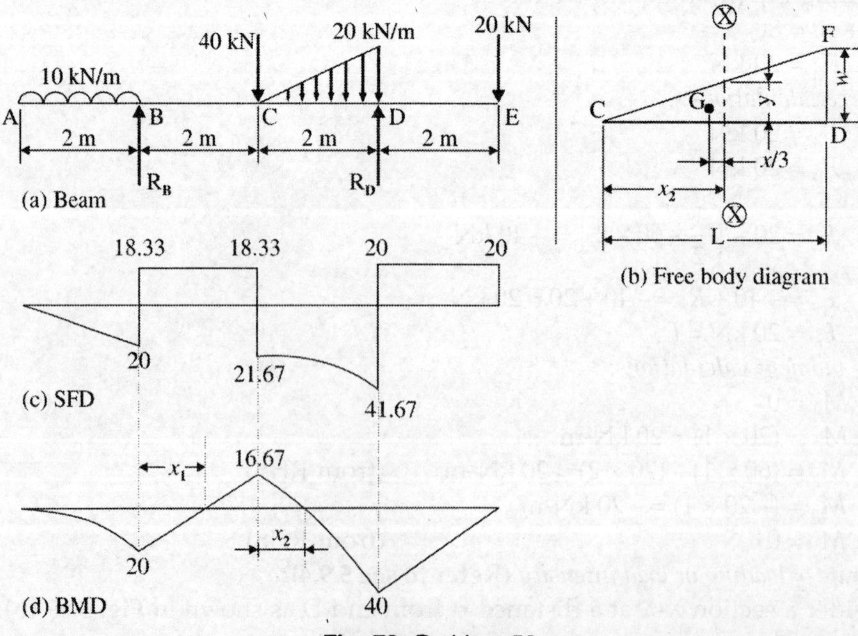

Fig. 70: Problem 53

Solution:
Reactions at supports:

$$R_B + R_D = 20 + 40 + \left(\frac{1}{2} \times 20 \times 2\right) + (10 \times 2) = 100 \text{ kN} \qquad \text{... Eq. (i)}$$

Taking moments about B and equating to zero, we have

$$R_D \times 4 = (20 \times 6) + \left[\left(\frac{1}{2} \times 20 \times 2\right) \times \left(\frac{2 \times 2}{3} + 2\right)\right] + (40 \times 2) - (10 \times 2) \times \left(\frac{2}{2}\right)$$

$$R_D = 61.67 \text{ kN} \qquad \text{... Eq. (ii)}$$

Substituting Eq. (ii) in Eq. (i), we have

$$R_B + 61.67 = 100$$

$$R_B = 38.33 \text{ kN} \qquad \text{... Eq. (iii)}$$

Shear force calculations:

$$F_A = 0 \text{ kN}$$
$$F_{A-B} = 0 - (10 \times 2) = -20 \text{ kN}$$
$$F_B = -20 + 38.33 = 18.33 \text{ kN}$$
$$F_C = 18.33 - 40 = -21.67 \text{ kN}$$

$$F_{C-D} = -21.67 - \left(\frac{1}{2} \times 20 \times 2\right) = -41.67 \text{ kN}$$

$$F_D = -41.67 + 61.67 = 20 \text{ kN}$$
$$F_E = 20 \text{ kN} = F_D$$

Bending moment calculations:

$$M_A = 0$$

$$M_B = -(10 \times 2) \times \left(\frac{2}{2}\right) = -20 \text{ kN-m}$$

$$M_C = -(10 \times 2) \times \left(\frac{2}{2} + 2\right) + (38.33 \times 2) = 16.67 \text{ kN-m}$$

$$M_D = -(20 \times 2) = -40 \text{ kN-m} \qquad \text{(from RHS)}$$
$$M_E = 0 \qquad \text{(from RHS)}$$

Point of contraflexure:

To find x_1:

$$\frac{x_1}{20} = \frac{2 - x_1}{16.67}$$

$$16.67 x_1 = 40 - 20 x_1$$

$$36.67 x_1 = 40$$

$$x_1 = 1.09 \text{ m from B}$$

To find x_2:

Consider a section X-X at a distance x_2 from end C, as shown in **Fig. 5.70(b).**

$$\frac{y}{w} = \frac{x_2}{L} \Rightarrow y = \frac{w x_2}{L} = \frac{20 x_2}{2} = 10 x_2 \qquad \text{... Eq. (iv)}$$

Bending moment at X-X from C is

$$M_{x2} = -(10 \times 2) \times \left(\frac{2}{2} + 2 + x_2\right) + R_B.(2 + x_2) - 40 x_2 - \frac{1}{2}\, y.x_2 \left(\frac{x_2}{3}\right) = 0 \quad \text{... Eq. (v)}$$

$$0 = -20 \times (3 + x_2) + 38.33 \times (2 + x_2) - 40x_2 - \frac{1}{2} \times 10\, x_2^2 \times \left(\frac{x_2}{3}\right)$$

$$0 = -60 - 20x_2 + 76.66 + 38.33x_2 - 40x_2 - 1.67\, x_2^3$$

$$0 = -1.67\, x_2^3 - 21.67x_2 + 16.66$$

$$x_2 = 0.74 \text{ m from C}$$

The SFD and BMD diagrams are shown in **Figs 5.70(c) & (d)** respectively.

54. Draw the shear force and bending moment diagrams for the overhanging beam shown in Fig. 5.71(a).

Solution:

Reactions at supports:

$$R_A + R_C = 20 \text{ kN} \qquad \dots \text{ Eq. (i)}$$

Taking moments about A and equating to zero, we have

$$R_C \times 3 = (20 \times 4) + 10$$
$$R_C = 30 \text{ kN} \qquad \dots \text{ Eq. (ii)}$$

Substituting Eq. (ii) in Eq. (i), we have

$$R_A + 30 = 20$$
$$R_A = -10 \text{ kN} \quad \text{(opposite side)}$$
$$\dots \text{ Eq. (iii)}$$

Shear force calculations:

$$F_A = R_A = -10 \text{ kN}$$
$$F_B = -10 - 0 = -10 \text{ kN remains}$$

constant up to C

$$F_C = -10 + 30 = 20 \text{ kN}$$
$$F_D = 20 \text{ kN} = F_C$$

Bending moment calculations:

$$M_A = 0$$
$$M_{A-B} = -(10 \times 2) = -20 \text{ kN-m}$$
$$M_B = -20 + 10 = -10 \text{ kN-m}$$
$$M_C = -(20 \times 1) = -20 \text{ kN-m}, \; M_D = 0$$

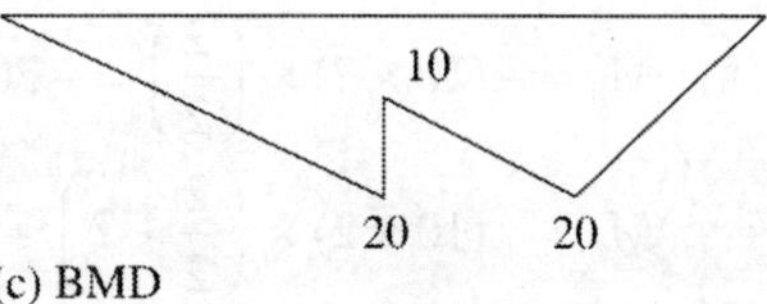

Fig. 71: Problem 54

The SFD and BMD diagrams are shown in **Figs 5.71(b) & (c)** respectively.

55. Draw SFD and BMD for the beam shown in Fig. 5.72(a). Indicate point of contraflexure, if any.

VTU – Dec. 15/ Jan. 16 – 14 Marks

Solution:

Reactions at supports:

$$R_A + R_B = 30 + (2 \times 1) = 32 \text{ kN} \qquad \dots \text{ Eq. (i)}$$

Taking moments about A and equating to zero, we have

$$R_B \times 7 = (30 \times 2) + 10 + (2 \times 1) \times \left(\frac{1}{2} + 7\right)$$

$$R_B = 12.14 \text{ kN} \qquad \dots \text{ Eq. (ii)}$$

Substituting Eq. (ii) in Eq. (i), we have

$$R_A + 12.14 = 32$$
$$R_A = 19.86 \text{ kN} \qquad \dots \text{ Eq. (iii)}$$

Shear force calculations:
$$F_A = R_A = 19.86 \text{ kN}$$
$$F_C = 19.86 - 30 = -10.14 \text{ kN}$$
$$\text{remains constant up to B}$$
$$F_B = -10.14 + 12.14 = 2 \text{ kN}$$
$$F_E = 2 - (2 \times 1) = 0 \text{ kN}$$

Bending moment calculations:
$$M_A = 0$$
$$M_C = (19.86 \times 2) = 39.72 \text{ kN-m}$$
$$M_{C-D} = (19.86 \times 5) - (30 \times 3) = 9.30 \text{ kN-m}$$
$$M_D = 9.30 + 10 = 19.30 \text{ kN-m}$$
$$M_B = -(2 \times 1) \times \left(\frac{1}{2}\right) = -1 \text{ kN-m}$$
$$M_E = 0$$

Point of contraflexure:
$$M_{max} = -(2 \times 1) \times \left(\frac{1}{2} + x\right) + 12.14x = 0$$
$$0 = -1 - 2x + 12.14x$$
$$1 = 10.14x$$
$$x = 0.098 \text{ m from B}$$

The SFD and BMD diagrams are shown in **Figs 5.72(b) & (c)** respectively.

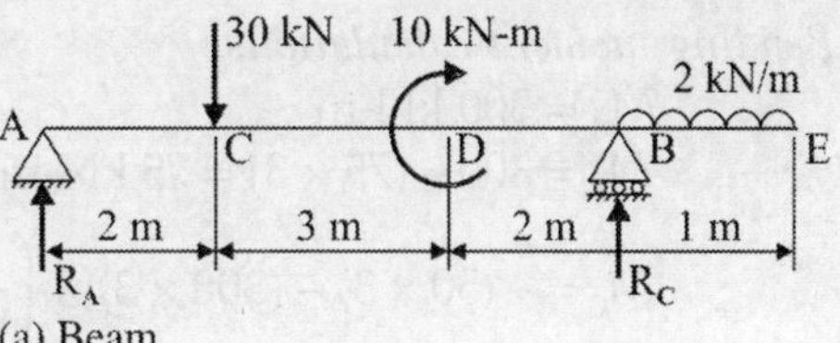

(a) Beam

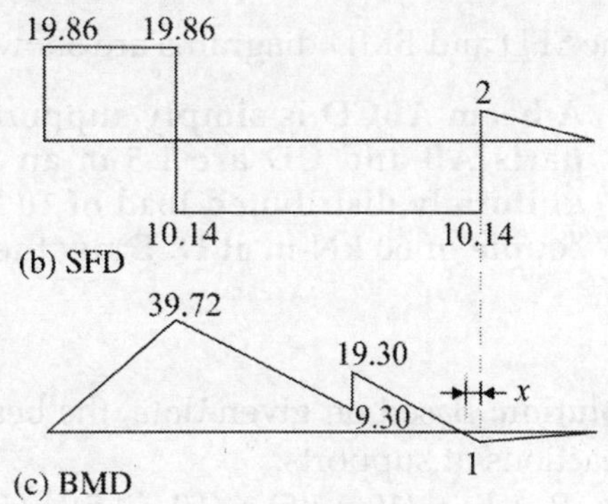

(b) SFD

(c) BMD

Fig. 72: Problem 55

56. For the beam shown in Fig. 5.73(a), draw the shear force and bending moment diagram. Mark the value at salient points.

Solution:
Reactions at supports:
$$R_A + R_C = 50 + (300 \times 6) = 1850 \text{ kN}$$
$$\ldots \text{ Eq. (i)}$$

Taking moments about A and equating to zero, we have

$$R_C \times 6 = (50 \times 9) + (300 \times 6) \times \left(\frac{6}{2} + 3\right) + 300$$

$$R_C = 1925 \text{ kN} \qquad \ldots \text{ Eq. (ii)}$$

Substituting Eq. (ii) in Eq. (i), we have
$$R_A + 1925 = 1850$$
$$R_A = -75 \text{ kN} \qquad \ldots \text{ Eq. (iii)}$$

Shear force calculations:
$$F_A = R_A = -75 \text{ kN}$$
$$F_B = -75 + 0 = -75 \text{ kN}$$
$$\text{remains constant up to B}$$
$$F_{B-C} = -75 - (300 \times 3) = -975 \text{ kN}$$
$$F_C = -975 + 1925 = 950 \text{ kN}$$
$$F_{C-D} = 950 - (300 \times 3) = 50 \text{ kN}$$
$$F_D = 50 \text{ kN} = F_{C-D}$$

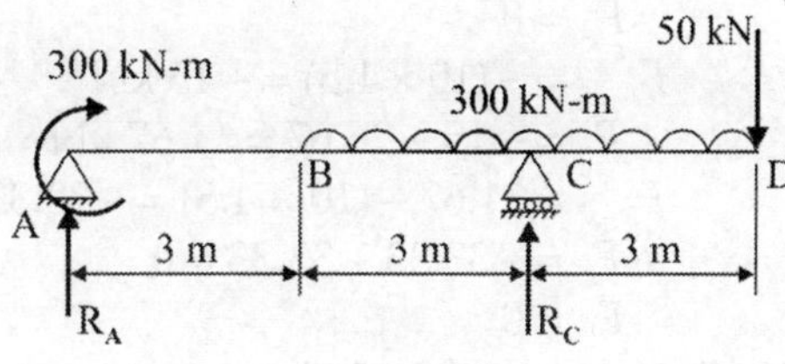

(a) Beam

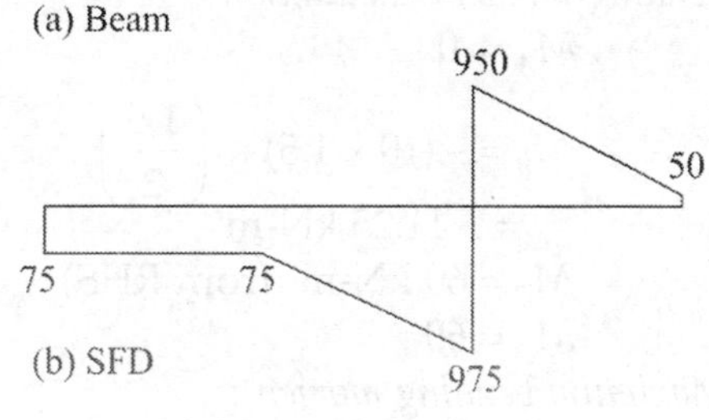

(b) SFD

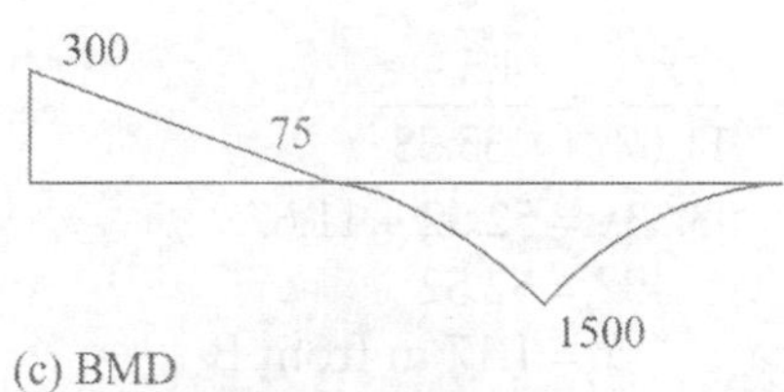

(c) BMD

Fig. 73: Problem 56

Bending moment calculations:

$$M_A = 300 \text{ kN-m}$$
$$M_B = 300 - (75 \times 3) = 75 \text{ kN-m}$$
$$M_C = -(50 \times 3) - (300 \times 3) \times \left(\frac{3}{2}\right) = -1500 \text{ kN-m (from RHS)}$$
$$M_D = 0$$

The SFD and BMD diagrams are shown in **Figs 5.73(b) & (c)** respectively.

57. **A beam ABCD is simply supported at B and C, 4.5 m apart and overhanging parts AB and CD are 1.5 m an 2 m long respectively. The beam carries a uniformly distributed load of 10 kN/m between A and C. There is a clockwise couple of 60 kN-m at D. Draw the SFD and BMD and mark the salient points.**

VTU – Dec. 15/ Jan. 16 – 14 Marks

Solution: Based on given data, the beam is as shown in **Fig. 5.74(a)**.

Reactions at supports:

$$R_B + R_C = (10 \times 1.5) + (10 \times 4.5) = 60 \text{ kN} \qquad \text{... Eq. (i)}$$

Taking moments about A and equating to zero, we have

$$R_C \times 4.5 = 60 + (10 \times 4.5) \times \left(\frac{4.5}{2}\right) - (10 \times 1.5) \times \left(\frac{1.5}{2}\right)$$

$$R_C = 33.33 \text{ kN} \qquad \text{... Eq. (ii)}$$

Substituting Eq. (ii) in Eq. (i), we have

$$R_B + 33.33 = 60$$
$$R_A = 26.67 \text{ kN} \qquad \text{... Eq. (iii)}$$

Shear force calculations:

$$F_A = 0$$
$$F_{A-B} = -(10 \times 1.5) = -15 \text{ kN}$$
$$F_B = -15 + 26.67 = 11.67 \text{ kN}$$
$$F_{B-C} = 11.67 - (10 \times 4.5) = -33.33 \text{ kN}$$
$$F_C = -33.33 + 33.33 = 0$$
$$F_D = 0$$

Bending moment calculations:

$$M_A = 0$$
$$M_B = -(10 \times 1.5) \times \left(\frac{1.5}{2}\right)$$
$$= -11.25 \text{ kN-m}$$
$$M_C = 60 \text{ kN-m (from RHS)}$$
$$M_D = 60$$

Maximum bending moment:

$$\frac{x}{11.67} = \frac{4.5 - x}{33.33}$$
$$33.33x = 52.52 - 11.67x$$
$$45x = 52.52$$
$$x = 1.17 \text{ m from B}$$

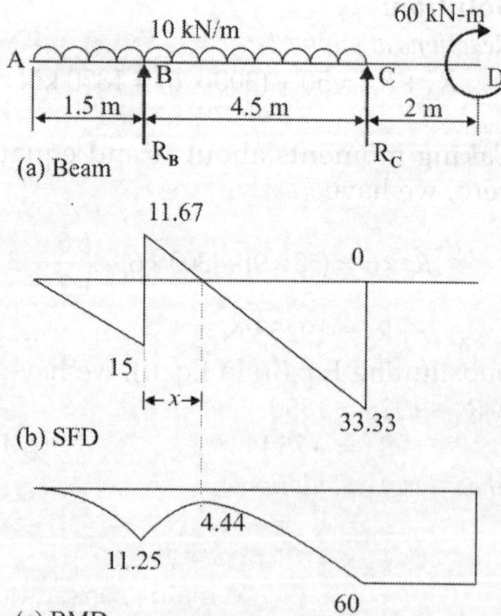

Fig. 74: Problem 57

The SFD and BMD diagrams are shown in **Figs 5.74(b) & (c)** respectively

58. For the beam shown in Fig. 5.75(a), determine the magnitude of load P acting at C such that the reaction at the supports A and B are equal. Draw the shear force and bending moment diagrams, indicating the values of salient points.

VTU – Dec. 2010 – 15 Marks, June/ July 2014 – 20 Marks;
(CV) June/ July 2008 – 14 Marks

Solution:

To find P: Since the reactions are equal, we have

$$R_A + R_B = P + (45 \times 4)$$
$$2R_B = 180 + P$$
$$R_B = 90 + 0.5P \qquad \dots \text{Eq. (i)}$$

Taking moments about A and equating to zero, we have

$$R_B \times 6 = 7P + 30 + (45 \times 4) \times \left(\frac{4}{2}\right)$$
$$6R_B = 7P + 390$$
$$6 \times (90 + 0.5P) = 7P + 390$$
$$540 + 3P = 7P + 390$$
$$P = 37.5 \text{ kN}$$

Reactions at supports:

$$R_B = 90 + (0.5 \times 37.5)$$
$$= 108.75 \text{ kN} = R_A$$

Shear force calculations:

$$F_A = 108.75 \text{ kN}$$
$$F_{A-D} = 108.75 - (45 \times 4) = -71.25 \text{ kN}$$
$$F_D = -71.25 \text{ kN}$$

remains constant up to B

$$F_B = -71.25 + 108.75 = 37.5 \text{ kN}$$
$$F_C = 37.5 \text{ kN} = P$$

Bending moment calculations:

$$M_A = 0$$
$$M_{A-D} = (108.75 \times 4) - (45 \times 4) \times \left(\frac{4}{2}\right) = 75 \text{ kN-m}$$
$$M_D = 75 + 30 = 105 \text{ kN-m}$$
$$M_B = -37.5 \times 1 = -37.5 \text{ kN-m}$$
$$M_C = 0$$

Maximum bending moment: Occurs at a point where shear force changes its sign.

$$\frac{x_1}{108.75} = \frac{4 - x_1}{71.25}$$
$$71.25x_1 = 435 - 108.75x_1$$
$$180x_1 = 435$$
$$x_1 = 2.42 \text{ m from A}$$

Point of contraflexure:

$$\frac{x_2}{37.5} = \frac{2 - x_2}{105}$$

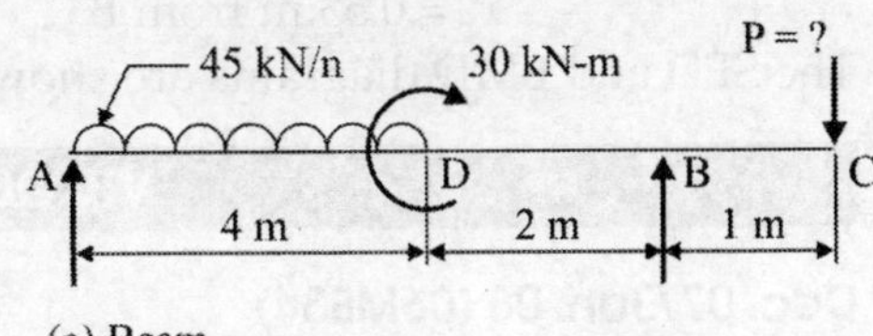

(a) Beam

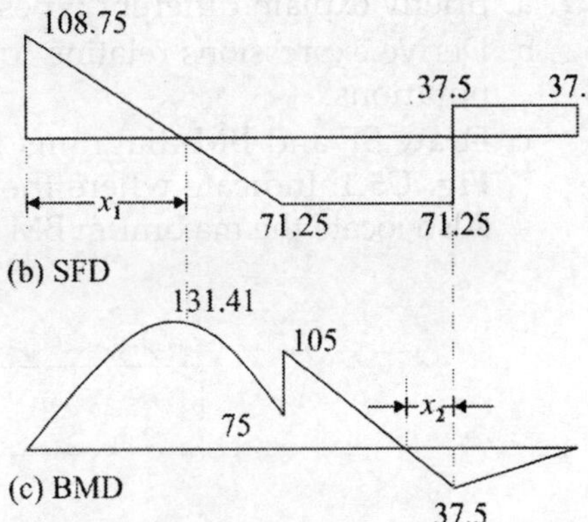

Fig. 75: Problem 58

$$105x_2 = 75 - 37.5x_2$$
$$142.50x_2 = 75$$
$$x_2 = 0.53 \text{ m from B}$$

Or
$$M_{max} = -37.5 \times (1 + x_2) + 108.75x_2$$
$$0 = -37.5 - 37.5x_2 + 108.75x_2$$
$$37.5 = 71.25x_2$$
$$x_2 = 0.53 \text{ m from B}$$

The SFD and BMD diagrams are shown in **Figs 5.75(b) & (c)** respectively.

VTU QUESTION PAPERS

Dec. 07/Jan. 08 (06ME34)

1. a. Briefly explain different types of beam supports. **(03 Marks)**
   b. Derive expressions relating load, shear force and bending moment with usual notations. **(05 Marks)**
   c. Draw SF and BM diagrams for the loading pattern on the beam shown in **Fig. U5.1**. Indicate where the inflexion and contraflexure points are located. Also locate the maximum BM and its magnitude. **(12 Marks)**

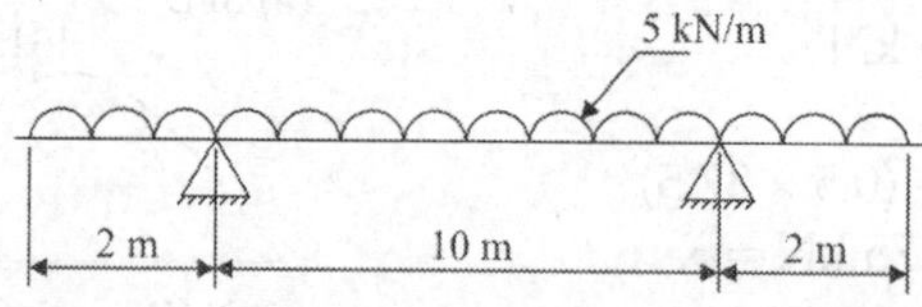

Fig. U5.1

June/July 2008 (06ME34)

2. a. Define shear force, bending moment, point of contraflexure and beam. **(04 Marks)**
   b. Draw shear force and bending moment diagram for the beam shown in **Fig. U5.2** indicating the principal values. **(16 Marks)**

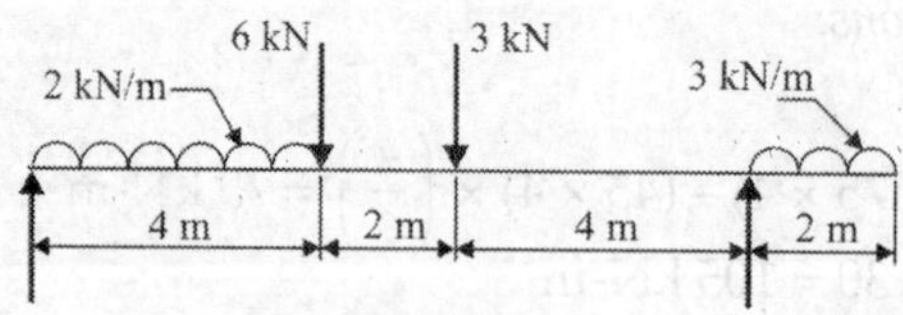

Fig. U5.2

Dec. 08/Jan. 09 (06ME34)

3. a. What are the different types of beams? Explain briefly. **(05 Marks)**
   b. For the beam shown in **Fig. U5.3**, draw shear force and bending moment diagrams. Locate the point of contraflexure, if any. **(15 Marks)**

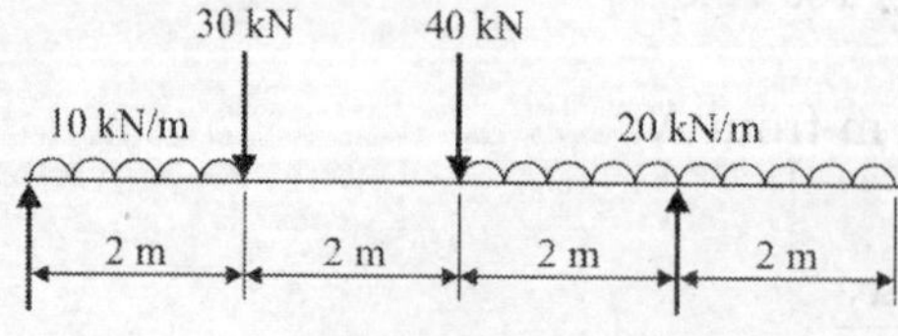

Fig. U5.3

June/July 2009 (06ME34)

4. Draw the shear force and bending moment diagrams for the overhanging beam shown in **Fig. U5.4**. **(20 Marks)**

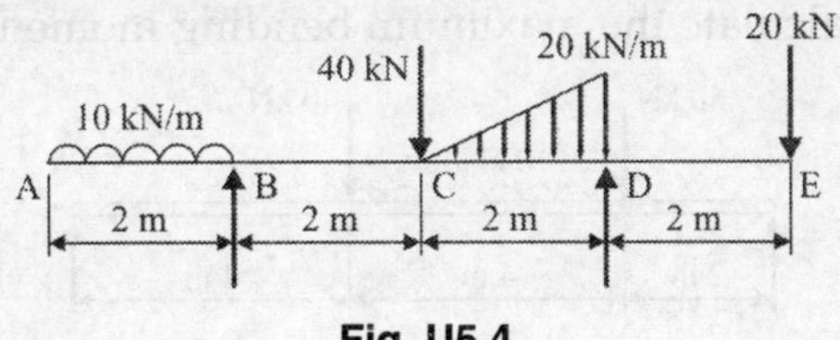

Fig. U5.4

Dec. 09/Jan. 10 (06ME34)

5. Draw the shear force and bending moment diagrams for the beam loaded as shown in **Fig. U5.5**. **(20 Marks)**

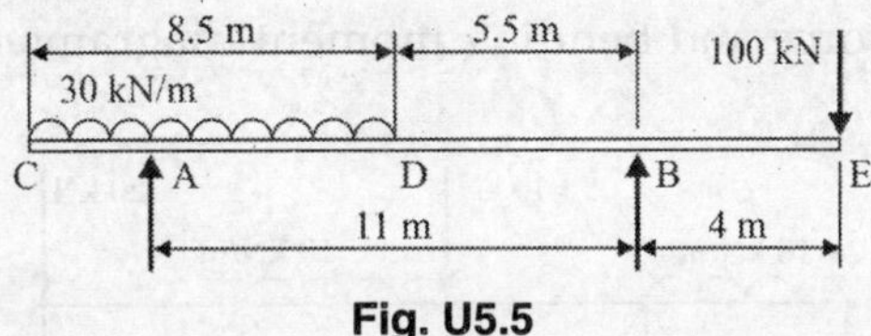

Fig. U5.5

May/June 2010 (06ME34)

6. a. Explain the terms:
    i. Sagging bending moment   ii. Hogging bending moment
    iii. Point of contraflexure. **(06 Marks)**
   b. Draw shear force and bending moment diagrams for the loading pattern on the beam shown in **Fig. U5.6**. Indicate where the inflexion and contraflexure points are located. Also locate the maximum bending moment with its magnitude. **(14 Marks)**

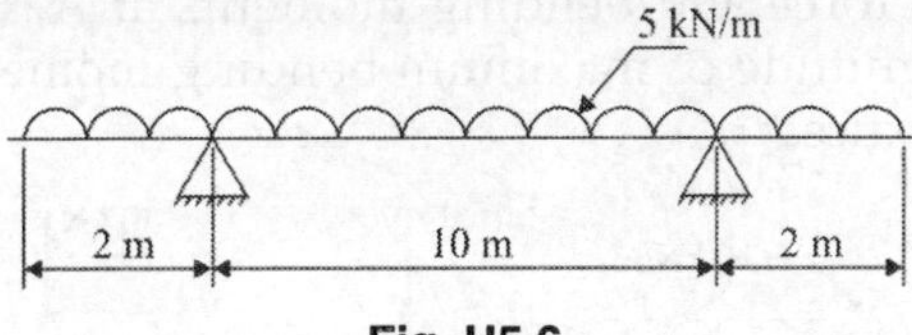

Fig. U5.6

Dec. 2010 (06ME34)

7. a. Obtain the relationship between shear force and bending moment. **(05 Marks)**
   b. For the beam shown in **Fig. U5.7**, determine the magnitude of load P acting at C such that the reaction at the supports A and B are equal. Draw the shear force and bending moment diagrams, indicating the values of salient points. **(15 Marks)**

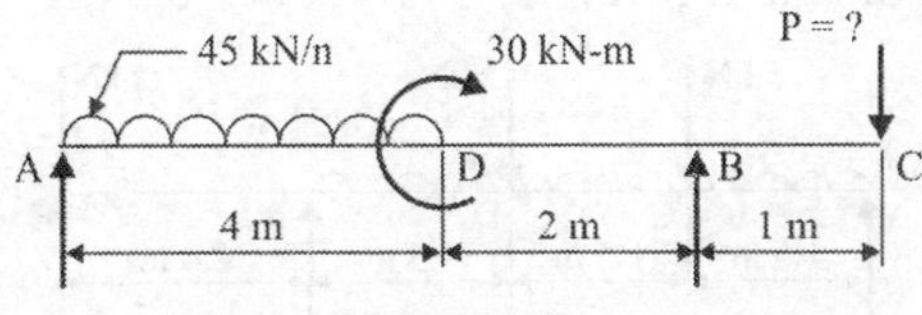

Fig. U5.7

June/July 2011 (06ME34)

8. a. Define shear force and bending moment. **(04 Marks)**

   b. Draw the shear force and bending moment diagrams for the beam shown in **Fig. U5.8**. Also calculate the maximum bending moment. **(16 Marks)**

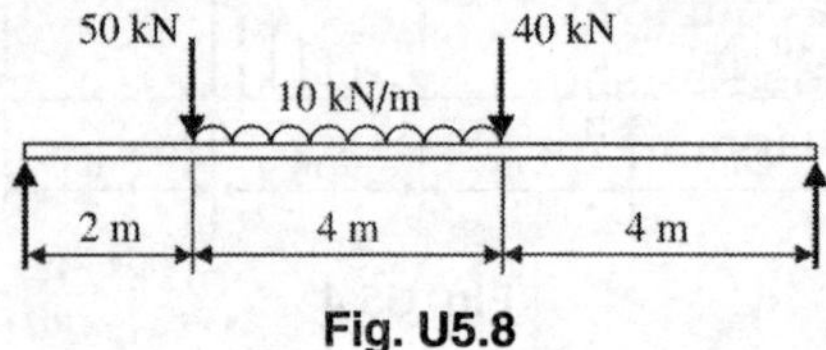

Fig. U5.8

Dec. 2011 (06ME34)

9. a. Classify beams (based on the type of supports) and loads and sketch them. **(06 Marks)**

   b. Draw the shear force and bending moment diagrams for the beam shown in **Fig. U5.9**. **(14 Marks)**

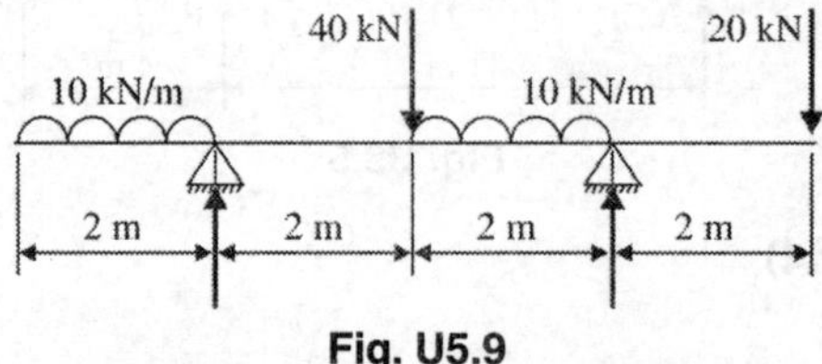

Fig. U5.9

Dec. 2011 (10ME34)

10. a. Derive an expression to establish a relationship between the intensity of load w, shear force F and bending moment M in the beam. **(06 Marks)**

   b. A beam 25 m long is supported at A and B and is loaded as shown in **Fig. U5.10**. Draw the shear force and bending moment diagrams for the beam computing shear force and bending moments at A, E, D B and C. Find the position and magnitude of maximum bending moment. Also determine the point of contraflexure. **(14 Marks)**

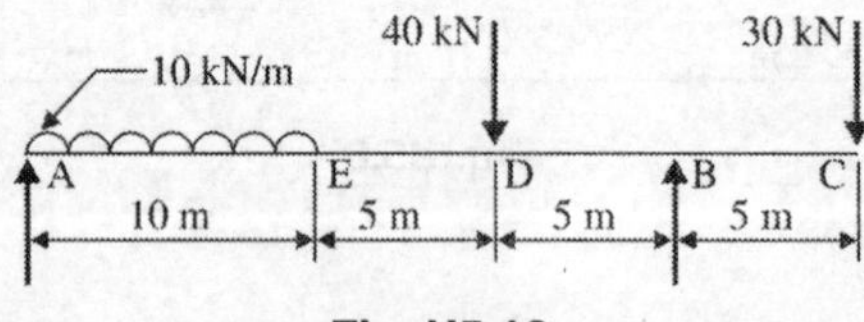

Fig. U5.10

June 2012 (06ME34)

11. a. Explain with neat diagram the sagging and hogging bending moment. **(04 Marks)**

   b. Draw the SFD and BMD for the loaded beam as shown in **Fig. U5.11**. Mark the salient values on the figure. **(16 Marks)**

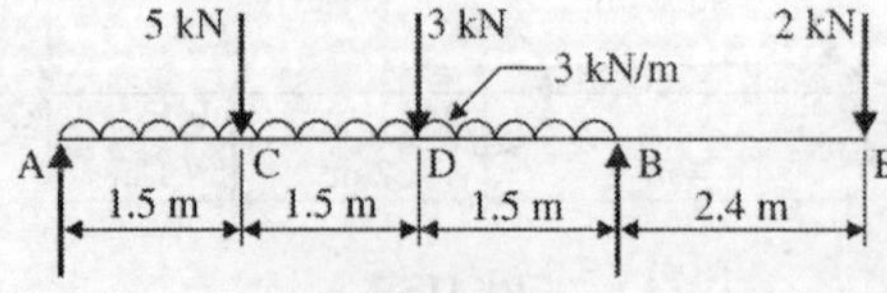

Fig. U5.11

June 2012 (10ME34)

12. a. Define: i. shear force   ii. bending moment   iii. point of contraflexure.
   (03 Marks)
   b. Draw the shear force and bending moment diagrams for a simply supported beam subjected to a couple at mid-span, as shown in **Fig. U5.12(a)**. **(05 Marks)**
   c. A cantilever is loaded as shown in **Fig. U5.12(b)**. Draw the shear force and bending moment diagrams for the beam. **(12 Marks)**

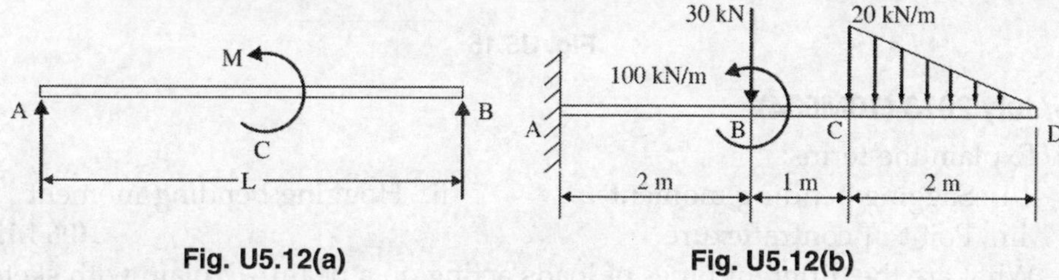

Fig. U5.12(a)   **Fig. U5.12(b)**

Dec. 2012 (10ME34)

13. a. A cantilever of length 2 m carries a uniformly distributed load of 1 kN/m run over a length of 1.5 m from the free end. Draw the shear force and bending moment diagram for the cantilever. **(06 Marks)**
   b. Draw the shear force and bending moment diagram for the overhanging beam carrying a uniformly distributed load of 2 kN/m over the entire length and a point load of 2 kN as shown in **Fig. U5.13**. Locate the point of contraflexure.
   (14 Marks)

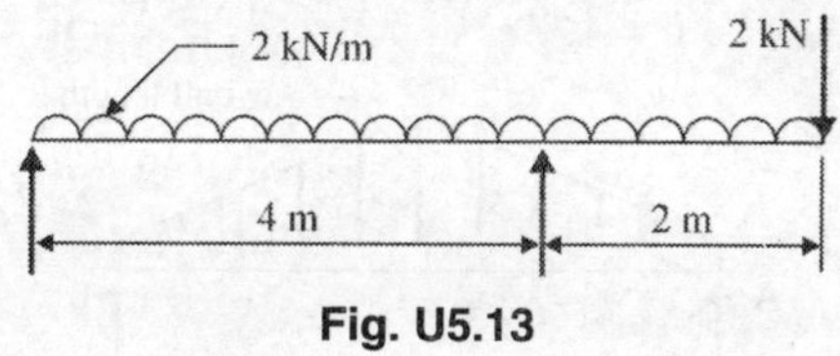

Fig. U5.13

Jan. 2013 (06ME34)

14. a. Define the following terms:
   i. shear force   ii. bending moment
   iii. shear force diagram   iv. bending moment diagram.
   (04 Marks)
   b. A beam is simply supported at its ends and carries uniformly distributed load of 20 per m length over its entire length. Derive expression for shear force and bending moment at an section at a distance 'X' from the left support. Draw the shear force and bending moment diagrams. **(08 Marks)**
   c. Draw the shear force and bending moment diagrams for the cantilever shown in **Fig. U5.14**. **(08 Marks)**

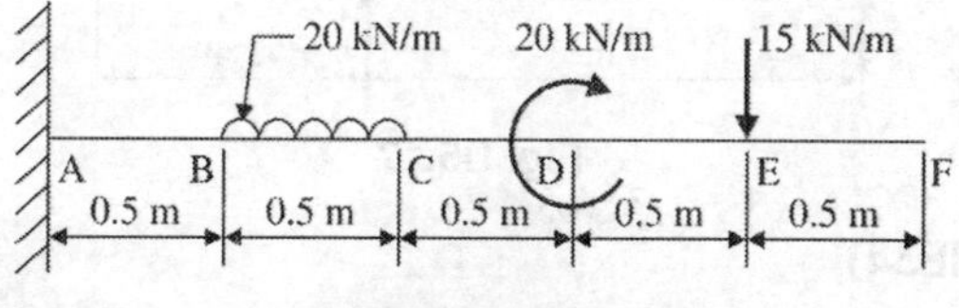

Fig. U5.14

June/July 2013 (06ME34)

15. Draw the shear force and bending moment diagrams for the beam shown in **Fig. U5.15**. Locate the point of contraflexure. **(20 Marks)**

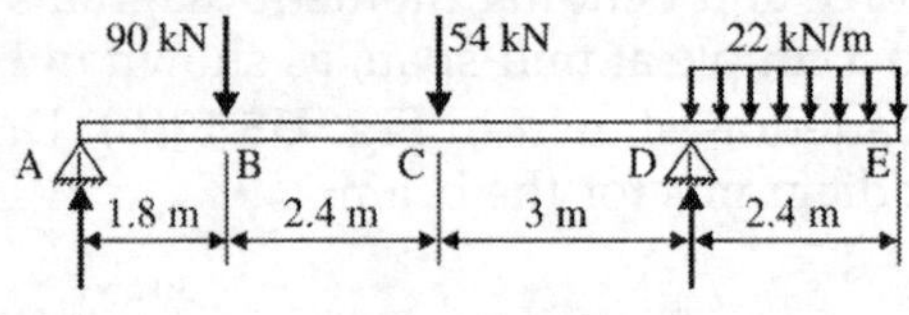

Fig. U5.15

June/July 2013 (10ME34)

16. a. Explain the terms:
   i. Sagging bending moment
   ii. Hogging bending moment
   iii. Point of contraflexure. **(06 Marks)**
   b. What are the different types of loads acting on a beam? Explain with sketches. **(06 Marks)**
   c. A simply supported beam of span 6 m is subjected to a concentrated load of 25 kN acting at a distance of 2 m from the left end. Also subjected to a uniformly distributed load of 10 kN/m over the entire span. Draw the bending moment and shear force diagrams indicating the maximum and minimum values. **(08 Marks)**

Dec. 13/Jan. 14 (06ME34)

17. Draw the bending moment and shear force diagrams for the beam shown in **Fig. U5.16** below. **(20 Marks)**

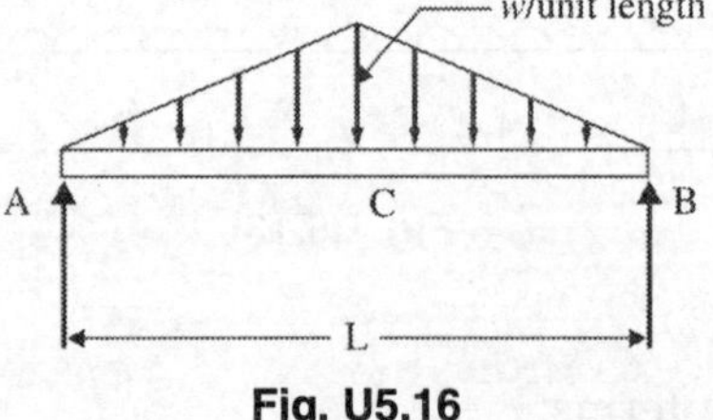

Fig. U5.16

Dec. 13/Jan. 14 (10ME34)

18. a. Define a beam. Explain with sketches, different types of beams. **(06 Marks)**
   b. Draw the shear force and bending moment diagrams for the overhanging beam carrying uniformly distributed load of 2 kN/m over the entire length and a point load of 2 kN as shown in **Fig. U5.17**. Locate the point of contraflexure. **(14 Marks)**

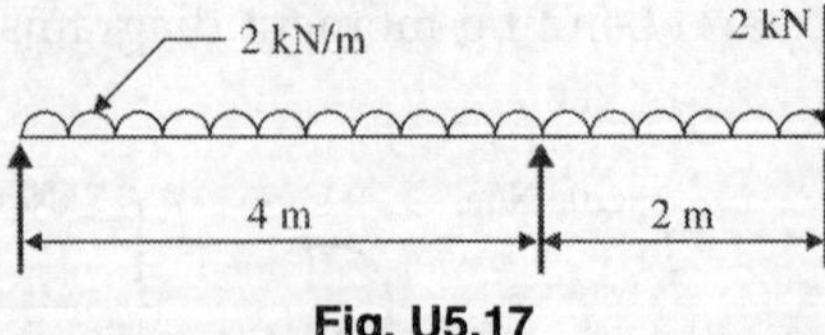

Fig. U5.17

June/July 2014 (06ME34)

19. For the beam shown in **Fig. U5.18**, determine the magnitude of load P acting at C such that the reaction at the supports A and B are equal. Draw the SF and BM

diagrams for the beam. Mark the salient points and their values on the diagram. Locate the point of contra flexure, if any. **(20 Marks)**

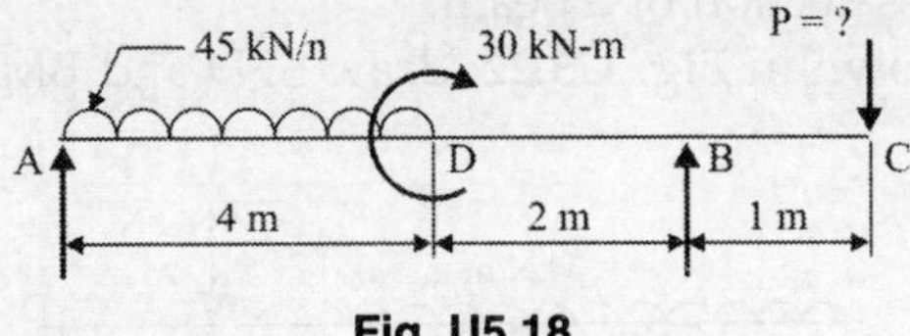

Fig. U5.18

June/July 2014 (10ME34)

20. a. Derive the relationship between load, shear force and bending moment.
(05 Marks)

b. Briefly explain the different types of loads. **(03 Marks)**

c. Draw SFD and BMD for the loading pattern on the beam shown in **Fig. U5.19**. Indicate the point of contraflexure. Also locate the maximum BM with its magnitude. **(12 Marks)**

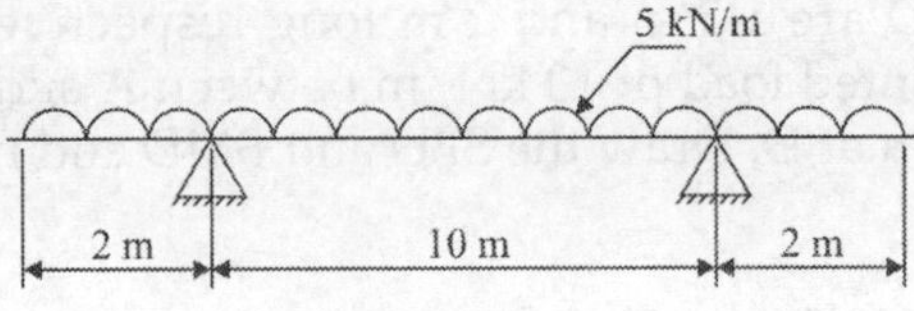

Fig. U5.19

Dec. 14/Jan. 15 (06ME34)

21. a. What are the different types of beams? Briefly explain. **(05 Marks)**

b. For the beam shown in **Fig. U5.20**, draw the shear force and bending moment diagrams. Clearly indicate the point of contra flexure. **(15 Marks)**

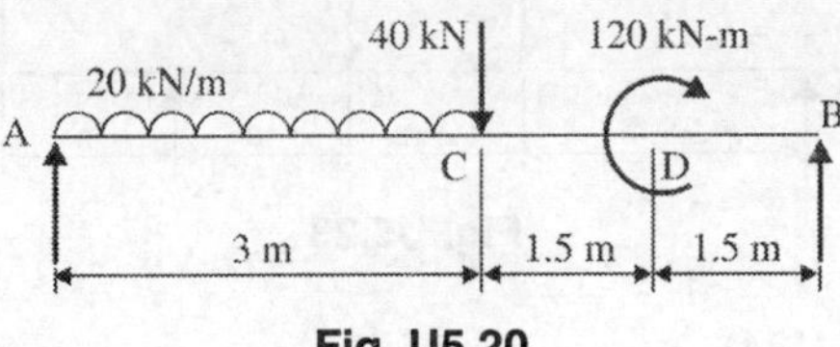

Fig. U5.20

Dec. 14/Jan. 15 (10ME34)

22. a. Derive expressions relating load, shear force and bending moment with usual notations. **(05 Marks)**

b. Draw the SFD and BMD for the overhanging beam shown in **Fig. U5.21**. Indicate all the significant values including point of contraflexure. **(15 Marks)**

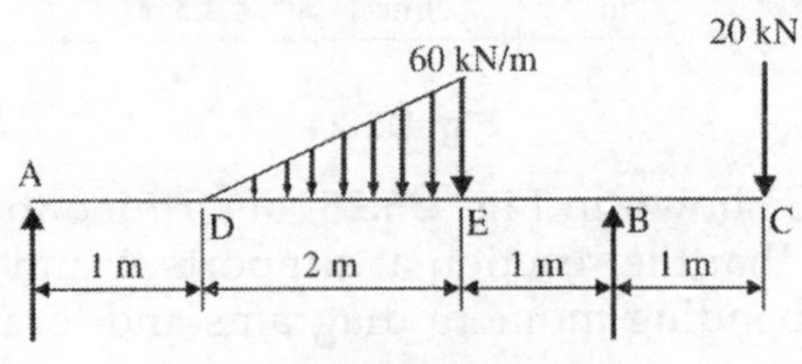

Fig. U5.21

June/July 15 (10ME34)

23. a. Establish the relationship between distributed load, shear force and bending moment at a cross-section of a beam. **(06 Marks)**

    b. For the beam shown in **Fig. U5.22**, draw SFD and BMD and mark the values of salient points. **(14 Marks)**

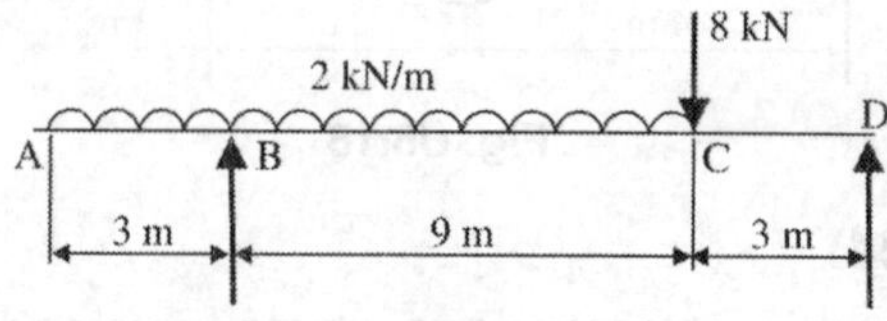

Fig. U5.22

Dec. 15/Jan. 16 (10ME/AU34)

24. a. Deduce the relationship between load (W), shear force (F) and bending moment (M). **(06 Marks)**

    b. A beam ABCD is simply supported at B and C, 4.5 m apart and overhanging parts AB and CD are 1.5 m and 2 m long respectively. The beam carries a uniformly distributed load of 10 kN/m between A and C. There is a clockwise couple of 60 kN-m at D. Draw the SFD and BMD and mark the salient points. **(14 Marks)**

June/July 2016 (10ME/AU34)

25. a. Derive an expression to establish a relationship between the intensity of load, shear force and bending moment. **(05 Marks)**

    b. Draw the shear force and bending moment diagram for the beam shown in **Fig. U5.23**. Locate the point of contra-flexure. **(15 Marks)**

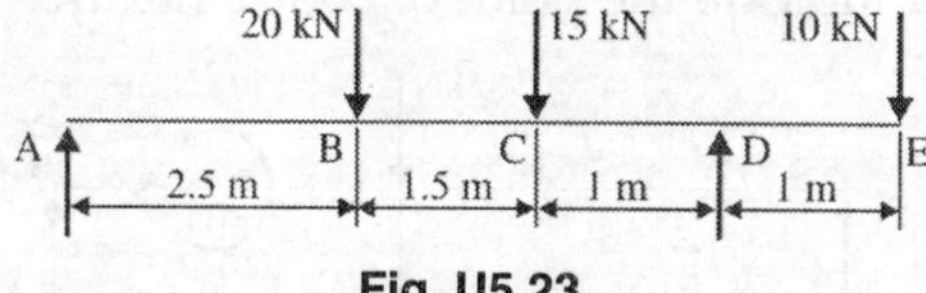

Fig. U5.23

DEC. 16/JAN. 17 (10ME/AU34)

26. a. Draw the shear force and bending moment diagrams for the cantilever beam shown in **Fig. U5.24**. **(08 Marks)**

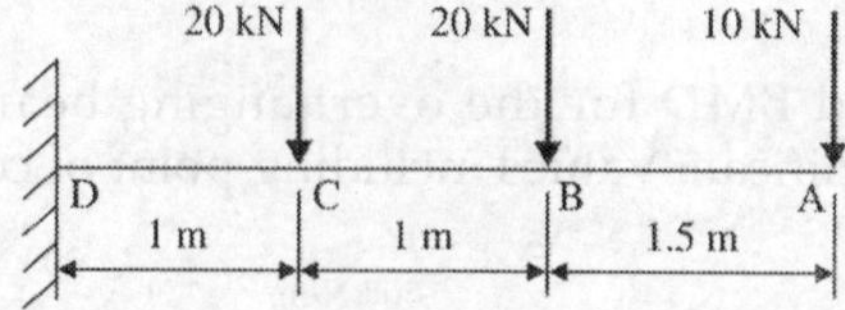

Fig. U5.24

    b. For the beam AC shown in **Fig. U5.25**, determine the magnitude of load P acting at C such that the reaction at supports A and B are equal. Draw the shear force and bending moment diagrams and locate the point of contra-flexure, if any. **(12 Marks)**

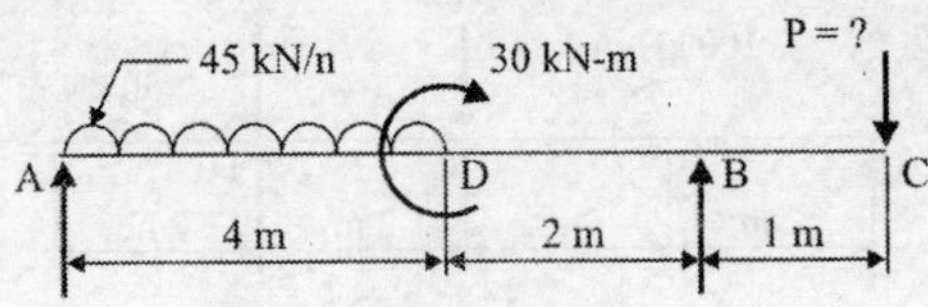

Fig. U5.25

Dec. 16/Jan. 17 (15ME/MA34)

27. Draw the SF and BM diagrams for the beam shown in **Fig. U5.26**.   **(16 Marks)**

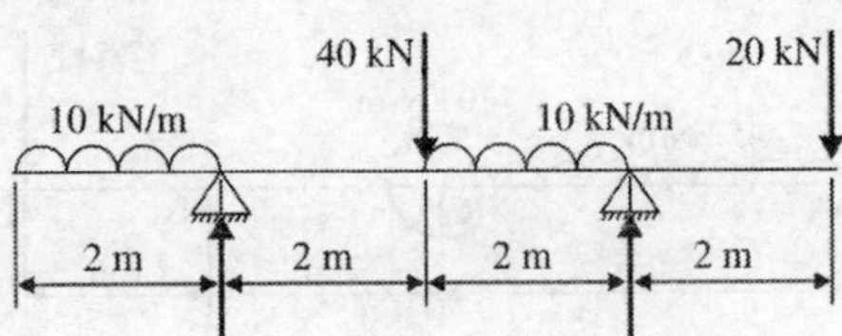

Fig. U5.26

June/July 2017 (15ME/MA34)

28. a. Define and explain the following terms:
   i. Shear force   ii. Bending moment
   iii. Shear force diagram   iv. Bending moment diagram   **(06 Marks)**
   b. Define and explain the following types of load:
   i. Concentrated load   ii. Uniformly distributed load
   iii. Uniformly varying load.   **(06 Marks)**
   c. A simply supported beam of length 6 m carries a point load of 3 kN and 6 kN at distances of 2 m and 4 m from the left end. Draw the shear force and bending moment diagrams for the beam.   **(08 Marks)**

June/July 2017 (15ME/MA34)

29. For the beam shown in **Fig. U5.27**, draw shear force and bending moment diagrams. Locate the point of contraflexure if any.   **(16 Marks)**

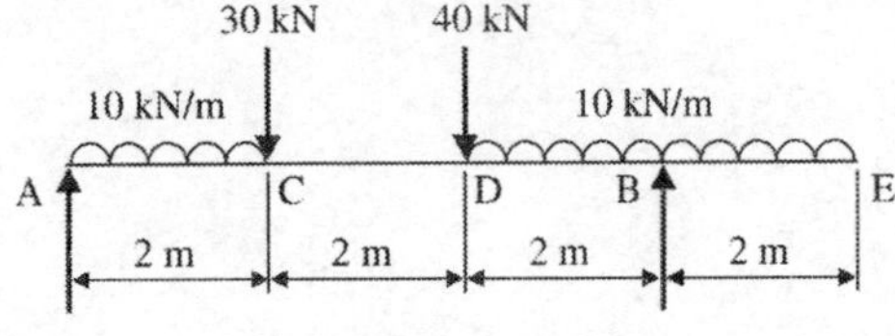

Fig. U5.27

Dec. 17/Jan. 18 (10ME/AU34)

30. a. Derive an expression to establish a relationship between the intensity of load W, shear force F and bending moment M in the beam.   **(06 Marks)**
   b. A beam 8 m long is simply supported at two points and loaded with two concentrated loads, UDL and a couple as shown in **Fig. U5.28**. Draw SF and BM diagrams.   **(14 Marks)**

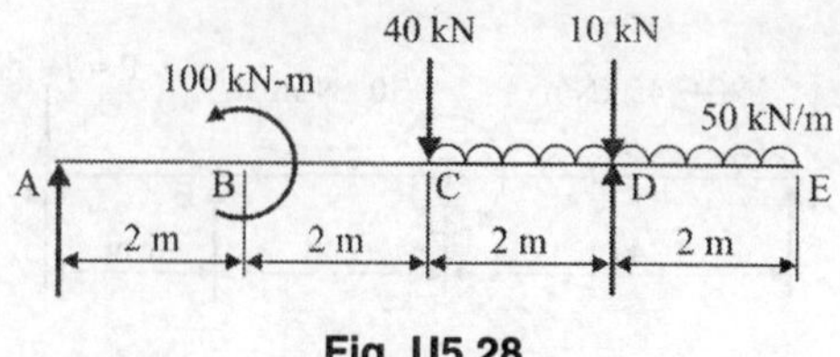

Fig. U5.28

Dec. 17/Jan. 18 (15ME/MA34)

31. For the beam shown in **Fig. U5.29** draw SFD ad BMD. Locate the point of contraflexure, if any. **(16 Marks)**

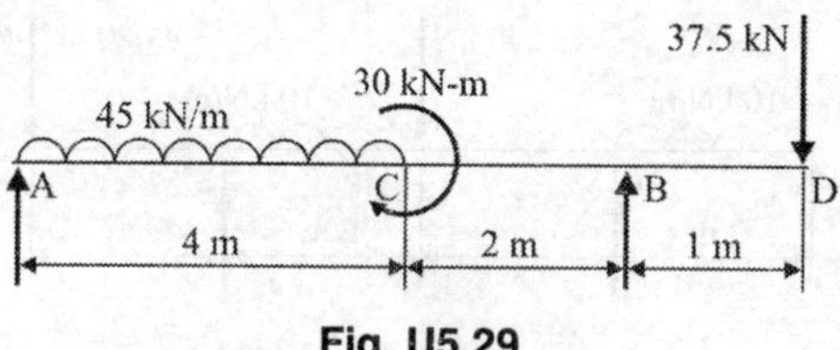

Fig. U5.29

32. Derive the relationship between load, shear force and bending moment for UDL. **(04 Marks)**

Bending Stresses in Beams

Chapter Outline

6.1 INTRODUCTION

A beam is a structural member whose length is large (longer than the width and the thickness) compared to its cross sectional area which is loaded and supported in the direction transverse to its axis. As discussed in chapter 5, when a straight beam is subjected to lateral loads, it is subjected to two actions: a bending moment and a shear force. Thus a beam section has to resist the action of bending moment (BM) and shear force (SF). This bending is resisted by the internal resistance set up by the cross-section of the beam, and the process of bending stops when it has developed full resistance to the BM and SF. The stresses produced at the section to resist the bending moment is known as *Bending stress or flexural stress or longitudinal stress* and that to resist the action of shearing force is known *shear stress or transverse stress*. The BM at any section represents the resultant moment, called the *moment of resistance* of internal stresses distributed over the section.

In this chapter the effect of bending stresses are discussed while the shear stresses are discussed in the next chapter.

6.2 PURE BENDING

A pure bending moment is one which is uniform along the length of the beam and is not accompanied by shear forces.

- An example of pure bending is a simply supported beam subjected to equal and opposite couples of same magnitude as shown in **Fig. 6.1**
- Another example is a cantilever beam AB subjected to a clockwise couple at the free end as shown in **Fig. 6.2** (Reproduced from Chapter 5 – **Fig. 5.9**).

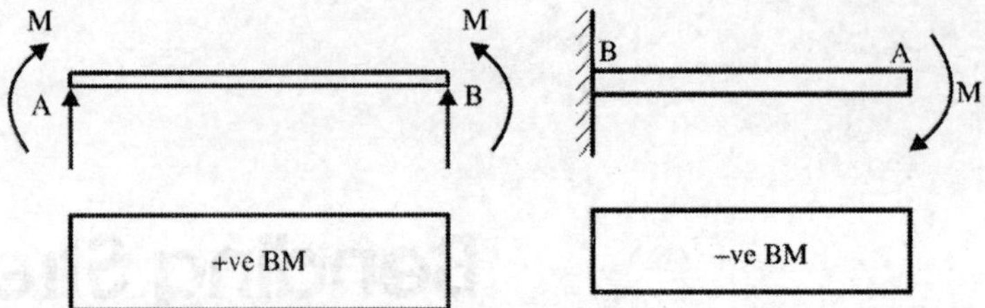

Fig. 6.1: Simply supported beam subjected to couples

Fig. 6.2: Cantilever beam with a couple at free end

If a beam is subjected to a pure bending moment, the outer fibres are in tension while the inner fibres are in compression which induces tensile and compressive stresses in the beam thereby producing a moment called the *moment of resistance* which is equal and opposite to the applied bending moment.

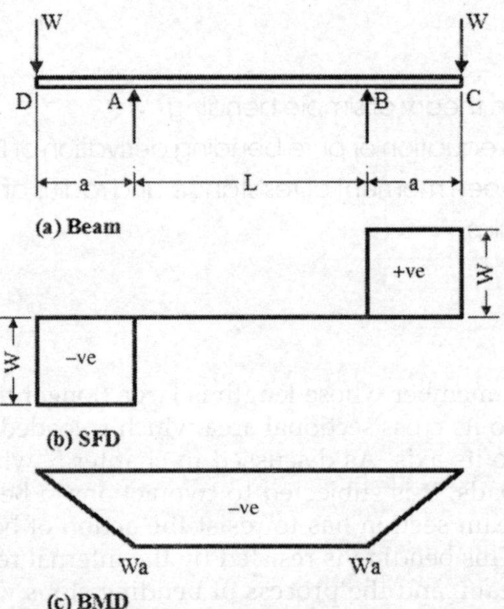

Fig. 6.3: Overhanging beam with point load at each end

On the other hand **Non-uniform** bending refers to flexure in the presence of shear forces, which means that the bending moment changes as we move along the axis of the beam.

Consider an overhanging beam shown in **Fig. 6.3**. It is observed that the bending moment is constant (i.e. shear force is zero) between the supports A and B. Hence the central region of this beam is in pure bending, while the regions of length a near the ends of the beam are in non-uniform bending because the bending moment varies and shear forces are present.

6.3 ASSUMPTIONS IN THEORY OF SIMPLE BENDING

- The beam in initially straight and unstressed.
- The stresses in the beam are within the elastic limit of its material, i.e. the material obeys Hooke's law.

- The material of the beam is homogeneous (i.e. uniform in density, strength, etc.) and isotropic (i.e. possesses same elastic property in all directions).
- Plane section remains plane even after bending (Bernoulli's assumption).
- The value of Young's modulus of the material of the beam is same in tension and compression.
- Every layer of the beam material is free to expand or contract longitudinally and laterally.
- The radius of curvature of the beam is very large compared to the cross section dimensions of the beam.
- The resultant force perpendicular to any cross-section of the beam is zero.

6.4 BENDING STRESS EQUATION OR PURE BENDING DERIVATION OF BERNOULLI'S EQUATION

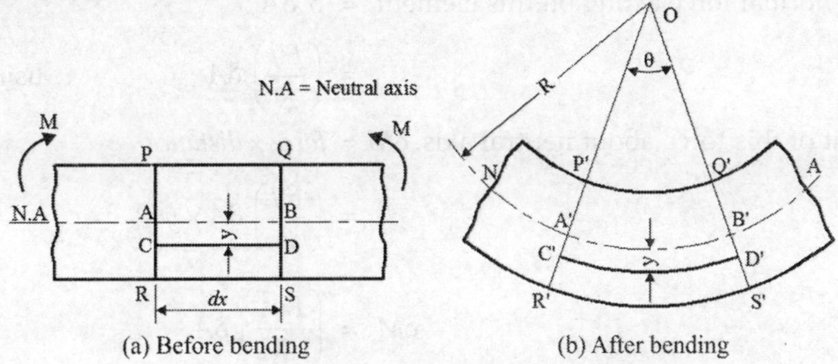

Fig. 6.4: Beam subjected to pure bending

Consider a portion of a beam PQRS as shown in **Fig. 6.4(a)** subjected to pure bending (M). Consider an element of length dx at a distance y from the neutral axis. Due to the applied moment, the beam takes the form as shown in **Fig. 6.4(b)** with O as center and the radius of curvature as R, such that the outer fibers are in tension while the inner fibers are in compression, i.e. layers above the neutral axis are in compression while layers below the neutral axis are in tension.

AB represents the neutral axis. Since there are no stresses acting on the neutral axis, there will be no change in the length of the element. Thus

$$AB = A'B' = R\theta \qquad \qquad \text{... Eq. (i)}$$

For the layer CD at a distance c from the neutral axis, we have $C'D' = (R + y)\theta$

Strain in layer CD, $\varepsilon = \dfrac{\text{Change in length}}{\text{Original length}}$

$$= \frac{C'D' - CD}{CD} = \frac{C'D'}{CD} - 1$$

$$= \frac{(R + y)\theta}{R\theta} - 1 \qquad \qquad \text{Since } CD = AB = A'B' = R\theta$$

$$= \frac{R + y - R}{R}$$

$\therefore$ Strain in layer CD, $\varepsilon = \dfrac{y}{R}$ $\qquad \qquad$ ... Eq. (ii)

But $\qquad E = \dfrac{\sigma}{\varepsilon}$

Strain $\qquad \varepsilon = \dfrac{\sigma}{E}$

Thus $\qquad \dfrac{\sigma}{E} = \dfrac{y}{R}$ $\hfill$ ...using Eq. (ii)

$\therefore \qquad \dfrac{\sigma}{y} = \dfrac{E}{R}$ $\hfill$ ... Eq. (iii)

6.5 RELATION BETWEEN MOMENT OF RESISTANCE AND RADIUS OF CURVATURE

Consider an elemental area δA at a distance y from the neutral axis as shown in **Fig. 6.5**.

The normal force acting on this element $= \sigma.\delta A$

$$= \left(\frac{Ey}{R}\right) \delta A \qquad \text{...using Eq. (iii)}$$

Moment of this force about neutral axis, $\delta M = force \times distance$

$$= \left(\frac{Ey}{R}\right) \delta A \times y$$

$$\delta M = \left(\frac{Ey^2}{R}\right) \delta A \qquad \text{... Eq. (iv)}$$

Thus total moment of resistance $\qquad M = \Sigma \delta M$

$$= \Sigma \left(\frac{Ey^2}{R}\right) \delta A$$

$$M = \left(\frac{E}{R}\right) \times \Sigma y^2 \delta A \qquad \text{... Eq. (v)}$$

Since $\Sigma y^2 \delta A$ is the moment of inertia (I) of the section about the neutral axis, we have

$$M = \left(\frac{E}{R}\right) I$$

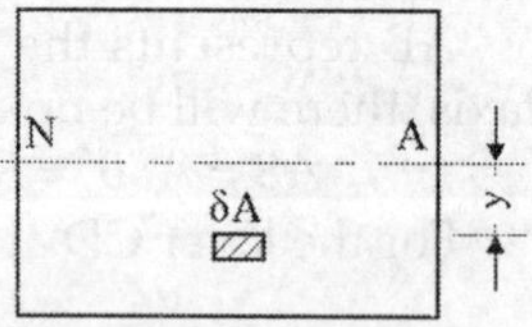

$$\therefore \quad \frac{M}{I} = \left(\frac{E}{R}\right) \qquad \text{... Eq. (vi)}$$

Fig. 6.5: Elemental area

Combining Eqs (iii) and (vi), we have $\qquad \dfrac{M}{I} = \dfrac{\sigma}{y} = \dfrac{E}{R}$ $\hfill$ ... (Eq. 6.1)

The value of y at the outer fibers of the beam is frequently denoted by c. At these outer fibers the bending stresses are maximum and the above equation may be written as

$$\frac{M}{I} = \frac{\sigma}{c} = \frac{E}{R} \qquad \text{... (Eq. 6.2)}$$

Eq. (6.2) is called the bending equation or the flexural equation.

$$M = \text{Bending moment}$$
$$I = \text{Moment of inertia}$$
$$\sigma \text{ or } \sigma_b = \text{Bending stress in the layer}$$
$$y \text{ or } c = \text{Distance of fiber considered from neutral axis}$$
$$E = \text{Young's modulus of the material of the beam}$$
$$R = \text{Radius of curvature}$$

The product of EI is called flexural rigidity.

6.6 SECTION MODULUS (Z)

We know that
$$\frac{M}{I} = \frac{\sigma}{c}$$

$$\sigma = \frac{Mc}{I} = \frac{M}{I/c}$$

$$\sigma = \frac{M}{Z}$$

where $Z = I/c$ is the section modulus

$$= \frac{\text{Moment of inertia about neutral axis}}{\text{Distance of extreme fiber from neutral axis}}$$

Section modulus is defined as the ratio of moment of inertia about the neutral axis to the distance of extreme fiber from neutral axis.

Table 6.1 gives the values of M.I and section modulus for various cross-sections.

The section modulus indicated in the table is given by taking the base of the section as reference.

Table 6.1: Properties of various cross-sections

Type	Section	Moment of inertia (I)	Distance to farthest point (c)	Section modulus
a.		$\dfrac{bh^3}{12}$	$\dfrac{h}{2}$	$\dfrac{bh^2}{6}$
b.		$\dfrac{(BH^3 - bh^3)}{12}$	$\dfrac{H}{2}$	$\dfrac{(BH^3 - bh^3)}{6H}$

Contd...

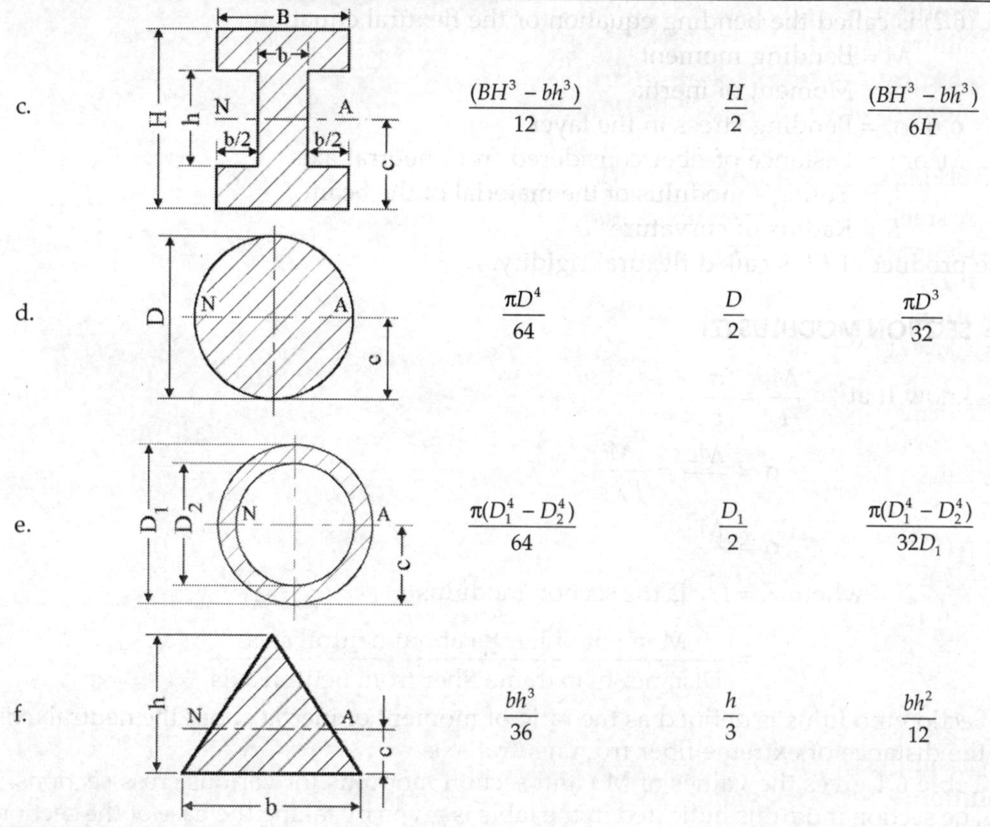

		Moment of Inertia	c	Section Modulus
c.		$\dfrac{(BH^3 - bh^3)}{12}$	$\dfrac{H}{2}$	$\dfrac{(BH^3 - bh^3)}{6H}$
d.		$\dfrac{\pi D^4}{64}$	$\dfrac{D}{2}$	$\dfrac{\pi D^3}{32}$
e.		$\dfrac{\pi(D_1^4 - D_2^4)}{64}$	$\dfrac{D_1}{2}$	$\dfrac{\pi(D_1^4 - D_2^4)}{32 D_1}$
f.		$\dfrac{bh^3}{36}$	$\dfrac{h}{3}$	$\dfrac{bh^2}{12}$

6.7 DEFINITIONS

- *Neutral axis:* In bending, fibers on one side of the beam are subjected to tension while those on the opposite side are in compression. There is a region within the beam cross-section at which the stress changes sign, i.e. where the stress is zero, and this is termed the neutral axis.

  The intersection of the neutral surface with any cross section of the beam perpendicular to its longitudinal axis is called the neutral axis.

- *Section modulus:* It is defined as the ratio of moment of inertia about the neutral axis to the distance of extreme fiber from neutral axis.

$$Z = \frac{\text{Moment of inertia about neutral axis}}{\text{Distance of extreme fiber from neutral axis}} = \frac{I}{c}$$

- *Moment of resistance:* If a beam is subjected to a pure bending moment, the outer fibres are in tension while the inner fibres are in compression which induces tensile and compressive stresses in the beam thereby producing a moment called the moment of resistance which is equal and opposite to the applied bending moment.

- *Modulus of rupture:* When a beam is loaded up to failure, the stresses in the beam section cannot be calculated by using the flexure formula. This is, however, done sometimes to compare strengths of beams of different materials. The stress calculated at rupture using the bending equation is known as the modulus of rupture. The stresses calculated are the maximum values in the section due to failure load.

- *Flexural rigidity or flexural stiffness:* The product of Young's modulus (E) and moment of inertia (I) is called flexural rigidity. It is represented as *EI*.

PROBLEMS ON CIRCULAR SECTION

1. **A steel wire of diameter 2 mm is bent is around a cylinder of radius 600 mm. Determine the normal strain developed in the wire. Also find the normal stress if E = 200 GPa.**

Solution: ε = ?, D = 2 mm, radius of cylinder = 600 mm, σ = ?, $E = 200 \times 10^3$ MPa.

Normal strain $\quad \varepsilon = \dfrac{y}{R} = \dfrac{c}{R} \qquad [c \text{ or } y]$

Here
$$c = D/2 = 2/2 = 1 \text{ mm}$$
$$R = c + \text{radius of cylinder} = 1 + 600 = 601 \text{ mm}$$

$$\varepsilon = \frac{1}{601} = 1.664 \times 10^{-3}$$

Normal stress $\quad \sigma = \varepsilon E = (1.664 \times 10^{-3}) \times 200 \times 10^3 = 332.78 \text{ MPa}$

Fig. 6.6: Problems 1 and 2

2. **A steel wire of diameter 5 mm is bent around a drum of radius 500 mm. Calculate the maximum bending stress and the bending moment in the wire, assuming E = 200 GPa.**

Solution: ε = ?, D = 5 mm, radius of cylinder = 500 mm, σ = ?, M = ?, $E = 200 \times 10^3$ MPa

Bending stress $\quad \sigma = \varepsilon E = E\left(\dfrac{c}{R}\right)$

Here $\quad c = D/2 = 5/2 = 2.5 \text{ mm}$
$$R = c + \text{radius of cylinder} = 2.5 + 500 = 502.5 \text{ mm}$$

$$\sigma = 200 \times 10^3 \times \frac{2.5}{502.5} = 995.02 \text{ MPa}$$

Bending moment $\quad M = \dfrac{EI}{R}$

But $\quad I = \dfrac{\pi D^4}{64} = \dfrac{\pi \times 5^4}{64} = 30.68 \text{ mm}^4$

$$M = \frac{(200 \times 10^3) \times 30.68}{502.5} = 12210.80 \text{ N-mm} = 12.21 \text{ N-m}$$

3. **A steel band saw is wrapped around a pulley of diameter 500 mm. The blade is 10 mm wide and 1 mm thick. If Young's modulus is 210 GPa, determine the bending stress developed in the blade.**

Solution: Diameter of pulley = 500 mm, b = 10 mm, h = 1 mm, $E = 210 \times 10^3$ MPa, σ = ?.

Bending stress $\sigma = \varepsilon E = E\left(\dfrac{c}{R}\right)$

Here $c = h/2 = 1/2 = 0.5\,\text{mm}$

$R = c + radius\ of\ cylinder = 0.5 + 250 = 250.5\,\text{mm}$

$$\sigma = 210 \times 10^3 \times \left(\dfrac{0.5}{250.5}\right) = 419.16\,\text{MPa}$$

4. **A steel plate of dimensions 10 mm × 4 mm is bent into a circular arc of radius 3 m. Calculate the maximum bending stress and the bending moment in the wire, assuming E = 200 GPa.**

Solution: $b = 10$ mm, $h = 4$ mm, radius of cylinder = 3000 mm, $\sigma = ?$, $M = ?$, $E = 200 \times 10^3$ MPa

Bending stress $\sigma = \varepsilon E = E\left(\dfrac{c}{R}\right)$

Here $c = h/2 = 4/2 = 2\,\text{mm}$

$R = c + radius\ of\ cylinder = 2 + 3000 = 3002\,\text{mm}$

$$\sigma = 200 \times 10^3 \times \left(\dfrac{2}{3002}\right) = 133.24\,\text{MPa}$$

Bending moment $M = \dfrac{EI}{R}$

But $I = \dfrac{bh^3}{12} = \dfrac{10 \times 4^3}{12} = 53.33\,\text{mm}^4$

$$M = \dfrac{(200 \times 10^3) \times 53.33}{3002} = 3553.19\,\text{N-mm} = 3.55\,\text{N-m}$$

5. **A thin steel of thickness 1 mm is bent into a circular arc subtending a central angle 55°. If arc length is 1 m, determine the maximum bending stress? Take E = 200 GPa.**

Solution: $h = 1$ mm, $\theta = 55° = 0.960$ rad., $L = 1000$ mm, $\sigma = ?$, $E = 200 \times 10^3$ MPa.

Bending stress $\sigma = \varepsilon E = E\left(\dfrac{c}{R}\right)$

Here $c = h/2 = 1/2 = 0.5\,\text{mm}$

Also $L = R\theta$

$R = 1000/0.960 = 1041.67\,\text{mm}$

$$\sigma = 200 \times 10^3 \times \left(\dfrac{0.5}{1041.767}\right) = 96\,\text{MPa}$$

6. **Calculate the maximum bending stress induced in a cast iron pipe of external diameter 40 mm, internal diameter 20 mm and of length 4 m when the pipe is simply supported at its ends and carries a point load of 80 N at its center.**

VTU – June/ July 2013 – 06 Marks

Solution: $\sigma = ?$, $D_1 = 40$ mm, $D_2 = 20$ mm, $L = 4000$ mm, $W = 80$ N.

Bending stress $\qquad \sigma = \dfrac{M}{Z}$

For a simply supported beam with point load at mid span

$$M = \frac{WL}{4} = \frac{80 \times 4000}{4} = 80000 \text{ N-mm}$$

Section modulus $Z = \dfrac{I}{c} = \dfrac{\pi\left(D_1^4 - D_2^4\right)}{32D_1} = \dfrac{\pi(40^4 - 20^4)}{32 \times 40} = 5890.49 \text{ mm}^3$

$$\sigma = \frac{80000}{5890.49} = 13.58 \text{ MPa}$$

7. **A simply supported beam of circular cross section having a diameter of 100 mm is subjected to two point loads of 10 kN each at a distance of 250 mm from each support. The effective span of the beam is 900 mm. Determine the maximum bending stress in the beam.**

Solution: $D = 100$ mm, $\sigma = ?$.

Based on the given data, the beam is as shown in **Fig. 6.7**.

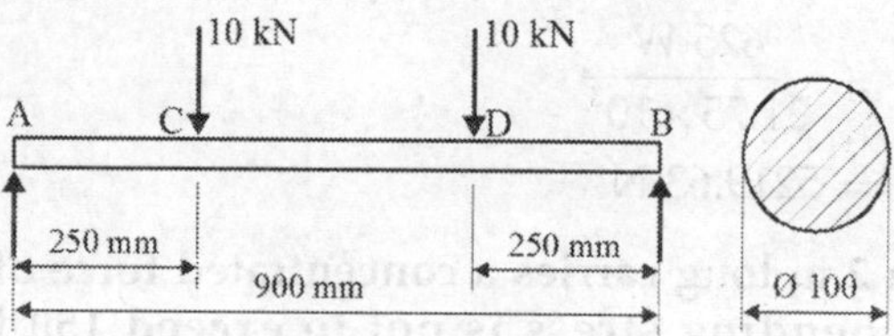

Fig. 6.7: Problem 7

Since the loading is symmetric, the reaction at the supports are $R_A = R_B = 10$ kN
The maximum bending moment is $M_C = M_D = 10 \times 250 = 2500$ kN-mm $= 2.5 \times 10^6$ N-mm

Bending stress $\qquad \sigma = \dfrac{M}{Z}$

But $\qquad Z = \dfrac{I}{c} = \dfrac{\pi D^3}{32} = \dfrac{\pi \times 100^3}{32} = 98.17 \times 10^3 \text{ mm}^3$

$$\sigma = \frac{2.5 \times 10^6}{98.17 \times 10^3} = 25.46 \text{ MPa}$$

8. **Repeat the above problem for a hollow shaft of external diameter 40 mm and inner diameter 25 mm.**

Solution: $D_1 = 100$ mm, $D_2 = 50$ mm, $L = 900$ mm, $\sigma = ?$.

Bending stress $\qquad \sigma = \dfrac{M}{Z}$

But $\qquad Z = \dfrac{I}{c} = \dfrac{\pi\left(D_1^4 - D_2^4\right)}{32D_1} = \dfrac{\pi(100^4 - 50^4)}{32 \times 100} = 92.04 \times 10^3 \text{ mm}^3$

$$\sigma = \frac{2.5 \times 10^6}{92.04 \times 10^3} = 27.16 \text{ MPa}$$

9. **A circular pipe of external diameter 70 mm and thickness 8 mm is used a simply supported beam over an effective span of 2.5 m. Find the maximum concentrated load that can be applied at the centre of the span if permissible stress in the tube is 150 MPa.**

VTU – June/ July 2017 – 10 Marks; Dec. 16/ Jan. 17 – 08 Marks

Solution: $D_1 = 70$ mm, $t = 8$ mm, $D_2 = D_1 - 2t = 70 - 16 = 54$ mm, $L = 2500$ mm, $W = ?$, $\sigma = 150$ MPa.

Bending stress $\qquad \sigma = \dfrac{M}{Z}$

For a simply supported beam with point load at mid span

$$M = \frac{WL}{4} = \frac{W \times 2500}{4} = 625\, W$$

Section modulus $Z = \dfrac{I}{c} = \dfrac{\pi\left(D_1^4 - D_2^4\right)}{32 D_1} = \dfrac{\pi(70^4 - 54^4)}{32 \times 70} = 21.75 \times 10^3 \text{ mm}^3$

$$150 = \frac{625\, W}{21.75 \times 10^3}$$

$$W = 5219.63 \text{ N}$$

10. **A cantilever beam 2 m long carries a concentrated force of 5 kN at its free end. If the maximum bending stress is not to exceed 150 MPa, determine the required diameter if the beam is circular.**

Solution: $L = 2000$ mm, $W = 5000$ N, $\sigma = 150$ MPa, $D = ?$.

Bending stress $\quad \sigma = \dfrac{M}{Z}$

For a cantilever beam with point load at free end
$$M = WL = 5000 \times 2000 = 10 \times 10^6 \text{ N-mm}$$

Section modulus $Z = \dfrac{I}{c} = \dfrac{\pi D^3}{32} = 0.09817\, D^3$

$$150 = \frac{10 \times 10^6}{0.09817\, D^3}$$

$$D = 87.90 \text{ mm} \approx 88 \text{ mm}$$

11. **A simply supported beam of circular cross section is subjected to two point loads of 10 kN each at a distance of 250 mm from each support. The effective span of the beam is 900 mm. If the maximum bending stress is not to exceed 125 MPa, determine the required diameters of the beam. The ratio of inner diameter to outer diameter is 0.5.**

Solution: $K = D_2/D_1 = 0.5$, $\sigma = 150$ MPa, $D_1, D_2 = ?$

Based on the given data, the beam is as shown in **Fig. 6.8**.

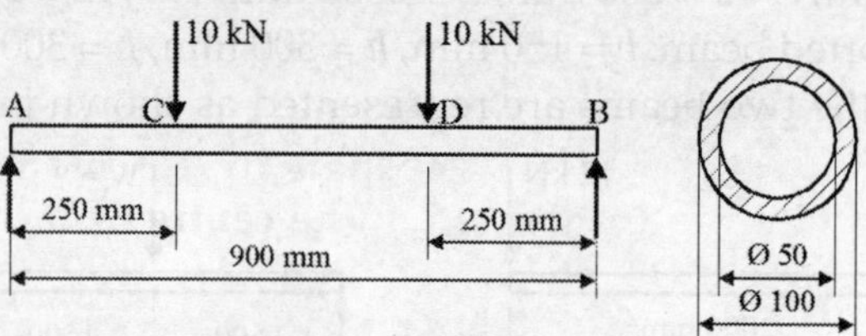

Fig. 6.8: Problem 11

Since the loading is symmetric, the reaction at the supports are $R_A = R_B = 10$ kN

The maximum bending moment is $M_C = M_D = 10 \times 250 = 2500$ kN-mm $= 2.5 \times 10^6$ N-mm

Bending stress $\quad \sigma = \dfrac{M}{Z}$

But $\qquad Z = \dfrac{I}{c} = \dfrac{\pi\left(D_1^4 - D_2^4\right)}{32 D_1} = \dfrac{\pi D_1^4(1 - 0.5^4)}{32 D_1} = 0.09204\, D_1^3$

$$125 = \dfrac{2.5 \times 10^6}{0.09204\, D_1^3}$$

$\qquad\qquad D_1 = 60.12$ mm

And $\qquad D_2 = 0.5 \times 60.12 = 30.06$ mm

12. **A hollow circular rod having outside diameter twice the inside diameter is used as a beam. It is observed from bending moment diagram of the beam that the maximum bending moment is 40 kN-m. If the allowable bending stress in the beam is restricted to 120 MPa, find the inside diameter of the beam.**

Solution: $D_1 = 2D_2 \Rightarrow K = D_2/D_1 = 0.5$, $M = 40 \times 10^6$ N-mm, $\sigma = 120$ MPa, $D_1, D_2 = ?$

Bending stress $\quad \sigma = \dfrac{M}{Z}$

But $\qquad Z = \dfrac{I}{c} = \dfrac{\pi\left(D_1^4 - D_2^4\right)}{32 D_1} = \dfrac{\pi D_1^4(1 - 0.5^4)}{32 D_1} = 0.09204\, D_1^3$

$$120 = \dfrac{40 \times 10^6}{0.09204\, D_1^3}$$

$\qquad\qquad D_1 = 153.57$ mm ≈ 154 mm

And $\qquad D_2 = 0.5 \times 154 = 77$ mm

PROBLEMS ON SQUARE CROSS-SECTION

13. **A cantilever of square section 200 mm × 200 mm, 2 m long just fails in flexure when a load of 12 kN is placed at its free end. A beam of the same material and having a rectangular cross-section 150 mm wide and 300 mm deep is simply supported over a span of 3 m. Calculate the minimum central load point required to break the beam.**

VTU – Dec. 16/ Jan. 17 – 08 Marks; June/ July 2013 – 08 Marks

Solution:

Case i: Cantilever beam, $b = h = 200$ mm, $L = 2000$ mm, $W = 12 \times 10^3$ N, $\sigma = ?$

Case ii: Simply supported beam: $b = 150$ mm, $h = 300$ mm, $L = 3000$ mm, $W = ?$

Based on given data the two beams are represented as shown in **Fig. 6.9**.

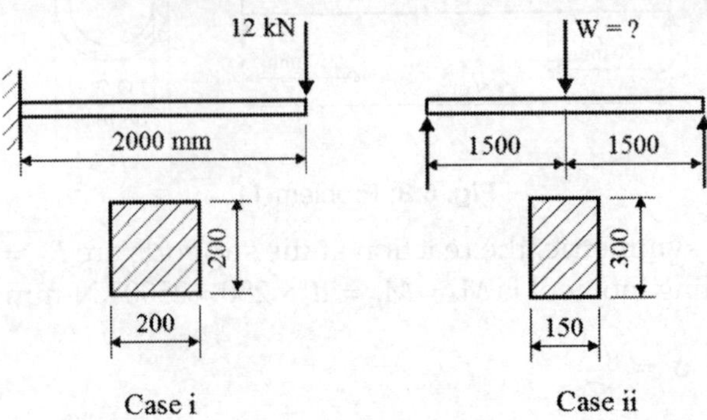

Fig. 6.9: Problem 13

Case i: Cantilever beam

Bending stress $\quad \sigma = \dfrac{M}{Z}$

For a cantilever beam with point load at free end

$$M = WL = 12 \times 10^3 \times 2000 = 24 \times 10^6 \text{ N-mm}$$

Section modulus $Z = \dfrac{I}{c} = \dfrac{bh^2}{6} = \dfrac{200 \times 200^2}{6} = 1.33 \times 10^6 \text{ mm}^3$

$$\sigma = (24 \times 10^6)/(1.33 \times 10^6) = 18 \text{ MPa}$$

Case ii: Simply supported beam

For a simply supported beam with point load at mid-span

$$M = \frac{WL}{4} = \frac{W \times 3000}{4} = 750 \, W$$

Section modulus $Z = \dfrac{I}{c} = \dfrac{bh^2}{6} = \dfrac{150 \times 300^2}{6} = 2.25 \times 10^6 \text{ mm}^3$

$$18 = \frac{750 \, W}{2.25 \times 10^6}$$

$$W = 54000 \text{ N} = 54 \text{ kN}$$

14. **A cantilever beam of square cross section 200 mm × 200 mm, 2 m long just fails in bending, when a load of 20 kN is placed at its free end. A beam of the same material having a rectangular cross section 150 mm × 300 mm, simply supported over a span of 3 m is to be used under uniformly distributed load w N/m. What can be the maximum value of w?**

VTU – Dec. 2010 – 12 Marks

Solution:

Case i: Cantilever beam, $b = h = 200$ mm, $L = 2000$ mm, $W = 20 \times 10^3$ N, $\sigma = ?$

Case ii: Simply supported beam: $b = 150$ mm, $h = 300$ mm, $L = 3000$ mm, $W = ?$

Based on given data the two beams are represented as shown in **Fig. 6.10**.

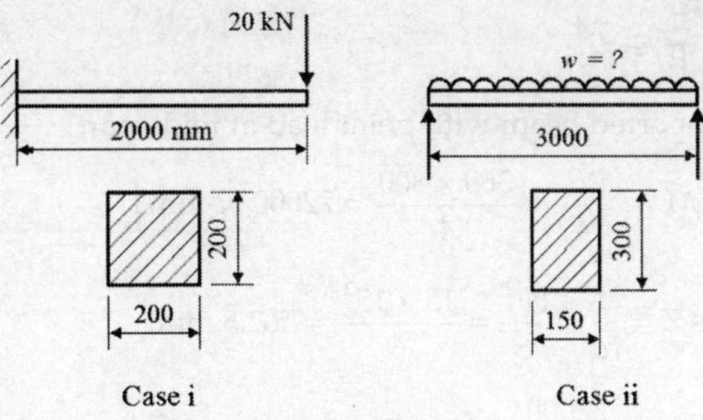

Fig. 6.10: Problem 14

Case i: Cantilever beam

Bending stress $\sigma = \dfrac{M}{Z}$

For a cantilever beam with point load at free end
$$M = WL = 20 \times 10^3 \times 2000 = 40 \times 10^6 \text{ N-mm}$$

Section modulus $Z = \dfrac{I}{c} = \dfrac{bh^2}{6} = \dfrac{200 \times 200^2}{6} = 1.33 \times 10^6 \text{ mm}^3$

$$\sigma = \frac{40 \times 10^6}{1.33 \times 10^6} = 30 \text{ MPa}$$

Case ii: Simply supported beam

For a simply supported beam with UDL over entire span,

$$M = \frac{wL^2}{8} = \frac{w \times 3000^2}{8} = (1.125 \times 10^6)\, w$$

Section modulus $Z = \dfrac{I}{c} = \dfrac{bh^2}{6} = \dfrac{150 \times 300^2}{6} = 2.25 \times 10^6 \text{ mm}^3$

$$30 = \frac{(1.125 \times 10^6)w}{2.25 \times 10^6}$$

$$W = 60 \text{ N/mm} = 60 \text{ kN/m}$$

15. **A simply supported cast iron square beam of 800 mm length and 15 mm × 15 mm in section fails on applying a load of 360 N at mid-span. Find the maximum uniformly distributed load that can be applied safely to a 40 mm wide, 75 mm deep and 1.6 m long cantilever made of same material.**

VTU – Dec. 13/ Jan. 14 – 08 Marks; [Similar: (CV) June/ July 2009 – 10 Marks]

Solution:

Case i: Simply supported beam: $b = h = 15$ mm, $L = 800$ mm, $W = 360$ N, $\sigma = ?$

Case ii: Cantilever beam, $b = 40$ mm, $h = 75$ mm, $L = 1600$ mm, $w = ?$

Case i: Simply supported beam

Bending stress $\sigma = \dfrac{M}{Z}$

For a simply supported beam with point load at mid-span

$$M = \frac{WL}{4} = \frac{360 \times 800}{4} = 72000 \text{ N-mm}$$

Section modulus $Z = \dfrac{I}{c} = \dfrac{bh^2}{6} = \dfrac{15 \times 15^2}{6} = 562.5 \text{ mm}^3$

$$\sigma = \frac{72000}{562.5} = 128 \text{ MPa}$$

Case ii: Cantilever beam

For a cantilever beam with UDL over entire span

$$M = \frac{wL^2}{2} = \frac{w \times 1600^2}{2} = (1.28 \times 10^6)\, w$$

Section modulus $Z = \dfrac{I}{c} = \dfrac{bh^2}{6} = \dfrac{40 \times 75^2}{6} = 37500 \text{ mm}^3$

$$128 = \frac{\left(1.28 \times 10^6\right) w}{37500}$$

$$w = 3.75 \text{ N/mm} = 3.75 \text{ kN/m}$$

16. **Compare the bending resistances of a beam with square cross-section placed with two sides horizontal to that with a diagonal horizontal for the same stress in each case.**

VTU – Jan 2004

Solution: Based on given data the two beams are represented as shown in **Fig. 6.11**.

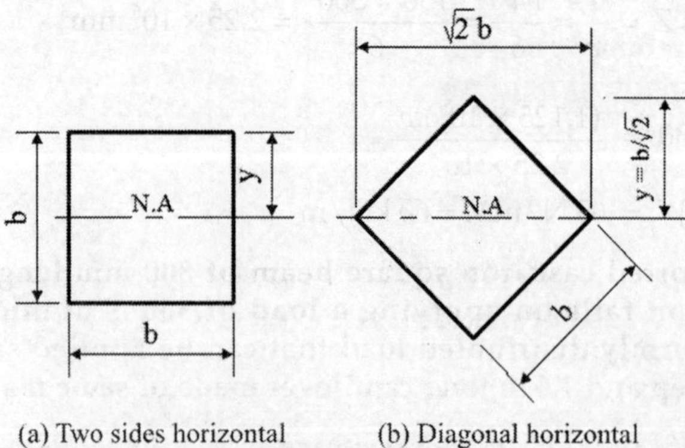

(a) Two sides horizontal   (b) Diagonal horizontal

Fig. 6.11: Problem 16

Case a: Two sides horizontal

Bending stress $\sigma = \dfrac{M}{Z}$

$$M = \sigma Z$$

$$\text{Section modulus } Z = \frac{I}{y} = \frac{b^4/12}{b/2} = \frac{b^3}{6}$$

$$\text{Moment of resistance } M_1 = \sigma \left(\frac{b^3}{6} \right)$$

Case b: Diagonal horizontal

MI about neutral axis = sum of MI of two triangles about neutral axis

$$\text{Bending stress } \quad \sigma = \frac{M}{Z}$$

$$I = 2\left(\frac{bh^3}{12} \right) = \frac{bh^3}{6}$$

$$= \frac{\left(\sqrt{2}b \right)\left(b/\sqrt{2} \right)^3}{6}$$

$$I = \frac{b^4}{12} \text{ and } y = \frac{b}{\sqrt{2}}$$

$$\text{Section modulus } Z = \frac{I}{y} = \frac{b^4/12}{b/\sqrt{2}} = \frac{\sqrt{2}b^3}{12}$$

$$\text{Moment of resistance } M_2 = \sigma \left(\frac{\sqrt{2}b^3}{12} \right)$$

$$\text{Thus} \qquad \frac{M_1}{M_2} = \frac{\sigma b^3/6}{\sigma \sqrt{2}b^3/12} = \sqrt{2}$$

17. Prove that the moment of resistance of a beam of square section with its diagonal in the plane of bending is increased by flattening the top and bottom corners, as shown in Fig. 6.12(a), and that the moment of resistance is a maximum when $y = 8b/9$.

Or Prove that the strength of a square section used as a beam to bend about a diagonal can be increased by flattening the comers in the plane of loading and that the maximum strength is obtained by removing one-ninth of the diagonal length, equally divided at the top and bottom.

Solution: Divide the given **Fig. 6.12 (a)** consisting of a rectangle and 4 triangles as shown in **Fig. 6.12(b)**.

$$\text{MI of each triangle about its base} = \frac{bh^3}{12} = \frac{y^4}{12}$$

$$\text{MI of rectangle about centroidal axis} = \frac{bh^3}{12} = \frac{2(b-y)(2y)^3}{12}$$

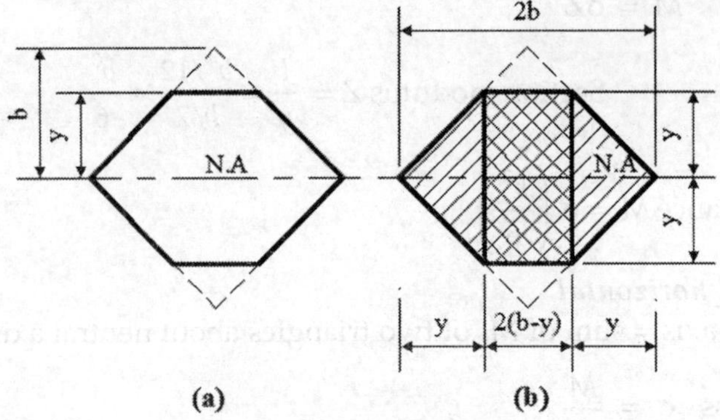

Fig. 6.12: Problem 17

$$\text{MI of the entire section} \ = \ \frac{2(b-y)(2y)^3}{12} + 4\left(\frac{y^4}{12}\right)$$

$$= \ \frac{4(b-y)y^3}{3} + \left(\frac{y^4}{3}\right)$$

$$= \ \frac{4by^3}{3} - \left(\frac{4y^4}{3}\right) + \left(\frac{y^4}{3}\right)$$

$$I \ = \ \frac{4by^3}{3} - y^4$$

$$\text{Section modulus } Z \ = \ \frac{I}{y} = \frac{(4by^3/3) - y^4}{y} = \frac{4by^2}{3} - y^3$$

$$\text{Bending stress} \quad \sigma \ = \ \frac{M}{Z}$$

$$M \ = \ \sigma Z = \sigma\left(\frac{4by^2}{3} - y^3\right)$$

For maximum value of moment of resistance,

$$\frac{dM}{dy} = 0$$

$$\frac{d}{dy}\left[\sigma\left(\frac{4by^2}{3} - y^3\right)\right] = 0$$

$$\frac{8by}{3} - 3y^2 = 0$$

$$\frac{8by}{3} = 3y^2$$

$$\frac{8b}{3} = 3y$$

$$y \ = \ \frac{8b}{9} \quad \text{thus proved.}$$

PROBLEMS ON RECTANGULAR CROSS-SECTION

18. A 250 mm × 150 mm rectangular beam is subjected to maximum bending moment of 750 kN-m. Determine:
  i.   Maximum stress in the beam
  ii. If the value of E for the beam material is 200 GPa, find out the radius of curvature for the portion of the beam where the bending moment is maximum.

Solution: $b = 150$ mm, $h = 250$ mm, $M = 750 \times 10^6$ N-mm, $\sigma = ?$, $E = 200$ GPa, $R = ?$

$$\text{Bending stress} \quad \sigma = \frac{M}{Z} = \frac{M}{bh^2/6} = \frac{750 \times 10^6}{150 \times 250^2/6} = 480 \text{ MPa}$$

$$\text{Also} \quad \frac{\sigma}{c} = \frac{E}{R}$$

$$R = \frac{Ec}{\sigma} = \frac{200 \times 10^3 \times (250/2)}{480} = 52083.33 \text{ mm}$$

19. A simply supported beam of span 4 m carries an UDL of 10 kN/m over the entire span. If the cross section of the beam is rectangular of 150 mm × 300 mm, determine the bending stress in the beam.

Solution: $L = 4000$ mm, $w = 10$ kN/m $= 10$ N/mm, $b = 150$ mm, $h = 300$ mm, $\sigma = ?$

$$\text{Bending stress} \quad \sigma = \frac{M}{Z} \qquad \qquad \text{... Eq. (i)}$$

For a simply supported beam with UDL over entire span

$$M = \frac{wL^2}{8} = \frac{10 \times 4000^2}{8} = 20 \times 10^6 \text{ N-mm}$$

$$\text{Section modulus} \quad Z = \frac{I}{c} = \frac{bh^2}{6} = \frac{150 \times 300^2}{6} = 2.25 \times 10^6 \text{ mm}^3$$

$$\text{Eq. (i) yields...} \quad \sigma = \frac{20 \times 10^6}{2.25 \times 10^6} = 8.89 \text{ MPa}$$

20. A beam of rectangular cross-section 50 mm wide and 100 mm deep is simply supported over a span of 1500 mm. It carries a concentrated load of 50 kN, 500 mm from the left support. Calculate the maximum tensile stress in the beam and indicate where it occurs.

Solution: $b = 50$ mm, $h = 100$ mm, $L = 1500$ mm, $W = 50 \times 10^3$ N, $\sigma = ?$

Based on given data the beam is represented as shown in **Fig. 6.13**.

Reactions at supports:

$$R_A + R_B = 50 \text{ kN} \qquad \qquad \text{... Eq. (i)}$$

Taking moments about A and equating to zero, we have

$$R_B \times 1500 = 50 \times 500$$

$$R_B = 16.67 \text{ kN} \qquad \qquad \text{... Eq. (ii)}$$

Substituting Eq. (ii) in Eq. (i), we have

$$R_A + 16.67 = 50$$

$$R_A = 33.33 \text{ kN} \qquad \qquad \text{... Eq. (iii)}$$

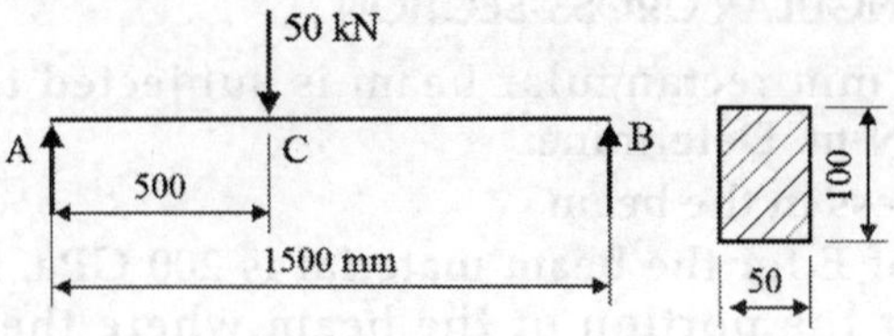

Fig. 6.13: Problem 20

Bending moment calculations:

$$M_A = 0$$
$$M_C = R_A \times 500 = 33.33 \times 500 = 16665 \text{ kN-mm}$$
$$M_B = 0 \qquad \text{(from RHS)}$$

Thus the maximum bending moment occurs at C.

$$\text{Bending stress} \quad \sigma = \frac{M}{Z} \qquad\qquad \ldots \text{Eq. (iv)}$$

$$\text{Section modulus } Z = \frac{I}{c} = \frac{bh^2}{6} = \frac{50 \times 100^2}{6} = 83.33 \times 10^3 \text{ mm}^3$$

$$\text{Eq. (iv) yields} \ldots \sigma = \frac{16665 \times 10^3}{83.33 \times 10^3} = 199.98 \text{ MPa}$$

$$\sigma \approx 200 \text{ MPa}$$

The maximum tensile occurs where the bending moment is maximum.

21. **A simply supported beam of span 6 m is subjected to a concentrated load of 25 kN acting at a distance of 2 m from the left end and a uniformly distributed load of 10 kN/m over the entire span. If the cross section of the beam is rectangular of 100 mm × 200 mm, determine the maximum tensile and compressive stresses developed in the beam due to bending.**

Solution: $L = 6000$ mm, $W = 25 \times 10^3$ N, $w = 10$ kN/m $= 10$ N/mm, $b = 100$ mm, $h = 200$ mm, $\sigma = ?$

Based on given data the beam is represented as shown in **Fig. 6.14**.

Reactions at supports:

$$R_A + R_B = 25 + (10 \times 6) = 85 \text{ kN} \qquad \ldots \text{Eq. (i)}$$

Taking moments about A and equating to zero, we have

$$R_B \times 6 = (25 \times 2) + \left[10 \times 6 \times \left(\frac{6}{2} \right) \right]$$

$$R_B = 38.33 \text{ kN} \qquad \ldots \text{Eq. (ii)}$$

Substituting Eq. (ii) in Eq. (i), we have

$$R_A + 38.33 = 85$$
$$R_A = 46.67 \text{ kN} \qquad \ldots \text{Eq. (iii)}$$

Shear force calculations:

$$F_A = R_A = 46.67 \text{ kN}$$
$$F_{A-C} = 46.67 - (10 \times 2) = 26.67 \text{ kN}$$

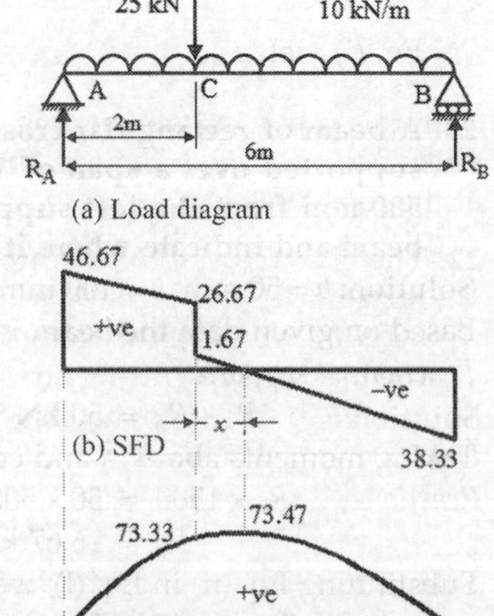

Fig. 6.14: Problem 21

$$F_C = 26.67 - 25 = 1.67 \text{ kN}$$
$$F_{C-B} = 1.67 - (10 \times 4) = -38.33 \text{ kN}$$
$$F_B = F_{C-B} = -38.33 \text{ kN} = R_B$$

Bending moment calculations:

$$M_A = 0$$

$$M_C = (6.67 \times 2) - \left[10 \times 6 \times \left(\frac{2}{2}\right)\right] = 73.34 \text{ kN} - \text{m}$$

$$M_B = (46.67 \times 6) - (25 \times 4) - \left[10 \times 6 \times \left(\frac{6}{2}\right)\right] = 0.02 \text{ kN} - \text{m} \approx 0$$

Or $\qquad\qquad M_B = 0 \qquad\qquad$ (from RHS)

Maximum bending moment:

$$\frac{x}{1.67} = \frac{4-x}{38.33}$$
$$38.33x = 1.67(4-x)$$
$$36.66x = 6.68$$
$$x = 0.167 \text{ m}$$
$$M_{\max} = [46.67 \times (2 + 0.167)] - (25 \times 0.167)$$
$$- \left[10 \times (2 + 0.167) \times \left(\frac{2 + 0.167}{2}\right)\right] = 73.47 \text{ kN-m}$$

Bending stress $\quad \sigma = \dfrac{M}{Z}$ $\qquad\qquad\qquad\qquad\qquad\qquad\qquad$ ... Eq. (iv)

Section modulus $Z = \dfrac{I}{c} = \dfrac{bh^2}{6} = \dfrac{100 \times 200^2}{6} = 666.67 \times 10^3 \text{ mm}^3$

Eq. (iv) yields... $\sigma = \dfrac{73.47 \times 10^6}{666.67 \times 10^3} = 110.21 \text{ MPa (Tensile stress)}$

$$\sigma = -\frac{M}{Z} = -110.21 \text{ MPa (Compressive stress)}$$

In this problem, the bending moment is positive; therefore, the maximum tensile stress occurs at the bottom of the beam and the maximum compressive stress occurs at the top.

22. The cross-section of a simply supported beam 5 m long consists of a hollow rectangular box as shown in the Fig. 6.15. The beam is loaded with a UDL of 6 kN/m over its entire length and a point load of 10 kN at its centre. Determine the maximum bending stress.

Solution: $L = 5000$ mm, $w = 6$ kN/m $= 6$ N/mm, $W = 10 \times 10^3$ N, $\sigma = ?$, $B = 250$ mm, $H = 500$ mm, $b = 200$ mm, $h = 450$ mm

Reactions at supports:

$$R_A + R_B = 10 + (6 \times 5) = 40 \text{ kN} \qquad\qquad\qquad\qquad \text{... Eq. (i)}$$

Taking moments about A and equating to zero, we have

$$R_B \times 5 = (10 \times 2.5) + \left[6 \times 5 \times \left(\frac{5}{2}\right)\right]$$

$$R_B = 20 \text{ kN} \qquad\qquad \text{... Eq. (ii)}$$

Substituting Eq. (ii) in Eq. (i), we have

$$R_A + 20 = 40$$
$$R_A = 20 \text{ kN} \qquad\qquad \text{... Eq. (iii)}$$

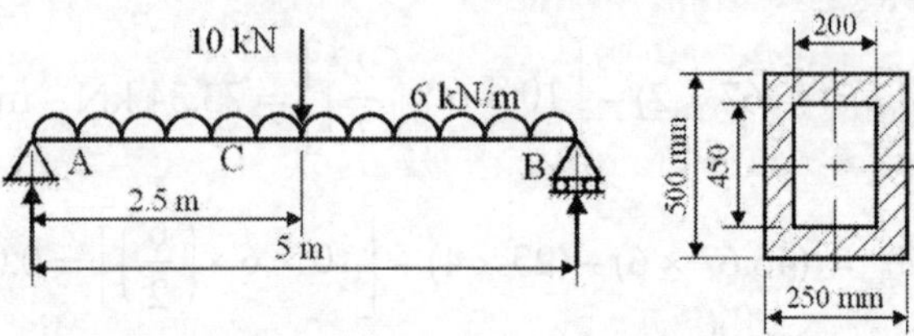

Fig. 6.15: Problem 22

Maximum bending moment:

Due to symmetry, maximum BM occurs at mid span, i.e. $x = 2.5$ m

$$M_{max} = [20 \times 2.5] - \left[6 \times 2.5 \times \left(\frac{2.5}{2}\right)\right] = 31.25 \text{ kN-m}$$

$$= 31.25 \times 10^6 \text{ N-mm}$$

Or

$$M_{max} = \left(\frac{wL^2}{8}\right) + \left(\frac{WL}{4}\right) = \left(\frac{6 \times 5^2}{8}\right) + \left(\frac{10 \times 5}{4}\right) = 31.25 \text{ kN-m}$$

$$= 31.25 \times 10^6 \text{ N-mm}$$

Bending stress $\quad \sigma = \dfrac{M}{Z} \qquad\qquad \text{... Eq. (iv)}$

Section modulus $Z = \dfrac{I}{c} = \dfrac{BH^3 - bh^3}{6H} = \dfrac{(250 \times 500^3) - (200 \times 450^3)}{6 \times 500} = 4.34 \times 10^6 \text{ mm}^3$

Eq. (iv) yields... $\sigma = \dfrac{31.25 \times 10^6}{4.34 \times 10^6} = 7.2 \text{ MPa}$

23. A wooden beam 10 m long has a rectangular cross section, 300 mm wide and 360 mm deep. It is simply supported and loaded with a uniformly distributed load over entire span. Find the safe intensity of load, if allowable bending stress is 10 MPa.

VTU – (CV) Dec. 2011 – 10 Marks

Solution: $L = 10000$ mm, $b = 300$ mm, $h = 360$ mm, $w = ?$, $\sigma = 10$ MPa

Bending stress $\quad \sigma = \dfrac{M}{Z} \qquad\qquad \text{... Eq. (i)}$

For a simply supported beam with UDL over entire span

$$M = \frac{wL^2}{8} = \frac{w \times 10000^2}{8} = (12.5 \times 10^6)w \text{ N-mm}$$

Section modulus $\quad Z = \dfrac{I}{c} = \dfrac{bh^2}{6} = \dfrac{300 \times 360^2}{6} = 6.48 \times 10^6 \text{ mm}^3$

Eq. (i) yields... $10 = \dfrac{(12.5 \times 10^6)w}{6.48 \times 10^6}$

$$w = 5.184 \text{ N/mm} = 5.184 \text{ kN/m}$$

24. A simply supported beam of span 5 m has a cross-section of 150 mm × 250 mm. If the permissible stress is 10 MPa, find:
(a) Maximum intensity of uniformly distributed load it can carry
(b) Maximum concentrated load W applied at 2 m from an end it can carry.

VTU – Dec. 16/ Jan. 17 – 10 Marks, June 2012 – 10 Marks

Solution: $L = 5000$ mm, $b = 150$ mm, $h = 250$ mm, $\sigma = 10$ MPa, a) $w = ?$, b) $W = ?$ at 2 m from an end

Bending stress $\sigma = \dfrac{M}{Z}$ ... Eq. (i)

Section modulus $Z = \dfrac{I}{c} = \dfrac{bh^2}{6} = \dfrac{150 \times 250^2}{6} = 1.56 \times 10^6 \text{ mm}^3$

Case a: For a simply supported beam with UDL over entire span

$$M = \frac{wL^2}{8} = \frac{w \times 5000^2}{8} = (3.125 \times 10^6)w \text{ N-mm}$$

Eq. (i) yields... $10 = \dfrac{(3.125 \times 10^6)w}{1.56 \times 10^6}$

$$w = 4.9 \text{ N/mm} \approx 5 \text{ kN/m}$$

Case b: For a simply supported beam with intermediate point load

$$M = \frac{Wab}{L} = \frac{W \times 2000 \times 3000}{5000} = (1200)W \text{ N-mm}$$

[here $a = 2$ m, $b = L - 2 = 3$ m]

Eq. (i) yields... $10 = \dfrac{(1200)W}{1.56 \times 106}$

$$W = 13000 \text{ N} = 13 \text{ kN}$$

25. Determine the maximum allowable span length L for a simple beam shown in Fig. 6.16. The beam is of rectangular cross section 140 mm × 240 mm subjected to a uniformly distributed load of $w = 6.5$ kN/m and the allowable bending stress is 8.2 MPa.

VTU – June/ July 2009 – 08 Marks

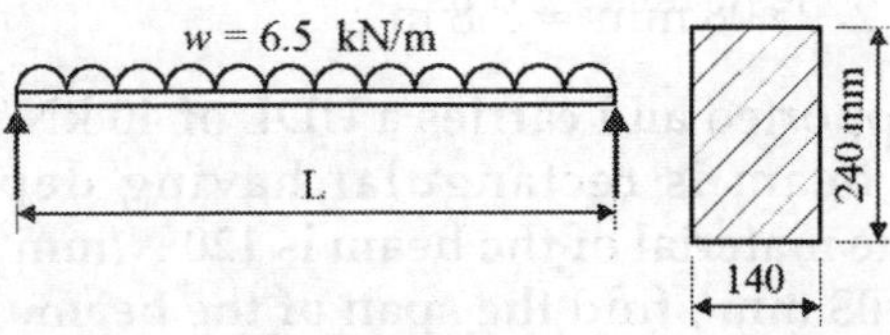

Fig. 6.16: Problem 25

Solution: $L = ?$, $b = 140$ mm, $h = 240$ mm, $w = 6.5$ kN/m $= 6.5$ N/mm, $\sigma = 8.2$ MPa

Bending stress $\quad \sigma = \dfrac{M}{Z}$ ... Eq. (i)

For a simply supported beam with UDL over entire span

$$M = \frac{wL^2}{8} = \frac{6.5L^2}{8} = (0.8125)\, L^2 \text{ N-mm}$$

Section modulus $Z = \dfrac{I}{c} = \dfrac{bh^2}{6} = \dfrac{140 \times 240^2}{6} = 1.344 \times 10^6 \text{ mm}^3$

Eq. (i) yields... $\quad 8.2 = \dfrac{(0.8125)L^2}{1.344 \times 10^6}$

$$L = 3682.94 \text{ mm} = 3.683 \text{ m}$$

26. Determine the maximum allowable span of length L for a simple beam as shown in Fig. 6.17. The rectangular beam of cross section 125 × 250 mm is subjected to a UDL of 8 kN/m. Allowable bending stress = 6 MPa.

VTU – Dec. 13/ Jan. 14 – 10 Marks

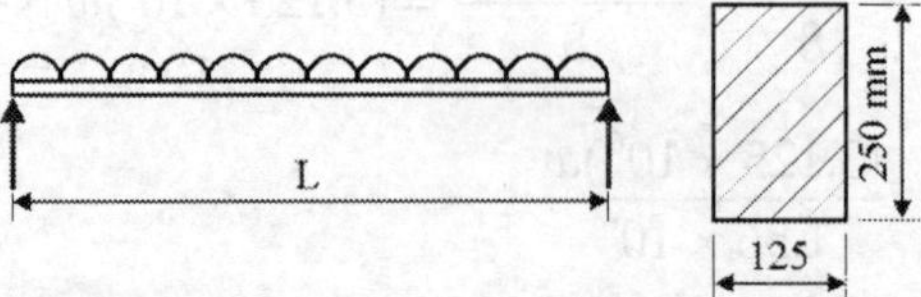

Fig. 6.17: Problem 26

Solution: $L = ?$, $b = 125$ mm, $h = 250$ mm, $w = 8$ kN/m $= 8$ N/mm, $\sigma = 6$ MPa.

Bending stress $\quad \sigma = \dfrac{M}{Z}$ ... Eq. (i)

For a simply supported beam with UDL over entire span

$$M = \frac{wL^2}{8} = \frac{40L^2}{8} = L^2$$

Section modulus $\quad Z = \dfrac{I}{c} = \dfrac{bh^2}{6} = \dfrac{125 \times 250^2}{6} = 1.30 \times 10^6 \text{ mm}^3$

Eq. (i) yields... $\quad 6 = \dfrac{L^2}{1.30 \times 10^6}$

$$L = 2795.08 \text{ mm} \approx 2.8 \text{ m}$$

27. A beam is simply supported and carries a UDL of 40 kN/m over the entire span. The section of the beam is rectangular having depth as 500 mm. If the maximum stress in the material of the beam is 120 N/mm^2 and moment of inertia of the section is 7 × 108 mm^4, find the span of the beam.

VTU – June/ July 2013 – 08 Marks

Solution: $w = 40\ \text{kN/m} = 40\ \text{N/mm}$, $h = 500\ \text{mm}$, $\sigma = 120\ \text{MPa}$, $I = 7 \times 10^8\ \text{mm}^4$, $L = ?$,

$$\text{Bending stress} \quad \sigma = \frac{M}{Z} \qquad \qquad \text{... Eq. (i)}$$

For a simply supported beam with UDL over entire span

$$M = \frac{wL^2}{8} = \frac{40L^2}{8} = 5L^2$$

$$\text{Section modulus} \quad Z = \frac{I}{c} = \frac{7 \times 10^8}{500/2} = 2.80 \times 10^6\ \text{mm}^3$$

$$\text{Eq. (i) yields...} \quad 120 = \frac{5L^2}{2.80 \times 10^6}$$

$$L = 8197.56\ \text{mm} \approx 8.2\ \text{m}$$

28. **A cantilever beam 4 m long is subjected to a uniformly distributed load of 10 kN/m. The allowable working stress in either tension or compression is 100 MPa. If the cross-section is to be rectangular, determine the dimensions, if the depth is twice the width.**

Solution: $L = 4000\ \text{mm}$, $w = 10\ \text{kN/m} = 10\ \text{N/mm}$, $h = 2b$, $\sigma_t = \sigma_c = 100\ \text{MPa}$, $b, h = ?$

$$\text{Bending stress} \quad \sigma = \frac{M}{Z} \qquad \qquad \text{... Eq. (i)}$$

For a cantilever beam UDL over entire span

$$M = \frac{wL^2}{2} = \frac{10 \times 4000^2}{2} = 80 \times 10^6\ \text{N-mm}$$

$$\text{Section modulus } Z = \frac{I}{c} = \frac{bh^2}{6} = \frac{b(2b)^2}{6} = 0.67\ b^3$$

$$\text{Eq. (i) yields...} 100 = \frac{80 \times 10^6}{0.67 b^3}$$

$$b = 106.08\ \text{mm} \approx 110\ \text{mm}$$

$$h = 2 \times 110 = 220\ \text{mm}$$

29. **In a beam of wood simply supported over a span of 6 m is loaded with a central point load of 60 kN. The width to depth ratio of the beam is 0.5. Determine cross section details of the beam if tensile and compressive stress in the beam not to exceed 8 N/mm^2 and 6 N/mm^2 respectively.**

Solution: $L = 6000\ \text{mm}$, $W = 60 \times 10^3\ \text{N}$, $b/h = 0.5$, $\sigma_t = 8\ \text{MPa}$, $\sigma_c = 6\ \text{MPa}$, $b, h = ?$

$$\text{Bending stress} \quad \sigma = \frac{M}{Z} \qquad \qquad \text{... Eq. (i)}$$

For a simply supported beam with point load at mid-span

$$M = \frac{WL}{4} = \frac{60 \times 10^3 \times 6000}{4} = 90 \times 10^6\ \text{N-mm}$$

Section modulus $Z = \dfrac{I}{c} = \dfrac{bh^2}{6} = \dfrac{bh^2}{6} = \dfrac{b(2b^2)}{6} = 0.67\,b^3$

As the section is symmetrical about the N.A (neutral axis), the lower value of stress is to be used.

$$6 = (90 \times 10^6)/(0.67\,b^3)$$
$$b = 281.85 \text{ mm} \approx 282 \text{ mm}$$
$$h = 2 \times 282 = 564 \text{ mm}$$

30. A beam of span 6 m is simply supported at its ends and carries a UDL of 12 kN/m over the entire span along with a point load of 6 kN at 3.5 m from the right support. Determine cross section details of the beam if the depth is twice the width and the stress is not to exceed 8 MPa.

Solution: $L = 6000$ mm, $w = 12$ kN/m $= 12$ N/mm, $W = 6 \times 10^3$ N at 3.5 m from right support, $b/h = 0.5$, $\sigma = 8$ MPa, $b,h = ?$

Based on given data the beam is represented as shown in **Fig. 6.18**.

Reactions at supports:

$$R_A + R_B = 6 + (12 \times 6) = 78 \text{ kN} \qquad \dots \text{Eq. (i)}$$

Taking moments about A and equating to zero, we have

$$R_B \times 6 = (6 \times 2.5) + \left[12 \times 6 \times \left(\frac{6}{2}\right) \right]$$
$$R_B = 38.50 \text{ kN} \qquad \dots \text{Eq. (ii)}$$

Substituting Eq. (ii) in Eq. (i), we have

$$R_A + 38.50 = 78$$
$$R_A = 39.50 \text{ kN} \qquad \dots \text{Eq. (iii)}$$

Shear force calculations:

$$F_A = R_A = 39.50 \text{ kN}$$
$$F_{A-C} = 39.50 - (12 \times 2.5) = 9.5 \text{ kN}$$
$$F_C = 9.5 - 6 = 3.5 \text{ kN}$$
$$F_{C-B} = 3.5 - (12 \times 3.5) = -38.50 \text{ kN}$$
$$F_B = F_{C-B} = -38.50 \text{ kN} = R_B$$

Bending moment calculations:

$$M_A = 0$$

$$M_C = (39.50 \times 2.5) - \left[12 \times 2.5 \times \left(\frac{2.5}{2}\right) \right]$$
$$= 61.25 \text{ kN-m}$$
$$M_B = 0 \qquad \text{(from RHS)}$$

Maximum bending moment:

$$\frac{x}{3.5} = \frac{3.5 - x}{38.50}$$
$$42\,x = 12.25$$
$$x = 0.29 \text{ m}$$

$$M_{max} = [39.50 \times (2.5 + 0.29)] - (6 \times 0.29) - \left[12 \times (2.5 + 0.29) \times \left(\frac{2.5 + 0.29}{2}\right) \right]$$

$$= 61.76 \text{ kN-m}$$

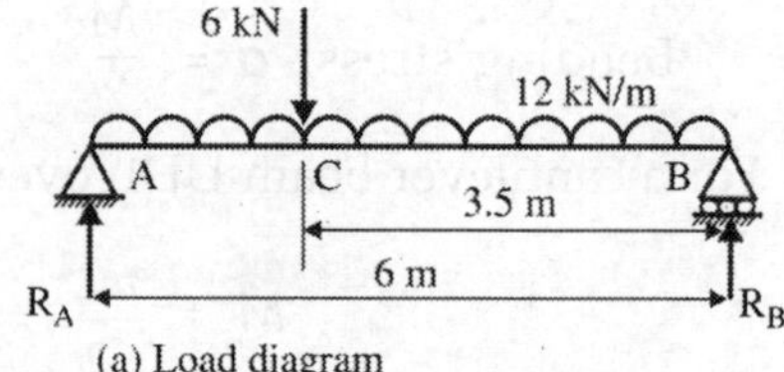

(a) Load diagram

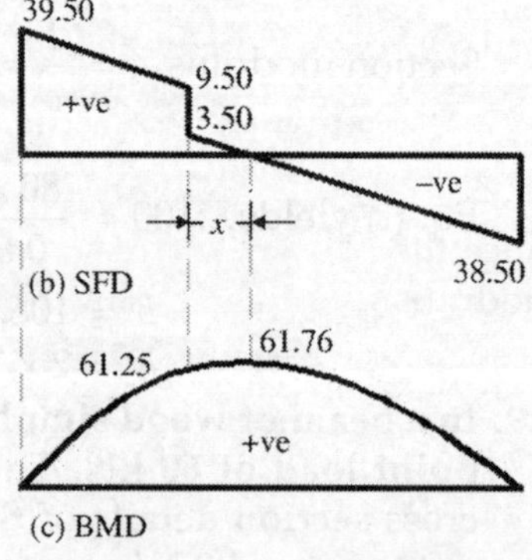

(b) SFD

(c) BMD

Fig. 6.18: Problem 30

Bending stress $\quad \sigma = \dfrac{M}{Z}$ $\qquad$ ... Eq. (iv)

Moment $\qquad M = M_{max} = 61.76$ kN-m

Section modulus $Z = \dfrac{I}{c} = \dfrac{bh^2}{6} = \dfrac{bh^2}{6} = \dfrac{b(2b^2)}{6} = 0.67\,b^3$

Eq. (iv) yields... $\qquad 8 = \dfrac{61.76 \times 10^6}{0.67\,b^3}$

$$b = 225.86 \text{ mm} \approx 230 \text{ mm}$$
$$h = 2 \times 230 = 460 \text{ mm}$$

31. Three beams have the same length, same allowable stress and same bending moment. The cross sections of the beams are square, circular and a rectangle with height equal to twice the width. Find the ratios of weights of circular and rectangular beams to that of square beam.

Solution: Based on given data the cross-sections are as shown in **Fig. 6.19**.

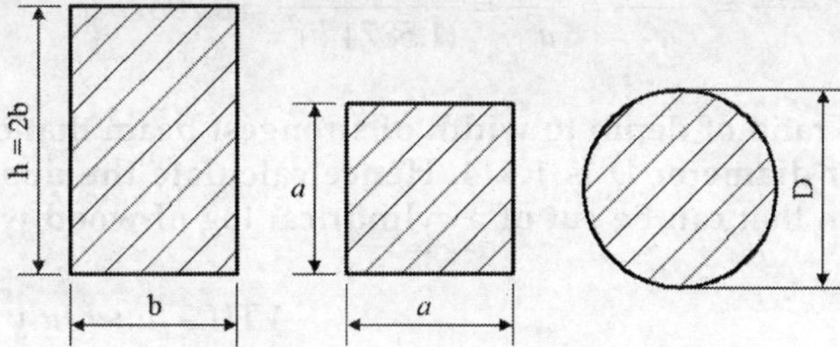

Fig. 6.19: Problem 31

Let $\qquad a$ = side of the square

$\qquad\qquad D$ = diameter of the circle

$\qquad\qquad b$ = width of rectangle

$\qquad\qquad D$ = depth or height of rectangle

Since the allowable stress and bending moment of the beams are same, their section modulus should also be same

i.e. $\qquad Z_{sq} = Z_{rec} = Z_{cir}$

$$Z_{sq} = \dfrac{a^3}{6} \qquad\qquad \text{... Eq. (i)}$$

$$Z_{rec} = \dfrac{bh^2}{6} = \dfrac{b(2b)^2}{6} = \dfrac{2b^3}{3} \qquad\qquad \text{... Eq. (ii)}$$

$$Z_{cir} = \dfrac{\pi D^3}{32} \qquad\qquad \text{... Eq. (iii)}$$

Equating Eqs (i) and (ii), we have

$$\dfrac{a^3}{6} = \dfrac{2b^3}{3}$$

$$\frac{a^3}{b^3} = 4$$

$$a = 1.5874\,b \qquad\qquad \text{... Eq. (iv)}$$

Equating Eqs (i) and (iii), we have

$$\frac{a^3}{6} = \frac{\pi D^3}{32}$$

$$\frac{a^3}{D^3} = 0.5890$$

$$D = 1.1930\,a \qquad\qquad \text{... Eq. (iv)}$$

$$\text{Now } \frac{W_{cir}}{W_{sq}} = \frac{\text{density} \times (\text{area} \times \text{length})}{\text{density} \times (\text{area} \times \text{length})} = \frac{A_{cir}}{A_{sq}} = \frac{\pi D^2/4}{a^2} = \frac{\pi(1.1930a)^2/4}{a^2}$$

$$= 1.1178$$

$$\frac{W_{rec}}{W_{sq}} = \frac{A_{rec}}{A_{sq}} = \frac{b(2b)}{a^2} = \frac{2b^2}{a^2} = \frac{2b^2}{(1.5874\,b)^2} = 0.7937$$

32. Prove that the ratio of depth to width of strongest beam that can be cut from a circular log of diameter D is 1.414. Hence calculate the depth and width of strongest beam that can be cut of a cylindrical log of wood whose diameter is 300 mm.

VTU – June/ July 2014 – 10 Marks

Solution:

Let $\qquad D =$ Diameter of log

$\qquad\qquad b =$ width of beam

$\qquad\qquad h =$ depth of beam

For a rectangular cross-section

$$Z = \frac{bh^2}{6}$$

From **Fig. 6.20**, $D^2 = b^2 + h^2$

$$h^2 = D^2 - b^2 \qquad\qquad \text{... Eq. (i)}$$

$$Z = \frac{b(D^2 - b^2)}{6} = \frac{bD^2 - b^3}{6} \qquad\qquad \text{... Eq. (ii)}$$

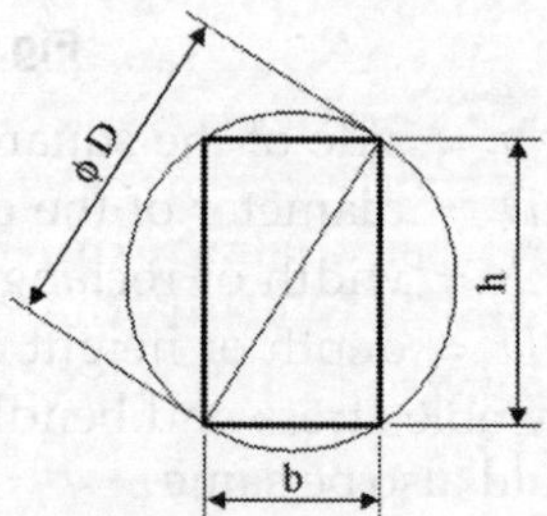

Fig. 6.20: Problem 32

For the strongest section,

$$\frac{dz}{db} = 0$$

$$\frac{d}{db}\left[\frac{bD^2 - b^3}{6}\right] = 0$$

$$D^2 - 3b^2 = 0 \qquad\qquad \text{... Eq. (iii)}$$

$$b^2 + h^2 - 3b^2 = 0 \qquad\qquad \text{... using Eq. (i)}$$

$$h^2 - 2b^2 = 0$$

$$\frac{h}{b} = \sqrt{2} = 1.414 \qquad \text{... Eq. (iv)}$$

Also from Eq. (iii)

$$D^2 - 3b^2 = 0$$
$$D^2 = 3b^2$$
$$\frac{D}{b} = \sqrt{3} \quad \text{or} \quad b = D/\sqrt{3} \qquad \text{... Eq. (v)}$$

Eq. (i) yields ...
$$h^2 = D^2 - b^2$$
$$= D^2 - (D/\sqrt{3})^2$$
$$= D^2 - \frac{D^2}{3}$$
$$h^2 = \frac{2D^2}{3}$$
$$h = D\sqrt{\frac{2}{3}} \qquad \text{... Eq. (vi)}$$

For $D = 300$ mm,

Eq. (v) yields ... $b = 300/\sqrt{3} = 173.21$ mm

Eq. (iv) yields ... $h = 1.414 \times 173.21 = 244.95$ mm

PROBLEMS ON T-SECTION

33. A T section has a flange of 200 mm × 50 mm. The web is also 200 mm × 50 mm. It is subjected to a bending moment of 15 kN-m. Draw the bending stress distribution across the section, indicating the salient values.

Solution: $M = 15 \times 10^6$ N-mm, $\sigma_t = ?$, $\sigma_C = ?$
Based on given data, T section is as shown in **Fig. 6.21(a)**.

To find $\bar{y}$:

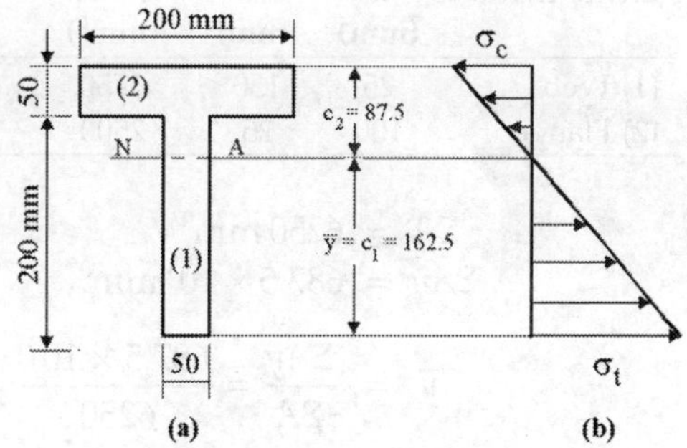

Fig. 6.21: Problem 33

Element No.	b (mm)	h (mm)	$A = bh$ (mm^2)	y (from base) = $(h/2) + x$ (mm)	Ay (mm^3)	$I_G = bh^3/12$ (mm^4)
(1) Web	50	200	10000	$(200/2) = 100$	1×10^6	33.33×10^6
(2) Flange	200	50	10000	$200 + (50/2) = 225$	2.25×10^6	2.08×10^6

x = distance of fiber considered from base

$$\Sigma A = 20000 \text{ mm}^2$$
$$\Sigma Ay = 3.25 \times 10^6 \text{ mm}^3$$
$$\bar{y} = \frac{\Sigma Ay}{\Sigma A} = \frac{3.25 \times 10^6}{20000} = 162.5 \text{ mm}$$

i.e. $\quad \bar{y} = c_1 = 162.5$ mm from base (tensile)

$c_2 = \Sigma h - c_1 = 250 - 162.5 = 87.5$ mm from top face (compressive)

Bending stress $\quad \sigma = \dfrac{M}{Z} = \dfrac{Mc}{I}$ $\qquad$ ... Eq. (i)

But $\quad I = I_1 + I_2$

$$= [I_{G1} + A_1(\bar{y} \sim y_1)^2] + [I_{G2} + A_2(\bar{y} \sim y_1)^2]$$

$$= \{33.33 \times 10^6 + [10000 \times (162.5 - 100)^2]\}$$
$$+ \{2.08 \times 10^6 + [10000 \times (225 - 162.5)^2]\}$$

$$I = 113.54 \times 10^6 \text{ mm}^4$$

Eq. (i) yields...

Tensile stress $\quad \sigma_t = \dfrac{Mc_1}{I} = \dfrac{(15 \times 10^6) \times 162.5}{113.54 \times 10^6} = 21.47$ MPa

Comp stress $\quad \sigma_c = \dfrac{Mc_2}{I} = \dfrac{(15 \times 10^6) \times 87.5}{113.54 \times 10^6} = 11.56$ MPa

The bending stress distribution is shown in **Fig. 6.21(b)**.

34. A beam of T-section as shown in Fig. 6.22 is subjected to a bending moment of 12 kN-m. Determine the maximum tensile and compressive stresses. Also determine the bending stress at point A.

Solution: $M = 12 \times 10^6$ N-mm, $\sigma_t = ?$, $\sigma_c = ?$

To find $\bar{y}$:

Element No.	b (mm)	h (mm)	$A = bh$ (mm²)	y (from base) = $(h/2) + x$ (mm)	Ay (mm³)	$I_G = bh^3/12$ (mm⁴)
(1) Web	25	150	3750	$(150/2) = 75$	281.25×10^6	7.03×10^6
(2) Flange	100	25	2500	$150 + (25/2) = 162.5$	406.25×10^6	1.30×10^5

x = distance of fiber considered from base

$\Sigma A = 6250$ mm²

$\Sigma Ay = 687.5 \times 10^3$ mm³

$$\bar{y} = \frac{\Sigma Ay}{\Sigma A} = \frac{687.5 \times 10^3}{6250} = 110 \text{ mm}$$

i.e. $\quad \bar{y} = c_1 = 110$ mm from base (tensile)

$c_2 = \Sigma h - c_1 = 175 - 110 = 65$ mm from top face (compressive)

Case a:

Bending stress $\quad \sigma = \dfrac{Mc}{I}$ $\qquad$ ... Eq. (i)

But $\quad I = I_1 + I_2$

$$= [I_{G1} + A_1(\bar{y} \sim y_1)^2] + [I_{G2} + A_2(\bar{y} \sim y_1)^2]$$

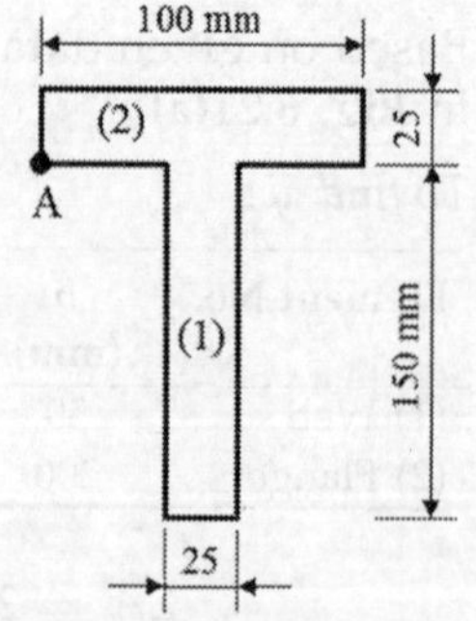

Fig. 6.22: Problem 34

$$= \{7.03 \times 10^6 + [3750 \times (110 - 75)^2]\}$$
$$+ \{1.30 \times 10^5 + [2500 \times (162.5 - 110)^2]\}$$
$$I = 18.64 \times 10^6 \text{ mm}^4$$

Eq. (i) yields...

Tensile stress $\quad \sigma_t = \dfrac{Mc_1}{I} = \dfrac{(12 \times 10^6) \times 110}{18.64 \times 10^6} = 70.82 \text{ MPa}$

Comp. stress $\quad \sigma_c = \dfrac{Mc_2}{I} = \dfrac{(12 \times 10^6) \times 65}{18.64 \times 10^6} = 41.85 \text{ MPa}$

Case b: Bending stress at A

Here $\qquad\qquad c = 175 - 110 - 25 = 40 \text{ mm}$

Or $\qquad\qquad c = 65 - 25 = 40 \text{ mm}$

$$\sigma = \frac{Mc}{I} = \frac{(12 \times 10^6) \times 40}{18.64 \times 10^6} = 25.75 \text{ MPa (Comp)}$$

35. A cast iron beam of T-section is shown in Fig. 6.23(a). The beam is simply supported on a span of 8 m. The beam caries a uniformly distributed load of 1.5 kN/m length over the entire span. Determine the maximum tensile and compressive stresses.

VTU – Dec. 2012 – 10 Marks

Solution: $L = 8000 \text{ mm}, w = 1.5 \text{ kN/m} = 1.5 \text{ N/mm}, \sigma_t = ?, \sigma_c = ?$

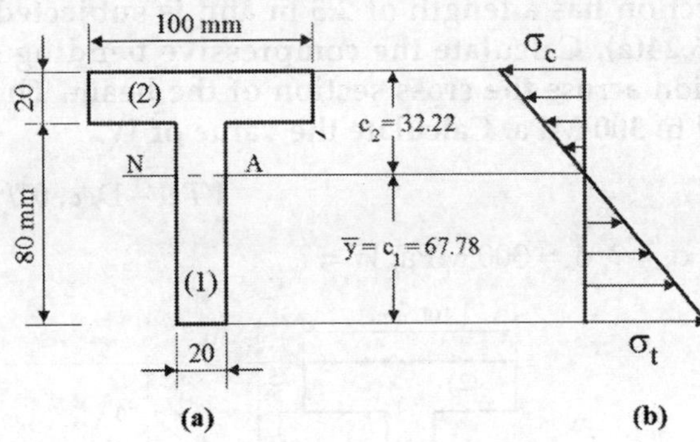

Fig. 6.23: Problem 35

To find $\overline{y}$:

Element No.	b (mm)	h (mm)	A = bh (mm²)	y (from base) = (h/2) + x (mm)	Ay (mm³)	$I_G = bh^3/12$ (mm⁴)
(1) Web	20	80	1600	(80/2) = 40	64×10^3	0.853×10^6
(2) Flange	100	20	2000	80 + (20/2) = 90	180×10^3	66.67×10^3

x = distance of fiber considered from base

$$\Sigma A = 3600 \text{ mm}^2$$
$$\Sigma Ay = 244 \times 10^3 \text{ mm}^3$$

$$\overline{y} = \frac{\Sigma Ay}{\Sigma A} = \frac{244 \times 10^3}{3600} = 67.78 \text{ mm}$$

i.e. $\bar{y} = c_1 = 67.78$ mm from base (Tensile)

$c_2 = \Sigma h - c_1 = 100 - 67.78 = 32.22$ mm from top face (Compressive)

Bending stress $\sigma = \dfrac{Mc}{I}$ ... Eq. (i)

For a simply supported beam with UDL over entire span,

$$M = \frac{wL^2}{8} = \frac{1.5 \times 8000^2}{8} = 12 \times 10^6 \text{ N-mm}$$

Also $I = I_1 + I_2$

$$= [I_{G1} + A_1(\bar{y} \sim y_1)^2] + [I_{G2} + A_2(\bar{y} \sim y_2)^2]$$
$$= \{0.853 \times 10^6 + [1600 \times (67.78 - 40)^2]\}$$
$$+ \{66.67 \times 10^3 + [2000 \times (90 - 67.78)^2]\}$$
$$I = 3.14 \times 10^6 \text{ mm}^4$$

Eq. (i) yields...

Tensile stress $\sigma_t = \dfrac{Mc_1}{I} = \dfrac{(12 \times 10^6) \times 67.78}{3.14 \times 10^6} = 259.03$ MPa

Comp stress $\sigma_c = \dfrac{Mc_2}{I} = \dfrac{(12 \times 10^6) \times 32.22}{3.14 \times 10^6} = 123.13$ MPa

The bending stress distribution is shown in **Fig. 6.23(b)**.

36. A beam of T section has a length of 2.5 m and is subjected to a point load as shown in Fig. 6.24(a). Calculate the compressive bending stress and plot the stress distribution across the cross section of the beam. The maximum tensile stress is limited to 300 MPa. Calculate the value of W.

VTU – Dec. 07/ Jan. 08 – 14 Marks

Solution: $L = 2.5$ m, $\sigma_c = ?$, $\sigma_t = 300$ MPa, $W = ?$

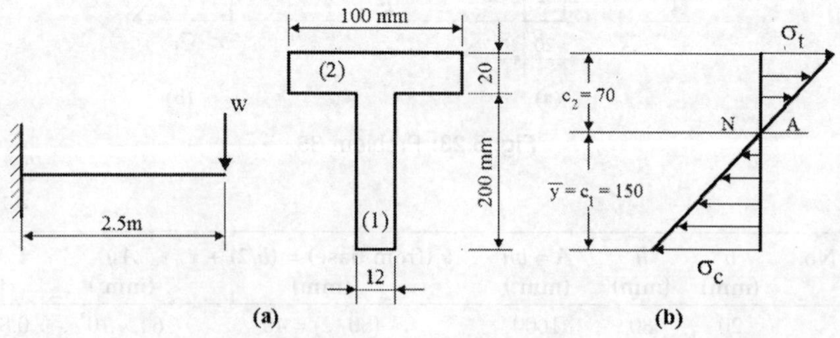

Fig. 6.24: Problem 36

To find $\bar{y}$:

Element No.	b (mm)	h (mm)	A = bh (mm²)	y (from base) = (h/2) + x (mm)	Ay (mm³)	$I_G = bh^3/12$ (mm⁴)
(1) Web	12	200	2400	(200/2) = 100	240 × 10³	8 × 10⁶
(2) Flange	100	20	2000	200 + (20/2) = 210	420 × 10³	66.67 × 10³

x = distance of fiber considered from base

$$\Sigma A = 4400 \text{ mm}^2$$
$$\Sigma Ay = 660 \times 10^3 \text{ mm}^3$$

$$\overline{y} = \frac{\Sigma Ay}{\Sigma A} = \frac{660 \times 10^3}{4400} = 150 \text{ mm}$$

i.e. $\overline{y} = c_1 = 150$ mm from base (Compressive)

$c_2 = \Sigma h - c_2 = 220 - 150 = 70$ mm from top face (Tensile)

Since the beam undergoes hogging BM, the upper layers are in tension while the bottom layers are in compression.

Bending stress $\sigma = \dfrac{Mc}{I}$ ... Eq. (i)

For a cantilever beam with point load at end span,

$$M = WL = 2500 \, W$$

Also $I = I_1 + I_2$

$$= [I_{G1} + A_1(\overline{y} \sim y_1)^2] + [I_{G2} + A_2(\overline{y} \sim y_1)^2]$$
$$= \{8 \times 10^6 + [2400 \times (150 - 100)^2]\}$$
$$\quad + \{66.67 \times 10^3 + [2000 \times (210 - 150)^2]\}$$
$$I = 21.27 \times 10^6 \text{ mm}^4$$

Eq. (i) yields...

Tensile stress $\sigma_t = \dfrac{Mc_2}{I}$

$$300 = \frac{(2500 \, W) \times 70}{21.27 \times 10^6}$$

$$W = 36.46 \times 10^3 \, N$$

Comp stress $\sigma_c = \dfrac{Mc_2}{I} = \dfrac{(2500 \times 36.46 \times 10^3) \times 150}{21.27 \times 10^6} = 642.81$ MPa

The bending stress distribution is shown in **Fig. 6.24(b)**.

37. A beam of T section has a length of 2 m and is subjected to a point load as shown in Fig. 6.25. Calculate the maximum value of W that the beam can carry if the limiting stresses in tension and compression are 90 MPa and 150 MPa respectively.

Solution: $L = 2$ m, $\sigma_t = 90$ MPa, $\sigma_c = 150$ MPa, $W = ?$

To find $\overline{y}$:

Element No.	b (mm)	h (mm)	$A = bh$ (mm^2)	y (from base) = $(h/2) + x$ (mm)	Ay (mm^3)	$I_G = bh^3/12$ (mm^4)
(1) Web	15	120	1800	$(120/2) = 60$	108×10^3	2.16×10^6
(2) Flange	120	20	2400	$120 + (20/2) = 130$	312×10^3	80×10^3

x = distance of fiber considered from base

$$\Sigma A = 4200 \text{ mm}^2$$
$$\Sigma Ay = 420 \times 10^3 \text{ mm}^3$$

$$\overline{y} = \frac{\Sigma Ay}{\Sigma A} = \frac{420 \times 10^3}{4200} = 100 \text{ mm}$$

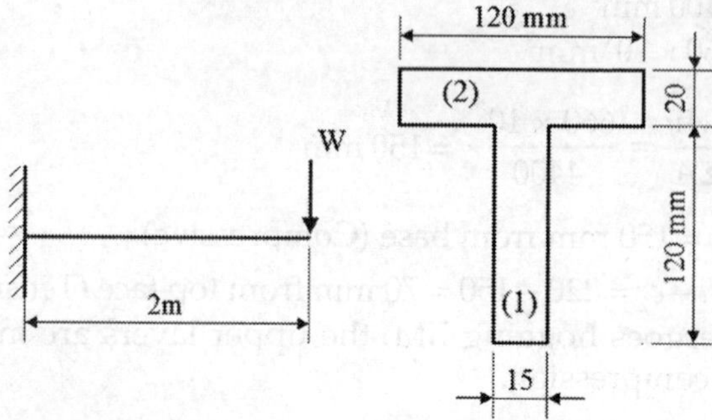

Fig. 6.25: Problem 37

i.e. $\quad \bar{y} = c_1 = 100$ mm from base (Compressive)

$\quad c_2 = \Sigma h - c_2 = 140 - 100 = 40$ mm from top face (Tensile)

Since the beam undergoes hogging BM, the upper layers are in tension while the bottom layers are in compression.

Bending stress $\quad \sigma = \dfrac{Mc}{I}$ $\qquad$ ... Eq. (i)

For a cantilever beam with point load at end span,

$$M = WL = 2000\,W$$

Also $\quad I = I_1 + I_2$

$$= [I_{G1} + A_1(\bar{y} \sim y_1)^2] + [I_{G2} + A_2(\bar{y} \sim y_2)^2]$$

$$= \{2.16 \times 10^6 + [1800 \times (100 - 60)^2]\}$$

$$+ \{80 \times 10^3 + [2400 \times (130 - 100)^2]\}$$

$$I = 7.28 \times 10^6 \text{ mm}^4$$

Eq. (i) yields...

Tensile stress $\quad \sigma_t = \dfrac{Mc_2}{I}$

$$90 = \frac{(2000\,W) \times 40}{7.28 \times 10^6}$$

$$W = 8190 \text{ N} \qquad \qquad \text{... Eq. (ii)}$$

Comp stress $\quad \sigma_c = \dfrac{Mc_1}{I}$

$$150 = \frac{(2000\,W) \times 100}{7.28 \times 10^6}$$

$$W = 5460 \text{ N} \qquad \qquad \text{... Eq. (iii)}$$

From Eqs (ii) and (iii), the maximum value of W is 5460 N (least value).

38. **A uniform T-section beam is 100 mm wide and 150 mm deep with a flange thickness of 25 mm and a web thickness of 12 mm. If the limiting bending stresses for the material of the beam are 80 MPa in compression and 160 MPa in tension, find the maximum UDL that the beam can carry over a simply supported span of 5 m.**

Solution: $\sigma_t = 160$ MPa, $\sigma_c = 80$ MPa, $w = ?$, $L = 5000$ mm

To find $\bar{y}$:

Element No.	b (mm)	h (mm)	$A = bh$ (mm²)	y (from base) $= (h/2) + x$ (mm)	Ay (mm³)	$I_G = bh^3/12$ (mm⁴)
(1) Web	12	125	1500	$(125/2) = 62.5$	93750	1.95×10^6
(2) Flange	100	25	2500	$125 + (25/2) = 137.5$	343750	130.21×10^3

x = distance of fiber considered from base

$$\Sigma A = 4000 \text{ mm}^2$$
$$\Sigma Ay = 437500 \text{ mm}^3$$

$$\bar{y} = \frac{\Sigma Ay}{\Sigma A} = \frac{437500}{4000} = 109.38 \text{ mm}$$

i.e. $\bar{y} = c_1 = 109.38$ mm from base (Tensile)

$$c_2 = \Sigma h - c_2 = 150 - 109.38 = 40.62 \text{ mm}$$
$$\text{from top face (Comp)}$$

Bending stress $\sigma = \dfrac{Mc}{I}$ ... Eq. (i)

For a simply supported beam with UDL over entire span,

Fig. 6.26: Problem 38

$$M = \frac{wL^2}{8} = \frac{w \times 5000^2}{8} = (3.125 \times 10^6)w$$

Also $I = I_1 + I_2$

$$= [I_{G1} + A_1(\bar{y} \sim y_1)^2] + [I_{G2} + A_2(\bar{y} \sim y_2)^2]$$
$$= \{1.95 \times 10^6 + [1500 \times (109.38 - 62.5)^2]\}$$
$$+ \{130.21 \times 10^3 + [2500 \times (137.5 - 109.38)^2]\}$$
$$I = 7.35 \times 10^6 \text{ mm}^4$$

Eq. (i) yields...

Tensile stress $\sigma_t = \dfrac{Mc_1}{I}$

$$160 = \frac{(3.125 \times 10^6)w \times 109.38}{7.35 \times 10^6}$$

$$w = 3.44 \text{ N/mm} = 3.44 \text{ kN/m} \qquad \text{... Eq. (ii)}$$

Comp stress $\sigma_c = \dfrac{Mc_2}{I}$

$$80 = \frac{(3.125 \times 10^6)w \times 40.62}{7.35 \times 10^6}$$

$$w = 4.63 \text{ N/mm} = 4.63 \text{ kN/m} \qquad \text{... Eq. (iii)}$$

From Eqs (ii) and (iii), the maximum value of w is 3.44 kN/m (least value).

PROBLEMS ON I-SECTION

39. At a given position in a beam of uniform I-section is subjected to a bending moment of 100 kN-m. Plot the variation of bending stress across the section. [Refer Fig. 6.27(a)]

VTU – June/ July 2014 – 10 Marks

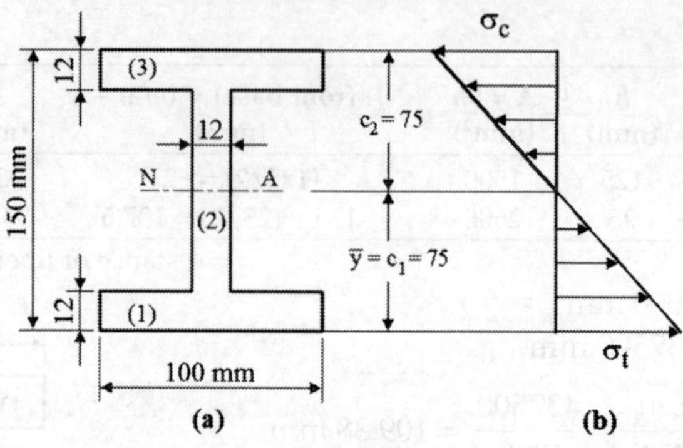

Fig. 6.27: Problem 39

Solution: $M = 100 \times 10^6$ N-mm, $\sigma_t = ?$, $\sigma_C = ?$

To find $\overline{y}$:

Element No.	b (mm)	h (mm)	$A = bh$ (mm²)	y (from base) = $(h/2) + x$ (mm)	Ay (mm³)	$I_G = bh^3/12$ (mm⁴)
(1) Bottom flange	100	12	1200	$(12/2) = 6$	7200	14.40×10^3
(2) Web	12	126	1512	$12 + (126/2) = 75$	113.4×10^3	2×10^6
(3) Top flange	100	12	1200	$12 + 126 + (12/2) = 144$	172.8×10^3	14.40×10^3

x = distance of fiber considered from base

$$\Sigma A = 3912 \text{ mm}^2$$
$$\Sigma Ay = 293.4 \times 10^3 \text{ mm}^3$$

$$\overline{y} = \frac{\Sigma Ay}{\Sigma A} = \frac{293.4 \times 10^3}{3912} = 75 \text{ mm}$$

i.e. $\overline{y} = c_1 = 75$ mm from base (Tensile)

$$c_2 = \Sigma h - c_1 = 150 - 75 = 75 \text{ mm from top face (Comp)}$$

Note: Since the I- section has equal flanges, $c_1 = c_2 = 75$ mm

Bending stress $\sigma = \dfrac{M}{Z} = \dfrac{Mc}{I}$ ... Eq. (i)

But $I = I_1 + I_2 + I_3$

$$= [I_{G1} + A_1(\overline{y} \sim y_1)^2] + [I_{G2} + A_2(\overline{y} \sim y_2)^2] + [I_{G3} + A_3(\overline{y} \sim y_3)^2]$$

$$= \{14.40 \times 10^3 + [1200 \times (75 - 6)^2]\} + \{2 \times 10^6 + [1512 \times (75 - 75)^2]\}$$
$$+ \{14.40 \times 10^3 + [1200 \times (144 - 75)^2]\}$$

$$I = 13.46 \times 10^6 \text{ mm}^4$$

OR $I = \dfrac{(BH^3 - bh^3)}{12}$, for symmetrical I section

$$= \frac{(100 \times 150^3 - 88 \times 126^3)}{12}$$

$$I = 13.46 \times 10^6 \text{ mm}^4$$

Eq. (i) yields...

Tensile stress $\quad \sigma_t = \dfrac{Mc_1}{I} = \dfrac{(100 \times 10^6) \times 75}{13.46 \times 10^6} = 557.21 \text{ MPa}$

Comp stress $\quad \sigma_c = \dfrac{Mc_2}{I} = \dfrac{(100 \times 10^6) \times 75}{13.46 \times 10^6} = 557.21 \text{ MPa}$

Since $c_1 = c_2$, we have $\sigma_t = \sigma_c = 557.21$ MPa
The bending stress distribution is shown in **Fig. 6.27(b)**.

40. **A beam of an I-section consists of 180 mm × 15 mm flanges and a web of 280 mm × 15 mm thickness. It is subjected to a bending moment of 120 kN-m. Sketch the bending stress distribution along the depth of the section.**

Solution: $M = 120 \times 10^6$ N-mm, $\sigma_t = ?$, $\sigma_c = ?$
Based on given data, I-section is as shown in **Fig. 6.28(a)**.

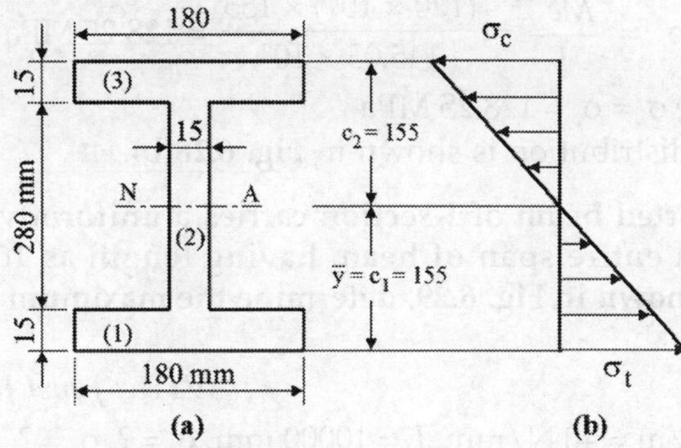

Fig. 6.28: Problem 40

To find $\bar{y}$:

Element No.	b (mm)	h (mm)	A = bh (mm²)	y (from base) = (h/2) + x (mm)	Ay (mm³)
(1) Bottom flange	180	15	2700	(15/2) = 7.5	20250
(2) Web	15	280	4200	15 + (280/2) = 155	651000
(3) Top flange	180	15	2700	15 + 280 + (15/2) = 302.5	816750

x = distance of fiber considered from base

$$\Sigma A = 9600 \text{ mm}^2$$
$$\Sigma Ay = 1.49 \times 10^6 \text{ mm}^3$$

$$\bar{y} = \frac{\Sigma Ay}{\Sigma A} = \frac{1.49 \times 10^6}{9600} = 155 \text{ mm}$$

i.e. $\qquad \bar{y} = c_1 = 155$ mm from base (Tensile)

$\qquad c_2 = \Sigma h - c_1 = 310 - 155 = 155$ mm from top face (Compressive)

Note: Since the I- section has equal flanges, $c_1 = c_2 = 155$ mm

Bending stress $\sigma = \dfrac{M}{Z} = \dfrac{Mc}{I}$ ... Eq. (i)

But

$$I = I_1 + I_2 + I_3$$

$$= [I_{G1} + A_1(\bar{y} \sim y_1)^2] + [I_{G2} + A_2(\bar{y} \sim y_2)^2] + [I_{G3} + A_3(\bar{y} \sim y_3)^2]$$

$$= \{50625 + [2700 \times (155 - 7.5)^2]\}$$

$$+ \{27.44 \times 10^6 + [4200 \times (155 - 155)^2]\}$$

$$+ \{50625 + [2700 \times (302.5 - 155)^2]\}$$

$$I = 145.03 \times 10^6 \text{ mm}^4$$

OR $I = \dfrac{(BH^3 - bh^3)}{12} = \dfrac{(180 \times 310^3 - 165 \times 280^3)}{12} = 145.03 \times 10^6 \text{ mm}^4$

Eq. (i) yields...

Tensile stress $\sigma_t = \dfrac{Mc_1}{I} = \dfrac{(120 \times 10^6) \times 155}{145.03 \times 10^6} = 128.25 \text{ MPa}$

Comp stress $\sigma_c = \dfrac{Mc_2}{I} = \dfrac{(120 \times 10^6) \times 155}{145.03 \times 10^6} = 128.25 \text{ MPa}$

Since $c_1 = c_2$, we have $\sigma_t = \sigma_c = 128.25$ MPa

The bending stress distribution is shown in **Fig. 6.28(b)**.

41. **A simply supported beam of I-section carries a uniformly distributed load of 40 kN/m run on entire span of beam having length as 10 m. If I section has dimensions as shown in Fig. 6.29, determine the maximum stress produced due to bending.**

VTU – June/ July 2011 – 08 Marks

Solution: $w = 40 \text{ kN/m} = 40 \text{ N/mm}$, $L = 10000$ mm, $\sigma_t = ?$, $\sigma_c = ?$

To find $\bar{y}$:

Element No.	b (mm)	h (mm)	$A = bh$ (mm^2)	y (from base) = $(h/2) + x$ (mm)	Ay (mm^3)
(1) Bottom flange	200	20	4000	$(20/2) = 10$	40000
(2) Web	10	360	3600	$20 + (360/2) = 200$	720×10^3
(3) Top flange	200	20	4000	$20 + 360 + (20/2) = 390$	1.56×10^6

x = distance of fiber considered from base

$$\Sigma A = 11600 \text{ mm}^2$$

$$\Sigma Ay = 2.32 \times 10^6 \text{ mm}^3$$

$$\bar{y} = \frac{\Sigma Ay}{\Sigma A} = \frac{2.32 \times 10^6}{11600} = 200 \text{ mm}$$

i.e. $\bar{y} = c_1 = 200$ mm from base (Tensile)

$c_2 = \Sigma h - c_1 = 400 - 200 = 200$ mm

from top face (Compressive)

Note: Since the I- section has equal flanges, $c_1 = c_2 = 200$ mm

Bending stress $\sigma = \dfrac{M}{Z} = \dfrac{Mc}{I}$ ... Eq. (i)

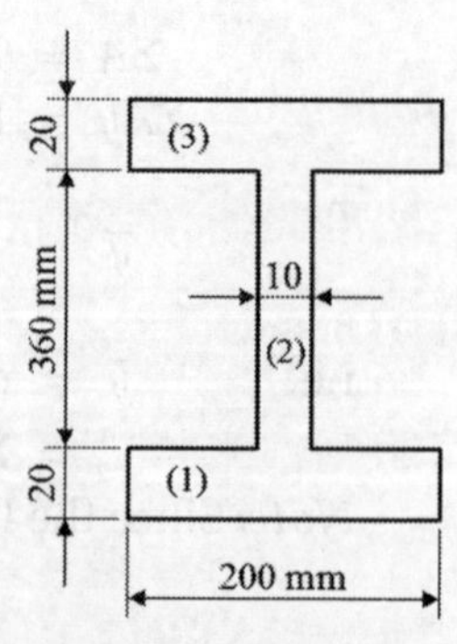

Fig. 6.29: Problem 41

For a simply supported beam with UDL over entire span,

$$M = \frac{wL^2}{8} = \frac{40 \times 10000^2}{8} = 500 \times 10^6 \text{ N-mm}$$

$$I = \frac{(BH^3 - bh^3)}{12} = \frac{(200 \times 400^3 - 190 \times 360^3)}{12} = 328 \times 10^6 \text{ mm}^4$$

Eq. (i) yields…

Tensile stress $\quad \sigma_t = \dfrac{Mc_1}{I} = \dfrac{(500 \times 10^6) \times 200}{328 \times 10^6} = 304.88 \text{ MPa}$

Comp stress $\quad \sigma_c = \dfrac{Mc_2}{I} = \dfrac{(500 \times 10^6) \times 200}{328 \times 10^6} = 304.88 \text{ MPa}$

Since $c_1 = c_2$, we have $\sigma_t = \sigma_c = 304.88$ MPa

42. A uniform I-section beam is 100 mm wide and 150 mm deep with a flange thickness of 25 mm and web thickness of 12 mm. The beam is simply supported over a span of 5 m. It carries a uniformly distributed load of intensity 83.4 kN/m throughout its length. Determine the bending stress in the beam and plot the stress distribution across its cross section.

Solution: $w = 83.4 \text{ kN/m} = 83.4 \text{ N/mm}$, $L = 5000 \text{ mm}$, $\sigma_t = ?$, $\sigma_c = ?$
Based on given data, I section is as shown in **Fig. 6.30(a)**.

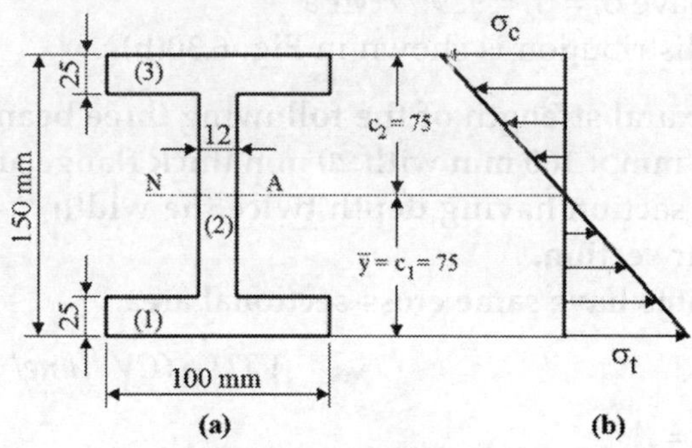

Fig. 6.30: Problem 42

To find $\bar{y}$:

Element No.	b (mm)	h (mm)	A = bh (mm²)	y (from base) = (h/2) + x (mm)	Ay (mm³)
(1) Bottom flange	100	25	2500	(25/2) = 12.5	31250
(2) Web	12	100	1200	25 + (100/2) = 75	90000
(3) Top flange	100	25	2500	25 + 100 + (25/2) = 137.5	3437500

x = distance of fiber considered from base

$$\Sigma A = 6200 \text{ mm}^2$$
$$\Sigma Ay = 465000 \text{ mm}^3$$

$$\bar{y} = \frac{\Sigma Ay}{\Sigma A} = \frac{465000}{6200} = 75 \text{ mm}$$

i.e. $\bar{y} = c_1 = 75$ mm from base (Tensile)

$$c_2 = \Sigma h - c_1 = 150 - 75 = 75 \text{ mm}$$

from top face (Compressive)

Note: Since the I-section has equal flanges [is symmetric about Y axis], $c_1 = c_2 = 75$ mm

Bending stress $\sigma = \dfrac{M}{Z} = \dfrac{Mc}{I}$ ... Eq. (i)

For a simply supported beam with UDL over entire span,

$$M = \frac{wL^2}{8} = \frac{83.4 \times 5000^2}{8} = 260.63 \times 10^6 \text{ N-mm}$$

$$I = \frac{(BH^3 - bh^3)}{12} = \frac{(100 \times 150^3 - 88 \times 100^3)}{12} = 20.80 \times 10^6 \text{ mm}^4$$

Eq. (i) yields...

Tensile stress $\sigma_t = \dfrac{Mc_1}{I} = \dfrac{(260.63 \times 10^6) \times 75}{20.80 \times 10^6} = 939.77$ MPa

Comp stress $\sigma_c = \dfrac{Mc_2}{I} = \dfrac{(260.63 \times 10^6) \times 75}{20.80 \times 10^6} = 939.77$ MPa

Since $c_1 = c_2$, we have $\sigma_t = \sigma_c = 939.77$ MPa

The bending stress distribution is shown in **Fig. 6.30(b)**.

43. **Compare the flexural strength of the following three beams:**
    (a) **I-section 320 mm × 160 mm with 20 mm thick flange and 13 mm thick web.**
    (b) **Rectangular section having depth twice the width**
    (c) **Solid circular section.**
    All the three beams have same cross-sectional area.

VTU – (CV) June/ July 2014 – 12 Marks

Solution: $A_{I-sec} = A_{rec} = A_{Cir}$

Based on given data, the beams are as shown in **Fig. 6.31.**

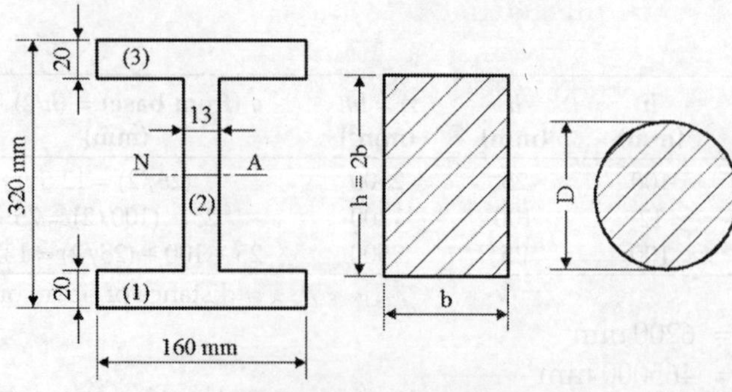

Fig. 6.31: Problem 43

Case a: I - section

Cross-sectional area $\qquad A_{I-sec} = (160 \times 20) + (13 \times 280) + (160 \times 20) = 10040 \text{ mm}^2$

MI about neutral axis (NA) $\qquad I = \dfrac{(BH^3 - bh^3)}{12} = \dfrac{(160 \times 320^3 - 147 \times 280^3)}{12}$

$$= 168 \times 10^6 \text{ mm}^4$$

Section modulus $\qquad Z_{I-sec} = \dfrac{I}{c} = \dfrac{I}{H/2} = \dfrac{168 \times 10^6}{320/2} = 1.05 \times 10^6 \text{ mm}^4$

Case b: Rectangular section

Cross-sectional area $\qquad A_{rec} = bh = b(2b) = 2b^2$

Since areas are same $\qquad A_{rec} = A_{I-sec}$

$\qquad\qquad 2b^2 = 10040$

$\qquad\qquad b = 70.85 \text{ mm} \approx 72 \text{ mm}$

$\qquad\qquad h = 2 \times 72 = 144 \text{ mm}$

Section modulus $\qquad Z_{rec} = \dfrac{bh^2}{6} = \dfrac{72 \times 144^2}{6} = 2.49 \times 10^5 \text{ mm}^3$

Case c: Circular section

Cross-sectional area $\qquad A_{cir} = \pi D^2/4$

Since areas are same $\qquad A_{cir} = A_{I-sec}$

$\qquad\qquad \pi D^2/4 = 10040$

$\qquad\qquad D = 113.06 = 115 \text{ mm}$

Section modulus $\qquad Z_{cir} = \dfrac{\pi D^3}{32} = \dfrac{\pi \times 115^3}{32} = 149.31 \times 10^3 \text{ mm}^3$

Flexural strengths:

$$\dfrac{Z_{I-sec}}{Z_{rec}} = \dfrac{1.05 \times 10^6}{2.49 \times 10^5} = 4.217$$

$$\dfrac{Z_{I-sec}}{Z_{cir}} = \dfrac{1.05 \times 10^6}{149.31 \times 10^3} = 7.032$$

44. **An I-section girder, 200 mm wide by 300 mm deep, with flange and web of thickness 20 mm is used as a simply supported beam over a span of 7 m. The girder carries a distributed load of 5 kN/m and a concentrated load of 20 kN at mid-span. Determine the maximum stress set-up in the girder.**

Solution: $L = 7000 \text{ mm}$, $w = 5 \text{ kN/m} = 5 \text{ N/mm}$, $W = 20 \times 10^3 \text{ N}$, $\sigma_t = ?$, $\sigma_c = ?$

Based on given data, I-section is as shown in **Fig. 6.32**.

To find $\bar{y}$:

Element No.	b (mm)	h (mm)	$A = bh$ (mm^2)	y (from base) = $(h/2) + x$ (mm)	Ay (mm^3)
(1) Bottom flange	200	20	4000	$(20/2) = 10$	40000
(2) Web	20	260	5200	$20 + (260/2) = 150$	780×10^3
(3) Top flange	200	20	4000	$20 + 260 + (20/2) = 290$	1.16×10^6

x = distance of fiber considered from base

$$\Sigma A = 13200 \text{ mm}^2$$

$$\Sigma Ay = 1.98 \times 10^6 \text{ mm}^3$$

$$\bar{y} = \frac{\Sigma Ay}{\Sigma A} = \frac{1.98 \times 10^6}{13200} = 150 \text{ mm}$$

i.e. $\bar{y} = c_1 = 150$ mm from base (Tensile)

$$c_2 = \Sigma h - c_1 = 300 - 150 = 150 \text{ mm}$$

from top face (Compressive)

Note: Since the I-section has equal flanges [is symmetric about Y axis], $c_1 = c_2 = 150$ mm

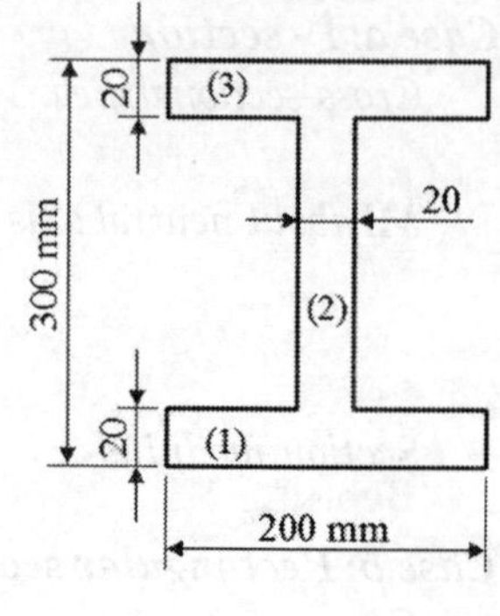

Fig. 6.32: Problem 44

Bending stress $\sigma = \dfrac{M}{Z} = \dfrac{Mc}{I}$ ... Eq. (i)

For a simply supported beam with UDL over entire span,

$$M = \left(\frac{wL^2}{8}\right) + \left(\frac{WL}{4}\right) = \left(\frac{5 \times 7^2}{8}\right) + \left(\frac{20 \times 7}{4}\right) = 65.63 \text{ kN-m}$$

$$= 65.63 \times 10^6 \text{ N-mm}$$

$$I = \frac{(BH^3 - bh^3)}{12} = \frac{(200 \times 300^3 - 180 \times 260^3)}{12} = 1.86 \times 10^8 \text{ mm}^4$$

Eq. (i) yields...

Tensile stress $\sigma_t = \dfrac{Mc_1}{I} = \dfrac{(65.63 \times 10^6) \times 150}{1.86 \times 10^8} = 52.93 \text{ MPa}$

Comp stress $\sigma_c = \dfrac{Mc_2}{I} = \dfrac{(65.63 \times 10^6) \times 150}{1.86 \times 10^8} = 52.93 \text{ MPa}$

Since $c_1 = c_2$, we have $\sigma_t = \sigma_c = 52.93$ MPa

45. A beam simply supported at ends and having cross-section as shown in Fig. 6.33 is loaded with a UDL over a span of 8 m. The allowable bending stress in tension is 30 MPa and that in compression is 45 MPa. Determine the maximum value of UDL, the beam can carry.

VTU – Dec. 16/ Jan. 17 – 12 Marks; [similar: (ME) June/ July 2013 – 15 Marks

Solution: $L = 8000$ mm, $\sigma_t = 30$ MPa, $\sigma_c = 45$ MPa, $W = ?$

To find $\bar{y}$:

Element No.	b (mm)	h (mm)	A = bh (mm²)	y (from base) = (h/2) + x (mm)	Ay (mm³)	$I_G = bh^3/12$ (mm⁴)
(1) Bottom flange	120	50	6000	(50/2) = 25	150 × 10³	1.25 × 10⁶
(2) Web	30	120	3600	50 + (120/2) = 110	396 × 10³	4.32 × 10⁶
(3) Top flange	100	30	3000	50 + 120 + (30/2) = 185	555 × 10³	225 × 10³

x = distance of fiber considered from base

$$\Sigma A = 12600 \text{ mm}^2$$

$$\Sigma Ay = 1.101 \times 10^6 \text{ mm}^3$$

$$\bar{y} = \frac{\Sigma Ay}{\Sigma A} = \frac{1.101 \times 10^6}{12600} = 87.38 \text{ mm}$$

i.e. $\bar{y} = c_1 = 87.38$ mm from base (Tensile)

$$c_2 = \Sigma h - c_1 = 200 - 87.38 = 112.62 \text{ mm}$$

from top face (Compressive)

Bending stress $\sigma = \dfrac{M}{Z} = \dfrac{Mc}{I}$ ... Eq. (i)

But $I = I_1 + I_2 + I_3$

Fig. 6.33: Problem 45

$$= [I_{G1} + A_1(\bar{y} \sim y_1)^2] + [I_{G2} + A_2(\bar{y} \sim y_2)^2] + [I_{G3} + A_3(\bar{y} \sim y_3)^2]$$

$$= \{1.25 \times 10^6 + [6000 \times (87.38 - 25)^2]\}$$
$$+ \{4.32 \times 10^6 + [3600 \times (110 - 87.38)^2]\}$$
$$+ \{225 \times 10^3 + [3000 \times (185 - 87.38)^2]\}$$

$$I = 59.57 \times 10^6 \text{ mm}^4$$

Tensile stress $\sigma_t = \dfrac{Mc_1}{I}$

$$30 = \frac{(8 \times 10^6)w \times 87.38}{59.57 \times 10^6}$$

$$w = 2.56 \text{ N/mm} = 2.56 \text{ kN/m} \qquad \text{... Eq. (ii)}$$

Comp stress $\sigma_c = \dfrac{Mc_2}{I}$

$$30 = \frac{(8 \times 10^6)w \times 112.62}{59.57 \times 10^6}$$

$$w = 2.98 \text{ N/mm} = 2.98 \text{ kN/m} \qquad \text{... Eq. (iii)}$$

From Eqs (ii) and (iii), the maximum value of w is 2.56 kN/m (least value).

46. A cast iron beam has an I section with a top flange 80 mm × 40 mm, web 120 mm × 20 mm and bottom flange 160 mm × 40 mm. If the tensile stress is not to exceed 30 MPa and the compressive stress 90 MPa, what is the uniformly distributed load the beam can carry over a simply supported span of 6 m, if the large flange is in tension.

VTU – Dec. 2011 – 10 Marks

Solution: $L = 6000$ mm, $\sigma_t = 30$ MPa, $\sigma_c = 90$ MPa, $w = ?$

Based on given data, I section is as shown in **Fig. 6.32**.

To find $\bar{y}$:

Element No.	b (mm)	h (mm)	$A = bh$ (mm²)	y (from base) = $(h/2) + x$ (mm)	Ay (mm³)	$I_G = bh^3/12$ (mm⁴)
(1) Bottom flange	160	40	6400	$(40/2) = 20$	128×10^3	853.33×10^3
(2) Web	20	120	2400	$40 + (120/2) = 100$	240×10^3	2.88×10^6
(3) Top flange	80	40	3200	$40 + 120 + (40/2) = 180$	576×10^3	426.67×10^3

x = distance of fiber considered from base

$$\Sigma A = 12000 \text{ mm}^2$$
$$\Sigma Ay = 944 \times 10^3 \text{ mm}^3$$

$$\bar{y} = \frac{\Sigma Ay}{\Sigma A} = \frac{944 \times 10^3}{12000} = 78.67 \text{ mm}$$

i.e. $\bar{y} = c_1 = 78.67$ mm from base (Tensile)

$c_2 = \Sigma h - c_1 = 200 - 78.67 = 121.33$ mm
from top face (Compressive)

Bending stress $\sigma = \dfrac{M}{Z} = \dfrac{Mc}{I}$ ... Eq. (i)

For a simply supported beam with UDL over entire span,

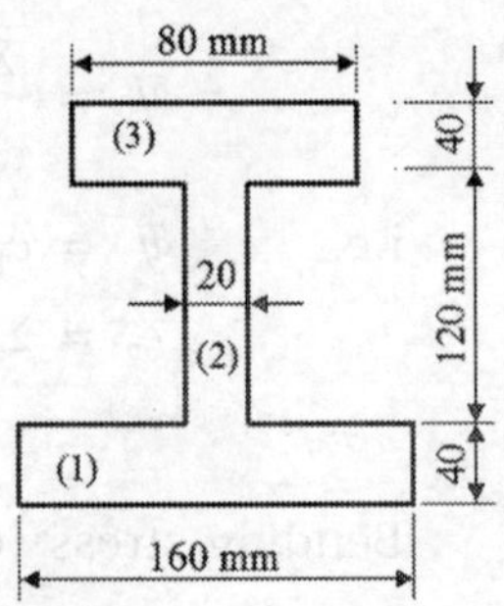

Fig. 6.34: Problem 46

$$M = \frac{wL^2}{8} = \frac{w \times 6000^2}{8} = (4.5 \times 10^6)w$$

Also $I = I_1 + I_2 + I_3$

$$= [I_{G1} + A_1(\bar{y} \sim y_1)^2] + [I_{G2} + A_2(\bar{y} \sim y_2)^2] + [I_{G3} + A_3(\bar{y} \sim y_3)^2]$$

$$= \{853.33 \times 10^3 + [6400 \times (78.67 - 20)^2]\}$$
$$+ \{2.88 \times 10^6 + [2400 \times (100 - 78.67)^2]\}$$
$$+ \{426.67 \times 10^3 + [3200 \times (180 - 78.67)^2]\}$$

$$I = 60.14 \times 10^6 \text{ mm}^4$$

Tensile stress $\sigma_t = \dfrac{Mc_1}{I}$

$$30 = \frac{(4.5 \times 10^6)w \times 78.67}{60.14 \times 10^6}$$

$$w = 5.10 \text{ N/mm} = 5.10 \text{ kN/m} \qquad \text{... Eq. (ii)}$$

Comp stress $\sigma_c = \dfrac{Mc_2}{I}$

$$90 = \frac{(4.5 \times 10^6)w \times 121.33}{60.14 \times 10^6}$$

$$w = 9.91 \text{ N/mm} = 9.91 \text{ kN/m} \qquad \text{... Eq. (iii)}$$

From Eqs (ii) and (iii), the maximum value of w is 5.10 kN/m (least value).

47. A cast iron beam of I-section is as shown in Fig. 6.35. The beam is simply supported on a span of 5. If the tensile stress is not to exceed 20 N/mm², find the safe uniformly distributed load, which the beam can carry. Also find the maximum compressive stress.

VTU – Jan. 2013 – 10 Marks

Solution: $L = 5000$ mm, $\sigma_t = 20$ MPa, $w = ?$, $\sigma_c = ?$

To find $\bar{y}$:

Element No.	b (mm)	h (mm)	$A = bh$ (mm²)	y (from base) $= (h/2) + x$ (mm)	Ay (mm³)	$I_G = bh^3/12$ (mm⁴)
(1) Bottom flange	160	40	6400	$(40/2) = 20$	128×10^3	853.33×10^3
(2) Web	20	200	4000	$40 + (200/2) = 140$	560×10^3	13.33×10^6
(3) Top flange	80	20	1600	$40 + 200 + (20/2) = 250$	400×10^3	53.33×10^3

x = distance of fiber considered from base

$$\Sigma A = 12000 \text{ mm}^2$$
$$\Sigma Ay = 1.09 \times 10^6 \text{ mm}^3$$

$$\bar{y} = \frac{\Sigma Ay}{\Sigma A} = \frac{1.09 \times 10^6}{12000} = 90.83 \text{ mm}$$

i.e. $\bar{y} = c_1 = 90.83$ mm from base (Tensile)

$$c_2 = \Sigma h - c_1 = 260 - 90.83 = 169.17 \text{ mm}$$
from top face (Compressive)

Bending stress $\quad \sigma = \dfrac{M}{Z} = \dfrac{Mc}{I} \qquad$ ... Eq. (i)

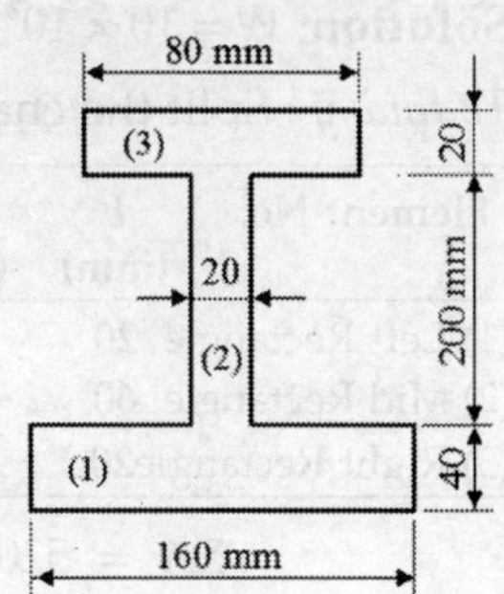

Fig. 6.35: Problem 47

For a simply supported beam with UDL over entire span,

$$M = \frac{wL^2}{8} = \frac{w \times 5000^2}{8} = (3.125 \times 10^6)w$$

Also
$$\begin{aligned}
I &= I_1 + I_2 + I_3 \\
&= [I_{G1} + A_1(\bar{y} \sim y_1)^2] + [I_{G2} + A_2(\bar{y} \sim y_2)^2] + [I_{G3} + A_3(\bar{y} \sim y_3)^2] \\
&= \{853.33 \times 10^3 + [6400 \times (90.83 - 20)^2]\} \\
&\quad + \{13.33 \times 10^6 + [4000 \times (140 - 90.83)^2]\} \\
&\quad + \{53.33 \times 10^3 + [1600 \times (250 - 90.83)^2]\} \\
I &= 96.55 \times 10^6 \text{ mm}^4
\end{aligned}$$

Tensile stress $\quad \sigma_t = \dfrac{Mc_1}{I}$

$$20 = \frac{(3.125 \times 10^6)w \times 90.83}{96.55 \times 10^6}$$

$$W = 6.80 \text{ N/mm} = 6.80 \text{ kN/m} \qquad\qquad \text{... Eq. (ii)}$$

Comp stress $\quad \sigma_c = \dfrac{Mc_2}{I} = \dfrac{(3.125 \times 10^6)w \times 6.80 \times 169.17}{96.55 \times 10^6} = 37.23 \text{ MPa}$

PROBLEMS ON C-SECTION

48. Determine the maximum tensile and compressive stresses for the channel shown in Fig. 6.36 (a).

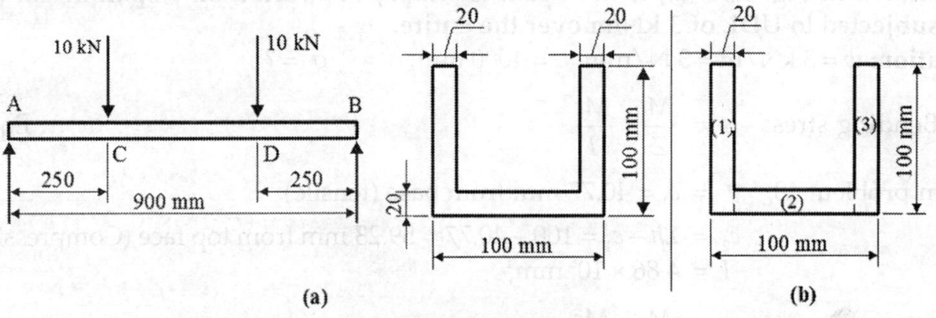

(a)

(b)

Fig. 6.36: Problem 48

Solution: $W = 10 \times 10^3$ N, $\sigma_t = ?$, $\sigma_c = ?$

To find $\bar{y}$: Split the channel into three rectangles as shown in **Fig. 6.36(b)**.

Element No.	b (mm)	h (mm)	$A = bh$ (mm^2)	y (from base) = $(h/2) + x$ (mm)	Ay (mm^3)	$I_G = bh^3/12$ (mm^4)
(1) Left Rectangle	20	100	2000	$(100/2) = 50$	100×10^3	1.67×10^6
(2) Mid Rectangle	60	20	1200	$(20/2) = 10$	12×10^3	40×10^3
(3) Right Rectangle	20	100	2000	$(100/2) = 50$	100×10^3	1.67×10^6

$$\Sigma A = 5200 \text{ mm}^2$$
$$\Sigma Ay = 212 \times 10^3 \text{ mm}^3$$

$$\bar{y} = \frac{\Sigma Ay}{\Sigma A} = \frac{212 \times 10^3}{5200} = 40.77 \text{ mm}$$

i.e. $\bar{y} = c_1 = 40.77$ mm from base (Tensile)

$c_2 = \Sigma h - c_1 = 100 - 40.77 = 59.23$ mm from top face (Compressive)

Bending stress $\sigma = \dfrac{M}{Z} = \dfrac{Mc}{I}$ ... Eq. (i)

Since the loading is symmetric, the reactions at the supports are $R_A = R_B = 10$ kN

The maximum bending moment is $M_C = M_D = 10 \times 250 = 2500$ kN-mm $= 2.5 \times 10^6$ N-mm

Also $I = I_1 + I_2 + I_3$

$$= [I_{G1} + A_1(\bar{y} \sim y_1)^2] + [I_{G2} + A_2(\bar{y} \sim y_2)^2] + [I_{G3} + A_3(\bar{y} \sim y_3)^2]$$
$$= \{1.67 \times 10^6 + [2000 \times (50 - 40.77)^2]\}$$
$$+ \{40 \times 10^3 + [1200 \times (40.77 - 10)^2]\}$$
$$+ \{1.67 \times 10^6 + [2000 \times (50 - 40.77)^2]\}$$

$$I = 4.86 \times 10^6 \text{ mm}^4$$

Tensile stress $\sigma_t = \dfrac{Mc_1}{I} = \dfrac{(2.5 \times 10^6) \times 40.77}{4.86 \times 10^6} = 20.97$ MPa

Comp stress $\sigma_c = \dfrac{Mc_2}{I} = \dfrac{(2.5 \times 10^6) \times 59.23}{4.86 \times 10^6} = 30.47$ MPa

49. Determine the maximum tensile and compressive stresses for the channel shown in Fig. 6.36 (a), if the beam is simply supported on a span of 4m and subjected to UDL of 3 kN/m over the entire.

Solution: $w = 3$ kN/m $= 3$ N/mm, $L = 4000$ mm, $\sigma_t = ?$, $\sigma_c = ?$

Bending stress $\sigma = \dfrac{M}{Z} = \dfrac{Mc}{I}$ ... Eq. (i)

From problem 48, $\bar{y} = c_1 = 40.77$ mm from base (tensile)

$c_2 = \Sigma h - c_1 = 100 - 40.77 = 59.23$ mm from top face (Compressive)

$I = 4.86 \times 10^6$ mm^4

Bending stress $\sigma = \dfrac{M}{Z} = \dfrac{Mc}{I}$ ... Eq. (i)

For a simply supported beam with UDL over entire span,

$$M = \frac{wL^2}{8} = \frac{3 \times 4000^2}{8} = 6 \times 10^6 \text{ N-mm}$$

Eq. (i) yields...

Tensile stress $\quad \sigma_t = \dfrac{Mc_1}{I} = \dfrac{(6 \times 10^6) \times 40.77}{4.86 \times 10^6} = 50.33 \text{ MPa}$

Comp stress $\quad \sigma_c = \dfrac{Mc_2}{I} = \dfrac{(6 \times 10^6) \times 59.23}{4.86 \times 10^6} = 73.12 \text{ MPa}$

50. A simply supported beam with cross-section as shown in Fig. 6.37(a) carries point loads 'W'. Determine the maximum value of W taking allowable bending stresses in compression as 70 N/mm² and that in tension as 40 N/mm².

VTU – June/ July 2011 – 12 Marks

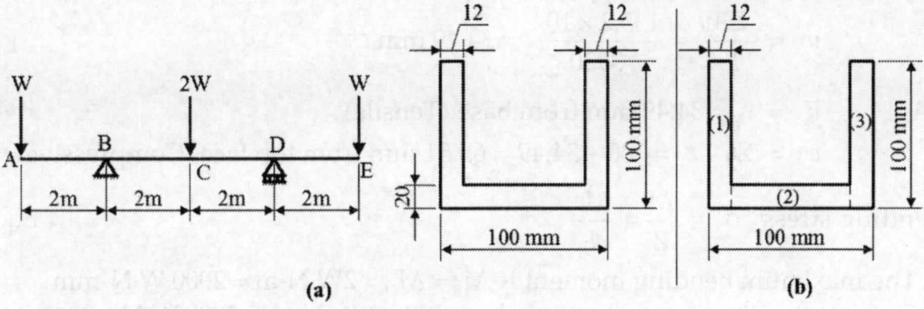

Fig. 6.37: Problem 50

Solution: $\sigma_t = 40$ MPa, $\sigma_c = 70$ MPa, $W = ?$

Reactions at supports:

$$R_B + R_D = W + 2W + W = 4W \qquad \ldots \text{Eq. (i)}$$

Taking moments about B and equating to zero, we have

$$R_D \times 4 = (2W \times 2) + (W \times 6) - (W \times 2)$$
$$4R_D = 8W$$
$$R_D = 2W \qquad \qquad \ldots \text{Eq. (ii)}$$

Substituting Eq. (ii) in Eq. (i), we have

$$R_B + 2W = 4W$$
$$R_B = 2W \qquad \qquad \ldots \text{Eq. (iii)}$$

Here the reactions are equal as the beam is symmetrically loaded.

Shear force calculations:

$$F_A = -W$$
$$F_B = -W + 2W = W$$
$$F_C = W - 2W = -W$$
$$F_D = -W + 2W = W$$
$$F_E = F_D = W$$

Bending moment calculations:

$$M_A = 0$$
$$M_B = -2W \text{ N-m}$$
$$M_C = -4W + (2W \times 2) = 0$$
$$M_D = -2W \text{ N-m}$$
$$M_E = 0 \qquad \text{(from RHS)}$$

To find $\bar{y}$: Split the channel into three rectangles as shown in **Fig. 6.37(b)**.

Element No.	b (mm)	h (mm)	$A = bh$ (mm^2)	y (from base) = $(h/2) + x$ (mm)	Ay (mm^3)	$I_G = bh^3/12$ (mm^4)
(1) Left Rectangle	12	100	1200	$(100/2) = 50$	60×10^3	1×10^6
(2) Mid Rectangle	76	20	1520	$(20/2) = 10$	15.2×10^3	50.67×10^3
(3) Right Rectangle	12	100	1200	$(100/2) = 50$	60×10^3	1×10^6

$$\Sigma A = 3920 \text{ mm}^2$$
$$\Sigma Ay = 135.2 \times 10^3 \text{ mm}^3$$

$$\bar{y} = \frac{\Sigma Ay}{\Sigma A} = \frac{135.2 \times 10^3}{3920} = 34.49 \text{ mm}$$

i.e. $\quad \bar{y} = c_1 = 34.49$ mm from base (Tensile)

$$c_2 = \Sigma h - c_1 = 100 - 34.49 = 65.51 \text{ mm from top face (Compressive)}$$

Bending stress $\quad \sigma = \dfrac{M}{Z} = \dfrac{Mc}{I}$ $\qquad\qquad$ ... Eq. (iv)

The maximum bending moment is $M_B = M_D = 2W$ N-m = 2000 W N-mm

OR $\quad$ Since the loading is symmetrical, max. $BM = 2W$ N-m = 2000 W N-mm

Also $\quad I = I_1 + I_2 + I_3$

$$= [I_{G1} + A_1(\bar{y} \sim y_1)^2] + [I_{G2} + A_2(\bar{y} \sim y_2)^2] + [I_{G3} + A_3(\bar{y} \sim y_3)^2]$$
$$= \{1 \times 10^6 + [1200 \times (50 - 34.49)^2]\}$$
$$+ \{50.67 \times 10^3 + [1520 \times (34.49 - 10)^2]\}$$
$$+ \{1 \times 10^6 + [1200 \times (50 - 34.49)^2]\}$$
$$I = 3.54 \times 10^6 \text{ mm}^4$$

Eq. (iv) yields...

Tensile stress $\quad \sigma_t = \dfrac{Mc_1}{I}$

$$40 = \frac{2000W \times 34.49}{3.45 \times 10^6}$$

$$W = 2052.77 \text{ N} \qquad\qquad \text{... Eq. (v)}$$

Comp stress $\quad \sigma_c = \dfrac{Mc_2}{I}$

$$70 = \frac{2000W \times 65.51}{3.45 \times 10^6}$$

$$W = 1891.31 \text{ N} \qquad\qquad \text{... Eq. (vi)}$$

From Eqs (v) and (vi), the maximum value of W is 1891.31 N (least value).

PROBLEMS ON ANGLES

51. An unequal angle section as shown in Fig. 6.38 is used as a simply supported beam over a span of 2 m and uniformly distributed load of 10 kN/m, inclusive of its own weight. Determine the maximum tensile and compressive stresses in the section.

VTU – June/July 2008 – 10 Marks

Solution: $L = 2000$ mm, $w = 10$ kN/m $= 10$ N/mm, $\sigma_t = ?$, $\sigma_c = ?$

To find $\bar{y}$: Split the channel into three rectangles as shown in **Fig. 6.37(b)**.

Element No.	b (mm)	h (mm)	$A = bh$ (mm²)	y (from base) $= (h/2) + x$ (mm)	Ay (mm³)	$I_G = bh^3/12$ (mm⁴)
(1) Left Rectangle	12.5	107.5	1343.75	$(107.5/2) = 53.75$	72.23×10^3	1.29×10^6
(2) Mid Rectangle	100	12.5	1250	$107.5 + (12.5/2) = 113.75$	142.18×10^3	16.28×10^3

$$\Sigma A = 2593.75 \text{ mm}^2$$
$$\Sigma Ay = 214.45 \times 10^3 \text{ mm}^3$$

$$\bar{y} = \frac{\Sigma Ay}{\Sigma A} = \frac{214.45 \times 10^3}{2593.75} = 82.66 \text{ mm}$$

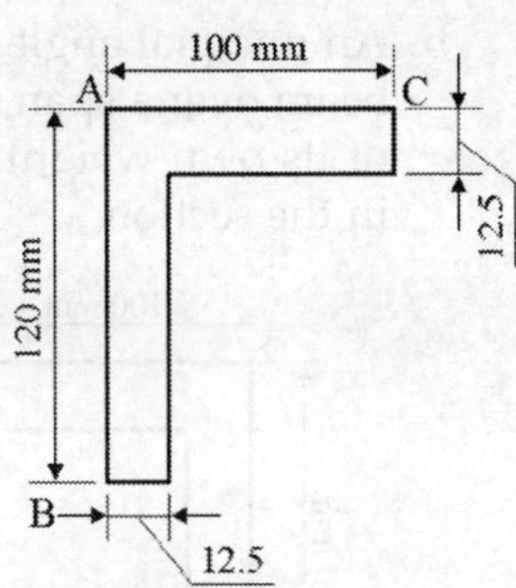

Fig. 6.38: Problem 51

i.e. $\bar{y} = c_1 = 82.66$ mm from base (Tensile)

$$c_2 = \Sigma h - c_1 = 100 - 82.66 = 37.34 \text{ mm}$$
from top face (Compressive)

Bending stress $\sigma = \dfrac{M}{Z} = \dfrac{Mc}{I}$ ... Eq. (iv)

For a simply supported beam with UDL over entire span,

$$M = \frac{wL^2}{8} = \frac{10 \times 2000^2}{8} = 5 \times 10^6 \text{ N-mm}$$

Also $I = I_1 + I_2 + I_3$

$$= [I_{G1} + A_1(\bar{y} \sim y_1)^2] + [I_{G2} + A_2(\bar{y} \sim y_2)^2]$$
$$= \{1.29 \times 10^6 + [1343.75 \times (82.66 - 53.75)^2]\}$$
$$+ \{16.28 \times 10^3 + [1250 \times (113.75 - 82.66)^2]\}$$
$$I = 3.64 \times 10^6 \text{ mm}^4$$

Eq. (iv) yields...

Tensile stress $\sigma_t = \dfrac{Mc_1}{I} = \dfrac{(5 \times 10^6) \times 82.66}{3.64 \times 10^6} = 113.54$ MPa

Comp stress $\sigma_c = \dfrac{Mc_2}{I} = \dfrac{(5 \times 10^6) \times 37.34}{3.64 \times 10^6} = 51.29$ MPa

VTU QUESTION PAPERS

Dec. 07/Jan. 08 (06ME34)

1. A beam of T-section has a length of 2.5 m and is subjected to a point load as shown in **Fig. U6.1**. Calculate the compressive bending stress and plot the stress distribution across the cross-section of the beam. The maximum tensile stress is limited to 300 MPa. Calculate the value of W. **(14 Marks)**

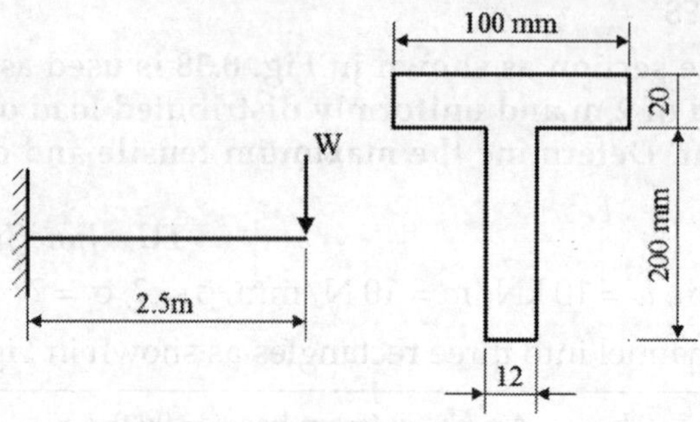

Fig. U6.1

June/July 2008 (06ME34)

2. a. Explain neutral axis and modulus of section as applied to beam. **(04 Marks)**

   b. An unequal angle section as shown in **Fig. U6.2** is used as a simply supported beam over a span of 2 m and uniformly distributed load of 10 kN/m, inclusive of its own weight. Determine the maximum tensile and compressive stresses in the section **(10 Marks)**

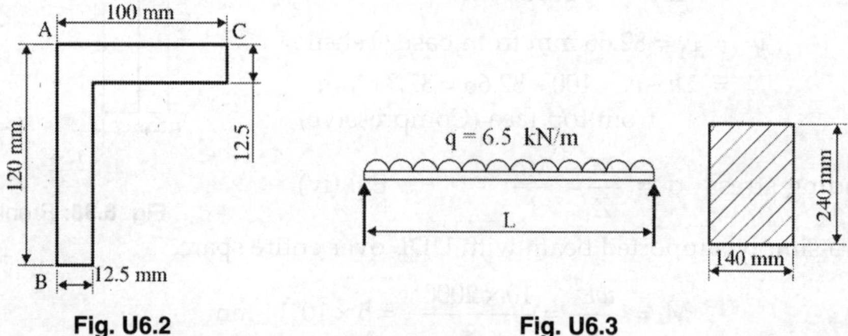

Fig. U6.2   Fig. U6.3

June/July 2009 (06ME34)

3. a. State the assumptions made in developing the theory of simple bending. **(04 Marks)**

   b. Derive an expression for the bending stress and the radius of curvature for a straight beam subjected to pure bending. **(08 Marks)**

   c. Determine the maximum allowable span length L for a simple beam shown in **Fig. U6.3**. The beam is of rectangular cross section 140 mm × 240 mm subjected to a uniformly distributed load q = 6.5 kN/m and the allowable bending stress is 8.2 MPa. **(08 Marks)**

Dec. 09/Jan. 10 (06ME34)

4. Prove the relations $\dfrac{M}{I} = \dfrac{\sigma}{Y} = \dfrac{E}{R}$ with usual notations. **(10 Marks)**

Dec. 2010 (06ME34)

5. A cantilever beam of square cross section 200 mm × 200 mm, 2 m long just fails in bending, when a load f 20 kN is placed at its free end. A beam of the same material having a rectangular cross section 150 mm × 300 mm, simply supported

over a span of 3 m is to be used under uniformly distributed load w N/m. What can be the maximum value of w? **(12 Marks)**

June/July 2011 (06ME34)

6. a. Derive an expression for the bending stress and radius of curvature for a straight beam subjected to pure bending. Also state the assumptions made in the theory of simple bending. **(12 Marks)**

   b. A simply supported beam of I- section carries a uniformly distributed load of 40 kN/m run on entire span of beam having length as 10 m. If I section is having dimensions s shown in **Fig. U6.4**, determine the maximum stress produced due to bending. **(08 Marks)**

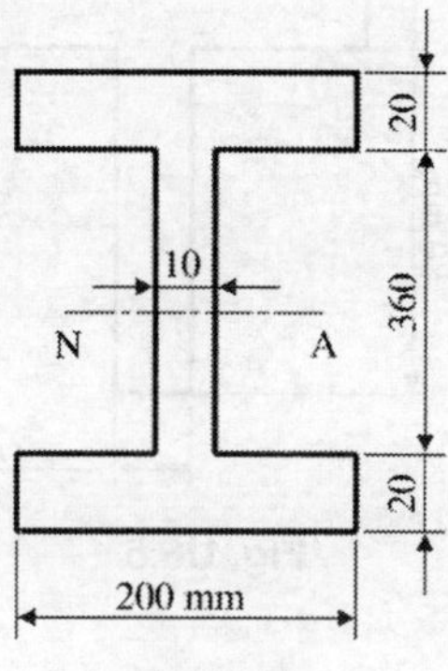

Fig. U6.4

Dec. 2011 (06ME34)

7. a. State the assumptions made in theory of simple bending. **(04 Marks)**

   b. Derive an expression for the relationship between bending stress and radius of curvature of a beam. **(06 Marks)**

   c. A cast iron beam has an I section with a top flange 80 mm × 40 mm, web 120 mm × 20 mm and bottom flange 160 mm × 40 mm. If the tensile stress is not to exceed 30 N/mm^2 and the compressive stress 90 N/mm^2, what is the uniformly distributed load the beam can carry over a simply supported span of 6 m, if the large flange is in tension. **(10 Marks)**

Dec. 2011 (10ME34)

8. a. State the assumptions made in the theory of simple bending. **(05 Marks)**

   b. A uniform I-section beam is 100 mm wide and 150 mm deep with a flange thickness of 25 mm and web thickness of 12 mm. The beam is simply supported over a span of 5 m. It carries a uniformly distributed load of intensity 83.4 kN/m throughout its length. Determine the bending stress in the beam and plot the stress distribution across its cross section. **(15 Marks)**

June 2012 (06ME34)

9. Explain:　　　　i. Section modulus　　　ii. Flexural rigidity **(04 Marks)**

June 2012 (10ME34)

10. A simply supported beam of span 5 m has a cross section 150 mm × 250 mm. if the permissible stress is 10 N/mm^2, find:

   i. Maximum intensity of uniformly distributed load it can carry.

ii. The maximum concentrated load P applied at 2 m from one end it can carry.
(10 Marks)

Dec. 2012 (10ME34)

11. A cast iron beam of T-section is shown in **Fig. U6.5**. The beam is simply supported on a span of 8 m. The beam caries a uniformly distributed load of 1.5 kN/m length over the entire span. Determine the maximum tensile and compressive stresses. **(10 Marks)**

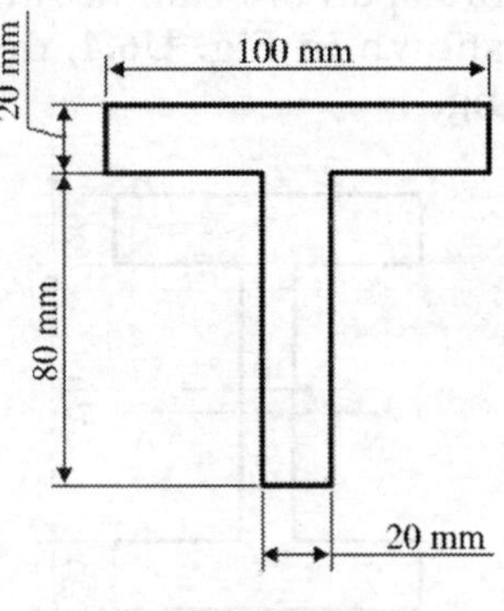

Fig. U6.5

Jan. 2013 (06ME34)

12. A cast iron beam of I-section is as shown in **Fig. U6.6**. The beam is simply supported on a span of 5 m. If the tensile stress is not to exceed 20 N/mm², find the safe uniformly distributed load, which the beam can carry. Also find the maximum compressive stress. **(10 Marks)**

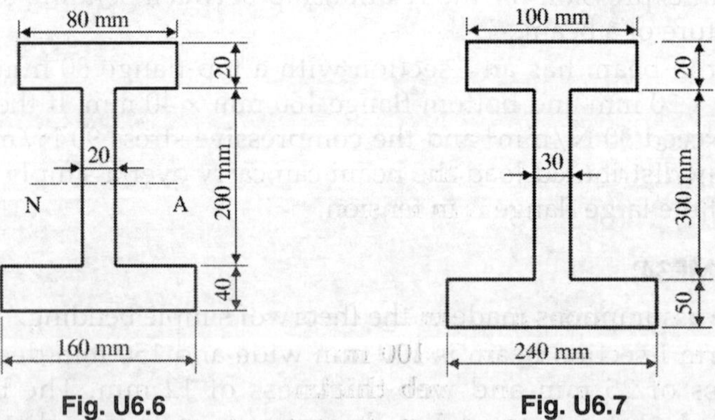

Fig. U6.6   **Fig. U6.7**

June/July 2013 (06ME34)

13. A simply supported beam of I-section as shown in **Fig. U6.7** is subjected to uniformly distributed load. Find the load per meter length of the beam, if the beam length is 4 m and the allowable stress in tension is 24 MPa. **(15 Marks)**

June/July 2013 (10ME34)

14. a. Enumerate the assumptions made in the theory of simple bending. **(04 Marks)**
    b. A cantilever of square section 200 mm × 200 mm, 2 m long just fails in flexure when a load of 12 kN is placed at its free end. A beam of same material and

having a rectangular cross section 150 mm wide and 300 mm deep is simply supported over a span of 3 m. Calculate the minimum central concentrated load required to break the beam. **(08 Marks)**

Dec. 13/Jan. 14 (06ME34)

15. a. Prove that the relation $\dfrac{M}{I} = \dfrac{\sigma}{y} = \dfrac{E}{R}$, with usual notations. **(10 Marks)**

  b. Determine the maximum allowable span of length L for a simple beam as shown in **Fig. U6.8**. The rectangular beam of cross section 125×250 mm is subjected to a UDL of 8 kN/m. Allowable bending stress = 6 MPa. **(10 Marks)**

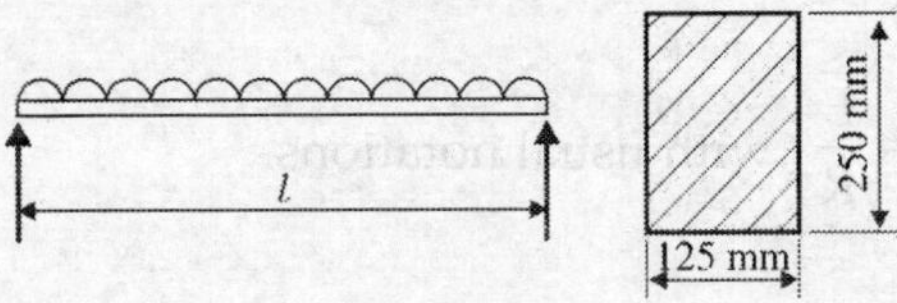

Fig. U6.8

Dec. 13/Jan. 14 (10ME34)

16. a. State the assumptions made in the theory of simple bending. **(02 Marks)**

  b. A simply supported cast iron square beam of 800 mm length and 15 mm × 15 mm in section fails on applying a load of 360 N at mid-span. Find the maximum uniformly distributed load that can be applied safely to a 40 mm wide, 75 mm deep and 1.6 m long cantilever made of same material.

  (08 Marks)

June/July 2014 (06ME34)

17. Prove that the ratio of depth to width of strongest beam that can be cut from a circular log of diameter d is 1.414. Hence calculate the depth and width of strongest beam that can be cut of a cylindrical log of wood whose diameter is 300 mm. **(10 Marks)**

June/July 2014 (10ME34)

18. a. What are the assumptions made in the theory of bending? **(04 Marks)**

  b. At a given position in a beam of uniform I-section is subjected to a bending moment of 100 kN-m. Plot the variation of bending stress across the section. [Refer **Fig. U6.9**]

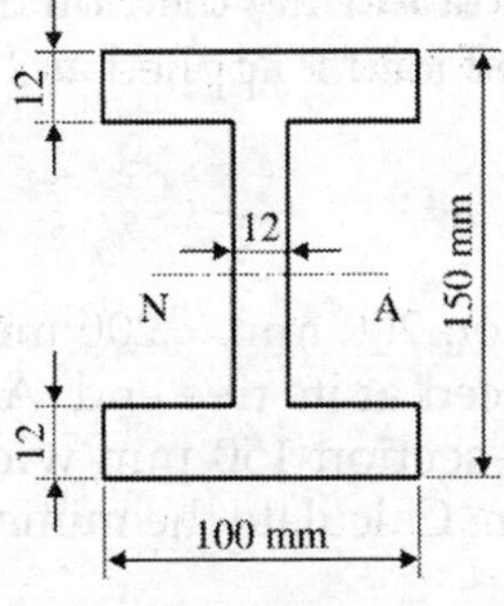

Fig. U6.9

Dec. 14/ Jan. 15 (06ME34)

19. Prove the relation $\dfrac{M}{I} = \dfrac{\sigma}{y} = \dfrac{E}{R}$ with usual notations. **(10 Marks)**

Dec. 14/Jan. 15 (10ME34)

20. a. What are the assumptions made in simple theory of bending? **(04 Marks)**
    b. Derive an expression for relationship between bending stress and radius of curvature. **(06 Marks)**

June/July 15 (10ME34)

21. Prove that $\dfrac{M}{I} = \dfrac{\sigma}{y} = \dfrac{E}{R}$ with usual notations. **(10 Marks)**

Dec. 15/Jan. 16 (10ME/AU34)

22. a. Enumerate the assumptions made in theory of pure bending. Write the bending equation with usual notations. **(06 Marks)**
    b. A beam of an I-section consists of 180 mm × 15 mm flanges and a web of 280 mm × 15 mm thickness. It is subjected to a bending moment of 120 kN-m. Sketch the bending stress distribution along the depth of the section. **(06 Marks)**

June/July 2016 (10ME/AU34)

23. a. List the assumptions made in simple bending theory and establish the relationship between bending stress and radius of curvature. **(10 Marks)**
    b. A uniform I-section beam is 100 mm wide and 150 mm deep with a flange thickness of 25 mm and web thickness of 100 mm. The beam is simply supported over a span of 5 m and carries a udl of 83.4 kN/m throughout its length. Determine the bending stress in the beam. **(10 Marks)**

Dec. 16/Jan. 17 (10ME/AU34)

24. a. Derive the bending equation $\dfrac{M}{I} = \dfrac{\sigma}{y} = \dfrac{E}{R}$ **(10 Marks)**
    b. A simply supported beam of span 5 m has a cross-section of 150 mm × 250 mm. If the permissible stress is 10 MPa, find:
    i. Maximum intensity of uniformly distributed load it can carry
    ii. Maximum concentrated load P applied at 2 m from an end it can carry. **(10 Marks)**

Dec. 16/Jan. 17 (15ME/MA34)

25. A cantilever of square section 200 mm × 200 mm, 2 m long just fails in flexure when a load of 12 kN is placed at its free end. A beam of the same material and having a rectangular cross-section 150 mm wide and 300 mm deep is simply supported over a span of 3 m. Calculate the minimum control load point required to break the beam. **(08 Marks)**

June/July 2017 (15ME/MA34)

26. a. What do you mean by "simple bending"? What are the assumptions made in theory of simple bending? **(07 Marks)**

b. A cantilever of length 2 m fails when a load of 2 kN is applied at the free end. If the section of the beam is 40 mm × 60 mm, find the stress at failure. **(05 Marks)**

c. An I-section beam 350 mm × 150 mm has a web thickness of 10 mm and a flange thickness of 20 mm. If the shear force acting on the beam is 40 kN, find the maximum shear stress developed in the I-section. **(08 Marks)**

June/July 2017 (15ME/MA34)

27. Derive a relationship between bending stress and radius of curvature. **(08 Marks)**

Dec. 17/Jan. 18 (15ME/MA34)

28. List the assumptions made in theory of pure bending. Write the bending equation with usual notations with their meanings. **(06 Marks)**

Shear Stresses in Beams

Chapter Outline

7.1 INTRODUCTION

In *chapter 5*, we have observed that when a beam is subjected to lateral loads, both bending moments and shear forces act on the cross-sections. The stresses produced at this section to resist the bending moment is known as *bending stress or flexural stress or longitudinal stress* and that to resist the action of shearing force is known *shear stress or transverse stress*. The effect of bending stresses has been discussed in *chapter 6*. In this chapter we will discuss the effect of shear or transverse stress.

As observed in chapter 5, this shear force tends to produce relative sliding between adjacent vertical sections of the beam and is always accompanied by *complementary shear stress* which is equal in magnitude at any point in the beam. *[chapter 3, sub-section 3.6]*. Thus for beams in bending, shear stresses are set up both horizontally and vertically.

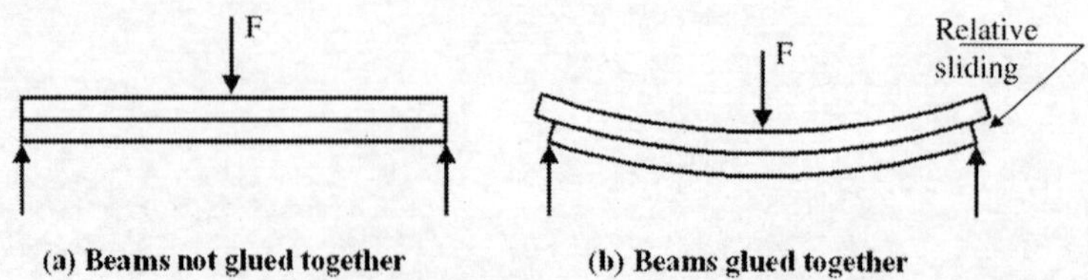

Fig. 7.1: Bending of beams

The existence of horizontal shear stresses in a beam can be explained as follows: Consider two beams of rectangular cross-section on simple supports subjected to a load *F* as shown in **Fig. 7.1(a)**. If friction between the beams is small, the beams will bend independently as indicated in **Fig. 7.1(b)** and therefore the bottom surface of the upper beam will slide relative to the top surface of the lower beam.

On the other hand, if the two beams are glued along the contact surface, so that they become a single solid beam of depth equal to the combined depths of the initial two beams then shear stresses must develop along the glued surface in order to prevent the sliding. Because of the presence of these shear stresses, the single solid beam is much stiffer and stronger than the two separate beams.

For an element at either the top or bottom surface, however there can be no vertical shears if the surface is free or unloaded and hence the horizontal shear is also zero. i.e. $\tau = 0$, when $y = \pm h/2$

7.2 SHEAR STRESS DISTRIBUTION IN A LOADED BEAM

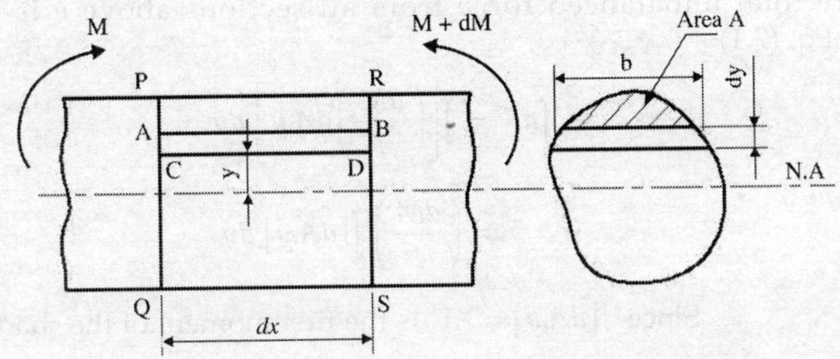

Fig. 7.2: Shear stress due to bending

Assumptions

- Modulus of Elasticity is same in tension and in compression.
- The shear stress is uniformly distributed over the width. [i.e. the average shear stress is calculated across the width]
- The material should be linearly elastic.

Consider the portion of a beam PQRS of length dx as shown in **Fig. 7.2(a)**, and an element ABCD at a distance y from the neutral axis (N.A). In general the bending moment changes slightly as we move from one section to an adjacent section of the beam.

$$
\begin{aligned}
\text{Let} \quad M &= \text{Bending moment on section PQ} \\
(M + dM) &= \text{Bending moment on section RS} \\
F &= \text{Shear force on section PQ} \\
(F + dF) &= \text{Shear force on section RS} \\
\sigma &= \text{Bending stress section PQ} \\
(\sigma + d\sigma) &= \text{Bending stress on section RS} \\
I &= \text{Moment of inertia about N.A} \\
y \text{ or } c &= \text{Distance of fiber considered from neutral axis} \\
\tau &= \text{shear stress}
\end{aligned}
$$

Now bending stress at section PQ $\qquad \sigma = \dfrac{M}{Z} = \dfrac{My}{I}$

Bending stress at section RS $\qquad (\sigma + d\sigma) = \dfrac{(M + dM)y}{I}$

Longitudinal force on the element AC $\qquad = \sigma.dA = \left(\dfrac{M}{I}\right)dA.y$

Longitudinal force on the element BD $= (\sigma + d\sigma).dA = \left(\dfrac{M + dM}{I}\right)dA.y$

Since the two forces are acting on the same line but in opposite direction, there will be an unbalanced force on the strip.

i.e. net unbalanced force on the strip $\quad dF = \left(\dfrac{M + dM}{I}\right)dA.y - \left(\dfrac{M}{I}\right)dA.y$

$$dF = \left(\dfrac{dM}{I}\right)dA.y \qquad \text{... (Eq. 7.1)}$$

Therefore total unbalanced force from all sections above y is obtained by integrating Eq. (7.1)

$$\int dF = \int \left[\left(\dfrac{dM}{I}\right)dA.y\right] dy$$

$$= \left(\dfrac{dM}{I}\right) \int [dA.y]\, dy$$

Since $\int [dA.y] = A\bar{y}$ is the first moment of the shaded area with respect to the neutral axis

$$F = \left(\dfrac{dM}{I}\right)A\bar{y} \qquad \text{... (Eq. 7.2)}$$

If τ is the shear stress, then $\quad \tau = \dfrac{F}{A} = \dfrac{(dM/I)\, A\bar{y}}{b.dx}$

$$= \left(\dfrac{dM}{I}\right)\left(\dfrac{A\bar{y}}{b.dx}\right)$$

$$\text{Since} \left(\dfrac{dM}{dx}\right) = F$$

$$\tau = \left(\dfrac{F}{Ib}\right)A\bar{y} \qquad \text{... (Eq. 7.3)}$$

$\bar{y} = $ Distance of CG of area A above NA

Eq. (7.3) is known as the shear formula

Limitations on the use of shear formula

- Valid only for prismatic beams of linearly elastic materials with small deflections.
- Not applicable to sections of triangular or semicircular shape (non-prismatic beams).
- Shear stresses must be uniform across the width of the cross section.
- Not applicable to edges of the cross section that intersects the boundary of the member at an angle other than 90°.
- The shear formula should not be used to determine the shear stress web-flange junction as in T and I sections, since stress concentration occurs whenever cross-section changes suddenly.

7.3 SHEAR STRESS DISTRIBUTION IN A RECTANGLE

VTU – Mech.: Dec. 15/ Jan. 16 – 08 Marks;
June/ July 2014 – 10 Marks; Dec. 13/ Jan. 14 – 10 Marks;
June/ July 2013 – 05 Marks; Jan. 2013 – 10 Marks; May/ June 2010 – 06 Marks;
June/ July 2008 –06 Marks; Dec.07/ Jan.08 – 06 Marks
Civil: June/ July 2014 – 10 Marks, June/ July 2013 – 06 Marks,
Jan. 2013 – 10 Marks; June 2012 – 10 Marks,
Dec. 2011 – 08 Marks, May/ June 2010 – 06 Marks; June/ July 2008 –06 Marks,
Dec.07/ Jan.08 – 05 Marks, Dec.08/ Jan.09 – 12 Marks

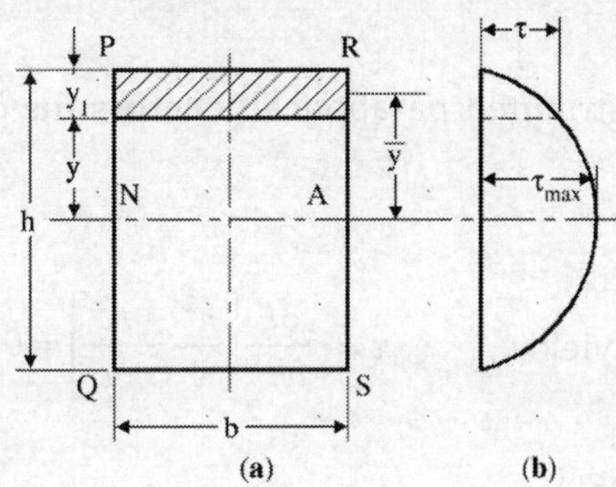

Fig. 7.3: Shear stress distribution over a rectangle

Consider a rectangular cross-section PQRS as shown in **Fig. 7.3(a)**.

Let b = width of the beam

h = height or depth of the beam

y = distance of fiber considered above neural axis (N.A)

$\bar{y}$ = distance of CG of area A above N.A

y_1 = depth of section considered

τ = shear stress

We know that shear stress at any height y above the N.A is

$$\tau = \left(\frac{F}{Ib}\right) A\bar{y} \qquad \text{... Eq. (i)}$$

Area of shaded portion $\quad A = by_1 = b\left(\frac{h}{2} - y\right) \qquad \text{... Eq. (ii)}$

Distance of CG $\quad \bar{y} = y + \frac{y_1}{2} = y + \frac{1}{2}\left(\frac{h}{2} - y\right) = y + \left(\frac{h}{4} - \frac{y}{2}\right) = \left(\frac{y}{2} + \frac{h}{4}\right)$

$$\text{... Eq. (iii)}$$

Substituting Eqs (ii) and (iii) in (i), we have

$$\tau = \frac{F}{Ib}\left[b\left(\frac{h}{2} - y\right)\left(\frac{y}{2} + \frac{h}{4}\right)\right]$$

$$= \frac{F}{I}\left[\frac{hy}{4} - \frac{y^2}{2} + \frac{h^2}{8} - \frac{hy}{4}\right]$$

$$= \frac{F}{I}\left[\frac{h^2}{8} - \frac{y^2}{2}\right]$$

$$\tau = \frac{F}{2I}\left[\frac{h^2}{4} - y^2\right] \qquad \text{... (Eq. 7.4)}$$

Substituting $I = \dfrac{bh^3}{12}$

$$\tau = \frac{6F}{bh^3}\left[\frac{h^2}{4} - y^2\right] \qquad \text{... (Eq. 7.5)}$$

The shear stress is distributed parabolically across the depth of the section, as shown in **Fig. 7.3(b)**.

Boundary conditions

- At $y = h/2$, (Eq. 7.5) yields... $\qquad \tau = \dfrac{6F}{bh^3}\left[\dfrac{h^2}{4} - \dfrac{h^2}{4}\right] = 0 \qquad$ ... (Eq. 7.6)

- At neutral axis, $y = 0$

(Eq. 7.5) yields... $\qquad \tau_{max} = \dfrac{6F}{bh^3}\left[\dfrac{h^2}{4} - 0\right] = \dfrac{3F}{2bh}$

$$\tau_{max} = \frac{3F}{2A} = 1.5\tau_{avg}$$

Since $\tau_{avg} = F/A \qquad$ ... (Eq. 7.7)

Thus the shear stress in a rectangular section is 50% greater than the average shear stress on the cross-section.

7.4 SHEAR STRESS DISTRIBUTION IN AN I-SECTION

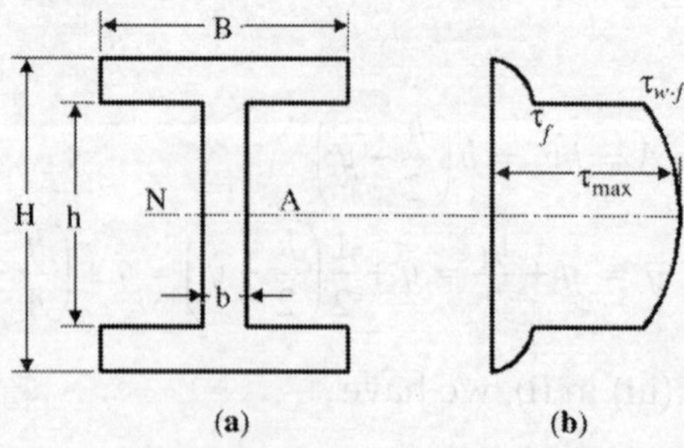

Fig. 7.4: Shear stress distribution over an I section

Consider an I-section as shown in **Fig. 7.4(a)**. When an I-section is subjected to shear force, shear stresses are developed throughout the cross section. The distribution of shear stresses is much more complicated than that observed in a rectangular beam. The shear stresses in the flanges of the beam act in both vertical and horizontal directions The shear stresses in the web of a wide-flange beam act only in the vertical direction and are larger than the stresses in the flanges.

Let $\quad B$ = Overall width of the section

$\quad\quad\quad\quad H$ = Overall depth of the section

$\quad\quad\quad\quad b$ = width of the web

$\quad\quad\quad\quad h$ = height or depth of the web

$\quad\quad\quad\quad y$ = distance of fiber considered above neural axis (N.A)

$\quad\quad\quad\quad \overline{y}$ = distance of CG of area A above N.A

$\quad\quad\quad\quad \tau$ = shear stress

We know that shear stress at any height y above the N.A is

$$\tau = \left(\frac{F}{Ib}\right)A\overline{y} \qquad\qquad \dots \text{Eq. (i)}$$

Case a: Shear stress in the flange: (y > h/2) (Fig. 7.5)

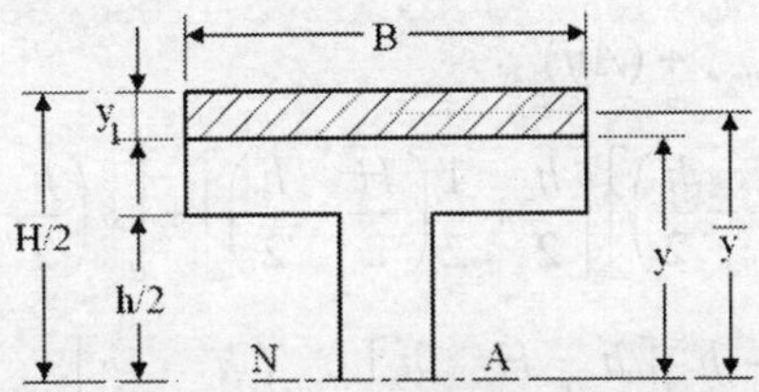

Fig. 7.5: Shear stress in the flange

Area of shaded portion $\quad A = By_1 = B\left(\frac{H}{2} - y\right) \qquad\qquad \dots \text{Eq. (ii)}$

Distance of CG $\quad \overline{y} = y + \dfrac{y_1}{2} = y + \dfrac{1}{2}\left(\dfrac{H}{2} - y\right) = y + \left(\dfrac{H}{4} - \dfrac{y}{2}\right) = \left(\dfrac{y}{2} + \dfrac{H}{4}\right)$

$$\dots \text{Eq. (iii)}$$

Substituting Eqs (ii) and (iii) in (i) we have

$$\tau_f = \frac{F}{IB}\left[B\left(\frac{H}{2} - y\right)\left(\frac{y}{2} + \frac{H}{4}\right)\right] \qquad \dots \text{for flange, width} = B$$

$$= \frac{F}{I}\left[\frac{Hy}{4} - \frac{y^2}{2} + \frac{H^2}{8} - \frac{Hy}{4}\right]$$

$$= \frac{F}{I}\left[\frac{H^2}{8} - \frac{y^2}{2}\right]$$

$$\tau_f = \frac{F}{2I}\left[\frac{H^2}{4} - y^2\right] \qquad\qquad \dots \text{(Eq. 7.8)}$$

Boundary conditions:

- At upper edge of flange: $y = H/2$

  (Eq. 7.8) yields... $\quad \tau_f = 0 \qquad\qquad\qquad \dots \text{(Eq. 7.9)}$

- At lower edge of flange: $y = h/2$

  (Eq. 7.8) yields... $\quad \tau_f = \dfrac{F}{2I}\left[\dfrac{H^2}{4} - \dfrac{h^2}{4}\right]$

$$\tau_f = \frac{F}{8I}\left(H^2 - h^2\right) \qquad \ldots \text{(Eq. 7.10)}$$

Case b: Shear stress in the web (Fig. 7.6)

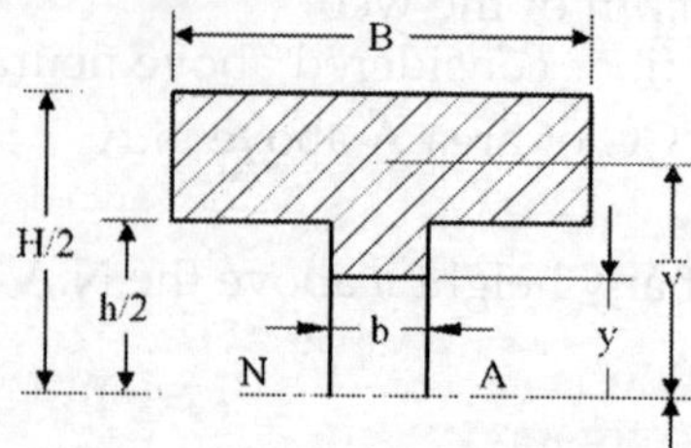

Fig. 7.6: Shear stress in the web

In this case, $A\overline{y} = (A\overline{y})_{flange} + (A\overline{y})_{web}$

$$= \left[B\left(\frac{H}{2} - \frac{h}{2}\right)\right]\left[\frac{h}{2} + \frac{1}{2}\left(\frac{H}{2} - \frac{h}{2}\right)\right] + \left[b\left(\frac{h}{2} - y\right)\right]\left[y + \frac{1}{2}\left(\frac{h}{2} - y\right)\right]$$

$$= B\left(\frac{H-h}{2}\right)\left[\frac{h}{2} + \frac{H}{4} - \frac{h}{4}\right] + b\left(\frac{h}{2} - y\right)\left[y + \frac{h}{4} - \frac{y}{2}\right]$$

$$= B\left(\frac{H-h}{2}\right)\left[\frac{1}{2}\left(\frac{H}{2} + \frac{h}{2}\right)\right] + b\left(\frac{h}{2} - y\right)\left[\frac{y}{2} + \frac{h}{4}\right]$$

$$= \frac{B}{2}\left(\frac{H-h}{2}\right)\left(\frac{H+h}{2}\right) + b\left(\frac{h}{2} - y\right)\left[\frac{1}{2}\left(\frac{h}{2} + y\right)\right]$$

$$= \frac{B}{8}\left(H^2 - h^2\right) + \frac{b}{2}\left(\frac{h}{2} - y\right)\left(\frac{h}{2} + y\right)$$

$$A\overline{y} = \frac{B}{8}\left(H^2 - h^2\right) + \frac{b}{2}\left(\frac{h^2}{4} - y^2\right) \qquad \ldots \text{Eq. (iv)}$$

Substituting Eq. (iv) in Eq. (i) we have

$$\tau_w = \frac{F}{Ib}\left[\frac{B}{8}\left(H^2 - h^2\right) + \frac{b}{2}\left(\frac{b^2}{4} - y^2\right)\right] \qquad \ldots \text{for web, width } b \ldots \text{(Eq. 7.11)}$$

Boundary conditions:
- At the junction of web and bottom of top flange: $y = h/2$

(Eq. 7.11) yields... $\tau_{w-f} = \dfrac{F}{Ib}\left[\dfrac{B}{8}\left(H^2 - h^2\right) + \dfrac{b}{2}\left(\dfrac{b^2}{4} - \dfrac{h^2}{4}\right)\right]$

$$\tau_{w-f} = \frac{FB}{8Ib}\left(H^2 - h^2\right) \qquad \ldots \text{(Eq. 7.12)}$$

At neutral axis, $\qquad y = 0$

(Eq. 7.11) yields... $\tau_{max} = \dfrac{F}{Ib}\left[\dfrac{B}{8}\left(H^2 - h^2\right) + \dfrac{b}{2}\left(\dfrac{h^2}{4} - 0\right)\right]$

$\qquad\qquad = \dfrac{F}{Ib}\left[\dfrac{B}{8}\left(H^2 - h^2\right) + \dfrac{bh^2}{8}\right]$

$\qquad \tau_{max} = \dfrac{F}{8Ib}\left[B(H^2 - h^2) + bh^2\right]$ ... (Eq. 7.13)

The shear stress distribution is as shown in **Fig. 7.4(b)**.
Note: Shear stress in the web may also be found as follows:
(Eq. 7.10) divided by (Eq. 7.12) gives

$$\frac{\tau_{f-low}}{\tau_{f-up}} = \frac{F(H^2 - h^2)/8I}{FB(H^2 - h^2)/8Ib} = \frac{b}{B}$$

Or $\qquad\qquad \tau_{w-f} = \tau_w = \left(\dfrac{B}{b}\right)\tau_f$ ... (Eq. 7.13a)

7.5 SHEAR STRESS DISTRIBUTION IN A T-SECTION

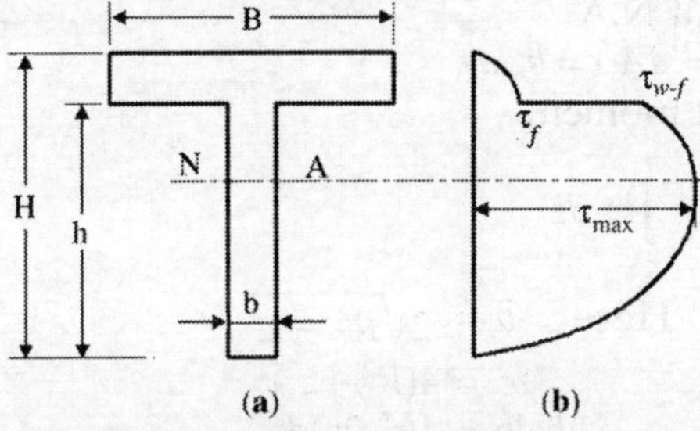

Fig. 7.7: Shear stress distribution over a T-section

Consider a T-section as shown in **Fig. 7.7(a)**. The procedure for finding the shear stress distribution is same as that of I-section. The shear stress distribution diagram is as shown in **Fig. 7.7(b)**.

7.6 SHEAR STRESS DISTRIBUTION IN A CIRCULAR SECTION

VTU – June 2012 – 10 Marks; Jan. 2013 – 10 Marks; (CV) Jan. 2013 – 10 Marks

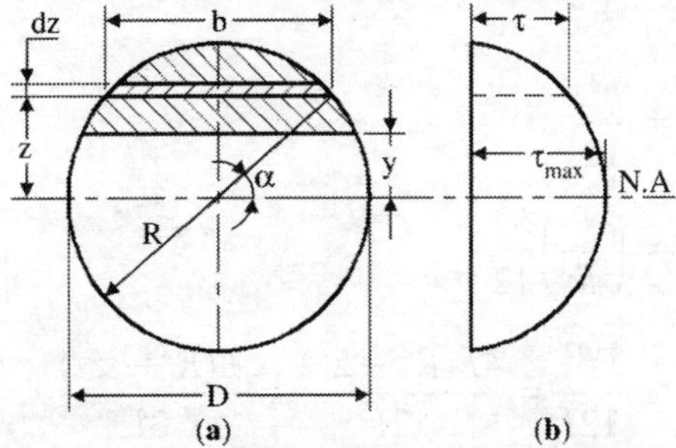

Fig. 7.8: Shear stress distribution over a circular section

Consider a circular section as shown in **Fig. 7.8(a)**.

Let $\quad D$ = Diameter of the circle

$\quad\quad R$ = Radius of circle

$\quad\quad b$ = width of the strip

$\quad\quad z$ = distance of fiber considered above neural axis (N.A)

$\quad\quad \bar{y}$ = distance of CG of area A above N.A

$\quad\quad \tau$ = shear stress

We know that shear stress at any height y above the N.A is

$$\tau = \left(\frac{F}{Ib}\right) A\bar{y} \qquad\qquad \text{... Eq. (i)}$$

Consider a strip of thickness dz at a distance z from N.A and of area dA

From **Fig. 7.8(a)**, $\quad \sin\alpha = \dfrac{z}{R} \Rightarrow z = R\sin\alpha = y \qquad\qquad \text{... Eq. (ii)}$

$$\cos\alpha = \frac{b/2}{R} \Rightarrow b = 2R\cos\alpha \qquad\qquad \text{... Eq. (iii)}$$

$$\frac{b}{2} = \sqrt{R^2 - z^2} \Rightarrow b = 2\sqrt{R^2 - z^2} \qquad\qquad \text{... Eq. (iv)}$$

Area of the strip $\quad dA = b.dz \qquad\qquad\qquad\qquad\qquad\qquad \text{... Eq. (v)}$

Moment of this area about N.A

$$A = dA.z = bz.dz$$

For shaded portion, total moment

$$A\bar{y} = \int_{z}^{R} bz.dz \qquad\qquad \text{... Eq. (vi)}$$

$$\text{Here} \quad b = 2\sqrt{R^2 - z^2}$$

$$b^2 = 4(R^2 - z^2)$$

$$2b.db = 4(-2z)dz$$

$$z.dz = -\frac{1}{4} b.db$$

$$\text{When} \quad z = R, b = 0; z = z, b = b$$

$$A\bar{y} = \int_{b}^{0} -\frac{1}{4} b^2.db$$

$$= \frac{1}{4}\int_{0}^{b} b^2.db$$

$$A\bar{y} = \frac{b^3}{12}$$

Eq. (i) yields... $\quad\quad \tau = \left(\dfrac{F}{Ib}\right)\dfrac{b^3}{12}$

$$= \frac{Fb^2}{12I} = \frac{4F(R^2 - z^2)}{12I} = \frac{F(R^2 - z^2)}{3I} \qquad \text{... using Eq. (iv)}$$

$$= \frac{F}{3I}\left(R^2 - y^2\right) \qquad\qquad \text{... since } y = z, \text{ from Eq. (ii)}$$

$$\tau = \frac{4F}{3\pi R^4}\left[R^2 - y^2\right]$$

$$\tau = \frac{4F}{3\pi R^2}\left[1 - \left(\frac{y}{R}\right)^2\right] \quad \text{or} \quad \tau = \frac{16F}{3\pi D^2}\left[1 - \frac{4y^2}{D^2}\right] \qquad \text{... (Eq. 7.14)}$$

Hence shear stress varies parabolically with depth
Boundary conditions:
   At $y = R$, (Eq. 7.14) yields... $\tau = 0$ ... (Eq. 7.15)

   At N.A, $y = 0$, (Eq. 7.14) yields... $\tau_{max} = \dfrac{4F}{3\pi R^2}$ ... (Eq. 7.16)

$$\text{Since } \tau_{avg} = \frac{F}{A} = \frac{F}{\pi R^2}$$

$$\therefore \quad \tau_{max} = \frac{4}{3}\,\tau_{avg} \qquad \text{... (Eq. 7.17)}$$

PROBLEMS ON CIRCULAR CROSS-SECTION

1. **A cantilever beam of length 1 m has a circular cross section of diameter 300 mm. Determine the concentrated load the can be applied at the free end to produce a maximum shear of 1.5 MPa.**

VTU – Dec. 2010 – 08 Marks

Solution: $L = 1000$ mm, $D = 300$ mm, $W = ?$, $\tau_{max} = 1.5$ MPa

$$\text{Shear stress} \quad \tau_{max} = \frac{4F}{3\pi R^2}$$

For a cantilever beam with point load at free end, shear force $F = W$

$$1.5 = \frac{4W}{3\pi \times (300/2)^2}$$

$$W = 7952.56 \text{ N}$$

PROBLEMS ON RECTANGULAR CROSS-SECTION

2. **A simply supported beam of span 4 m carries an UDL of 25 kN/m over the entire span. If the cross section of the beam is rectangular of 150 mm × 300 mm, determine the stress at a distance of 50 mm above neutral axis. Also sketch the shear stress distribution.**

Solution: $L = 4000$ mm, $w = 25$ kN/m, $b = 150$ mm, $h = 300$ mm, $\tau = ?$

Based on given data, the hollow box is s shown in **Fig. 7.9(a)**.

$$\text{Average stress} \quad \tau_{avg} = \frac{F}{A}$$

For a simply supported beam with UDL over entire span

$$F = \frac{wL}{2} = \frac{25 \times 4}{2} = 50 \text{ kN}$$

$$\tau_{avg} = \frac{50 \times 10^3}{150 \times 300} = 1.11 \text{ MPa}$$

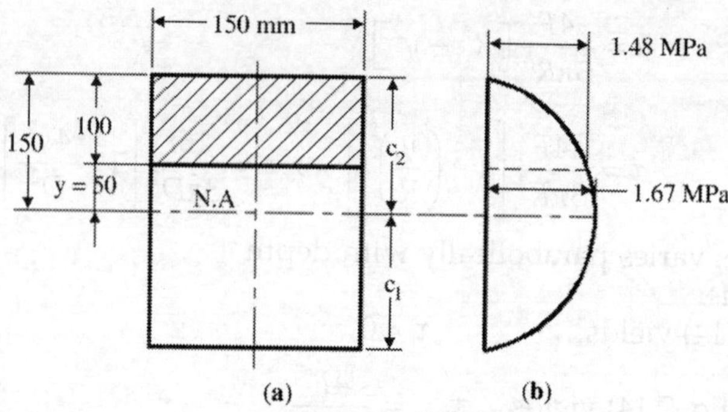

Fig. 7.9: Problem 2

Maximum shear stress $\quad \tau_{max} = 1.5\tau_{avg} = 1.5 \times 1.11 = 1.67$ MPa

Shear stress at any distance y

$$\tau = \left(\frac{F}{Ib}\right) A\overline{y} \qquad \qquad \dots \text{Eq. (i)}$$

Due to symmetry, $\qquad c_1 = c_2 = c = \dfrac{h}{2} = \dfrac{300}{2} = 150$ mm

Area $\qquad A = b(c_2 - y) = 150 \times (150 - 50) = 15000$ mm^2

Distance of CG $\qquad \overline{y} = y + \dfrac{(c_2 - y)}{2} = 50 + \dfrac{150 - 50}{2} = 100$ mm

MI of entire section $\qquad I = \dfrac{bh^3}{12} = \dfrac{150 \times 300^3}{12} = 337.5 \times 10^6$ mm^4

Eq. (i) yields... $\qquad \tau = \dfrac{50 \times 10^3}{337.5 \times 10^6 \times 150} \times 15000 \times 100$

$$\tau = 1.48 \text{ MPa}$$

OR   Shear stress at any distance y

$$\tau = \frac{6F}{bh^3}\left[\frac{h^2}{4} - y^2\right]$$

$$= \frac{6 \times 50 \times 10^3}{150 \times 300^3}\left[\frac{300^2}{4} - 50^2\right]$$

Here $y = 50$ mm above N.A

$$\tau = 1.48 \text{ MPa}$$

The shear stress distribution is as shown in **Fig. 7.9(b)**.

3. **A hollow box section 120 mm wide, 200 mm deep is having a uniform wall thickness of 10 mm. Obtain the shear stress variation across the cross-section. Shear force at the section is 120 kN.**

VTU – (CV) June/ July 2009 –10 Marks

Solution: $F = 120 \times 10^3$ N, $\tau = ?$

Based on given data, the hollow box is as shown in **Fig. 7.10(a)**.

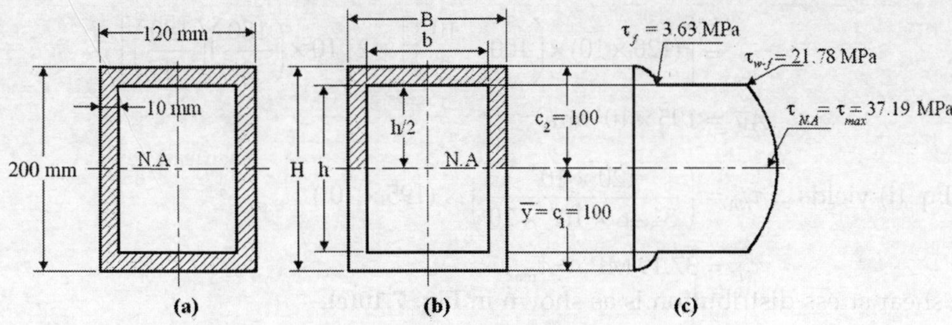

Fig. 7.10: Problem 3

From **Fig. 7.10(b)**, $\qquad B = 120$ mm, $H = 200$ mm, $t = 10$ mm.

$$b = B - 2t = 120 - (2 \times 10) = 100 \text{ mm}$$

$$h = H - 2t = 200 - (2 \times 10) = 180 \text{ mm}$$

Shear stress $\qquad\qquad \tau = \left(\dfrac{F}{Ib'}\right)A\overline{y}$ $\qquad\qquad\qquad\qquad\qquad$ ... Eq. (i)

Due to symmetry, $\qquad c_1 = c_2 = c = \dfrac{H}{2} = \dfrac{200}{2} = 100$ mm

a. *Shear stress at boundaries is zero*

b. *Shear stress at the bottom of flange:* Here $b' = B = 120$ mm

$$A\overline{y} = (Bt)\left(c_2 - \frac{t}{2}\right) = (120 \times 10) \times \left(100 - \frac{10}{2}\right) = 114 \times 10^3 \text{ mm}^3$$

$$I = \frac{(BH^3 - bh^3)}{12} = \frac{(120 \times 200^3 - 100 \times 180^3)}{12} = 31.46 \times 10^6 \text{ mm}^4$$

Eq. (i) yields... $\qquad \tau_f = \left(\dfrac{120 \times 10^3}{31.46 \times 10^6 \times 120}\right) \times (114 \times 10^3)$

$$\tau_f = 3.63 \text{ MPa}$$

c. *Shear stress at the junction of web and flange:* Here $b' = 2t = 20$ mm

$$[2t = \text{two web thickness}]$$

$$A\overline{y} = (Bt)\left(c_2 - \frac{t}{2}\right) = (120 \times 10) \times \left(100 - \frac{10}{2}\right) = 114 \times 10^3 \text{ mm}^3$$

Eq. (i) yields... $\tau_{w-f} = \left(\dfrac{120 \times 10^3}{31.46 \times 10^6 \times 20}\right) \times (114 \times 10^3) = 21.78$ MPa

or $\qquad \tau_{w-f} = \left(\dfrac{B}{b'}\right)\tau_f = \left(\dfrac{120}{20}\right) \times 3.63 = 21.78$ MPa

d. *Shear stress at neutral axis:* Here $b' = 2t = 20$ mm $\qquad [2t = \text{two web thickness}]$

$$A\overline{y} = (A\overline{y})_{flange} + (A\overline{y})_{web}$$

$$= (Bt)\left(c_2 - \frac{t}{2}\right) + 2\,[t(h/2) \times (h/4)]$$

$$= \left[(120 \times 10) \times \left(100 - \frac{10}{2} \right) \right] + 2 \left[10 \times \left(\frac{180}{2} \right) \left(\frac{180}{4} \right) \right]$$

$$A\bar{y} = 195 \times 10^3 \, \text{mm}^3$$

Eq. (i) yields... $\tau_{NA} = \left(\dfrac{120 \times 10^3}{31.46 \times 10^6 \times 20} \right) \times (195 \times 10^3)$

$$\tau_{NA} = 37.19 \, \text{MPa} = \tau_{max}$$

The shear stress distribution is as shown in **Fig. 7.10(c)**.

4. **A hollow square aluminum box beam has the cross section shown in Fig. 7.11(a). Calculate the maximum and minimum shear stresses in the webs of the beam due to a shear force of 80 kN.**

Solution: $F = 80 \times 10^3 \, \text{N}, \tau = ?$

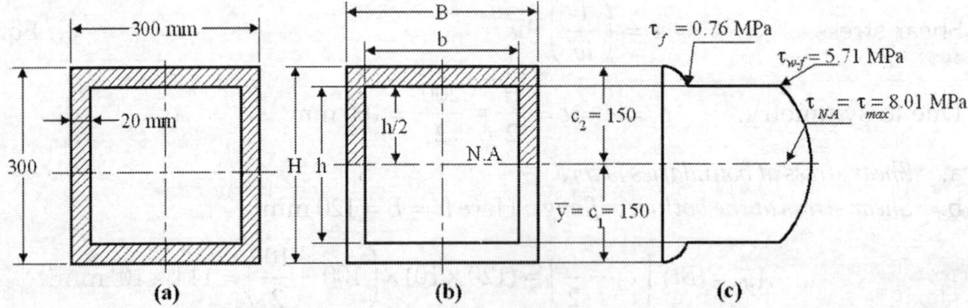

Fig. 7.11: Problem 4

From **Fig. 7.11(b)**, $B = h = 300 \, \text{mm}, t = 20 \, \text{mm}.$

$$b = h = B - 2t = 300 - 2 \times 20 = 260 \, \text{mm}$$

Shear stress $\qquad \tau = \left(\dfrac{F}{Ib'} \right) A\bar{y} \qquad\qquad$ ... Eq. (i)

Due to symmetry, $c_1 = c_2 = c = \dfrac{H}{2} = \dfrac{300}{2} = 150 \, \text{mm}$

a. *Shear stress at boundaries is zero*

b. *Shear stress at the bottom of flange:* Here $b' = B = 300 \, \text{mm}$

$$A\bar{y} = (Bt) \left(c_2 - \frac{t}{2} \right) = (300 \times 20) \times \left(150 - \frac{20}{2} \right) = 840 \times 10^3 \, \text{mm}^3$$

$$I = \frac{(BH^3 - bh^3)}{12} = \frac{(300 \times 300^3 - 260 \times 260^3)}{12} = 294.18 \times 10^6 \, \text{mm}^4$$

Eq. (i) yields... $\tau_f = \left(\dfrac{80 \times 10^3}{294.18 \times 10^6 \times 300)} \right) \times (840 \times 10^3)$

$$\tau_f = 0.76 \, \text{MPa}$$

c. *Shear stress at the junction of web and flange:* Here $b' = 2t = 40 \, \text{mm}$

$$[2t = \text{two web thickness}]$$

$$A\bar{y} = (Bt)\left(c_2 - \frac{t}{2}\right) = (300 \times 20) \times \left(150 - \frac{20}{2}\right) = 840 \times 10^3 \text{ mm}^3$$

Eq. (i) yields... $\tau_{w-f} = \left(\dfrac{80 \times 10^3}{294.18 \times 10^6 \times 300}\right) \times (840 \times 10^3) = 5.71$ MPa

or $\qquad \tau_{w-f} = \left(\dfrac{B}{b'}\right)\tau_f = \left(\dfrac{300}{40}\right) \times 0.76 = 5.7$ MPa

d. *Shear stress at neutral axis:* Here $b' = 2t = 40$ mm $\qquad$ [2t = two web thickness]

$$A\bar{y} = (A\bar{y})_{flange} + (A\bar{y})_{web}$$

$$= (Bt)\left(c_2 - \frac{t}{2}\right) + 2\,[t(h/2) \times (h/4)]$$

$$= \left[(300 \times 20) \times \left(150 - \frac{20}{2}\right)\right] + 2\left[20 \times \left(\frac{260}{2}\right)\left(\frac{260}{4}\right)\right]$$

$$A\bar{y} = 1178 \times 10^3 \text{ mm}^3$$

Eq. (i) yields... $\tau_{NA} = \left(\dfrac{80 \times 10^3}{294.18 \times 10^6 \times 40)}\right) \times (1178 \times 10^3)$

$$\tau_{NA} = 8.01 \text{ MPa} = \tau_{max}$$

The shear stress distribution is as shown in **Fig. 7.11(c)**.

5. **A simply supported beam is subjected to a shear force of 35 kN. If the cross section of the beam is a rectangle of 150 mm × 450 mm, determine:**
   (a) **The magnitude of the shear stress in the beam at 150 mm from top edge.**
   (b) **The magnitude of the shear stress in the beam at 100 mm from bottom edge.**
   (c) **The maximum shear stress that occurs in the beam at any location.**
   (d) **The maximum bending stress in the beam at any location, if the maximum BM is 40 kN-m.**

Solution: $F = 35 \times 10^3$ N, $M_{max} = 40 \times 10^3$ N-mm, $b = 150$ mm, $h = 450$ mm, $\tau = ?$, $\sigma = ?$

Based on given data, the hollow box is as shown in **Fig. 7.12(a)**.

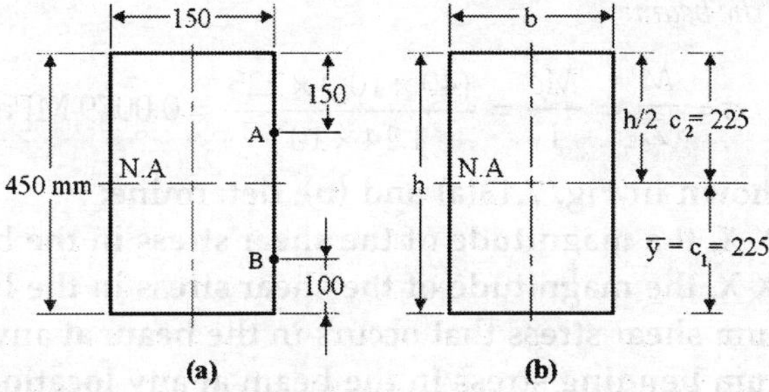

Fig. 7.12: Problem 5

Shear stress $\qquad \tau = \left(\dfrac{F}{Ib}\right) A\bar{y}$ $\qquad\qquad\qquad$ ... Eq. (i)

Due to symmetry, $\quad c_1 = c_2 = c = \dfrac{h}{2} = \dfrac{450}{2} = 225 \text{ mm}$

$$I = \frac{bh^3}{12} = \frac{(150 \times 450^3)}{12} = 1.14 \times 10^9 \text{ mm}^4$$

a. *Shear stress in the beam at $h_2 = 150$ mm from top edge:*

$$A\bar{y} = (bh_2)\left(c_2 - \frac{h_2}{2}\right) = (150 \times 150) \times \left(225 - \frac{150}{2}\right) = 3.38 \times 10^6 \text{ mm}^3$$

Eq. (i) yields... $\qquad \tau = \left(\dfrac{35 \times 10^3}{1.14 \times 10^9 \times 150}\right) \times (3.38 \times 10^6)$

$$\tau = 0.69 \text{ MPa}$$

b. *Shear stress in the beam at $h_1 = 100$ mm from bottom edge:*

$$A\bar{y} = (bh_1)\left(c_2 - \frac{h_1}{2}\right) = (150 \times 100) \times \left(225 - \frac{100}{2}\right) = 2.63 \times 10^6 \text{ mm}^3$$

Eq. (i) yields... $\qquad \tau = \left(\dfrac{35 \times 10^3}{1.14 \times 10^9 \times 150}\right) \times (2.63 \times 10^6)$

$\qquad$ or $\qquad\qquad \tau = 0.538 \text{ MPa}$

c. *Maximum shear stress:*

Maximum shear stress at N.A i.e. $\dfrac{h}{2} = 225$ mm

$$A\bar{y} = (bh)\left(\frac{h}{2}\right) = (150 \times 225) \times \left(\frac{225}{2}\right) = 3.8 \times 10^6 \text{ mm}^3$$

Eq. (i) yields... $\quad \tau = \left(\dfrac{35 \times 10^3}{1.14 \times 10^9 \times 150}\right) \times (3.8 \times 10^6)$

$$\tau = 0.78 \text{ MPa}$$

d. *Bending stress in the beam:*

$$\sigma = \frac{M}{Z} = \frac{Mc}{I} = \frac{(40 \times 10^3) \times 225}{1.14 \times 10^9} = 0.0079 \text{ MPa}$$

6. For the beam shown in Fig. 7.13(a) and (b), determine:

(a) At section X-X, the magnitude of the shear stress in the beam at point A.

(b) At section X-X, the magnitude of the shear stress in the beam at point B.

(c) The maximum shear stress that occurs in the beam at any location.

(d) The maximum bending stress in the beam at any location.

Solution: $w = 15 \text{ kN/m} = 15 \text{ N/mm}$, $L = 6000 \text{ m}$, $b = 100 \text{ mm}$, $h = 400 \text{ mm}$, $\tau = ?$, $\sigma = ?$.

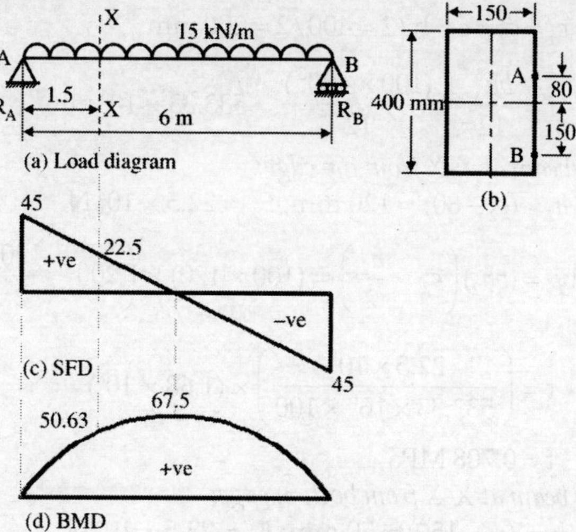

Fig. 7.13: Problem 6

Reactions at supports:
$$R_A + R_B = (15 \times 6) = 90 \text{ kN} \qquad \text{... Eq. (i)}$$
Taking moments about A aand equating to zero, we have

$$R_B \times 6 = \left[15 \times 6 \times \left(\frac{6}{2} \right) \right]$$

$$R_B = 45 \text{ kN} \qquad \text{... Eq. (ii)}$$
Substituting Eq. (ii) in Eq. (i), we have
$$R_A + 45 = 90$$
$$R_A = 45 \text{ kN} \qquad \text{... Eq. (iii)}$$
Shear force calculations:
$$F_A = R_A = 45 \text{ kN}$$
$$F_X = 45 - (15 \times 1.5) = 22.5 \text{ kN}$$
$$F_{X-B} = 22.5 - (15 \times 4.5) = -45 \text{ kN}$$
$$F_B = F_{X-B} = -45 \text{ kN} = R_B$$
Bending moment calculations:
$$M_A = 0$$

$$M_X = (45 \times 1.5) - \left[15 \times 1.5 \times \left(\frac{1.5}{2} \right) \right] = 50.63 \text{ kN-m}$$

$$M_B = 0$$

Maximum bending moment:
Since the beam is symmetric, maximum bending moment occurs at mid-span i.e.
$x = 3$ m

$$M_{max} = [45 \times 3] - \left[15 \times 3 \times \left(\frac{3}{2} \right) \right] = 67.5 \text{ kN-m}$$

The SFD and BMD diagrams are shown in **Figs 7.13(c) & (d)** respectively.

Shear stress $\qquad \tau = \left(\frac{F}{Ib} \right) A\bar{y} \qquad \text{... Eq. (iv)}$

Due to symmetry, $\quad c_1 = c_2 = c = h/2 = 400/2 = 200$ mm

$$I = \frac{bh^3}{12} = \frac{(100 \times 400^3)}{12} = 533.33 \times 10^6 \text{ mm}^4$$

a. *Shear stress in the beam at X-X from top edge:*

Here $\qquad h_2 = (c_2 - 80) = 120$ mm; $F_X = 22.5 \times 10^3$ N

$$A\bar{y} = (bh_2)\left(c_2 - \frac{h_2}{2}\right) = (100 \times 120) \times \left(200 - \frac{120}{2}\right) = 1.68 \times 10^6 \text{ mm}^3$$

Eq. (iv) yields... $\tau = \left(\dfrac{22.5 \times 10^3}{533.33 \times 16^6 \times 100}\right) \times (1.68 \times 10^6)$

$$\tau = 0.708 \text{ MPa}$$

b. *Shear stress in the beam at X-X from bottom edge:*

Here $\qquad h_2 = (c_2 - 150) = 50$ mm; $F_X = 22.5 \times 10^3$ N

$$A\bar{y} = (bh_1)\left(c_2 - \frac{h_1}{2}\right) = (100 \times 50) \times \left(200 - \frac{50}{2}\right) = 875 \times 10^3 \text{ mm}^3$$

Eq. (iv) yields... $\tau = \left(\dfrac{22.5 \times 10^3}{533.33 \times 16^6 \times 100}\right) \times (875 \times 10^3)$

$$\tau = 0.369 \text{ MPa}$$

c. *Maximum shear stress:*

Maximum shear stress occurs at N.A i.e. $\dfrac{h}{2} = 200$ mm,

$$F_{max} = 45 \times 10^3 \text{ N} \qquad\qquad\qquad \text{... From \textbf{Fig. 7.13(c)}}$$

$$A\bar{y} = (bh)\left(\frac{h}{2}\right) = (100 \times 200) \times \left(\frac{200}{2}\right) = 2 \times 10^6 \text{ mm}^3$$

Eq. (iv) yields... $\tau = \left(\dfrac{45 \times 10^3}{533.33 \times 10^6 \times 100}\right) \times (2 \times 10^6)$

$$\tau = 1.687 \text{ MPa} = \tau_{max}$$

d. *Bending stress in the beam:*

$$M_{max} = 67.5 \times 10^6 \text{ N-mm} \qquad\qquad \text{... From \textbf{Fig. 7.13(d)}}$$

$$\sigma = \frac{M}{Z} = \frac{Mc}{I} = \frac{(67.5 \times 10^6) \times 200}{533.33 \times 10^6} = 25.3 \text{ MPa}$$

7. Compute the bending stress and shear stress at point C, shown in Fig. 7.14(a).

VTU – (CV) Dec. 10 – 10 Marks

Solution: $w = 80$ kN/m $= 80$ N/mm, $L = 1800$ mm, $b = 150$ mm, $h = 600$ mm, $\tau = ?$, $\sigma = ?$.

Reactions at supports:

$$R_A + R_B = (80 \times 1.8) = 144 \text{ kN} \qquad\qquad\qquad \text{... Eq. (i)}$$

Taking moments about A and equating to zero, we have

$$R_B \times 1.8 = \left[80 \times 1.8 \times \left(\frac{1.8}{2}\right)\right]$$

$$R_B = 72 \text{ kN} \qquad \dots \text{ Eq. (ii)}$$

Substituting Eq. (ii) in Eq. (i), we have

$$R_A + 72 = 144$$

$$R_A = 72 \text{ kN} \qquad \dots \text{ Eq. (iii)}$$

Shear force calculations:

$$F_A = R_A = 72 \text{ kN}$$

$$F_C = 72 - (80 \times 0.6) = 24 \text{ kN}$$

$$F_{C-B} = 24 - (80 \times 1.2) = -72 \text{ kN}$$

$$F_B = F_{C-B} = -72 \text{ kN} = R_B$$

Bending moment calculations:

$$M_A = 0$$

$$M_C = (72 \times 0.6) - \left[80 \times 0.6 \times \left(\frac{0.6}{2}\right)\right]$$

$$= 28.8 \text{ kN-m}$$

$$M_B = 0$$

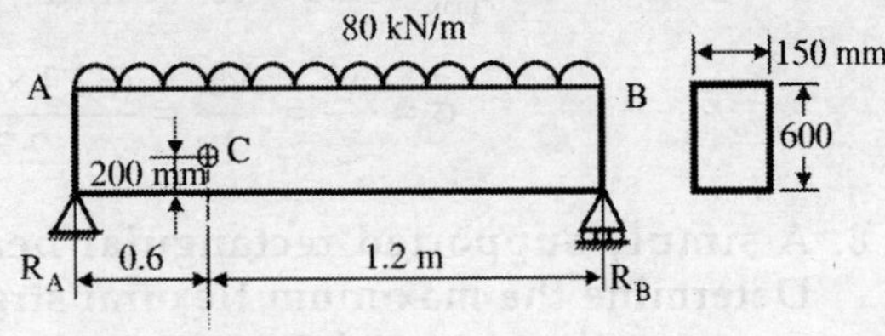

Fig. 7.14: Problem 7

Maximum bending moment:

Since the beam is symmetric, maximum bending moment occurs at mid-span i.e. $x = 0.9$ m

$$M_{\text{max}} = [72 \times 0.9] - \left[80 \times 0.9 \times \left(\frac{0.9}{2}\right)\right] = 32.4 \text{ kN-m}$$

The SFD and BMD diagrams are shown in **Figs 7.14(b) & (c)** respectively.

$$\text{Shear stress} \qquad \tau = \left(\frac{F}{Ib}\right) A\overline{y} \qquad \dots \text{ Eq. (iv)}$$

Due to symmetry, $\quad c_1 = c_2 = \dfrac{h}{2} = \dfrac{600}{2} = 300$ mm

$$I = \frac{bh^3}{12} = \frac{(150 \times 600^3)}{12} = 2.7 \times 10^9 \text{ mm}^4$$

a. *Shear stress in the beam at C from bottom edge:*

Here $\qquad h_1 = 200$ mm; $F_C = 24 \times 10^3$ N

$$A\overline{y} = (bh_1)\left(c_2 - \frac{h_1}{2}\right) = (150 \times 200) \times \left(300 - \frac{200}{2}\right) = 6 \times 10^6 \text{ mm}^3$$

Eq. (iv) yields... $\tau = \left(\dfrac{24 \times 10^3}{2.7 \times 10^9 \times 150}\right) \times (6 \times 10^6)$

$$\tau = 0.356 \text{ MPa}$$

b. *Bending stress in the beam at C from bottom edge:*

Here $\qquad c = (c_1 - 200) = (300 - 200) = 100$ mm

$$M_{max} = 32.4 \times 10^6 \text{ N-mm} \qquad \text{... From Fig. 7.16(c)}$$

$$\sigma = \frac{M}{Z} = \frac{Mc}{I} = \frac{(32.4 \times 10^6) \times 100}{2.7 \times 10^9} = 1.2 \text{ MPa}$$

8. **A simply supported rectangular beam is loaded as shown in Fig. 7.15(a). Determine the maximum flexural stresses and maximum shearing stress at a cross section located 2 m from the left support. Sketch the flexural and shearing stress distributions at the specified cross section.**

VTU – (CV) Dec. 13/ Jan. 14 – 12 Marks

Solution: $L = 6000$ mm, $W = 20 \times 10^3$ N, $w = 10$ kN/m $= 10$ N/mm, $b = 200$ mm, $h = 300$ mm, $\sigma = ?, \tau = ?,$

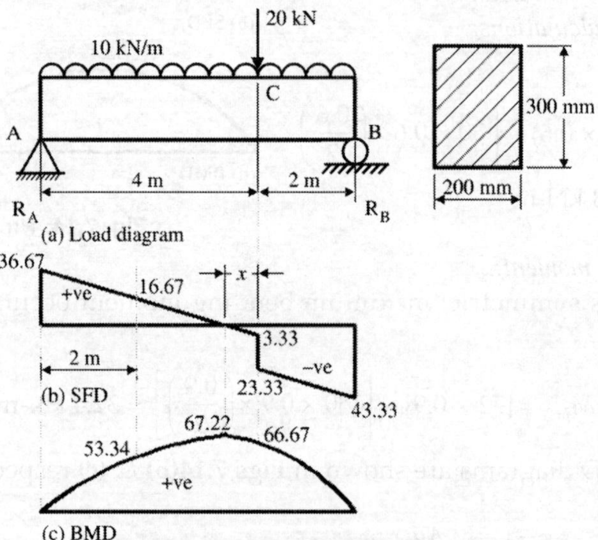

Fig. 7.15: Problem 8

Reactions at supports:

$$R_A + R_B = 20 + (10 \times 6) = 80 \text{ kN} \qquad \text{... Eq. (i)}$$

Taking moments about A and equating to zero, we have

$$R_B \times 6 = (20 \times 4) + \left[10 \times 6 \times \left(\frac{6}{2} \right) \right]$$

$$R_B = 43..33 \text{ kN} \qquad \text{... Eq. (ii)}$$

Substituting Eq. (ii) in Eq. (i), we have

$$R_A + 43.33 = 80$$

$$R_A = 36.67 \text{ kN} \qquad \text{... Eq. (iii)}$$

Shear force calculations:

$$F_A = R_A = 36.67 \text{ kN}$$

$$F_{A-C} = 36.67 - (10 \times 4) = -3.33 \text{ kN}$$

$$F_C = -3.33 - 20 = -23.33 \text{ kN}$$

$$F_{C-B} = -23.33 - (10 \times 2) = -43.33 \text{ kN}$$

$$F_B = F_{C-B} = -43.33 \text{ kN} = R_B$$

Bending moment calculations:

$$M_A = 0$$

$$M_C = (36.67 \times 4) - \left[10 \times 4 \times \left(\frac{4}{2}\right)\right] = 66.67 \text{ kN-m}$$

$$M_B = 0$$

Maximum bending moment:

$$\frac{x}{3.33} = \frac{4-x}{36.67}$$

$$36.67x = 3.33 \times (4-x)$$

$$40x = 13.32$$

$$x = 0.33 \text{ m}$$

$$M_{max} = [36.67 \times (4-0.33)] - \left[(10 \times (4-0.33)) \times \left(\frac{4-0.33}{2}\right)\right] = 67.23 \text{ kN-m}$$

The SFD and BMD diagrams are shown in **Figs 7.15(b) & (c)** respectively

Stresses at 2 m from left support:

Bending stress $\quad \sigma = \dfrac{M}{Z}$ $\hspace{4cm}$ ... Eq. (iv)

Due to symmetry, $\quad c_1 = c_2 = \dfrac{H}{2} = \dfrac{300}{2} = 150 \text{ mm}$

$$I = \frac{bh^3}{12} = \frac{(200 \times 300^3)}{12} = 450 \times 10^6 \text{ mm}^4$$

Section modulus $\quad Z = \dfrac{I}{c} = \dfrac{450 \times 10^6}{150} = 3 \times 10^6 \text{ mm}^3$

Or $\qquad Z = \dfrac{I}{c} = \dfrac{bh^2}{6} = \dfrac{200 \times 300^2}{6} = 3 \times 10^6 \text{ mm}^3$

$$M = R_A \, l - wl\left(\frac{l}{2}\right) \hspace{3cm} \text{Here } l = 2 \text{ m from left support}$$

$$= (36.67 \times 2) - (10 \times 2)\left(\frac{2}{2}\right)$$

$$M = 53.34 \text{ kN-m}$$

Eq. (iv) yields... $\sigma = \dfrac{53.34 \times 10^6}{3 \times 10^6} = 17.78 \text{ MPa (Tensile stress)}$

Maximum shear stress

$$\tau = \left(\frac{F}{Ib}\right) A\bar{y} \hspace{4cm} \text{... Eq. (v)}$$

Maximum shear stress occurs at N.A i.e. $\dfrac{h}{2} = 150 \text{ mm}$,

$$F = R_A - wl = 36.67 - (10 \times 2) = 16.67 \text{ kN}$$

$$\text{Here } l = 2 \text{ m from left support}$$

$$A\bar{y} = (bh)\left(\frac{h}{2}\right) = (200 \times 150) \times \left(\frac{150}{2}\right) = 2.25 \times 10^6 \text{ mm}^3$$

Eq. (v) yields... $\quad \tau = \left(\dfrac{16.67 \times 10^3}{450 \times 10^6 \times 200}\right) \times (2.25 \times 10^6)$

$$\tau = 0.416 \text{ MPa} = \tau_{max}$$

The flexural and shearing stress distributions diagrams are shown in **Figs 7.16**.

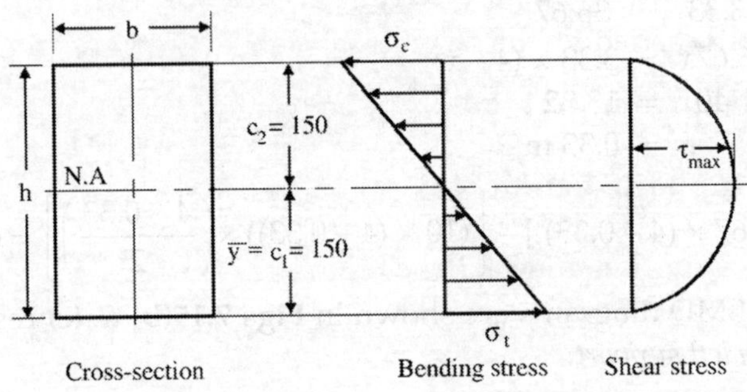

Fig. 7.16: Stress distribution diagrams Problem 8

9. **A simply supported wooden beam of span 1.3 m having a cross section 150 mm wide by 250 mm deep carries a point load W at the centre. The permissible stress is 7 N/mm^2 in bending and 1 N/mm^2 in shearing. Determine the safe load W.**

VTU – (CV) Dec.08/ Jan.09 – 12 Marks

Solution: $L = 1300$ mm, $b = 150$ mm, $h = 250$ mm, $\sigma = 7$ MPa, $\tau = 1$ MPa, $W = ?$.

For a simply supported beam subjected to point load at mid-span

$$F = \frac{W}{2} = 0.5\,W$$

$$M = \frac{WL}{4} = \frac{1300\,W}{4} = 325\,W$$

a. Based on bending stress:

Bending stress $\qquad \sigma = \dfrac{M}{Z}$ $\hfill$ ... Eq. (i)

Due to symmetry, $\quad c_1 = c_2 = \dfrac{h}{2} = \dfrac{250}{2} = 125 \text{ mm}$

$$I = \frac{bh^3}{12} = \frac{(150 \times 250^3)}{12} = 195.31 \times 10^6 \text{ mm}^4$$

Section modulus $\quad Z = \dfrac{I}{c} = \dfrac{195.31 \times 10^6}{125} = 1.563 \times 10^6 \text{ mm}^3$

Eq. (i) yields... $\quad 7 = \dfrac{325W}{1.563 \times 10^6}$

$\qquad\qquad\qquad\quad W = 33.65 \times 10^3 \text{ N}$ $\hfill$ ... Eq. (ii)

b. *Based on shear stress:*

Max. shear stress $\quad \tau_{max} = 1.5\tau_{avg} = 1.5\left(\dfrac{F}{A}\right)$

Here $\qquad\qquad \tau = \tau_{max}$

$\therefore \quad 1 = 1.5\left(\dfrac{0.5W}{150 \times 250}\right)$

$\qquad\qquad W = 50 \times 10^3\,\text{N}$ $\qquad\qquad\qquad\qquad$ ... Eq. (iii)

From Eqs (ii) and (iii), the safe load is $W = 33.65$ kN (minimum value) and maximum load carried by the beam is $W = 50$ kN (Maximum value)

10. **Using the data from previous problem, determine the value of load if the beam is:**
    (a) Simply supported and carries an eccentric point load at 0.25 m from left support.
    (b) Simply supported and carries a UDL of w N/m over the entire span.
    (c) Cantilever and carries a point load at free end.
    (d) Cantilever and carries a UDL of w N/m over the entire span.

Solution: $L = 1300$ mm, $b = 150$ mm, $h = 250$ mm, $\sigma = 7$ MPa, $\tau = 1$ MPa, $W = ?$.

From **problem 9**, we have

$\qquad\qquad c_1 = c_2 = 125$ mm, $I = 195.31 \times 10^6$ mm^4, $Z = 1.563 \times 10^6$ mm^3

Case a: Simply supported and carries an eccentric point load at 0.25 m from left support

$$F_A = \frac{Wb}{L} = \frac{W(1300 - 250)}{1300} = 0.81\,W$$

$$F_B = \frac{Wa}{L} = \frac{W \times 250}{1300} = 0.19\,W$$

$$M = \frac{Wab}{L} = \frac{W \times 250 \times (1300 \times 250)}{1300} = 201.92\,W$$

a. *Based on bending stress:*

Bending stress $\qquad \sigma = \dfrac{M}{Z}$

$$7 = \frac{201.92\,W}{1.563 \times 10^6}$$

$\qquad\qquad W = 54.18 \times 10^3\,\text{N}$ $\qquad\qquad\qquad\qquad$ ... Eq. (a)

b. *Based on shear stress:*

Max. shear stress $\quad \tau_{max} = 1.5\tau_{avg} = 1.5\left(\dfrac{F}{A}\right)$

$\qquad\qquad\qquad\qquad$ Here $\tau = \tau_{max}$, and $F = F_A$ maximum value

$$1 = 1.5\left(\frac{0.81\,W}{150 \times 250}\right)$$

$\qquad\qquad W = 30.86 \times 10^3\,\text{N}$ $\qquad\qquad\qquad\qquad$ ... Eq. (b)

From Eqs (a) and (b), the safe load is $W = 30.86$ kN (minimum value) and maximum load carried by the beam is $W = 54.18$ kN (Maximum value)

Case b: Simply supported and carries a UDL of w N/m over the entire span.

$$F = \frac{wL}{2} = \frac{w \times 1300}{2} = 650\,w$$

$$M = \frac{wL^2}{8} = \frac{w \times 1300^2}{8} = 211250\,w$$

a. *Based on bending stress:*

Bending stress $\qquad \sigma = \dfrac{M}{Z}$

$$7 = \frac{211250\,w}{1.563 \times 10^6}$$

$$w = 51.79 \text{ N/mm} = 51.79 \text{ kN/m} \qquad\qquad \dots \text{Eq. (c)}$$

b. *Based on shear stress:*

Max. shear stress $\quad \tau_{max} = 1.5\tau_{avg} = 1.5\left(\dfrac{F}{A}\right)$ $\qquad\qquad$ Here $\tau = \tau_{max}$

$$1 = 1.5\left(\frac{650\,W}{150 \times 250}\right)$$

$$w = 38.46 \text{ N/mm} = 38.46 \text{ kN/m} \qquad\qquad \dots \text{Eq. (d)}$$

From Eqs (c) and (d), the safe value of UDL is $w = 38.46$ kN/m (minimum value) and maximum UDL carried by the beam is $w = 51.79$ kN/m (Maximum value)

Case c: Cantilever and carries a point load at free end.

$$F = W$$
$$M = WL = 1300\,W$$

a. *Based on bending stress:*

Bending stress $\qquad \sigma = \dfrac{M}{Z}$

$$7 = \frac{1300\,W}{1.563 \times 10^6}$$

$$W = 8416.15 \text{ N} \qquad\qquad\qquad\qquad\qquad \dots \text{Eq. (e)}$$

b. *Based on shear stress:*

Max. shear stress $\quad \tau_{max} = 1.5\tau_{avg} = 1.5\,(F/A)$ $\qquad\qquad$ Here $\tau = \tau_{max}$

$$1 = 1.5\left(\frac{W}{150 \times 250}\right)$$

$$W = 25 \times 10^3 \text{ N} \qquad\qquad\qquad\qquad \dots \text{Eq. (f)}$$

From Eqs (e) and (f), the safe load is $W = 8.416$ kN (minimum value) and maximum load carried by the beam is $W = 25$ kN (Maximum value)

Case d: Cantilever and carries a UDL of w N/m over the entire span.

$$F = wL = 1300\,w$$

$$M = \frac{wL^2}{2} = \frac{w \times 1300^2}{2} = 845000\,w$$

a. *Based on bending stress:*

Bending stress $\qquad \sigma = \dfrac{M}{Z}$

$$7 = \frac{845000\,w}{1.563 \times 10^6}$$

$$w = 12.95 \text{ N/mm} = 12.95 \text{ kN/m} \qquad \qquad \dots \text{Eq. (g)}$$

b. *Based on shear stress:*

Max. shear stress $\quad \tau_{max} = 1.5\tau_{avg} = 1.5\left(\dfrac{F}{A}\right) \qquad\qquad$ Here $\tau = \tau_{max}$

$$1 = 1.5\left(\frac{1300\,w}{150 \times 250}\right)$$

$$w = 19.23 \text{ N/mm} = 19.23 \text{ kN/m} \qquad\qquad \dots \text{Eq. (h)}$$

From Eqs (g) and (h), the safe value of UDL is w = 12.95 kN/m (minimum value) and maximum UDL carried by the beam is w = 19.23 kN/m (Maximum value)

11. A beam of square cross-section is subjected to a shear force F so placed that one of its diagonals is horizontal. Draw the shear stress distribution for the section and find the maximum shear stress.

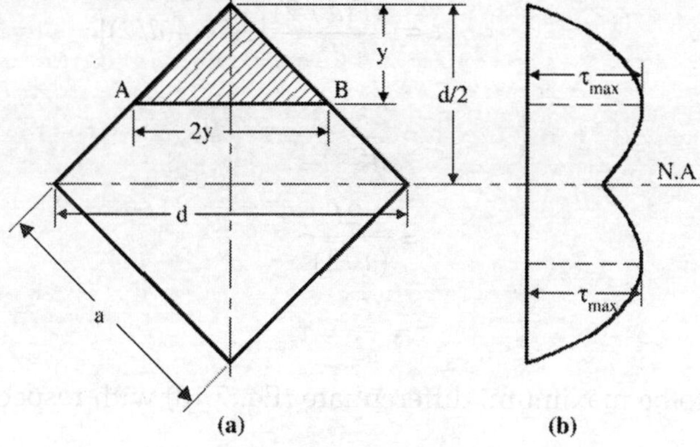

Fig. 7.17: Problem 11

Solution:
Consider a square with one of its diagonal horizontal, as shown in **Fig. 7.17(a)**.

Let $\qquad a$ = length of side

$\qquad\qquad d$ = length of the diagonal

We know that shear stress at any height y above the N.A is

$$\tau = \left(\frac{F}{Ib}\right)A\bar{y} \qquad\qquad \dots \text{Eq. (i)}$$

At any distance y from the apex, width $AB = 2y$

Area of shaded portion $\qquad\qquad A = \dfrac{1}{2}\,2y.y \qquad\qquad \dots \text{Eq. (ii)}$

Distance of CG
$$\bar{y} = \frac{d}{2} - \frac{2y}{3} \qquad \ldots \text{Eq. (iii)}$$

MI about N.A
$$I = 2\left[\frac{d(d/2)^3}{12}\right] = \frac{d^4}{48} \qquad \ldots \text{Eq. (iv)}$$

Diagonal length
$$d = \sqrt{a^2 + a^2} = a\sqrt{2} \qquad \ldots \text{Eq. (v)}$$

Substituting Eqs (ii), (iii) and (iv) in (i), we have

$$\tau = \frac{F}{(d^4/48)2y}\left[\frac{1}{2}\,2y.y\left(\frac{d}{2} - \frac{2y}{3}\right)\right] \qquad \text{Here } b = 2y$$

$$= \frac{24Fy}{d^4}\left(\frac{3d - 4y}{6}\right)$$

$$\tau = \frac{4Fy}{d^4}(3d - 4y) \qquad \ldots \text{(Eq. 7.18)}$$

The shear stress is distributed parabolically as shown in **Fig. 7.17(b)**.
The first term increases with increase in value of y, the second term decreases with increasing value of y across the depth of the section.

Boundary conditions:

At $y = 0$, (Eq. 7.18) yields... $\qquad \tau = 0 \qquad \ldots \text{(Eq. 7.19)}$

At $y = d/2$

(Eq. 7.18) yields...
$$\tau = \frac{4F(d/2)}{d^4}[3d - 4(d/2)]$$

$$= \frac{2F}{d^2}$$

$$= \frac{2F}{(a\sqrt{2})^2} \qquad \ldots \text{Using (Eq. v)}$$

$$\tau = \frac{F}{a^2} = \tau_{avg} \qquad \ldots \text{(Eq. 7.20)}$$

For shear stress to be maximum, differentiate (Eq. 7.18) with respect to y and equate to zero

i.e.
$$\frac{d\tau}{dy} = 0$$

$$\frac{d}{dy}\left[\frac{4Fy}{d^4}(3d - 4y)\right] = 0$$

$$\frac{d}{dy}[y(3d - 4y)] = 0$$

$$3d - 8y = 0$$

$$y = \frac{3d}{8} \qquad \ldots \text{(Eq. 7.21)}$$

Substituting the above value of y in (Eq. 7.18), we have

$$\tau_{max} = \frac{4F}{d^4}\left(\frac{3d}{8}\right)\left[3d - 4\left(\frac{3d}{8}\right)\right]$$

$$= \frac{3F}{2d^3}\left[3d - \left(\frac{3d}{2}\right)\right]$$

$$= \frac{9F}{4d^2}$$

$$= \frac{9F}{4(a\sqrt{2})^2} = \frac{9F}{8a^2} \qquad\qquad \text{... Using (Eq. v)}$$

$$\tau_{max} = \frac{9}{8}\,\tau_{avg} \qquad\qquad \text{... (Eq. 7.22)}$$

12. **A simply supported beam of rectangular cross section carries a UDL over the entire span. If the allowable stresses in bending and shear are σ and τ, respectively, derive an expression for the length of the beam.**

    If the allowable bending and shear stresses are 8 MPa and 2 MPa respectively, find the ratio of length to depth.

Solution: Case 1: L = ? Case 2: $\sigma = 8$ MPa, $\tau = 2$ MPa, $\dfrac{L}{h}$ = ?

Let σ = Bending stress in the layer τ = Shear stress
           b = width of section h = depth of section
           L = Length of the beam M = bending moment
           Z = Section modulus I = Moment of inertia
           F = Shear force w = uniformly distributed load
           A = cross sectional area

Case 1: To find L

 a. *Based on bending stress:*

Bending stress $\sigma = \dfrac{M}{Z}$ $\qquad\qquad$ ... Eq. (i)

For a simply supported beam with UDL over entire span

Shear force $F = \dfrac{wL}{2}$

Bending moment $M = \dfrac{wL^2}{8}$

MI of entire section $I = \dfrac{bh^3}{12}$

Section modulus $Z = \dfrac{bh^2}{6}$

Eq. (i) yields... $\sigma = \dfrac{wL^2/8}{bh^2/6} = \dfrac{3wL^2}{4bh^2}$

$$w = \dfrac{4\sigma bh^2}{3L^2} \qquad\qquad \text{... Eq. (ii)}$$

b. *Based on shear stress:*

Avg. shear stress $\quad \tau_{max} = \dfrac{3F}{2A} = \dfrac{3(wL/2)}{2(bh)} = \dfrac{3wL}{4bh}$

$$w = \frac{4\tau_{max}bh}{3L} \qquad \text{... Eq. (iii)}$$

Equating Eqs (ii) and (iii), we have

$$\frac{4\sigma bh^2}{3L^2} = \frac{4\tau_{max}bh}{3L}$$

$$\frac{\sigma h}{L} = \tau_{max}$$

$$L = \left(\frac{\sigma}{\tau_{max}}\right)h \qquad \text{... Eq. (iv)}$$

If actual length $\quad L_{act} < L$, the shear stress governs the design and
If $\qquad\qquad L_{act} > L$ the bending stress governs the design.

Case 2: To find L/h:

Eq. (iv) yields... $\quad \dfrac{L}{h} = \left(\dfrac{8}{2}\right) = 4$

13. Repeat the above problem for a simply supported beam with point load at mid-span. If the allowable bending and shear stresses are 12 MPa and 1 MPa respectively, find the ratio of length to depth.

Solution: Case 1: $L = ?$ Case 2: $\sigma = 12$ MPa, $\tau = 1$ MPa, $L/h = ?$

Let W = Point load , $\qquad\qquad$ *Other parameters being same as in Problem 12.*

Case 1: To find L

a. *Based on bending stress:*

Bending stress $\qquad \sigma = \dfrac{M}{Z} \qquad\qquad\qquad\qquad$ ... Eq. (i)

For a simply supported beam with point load at mid-span

Shear force $\qquad F = \dfrac{W}{2}$

Bending moment $\qquad M = \dfrac{WL}{4}$

Eq. (i) yields... $\qquad \sigma = \dfrac{WL/4}{bh^2/6} = \dfrac{3WL}{2bh^2}$

$$W = \frac{2\sigma bh^2}{3L} \qquad \text{... Eq. (ii)}$$

b. *Based on shear stress:*

Avg. shear stress $\quad \tau_{max} = \dfrac{3F}{2A} = \dfrac{3(W/2)}{2(bh)} = \dfrac{3W}{4bh}$

$$W = \frac{4\tau_{max}bh}{3} \qquad \text{... Eq. (iii)}$$

Equating Eqs (ii) and (iii), we have

$$\frac{2\sigma bh^2}{3L} = \frac{4\tau_{max}bh}{3}$$

$$\frac{\sigma h}{L} = 2\tau_{max}$$

$$L = \left(\frac{\sigma}{2\tau_{max}}\right)h \qquad \ldots \text{Eq. (iv)}$$

Case 2: To find L/h:

Eq. (iv) yields... $\dfrac{L}{h} = \left(\dfrac{12}{2 \times 1}\right) = 6$

PROBLEMS ON T SECTION

14. **A T-shaped cross section of a beam Fig. 7.18(a) is subjected to a vertical shear force of 100 kN. Calculate the shear stress at the neutral axis and at the junction of the web and the flange. M.I about the horizontal neutral axis is 0.0001134 m⁴.**

VTU – Dec. 09/ Jan. 10 – 10 Marks; [Similar: Dec. 14/ Jan. 15 – 10 Marks]

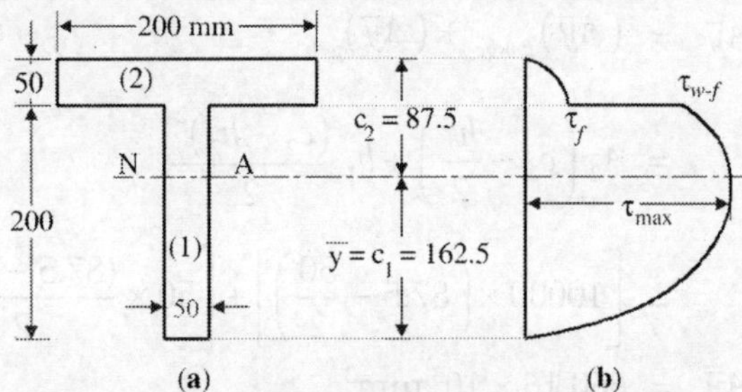

Fig. 7.18: Problem 14

Solution: $F = 100 \times 10^3$ N, $\tau = ?$, $I = 0.0001134$ m⁴ $= 113.4 \times 10^6$ mm⁴

To find $\overline{y}$:

Element No.	b (mm)	h (mm)	A = bh (mm²)	y (from base) = (h/2) + x (mm)	Ay (mm³)
(1) Web	50	200	10000	(200/2) = 100	1×10^6
(2) Flange	200	50	10000	200 + (50/2) = 225	2.25×10^6

x = distance of fiber considered from base

$$\Sigma A = 20000 \text{ mm}^2$$
$$\Sigma Ay = 3.25 \times 10^6 \text{ mm}^3$$

$$\overline{y} = \frac{\Sigma Ay}{\Sigma A} = \frac{3.25 \times 10^6}{20000} = 162.5 \text{ mm}$$

i.e. $\quad \overline{y} = c_1 = 162.5$ mm from base (Tensile)

$\quad c_2 = \Sigma h - c_1 = 250 - 162.5 = 87.5$ mm from top face (Compressive)

Shear stress $\qquad \tau = \left(\dfrac{F}{Ib'}\right) A\bar{y}$ $\qquad\qquad$ ... Eq. (i)

a. *Shear stress at boundaries is zero.*

b. *Shear stress at the bottom of flange:* Here $b' = b_2 = 200$ mm

$$A\bar{y} = A_2\left(c_2 - \frac{h_2}{2}\right) = 10000 \times \left(87.5 - \frac{50}{2}\right) = 625 \times 10^3 \text{ mm}^3$$

Eq. (i) yields... $\qquad \tau_f = \left(\dfrac{100 \times 10^3}{113.4 \times 10^6 \times 200}\right) \times (625 \times 10^3) = 2.76$ MPa

c. *Shear stress at the junction of web and flange:* Here $b' = b_1 = 50$ mm

$$A\bar{y} = A_2\left(c_2 - \frac{h_2}{2}\right) = 10000 \times \left(87.5 - \frac{50}{2}\right) = 625 \times 10^3 \text{ mm}^3$$

Eq. (i) yields... $\qquad \tau_{w-f} = \left(\dfrac{100 \times 10^3}{113.4 \times 10^6 \times 50}\right) \times (625 \times 10^3) = 11.02$ MPa

Or $\qquad\qquad \tau_{w-f} = \left(\dfrac{b_2}{b_1}\right)\tau_f = \left(\dfrac{200}{50}\right) \times 2.756 = 11.02$ MPa

d. *Shear stress at neutral axis:* Here $b' = b_1 = 50$ mm

$$A\bar{y} = \left(A\bar{y}\right)_{flange} + \left(A\bar{y}\right)_{web}$$

$$= A_2\left(c_2 - \frac{h_2}{2}\right) + b_1\frac{\left(c_2 - h_2\right)^2}{2}$$

$$= \left[10000 \times \left(87.5 - \frac{50}{2}\right)\right] + \left[50 \times \frac{(87.5 - 50)^2}{2}\right]$$

$$A\bar{y} = 660.16 \times 10^3 \text{ mm}^3$$

Eq. (i) yields... $\qquad \tau_{NA} = \left(\dfrac{100 \times 10^3}{113.4 \times 10^6 \times 50}\right) \times (660.16 \times 10^3)$

$$\tau_{NA} = 11.64 \text{ MPa} = \tau_{max}$$

The shear stress distribution is as shown in **Fig. 7.18(b)**.

15. A cross section of the beam is as shown in Fig. 7.19(a). The shear force on the section is 400 kN. Estimate the shear stress at various points and plot the shear stress distribution diagram.

VTU – (CV) Dec.07/ Jan.08 – 10 Marks

Solution: $F = 400 \times 10^3$ N, $\tau = ?$.

To find $\bar{y}$:

Element No.	b (mm)	h (mm)	$A = bh$ (mm^2)	y (from base) = $(h/2) + x$ (mm)	Ay (mm^3)	$I_G = bh^3/12$ (mm^4)
(1) Web	15	160	2400	$(160/2) = 80$	192×10^3	5.12×10^6
(2) Flange	160	15	2400	$160 + (15/2) = 167.5$	402×10^3	45×10^3

x = distance of fiber considered from base

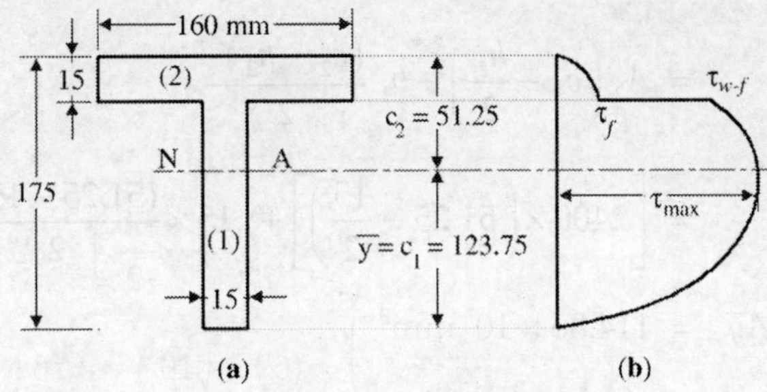

Fig. 7.19: Problem 15

$$\Sigma A = 4800 \text{ mm}^2$$
$$\Sigma Ay = 594 \times 10^3 \text{ mm}^3$$

$$\bar{y} = \frac{\Sigma Ay}{\Sigma A} = \frac{594 \times 10^3}{4800} = 123.75 \text{ mm}$$

i.e. $\quad \bar{y} = c_1 = 123.75$ mm from base (Tensile)

$\quad c_2 = \Sigma h - c_1 = 175 - 123.75 = 51.25$ mm from top face (Compressive)

Shear stress $\qquad \tau = \left(\dfrac{F}{Ib'}\right)A\bar{y}$ $\qquad\qquad\qquad\qquad$ ... Eq. (i)

$$I = I_1 + I_2$$
$$= [I_{G1} + A_1(\bar{y} \sim y_1)^2] + [I_{G2} + A_2(\bar{y} \sim y_2)^2]$$
$$= \{5.12 \times 10^6 + [2400 \times (123.75 - 80)^2]\}$$
$$\qquad + \{45 \times 10^3 + [2400 \times (123.75 - 167.5)^2]\}$$
$$I = 14.35 \times 10^6 \text{ mm}^4$$

a. *Shear stress at boundaries is zero.*

b. *Shear stress at the bottom of flange:* Here $b' = b_2 = 160$ mm

$$A\bar{y} = A_2\left(c_2 - \frac{h_2}{2}\right) = 2400 \times \left(51.25 - \frac{15}{2}\right) = 105 \times 10^3 \text{ mm}^3$$

Eq. (i) yields... $\qquad \tau_f = \left(\dfrac{400 \times 10^3}{14.35 \times 10^6 \times 160}\right) \times (105 \times 10^3) = 18.293$ MPa

c. *Shear stress at the junction of web and flange:* Here $b' = b_1 = 15$ mm

$$A\bar{y} = A_2\left(c_2 - \frac{h_2}{2}\right) = 2400 \times \left(51.25 - \frac{15}{2}\right) = 105 \times 10^3 \text{ mm}^3$$

Eq. (i) yields... $\qquad \tau_{w-f} = \left(\dfrac{400 \times 10^3}{14.35 \times 10^6 \times 15}\right) \times (10^5 \times 10^3) = 195.12$ MPa

Or $\qquad\qquad \tau_{w-f} = \left(\dfrac{b_2}{b_1}\right)\tau_f = \left(\dfrac{160}{15}\right) \times 18.296 = 195.12$ MPa

d. *Shear stress at neutral axis:* Here $b' = b_1 = 15$ mm

$$A\bar{y} = \left(A\bar{y}\right)_{flange} + \left(A\bar{y}\right)_{web}$$

$$= A_2 \left(c_2 - \frac{h_2}{2} \right) + b_1 \frac{(c_2 - h_2)^2}{2}$$

$$= \left[2400 \times \left(51.25 - \frac{15}{2} \right) \right] + \left[15 \times \frac{(51.25 - 15)^2}{2} \right]$$

$$A\bar{y} = 114.86 \times 10^3 \text{ mm}^3$$

Eq. (i) yields... $\quad \tau_{NA} = \left(\dfrac{400 \times 10^3}{14.35 \times 10^6 \times 15} \right) \times (114.86 \times 10^3)$

$$\tau_{NA} = 213.44 \text{ MPa} = \tau_{max}$$

The shear stress distribution is as shown in **Fig. 7.19(b)**.

16. **The T-section shown in Fig. 7.20(a) is subjected to shear force of 100 kN. Draw shear stress distribution diagram and find the maximum shear stress.**

VTU – Civil: Dec. 15/ Jan. 16 – 12 Marks, [Similar: June 2012 – 15 Marks; Dec. 2011 – 10 Marks; Dec. 10 – 10 Marks]

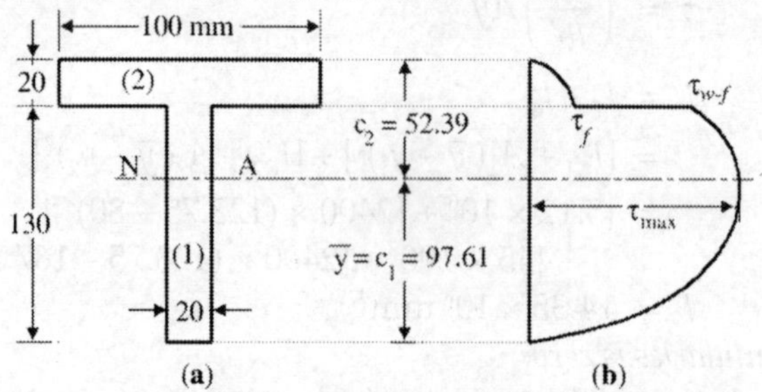

Fig. 7.20: Problem 16

Solution: $F = 100 \times 10^3$ N, $\tau = ?$

To find $\bar{y}$:

Element No.	b (mm)	h (mm)	A = bh (mm²)	y (from base) = (h/2) + x (mm)	Ay (mm³)	$I_G = bh^3/12$ (mm⁴)
(1) Web	20	130	2600	(130/2) = 65	169 × 10³	3.66 × 10⁶
(2) Flange	100	20	2000	130 + (20/2) = 140	280 × 10³	66.67 × 10³

x = distance of fiber considered from base

$$\Sigma A = 4600 \text{ mm}^2$$
$$\Sigma Ay = 449 \times 10^3 \text{ mm}^3$$

$$\bar{y} = \frac{\Sigma Ay}{\Sigma A} = \frac{449 \times 10^6}{4600} = 97.61 \text{ mm}$$

i.e. $\quad \bar{y} = c_1 = 97.61$ mm from base (Tensile)

$\quad c_2 = \Sigma h - c_1 = 150 - 97.61 = 52.39$ mm from top face (Compressive)

Shear stress $\quad \tau = \left(\dfrac{F}{Ib'} \right) A\bar{y} \quad\quad$ ... Eq. (i)

$$I = I_1 + I_2$$

$$= [I_{G1} + A_1(\bar{y} \sim y_1)^2] + [I_{G2} + A_2(\bar{y} \sim y_2)^2]$$

$$= \{3.66 \times 10^6 + [2600 \times (97.61 - 65)^2]\}$$
$$+ \{66.67 \times 10^3 + [2000 \times (97.61 - 140)^2]\}$$

$$I = 10.08 \times 10^6 \text{ mm}^4$$

a. *Shear stress at boundaries is zero.*

b. *Shear stress at the bottom of flange:* Here $b' = b_2 = 100$ mm

$$A\bar{y} = A_2\left(c_2 - \frac{h_2}{2}\right) = 2000 \times \left(52.39 - \frac{20}{2}\right) = 84.78 \times 10^3 \text{ mm}^3$$

Eq. (i) yields... $\quad \tau_f = \left(\dfrac{100 \times 10^3}{10.08 \times 10^6 \times 100}\right) \times (84.78 \times 10^3) = 8.41$ MPa

c. *Shear stress at the junction of web and flange:* Here $b' = b_1 = 20$ mm

$$A\bar{y} = A_2\left(c_2 - \frac{h_2}{2}\right) = 2000 \times \left(52.39 - \frac{20}{2}\right) = 84.78 \times 10^3 \text{ mm}^3$$

Eq. (i) yields... $\quad \tau_{w-f} = \left(\dfrac{100 \times 10^3}{10.08 \times 10^6 \times 20}\right) \times (84.78 \times 10^3) = 42.05$ MPa

Or $\qquad \tau_{w-f} = \left(\dfrac{b_2}{b_1}\right) \tau_f = \left(\dfrac{100}{20}\right) \times 8.41 = 42.05$ MPa

d. *Shear stress at neutral axis:* Here $b' = b_1 = 20$ mm

$$A\bar{y} = \left(A\bar{y}\right)_{flange} + \left(A\bar{y}\right)_{web}$$

$$= A_2\left(c_2 - \frac{h_2}{2}\right) + b_1 \frac{(c_2 - h_2)^2}{2}$$

$$= \left[2000 \times \left(52.39 - \frac{20}{2}\right)\right] + \left[20 \times \frac{(52.39 - 20)^2}{2}\right]$$

$$A\bar{y} = 95.27 \times 10^3 \text{ mm}^3$$

Eq. (i) yields... $\quad \tau_{NA} = \left(\dfrac{100 \times 10^3}{10.08 \times 10^6 \times 20}\right) \times (95.27 \times 10^3)$

$$\tau_{NA} = 47.25 \text{ MPa} = \tau_{max}$$

The shear stress distribution is as shown in **Fig. 7.20(b)**.

17. **A 'T'-section of flange 120 mm × 12 mm and overall depth 200 mm, with web 12 mm thick is loaded such that, at a section it has a moment of 20 kN-m and shear force of 120 kN. Sketch the bending and shear stress distribution diagram, marking the salient values.**

VTU – May/ June 2010 – 14 Marks; (CV) June/ July 2008 –14 Marks

Solution: $F = 120 \times 10^3$ N, $M = 20 \times 10^6$ N-mm, $\sigma = ?, \tau = ?$.

Based on given data, T section is as shown in **Fig. 7.21(a)**.

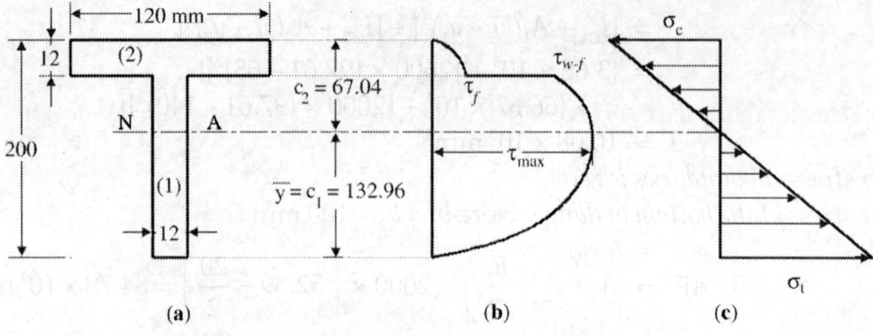

Fig. 7.21: Problem 17

To find $\overline{y}$:

Element No.	b (mm)	h (mm)	$A = bh$ (mm²)	y (from base) = $(h/2) + x$ (mm)	Ay (mm³)	$I_G = bh^3/12$ (mm⁴)
(1) Web	12	188	2256	(188/2) = 94	212064	6.645×10^6
(2) Flange	120	12	1440	188 + (12/2) = 194	279360	17.28×10^3

x = distance of fiber considered from base

$$\Sigma A = 3696 \text{ mm}^2$$
$$\Sigma Ay = 491424 \text{ mm}^3$$

$$\overline{y} = \frac{\Sigma Ay}{\Sigma A} = \frac{491424}{3696} = 132.96 \text{ mm}$$

i.e. $\quad \overline{y} = c_1 = 132.96$ mm from base (Tensile)

$\quad c_2 = \Sigma h - c_1 = 200 - 132.96 = 67.04$ mm from top face (Compressive)

Shear stress $\qquad \tau = \left(\dfrac{F}{Ib'}\right) A\overline{y}$ $\qquad\qquad\qquad$ ... Eq. (i)

$$I = I_1 + I_2$$
$$= [I_{G1} + A_1(\overline{y} \sim y_1)^2] + [I_{G2} + A_2(\overline{y} \sim y_2)^2]$$
$$= \{6.645 \times 10^6 + [2256 \times (132.96 - 94)^2]\}$$
$$\quad + \{17.28 \times 10^3 + [1440 \times (132.96 - 194)^2]\}$$
$$I = 15.452 \times 10^6 \text{ mm}^4$$

a. *Shear stress at boundaries is zero.*

b. *Shear stress at the bottom of flange:* **Here** $b' = b_2 = 120$ mm

$$A\overline{y} = A_2\left(c_2 - \frac{h_2}{2}\right) = 1440 \times \left(67.04 - \frac{12}{2}\right) = 87.90 \times 10^3 \text{ mm}^3$$

Eq. (i) yields... $\qquad \tau_f = \left(\dfrac{120 \times 10^3}{15.452 \times 10^6 \times 120}\right) \times (87.90 \times 10^3) = 5.69$ MPa

c. *Shear stress at the junction of web and flange:* **Here** $b' = b_1 = 12$ mm

$$A\overline{y} = A_2\left(c_2 - \frac{h_2}{2}\right) = 1440 \times \left(67.04 - \frac{12}{2}\right) = 87.90 \times 10^3 \text{ mm}^3$$

Eq. (i) yields... $\qquad \tau_{w-f} = \left(\dfrac{120 \times 10^3}{15.452 \times 10^6 \times 12}\right) \times (87.90 \times 10^3) = 56.88$ MPa

Or
$$\tau_{w-f} = \left(\frac{b_2}{b_1}\right)\tau_f = \left(\frac{120}{12}\right)\times 5.69 = 56.88\,\text{MPa}$$

d. *Shear stress at neutral axis:* Here $b' = b_1 = 12$ mm

$$A\bar{y} = (A\bar{y})_{flange} + (A\bar{y})_{web}$$

$$= A_2\left(c_2 - \frac{h_2}{2}\right) + b_1\frac{(c_2 - h_2)^2}{2}$$

$$= \left[1440\times\left(67.04 - \frac{12}{2}\right)\right] + \left[12\times\frac{(67.04 - 12)^2}{2}\right]$$

$$A\bar{y} = 106.08 \times 10^3\,\text{mm}^3$$

Eq. (i) yields... $\tau_{NA} = \left(\dfrac{120\times 10^3}{15.452\times 10^6 \times 12}\right) \times (106.08\times 10^3)$

$$\tau_{NA} = 68.65\,\text{MPa} = \tau_{max}$$

The shear stress distribution is as shown in **Fig. 7.21(b)**.

b. *Bending stresses:*

Bending stress $\quad \sigma = \dfrac{M}{Z} = \dfrac{Mc}{I} \qquad\qquad\qquad$ ... Eq. (ii)

Tensile stress $\quad \sigma_t = \dfrac{Mc_1}{I} = \dfrac{(20\times 10^6)\times 132.96}{15.452\times 10^6} = 172.10\,\text{MPa}$

Comp. stress $\quad \sigma_c = \dfrac{Mc_2}{I} = \dfrac{(20\times 10^6)\times 67.04}{15.452\times 10^6} = 86.77\,\text{MPa}$

The bending stress distribution is shown in **Fig. 7.21(c)**.

18. **A beam consists of T-section having flange of (125 × 25) mm and web of section (175 × 25) mm. Beam is simply supported, and carries a udl of 30 kN/m over a span of 4 m. Calculate the bending stress and shear stress across the section. Draw the shear stress distribution diagram for bending stress and shear stress at various points on the beam.**

VTU – (CV) June 2012 – 14 Marks

Solution: $w = 30\,\text{kN/m} = 30\,\text{N/mm}$, $L = 4000\,\text{mm}$, $\sigma = ?$, $\tau = ?$.

Based on given data, the beam and its cross section is as shown in **Fig. 7.22(a) & (b)** respectively.

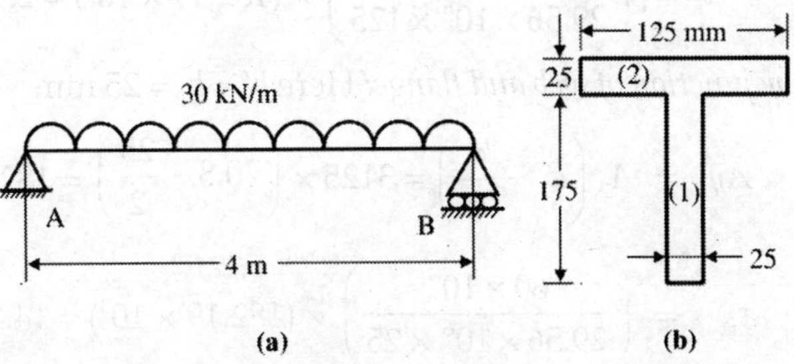

Fig. 7.22: Problem 18

Reactions at supports:

For symmetrical loading $R_A = R_B = \dfrac{30 \times 4}{2} = 60$ kN

Thus the maximum shear force in the beam is $F = 60$ kN $= 60 \times 10^3$ N

Maximum bending moment $M = \dfrac{30 \times 4^2}{8} = 60$ kN-m $= 60 \times 10^6$ N-mm

To find $\bar{y}$:

Element No.	b (mm)	h (mm)	$A = bh$ (mm²)	y (from base) = $(h/2) + x$ (mm)	Ay (mm³)	$I_G = bh^3/12$ (mm⁴)
(1) Web	25	175	4375	$(175/2) = 87.5$	3.83×10^5	11.17×10^6
(2) Flange	125	25	3125	$175 + (25/2) = 187.5$	5.86×10^5	1.63×10^5

x = distance of fiber considered from base

$$\Sigma A = 7500 \text{ mm}^2$$
$$\Sigma Ay = 9.69 \times 10^5 \text{ mm}^3$$

$$\bar{y} = \frac{\Sigma Ay}{\Sigma A} = \frac{9.69 \times 10^5}{7500} = 129.2 \text{ mm}$$

i.e. $\bar{y} = c_1 = 129.2$ mm from base (Tensile)

$c_2 = \Sigma h - c_1 = 200 - 129.2 = 70.8$ mm from top face (Compressive)

a. Shear stresses:

Shear stress $\qquad \tau = \left(\dfrac{F}{Ib'}\right) A\bar{y}$ $\qquad\qquad$ ... Eq. (i)

$$I = I_1 + I_2$$
$$= [I_{G1} + A_1(\bar{y} \sim y_1)^2] + [I_{G2} + A_2(\bar{y} \sim y_2)^2]$$
$$= \{11.17 \times 10^6 + [4375 \times (129.2 - 87.5)^2]\}$$
$$+ \{1.63 \times 10^5 + [3125 \times (129.2 - 187.5)^2]\}$$
$$I = 29.56 \times 10^6 \text{ mm}^4$$

a. *Shear stress at boundaries is zero.*

b. *Shear stress at the bottom of flange:* Here $b' = b_2 = 125$ mm

$$A\bar{y} = A_2\left(c_2 - \frac{h_2}{2}\right) = 3125 \times \left(70.8 - \frac{25}{2}\right) = 182.19 \times 10^3 \text{ mm}^3$$

Eq. (i) yields... $\tau_f = \left(\dfrac{60 \times 10^3}{29.56 \times 10^6 \times 125}\right) \times (182.19 \times 10^3) = 2.96$ MPa

c. *Shear stress at the junction of web and flange:* Here $b' = b_1 = 25$ mm

$$A\bar{y} = A_2\left(c_2 - \frac{h_2}{2}\right) = 3125 \times \left(70.8 - \frac{25}{2}\right) = 182.19 \times 10^3 \text{ mm}^3$$

Eq. (i) yields... $\tau_{w-f} = \left(\dfrac{60 \times 10^3}{29.56 \times 10^6 \times 25}\right) \times (182.19 \times 10^3) = 14.80$ MPa

Or $$\tau_{w-f} = \left(\frac{b_2}{b_1}\right)\tau_f = \left(\frac{125}{25}\right)\times 2.96 = 14.80\ \text{MPa}$$

d. *Shear stress at neutral axis:* Here $b' = b_1 = 25\ \text{mm}$

$$A\overline{y} = \left(A\overline{y}\right)_{flange} + \left(A\overline{y}\right)_{web}$$

$$= A_2\left(c_2 - \frac{h_2}{2}\right) + b_1\frac{\left(c_2 - h_2\right)^2}{2}$$

$$= \left[3125\times\left(70.8 - \frac{25}{2}\right)\right] + \left[25\times\frac{(70.8-25)^2}{2}\right]$$

$$A\overline{y} = 208.41\times 10^3\ \text{mm}^3$$

Eq. (i) yields... $$\tau_{NA} = \left(\frac{60\times 10^3}{29.56\times 10^6\times 25}\right)\times(208.41\times 10^3)$$

$$\tau_{NA} = 16.92\ \text{MPa} = \tau_{max}$$

The shear stress distribution is as shown in **Fig. 7.23(b)**.

b. *Bending stresses:*

Bending stress $$\sigma = \frac{M}{Z} = \frac{Mc}{I} \qquad\qquad \text{... Eq. (ii)}$$

Tensile stress $$\sigma_t = \frac{Mc_1}{I} = \frac{(60\times 10^6)\times 129.2}{29.56\times 10^6} = 262.25\ \text{MPa}$$

Comp. stress $$\sigma_c = \frac{Mc_2}{I} = \frac{(60\times 10^6)\times 70.8}{29.56\times 10^6} = 143.71\ \text{MPa}$$

The bending stress distribution is shown in **Fig. 7.23(c)**.

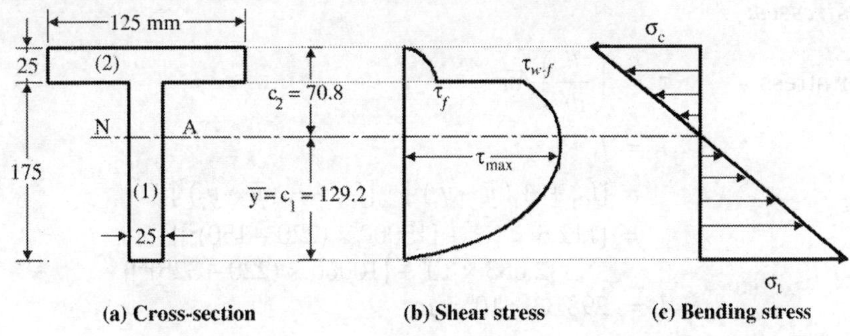

Fig. 7.23: Stress distribution diagrams (Problem 18)

19. **A simply supported beam of span 6m has a cross section as shown in Fig. 7.24(a) and carries two point loads each of 30 kN at a distance of 2 m form each support. Calculate the bending stress and shear stress for maximum values of bending moment and shear force respectively. Draw neat diagram of bending stress and shear stress distribution across the section.**

VTU – Civil: June/ July 2016 – 14 Marks, Dec. 2011 – 12 Marks

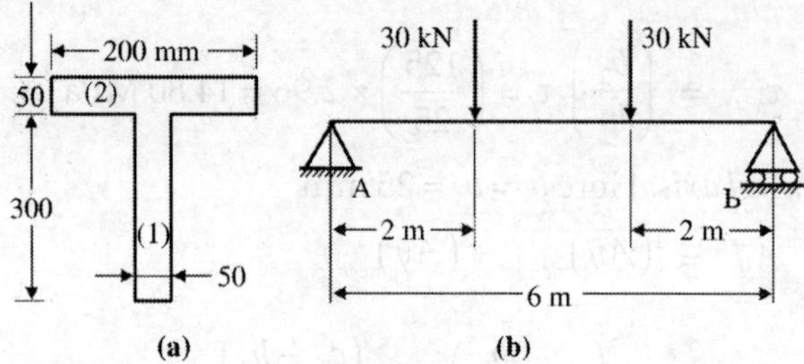

Fig. 7.24: Problem 19

Solution: $W = 30$ kN, $L = 6000$ mm, $\sigma = ?$, $\tau = ?$.

Based on given data, the beam is as shown in **Fig. 7.24(b)**.

Reactions at supports:

For symmetrical loading $R_A = R_B = 30$ kN

Thus the maximum shear force in the beam is $F = 30$ kN $= 30 \times 10^3$ N

Maximum bending moment $M = (30 \times 3) - (30 \times 1) = 60$ kN-m $= 60 \times 10^6$ N-mm

To find $\bar{y}$:

Element No.	b (mm)	h (mm)	$A = bh$ (mm^2)	y (from base) = $(h/2) + x$ (mm)	Ay (mm^3)	$I_G = bh^3/12$ (mm^4)
(1) Web	50	300	15000	$(300/2) = 150$	2.25×10^6	112.5×10^6
(2) Flange	200	50	10000	$300 + (50/2) = 325$	3.25×10^6	2.083×10^6

x = distance of fiber considered from base

$$\Sigma A = 2500 \text{ mm}^2$$
$$\Sigma Ay = 5.5 \times 10^6 \text{ mm}^3$$

$$\bar{y} = \frac{\Sigma Ay}{\Sigma A} = \frac{5.50 \times 10^6}{25000} = 220 \text{ mm}$$

i.e. $\quad \bar{y} = c_1 = 220$ mm from base (Tensile)

$\quad c_2 = \Sigma h - c_1 = 350 - 220 = 130$ mm from top face (Compressive)

a. Shear stresses:

Shear stress $\quad \tau = \left(\dfrac{F}{Ib'}\right) A\bar{y}$ $\qquad$ ... Eq. (i)

$$I = I_1 + I_2$$
$$= [I_{G1} + A_1(\bar{y} \sim y_1)^2] + [I_{G2} + A_2(\bar{y} \sim y_2)^2]$$
$$= \{112.5 \times 10^6 + [15000 \times (220 - 150)^2]\}$$
$$\quad + \{2.083 \times 10^6 + [10000 \times (220 - 325)^2]\}$$
$$I = 298.33 \times 10^6 \text{ mm}^4$$

a. *Shear stress at boundaries is zero.*

b. *Shear stress at the bottom of flange:* Here $b' = b_2 = 200$ mm

$$A\bar{y} = A_2\left(c_2 - \frac{h_2}{2}\right) = 10000 \times \left(130 - \frac{50}{2}\right) = 1.05 \times 10^6 \text{ mm}^3$$

Eq. (i) yields... $\quad \tau_f = \left(\dfrac{30 \times 10^3}{298.33 \times 10^6 \times 200}\right) \times (1.05 \times 10^6) = 0.53$ MPa

c. *Shear stress at the junction of web and flange:* Here $b' = b_1 = 50$ mm

$$A\bar{y} = A_2\left(c_2 - \frac{h_2}{2}\right) = 10000 \times \left(130 - \frac{50}{2}\right) = 1.05 \times 10^6 \text{ mm}^3$$

Eq. (i) yields...
$$\tau_{w-f} = \left(\frac{30 \times 10^3}{298.33 \times 10^6 \times 200}\right) \times (1.05 \times 10^6) = 2.11 \text{ MPa}$$

Or
$$\tau_{w-f} = \left(\frac{b_2}{b_1}\right)\tau_f = \left(\frac{200}{50}\right) \times 0.53 = 2.11 \text{ MPa}$$

d. *Shear stress at neutral axis:* Here $b' = b_1 = 50$ mm

$$A\bar{y} = \left(A\bar{y}\right)_{flange} + \left(A\bar{y}\right)_{web}$$

$$= A_2\left(c_2 - \frac{h_2}{2}\right) + b_1\frac{\left(c_2 - h_2\right)^2}{2}$$

$$= \left[10000 \times \left(130 - \frac{50}{2}\right)\right] + \left[50 \times \frac{(130-50)^2}{2}\right]$$

$$A\bar{y} = 1.21 \times 10^6 \text{ mm}^3$$

Eq. (i) yields...
$$\tau_{NA} = \left(\frac{30 \times 10^3}{298.33 \times 10^6 \times 50}\right) \times (1.21 \times 10^6)$$

$$\tau_{NA} = 16.92 \text{ MPa} = \tau_{max}$$

The shear stress distribution is as shown in **Fig. 7.25(b)**.

b. *Bending stresses:*

Bending stress
$$\sigma = \frac{M}{Z} = \frac{Mc}{I} \qquad\qquad \text{... Eq. (ii)}$$

Tensile stress
$$\sigma_t = \frac{Mc_1}{I} = \frac{(60 \times 10^6) \times 220}{298.33 \times 10^6} = 44.25 \text{ MPa}$$

Comp. stress
$$\sigma_c = \frac{Mc_2}{I} = \frac{(60 \times 10^6) \times 130}{298.33 \times 10^6} = 26.15 \text{ MPa}$$

The bending stress distribution is shown in **Fig. 7.25(c)**.

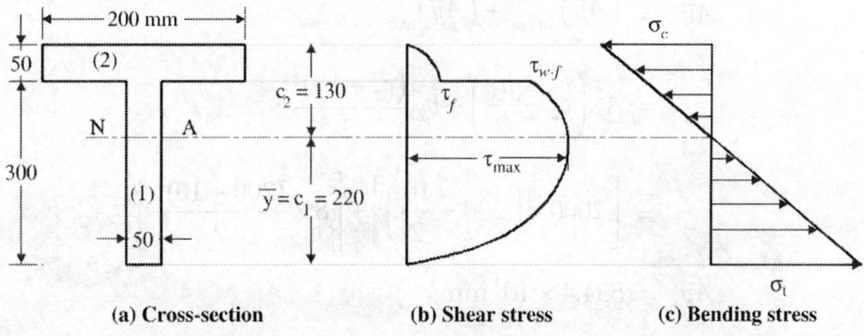

Fig. 7.25: Stress distribution diagrams (Problem 19)

PROBLEMS ON I SECTION

20. An I section has the following dimensions. Flanges 200 mm × 10 mm; web 380 mm × 8 mm. The maximum shear stress developed in the beam is 20 N/mm². Find the force to which the beam is subjected to?

VTU – Dec. 14/ Jan. 15 – 10 Marks

Solution: $\tau_{max} = 20 \text{ N/mm}^2$, $W = ?$

Based on given data, the cross section is as shown in **Fig. 7.26**.

To find $\bar{y}$:

Element No.	b (mm)	h (mm)	$A = bh$ (mm²)	y (from base) = $(h/2) + x$ (mm)	Ay (mm³)	$I_G = bh^3/12$ (mm⁴)
(1) Bottom flange	200	10	2000	$(10/2) = 5$	10×10^3	16.67×10^3
(2) Web	8	380	3040	$10 + (380/2) = 200$	608×10^3	36.58×10^6
(3) Top flange	200	10	2000	$10 + 380 + (10/2) = 395$	790×10^3	16.67×10^3

x = distance of fiber considered from base

$$\Sigma A = 7040 \text{ mm}^2$$
$$\Sigma Ay = 1408 \times 10^3 \text{ mm}^3$$

$$\bar{y} = \frac{\Sigma Ay}{\Sigma A} = \frac{1408 \times 10^3}{7040} = 200 \text{ mm}$$

i.e. $\quad \bar{y} = c_1 = 200 \text{ mm from base (Tensile)}$

$$c_2 = \Sigma h - c_1 = 400 - 200 = 200 \text{ mm}$$
$$\text{from top face (Compressive)}$$

Note: Since the I-section has equal flanges, $c_1 = c_2 = 200 \text{ mm}$

Shear stress $\quad \tau = \left(\dfrac{F}{Ib'}\right) A\bar{y} \qquad$ ... Eq. (i)

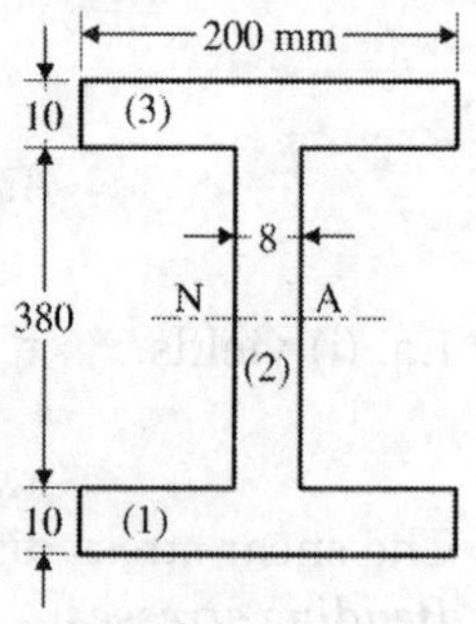

Fig. 7.26: Problem 20

But $\quad I = \dfrac{(BH^3 - bh^3)}{12}$, for symmetrical I section

$$= \frac{(200 \times 400^3 - 192 \times 380^3)}{12}$$

$$I = 188.71 \times 10^6 \text{ mm}^4$$

Since maximum shear stress occurs at neutral axis: Here $b' = b_2 = 8 \text{ mm}$

$$A\bar{y} = \left(A\bar{y}\right)_{flange} + \left(A\bar{y}\right)_{web}$$

$$= A_3 \left(c_2 - \frac{h_3}{2}\right) + b_2 \frac{(c_2 - h_3)^2}{2}$$

$$= \left[2000 \times \left(200 - \frac{10}{2}\right)\right] + \left[8 \times \frac{(200 - 10)^2}{2}\right]$$

$$A\bar{y} = 534.4 \times 10^3 \text{ mm}^3$$

Eq. (i) yields... $20 = \left(\dfrac{F}{188.71 \times 10^6 \times 8}\right) \times (534.4 \times 10^3)$

$$F = 56500 \text{ N} = 56.5 \text{ kN} = W$$

21. A rolled I-section of size 50 mm × 75 mm is used as a beam, with an effective span of 3m. The flanges are 5 mm thick and the web is 3.75 mm thick. Calculate the uniformly distributed load the beam can carry if the maximum intensity of shear stress induced is limited to 40 N/mm².

VTU – June/ July 2013 – 08 Marks

Solution: $\tau_{max} = 40 \text{ N/mm}^2$, $w = ?$, $L = 3000$ mm
Based on given data, the cross section is as shown in **Fig. 7.27**.

To find $\bar{y}$:

Element No.	b (mm)	h (mm)	$A = bh$ (mm²)	y (from base) = $(h/2) + x$ (mm)	Ay (mm³)	$I_G = bh^3/12$ (mm⁴)
(1) Bottom flange	50	5	250	$(5/2) = 2.5$	625	520.83
(2) Web	3.75	65	243.75	$5 + (65/2) = 37.5$	9140.63	85.82×10^3
(3) Top flange	50	5	250	$5 + 65 + (5/2) = 72.5$	18125	520.83

x = distance of fiber considered from base

$$\Sigma A = 743.75 \text{ mm}^2$$
$$\Sigma Ay = 27890.63 \text{ mm}^3$$

$$\bar{y} = \frac{\Sigma Ay}{\Sigma A} = \frac{27890.63}{743.75} = 37.5 \text{ mm}$$

i.e. $\bar{y} = c_1 = 37.5$ mm from base (Tensile)

$c_2 = \Sigma h - c_1 = 75 - 37.5 = 37.5$ mm
from top face (Compressive)

Note: Since the I-section has equal flanges, $c_1 = c_2 = 37.5$ mm

Shear stress $\tau = \left(\dfrac{F}{Ib'}\right) A\bar{y}$ ... Eq. (i)

Fig. 7.27: Problem 21

But $I = \dfrac{(BH^3 - bh^3)}{12}$, for symmetrical I section

$$= \frac{(50 \times 75^3 - 46.25 \times 65^3)}{12}$$

$$I = 699.96 \times 10^3 \text{ mm}^4$$

Since maximum shear stress occurs at neutral axis: Here $b' = b_2 = 3.75$ mm

$$A\bar{y} = \left(A\bar{y}\right)_{flange} + \left(A\bar{y}\right)_{web}$$

$$= A_3\left(c_2 - \frac{h_3}{2}\right) + b_2 \frac{(c_2 - h_3)^2}{2}$$

$$= \left[250 \times \left(37.5 - \frac{5}{2}\right)\right] + \left[3.75 \times \frac{(37.5 - 5)^2}{2}\right]$$

$$A\bar{y} = 10.73 \times 10^3 \text{ mm}^3$$

Eq. (i) yields... $40 = \left(\dfrac{F}{699.36 \times 10^3 \times 3.75}\right) \times (10.73 \times 10^3)$

$$F = 9776.73 \text{ N}$$

For a simply supported beam with UDL over entire span

$$F = \frac{wL}{2}$$

$$9776.73 = \frac{w \times 3}{2}$$

$$w = 6517.82 \text{ N/m}$$

22. Draw shear stress distribution for an I-shaped section of a beam as shown in Fig. 7.28(a). The shear force on this section is 200 kN.

VTU – June 2012 – 16 Marks; [Similar: June/ July 15 – 10 Marks]

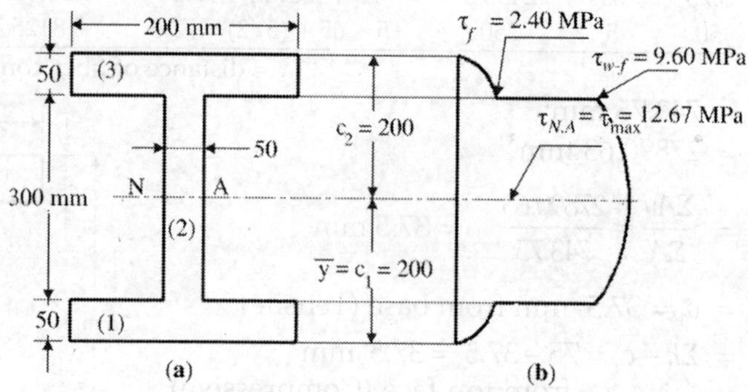

Fig. 7.28: Problem 22

Solution: $F = 200 \times 10^3$ N, $\tau = ?$

To find $\bar{y}$:

Element No.	b (mm)	h (mm)	$A = bh$ (mm²)	y (from base) = $(h/2) + x$ (mm)	Ay (mm³)	$I_G = bh^3/12$ (mm⁴)
(1) Bottom flange	200	50	10000	$(50/2) = 25$	250×10^3	2.08×10^6
(2) Web	50	300	15000	$50 + (300/2) = 200$	3×10^6	112.5×10^6
(3) Top flange	200	50	10000	$50 + 300 + (50/2) = 375$	3.75×10^6	2.08×10^6

x = distance of fiber considered from base

$$\Sigma A = 35 \times 10^3 \text{ mm}^2$$

$$\Sigma Ay = 7 \times 10^6 \text{ mm}^3$$

$$\bar{y} = \frac{\Sigma Ay}{\Sigma A} = \frac{7 \times 10^6}{35 \times 10^3} = 200 \text{ mm}$$

i.e. $\bar{y} = c_1 = 200$ mm from base (Tensile)

$c_2 = \Sigma h - c_1 = 400 - 200 = 200$ mm from top face (Compressive)

Note: Since the I-section has equal flanges, $c_1 = c_2 = 200$ mm

Shear stress $\tau = \left(\dfrac{F}{Ib'}\right) A\bar{y}$ ... Eq. (i)

But $\qquad I = \dfrac{(BH^3 - bh^3)}{12}$, for symmetrical I section

$$= \dfrac{(200 \times 400^3 - 150 \times 300^3)}{12}$$

$$I = 729.17 \times 10^6 \text{ mm}^4$$

Shear stress $\qquad \tau = \left(\dfrac{F}{Ib'}\right) A\bar{y}$ $\qquad\qquad$ ... Eq. (i)

a. *Shear stress at boundaries is zero.*

b. *Shear stress at the bottom of top flange:* Here $b' = b_3 = 200$ mm

$$A\bar{y} = A_3 \left(c_2 - \dfrac{h_3}{2}\right) = 10000 \times \left(200 - \dfrac{50}{2}\right) = 1.75 \times 10^6 \text{ mm}^3$$

Eq. (i) yields... $\qquad \tau_f = \left(\dfrac{200 \times 10^3}{729.17 \times 10^6 \times 200}\right) \times (1.75 \times 10^6) = 2.40 \text{ MPa}$

c. *Shear stress at the junction of web and top flange:* Here $b' = b_2 = 50$ mm

$$A\bar{y} = A_3 \left(c_2 - \dfrac{h_3}{2}\right) = 10000 \times \left(200 - \dfrac{50}{2}\right) = 1.75 \times 10^6 \text{ mm}^3$$

Eq. (i) yields... $\qquad \tau_{w-f} = \left(\dfrac{200 \times 10^3}{729.17 \times 10^6 \times 50}\right) \times (1.75 \times 10^6) = 9.60 \text{ MPa}$

Or $\qquad \tau_{w-f} = \left(\dfrac{b_3}{b_2}\right) \tau_f = \left(\dfrac{200}{50}\right) \times 2.40 = 9.60 \text{ MPa}$

d. *Shear stress at neutral axis:* Here $b' = b_2 = 50$ mm

$$A\bar{y} = \left(A\bar{y}\right)_{flange} + \left(A\bar{y}\right)_{web}$$

$$= A_3 \left(c_2 - \dfrac{h_3}{2}\right) + b_2 \dfrac{(c_2 - h_3)^2}{2}$$

$$= \left[10000 \times \left(200 - \dfrac{50}{2}\right)\right] + \left[50 \times \dfrac{(200 - 50)^2}{2}\right]$$

$$A\bar{y} = 2.31 \times 10^6 \text{ mm}^3$$

Eq. (i) yields... $\qquad \tau_{NA} = \left(\dfrac{200 \times 10^3}{729.17 \times 10^6 \times 50}\right) \times (2.31 \times 10^6)$

$$\tau_{NA} = 12.67 \text{ MPa} = \tau_{max}$$

The shear stress distribution is as shown in **Fig. 7.28(b)**.

23. **An I-section beam 350 mm × 150 mm has a web thickness of 10 mm and a flange thickness of 20 mm. If the shear force acting on the beam is 40 kN, find the maximum shear stress developed in the I-section.**

VTU – June/ July 2017 – 08 Marks

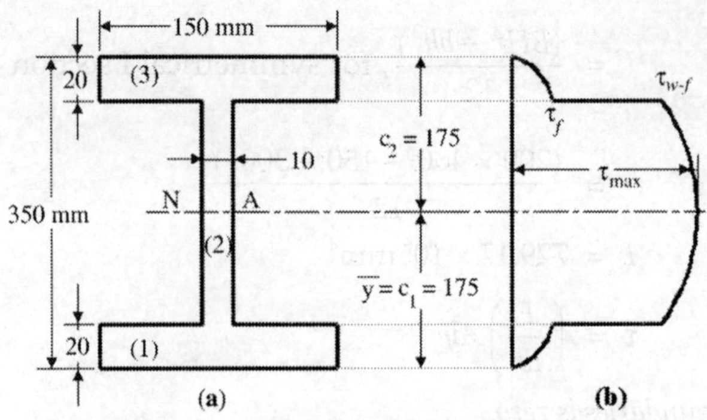

Fig. 7.29: Problem 23

Solution: $F = 40 \times 10^3$ N, $\tau = ?$

Based on given data, the cross section is as shown in **Fig. 7.29(a)**.

To find $\bar{y}$:

Element No.	b (mm)	h (mm)	$A = bh$ (mm^2)	y (from base) = $(h/2) + x$ (mm)	Ay (mm^3)	$I_G = bh^3/12$ (mm^4)
(1) Bottom flange	150	20	3000	$(20/2) = 10$	30×10^3	1×10^5
(2) Web	10	310	3100	$20 + (310/2) = 175$	542.5×10^3	24.82×10^6
(3) Top flange	150	20	3000	$20 + 310 + (20/2) = 340$	1.02×10^6	1×10^5

x = distance of fiber considered from base

$$\Sigma A = 9100 \text{ mm}^2$$
$$\Sigma Ay = 1592500 \text{ mm}^3$$

$$\bar{y} = \frac{\Sigma Ay}{\Sigma A} = \frac{1592500}{9100} = 175 \text{ mm}$$

i.e. $\quad \bar{y} = c_1 = 175$ mm from base (Tensile)

$\quad\quad c_2 = \Sigma h - c_1 = 350 - 175 = 175$ mm from top face (Compressive)

Note: Since the I-section has equal flanges, $c_1 = c_2 = 175$ mm

Shear stress $\quad \tau = \left(\dfrac{F}{Ib'}\right) A\bar{y}$ $\quad\quad\quad\quad$ ... Eq. (i)

But $\quad I = \dfrac{(BH^3 - bh^3)}{12}$, for symmetrical I section

$$= \frac{(150 \times 350^3 - 140 \times 310^3)}{12}$$

$$I = 188.38 \times 10^6 \text{ mm}^4$$

Shear stress $\quad \tau = \left(\dfrac{F}{Ib'}\right) A\bar{y}$ $\quad\quad\quad\quad$ ... Eq. (i)

a. *Shear stress at boundaries is zero.*

b. *Shear stress at the bottom of top flange:* Here $b' = b_3 = 150$ mm

$$A\bar{y} = A_3 \left(c_2 - \frac{h_3}{2}\right) = 3000 \times \left(175 - \frac{20}{2}\right) = 495 \times 10^3 \text{ mm}^3$$

Eq. (i) yields... $\quad \tau_f = \left(\dfrac{40 \times 10^3}{188.38 \times 10^6 \times 150} \right) \times (495 \times 10^3) = 0.70 \text{ MPa}$

c. *Shear stress at the junction of web and top flange:* Here $b' = b_2 = 10$ mm

$$A\overline{y} = A_3 \left(c_2 - \frac{h_3}{2} \right) = 3000 \times \left(175 - \frac{20}{2} \right) = 495 \times 10^3 \text{ mm}^3$$

Eq. (i) yields... $\quad \tau_{w-f} = \left(\dfrac{40 \times 10^3}{188.38 \times 10^6 \times 10} \right) \times (495 \times 10^3) = 10.51 \text{ MPa}$

Or $\quad\quad \tau_{w-f} = \left(\dfrac{b_3}{b_2} \right) \tau_f = \left(\dfrac{150}{10} \right) \times 0.70 = 10.5 \text{ MPa}$

d. *Shear stress at neutral axis:* Here $b' = b_2 = 10$ mm

$$A\overline{y} = \left(A\overline{y} \right)_{flange} + \left(A\overline{y} \right)_{web}$$

$$= A_3 \left(c_2 - \frac{h_3}{2} \right) + b_2 \frac{(c_2 - h_3)^2}{2}$$

$$= \left[3000 \times \left(175 - \frac{20}{2} \right) \right] + \left[10 \times \frac{(175 - 20)^2}{2} \right]$$

$$A\overline{y} = 615125 \text{ mm}^3$$

Eq. (i) yields... $\quad \tau_{NA} = \left(\dfrac{40 \times 10^3}{188.38 \times 10^6 \times 10} \right) \times (615125)$

$$\tau_{NA} = 13.06 \text{ MPa} = \tau_{max}$$

The shear stress distribution is as shown in **Fig. 7.29(b)**

24. **The cross-section of a beam is shown in Fig. 7.30(a). The shear force on the section is 410 kN. Estimate the shear stresses at various points and plot the shear distribution diagram.**

VTU – June/ July 2015 – 14 Marks

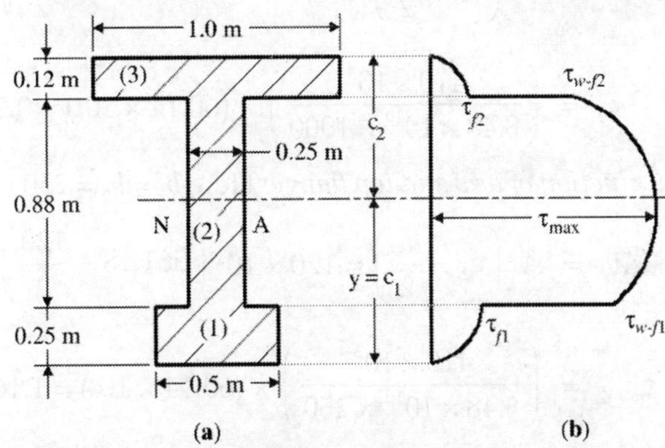

Fig. 7.30: Problem 24

Solution: $F = 410 \times 10^3$ N, $\tau = ?$

Based on given data, the cross section is as shown in **Fig. 7.29(a)**.

To find $\bar{y}$:

Element No.	b (mm)	h (mm)	$A = bh$ (mm^2)	y (from base) = $(h/2) + x$ (mm)	Ay (mm^3)	$I_G = bh^3/12$ (mm^4)
(1) Bottom flange	500	250	125×10^3	$(250/2) = 125$	0.16×10^8	6.51×10^8
(2) Web	250	880	220×10^3	$250 + (880/2) = 690$	1.52×10^8	142×10^8
(3) Top flange	1000	120	120×10^3	$250 + 880 + (120/2) = 1190$	1.43×10^8	1.44×10^8

x = distance of fiber considered from base

$$\Sigma A = 465 \times 10^3 \text{ mm}^2$$
$$\Sigma Ay = 3.11 \times 10^8 \text{ mm}^3$$

$$\bar{y} = \frac{\Sigma Ay}{\Sigma A} = \frac{3.11 \times 10^8}{465 \times 10^3} = 688.82 \text{ mm}$$

i.e. $\bar{y} = c_1 = 688.82$ mm from base (Tensile)

$c_2 = \Sigma h - c_1 = 1250 - 688.82 = 561.18$ mm from top face (Compressive)

Note: Since the I-section has unequal flanges, $c_1 \neq c_2$

Shear stress $\qquad \tau = \left(\dfrac{F}{Ib'}\right) A\bar{y}$ $\qquad\qquad$ ... Eq. (i)

$$I = I_1 + I_2 + I_3$$
$$= [I_{G1} + A_1(\bar{y} \sim y_1)^2] + [I_{G2} + A_2(\bar{y} \sim y_2)^2] + [I_{G3} + A_3(\bar{y} \sim y_3)^3]$$
$$= \{6.51 \times 10^8 + [125 \times 10^3 \times (688.82 - 125)^2]\}$$
$$+ \{142 \times 10^8 + [220 \times 10^3 \times (688.82 - 690)^2]\}$$
$$+ \{1.44 \times 10^8 + [120 \times 10^3 \times (688.82 - 1190)^2]\}$$
$$I = 8.48 \times 10^{10} \text{ mm}^4$$

Shear stress $\qquad \tau = \left(\dfrac{F}{Ib'}\right) A\bar{y}$ $\qquad\qquad$ ... Eq. (i)

a. *Shear stress at boundaries is zero.*

b. *Shear stress at the bottom of top flange:* Here $b' = b_3 = 1000$ mm

$$A\bar{y} = A_3\left(c_2 - \frac{h_3}{2}\right) = 120 \times 10^3 \left(561.18 - \frac{120}{2}\right) = 60.14 \times 10^6 \text{ mm}^3$$

Eq. (i) yields... $\quad \tau_{f2} = \left(\dfrac{410 \times 10^3}{8.48 \times 10^{10} \times 1000}\right) \times (60.14 \times 10^6) = 0.29$ MPa

c. *Shear stress at the junction of web and top flange:* Here $b' = b_2 = 250$ mm

$$A\bar{y} = A_3\left(c_2 - \frac{h_3}{2}\right) = 120 \times 10^3 \left(561.18 - \frac{120}{2}\right) = 60.14 \times 10^6 \text{ mm}^3$$

Eq. (i) yields... $\quad \tau_{w-f)2} = \left(\dfrac{410 \times 10^3}{8.48 \times 10^{10} \times 250}\right) \times (60.14 \times 10^6) = 1.16$ MPa

Or $\qquad \tau_{w-f)2} = \left(\dfrac{b_3}{b_2}\right)\tau_f = \left(\dfrac{1000}{250}\right) \times 0.29 = 1.16\,\text{MPa}$

d. *Shear stress at neutral axis:* Here $b' = b_2 = 250$ mm

$$A\overline{y} = \left(A\overline{y}\right)_{flange} + \left(A\overline{y}\right)_{web}$$

$$= A_3\left(c_2 - \dfrac{h_3}{2}\right) + b_2\dfrac{\left(c_2 - h_3\right)^2}{2}$$

$$= \left[120 \times 10^3 \times \left(561.18 - \dfrac{120}{2}\right)\right] + \left[250 \times \dfrac{(561.18 - 120)^2}{2}\right]$$

$$A\overline{y} = 84.47 \times 10^6\,\text{mm}^3$$

Eq. (i) yields... $\quad \tau_{NA} = \left(\dfrac{410 \times 10^3}{8.48 \times 10^{10} \times 250}\right) \times (84.47 \times 10^6)$

$$\tau_{NA} = 1.63\,\text{MPa} = \tau_{max}$$

e. *Shear stress at the top of bottom flange:* Here $b' = b_1 = 500$ mm

$$A\overline{y} = A_1\left(c_1 - \dfrac{h_1}{2}\right) = 125 \times 10^3\left(688.82 - \dfrac{250}{2}\right) = 70.48 \times 10^6\,\text{mm}^3$$

Eq. (i) yields... $\quad \tau_{f1} = \left(\dfrac{410 \times 10^3}{8.48 \times 10^{10} \times 500}\right) \times (70.48 \times 10^6) = 0.68\,\text{MPa}$

f. *Shear stress at the junction of web and bottom flange:* Here $b' = b_2 = 250$ mm

$$A\overline{y} = A_1\left(c_1 - \dfrac{h_1}{2}\right) = 125 \times 10^3\left(688.82 - \dfrac{250}{2}\right) = 70.48 \times 10^6\,\text{mm}^3$$

Eq. (i) yields... $\quad \tau_{w-f)1} = \left(\dfrac{410 \times 10^3}{8.48 \times 10^{10} \times 250}\right) \times (70.48 \times 10^6) = 1.36\,\text{MPa}$

Or $\qquad \tau_{w-f)1} = \left(\dfrac{b_1}{b_2}\right)\tau_f = \left(\dfrac{500}{250}\right) \times 0.68 = 1.36\,\text{MPa}$

The shear stress distribution is as shown in **Fig. 7.30(b)**.

25. **A beam with I-section as shown in Fig. 7.31(a), is subjected to a bending moment of 120 kN-m and a shear force of 60 kN. Sketch the bending stress and shear stress diagram.**

VTU – June/ July 15 – 10 Marks;
[Civil: June/ July 2014 – 16 Marks,
Dec. 2012 – 10 Marks, Dec. 09/ Jan. 10 – 15 Marks]

Solution: $F = 60 \times 10^3$ N, $M = 120 \times 10^6$ N-mm $\tau = ?$, $\sigma = ?$

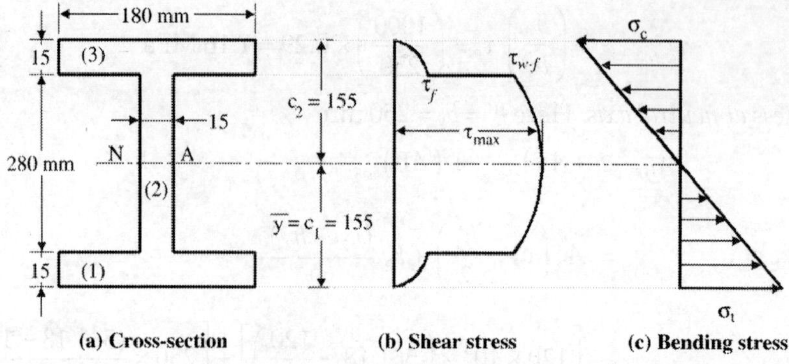

(a) Cross-section   **(b) Shear stress**   **(c) Bending stress**

Fig. 7.31: Problem 25

To find $\bar{y}$:

Element No.	b (mm)	h (mm)	$A = bh$ (mm²)	y (from base) = $(h/2) + x$ (mm)	Ay (mm³)	$I_G = bh^3/12$ (mm⁴)
(1) Bottom flange	180	15	2700	$(15/2) = 7.5$	20.25×10^3	50625
(2) Web	15	280	4200	$15 + (280/2) = 155$	651×10^3	27.44×10^6
(3) Top flange	180	15	2700	$15 + 280 + (15/2) = 302.5$	816.75×10^3	50625

x = distance of fiber considered from base

$$\Sigma A = 9600 \text{ mm}^2$$
$$\Sigma Ay = 1.488 \times 10^6 \text{ mm}^3$$

$$\bar{y} = \frac{\Sigma Ay}{\Sigma A} = \frac{1.488 \times 10^6}{9600} = 155 \text{ mm}$$

i.e. $\bar{y} = c_1 = 155$ mm from base (Tensile)

$$c_2 = \Sigma h - c_1 = 310 - 155 = 155 \text{ mm from top face (Compressive)}$$

Note: Since the I-section has equal flanges, $c_1 = c_2 = 155$ mm

Shear stress $\tau = \left(\dfrac{F}{Ib'}\right) A\bar{y}$ ... Eq. (i)

But $I = \dfrac{(BH^3 - bh^3)}{12}$, for symmetrical I-section

$$= \frac{(180 \times 310^3 - 165 \times 280^3)}{12}$$

$$I = 145.03 \times 10^6 \text{ mm}^4$$

a. *Shear stresses:*

Shear stress $\tau = \left(\dfrac{F}{Ib'}\right) A\bar{y}$ ... Eq. (i)

a. *Shear stress at boundaries is zero.*

b. *Shear stress at the bottom of top flange:* Here $b' = b_3 = 180$ mm

$$A\bar{y} = A_3 \left(c_2 - \frac{h_3}{2}\right) = 2700 \times \left(155 - \frac{15}{2}\right) = 398.25 \times 10^3 \text{ mm}^3$$

Eq. (i) yields... $\tau_f = \left(\dfrac{60 \times 10^3}{145.03 \times 10^6 \times 180}\right) \times (398.25 \times 10^3) = 0.915 \text{ MPa}$

c. *Shear stress at the junction of web and top flange:* Here $b' = b_2 = 15$ mm

$$A\overline{y} = A_3\left(c_2 - \frac{h_3}{2}\right) = 2700 \times \left(155 - \frac{15}{2}\right) = 398.25 \times 10^3 \text{ mm}^3$$

Eq. (i) yields... $\tau_{w-f} = \left(\dfrac{60 \times 10^3}{145.03 \times 10^6 \times 15}\right) \times (398.25 \times 10^3) = 10.98 \text{ MPa}$

Or $\tau_{w-f} = \left(\dfrac{b_3}{b_2}\right)\tau_f = \left(\dfrac{180}{15}\right) \times 0.915 = 10.98 \text{ MPa}$

d. *Shear stress at neutral axis:* Here $b' = b_2 = 15$ mm

$$A\overline{y} = \left(A\overline{y}\right)_{flange} + \left(A\overline{y}\right)_{web}$$

$$= A_3\left(c_2 - \frac{h_3}{2}\right) + b_2\frac{\left(c_2 - h_3\right)^2}{2}$$

$$= \left[2700 \times \left(155 - \frac{15}{2}\right)\right] + \left[15 \times \frac{(155 - 15)^2}{2}\right]$$

$$A\overline{y} = 545.25 \times 10^3 \text{ mm}^3$$

Eq. (i) yields... $\tau_{NA} = \left(\dfrac{60 \times 10^3}{145.03 \times 10^6 \times 15}\right) \times (545.25 \times 10^3)$

$$\tau_{NA} = 15.04 \text{ MPa} = \tau_{max}$$

The shear stress distribution is as shown in **Fig. 7.31(b)**.

b. *Bending stresses:*

Bending stress $\sigma = \dfrac{M}{Z} = \dfrac{Mc}{I}$ ... Eq. (ii)

Tensile stress $\sigma_t = \dfrac{Mc_1}{I} = \dfrac{(120 \times 10^6) \times 155}{145.03 \times 10^6} = 128.25 \text{ MPa}$

Comp. stress $\sigma_c = \dfrac{Mc_2}{I} = \dfrac{(120 \times 10^6) \times 155}{145.03 \times 10^6} = 128.25 \text{ MPa}$

The bending stress distribution is shown in **Fig. 7.31(c)**.

26. **A beam with an I- section consists of 200 mm × 20 mm flanges and a web of 300 mm depth, 20 mm thickness. It is subjected to bending moment of 100 kN-m and a shear force of 50 kN. Sketch the bending moment and shear force distribution along the depth of the section.**

VTU – (CV) June/ July 2013 – 10 Marks; [similar: May/ June 2010 – 08 Marks]

Solution: $F = 50 \times 10^3$ N, $M = 100 \times 10^6$ N-mm $\tau = ?$, $\sigma = ?$

Based on given data, the cross section is as shown in **Fig. 7.32(a)**.

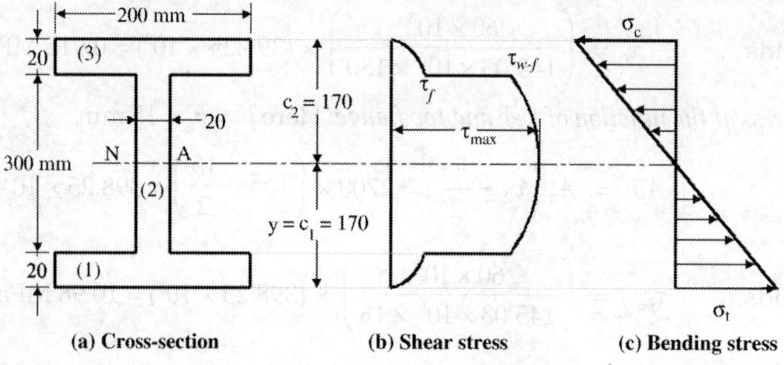

(a) Cross-section   **(b) Shear stress**   **(c) Bending stress**

Fig. 7.32: Problem 26

To find $\bar{y}$:

Element No.	b (mm)	h (mm)	A = bh (mm²)	y (from base) = (h/2) + x (mm)	Ay (mm³)	$I_G = bh^3/12$ (mm⁴)
(1) Bottom flange	200	20	4000	(20/2) = 10	40 × 10³	133.33 × 10³
(2) Web	20	300	6000	20 + (300/2) = 170	1.02 × 10⁶	45 × 10⁶
(3) Top flange	200	20	4000	20 + 300 + (20/2) = 330	1.32 × 10⁶	133.33 × 10³

x = distance of fiber considered from base

$$\Sigma A = 14000 \text{ mm}^2$$
$$\Sigma Ay = 2.38 \times 10^6 \text{ mm}^3$$

$$\bar{y} = \frac{\Sigma Ay}{\Sigma A} = \frac{2.38 \times 10^6}{14000} = 170 \text{ mm}$$

i.e. $\bar{y} = c_1 = 170$ mm from base (Tensile)

$c_2 = \Sigma h - c_1 = 340 - 170 = 170$ mm from top face (Compressive)

Note: Since I-section has equal flanges, $c_1 = c_2 = 170$ mm

Shear stress $\tau = \left(\dfrac{F}{Ib'}\right) A\bar{y}$ ... Eq. (i)

But $I = \dfrac{(BH^3 - bh^3)}{12}$, for symmetrical I section

$$= \frac{(200 \times 340^3 - 180 \times 300^3)}{12}$$

$$I = 250.06 \times 10^6 \text{ mm}^4$$

a. Shear stresses:

Shear stress $\tau = \left(\dfrac{F}{Ib'}\right) A\bar{y}$ ... Eq. (i)

a. Shear stress at boundaries is zero.

b. Shear stress at the bottom of top flange: Here $b' = b_3 = 200$ mm

$$A\bar{y} = A_3 \left(c_2 - \frac{h_3}{2}\right) = 4000 \times \left(170 - \frac{20}{2}\right) = 640 \times 10^3 \text{ mm}^3$$

Eq. (i) yields... $\tau_f = \left(\dfrac{50 \times 10^3}{250.06 \times 10^6 \times 200}\right) \times (640 \times 10^3) = 0.64 \text{ MPa}$

c. *Shear stress at the junction of web and top flange:* Here $b' = b_2 = 20$ mm

$$A\bar{y} = A_3\left(c_2 - \frac{h_3}{2}\right) = 4000 \times \left(170 - \frac{20}{2}\right) = 640 \times 10^3 \text{ mm}^3$$

Eq. (i) yields... $\tau_{w-f} = \left(\dfrac{50 \times 10^3}{250.06 \times 10^6 \times 20}\right) \times (640 \times 10^3) = 6.40$ MPa

Or $\qquad \tau_{w-f} = \left(\dfrac{b_3}{b_2}\right)\tau_f = \left(\dfrac{200}{20}\right) \times 0.64 = 10.98$ MPa

d. *Shear stress at neutral axis:* Here $b' = b_2 = 20$ mm

$$A\bar{y} = \left(A\bar{y}\right)_{flange} + \left(A\bar{y}\right)_{web}$$

$$= A_3\left(c_2 - \frac{h_3}{2}\right) + b_2\frac{\left(c_2 - h_3\right)^2}{2}$$

$$= \left[4000 \times \left(170 - \frac{20}{2}\right)\right] + \left[20 \times \frac{(170 - 20)^2}{2}\right]$$

$$A\bar{y} = 865 \times 10^3 \text{ mm}^3$$

Eq. (i) yields... $\tau_{NA} = \left(\dfrac{50 \times 10^3}{250.06 \times 10^6 \times 20}\right) \times (865 \times 10^3)$

$$\tau_{NA} = 8.65 \text{ MPa} = \tau_{max}$$

The shear stress distribution is as shown in **Fig. 7.32(b)**.

b. *Bending stresses:*

Bending stress $\qquad \sigma = \dfrac{M}{Z} = \dfrac{Mc}{I}$ $\qquad\qquad\qquad\qquad$ ... Eq. (ii)

Tensile stress $\qquad \sigma_t = \dfrac{Mc_1}{I} = \dfrac{(100 \times 10^6) \times 170}{250.06 \times 10^6} = 67.98$ MPa

Comp. stress $\qquad \sigma_c = \dfrac{Mc_2}{I} = \dfrac{(100 \times 10^6) \times 170}{250.06 \times 10^6} = 67.98$ MPa

The bending stress distribution is shown in **Fig. 7.32(c)**.

VTU QUESTION PAPERS

Dec. 07/Jan. 08 (06ME34)

1. Prove that the maximum traverse shear stress is 1.5 times the average shear stress in a beam of rectangular cross section. Plot the shear stress distribution. What assumptions are made? **(06 Marks)**

June/July 2008 (06ME34)

2. Prove that maximum shear stress in a rectangular section of width b and depth d is equal to 1.5 times of its average shear stress. **(06 Marks)**

Dec. 09/Jan. 10 (06ME34)

3. A T-shaped cross section of a beam **Fig. U7.1** is subjected to a vertical shear force of 100 kN. Calculate the shear stress at the neutral axis and at the junction of the web and the flange. M.I about the horizontal neutral axis is 0.0001134 m^4.

(10 Marks)

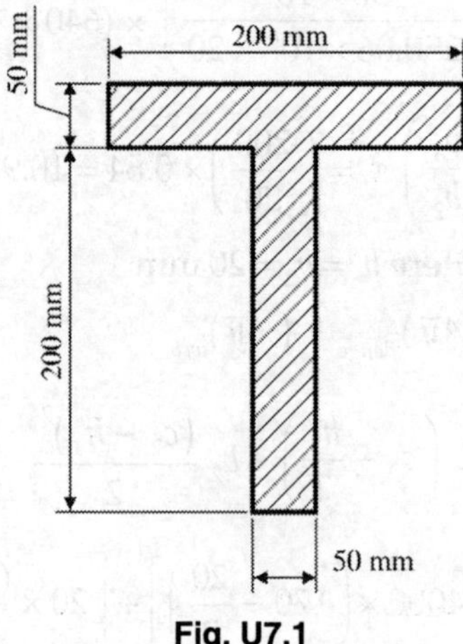

Fig. U7.1

May/June 2010 (06ME34)

4. a. Show that the maximum shear stress for a rectangular section is 1.5 times the average shear stress. **(06 Marks)**

   b. A 'T' section of flange 120 mm × 12 mm and overall depth 200 mm, with web 12 mm thick is loaded such that, at a section it has a moment of 20 kN-m and shear force of 120 kN. Sketch the bending and shear stress distribution diagram, marking the salient values. **(14 Marks)**

Dec. 2010 (06ME34)

5. A cantilever beam of length 1 m has a circular cross section of diameter 300 mm. Determine the concentrated load the can be applied at the free end to produce a maximum shear of 1.5 N/mm^2. **(08 Marks)**

June 2012 (06ME34)

6. Draw shear stress distribution for an I-shaped section of a beam as shown in **Fig. U7.2**. The shear force on this section is 200 kN. **(16 Marks)**

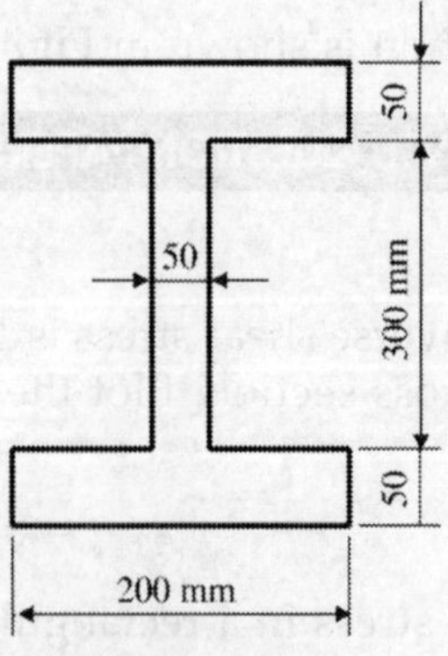

Fig. U7.2

June 2012 (10ME34)

7. Prove that the maximum shear stress in a circular section of a beam is 4/3 times the average shear stress. **(10 Marks)**

JAN. 2013 (06ME34)

8. Prove that the shear stress distribution in a circular section of beam which is subjected to shear force F is given by

$$\tau = \frac{16F}{3\pi d^2}\left(1 - \frac{4y^2}{d^2}\right)$$

where d = diameter of the section,

   y = distance between neutral axis to the section under consideration.
And show that the maximum shear stress is 4/3 times the average shear stress. **(10 Marks)**

June/July 2013 (06ME34)

9. Prove that the maximum shear stress in a rectangular section is 1.5 times the average shear stress. **(05 Marks)**

June/July 2013 (10ME34)

10. A rolled I-section of size 50 mm × 75 mm is used as a beam, with an effective span of 3 m. The flanges are 5 mm thick and the web is 3.75 mm thick. Calculate the uniformly distributed load the beam can carry if the maximum intensity of shear stress induced is limited to 40 N/mm^2. **(08 Marks)**

Dec. 13/Jan. 14 (10ME34)

11. Show that the shear stress across the rectangular section varies parabolically. Also show that the maximum shear stress is 1.5 times the average shear stress. Sketch the stress variation across the section. **(10 Marks)**

June/July 2014 (06ME34)

12. Prove that in case of a rectangular section of a beam, the maximum shear stress is 1.5 times the average shear stress. **(10 Marks)**

June/July 2014 (10ME34)

13. Prove that the maximum shear stress is 1.5 times the average shear stress in a beam of rectangular cross section. **(06 Marks)**

Dec. 14/Jan. 15 (06ME34)

14. The shear force acting on a section of a beam is 50 kN. The beam is of T-shaped having dimensions 100 mm × 100 mm × 20 mm as shown in **Fig. U7.3**. The moment of inertia about the neutral axis is 314.23 × 10^4 m^4. Calculate the shear stress at the neutral axis and at the junction of the web and flange. **(10 Marks)**

Dec. 14/Jan. 15 (10ME34)

15. An I section has the following dimensions. Flanges 200 mm × 10 mm; web 380 mm × 8 mm. The maximum shear stress developed in eh beam is 20 N/mm^2. Find the force to which the beam is subjected to? **(10 Marks)**

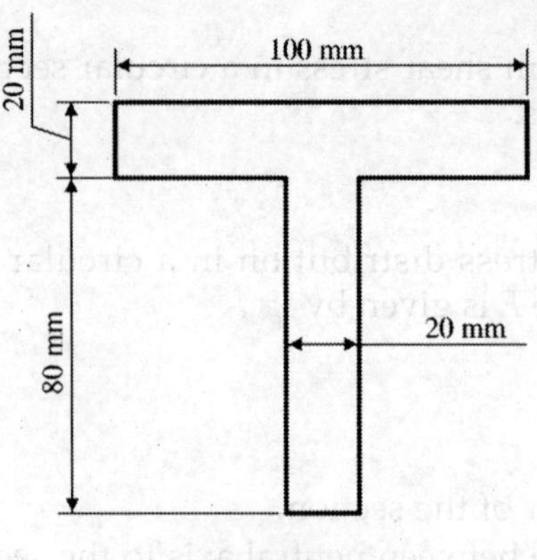

Fig. U7.3

June/July 15 (10ME34)

16. A beam of an I-section consists of 180 mm × 15 mm flanges and a web of 280 mm × 15 mm thickness. It is subjected to a shear force of 60 kN. Sketch the shear stress distribution along the depth of the section. **(10 Marks)**

Dec. 15/Jan. 16 (10ME/AU34)

17. Prove that in case of a rectangular section of a beam the maximum shear stress is 1.5 times the average shear stress. **(08 Marks)**

June/July 2017 (15ME/MA34)

18. An I-section beam 350 mm × 150 mm has a web thickness of 10 mm and a flange thickness of 20 mm. If the shear force acting on the beam is 40 kN, find the maximum shear stress developed in the I-section. **(08 Marks)**

Dec. 17/Jan. 18 (10ME/AU34)

19. Prove that the maximum shear stress is 1.5 times the average shear stress in a beam of rectangular cross-section. **(06 Marks)**

Deflection of Beams

Chapter Outline

8.1 INTRODUCTION

In the previous **chapters (6 and 7),** we have discussed the strength requirements based on bending and shear stresses developed in a beam. However, a design of beam is not complete until the deflection of the beam is determined for a particular load. For example excessive deflections can cause cracks in the buildings. Cars and aircraft must have sufficient rigidity to control structural vibrations. The deflection of beam depends upon the stiffness of the material, dimensions of the beams and the configuration of applied loads and supports.

8.2 EQUATIONS FOR DEFLECTION, SLOPE AND BENDING MOMENT OR DIFFERENTIAL EQUATION FOR DEFLECTION OF BEAMS OR EULER-BERNOULLI DEFLECTION EQUATION OR ELASTIC CURVE—DERIVATION OF DIFFERENTIAL EQUATION OF FLEXURE

VTU – Mech.: June/July 2017 – 10 Marks, June/July 2017 – 08 Marks, Dec. 15/Jan. 16 – 10 Marks, June/ July 15 – 10 Marks, Dec. 14/ Jan. 15 – 10 Marks, Dec. 14/Jan. 15 – 10 Marks, June/July 2014 – 06 Marks, Dec. 13/Jan. 14 – 05 Marks, June 2012 – 10 Marks, Dec. 08/Jan. 09 – 10 Marks, Dec. 07/Jan. 08 – 03 Marks. Civil: June/July 2017 – 06 Marks, Dec. 16/Jan. 17 – 08 Marks, Dec. 15/Jan. 16 – 06 Marks, June/July 2015 – 06 Marks, June/July 2014 – 06 Marks, June/July 2013 – 06 Marks, June 2012 – 08 Marks, Dec. 2011 – 06 Marks, June/July 2011 – 06 Marks, Dec. 09/Jan. 10 – 06 Marks, Dec. 2011 – 06 Marks, Dec.08/Jan.09 – 04 Marks, Dec.07/Jan.08 – 06 Marks]

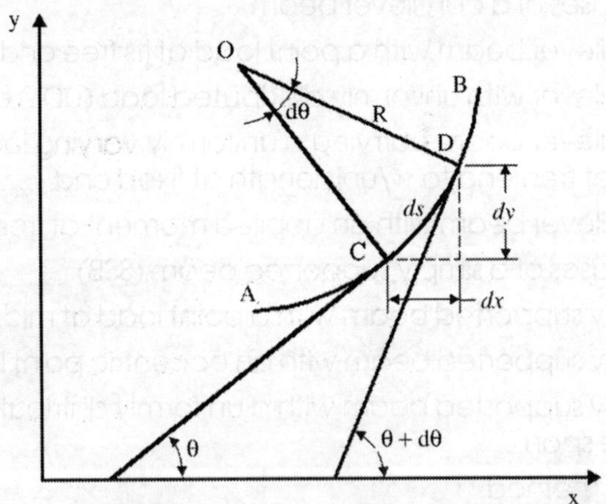

Fig. 8.1: Deflection curve of a beam

Fig. 8.1 represents a portion of a beam deflected under a given load. Consider an elemental length $CD = ds$ on the deflected curve. Let θ and $(\theta + d\theta)$ be the angles with x-axis made by the tangents at C and D respectively. Let O be the intersection point of these two tangents. Then O is called the center of curvature of the curve at any point between C and D.

From **Fig. 8.1**, arc length $\qquad ds = CD = R.d\theta$

$$R = \frac{ds}{d\theta} \qquad\qquad \text{... Eq. (i)}$$

If (x, y) are the coordinates at point C, then from **Fig. 8.1** we have

$$\tan\theta = \frac{dy}{dx}, \sin\theta = \frac{dy}{ds} \text{ and } \cos\theta = \frac{dx}{ds} \qquad \text{... Eq. (ii)}$$

Differentiating Eq. (ii) with respect to x, we have

$$(d^2y)/(dx^2) = \sec^2\theta \, \frac{d\theta}{dx}$$

$$= \sec^2\theta \, \frac{d\theta}{ds}\frac{ds}{dx}$$

$$= \sec^2\theta \, \frac{1}{R}\frac{1}{\cos\theta} \qquad \text{... using Eqs (i)and (ii)}$$

$$\frac{d^2y}{dx^2} = \sec^3\theta \, \frac{1}{R} \qquad \text{... Eq. (iii)}$$

$$\frac{1}{R} = \frac{d^2y/dx^2}{\sec^3\theta}$$

$$\frac{1}{R} = \frac{d^2y/dx^2}{(1+\tan^2\theta)^{3/2}} = \frac{d^2y/dx^2}{\left[1+(dy/dx)^2\right]^{3/2}}$$

Since the slope $\frac{dy}{dx}$ is a small quantity, negelcteing the term $\left(\frac{dy}{dx}\right)^2$, we have

$$\frac{1}{R} = \frac{d^2y}{dx^2} \qquad \text{... (Eq. 8.1)}$$

Now bending equation, $\qquad \dfrac{M}{I} = \dfrac{\sigma}{c} = \dfrac{E}{R}$

From which we have $\qquad \dfrac{1}{R} = \dfrac{M}{EI} \qquad \text{... (Eq. 8.2)}$

From Eqs (8.1) and (8.2), we have

$$\frac{M}{EI} = \frac{d^2y}{dx^2}$$

Or $\qquad\qquad M = EI\, \dfrac{d^2y}{dx^2} \qquad \text{... (Eq. 8.3)}$

Eq. (8.3) is called the differential equation for deflection or Euler–Bernoulli deflection equation.

Differentiating (Eq. 8.3), we have

Shear force $\qquad F = \dfrac{dM}{dx} = EI\,\dfrac{d^3y}{dx^3} \qquad$ since $\dfrac{dM}{dx} = F \qquad \text{... (Eq. 8.4)}$

Differentiating (Eq. 8.4), we have

Load intensity $\qquad W = \dfrac{dF}{dx} = EI\dfrac{d^4y}{dx^4} \qquad$ since $\dfrac{dF}{dx} = W \qquad$ ... (Eq. 8.5)

Other useful equations:

Deflection $\qquad\qquad\qquad = y \qquad\qquad\qquad\qquad\qquad$ ... (Eq. 8.6a)

Slope $\qquad\qquad\qquad \theta = \dfrac{dy}{dx} \qquad\qquad\qquad\qquad$ ... (Eq. 8.6b)

Moment $\qquad\qquad\qquad M = EI\dfrac{d^2y}{dx^2} \qquad\qquad\qquad$ ... (Eq. 8.6c)

Shear force $\qquad\qquad F = EI\dfrac{d^3y}{dx^3} \qquad\qquad\qquad$ ... (Eq. 8.6d)

Load intensity $\qquad\qquad W = EI\dfrac{d^4y}{dx^4} \qquad\qquad\qquad$ ... (Eq. 8.6e)

8.3 SIGN CONVENTIONS

- x is positive when measured towards right.
- y is positive when measured upwards and negative downwards (deflection).
- Clockwise rotation is taken as negative (slope).
- Sagging moment is taken as positive (moment).

8.4 ASSUMPTIONS IN DEFLECTION CURVE

VTU – (CV) May/June 2010 – 04 Marks

- Beam is straight and very large compared to its cross sectional dimensions.
- The value of Young's modulus of the material of the beam is same in tension and compression.
- Deflections and slopes are very small.
- Deflections caused by shearing action are negligibly small compared to bending.

8.5 METHODS FOR THE DETERMINATION OF BEAM DEFLECTIONS

- Double integration method.
- Macaulay's method or Singularity Functions.
- Moment area method or Mohr's method.
- Conjugate beam method or Method of elastic weights.
- Strain–Energy method (Castigliano's Theorem).
- Virtual work method.

8.6 DOUBLE INTEGRATION METHOD

The double integration method is a procedure to establish the equations for slope and deflection at points along the longitudinal axis (elastic curve) of a loaded beam. The equations are derived by integrating the differential equation of the elastic curve twice, hence the name *double integration*. The method assumes that all deformations are produced by moment.

We know that moment $\quad M = EI \dfrac{d^2y}{dx^2}$

Since the differential equation is of 2nd order we need two integrations
Integrating once we have

$$EI \frac{dy}{dx} = \int_0^x M + C_1 \qquad \qquad \text{... (Eq. 8.7)}$$

(Eq. 8.7) gives the *slope of the beam* at a given point.
Integrating again we have

$$EIy = \int_0^x \int_0^x M + C_1 x + C_2 \qquad \qquad \text{... (Eq. 8.8)}$$

(Eq. 8.8) gives the *deflection of the beam* at a given point.
Here C_1 and C_2 are constants and are to be evaluated using boundary conditions.
Useful boundary conditions:

- At fixed ends: $\qquad$ Deflection $y = 0 \qquad$ slope $\theta = \dfrac{dy}{dx} = 0$

- At simply supported or roller ends: $\quad$ Deflection $y = 0 \qquad$ slope $\theta = \dfrac{dy}{dx} \neq 0$

- For symmetrical beams: $\qquad$ Deflection $y = \dfrac{L}{2} \qquad$ slope $\theta = \dfrac{dy}{dx} = 0$

8.7 STANDARD CASES OF A CANTILEVER BEAM

8.7.1 Cantilever beam with a point load at its free end

VTU – Dec. 16/Jan. 17 – 08 Marks, Dec. 2011 – 08 Marks;
(CV) June/July 2014 – 06 Marks

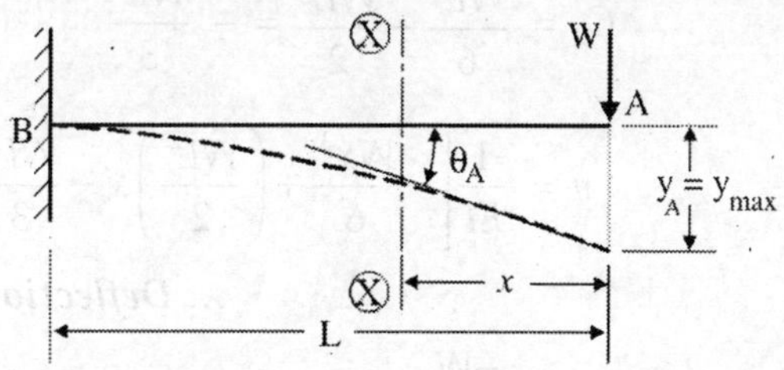

Fig. 8.2: Cantilever beam with point load at free end

Fig. 8.2 indicates a cantilever beam subjected to point load at free end.

Let
$\quad W \;=\;$ Point load at free end
$\quad L \;=\;$ Length of the beam
$\quad E \;=\;$ Young's modulus of the material of the beam
$\quad I \;=\;$ Moment of inertia
$\quad M_n \;=\;$ Bending moment at salient points
$\quad y \;=\;$ Deflection

$$\theta = \frac{dy}{dx} = \text{Slope}$$

Consider a section X-X at a distance x from free end A.

Bending moment at X-X is $\quad M_x = -W.x \qquad$ (Negative because of hogging)

$$\text{i.e. } EI\,\frac{d^2y}{dx^2} = -W.x$$

Integrating once we have $EI\,\dfrac{dy}{dx} = -\dfrac{Wx^2}{2} + C_1 \qquad\qquad$ ... Eq. (i)

Integrating again we have $\quad EIy = -\dfrac{Wx^3}{6} + C_1 x + C_2 \qquad$ ... Eq. (ii)

Boundary conditions:

At B: $x = L$, $\dfrac{dy}{dx} = 0$:

Eq. (i) yields... $\qquad\qquad 0 = -\dfrac{WL^2}{2} + C_1$

$$C_1 = \frac{WL^2}{2} \qquad\qquad\text{... Eq. (iii)}$$

Substituting C_1 in Eq. (i) we get

$$EI\,\frac{dy}{dx} = -\frac{Wx^2}{2} + \frac{WL^2}{2} \qquad \textbf{\textit{... Slope equation}} \text{ (Eq. 8.9a)}$$

Or $\qquad\qquad \dfrac{dy}{dx} = \theta = \dfrac{W}{2EI}\left(L^2 - x^2\right) \qquad$ ... (Eq. 8.9b)

At B: $x = L$, $y = 0$:

Eq. (ii) yields... $\qquad 0 = -\dfrac{WL^3}{6} + \left(\dfrac{WL^2}{2}\right)L + C_2 \qquad$ ... using (Eq. iii)

$$C_2 = \frac{WL^3}{6} - \frac{WL^3}{2} = -\frac{WL^3}{3} \qquad\qquad\text{... Eq. (iv)}$$

Eq. (ii) yields... $\qquad y = \dfrac{1}{EI}\left[-\dfrac{Wx^3}{6} + \left(\dfrac{WL^2}{2}\right)x - \dfrac{WL^3}{3}\right]$

$$\textbf{\textit{... Deflection equation}} \text{ (Eq. 8.10a)}$$

Or $\qquad\qquad y = \dfrac{-W}{6EI}\left[x^3 - 3L^2x + 2L^3\right] \qquad$ ... (Eq. 8.10b)

(Eq. 8.10) gives the deflection at all values of x.

Maximum slope and deflection: It occurs at the free end of the beam, where $x = 0$.

(Eq. 8.9) yields... $\qquad \dfrac{dy}{dx} = \theta_A = \theta_{\max} = \dfrac{WL^2}{2EI} \qquad$ ... (Eq. 8.11)

(Eq. 8.10) yields... $\qquad y_A = y_{\max} = -\dfrac{WL^3}{3EI} \qquad$ ... (Eq. 8.12)

Negative sign indicates that deflection is downwards

8.7.2 Cantilever beam with uniformly distributed load (UDL) over entire span

VTU – June/July 2016 – 10 Marks, June 2012 – 08 Marks;[Civil: June 2012 – 06 Marks, June/July 2009 – 06 Marks

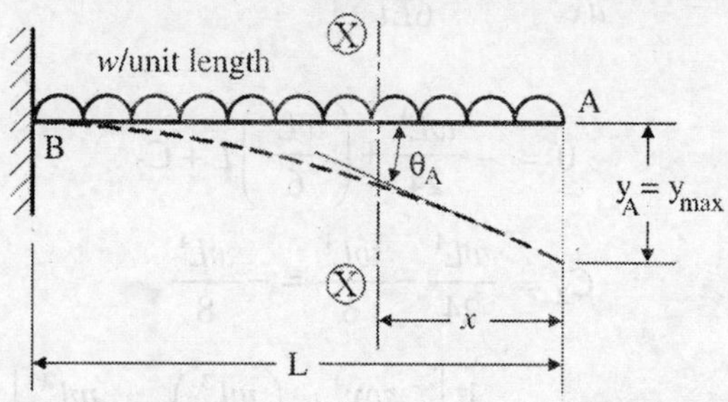

Fig. 8.3: Cantilever beam with UDL over entire span

Fig. 8.3 indicates a cantilever beam subjected to uniformly distributed load over entire span.

Let
w = Uniformly distributed load per unit length
L = Length of the beam
E = Young's modulus of the material of the beam
I = Moment of inertia
M_n = Bending moment at salient points
y = Deflection

$$\theta = \frac{dy}{dx} = \text{Slope}$$

Consider a section X-X at a distance x from free end A.

Bending moment at X-X is $\quad M_x = -wx\left(\frac{x}{2}\right) = -\left(\frac{wx^2}{2}\right)$

(Negative because, hogging)

i.e. $\qquad EI\frac{d^2y}{dx^2} = -\left(\frac{wx^2}{2}\right)$

Integrating once we have $EI\dfrac{dy}{dx} = -\dfrac{wx^3}{6} + C_1$ ... Eq. (i)

Integrating again we have $\quad EIy = -\dfrac{wx^4}{24} + C_1x + C_2$ ... Eq. (ii)

Boundary conditions:

At B: $x = L$, $\dfrac{dy}{dx} = 0$:

Eq. (i) yields... $\qquad 0 = -\dfrac{wL^3}{6} + C_1$

$$C_1 = \frac{wL^3}{6}$$ ... Eq. (iii)

Substituting C_1 in Eq. (i) we get

$$EI\frac{dy}{dx} = -\frac{wx^3}{6} + \frac{wL^3}{6} \qquad \textit{... \textbf{Slope equation}} \text{ (Eq. 8.13a)}$$

Or
$$\frac{dy}{dx} = \theta = \frac{w}{6EI}(L^3 - x^3) \qquad \text{... (Eq. 8.13b)}$$

At B: $x = L$, $y = 0$:

Eq. (ii) yields...
$$0 = -\frac{wL^4}{24} + \left(\frac{wL^3}{6}\right)L + C_2 \qquad \text{... using (Eq. iii)}$$

$$C_2 = \frac{wL^4}{24} - \frac{wL^4}{6} = -\frac{wL^4}{8} \qquad \text{... Eq. (iv)}$$

Eq. (ii) yields...
$$y = \frac{1}{EI}\left[-\frac{wx^4}{24} + \left(\frac{wL^3}{6}\right)x - \frac{wL^4}{8}\right]$$

$$\textit{... \textbf{Deflection equation}} \text{ (Eq. 8.14a)}$$

Or
$$y = \frac{-w}{24EI}\left[x^4 - 4L^3x + 3L^4\right] \qquad \text{... (Eq. 8.14b)}$$

Maximum slope and deflection: It occurs at the free end of the beam, where $x = 0$.

(Eq. 8.13) yields...
$$\frac{dy}{dx} = \theta_A = \theta_{max} = \frac{wL^3}{6EI} \qquad \text{... (Eq. 8.15)}$$

(Eq. 8.14) yields...
$$y_A = y_{max} = -\frac{wL^4}{8EI} \qquad \text{... (Eq. 8.16)}$$

Negative sign indicates that deflection is downwards

8.7.3 Cantilever beam carrying a uniformly varying load (UVL) from zero at free end to w/unit length at fixed end

VTU – Jan. 2013 – 10 Marks

Fig. 8.4 indicates a cantilever beam subjected to uniformly varying load of intensity 0 at free end to w/unit length at fixed end.

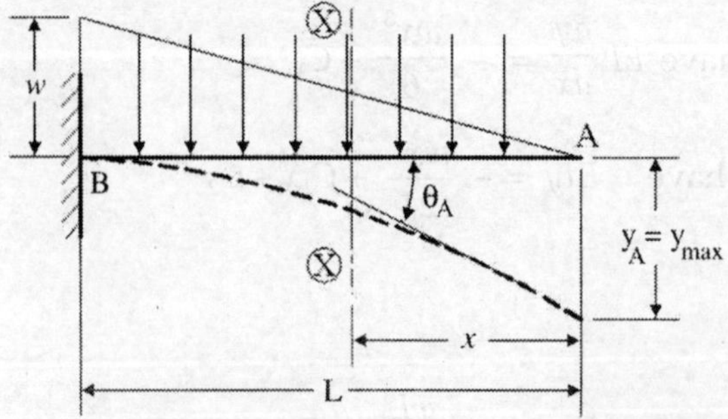

Fig. 8.4: Cantilever beam with UVL over entire span
(Zero at free end to w/unit length at fixed end)

Let
$$w = \text{Uniformly distributed load per unit length}$$
$$L = \text{Length of the beam}$$

$$E = \text{Young's modulus of the material of the beam}$$
$$I = \text{Moment of inertia}$$
$$M_n = \text{Bending moment at salient points}$$
$$y = \text{Deflection}$$

$$\theta = \frac{dy}{dx} = \text{Slope}$$

From sub-section 5.8.3, we have

Bending moment at X-X is $\qquad M_x = -\left(\dfrac{wx^3}{6L}\right)$

(Negative because, hogging)

i.e. $\qquad\qquad EI\dfrac{d^2y}{dx^2} = -\left(\dfrac{wx^3}{6L}\right)$

Integrating once we have $EI\dfrac{dy}{dx} = -\dfrac{wx^4}{24L} + C_1$ $\qquad\qquad$ ... Eq. (i)

Integrating again we have $\quad EIy = -\dfrac{wx^5}{120L} + C_1x + C_2$ $\qquad\qquad$ ... Eq. (ii)

Boundary conditions:

At B: $x = L$, $\dfrac{dy}{dx} = 0$:

Eq. (i) yields... $\qquad\qquad\qquad 0 = -\dfrac{wL^4}{24L} + C_1$

$$C_1 = \frac{wL^3}{24} \qquad\qquad\qquad ... \text{Eq. (iii)}$$

Substituting C_1 in Eq. (i) we get

$$EI\frac{dy}{dx} = -\frac{wx^4}{24L} + \frac{wL^3}{24} \qquad ... \textit{Slope equation } \text{(Eq. 8.17a)}$$

Or $\qquad\qquad \dfrac{dy}{dx} = \theta = \dfrac{w}{24EI}(L^3 - x^4) \qquad\qquad ... \text{(Eq. 8.17b)}$

At B: $x = L$, $y = 0$:

Eq. (ii) yields... $\qquad\qquad 0 = -\dfrac{wL^5}{120L} + \left(\dfrac{wL^3}{24}\right)L + C_2 \qquad ... \text{using (Eq. iii)}$

$$C_2 = \frac{wL^4}{120} - \frac{wL^4}{24} = -\frac{wL^4}{30} \qquad\qquad ... \text{Eq. (iv)}$$

Eq. (ii) yields... $\qquad\qquad y = \dfrac{1}{EI}\left[-\dfrac{wx^5}{120L} + \left(\dfrac{wL^3}{24}\right)x - \dfrac{wL^4}{30}\right]$

$$... \textit{Deflection equation } \text{(Eq. 8.18a)}$$

$$\text{Or} \qquad y = \frac{-w}{120EIL}\left[x^5 - 5L^4x + 4L^5\right] \qquad \text{... (Eq. 8.18b)}$$

Maximum slope and deflection: It occurs at the free end of the beam, where $x = 0$.

(Eq. 8.17) yields...
$$\frac{dy}{dx} = \theta_A = \theta_{max} = \frac{wL^3}{24EI} \qquad \text{... (Eq. 8.19)}$$

(Eq. 8.18) yields...
$$y_A = y_{max} = -\frac{wL^4}{30EI} \qquad \text{... (Eq. 8.20)}$$

Negative sign indicates that deflection is downwards

8.7.4 Cantilever beam with an applied moment at free end

Fig. 8.5 indicates a cantilever beam subjected to a CW couple at free end.

Let M = couple
L = Length of the beam
E = Young's modulus of the material of the beam
I = Moment of inertia
y = Deflection

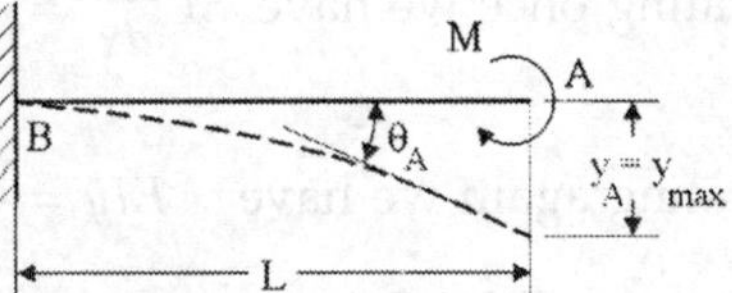

Fig. 8.5: Cantilever beam with a couple

$$\theta = \frac{dy}{dx} = \text{Slope}$$

At every section in the beam the bending moment will be $- M$ which remains constant throughout as shown in **Fig. 5.9(c)**.

Bending moment at X-X is $M_x = - M$ (Negative because, hogging)

i.e.
$$EI \frac{d^2y}{dx^2} = - M$$

Integrating once we have $EI \dfrac{dy}{dx} = -Mx + C_1$ ... Eq. (i)

Integrating again we have $EIy = -\dfrac{Mx^2}{2} + C_1x + C_2$ ... Eq. (ii)

Boundary conditions:

At B: $x = L$, $\dfrac{dy}{dx} = 0$:

Eq. (i) yields...
$$0 = -ML + C_1$$
$$C_1 = ML \qquad \text{... Eq. (iii)}$$

Substituting C_1 in Eq. (i) we get

$$EI \frac{dy}{dx} = -Mx + ML \qquad \text{... } \textit{Slope equation } \text{(Eq. 8.21a)}$$

$$\text{Or} \qquad \frac{dy}{dx} = \theta = \frac{M}{MI}(L - x) \qquad \text{... (Eq. 8.21b)}$$

At B: $x = L$, $y = 0$:

Eq. (ii) yields... $$0 = -\frac{ML^2}{2} + (ML)L + C_2 \qquad \text{... using (Eq. iii)}$$

$$C_2 = \frac{ML^2}{2} - ML^2 = -\frac{ML^2}{2} \qquad \text{... Eq. (iv)}$$

Eq. (ii) yields... $$y = \frac{1}{EI}\left[-\frac{Mx^2}{2} + (ML)x - \frac{ML^2}{2}\right]$$

... ***Deflection equation*** (Eq. 8.22a)

Or $$y = \frac{-M}{2EI}\left[x^2 - 2Lx + L^2\right] \qquad \text{... (Eq. 8.22b)}$$

Maximum slope and deflection: It occurs at the free end of the beam, where $x = 0$.

(Eq. 8.21) yields... $$\frac{dy}{dx} = \theta_A = \theta_{max} = \frac{ML}{EI} \qquad \text{... (Eq. 8.23)}$$

(Eq. 8.22) yields... $$y_A = y_{max} = -\frac{ML^2}{2EI} \qquad \text{... (Eq. 8.24)}$$

Negative sign indicates that deflection is downwards

Note: If several loads are acting on the beam, then using the principle of superposition, the total deflection may be obtained by summing up the individual load cases.

1. **Determine the slope and deflection at the free end of a cantilever beam subjected to a load of 10 kN. The span of beam is 2 m. Assume $E = 200$ GPa and $I = 80 \times 10^6$ mm^4. Also determine the deflection and slope at every 0.5 m.**

Solution: $\theta_{max} = ?$, $y_{max} = ?$, $W = 10 \times 10^3$ N, $L = 2000$ mm, $E = 200 \times 10^3$ MPa, $I = 80 \times 10^6$ mm^4.

a. *Maximum slope and deflection*

Maximum slope $$\theta_{max} = \frac{WL^2}{2EI} = \frac{10 \times 10^3 \times 2000^2}{2 \times (200 \times 10^3) \times (80 \times 10^6)} = 0.0013 \text{ rad}$$

Maximum deflection $$y_{max} = \frac{WL^3}{3EI} = \frac{10 \times 10^3 \times 2000^3}{3 \times (200 \times 10^3) \times (80 \times 10^6)} = 1.667 \text{ mm}$$

(Downward)

b. *Slope and deflection at every 0.5 m:*

Distance from free end	Slope equation	Deflection equation
x	$\dfrac{dy}{dx} = \theta = \dfrac{W}{2EI}(L^2 - x^2)$	$y = \dfrac{-W}{6EI}\left[x^3 - 3L^2x + 2L^3\right]$
mm	rad	mm
0	0.0013	$- 1.667$
500	0.0012	$- 1.055$
1000	0.0009	$- 0.521$
1500	0.0005	$- 0.143$
2000	0	0

2. A cantilever of length 2.5 m carries a uniformly distributed load of 16.4 kN/m over the entire length. If the moment of inertia of the beam is 7.95×10^7 mm⁴ and $E = 2 \times 10^5$ N/mm², determine the deflection at the free end. Derive the equation used.

VTU – Dec. 2012 – 10 Marks

Solution: $L = 2500$mm, $w = 16.4$ kN/m $= 16.4$ N/mm, $I = 7.95 \times 10^7$ mm⁴, $E = 2 \times 10^5$ N/mm² $y = ?$

For a cantilever beam with UDL over entire span

Deflection at free end, $y = y_{max} = \dfrac{wL^4}{8EI} = \dfrac{16.4 \times 2500^4}{8 \times (2 \times 10^5) \times (7.95 \times 10^7)} = 5.036$ mm

(Downward)

For derivation, refer *Sec. 8.7.2*

3. For the above problem, determine the deflection and slope at every 0.5 m.
Solution:

Distance from free end	Slope equation	Deflection equation
x	$\dfrac{dy}{dx} = \theta = \dfrac{W}{6EI}(L^3 - x^3)$	$y = \dfrac{-W}{24EI}\left[x^4 - 3L^3x + 2L^4\right]$
mm	rad	mm
0	0.0027	-5.036
500	0.0027	-3.696
1000	0.0025	-2.393
1500	0.0021	-1.225
2000	0.0013	-0.352
2500	0	0

4. A cantilever 120 mm wide and 200 mm deep is 2.5 m long. What is the uniformly distributed load which the beam can carry in order to have a deflection of 5 mm at the free end? Take $E = 200$ GPa.

VTU – Dec. 13/Jan. 14 – 04 Marks

Solution: $b = 120$ mm, $h = 200$ mm, $L = 2500$ mm, $w = ?$, $y = 5$ mm, $E = 2 \times 10^5$ MPa.

For a rectangular section, $I = \dfrac{bh^3}{12} = \dfrac{120 \times 200^3}{12} = 80 \times 10^6$ mm⁴

For a cantilever beam with UDL over entire span

Deflection at free end, $y = y_{max} = \dfrac{wL^4}{8EI}$

$$5 = \dfrac{w \times 2500^4}{8 \times (2 \times 10^5) \times (80 \times 10^6)}$$

$$\therefore \quad w = 16.384 \text{ N/mm} = 16.384 \text{ kN/m}$$

5. Determine the deflection at the free end of a cantilever beam loaded as shown in Fig. 8.6. Take $E = 200$ GPa, $I = 150 \times 10^6$ mm⁴. Also determine the deflection at every 0.5 m.

Solution: $y = ?$, $E = 200 \times 10^3$ MPa, $I = 150 \times 10^6$ mm⁴, $L = 3000$ mm, $w = 15$ kN/m $= 15$ N/mm, $W = 25 \times 10^3$ N.

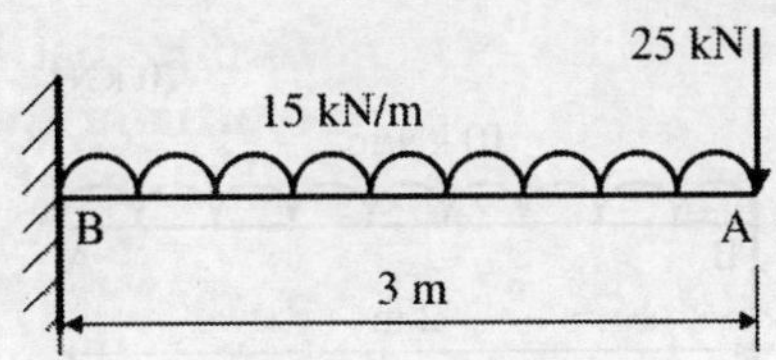

Fig. 8.6: Problem 5

Let suffix '1' refer to point load parameters and suffix '2' refer to UDL parameters.
Using the principal of superposition,
Total deflection, $\qquad y = y_1 + y_2$ $\qquad\qquad$ ... Eq. (i)
For a cantilever beam with point load at free end

$$y_1 = \frac{WL^3}{3EI} = \frac{25 \times 10^3 \times 3000^3}{3 \times (200 \times 10^3) \times (150 \times 10^6)} = 7.50 \text{ mm}$$

(Downward)

For a cantilever beam with UDL over entire span

$$y_2 = \frac{wL^4}{8EI} = \frac{15 \times 3000^4}{8 \times (200 \times 10^3) \times (150 \times 10^6)} = 5.0625 \text{ mm}$$

(Downward)

Eq. (i) yields ... $\qquad y = 7.5 + 5.0625 = 12.5625 \text{ mm}$ $\qquad$ (Downward)

Deflection at every 0.5 m:

Distance from free end	Deflection equation (Point load)	Deflection equation (UDL)	Total deflection $y = y_1 + y_2$
x	$y_1 = \dfrac{-W}{6EI}\left[x^3 - 3L^2x + 2L^3\right]$	$y_2 = \dfrac{-W}{24EI}\left[x^4 - 4L^3x + 3L^4\right]$	
mm	rad	mm	
0	-7.50	-5.063	-12.563
500	-5.642	-3.939	-9.581
1000	-3.889	-2.833	-6.722
1500	-2.344	-1.793	-4.137
2000	-1.111	-0.896	-2.007
2500	-0.295	-0.251	-0.546
3000	0	0	0

6. **A 2 m long cantilever is subjected to a UDL of 10 kN/m throughout its length and has a vertically downward point load of 20 kN at its free end. Taking E = 200 GPa and minimum deflection as 0.3 mm, determine the width and depth of the rectangular section. Depth of the section is twice the width.**

VTU – June/July 2017 – 06 Marks; (CV) Jan. 2013 – 10 Marks

Solution: $L = 2000$ mm, $w = 10$ kN/m $= 10$ N/mm, $W = 20 \times 10^3$ N, $E = 200 \times 10^3$ MPa, $y = -0.3$ mm, $h = 2b$, $b = ?$, $h = ?$
Based on given data, the problem is as shown in **Fig. 8.7**
Let suffix '1' refer to point load parameters and suffix '2' refer to UDL parameters.
Using the principal of superposition,
$$y = y_1 + y_2 \qquad\qquad\qquad ... \text{Eq. (i)}$$

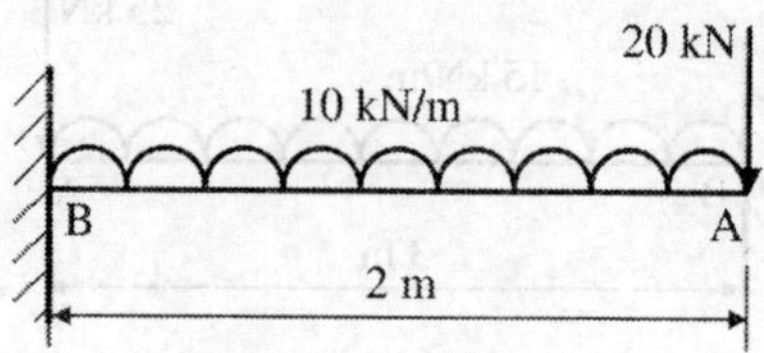

Fig. 8.7: Problem 6

For a cantilever beam with point load at free end

$$y_1 = \frac{WL^3}{3EI} = \frac{20 \times 10^3 \times 2000^3}{3 \times (200 \times 10^3) \times I} = \frac{266.67 \times 10^6}{I}$$

For a cantilever beam with UDL over entire span

$$y_2 = \frac{wL^4}{8EI} = \frac{10 \times 2000^4}{8 \times (200 \times 10^3) \times I} = \frac{100 \times 10^6}{I}$$

Eq. (i) yields ...
$$0.3 = \frac{266.67 \times 10^6}{I} + \frac{100 \times 10^6}{I}$$

$$I = 1.22 \times 10^9 \text{ mm}^4$$

For a rectangular section, $\qquad I = \dfrac{bh^3}{12}$

$$1.22 \times 10^9 = \frac{b(2b)^3}{12} \Rightarrow b = 207 \text{ mm} \quad \text{and} \quad h = 414 \text{ mm}$$

7. **Find the deflection of a cantilever beam subjected to eccentric point load as shown in Fig. 8.8.**

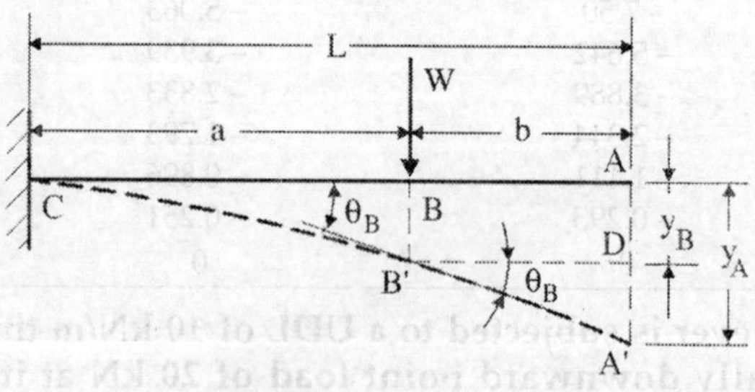

Fig. 8.8: Problem 7

Let
$$
\begin{aligned}
W &= \text{Eccentric point load} \\
L &= \text{Length of the beam} \\
M_n &= \text{Bending moment at salient points} \\
y_B &= \text{Deflection at B} \\
\theta_B &= \text{Slope at B}
\end{aligned}
$$

From *Sec. 8.7.1*

Maximum slope, $\qquad \dfrac{dy}{dx} = \theta_{max} = \dfrac{WL^2}{2EI}$ $\qquad$ ... using (Eq. 8.11)

Maximum deflection, $\qquad y_{max} = \dfrac{WL^3}{3EI}$ $\qquad$ (neglecting sign) ... using (Eq. 8.12)

Comparing the above equations with respect to **Fig. 8.8**, we have

$$\theta_B = \frac{Wa^2}{2EI} \quad \text{and} \quad y_B = \frac{Wa^3}{3EI} \qquad \text{... (Eq. 8.25)}$$

Since the portion AB is not subjected to any moment, it remains straight and hence $\theta_A = \theta_B$

$$\text{Slope at A} = \theta_A = \theta_B = \frac{Wa^2}{2EI} \qquad \text{... (Eq. 8.26)}$$

Thus deflection at A, $\quad y_A = AD + DA' = y_B + (y_A - y_B)$

$$\text{From } \Delta A'B'D \quad \tan \theta_B = \frac{(y_A - y_B)}{b}$$

$$\theta_B = \frac{(y_A - y_B)}{b}$$

$$[\tan \theta_B \approx \theta_B, \text{ since } \theta_B \text{ is very small}]$$

$$(y_A - y_B) = \theta_B . b$$

$$\therefore \quad y_A = y_B + \theta_B . b$$

$$y_A = \frac{Wa^3}{3EI} + \frac{Wa^2}{2EI} . b$$

$$y_A = \frac{Wa^3}{3EI} + \frac{Wa^2}{2EI} .(L - a) \quad \text{since } L = a + b \qquad \text{... (Eq. 8.27a)}$$

Or $\qquad y_A = \frac{W}{6EI} [3a^2 L - a^3] \qquad \text{(Downward)} \qquad \text{... (Eq. 8.27b)}$

Or $\qquad y_A = y_{max} = \frac{Wa^2}{6EI} [3L - a] \qquad \text{(Downward)} \qquad \text{... (Eq. 8.27c)}$

8. For the cantilever beam shown in Fig. 8.9. If $E = 200$ GPa and $I = 150 \times 10^6$ mm^4, determine
(a) Deflection and slope at load point
(b) Maximum slope and maximum deflection.

Solution: $\theta_B = ?$, $y_B = ?$, $\theta_{max} = ?$, $y_{max} = ?$, $W = 20 \times 10^3$ N, $L = 3500$ mm, $a = 2500$ mm, $b = 1000$ mm, $E = 200 \times 10^3$ MPa, $I = 150 \times 10^6$ mm^4.

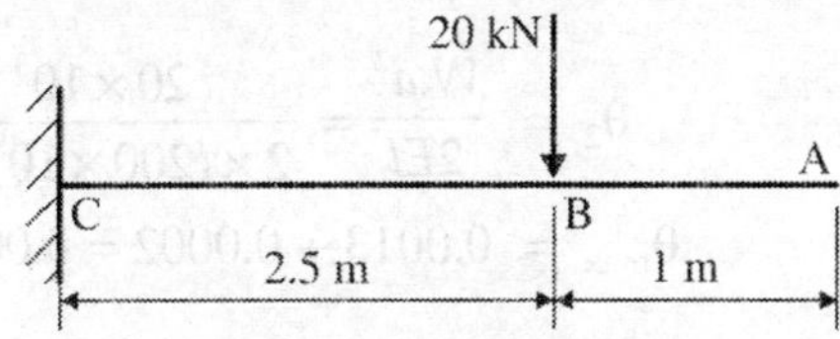

Fig. 8.9: Problem 8

a. *Slope and deflection at load point:*

$$\text{Slope} \qquad \theta_B = \frac{Wa^2}{2EI} = \frac{20 \times 10^3 \times 2500^2}{2 \times (200 \times 10^3) \times (150 \times 10^6)} = 0.0021 \text{ rad}$$

$$\text{Deflection} \qquad y_B = \frac{Wa^3}{3EI} = \frac{20 \times 10^3 \times 2500^3}{3 \times (200 \times 10^3) \times (150 \times 10^6)} = 3.472 \text{ mm}$$

$$\text{(Downward)}$$

b. *Maximum slope and deflection*

Slope
$$\theta_A = \theta_B = \frac{Wa^2}{2EI} = \frac{20 \times 10^3 \times 2500^2}{2 \times (200 \times 10^3) \times (150 \times 10^6)} = 0.0021 \text{ rad}$$

Deflection
$$y_A = y_{max} = \frac{Wa^2}{6EI}[3L - a]$$

$$y_A = y_{max} = \frac{20 \times 10^3 \times 2500^2}{2 \times (200 \times 10^3) \times (150 \times 10^6)} [(3 \times 3500) - 2500]$$

$$= 5.56 \text{ mm} \quad \text{(Downward)}$$

9. **A cantilever beam 5 m long is subjected to two point loads of 50 kN and 20 kN at distance of 3 m and 5 m from the fixed end respectively. If the moment of inertia is 3×10^8 and $E = 200$ GPa, determine the slope and deflection at the free end.**

Solution: *Let suffix '1' refer to end load parameters and suffix '2' refer to eccentric load parameters.*

Based on given data, the problem is as shown in **Fig. 8.10**.

$W_1 = 10 \times 10^3$ N, $W_2 = 20 \times 10^3$ N, $a = 1000$ mm, $b = 3000$ mm, $E = 200 \times 10^3$ MPa, $I = 3 \times 10^8$ mm^4, $L = 4000$ mm. $\theta_{max} = ?$, $y_{max} = ?$

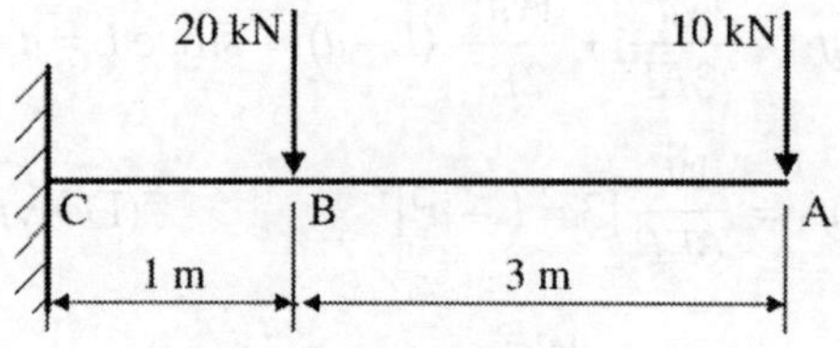

Fig. 8.10: Problem 9

a. *Slope:*

Total slope, $\qquad \theta_{max} = \theta_1 + \theta_2 \qquad$ ... Eq. (i)

For a cantilever beam with point load at free end

$$\theta_1 = \frac{W_1 L^2}{2EI} = \frac{10 \times 10^3 \times 4000^2}{2 \times (200 \times 10^3) \times (3 \times 10^8)} = 0.0013 \text{ rad}$$

For a cantilever beam with eccentric point load

$$\theta_2 = \frac{W_2 a^2}{2EI} = \frac{20 \times 10^3 \times 1000^2}{2 \times (200 \times 10^3) \times (3 \times 10^8)} = 0.0002 \text{ rad}$$

Eq. (i) yields ... $\qquad \theta_{max} = 0.0013 + 0.0002 = 0.0015 \text{ rad}$

b. *Deflection:*

Total deflection, $\qquad y_{max} = y_1 + y_2 \qquad$ ... Eq. (ii)

For a cantilever beam with point load at free end

$$y_1 = \frac{W_1 L^3}{3EI} = \frac{10 \times 10^3 \times 4000^3}{3 \times (200 \times 10^3) \times (3 \times 10^8)} = 3.555 \text{ mm}$$

For a cantilever beam with eccentric point load

$$y_2 = \frac{W_2 a^2}{6EI}[3L - a]$$

$$= \frac{20 \times 10^3 \times 1000^2}{6 \times (200 \times 10^3) \times (3 \times 10^8)} \left[(3 \times 4000) - 1000 \right]$$

$$y_2 = 0.611 \text{ mm}$$

Eq. (ii) yields ... $\quad y_{max} = 3.555 + 0.611 = 4.166 \text{ mm} \qquad \text{(Downward)}$

10. Explain the terms: **(a) Slope** **(b) Deflection** **(c) Deflection curve**

VTU – Civil: June/July 2016 – 06 Marks, June/July 2013 – 04 Marks, June/July 2013 – 04 Marks, Dec. 2012 – 06 Marks, May/June 2010 – 06 Marks

Solution:
Slope at any section is the angle made by the tangent drawn at the corresponding section in the beam. It is generally represented as tan θ measured with horizontal. Since the allowable deflection is very small, tan θ ≈ θ.

$$\text{Slope } \theta = \frac{dy}{dx}$$

Deflection at any section of a beam is the vertical displacement of the neutral layer of the beam at that section due to bending. It is represented as y.

Deflection curve: When the neutral layer of the beam is loaded it will bend in to a curve. This curve is known as deflection curve or Elastic curve.

11. Find the deflection of a cantilever loaded with a UDL of partial length a from the fixed end as shown in Fig. 8.11.

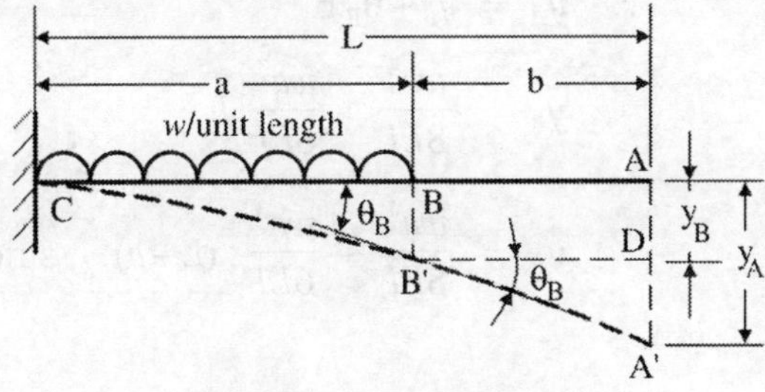

Fig. 8.11: Problem 8

Solution:
Fig. 8.11 indicates a cantilever beam subjected to uniformly distributed load over a span of 'a' from fixed end.

Let $\quad w$ = Uniformly distributed load per unit length
$\quad L$ = Length of the beam
$\quad a$ = Spread of UDL
$\quad E$ = Young's modulus of the material of the beam
$\quad I$ = Moment of inertia
$\quad M_n$ = Bending moment at salient points
$\quad y$ = Deflection

$$\theta \;=\; \frac{dy}{dx} = \text{Slope}$$

From **Sec. 8.7.2**

Maximum slope, $\dfrac{dy}{dx} = \theta_{max} = \dfrac{wL^3}{6EI}$ ... using (Eq. 8.15)

Maximum deflection, $y_{max} = \dfrac{wL^4}{8EI}$ (neglecting sign) ... using (Eq. 8.16)

Comparing the above equations with respect to **Fig. 8.11**, we have

$$\theta_B = \dfrac{wa^3}{6EI} \quad \text{and} \quad y_B = \dfrac{wa^4}{8EI} \qquad \text{... (Eq. 8.28)}$$

Since the portion AB is not subjected to any moment, it remains straight and hence $\theta_A = \theta_B$

Slope at $A = \theta_A = \theta_B = \dfrac{wa^3}{6EI}$ ... (Eq. 8.29)

Thus deflection at A, $y_A = AD + DA' = y_B + (y_A - y_B)$

From $\Delta A'B'D$ $\quad \tan \theta_B = \dfrac{(y_A - y_B)}{b}$

$$\theta_B = \dfrac{(y_A - y_B)}{b}$$

[$\tan \theta_B \approx \theta_B$ since θ_B is very small]
$$(y_A - y_B) = \theta_B.b$$

$\therefore \quad y_A = y_B + \theta_B.b$

$$y_A = \dfrac{wa^4}{8EI} + \dfrac{wa^3}{6EI}.b$$

$$y_A = \dfrac{wa^4}{8EI} + \dfrac{wa^3}{6EI} \cdot (L - a) \quad \text{since} \ L = a + b$$

... (Eq. 8.30a)

Or $\quad y_A = \dfrac{w}{24EI}\left[4a^3L - a^4\right]$ (Downward) ... (Eq. 8.30b)

Or $\quad y_A = y_{max} = \dfrac{wa^3}{24EI}\left[4L - a\right]$ (Downward)

... (Eq. 8.30c)

12. **A cantilever beam of span 5 m is subjected to a UDL of 6 kN/m over a length of 2 m from the fixed end as shown in Fig. 8.12. Determine the slope and deflection at point B. Also find the maximum slope and deflection at the free end of a cantilever beam. Take $E = 200$ GPa, $I = 150 \times 10^6$ mm^4.**

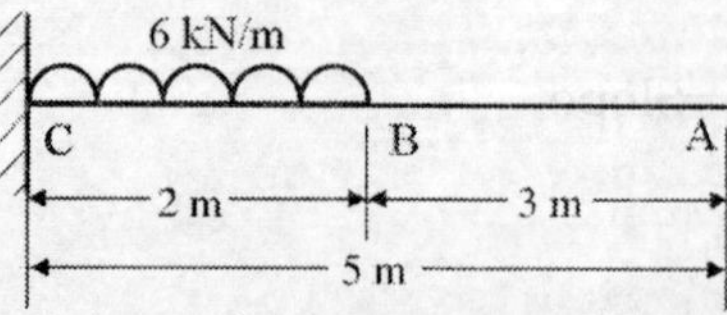

Fig. 8.12: Problem 12

Solution: $L = 5000$ mm, $w = 6$ kN/m $= 6$ N/mm, $a = 2000$ mm, $E = 200 \times 10^3$ MPa, $I = 150 \times 10^6$ mm^4, $\theta_B = ?$ $y_B = ?$, $\theta_{max} = ?$, $y_{max} = ?$

Slope at B
$$\theta_B = \frac{wa^3}{6EI} = \frac{6 \times 2000^3}{6 \times (200 \times 10^3) \times (150 \times 10^6)} = 0.0003 \text{ rad}$$

Deflection at B
$$y_B = \frac{wa^4}{8EI} = \frac{6 \times 2000^4}{8 \times (200 \times 10^3) \times (150 \times 10^6)} = 0.4 \text{ mm}$$

(Downward)

Maximum slope
$$\theta_{max} = \theta_A = \theta_B = \frac{wa^3}{6EI} = \frac{6 \times 2000^3}{6 \times (200 \times 10^3) \times (150 \times 10^6)} = 0.0003 \text{ rad}$$

Maximum deflection
$$y_{max} = y_A = \frac{wa^3}{24EI}[4L - a] = \frac{6 \times 2000^3 \times [(4 \times 5000) - 2000]}{24 \times (200 \times 10^3) \times (150 \times 10^6)}$$

$$= 1.2 \text{ mm} \qquad \text{(Downward)}$$

13. Find the deflection of a cantilever loaded with a UDL of partial length a from the free end as shown in Fig. 8.13(a).

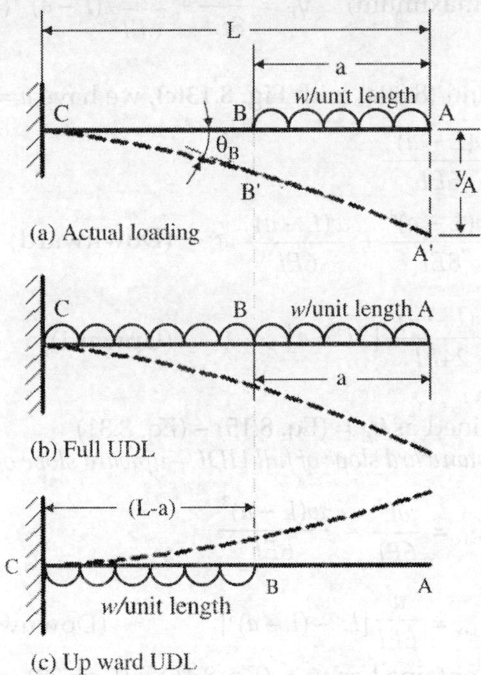

Fig. 8.13: Problem 13

Solution: Fig. 8.13(a) indicates a cantilever beam subjected to uniformly distributed load over a span of 'a' from free end.

Let
w = Uniformly distributed load per unit length
L = Length of the beam
a = Spread of UDL
E = Young's modulus of the material of the beam
I = Moment of inertia

$$M_n = \text{Bending moment at salient points}$$
$$y = \text{Deflection}$$

$$\theta = \frac{dy}{dx} = \text{Slope}$$

The slope and deflection at free end is obtained by taking the differences of **Fig. 8.13(b)** and **Fig. 8.13(c)**.

For **Fig. 8.13(b)**, from **sec. 8.7.2**, we have

Slope at free end (maximum) $\qquad \theta_{max} = \dfrac{wL^3}{6EI}$ $\qquad\qquad$ ... using (Eq. 8.15)

Deflection at free end (maximum) $y_{max} = \dfrac{wL^4}{8EI}$ $\quad$ (neglecting sign) ... using (Eq. 8.16)

For **Fig. 8.11,** from Problem 11, we have

Slope at free end (maximum) $\qquad \theta_B = \dfrac{wa^3}{6EI}$ $\qquad\qquad$ ... using (Eq. 8.29)

Deflection at free end (maximum) $\quad y_B = \dfrac{wa^4}{8EI} + \dfrac{wa^3}{6EI}.(L-a)$ $\quad$ (Downward)

$\qquad\qquad\qquad\qquad\qquad\qquad\qquad\qquad\qquad\qquad\qquad$ ... using (Eq. 8.30a)

Comparing Eqs (8.28) and (8.30a) with **Fig. 8.13(c)**, we have $a = (L - a)$

$$\theta_B = \frac{w(L-a)^3}{6EI} \qquad\qquad\qquad\qquad ... \text{(Eq. 8.31)}$$

$$y_B = \frac{w(L-a)^4}{8EI} + \frac{w(L-a)^3}{6EI}.a \qquad \text{(Downward)} \qquad ... \text{(Eq. 8.32a)}$$

Or $\qquad y_B = \dfrac{w(L-a)^3}{24EI}\left[3L + a\right]$ $\qquad$ (Upward) $\qquad\qquad$ ... (Eq. 8.32b)

Thus total slope is obtained as $\theta_A = $ (Eq. 8.15) – (Eq. 8.31)

$\qquad\qquad\qquad$ *= Downward slope of full UDL – upward slope of partial UDL*

$$\theta_A = \theta_{max} = \frac{wL^3}{6EI} - \frac{w(L-a)^3}{6EI} \qquad\qquad ... \text{(Eq. 8.33a)}$$

Or $\qquad \theta_A = \theta_{max} = \dfrac{w}{6EI}\left[L^3 - (L-a)^3\right]$ $\qquad$ (Downward) $\quad$ ... (Eq. 8.33b)

Thus total deflection is obtained as $y_A = $ (Eq. 8.16) – (Eq.8.32)

$$y_A = y_{max} = \frac{wL^4}{8EI} - \left[\frac{w(L-a)^4}{8EI} + \frac{w(L-a)^3}{6EI}\cdot a\right] \qquad ... \text{(Eq. 8.34a)}$$

$$= \frac{wL^4}{8EI} - \left[\frac{w(L-a)^3}{24EI}(3L+a)\right]$$

Or $\qquad y_A = y_{max} = \dfrac{w}{24EI}\left\{3L^4 - \left[(L-a)^3(3L+a)\right]\right\}$ (Downward) ... (Eq. 8.34b)

14. **A cantilever beam 4 m long is subjected to a uniformly distributed load of 10 kN/m over a length of 2 m from the free end. If the cross section is rectangular of 200 mm wide by 400 mm thick, determine the slope and deflection at the free end. Also determine the slope and deflection at the end of UDL (2 m from free end). Take E = 200 GPa.**

Solution: L = 4000 mm, a = 2000 mm, w = 10 kN/m = 10 N/mm, b = 200 mm, h = 400 mm, E = 200 × 10^3 MPa, θ_{max} = ?, y_{max} = ?, θ_B = ? y_B = ?.

Based on given data, the problem is as shown in **Fig. 8.14**.

For a rectangular cross-section, $\quad I = \dfrac{bh^3}{12} = \dfrac{200 \times 400^3}{12}$

$$I = 1.067 \times 10^9 \text{ mm}^4$$

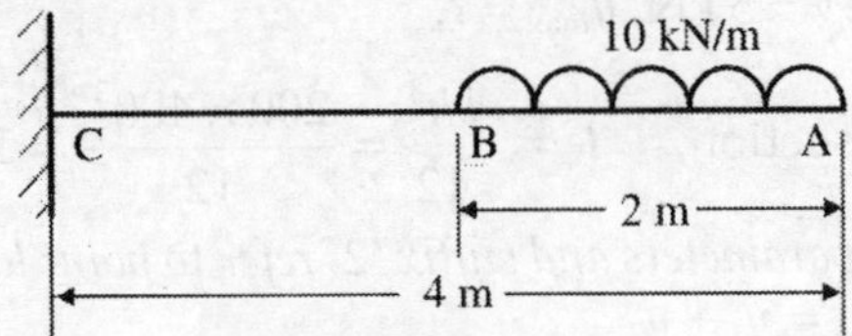

Fig. 8.14: Problem 14

Maximum parameters:

Maximum slope $\quad \theta_{max} = \theta_A = \dfrac{w}{6EI}[L^3 - (L-a)^3]$

$$= \dfrac{10 \times [4000^3 - (4000 - 2000)^3]}{6 \times (200 \times 10^3) \times (1.067 \times 10^9)}$$

$$\theta_{max} = \theta_A = 0.4374 \times 10^{-3} \text{ rad}$$

Maximum deflection $\quad y_{max} = y_A = \dfrac{w}{24EI}\{3L^4 - [(L-a)^3(3L+a)]\}$

$$= \dfrac{10 \times \{3 \times 4000^4 - [(4000 - 2000)^3 \times (3 \times 4000 + 2000)]\}}{24 \times (200 \times 10^3) \times (1.067 \times 10^9)}$$

$$y_{max} = y_A = 1.281 \text{ mm} \ \text{(Downward)}$$

Specific parameters:

Slope at B $\quad \theta_B = \dfrac{w(L-a)^3}{6EI} = \dfrac{10 \times (4000 - 2000)^3}{6 \times (200 \times 10^3) \times (1.067 \times 10^9)}$

$$= 6.25 \times 10^5 \text{ rad}$$

Deflection at B $\quad y_B = \dfrac{w(L-a)^3}{24EI}[3L+a]$

$$= \dfrac{10 \times (4000 - 2000)^3 \times (3 \times 4000 + 2000)}{24 \times (200 \times 10^3) \times (1.067 \times 10^9)}$$

$$= 0.2187 \text{ mm} \quad \text{(Downward)}$$

15. **A cantilever beam is loaded as shown in Fig. 8.15. If the cross section is rectangular of 200 mm wide by 400 mm thick, determine the deflection at the free end. Take E = 200 GPa.**

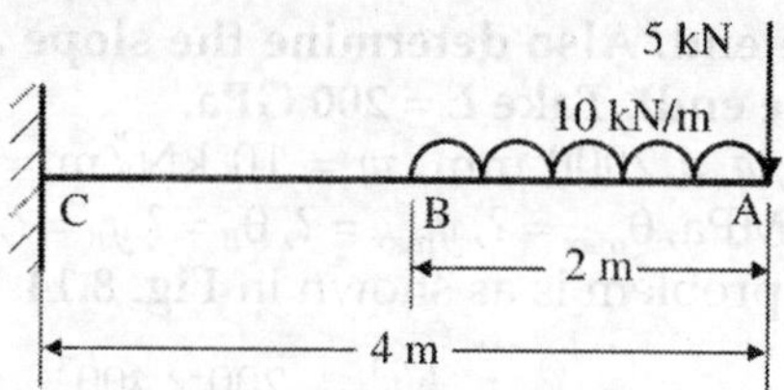

Fig. 8.15: Problem 15

Solution: L = 4000 mm, a = 2000 mm, w = 10 kN/m = 10 N/mm, b = 200 mm, h = 400 mm, E = 200 × 10^3 MPa, W = 5 kN, y_{max} = ?.

For a rectangular cross-section, $\quad I = \dfrac{bh^3}{12} = \dfrac{200 \times 400^3}{12} = 1.067 \times 10^9 \text{ mm}^4$

Let suffix '1' refer to UDL parameters and suffix '2' refer to point load parameters.

Total deflection, $\quad y_{max} = y_1 + y_2$ ... Eq. (i)

For a cantilever beam with point load at free end, maximum deflection

$$y_1 = \frac{WL^3}{3EI} = \frac{5 \times 10^3 \times 4000^3}{3 \times (200 \times 10^3) \times (1.067 \times 10^9)} = 0.5 \text{ mm}$$

For a cantilever beam with partial UDL from free end, maximum deflection

$$y_2 = \frac{w}{24EI} \{3L^4 - [(L-a)^3\,(3L+a)]\}$$

$$= \frac{10 \times \{3 \times 4000^4 - [(4000-2000)^3 \times (3 \times 4000 + 2000)]\}}{24 \times (200 \times 10^3) \times (1.067 \times 10^9)}$$

$$y_2 = 1.281 \text{ mm}$$

Eq. (i) yields ... $\quad y_{max} = 0.5 + 1.281 = 1.781 \text{ mm} \quad$ (Downward)

8.8 STANDARD CASES OF A SIMPLY SUPPORTED BEAM

8.8.1 Simply supported beam with a point load at mid-span

VTU – Mech.: June/July 2013 – 10 Marks;
Dec. 2011 – 10 Marks; June/July 2011 – 08 Marks,
June/July 2009 – 08 Marks
[Civil: June/July 2013 – 10 Marks,
Dec.12 – 04 Marks, Dec.08/Jan.09 – 06 Marks]

Fig. 8.16 indicates a simply supported beam subjected to point load at mid-span.

Let
$\quad\quad W$ = Point load
$\quad\quad L$ = Length of the beam
$\quad\quad F_n$ = Shear force at salient points
$\quad\quad M_n$ = Bending moment at salient points
$\quad\quad R_A$ = Reaction at support A
$\quad\quad R_B$ = Reaction at support B

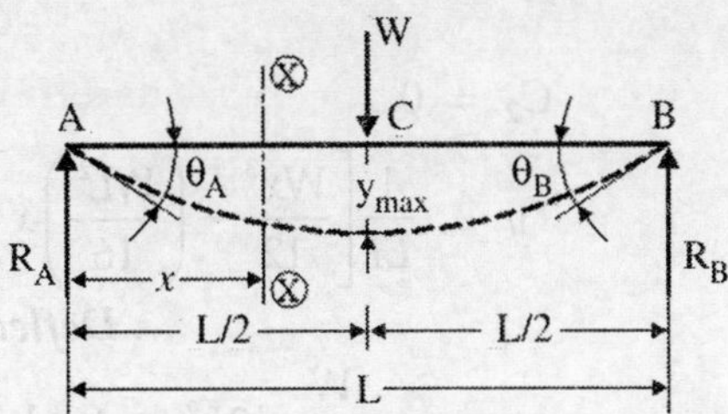

Fig. 8.16: Simply supported beam with point load at mid span

Reactions at supports:

$$R_A + R_B = W \qquad \text{... Eq. (a)}$$

Taking moments about A and equating to zero, we have

$$R_B L = W(L/2)$$

$$R_B = \frac{W}{2} \qquad \text{... Eq. (b)}$$

Substituting Eq. (b) in Eq. (a), we have

$$R_A + (W/2) = W$$

$$R_A = \frac{W}{2} \qquad \text{... Eq. (c)}$$

Here the reactions are equal as the beam is symmetrically loaded.
Consider a section X-X at a distance x from left support A.

Bending moment at X-X is $\qquad M_x = R_A \cdot x = \left(\dfrac{W}{2}\right) x \qquad$ (Positive because, sagging)

i.e. $\qquad EI \dfrac{d^2y}{dx^2} = \left(\dfrac{W}{2}\right) x$

Integrating once we have $\qquad EI \dfrac{dy}{dx} = \dfrac{Wx^2}{4} + C_1 \qquad \text{... Eq. (i)}$

Integrating again we have $\qquad EIy = \dfrac{Wx^3}{12} + C_1 x + C_2 \qquad \text{... Eq. (ii)}$

Boundary conditions:

At $x = \dfrac{L}{2}$, $\dfrac{dy}{dx} = 0$:

Eq. (i) yields... $\qquad 0 = \dfrac{WL^2}{16} + C_1$

$$C_1 = -\dfrac{WL^2}{16} \qquad \text{... Eq. (iii)}$$

Substituting C_1 in Eq. (i) we get

$$EI \dfrac{dy}{dx} = \dfrac{Wx^2}{4} - \dfrac{WL^2}{16} \qquad \text{... \textbf{\textit{Slope equation}} (Eq. 8.35a)}$$

Or $\qquad \dfrac{dy}{dx} = \theta = \dfrac{W}{16EI}(4x^2 - L^2) \qquad \text{... (Eq. 8.35b)}$

At $x = 0$, $y = 0$:

Eq. (ii) yields... $\qquad C_2 = 0 \qquad$ ... using (Eq. iii)

Eq. (ii) yields...

$$y = \frac{1}{EI}\left[\frac{Wx^3}{12} - \left(\frac{WL^2}{16}\right)x\right]$$

... *Deflection equation* (Eq. 8.36a)

Or

$$y = -\frac{W}{48EI}[3L^2x - 4x^3] \qquad \text{... (Eq. 8.36b)}$$

Maximum slope and deflection:

Maximum slope occurs at $x = 0$

(Eq. 8.35) yields...

$$\theta_A = \theta_{max} = -\frac{WL^2}{16EI} \qquad \text{... (Eq. 8.37a)}$$

Negative sign indicates that rotation from x-axis is in CW direction

Due to symmetry

$$\theta_B = \theta_{max} = \frac{WL^2}{16EI} \qquad \text{... (Eq. 8.37b)}$$

Positive sign indicates that rotation from x-axis is in CCW direction

Maximum deflection occurs at mid-span of the beam, where $x = \dfrac{L}{2}$

(Eq. 8.36) yields...

$$y_{max} = \frac{-W}{48EI}\left[3L^2\left(\frac{L}{2}\right) - 4\left(\frac{L}{2}\right)^3\right]$$

$$y_{max} = -\frac{WL^3}{48EI} \qquad \text{... (Eq. 8.38)}$$

Negative sign indicate that deflection is downwards

8.8.2 Simply supported beam subjected to eccentric point load

Fig. 8.17 indicates a simply supported beam subjected to an eccentric point load.

Let

$\qquad W \ = \ $ Point load

$\qquad L \ = \ $ Length of the beam

$\qquad F_n \ = \ $ Shear force at salient points

$\qquad M_n \ = \ $ Bending moment at salient points

$\qquad R_A \ = \ $ Reaction at support A

$\qquad R_B \ = \ $ Reaction at support B

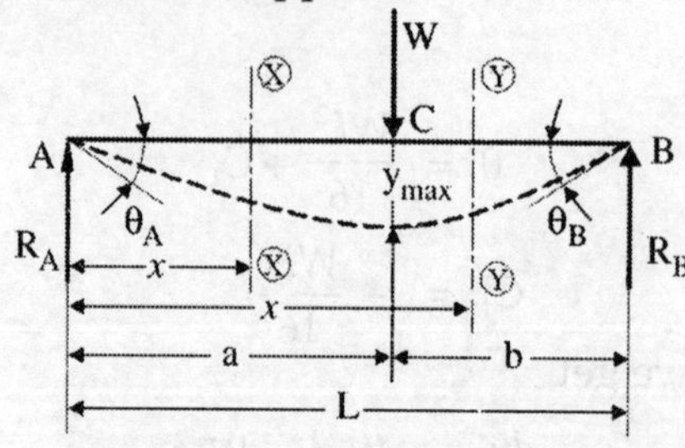

Fig. 8.17: Simply supported beam with eccentric point load

Reactions at supports:

$$R_A + R_B = W \qquad \text{... Eq. (a)}$$

Taking moments about A and equating to zero, we have

$$R_B L = Wa$$

$$R_B = \frac{Wa}{L} \qquad \qquad \text{... Eq. (b)}$$

Substituting Eq. (b) in Eq. (a), we have

$$R_A + \frac{Wa}{L} = W$$

$$R_A = W - \frac{Wa}{L} = \frac{WL - Wa}{L} = \frac{W(L-a)}{L}$$

$$R_A = \frac{Wb}{L} \qquad (\because L-a=b) \qquad \text{... Eq. (c)}$$

Region AC: $\qquad \qquad 0 < x < a$

Consider a section X-X at a distance x from end A.

Bending moment at X-X is $\qquad M_x = R_A.x = \left(\frac{Wb}{L}\right) x$ (Positive because, sagging)

i.e. $\qquad \qquad EI\dfrac{d^2y}{dx^2} = \left(\dfrac{Wb}{L}\right) x$

Integrating once we have $\qquad EI\dfrac{dy}{dx} = \dfrac{Wbx^2}{2L} + C_1 \qquad \qquad \text{... Eq. (i)}$

Integrating again we have $\qquad EIy = \dfrac{Wbx^3}{6L} + C_1 x + C_2 \qquad \qquad \text{... Eq. (ii)}$

Eqs (i) and (ii) give the slope and deflection of the beam in the portion AC only.

Region CB: $\qquad \qquad a < x < L$

Consider a section Y-Y at a distance x from left support A.

Bending moment at Y-Y is $\qquad M_x = R_A.x - W(x-a) = \left(\dfrac{Wb}{L}\right) x - W(x-a)$

i.e. $\qquad \qquad EI\dfrac{d^2y}{dx^2} = \left(\dfrac{Wb}{L}\right) x - W(x-a)$

Integrating once we have $\qquad EI\dfrac{dy}{dx} = \dfrac{Wbx^2}{2L} - \dfrac{W(x-a)^2}{2} + C_3 \qquad \qquad \text{... Eq. (iii)}$

Integrating again we have $\qquad EIy = \dfrac{Wbx^3}{6L} - \dfrac{W(x-a)^3}{6} + C_3 x + C_4 \qquad \qquad \text{... Eq. (iv)}$

Eqs (iv) and (v) give the slope and deflection of the beam in the portion CB only.

Since we have 4 constants of integration, we need 4 boundary conditions to evaluate them. The boundary conditions are:

- at $x = 0$, $y = 0$ in segment AC [in Eq. (ii)]
- at $x = L$, $y = 0$ in segment CB [in Eq. (iv)]
- at $x = a$, slope dy/dx should be same for both segments [in Eqs (i) & (iii)]
- at $x = a$, deflection y should be same for both segments [in Eqs (ii) & (iv)]

From the first condition, we have $C_2 = 0$ ... Eq. (v), using (Eq. ii)

From the second condition, $0 = \dfrac{WbL^3}{6L} - \dfrac{W(L-a)^3}{6} + C_3 L + C_4$

$$0 = \dfrac{WbL^3}{6} - \dfrac{W(L-a)^3}{6} + C_3 L + C_4$$

... Eq. (vi), using (Eq. iv)

From the third condition, $\dfrac{Wba^2}{2L} + C_1 = \dfrac{Wba^2}{2L} - 0 + C_3$ ... Eq. (vii), using Eqs (i) & (iii)

$$C_1 = C_3 \qquad\qquad \text{... Eq. (viii)}$$

From the fourth condition,

$$\dfrac{Wba^3}{6L} + C_1 a + C_2 = \dfrac{Wba^3}{6L} - \dfrac{W(a-a)^3}{6} + C_3 a + C_4 \quad \text{... Eq. (ix), using Eqs (i) & (iv)}$$

$$C_4 = 0 \qquad\qquad \text{... Eq. (x), using Eqs (v) & (viii)}$$

Substituting Eqs (viii) & (x) in Eq. (vi), yields

$$0 = \dfrac{WbL^2}{6} - \dfrac{W(L-a)^3}{6} + C_1 L + 0$$

$$C_1 L = -\dfrac{WbL^2}{6} + \dfrac{W(L-a)^3}{6}$$

$$= -\dfrac{WbL^2}{6} + \dfrac{Wb^3}{6} \qquad\qquad \text{Since } L - a = b$$

$$C_1 = \dfrac{-Wb(L^2 - b^2)}{6L} = C_3 \quad \text{... Eq. (xi), using Eq. (viii)}$$

Substituting these constants in Eqs (i) to (iv), we have
Region AC: $\qquad 0 < x < a$

Eq. (i) yields... $EI\dfrac{dy}{dx} = \dfrac{Wbx^2}{2L} - \dfrac{Wb(L^2 - b^2)}{6L} = \dfrac{-Wb(L^2 - b^2 - 3x^2)}{6L}$ ... Eq. (A)

Eq. (ii) yields... $EIy = \dfrac{Wbx^3}{6L} - \dfrac{Wbx(L^2 - b^2)}{6L} = \dfrac{-Wbx(L^2 - b^2 - x^2)}{6L}$ ... Eq. (B)

at $x = 0$, we get slope at A

Eq. (A) yields... $EI\theta_A = \dfrac{-Wb(L^2 - b^2)}{6L}$

$$\theta_A = \dfrac{-Wb(L^2 - b^2)}{6EIL} = -\dfrac{Wab(L + b)}{6EIL} \text{ (Clockwise)... (Eq. 8.39)}$$

Deflection under the load:

At $x = a$, Eq. (B) yields... $EIy_C = \dfrac{-Wba(L^2 - b^2 - a^2)}{6L}$

$$= \frac{-Wba[(L+b)(L-b)-a^2]}{6L} = \frac{-Wba[a(L+b)-a^2]}{6L}$$

$$= \frac{-Wba^2[(L+b)-a]}{6L} = \frac{-Wba^2[2b]}{6L} \qquad \text{Since } L-a=b$$

$$y_C = \frac{-Wa^2b^2}{3EIL} \qquad\qquad \ldots \text{(Eq. 8.40)}$$

Region AC: $\quad a < x < L$

Eq. (iii) yields... $\qquad EI\frac{dy}{dx} = \frac{Wbx^2}{2L} - \frac{W(x-a)^2}{2} - \frac{Wb(L^2-b^2)}{6L} \qquad \ldots \text{Eq. (C)}$

Eq. (iv) yields... $\qquad EIy = \frac{Wbx^3}{6L} - \frac{W(x-a)^3}{6} - \frac{Wbx(L^2-b^2)}{6L} \qquad \ldots \text{Eq. (D)}$

at $x = L$, we get slope at B

Eq. (C) yields... $\qquad EI\theta_B = \frac{WbL^2}{2L} - \frac{W(L-a)^2}{2} - \frac{Wb(L^2-b^2)}{6L}$

$$= \frac{WbL}{2} - \frac{Wb^2}{2} - \frac{Wb(L^2-b^2)}{6L} \qquad \text{Since } b=L-a$$

$$= Wb\left[\frac{L}{2} - \frac{b}{2} - \frac{(L^2-b^2)}{6L}\right]$$

$$= Wb\left[\frac{a+b}{2} - \frac{b}{2} - \frac{(L+b)(L-b)}{6L}\right] \qquad \text{Since } L=a+b$$

$$= Wb\left[\frac{a+b}{2} - \frac{b}{2} - \frac{a(L+b)}{6L}\right]$$

$$= Wb\left[\frac{a}{2} - \frac{a}{6} - \frac{ab}{6L}\right] = Wb\left[\frac{a}{3} - \frac{ab}{6L}\right]$$

$$= \frac{Wab}{6L}[2L-b)] = \frac{Wab}{6L}[L+(L-b)]$$

$$\therefore \quad \theta_B = \frac{Wab(L+a)}{6EIL} = \frac{Wa(L^2-a^2)}{6EIL}$$

$$\text{(Counter clockwise)} \qquad \ldots \text{(Eq. 8.41)}$$

Maximum deflection: This depends upon the values of a and b.

If $a > b$, then maximum deflection occurs in segment AC.

If $a < b$, then maximum deflection occurs in segment CB.

Consider $a > b$.

For maximum deflection $\frac{dy}{dx} = 0$

From Eq. (A) we have
$$0 = \frac{-Wb(L^2 - b^2 - 3x^2)}{6L}$$
$$0 = L^2 - b^2 - 3x^2$$
$$x = \sqrt{\frac{L^2 - b^2}{3}} \qquad \text{... (Eq. 8.42)}$$

From Eq. (B), we have
$$EIy_{max} = \left(\frac{-Wb}{6L}\right)\left(\sqrt{\frac{L^2 - b^2}{3}}\right)\left[\left(L^2 - b^2\right) - \frac{L^2 - b^2}{3}\right]$$
$$= \left(\frac{-Wb}{6L}\right)\left(\sqrt{\frac{L^2 - b^2}{3}}\right)\left[\frac{2\left(L^2 - b^2\right)}{3}\right] = \frac{-Wb}{9L}\left(\frac{L^2 - b^2}{3}\right)^{3./2}$$
$$y_{max} = \frac{-Wb(L^2 - b^2)^{3/2}}{9\sqrt{3}EIL} \qquad \text{... (Eq. 8.43)}$$

Negative sign indicate that deflection is downwards

Note: From the above derivation, it is observed that for a single eccentric point load, the double integration method is too complex. Now if there are two concentrated loads, then there would be 3 segments and 6 constants on integration; further we would require 6 conditions to evaluate these constants, which in turn increases the complexity of the problem. For this reason Double integration method is not preferred.

8.8.3 Simply supported beam with uniformly distributed load (UDL) over entire span

VTU – Mech.: Dec. 16/Jan. 17 – 10 Marks,
June/July 2013- 10 Marks, June/July 2014 – 10 Marks,
June/July 2008 – 05 Marks
[Civil: VTU – Dec.13/Jan.14 – 08 Marks, Dec.13/
Jan.14 – 06 Marks, Dec.07/Jan.08 – 14 Marks]

Fig. 8.18 indicates a simply supported beam subjected to UDL over the entire span.

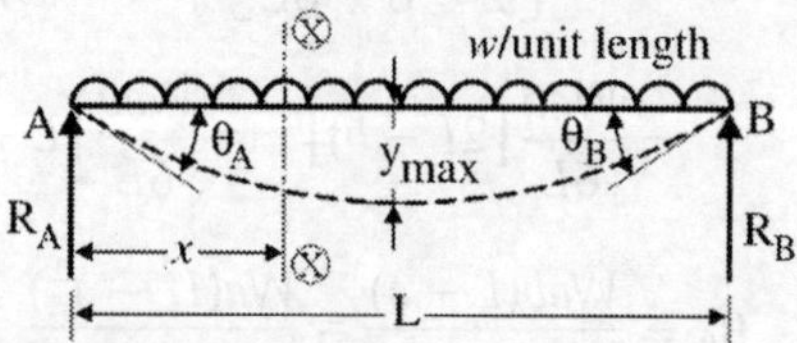

Fig. 8.18: Simply supported beam with UDL over entire span

Let
    w = Uniformly distributed load per unit length
    L = Length of the beam
    F_n = Shear force at salient points
    M_n = Bending moment at salient points
    R_A = Reaction at support A
    R_B = Reaction at support B

Reactions at supports:
$$R_A + R_B = wL \qquad \text{... Eq. (a)}$$

Taking moments about A and equating to zero, we have

$$R_B L = wL \left(\frac{1}{2}\right)$$

$$R_B = \frac{wL}{2} \qquad \qquad \text{... Eq. (b)}$$

Substituting Eq. (b) in Eq. (a), we have

$$R_A + \frac{wL}{2} = wL$$

$$R_A = \frac{wL}{2} \qquad \qquad \text{... Eq. (iii)}$$

Here the reactions are equal as the beam is symmetrically loaded.
Consider a section X-X at a distance x from free end A.

Shear force at X-X is
$$F_x = R_A - wx = \left(\frac{wL}{2}\right) - wx$$

Bending moment at X-X is
$$M_x = R_A.x - wx\left(\frac{x}{2}\right) = \left(\frac{wL}{2}\right)x - \left(\frac{wx^2}{2}\right)$$

i.e.
$$EI\frac{d^2y}{dx^2} = \left(\frac{wL}{2}\right)x - \left(\frac{wx^2}{2}\right)$$

Integrating once we have
$$EI\frac{dy}{dx} = \frac{wLx^2}{4} - \left(\frac{wx^3}{6}\right) + C_1 \qquad \text{... Eq. (i)}$$

Integrating again we have
$$EIy = \frac{wLx^3}{12} - \left(\frac{wx^4}{24}\right) + C_1 x + C_2 \qquad \text{... Eq. (ii)}$$

Boundary conditions:

At $x = \dfrac{L}{2}, \dfrac{dy}{dx} = 0$:

Eq. (i) yields...
$$0 = \left(\frac{wL}{4}\right)\left(\frac{L}{2}\right)^2 - \left(\frac{w}{6}\right)\left(\frac{L}{2}\right)^3 + C_1$$

$$C_1 = -\frac{wL^3}{24} \qquad \qquad \text{... Eq. (iii)}$$

Substituting C_1 in Eq. (i) we get

$$EI\frac{dy}{dx} = \frac{wLx^2}{4} - \left(\frac{wx^3}{6}\right) - \left(\frac{wL^3}{24}\right)$$

$$\text{... } \textit{Slope equation} \text{ (Eq. 8.44a)}$$

Or
$$\frac{dy}{dx} = \theta = \frac{w}{24EI}\left(6Lx^2 - 4x^3 - L^3\right) \qquad \text{... (Eq. 8.44b)}$$

At $x = 0$, $y = 0$:

Eq. (ii) yields... $\qquad\qquad C_2 = 0$ $\qquad\qquad\qquad$ ... using (Eq. iii)

Eq. (ii) yields... $\qquad EIy = \left[\dfrac{wLx^3}{12} - \left(\dfrac{wx^4}{24} \right) - \left(\dfrac{wL^3}{24} \right) x \right]$

$\qquad\qquad\qquad\qquad\qquad\qquad\qquad$ ... ***Deflection equation*** (Eq. 8.45a)

Or $\qquad\qquad\qquad\qquad y = \dfrac{-wx}{24EI} \left[L^3 - 2Lx^2 + x^3 \right]$ $\qquad$ ... (Eq. 8.45b)

Maximum slope and deflection:
Maximum slope occurs at $x = 0$

(Eq. 8.44) yields... $\qquad\qquad \theta_A = \theta_{\max} = - \dfrac{wL^3}{24EI}$ $\qquad\qquad$ ... (Eq. 8.46a)

$\qquad$ *Negative sign indicates that rotation from x-axis is in CW direction*

Due to symmetry $\qquad\qquad \theta_B = \theta_{\max} = \dfrac{wL^3}{24EI}$ $\qquad\qquad$ ... (Eq. 8.46b)

$\qquad$ *Positive sign indicates that rotation from x-axis is in CCW direction*

Maximum deflection occurs at mid-span of the beam, where $x = \dfrac{L}{2}$

(Eq. 8.45) yields... $\qquad y_{\max} = \left(\dfrac{-w}{24EI} \right)\left(\dfrac{L}{2} \right)\left[L^3 - 2L\left(\dfrac{L}{2} \right)^2 + \left(\dfrac{L}{2} \right)^3 \right]$

$\qquad\qquad\qquad\qquad\qquad y_{\max} = - \dfrac{5wL^4}{384EI}$ $\qquad\qquad\qquad$ ... (Eq. 8.47)

$\qquad$ *Negative sign indicate that deflection is downwards*

16. **A beam 3 m long, simply supported at its ends, is carrying a load W at the center. If the slope at the ends of the beam should not exceed 1°, find the deflection at the center of the beam.**

$\qquad\qquad\qquad\qquad\qquad\qquad\qquad$ *VTU – June/July 2013 (CV) – 06 Marks*

Solution: $L = 3000$ mm, $\theta = \theta_{\max} = 1° = 0.0175$ rad, $y_{\max} = ?$.

Slope at the supports $\qquad\qquad \theta_A = \theta_{\max} = \dfrac{WL^2}{16EI}$

$\qquad\qquad\qquad\qquad 0.0175 = \dfrac{WL^2}{16EI}$ $\qquad\qquad\qquad$ ... Eq. (i)

Maximum deflection $\qquad\qquad y_{\max} = \dfrac{WL^3}{48EI}$ $\qquad\qquad\qquad$ ... Eq. (ii)

Dividing Eq. (ii) by Eq. (i), we have

$\qquad\qquad\qquad \dfrac{y_{\max}}{0.0175} = \left(\dfrac{WL^3}{48EI} \right)\left(\dfrac{16EI}{WL^2} \right) = \dfrac{L}{3}$

$$y_{max} = \left(\frac{3000}{3}\right) \times 0.0175$$

$$y_{max} = 17.5\,\text{mm}$$

17. Determine the maximum slope and deflection for a simply supported beam of span 4 m carrying a UDL of 40 kN/m over the entire span. Take E = 200 GPa, I = 80 × 10^6 mm^4. Also determine the deflection at every 0.5 m

Solution: w = 40 kN/m = 40 N/mm, L = 4000 mm, θ_{max} = ?, y_{max} = ?, E = 200 × 10^3 MPa, I = 80 × 10^6 mm^4

For a simply supported beam with UDL over entire span

$$\text{Maximum slope } \theta_A = \theta_B = \theta_{max} = \frac{wL^3}{24EI} = \frac{40 \times 4000^3}{24 \times (200 \times 10^3) \times (80 \times 10^6)} = 0.0067\,\text{rad}$$

$$\text{Maximum deflection } y_{max} = \frac{5wL^4}{384EI} = \frac{5 \times 40 \times 4000^4}{384 \times (200 \times 10^3) \times (80 \times 10^6)} = 8.33\,\text{mm}$$

(Downward)

Displacement at every 0.5 m:

Distance from left support	Deflection
x	$y = \dfrac{-wx}{24EI}\left[x^3 - 2Lx^2 + x^3\right]$
mm	mm
0	0.0000
500	−3.236
1000	−5.938
1500	−7.715
2000	−8.333
2500	−7.715
3000	−5.938
3500	−3.236
4000	0.0000

18. A beam of uniform rectangular section 250 mm wide and 350 mm deep is simply supported at its ends. It carries an UDL of 12 kN/m over the entire span of 6m. If E = 1 × 10^4 N/mm^2, find

(a) Slope at the supports   (b) maximum deflection

VTU – (CV) June 2012 – 12 Marks

Solution: b = 250 mm, h = 350 mm, w = 12 kN/m = 12 N/mm, L = 6000 mm, E = 1 × 10^4 MPa, θ_{max} = ?, y_{max} = ?.

$$\text{Moment of inertia } I = \frac{bh^3}{12} = \frac{250 \times 350^3}{12} = 8.93 \times 10^8\,\text{mm}^4$$

For a simply supported beam with UDL over entire span

a. *Slope at the supports* $\theta_A = \theta_B = \theta_{max} = \dfrac{wL^3}{24EI}$

$$= \frac{12 \times 6000^3}{24 \times (1 \times 10^4) \times (8.93 \times 10^8)} = 0.0121\,\text{rad}$$

b. *Maximum deflection*
$$y_{max} = \frac{5wL^4}{384EI} = \frac{5 \times 12 \times 6000^4}{384 \times (1 \times 10^4) \times (8.93 \times 10^8)}$$
$$= 22.67 \text{ mm (Downward)}$$

19. A simply supported beam of span 6m is subjected to a concentrated load of 25 kN acting at mid-span and a uniformly distributed load of 10 kN/m over the entire span. If $E = 200 \times 10^3$ MPa, $I = 150 \times 10^6$ mm^4, determine:

(a) Maximum slope   (b) maximum deflection.

Solution: $L = 6000$ mm, $W = 25 \times 10^3$ N, $w = 10$ kN/m $= 10$ N/mm, $E = 200 \times 10^3$ MPa, $I = 150 \times 10^6$ mm^4, $\theta_{max} = ?$, $y_{max} = ?$.

Based on given data, the problem is as shown in **Fig. 8.19**

Let suffix '1' refer to point load parameters and suffix '2' refer to UDL parameters.

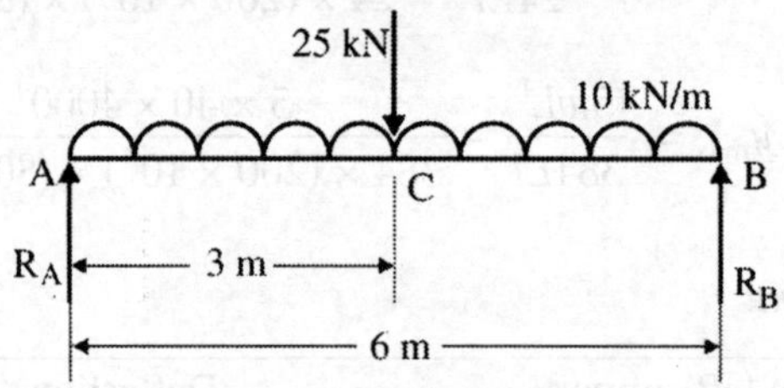

Fig. 8.19: Problem 19

Using the principal of superposition,

a. *Total slope:* $\theta_{max} = \theta_1 + \theta_2$ ... Eq. (i)

For a simply supported beam with point load at mid- span

$$\theta_1 = \frac{WL^2}{16EI} = \frac{25 \times 10^3 \times 6000^2}{16 \times (200 \times 10^3) \times (150 \times 10^6)} = 0.001875 \text{ rad}$$

For a simply supported beam with UDL over entire span

$$\theta_2 = \frac{wL^3}{24EI} = \frac{10 \times 6000^3}{24 \times (200 \times 10^3) \times (150 \times 10^6)} = 0.003 \text{ rad}$$

Eq. (i) yields ... $\theta_{max} = 0.001875 + 0.003 = 0.004875$ mm (Downward)

b. *Total deflection:* $y_{max} = y_1 + y_2$ ... Eq. (ii)

For a simply supported beam with point load at mid – span

$$y_1 = \frac{WL^3}{48EI} = \frac{25 \times 10^3 \times 6000^3}{48 \times (200 \times 10^3) \times (150 \times 10^6)} = 3.75 \text{ mm}$$

For a simply supported beam with UDL over entire span

$$y_2 = \frac{5wL^4}{384EI} = \frac{5 \times 10 \times 6000^4}{384 \times (200 \times 10^3) \times (150 \times 10^6)} = 5.625 \text{ mm}$$

Eq. (ii) yields ... $y_{max} = 3.75 + 5.625 = 9.375$ mm   (Downward)

20. A beam of length 5 m and of uniform rectangular section is simply supported at its ends. It carries a uniformly distributed load of 9 kN/m run over the entire length. Calculate the width and depth of the beam if permissible bending stress is 7 N/mm^2 and central deflection is not to exceed 1 cm. Take $E = 1 \times 10^4$ N/mm^2.

VTU – Dec. 14/Jan. 15 – 10 Marks, June/July 2014 – 10 Marks

Solution: $L = 5000$ mm, $w = 9$ kN/m $= 9$ N/mm, $b = ?$, $h = ?$, $\sigma = 7$ N/mm², $y = 10$ mm, $E = 1 \times 10^4$ N/mm².

Bending stress
$$\sigma = \frac{M}{Z} \qquad \text{... Eq. (i)}$$

For a simply supported beam with UDL over entire span

$$M = \frac{wL^2}{8} = \frac{9 \times 5000^2}{8} = 28.125 \times 10^6 \text{ N-mm}$$

Section modulus
$$Z = \frac{I}{c} = \frac{bh^2}{6}$$

Eq. (i) yields...
$$7 = \frac{28.125 \times 10^6}{bh^2 / 6}$$

$$bh^2 = 24.107 \times 10^6 \text{ mm}^3 \qquad \text{... Eq. (ii)}$$

For a simply supported beam with UDL over entire span

$$y_{max} = \frac{5wL^4}{384EI}$$

$$10 = \frac{5 \times 9 \times 5000^4}{384 \times (1 \times 10^4) \times (bh^3/12)}$$

$$bh^3 = 8.79 \times 10^9 \text{ mm}^4 \qquad \text{... Eq. (iii)}$$

Eq. (iii) divided by Eq. (ii) yields

$$\frac{bh^3}{bh^2} = \frac{8.79 \times 10^9}{24.107 \times 10^6}$$

$$h = 363.67 \text{ mm} \approx 365 \text{ mm}$$

Eq. (ii) yields...
$$b = \frac{24.107 \times 10^6}{365^2} = 181 \text{ mm}$$

21. **A steel girder of length 6 m acting as a beam carries a UDL of w N/m run throughout its length as shown in Fig. 8.20. If $I = 30 \times 10^{-6}$ m⁴ and depth is 270 mm, calculate:**
    (a) **Magnitude of w so that the maximum stress developed in the beam section does not exceed 72 MPa,**
    (b) **The slope and deflection in the beam at a distance of 1.8 m from one end. Take $E = 200$ GPa.**

VTU – June/July 2009 – 12 Marks

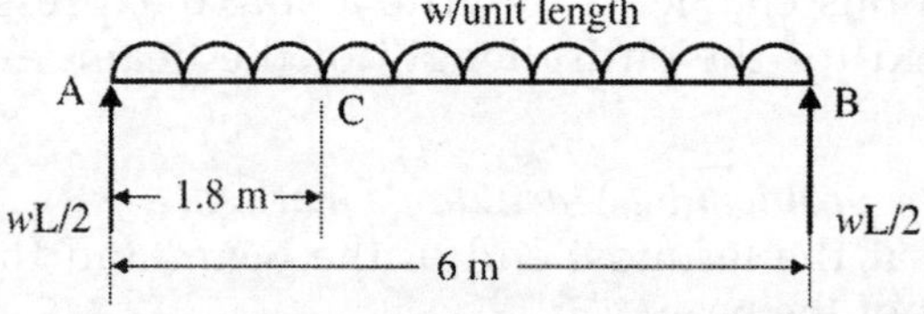

Fig. 8.20: Problem 21

Solution: $L = 6000$ mm, $I = 30 \times 10^{-6}$ m^4, $= 30 \times 10^6$ mm^4, $h = 270$ mm, $E = 2 \times 10^5$ MPa.

a) $w = ?$, $\sigma = 72$ MPa

b) $\theta_C = ?$, $y_C = ?$

a) *To find w:*

Bending stress $\qquad\qquad\qquad \sigma = \dfrac{M}{Z}$ $\qquad\qquad\qquad\qquad$ ... Eq. (i)

For a simply supported beam with UDL over entire span

$$M = \frac{wL^2}{8} = \frac{w \times 6000^2}{8} = (4.5 \times 10^6)w \text{ N-mm}$$

Section modulus $\qquad\qquad Z = \dfrac{I}{c} = \dfrac{30 \times 10^6}{270/2} = 222.22 \times 10^3 \text{ mm}^3$

$$\text{Here } c = y_{max} = h/2$$

Eq. (i) yields... $\qquad\qquad\qquad 72 = \dfrac{(4.5 \times 10^6)w}{222.22 \times 10^3}$

$$w = 3.556 \text{ N/mm} = 3.556 \text{ kN/m}$$

b) *To find* θ_C, y_C:

Slope equation $\qquad\qquad \theta = \dfrac{w}{24EI}(6Lx^2 - 4x^3 - L^3)$ $\quad$ ... using (Eq. 8.44b)

At $x = 1800$ mm, we have

$$\theta_C = \frac{3.556}{24 \times (2 \times 10^5) \times (30 \times 10^6)}[(6 \times 6000 \times 1800^2) - (4 \times 1800^3) - 6000^3]$$

$$\theta_C = -3.03 \times 10^{-3} \text{ rad}$$

Negative sign indicates that rotation from x-axis is in CW direction

Deflection equation $y = \dfrac{-wx}{24EI}[L^3 - 2Lx^2 + x^3]$

At C, $x = 1800$ mm, we have

$$y_C = \frac{-3.556 \times 1800}{24 \times (2 \times 10^5) \times (30 \times 10^6)}[6000^3 - (2 \times 6000 \times 1800^2) + 1800^3]$$

$$y_C = -8.13 \text{ mm} \qquad\qquad\qquad\qquad\qquad\qquad \text{(Downward)}$$

8.9 MACAULAY'S METHOD OR MACAULAY'S BRACKET FUNCTION OR METHOD OF SINGULARITY FUNCTIONS

Double Integration method is suitable for beams with single load, while Macaulay's method is suitable for beams with several loads. In Macaulay's method a single equation is formed for all loading on a beam. The equation is constructed in such a way that the constant of Integration apply to all portions of the beam. This *method is also called method of singularity functions or discontinuity functions.* Discontinuity functions enable us to write a single expression for the bending moment that is valid for the entire length of the beam, even if the loading is discontinuous.

Procedure to solve the problem by Macaulay's method:
- Take the origin at the leftmost end of the beam and the section in the last portion/segment of the beam.

- Write down the moment equation which is valid for all values of x, by taking a section between the last load and the other extreme end (*where* $x = L$), this must contain brackets $\langle ... \rangle$.

- Integrate the bracket terms $\langle x - a \rangle$ as follows:

  i.e. $\int \langle x - a \rangle \, dx$ will be $\dfrac{\langle x - a \rangle^2}{2} + C$ and not $\left(\dfrac{x^2}{2} - ax \right)$

- Obtains the constants of integration using boundary conditions. These constants are valid for all values of x.

- Depending on the value of x, if the term $\langle x - a \rangle$ is negative, the term should be neglected; i.e. if the expression $\langle ... \rangle$ becomes – ve after substituting the value of x, the term containing the factor $\langle x - a \rangle^n$ is to be omitted.

Example: Consider a simply supported beam subjected to loading as shown in **Fig. 8.21.**

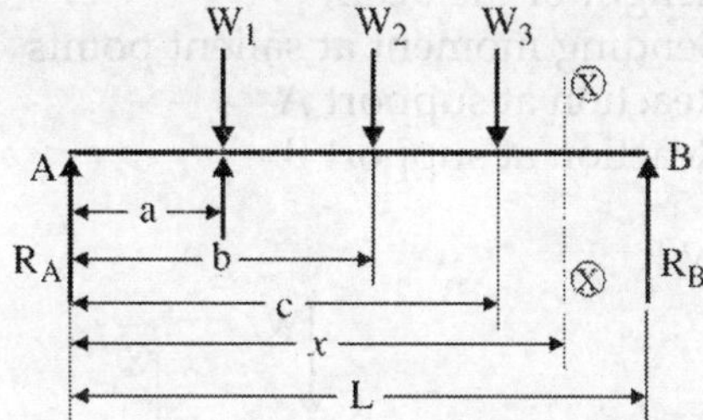

Fig. 8.21: Simply supported beam with point loads [Macaulay's method]

Consider a section X-X at a distance x from left support A such that it covers all the loads in the beam.

$$M_x = R_A.x \qquad \text{for } 0 < x < a$$
$$M_x = R_A.x - W_1(x - a) \qquad \text{for } a < x < b$$
$$M_x = R_A.x - W_1(x - a) - W_2(x - b) \qquad \text{for } b < x < c$$
$$M_x = R_A.x - W_1(x - a) - W_2(x - b) - W_3(x - c) \qquad \text{for } c < x < L$$

Thus for the entire beam,

$$M_x = R_A.x - W_1(x - a) - W_2(x - b) - W_3(x - c) \qquad ... \text{Eq. (i)}$$

In the above equation, it is to be noted that the term $(x - a)$ disappears when $x = a$, $(x - b)$ disappears when $x = b$ and $(x - c)$ disappears when $x \leq c$.

Using bracket functions, the bending moment equation for the beam is

$$M_x = R_A.\langle x \rangle - W_1 \langle x - a \rangle - W_2 \langle x - b \rangle - W_3 \langle x - c \rangle$$

i.e. $$EI \frac{d^2 y}{dx^2} = R_A.\langle x \rangle - W_1 \langle x - a \rangle - W_2 \langle x - b \rangle - W_3 \langle x - c \rangle \qquad ... \text{(Eq. 8.48a)}$$

Eq. (8.48a) is valid over the entire length of the beam and is called the *global bending moment equation* for the beam. Its integrals, representing the slope and deflection of the beam, are continuous functions. Thus, double integration of Eq. (8.48a) automatically assures continuity of deformation.

Integrating the above equation we have

$$EI\frac{dy}{dx} = R_A\frac{\langle x\rangle^2}{2} + C_1 - \frac{W_1\langle x-a\rangle^2}{2} - \frac{W_2\langle x-b\rangle^2}{2} - \frac{W_3\langle x-c\rangle^2}{2} \quad \ldots \text{(Eq. 8.48b)}$$

C_1 is the integration constant and should be written after the first term Integrating again we have

$$EIy = R_A\frac{\langle x\rangle^3}{6} + C_1x + C_2 - \frac{W_1\langle x-a\rangle^3}{6} - \frac{W_2\langle x-b\rangle^3}{6} - \frac{W_3\langle x-c\rangle^3}{6}$$

$$\ldots \text{(Eq. 8.48c)}$$

C_2 is the integration constant and should be written after $C_1\,x$

The constants of integration C_1 and C_2 are valid for all values of x and are obtained using boundary conditions.

8.9.1 Simply supported beam with an eccentric point load

Fig. 8.22 indicates a simply supported beam subjected to an eccentric point load.

Let
$\quad W$ = Point load
$\quad L$ = Length of the beam
$\quad M_n$ = Bending moment at salient points
$\quad R_A$ = Reaction at support A
$\quad R_B$ = Reaction at support B

Reactions at supports:
$$R_A + R_B = W \qquad\qquad \ldots \text{Eq. (a)}$$

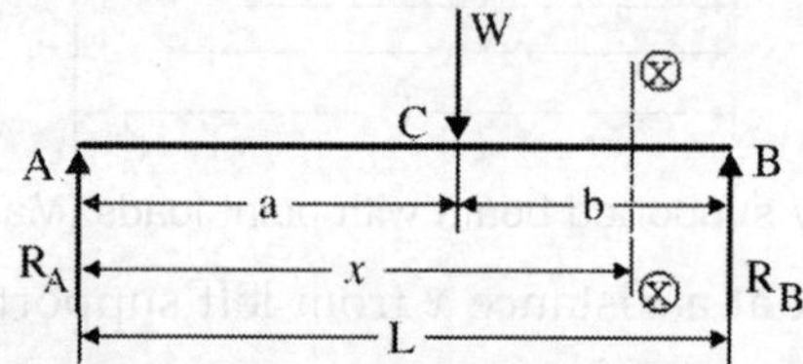

Fig. 8.22: SS beam with eccentric point load [Macaulay's method]

Taking moments about A and equating to zero, we have
$$R_B L = Wa$$
$$R_B = \frac{Wa}{L} \qquad\qquad \ldots \text{Eq. (b)}$$

Substituting Eq. (b) in Eq. (a), we have

$$R_A + \frac{Wa}{L} = W$$

$$R_A = W - \frac{Wa}{L} = \frac{WL - Wa}{L} = \frac{W(L-a)}{L}$$

$$R_A = \frac{Wb}{L} \qquad (\because \quad L - a = b) \qquad \ldots \text{Eq. (c)}$$

Consider a section X-X at a distance x from end A.

$$M_x = R_A.x - W(x-a) = \left(\frac{Wb}{L}\right)x - W(x-a)$$

i.e. $\qquad EI\dfrac{d^2y}{dx^2} = \left(\dfrac{Wb}{L}\right)x - W(x-a)$

Using bracket functions, the bending moment equation for the beam is

$$EI\dfrac{d^2y}{dx^2} = \left(\dfrac{Wb}{L}\right)\langle x\rangle - W\langle x-a\rangle$$

Integrating once we have $\quad EI\dfrac{dy}{dx} = \dfrac{Wb\langle x\rangle^2}{2L} + C_1 - \dfrac{W\langle x-a\rangle^2}{2}$ $\qquad$ ... Eq. (i)

Integrating again we have $\quad EIy = \dfrac{Wb\langle x\rangle^3}{6L} + C_1\langle x\rangle + C_2 - \dfrac{W\langle x-a\rangle^3}{6}$ $\qquad$ ... Eq. (ii)

Boundary conditions:

At $x = 0$, $y = 0$: Eq. (ii) yields... $\quad 0 = 0 + 0 + C_2 - \dfrac{W\langle 0-a\rangle^3}{6}$

$$C_2 = 0$$

$$\text{Ignore brackets containing negative value} \quad \text{... Eq. (iii)}$$

At $x = L$, $y = 0$: Eq. (ii) yields... $\quad 0 = \dfrac{WbL^3}{6L} + C_1 L + 0 - \dfrac{W\langle L-a\rangle^3}{6}$

$$C_1 L = -\dfrac{WbL^2}{6} + \dfrac{W\langle L-a\rangle^3}{6}$$

$$= -\dfrac{WbL^2}{6} + \dfrac{Wb^3}{6} \qquad (\because \;\; L-a = b)$$

$$C_1 = -\dfrac{Wb\left(L^2-b^2\right)}{6L} \qquad \text{... Eq. (iv)}$$

Substituting C_1 in Eq. (i) we get

$$EI\dfrac{dy}{dx} = \dfrac{Wb\langle x\rangle^2}{2L} - \dfrac{Wb(L^2-b^2)}{6L} - \dfrac{W\langle x-a\rangle^2}{2}$$

$$\text{... } \textbf{\textit{Slope equation}} \text{ (Eq. 8.49)}$$
$$\text{Same as Eq. (C) under Sec. 8.8.2}$$

Substituting C_1 and C_2 in Eq. (ii) we get

$$EIy = \dfrac{Wb\langle x\rangle^3}{6L} - \left[\dfrac{Wb\left(L^2-b^2\right)}{6L}\right]\langle x\rangle - \dfrac{W\langle x-a\rangle^3}{6}$$

$$\text{... } \textbf{\textit{Deflection equation}} \text{ (Eq. 8.50)}$$
$$\text{Same as Eq. (D) under Sec. 8.8.2}$$

At $x = 0$, we get slope at A

(Eq. 8.49) yields... $\qquad EI\theta_A = 0 - \dfrac{Wb(L^2-b^2)}{6L} - \dfrac{W\langle 0-a\rangle^2}{2}$

$$\text{Ignore brackets containing negative value}$$

$$\theta_A = -\frac{Wb(L^2 - b^2)}{6EIL} = -\frac{Wab(L + b)^2}{6EIL} \quad \text{(Clockwise)}$$

... (Eq. 8.51)

Same as (Eq. 8.39)

At $x = L$, we get slope at B

(Eq. 8.49) yields...

$$EI\theta_B = \frac{WbL^2}{2L} - \frac{Wb(L^2 - b^2)}{6L} - \frac{W\langle L - a\rangle^2}{2}$$

$$= \frac{WbL}{2} - \frac{Wb(L^2 - b^2)}{6L} - \frac{Wb^2}{2} \quad \text{Since } L - a = b$$

$$= Wb\left[\frac{L}{2} - \frac{b}{2} - \frac{(L^2 - b^2)}{6L}\right]$$

$$= Wb\left[\frac{a + b}{2} - \frac{b}{2} - \frac{(L + b)(L - b)}{6L}\right]$$

Since $L = a + b$

$$= Wb\left[\frac{a + b}{2} - \frac{b}{2} - \frac{a(L + b)}{6L}\right]$$

$$= Wb\left[\frac{a}{2} - \frac{a}{6} - \frac{ab}{6L}\right] = Wb\left[\frac{a}{3} - \frac{ab}{6L}\right]$$

$$= \frac{Wab}{6L}[2L - b] \quad = \frac{Wab}{6L}[L + (L - b)]$$

$$\theta_B = \frac{Wab(L + a)}{6EIL} = \frac{Wa(L^2 - a^2)}{6EIL}$$

(Counter clockwise)   ... (Eq. 8.52)

Same as (Eq. 8.41)

Deflection under the load:
at $x = a$, we get deflection under the load

(Eq. 8.50) yields...

$$EIy_C = \frac{Wba^3}{6L} - \left[\frac{Wb(L^2 - b^2)}{6}\right]a - 0$$

$$= \frac{-Wba[(L + b)(L - b) - a^2]}{6L} = \frac{-Wba[a(L + b) - a^2]}{6L}$$

$$= \frac{-Wba^2[(L + b) - a]}{6L} = \frac{-Wba^2[2b]}{6L} \quad \text{Since } L - a = b$$

$$y_C = \frac{-Wa^2b^2}{3EIL}$$

... (Eq. 8.53)

Same as (Eq. 8.40)

Maximum deflection: Maximum deflection may be obtained as discussed under Sec. 8.8.2

i.e.
$$y_{max} = \frac{-Wb(L^2 - b^2)^{3/2}}{9\sqrt{3}EIL}$$

Negative sign indicate that deflection is downwards

8.9.2 Simply supported beam with uniformly distributed load over entire span

VTU – (CV) Jan. 2013 – 10 Marks

Fig. 8.23 indicates a simply supported beam subjected to UDL over the entire span.

Let w = Uniformly distributed load per unit length
          L = Length of the beam
          F_n = Shear force at salient points
          M_n = Bending moment at salient points
          R_A = Reaction at support A
          R_B = Reaction at support B

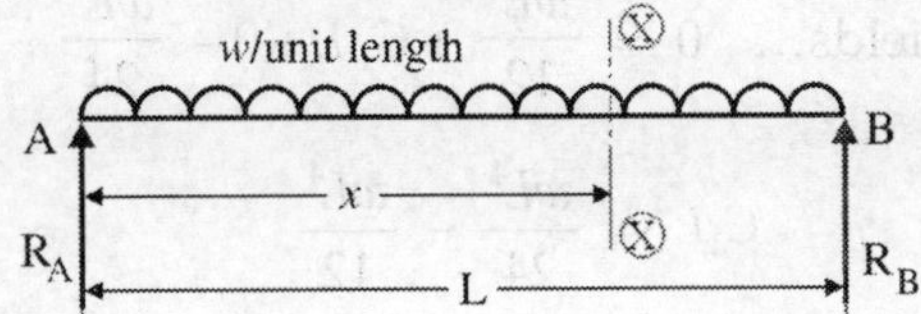

Fig. 8.23: SS beam with UDL over entire span [Macaulay's method]

Reactions at supports:
$$R_A + R_B = wL \qquad \text{... Eq. (a)}$$
Taking moments about A and equating to zero, we have

$$R_B L = wL\left(\frac{L}{2}\right)$$

$$R_B = \frac{wL}{2} \qquad \text{... Eq. (b)}$$

Substituting Eq. (b) in Eq. (a), we have

$$R_A + \frac{wL}{2} = wL$$

$$R_A = \frac{wL}{2} \qquad \text{... Eq. (c)}$$

Here the reactions are equal as the beam is symmetrically loaded.
Consider a section X-X at a distance x from free end A.

Shear force at X-X is
$$F_x = R_A - wx = \left(\frac{wL}{2}\right) - wx$$

Bending moment at X-X is
$$M_x = R_A.x - wx\left(\frac{x}{2}\right) = \left(\frac{wL}{2}\right)x - \left(\frac{wx^2}{2}\right)$$

i.e.
$$EI\frac{d^2y}{dx^2} = \left(\frac{wL}{2}\right)x - \left(\frac{wx^2}{2}\right)$$

Using bracket functions, the bending moment equation for the beam is

$$EI\frac{d^2y}{dx^2} = \left(\frac{wL}{2}\right)\langle x \rangle - \frac{w\langle x \rangle^2}{2}$$

Integrating once we have $\quad EI\frac{dy}{dx} = \frac{wL\langle x \rangle^2}{4} + C_1 - \frac{w\langle x \rangle^3}{6}$ $\qquad$ ... Eq. (i)

Integrating again we have $\quad EIy = \frac{wL\langle x \rangle^3}{12} + C_1\langle x \rangle + C_2 - \frac{w\langle x \rangle^4}{24}$ $\qquad$ ... Eq. (ii)

Boundary conditions:

At $x = 0$, $y = 0$: Eq. (ii) yields... $\quad 0 = 0 + 0 + C_2 - \frac{w\langle 0 - a \rangle^3}{6}$

$$C_2 = 0$$

[Ignore brackets containing negative value] $\qquad$ ... Eq. (iii)

At $x = L$, $y = 0$: Eq. (ii) yields... $\quad 0 = \frac{wL^4}{12} + C_1 L + 0 - \frac{wL^4}{24}$

$$C_1 L = \frac{wL^4}{24} - \frac{wL^4}{12}$$

$$C_1 = \frac{wL^3}{24} - \frac{wL^3}{12}$$

$$C_1 = -\frac{wL^3}{24} \qquad \text{... Eq. (iv)}$$

Substituting C_1 in Eq. (i) we get

$$EI\frac{dy}{dx} = \frac{wL\langle x \rangle^2}{4} - \frac{wL^3}{24} - \frac{w\langle x \rangle^3}{6}$$

$\qquad$ ... ***Slope equation*** (Eq. 8.54)
$\qquad$ Same as (Eq. 8.44a)

Substituting C_1 and C_2 in Eq. (ii) we get

$$EIy = \frac{wL\langle x \rangle^3}{12} - \frac{wL^3}{24}\langle x \rangle - \frac{w\langle x \rangle^4}{24}$$

$\qquad$ ... ***Deflection equation*** (Eq. 8.55)
$\qquad$ Same as (Eq. 8.45a)

At $x = 0$, we get slope at A

(Eq. 8.54) yields... $\qquad EI\theta_A = -\frac{wL^3}{24}$

$$\theta_A = -\frac{wL^3}{24EI} \qquad \text{(Clockwise)} \qquad \text{... (Eq. 8.56a)}$$

$\qquad$ Same as (Eq. 8.46a)

At $x = L$, we get slope at B

(Eq. 8.54) yields...

$$EI\theta_B = \frac{wL^3}{4} - \frac{wL^3}{24} - \frac{wL^3}{6}$$

$$\theta_B = \frac{wL^3}{24EI}$$

(Counter clockwise) ... (Eq. 8.55b)

Same as (Eq. 8.46b)

Maximum deflection:

Maximum deflection occurs at mid-span of the beam, where $x = \dfrac{L}{2}$

(Eq. 8.55) yields...

$$EIy_{max} = \frac{wL}{12}\left(\frac{L}{2}\right)^3 - \frac{wL^3}{24}\left(\frac{L}{2}\right) - \frac{w}{24}\left(\frac{L}{2}\right)^4$$

$$= \frac{wL^4}{12 \times 8} - \frac{wL^4}{24 \times 2} - \frac{wL^4}{24 \times 16}$$

$$= \frac{-wL^4}{24}\left[\frac{1}{16} + \frac{1}{2} - \frac{1}{4}\right]$$

$$y_{max} = -\frac{5wL^4}{384EI} \qquad \qquad \text{... (Eq. 8.56a)}$$

Same as (Eq. 8.47)

Negative sign indicate that deflection is downwards

22. **A simply supported beam of 5 m is subjected to a concentrated load of 25 kN at 3 m from left hand support. If $E = 200$ GPa and $I = 90 \times 10^6$ mm^4, calculate:**
    (a) **Slope at both ends**
    (b) **Deflection at load point**
    (c) **The position and magnitude of maximum deflection.**
    (d) **Slope at mid-span**

Solution: $W = 25 \times 10^3$ N, $L = 5000$ mm, $a = 3000$ mm, $b = 2000$ mm, $E = 200 \times 10^3$ MPa, $I = 90 \times 10^6$ mm^4.

a) θ_A , $\theta_B = ?$, b) $y_C = ?$, c) $x = ?$, $y_{max} = ?$, d) $\theta_{2500} = ?$

Based on given data, the problem is as shown in **Fig. 8.24**.

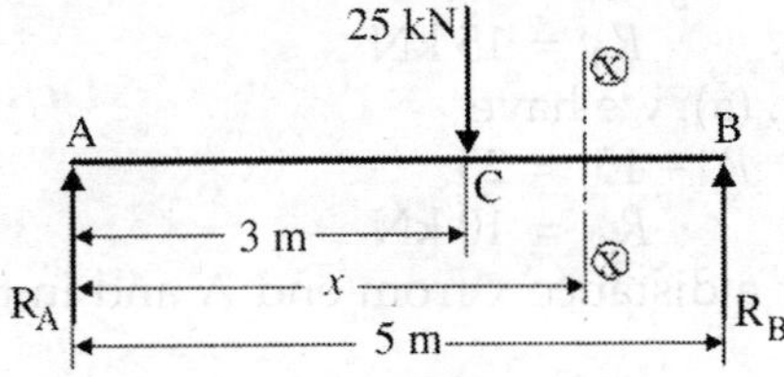

Fig. 8.24: Problem 22

Method 1: Using direct relations:

a. *Slope at both ends:*

Slope at A $\qquad \theta_A = -\dfrac{Wb(L^2 - b^2)}{6EIL} = -\dfrac{25 \times 10^3 \times 2000 \times (5000^2 - 2000^2)}{6 \times (200 \times 10^3) \times (90 \times 10^6) \times 5000}$

$$\theta_A = -0.00194 \text{ rad} \qquad\qquad \text{(Clockwise)}$$

Slope at B $\qquad \theta_B = \dfrac{Wa(L^2 - a^2)}{6EIL} = \dfrac{25 \times 10^3 \times 3000 \times (5000^2 - 3000^2)}{6 \times (200 \times 10^3) \times (90 \times 10^6) \times 5000}$

$$= 0.00222 \text{ rad} \qquad\qquad \text{(Counter clockwise)}$$

b. *Deflection at load point*

$$y_C = \dfrac{-Wa^2 b^2}{3EIL} = \dfrac{-25 \times 10^3 \times 3000^2 \times 2000^2}{3 \times (200 \times 10^3) \times 90 \times 10^6) \times 5000} = -3.33 \text{ mm}$$

c. *Position and magnitude of maximum deflection:*

Position of maximum deflection $x = \sqrt{\dfrac{L^2 - b^2}{3}} = \sqrt{\dfrac{5000^2 - 2000^2}{3}} = 2645.75 \text{ mm}$

Maximum deflection $y_{max} = \dfrac{-Wb(L^2 - b^2)^{3/2}}{9\sqrt{3}EIL} = \dfrac{25 \times 10^3 \times 2000 \times (5000^2 - 2000^2)^{3/2}}{9\sqrt{3} \times (200 \times 10^3) \times (90 \times 10^6) \times 5000}$

$$= -3.43 \text{ mm}$$

d. *Slope at mid-span*

Slope equation $EI\dfrac{dy}{dx} = \dfrac{Wb\langle x \rangle^2}{2L} - \dfrac{Wb(L^2 - b^2)}{6L} - \dfrac{W\langle x - a \rangle^2}{2}$ $\qquad$ ... using (Eq. 8.49)

Here $x = 2500$ mm at mid – span

Since $\langle x - a \rangle = \langle 2500 - 3000 \rangle = \langle -500 \rangle$, Ignore brackets containing negative value

$$\theta_{2500} = \dfrac{25 \times 10^3 \times 2000}{5000 \times (200 \times 10^3) \times (90 \times 10^6)} \left[\dfrac{\langle 2500 \rangle^2}{2} - \dfrac{(5000^2 - 2000^2)}{6} \right]$$

$$\theta_{2500} = -0.00021 \text{ rad}$$

Method 2: Using Macaulay's method

Reactions at supports:

$$R_A + R_B = 25 \text{ kN} \qquad\qquad\qquad \text{... Eq. (a)}$$

Taking moments about A and equating to zero, we have

$$R_B \times 5 = 25 \times 3$$
$$R_B = 15 \text{ kN} \qquad\qquad\qquad \text{... Eq. (b)}$$

Substituting Eq. (b) in Eq. (a), we have

$$R_A + 15 = 25$$
$$R_A = 10 \text{ kN} \qquad\qquad\qquad \text{... Eq. (c)}$$

Consider a section X-X at a distance x from end A and in the region CB as shown in **Fig. 8.24**.

Bending moment at X – X is $\quad M_x = R_A \cdot \langle x \rangle - W\langle x - 3000 \rangle$

i.e. $\qquad\qquad\qquad EI\dfrac{d^2 y}{dx^2} = 10 \times 10^3 \langle x \rangle - 25 \times 10^3 \langle x - 3000 \rangle$

Integrating once we have $\quad EI\dfrac{dy}{dx} = 5000\langle x \rangle^2 + C_1 - 12500\langle x - 3000 \rangle^2 \qquad$ ... Eq. (i)

Integrating again we have $\quad EIy = \dfrac{5000\langle x\rangle^3}{3} + C_1\langle x\rangle + C_2 - \dfrac{12500\langle x - 3000\rangle^3}{3}$

$$\dots \text{Eq. (ii)}$$

Boundary conditions:
At $x = 0, y = 0$:

Eq. (ii) yields... $\qquad\qquad 0 = 0 + 0 + C_2 - \dfrac{12500\langle 0 - 3000\rangle^3}{3}$

$$C_2 = 0$$

Ignore brackets containing negative value

At $x = L = 5000$ mm, $y = 0$:

Eq. (ii) yields... $\quad 0 = \dfrac{5000\langle 5000\rangle^3}{3} + C_1\langle 5000\rangle + 0 - \dfrac{12500\langle 5000 - 3000\rangle^3}{3}$

$$C_1 = -3.5 \times 10^{10}$$

Substituting C_1 in Eq. (i) we get

$$EI\frac{dy}{dx} = 5000\langle x\rangle^2 - 3.5 \times 10^{10} - 12500\langle x - 3000\rangle^2$$

$$\dots \textbf{\textit{Slope equation}} \text{ Eq. (iii)}$$

Substituting C_1 and C_2 in Eq. (ii) we get

$$EIy = \frac{5000\langle x\rangle^3}{3} - 3.5 \times 10^{10}\langle x\rangle - \frac{12500\langle x - 3000\rangle^3}{3}$$

$$\dots \textbf{\textit{Deflection equation}} \text{ Eq. (iv)}$$

a. *Slope at both ends:*
   At A, $x = 0$
   Eq. (iii) yields... $\qquad EI\theta_A = 0 - 3.5 \times 10^{10} - 0$

Ignore brackets containing negative value

$$\theta_A = -\frac{3.5 \times 10^{10}}{(200 \times 10^3) \times (90 \times 10^6)} = -0.00194 \text{ rad}$$

(Clockwise)

At B: $x = 5000$ mm

Eq. (iii) yields... $\qquad EI\theta_B = 5000\langle 5000\rangle^2 - 3.5 \times 10^{10} - 12500\langle 5000 - 3000\rangle^2$

$$\theta_B = -\frac{4 \times 10^{10}}{(200 \times 10^3) \times (90 \times 10^6)} = 0.00222 \text{ rad}$$

(Counter clockwise)

b. *Deflection at load point*
   At C, $x = 3000$ mm

Eq. (iv) yields... $\qquad EIy_C = \dfrac{5000\langle 3000\rangle^3}{3} - 3.5 \times 10^{10}\langle 3000\rangle - 0$

$$y_C = \frac{-6 \times 10^{13}}{(200 \times 10^3) \times (90 \times 10^6)} = -3.33 \text{ mm}$$

c. *Position and magnitude of maximum deflection:*

For maximum deflection $\dfrac{dy}{dx} = 0$

Eq. (iii) yields ...
$$0 = 5000x^2 - 3.5 \times 10^{10} - 12500(x - 3000)^2$$
$$0 = 0.4x^2 - 2.8 \times 10^6 - (x^2 + 9 \times 10^6 - 6000x)$$
$$0.6x^2 - 6000x + 11.8 \times 10^6 = 0$$
$$x = 2690.60 \text{ mm}$$

Eq. (iv) yields ...
$$EIy_{max} = \frac{5000 \langle 2690.60 \rangle^3}{3} - 3.5 \times 10^{10} \langle 2690.60 \rangle - 0$$

Ignore brackets containing negative value

$$y_{max} = \frac{-6.17 \times 10^{13}}{(200 \times 10^3) \times (90 \times 10^6)} = -3.43 \text{ mm}$$

d. *Slope at mid-span*
At $L/2$, $x = 2500$ mm

Eq. (iii) yields...
$$EI\theta_{2500} = 5000 \langle 2500 \rangle^2 - 3.5 \times 10^{10} - 0$$
$$\theta_{2500} = -0.00021 \text{ rad}$$

23. A simply supported beam of 6 m is subjected to a concentrated load of 18 kN at 4 m from left hand support as shown in Fig. 8.25. Calculate the position and magnitude of maximum deflection if $E = 200$ GPa and $I = 30 \times 10^6$ mm⁴.

VTU – Dec. 13/Jan. 14 – 10 Marks, June/July 2013 – 10 Marks

Solution: $W = 18 \times 10^3$ N, $L = 6000$ mm, $a = 4000$ mm, $b = 2000$ mm, $E = 200 \times 10^3$ MPa, $I = 30 \times 10^6$ mm⁴. $x = ?$, $y_{max} = ?$,

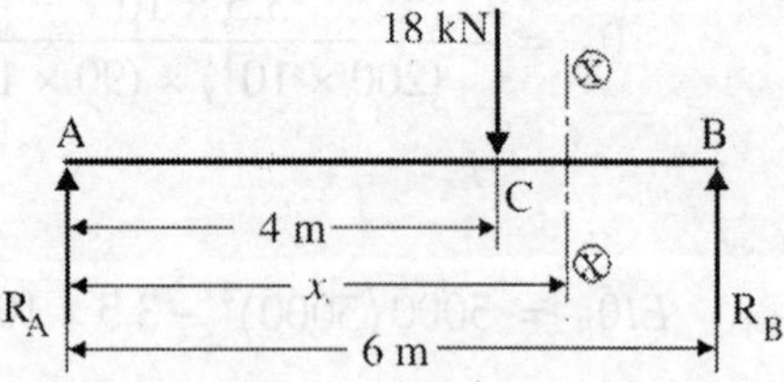

Fig. 8.25: Problem 23

Using Macaulay's method
Reactions at supports:
$$R_A + R_B = 18 \text{ kN} \qquad \qquad \text{... Eq. (a)}$$
Taking moments about A and equating to zero, we have
$$R_B \times 6 = 18 \times 4$$
$$R_B = 12 \text{ kN} \qquad \qquad \text{... Eq. (b)}$$
Substituting Eq. (b) in Eq. (a), we have
$$R_A + 12 = 18$$
$$R_A = 6 \text{ kN} \qquad \qquad \text{... Eq. (c)}$$
Consider a section X-X at a distance x from end A and in the region CB as shown in **Fig. 8.25**.

Bending moment at X-X is $\quad M_x = R_A \cdot \langle x \rangle - W \langle x - 4000 \rangle$

i.e. $\qquad\qquad\qquad EI \dfrac{d^2 y}{dx^2} = 6 \times 10^3 \langle x \rangle - 18 \times 10^3 \langle x - 4000 \rangle$

Integrating once we have $\quad EI \dfrac{dy}{dx} = 3000 \langle x \rangle^2 + C_1 - 9000 \langle x - 4000 \rangle^2 \qquad \ldots$ Eq. (i)

Integrating again we have $\quad EIy = 1000 \langle x \rangle^3 + C_1 \langle x \rangle + C_2 - 3000 \langle x - 4000 \rangle^3$

$$\ldots \text{Eq. (ii)}$$

Boundary conditions:
At $x = 0, y = 0$:
Eq. (ii) yields... $\qquad\qquad\qquad 0 = 0 + 0 + C_2 - 0$

$$C_2 = 0$$

Ignore brackets containing negative value

At $x = L = 6000$ mm, $y = 0$:

Eq. (ii) yields... $\qquad\qquad 0 = 1000 \langle 6000 \rangle^3 + C_1 \langle 6000 \rangle - 3000 \langle 6000 - 4000 \rangle^3$

$$C_1 = -3.2 \times 10^{10}$$

Substituting C_1 in Eq. (i) we get

$$EI \frac{dy}{dx} = 3000 \langle x \rangle^2 - 3.2 \times 10^{10} - 9000 \langle x - 4000 \rangle^2$$

$$\ldots \textbf{\textit{Slope equation}} \text{ Eq. (iii)}$$

Substituting C_1 and C_2 in Eq. (ii) we get

$$EIy = 1000 \langle x \rangle^3 - 3.2 \times 10^{10} - 3000 \langle x - 4000 \rangle^3$$

$$\ldots \textbf{\textit{Deflection equation}} \text{ Eq. (iv)}$$

For maximum deflection $\qquad \dfrac{dy}{dx} = 0$

Eq. (iii) yields ... $\qquad\qquad 0 = 3000 \langle x \rangle^2 - 3.2 \times 10^{10} - 9000 \langle x - 4000 \rangle^2$

$$0 = 0.33 x^2 - 3.55 \times 10^6 - (x^2 + 16 \times 10^6 - 8000x)$$

$$0.67 x^2 - 8000x + 19.55 \times 10^6 = 0$$

$$x = 3427.80 \text{ mm} = 3.42 \text{ m}$$

Eq. (iv) yields ... $\qquad EIy_{max} = 1000 \langle 3427.80 \rangle^3 - 3.2 \times 10^{10} \langle 3427.80 \rangle - 0$

Ignore brackets containing negative value

$$y_{max} = \frac{-6.94 \times 10^{13}}{(200 \times 10^3) \times (30 \times 10^6)} = -11.57 \text{ mm}$$

Note: On the other hand if we assume that the maximum deflection will be in the region AC (based on maximum BM), then we have

For maximum deflection $\qquad \dfrac{dy}{dx} = 0$

Eq. (iii) yields ... $\qquad\qquad 0 = 3000 \langle x \rangle^2 - 3.2 \times 10^{10} - 0$

$$x = 3266 \text{ mm}$$

Eq. (iv) yields ...
$$EIy_{max} = 1000\langle 3266 \rangle^3 - 3.2 \times 10^{10} \langle 3266 \rangle - 0$$

Ignore brackets containing negative value

$$y_{max} = \frac{-6.94 \times 10^{13}}{(200 \times 10^3) \times (30 \times 10^6)} = -11.61 \text{ mm}$$

24. A simply supported beam AB has a span of 5 m and carries a point load of 60 kN at a distance of 3m from left end A. Find the ratio of maximum deflection to the deflection under point load.

VTU – (CV) June/July 2014 – 14 Marks

Solution: $L = 5000$ mm, $W = 60 \times 10^3$ N, $a = 3000$ mm, $b = 2000$ mm, $\dfrac{y_{max}}{y_c} = ?$

Based on given data, the problem is as shown in **Fig. 8.26**.

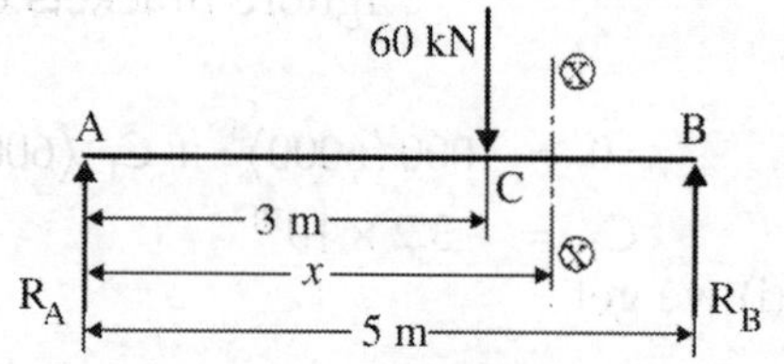

Fig. 8.26: Problem 24

Reactions at supports:

$$R_A + R_B = 60 \text{ kN} \qquad \qquad \text{... Eq. (a)}$$

Taking moments about A and equating to zero, we have
$$R_B \times 5 = 60 \times 3$$
$$R_B = 36 \text{ kN} \qquad \qquad \text{... Eq. (b)}$$

Substituting Eq. (b) in Eq. (a), we have
$$R_A + 36 = 60$$
$$R_A = 24 \text{ kN} \qquad \qquad \text{... Eq. (c)}$$

Consider a section X-X at a distance x from end A and in the region CB as shown in **Fig. 8.26**.

Bending moment at X-X is
$$M_x = R_A \cdot \langle x \rangle - W \langle x - 3000 \rangle$$

i.e.
$$EI\frac{d^2y}{dx^2} = 24 \times 10^3 \langle x \rangle - 60 \times 10^3 \langle x - 3000 \rangle$$

Integrating once we have
$$EI\frac{dy}{dx} = 12000\langle x \rangle^2 + C_1 - 30000 \langle x - 3000 \rangle^2 \qquad \text{... Eq. (i)}$$

Integrating again we have
$$EIy = 4000\langle x \rangle^3 + C_1\langle x \rangle + C_2 - 10000\langle x - 3000 \rangle^3 \qquad \text{... Eq. (ii)}$$

Boundary conditions:

At $x = 0$, $y = 0$:

Eq. (ii) yields...
$$0 = 0 + 0 + C_2 - 0$$
$$C_2 = 0$$

Ignore brackets containing negative value

At $x = L = 5000$ mm, $y = 0$:

Eq. (ii) yields...
$$0 = 4000\langle 5000 \rangle^3 + C_1\langle 5000 \rangle - 10000\langle 5000 - 3000 \rangle^3$$
$$C_1 = -8.4 \times 10^{10}$$

Substituting C_1 in Eq. (i) we get

$$EI\frac{dy}{dx} = 12000\langle x\rangle^2 - 8.4 \times 10^{10} - 30000\langle x - 3000\rangle^2$$

$$\dots \text{Eq. (iii)}$$

Substituting C_1 and C_2 in Eq. (ii) we get

$$EIy = 4000\langle x\rangle^3 - 8.4 \times 10^{10}\langle x\rangle - 10000\langle x - 3000\rangle^3$$

$$\dots \text{Eq. (iv)}$$

Deflection at load point:
At C, $x = 3000$ mm

Eq. (iv) yields... $\qquad EIy_C = 4000\langle 3000\rangle^3 - 8.4 \times 10^{10}\langle 3000\rangle - 0$

$$y_C = \frac{-1.44 \times 10^{14}}{EI}$$

Maximum deflection:

For maximum deflection $\frac{dy}{dx} = 0$

Eq. (iii) yields ... $\qquad 0 = 12000\langle x\rangle^2 - 8.4 \times 10^{10} - 30000\langle x - 3000\rangle^2$

$$0 = 0.4\,x^2 - 2.8 \times 10^6 - (x^2 + 9 \times 10^6 - 6000x)$$

$$0.6\,x^2 - 6000x + 11.8 \times 10^6 = 0$$

$$x = 2690.60 \text{ mm}$$

Eq. (iv) yields ... $\qquad EIy_{max} = 4000\langle 2690.60\rangle^3 - 8.4 \times 10^{10}\langle 2690.60\rangle$

$$- 10000\langle 2690.60 - 3000\rangle^3$$

Ignore brackets containing negative value

$$y_{max} = \frac{-1.48 \times 10^{14}}{EI} = -11.57 \text{ mm}$$

$$\frac{y_{max}}{y_C} = \frac{-1.48 \times 10^{14}/EI}{-1.44 \times 10^{14}/EI} = 1.027$$

25. **A beam of length 6 m is simply supported at its ends and carries two point loads of 40 kN at a distance of 1 m and 3 m respectively from the left support. By using Macaulay's method, determine:**
    (a) Deflection under each load
    (b) The point at which maximum deflection occurs.
    (c) Maximum deflection $\qquad$ Given $E = 2 \times 10^5$ N/mm^2 and $I = 85 \times 10^6$ mm^4.

VTU – Dec. 09/Jan. 10 – 20 Marks

Solution: $L = 6000$ mm, $W_1 = W_2 = 40 \times 10^3$ N, $x_1 = 1000$ mm, $x_2 = 3000$ mm, $E = 2 \times 10^5$ MPa, $I = 85 \times 10^6$ mm^4. a) y_C, $y_D = ?$, b) $x = ?$, c) $y_{max} = ?$
Based on given data, the problem is as shown in **Fig. 8.27**.
Reactions at supports:

$$R_A + R_B = 40 + 40 = 80 \text{ kN} \qquad \dots \text{Eq. (a)}$$

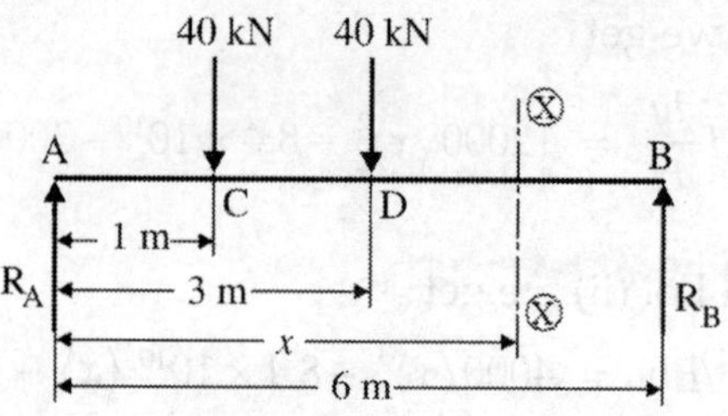

Fig. 8.27: Problem 25

Taking moments about A and equating to zero, we have

$$R_B \times 6 = (40 \times 3) + (40 \times 1)$$
$$R_B = 26.67 \text{ kN} \qquad \qquad \text{... Eq. (b)}$$

Substituting Eq. (b) in Eq. (a), we have

$$R_A + 26.67 = 80$$
$$R_A = 53.33 \text{ kN} \qquad \qquad \text{... Eq. (c)}$$

Consider a section X-X at a distance x from end A and in the region DB as shown in **Fig. 8.27**.

Bending moment at X – X is

$$M_x = R_A.\langle x \rangle - W_1 \langle x - 1000 \rangle - W_2 \langle x - 3000 \rangle$$

i.e.

$$EI \frac{d^2 y}{dx^2} = 53.33 \times 10^3 \langle x \rangle - 40 \times 10^3 \langle x - 1000 \rangle$$

$$- 40 \times 10^3 \langle x - 3000 \rangle$$

Integrating once we have

$$EI \frac{dy}{dx} = \frac{53.33 \times 10^3 \langle x \rangle^2}{2} + C_1 - 20000 \langle x - 1000 \rangle^2$$

$$- 20000 \langle x - 3000 \rangle^2 \qquad \qquad \text{... Eq. (i)}$$

Integrating again we have

$$EIy = \frac{53.33 \times 10^3 \langle x \rangle^3}{6} + C_1 \langle x \rangle + C_2$$

$$- \frac{20000 \langle x - 1000 \rangle^3}{3} - \frac{20000 \langle x - 3000 \rangle^3}{3}$$

$$\text{... Eq. (ii)}$$

Boundary conditions:

At $x = 0, y = 0$:

Eq. (ii) yields...

$$0 = 0 + 0 + C_2 - 0 - 0$$

Ignore brackets containing negative value

$$C_2 = 0$$

At $x = L = 6000$ mm, $y = 0$:

Eq. (ii) yields...

$$0 = \frac{53.33 \times 10^3 \langle 6000 \rangle^3}{6} + C_1 \langle 6000 \rangle - \frac{20000 \langle 6000 - 1000 \rangle^3}{3}$$

$$- \frac{20000 \langle 6000 - 3000 \rangle^3}{3}$$

$$C_1 = -1.51 \times 10^{11}$$

Substituting C_1 in Eq. (i) we get

$$EI\frac{dy}{dx} = \frac{53.33 \times 10^3 \langle x \rangle^2}{2} - 1.51 \times 10^{11} - 20000 \langle x - 1000 \rangle^2 - 20000 \langle x - 3000 \rangle^2$$

$$\dots \text{ Eq. (iii)}$$

Substituting C_1 and C_2 in Eq. (ii) we get

$$EIy = \frac{53.33 \times 10^3 \langle x \rangle^3}{6} - 1.51 \times 10^{11} \langle x \rangle - \frac{20000 \langle x - 1000 \rangle^3}{3} - \frac{20000 \langle x - 3000 \rangle^3}{3}$$

$$\dots \text{ Eq. (iv)}$$

a. *Deflection under each load*
   At C, x = 1000 mm

Eq. (iv) yields... $\quad EIy_C = \dfrac{53.33 \times 10^3 \langle 1000 \rangle^3}{6} - 1.51 \times 10^{11} \langle 1000 \rangle - 0 - 0$

$$y_C = (-1.42 \times 10^{14})/[(2 \times 10^5) \times (85 \times 10^6)] = -8.359 \text{ mm}$$

At D, $x = 3000$ mm

Eq. (iv) yields... $\quad EIy_D = \dfrac{53.33 \times 10^3 \langle 3000 \rangle^3}{6} - 1.51 \times 10^{11} \langle 3000 \rangle$

$$- \frac{20000 \langle 3000 - 1000 \rangle^3}{3} - 0$$

$$y_D = \frac{-2.66 \times 10^{14}}{(2 \times 10^5) \times (85 \times 10^6)} = -15.67 \text{ mm}$$

b. *The point at which maximum deflection occurs*

For maximum deflection $\dfrac{dy}{dx} = 0$

Eq. (iii) yields ... $\quad 0 = \dfrac{53.33 \times 10^3 \langle x \rangle^2}{6} - 1.51 \times 10^{11} - 20000 \langle x - 1000 \rangle^2$

$$- 20000 \langle x - 3000 \rangle^2$$

$$0 = 1.333x^2 - 7.55 \times 10^6 - (x^2 + 1 \times 10^6 - 2000x)$$

$$- (x^2 + 9 \times 10^6 - 6000x)$$

$$0.667x^2 - 8000x + 17.55 \times 10^6 = 0$$

$$x = 2890.21 \text{ mm}$$

c. *Maximum deflection*

Eq. (iv) yields ... $\quad EIy_{max} = \dfrac{53.33 \times 10^3 \langle 2890.21 \rangle^3}{6} - 1.51 \times 10^{11} \langle 2890.21 \rangle$

$$- \frac{20000 \langle 2890.21 - 1000 \rangle^3}{3} - 0$$

$$y_{max} = \frac{-2.21 \times 10^{14}}{(2 \times 10^5) \times (85 \times 10^6)} = -15.70 \text{ mm}$$

26. A beam of constant cross-section 10 m long is freely supported at its ends and loaded with two loads of 60 kN each at 3 m from either end. Find the slope at the support and the deflection under any one load. Take *EI* constant.

VTU – June/July 2015 – 14 Marks

Solution: $L = 10000$ mm, $W_1 = W_2 = 60 \times 10^3$ N, $x_1 = 3000$ mm, $x_2 = 7000$ mm a) θ_A, θ_B = ?, b) y_C or y_D = ?

Based on given data, the problem is as shown in **Fig. 8.28**.

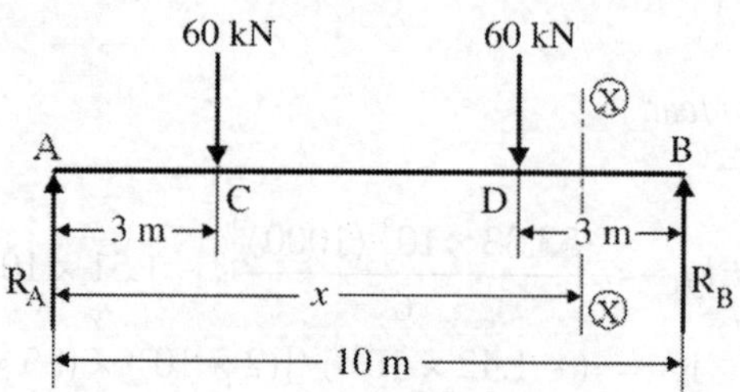

Fig. 8.28: Problem 26

Reactions at supports:

$$R_A + R_B = 60 + 60 = 120 \text{ kN} \qquad \text{... Eq. (a)}$$

Taking moments about A and equating to zero, we have

$$R_B \times 10 = (60 \times 7) + (60 \times 3)$$
$$R_B = 60 \text{ kN} \qquad \text{... Eq. (b)}$$

Substituting Eq. (b) in Eq. (a), we have

$$R_A + 60 = 120$$
$$R_A = 60 \text{ kN} \qquad \text{... Eq. (c)}$$

Consider a section X-X at a distance x from end A and in the region DB as shown in **Fig. 8.28**.

Bending moment at X-X is
$$M_x = R_A.\langle x \rangle - W_1 \langle x - 3000 \rangle - W_2 \langle x - 7000 \rangle$$

i.e.
$$EI \frac{d^2y}{dx^2} = 60 \times 10^3 \langle x \rangle - 60 \times 10^3 \langle x - 3000 \rangle$$
$$- 60 \times 10^3 \langle x - 7000 \rangle$$

Integrating once we have
$$EI \frac{dy}{dx} = 30000 \langle x \rangle^2 + C_1 - 30000 \langle x - 3000 \rangle^2$$
$$- 30000 \langle x - 7000 \rangle^2 \qquad \text{... Eq. (i)}$$

Integrating again we have
$$EIy = 10000 \langle x \rangle^3 + C_1 \langle x \rangle + C_2 - 10000 \langle x - 3000 \rangle^3$$
$$- 10000 \langle x - 7000 \rangle^3 \qquad \text{... Eq. (ii)}$$

Boundary conditions:
At $x = 0$, $y = 0$:
Eq. (ii) yields... $\qquad 0 = 0 + 0 + C_2 - 0 - 0 \qquad\qquad$ Ignore brackets containing negative value
$$C_2 = 0$$

At $x = L = 10000$ mm, $y = 0$:
Eq. (ii) yields... $\qquad 0 = 10000 \langle 10000 \rangle^3 + C_1 \langle 10000 \rangle + C_2$
$$- 10000 \langle 10000 - 3000 \rangle^3 - 10000 \langle 10000 - 7000 \rangle^3$$
$$C_1 = -6.30 \times 10^{11}$$

Substituting C_1 in Eq. (i) we get

$$EI\frac{dy}{dx} = 30000\langle x\rangle^2 - 6.30 \times 10^{11} - 30000\langle x - 3000\rangle^2 - 30000\langle x - 7000\rangle^2$$

$$\ldots \text{Eq. (iii)}$$

Substituting C_1 and C_2 in Eq. (ii) we get

$$EIy = 10000\langle x\rangle^3 - 6.30 \times 10^{11}\langle x\rangle - 10000\langle x - 3000\rangle^3 - 10000\langle x - 7000\rangle^3$$

$$\ldots \text{Eq. (iv)}$$

   a. *Slope at supports:*
   At A, $x = 0$
   Eq. (iii) yields... $\qquad EI\theta_A = 0 - 6.30 \times 10^{11} - 0 - 0$

$$\text{Ignore brackets containing negative value}$$

$$\theta_A = -\frac{6.30 \times 10^{11}}{EI} \qquad \text{(Clockwise)}$$

   At B, $x = 10000$ mm

   Eq. (iii) yields... $\qquad EI\theta_B = 30000\langle 10000\rangle^2 - 6.30 \times 10^{11}$

$$- 30000\langle 10000 - 3000\rangle^2$$

$$- 30000\langle 10000 - 7000\rangle^2$$

$$\theta_B = \frac{6.30 \times 10^{11}}{EI} \qquad \text{(Counter clockwise)}$$

   b. *Deflection under any one load:*
   At C, $x = 3000$ mm

   Eq. (iv) yields... $\qquad EIy_C = 10000\langle 3000\rangle^3 - 6.30 \times 10^{11}\langle 3000\rangle - 0 - 0$

$$y_C = \frac{-1.62 \times 10^{15}}{EI}$$

Note: Due to symmetrical loading $\quad y_C = y_D = \dfrac{-1.62 \times 10^{15}}{EI}$

27. **A beam of length 6 m is simply supported at its ends and carries two point loads of 48 kN and 40 kN at a distance of 1m and 3 m respectively from the left support. Find:**
    (a) **Deflection under each load**
    (b) **Point at which maximum deflection occurs and**
    (c) **Maximum deflection.** $\qquad$ Take $E = 2 \times 10^5$ **MPa and** $I = 85 \times 10^6$ **mm**^{4}**.**

VTU – June/July 2016 – 10 Marks, Dec. 2012 – 10 Marks; Dec. 2011 – 10 Marks
[Civil: Dec. 2012 – 10 Marks, June/July 2014 – 14 Marks]

Solution: $L = 6000$ mm, $W_1 = 48 \times 10^3$ N, $W_2 = 40 \times 10^3$ N, $x_1 = 1000$ mm, $x_2 = 3000$ mm, $E = 2 \times 10^5$ MPa, $I = 85 \times 10^6$ mm^4 a) y_A ,y_B = ?, b) x = ?, c) y_{max} = ?
Based on given data, the problem is as shown in **Fig. 8.29**.

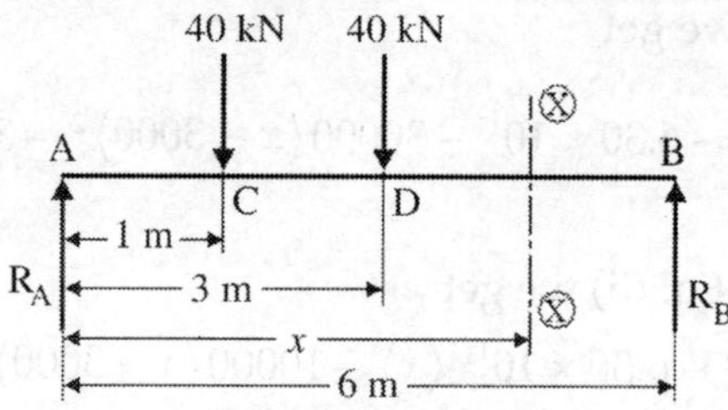

Fig. 8.29: Problem 27

Reactions at supports:

$$R_A + R_B = 48 + 40 = 88 \text{ kN} \qquad \text{... Eq. (a)}$$

Taking moments about A and equating to zero, we have

$$R_B \times 6 = (40 \times 3) + (48 \times 1)$$
$$R_B = 28 \text{ kN} \qquad \text{... Eq. (b)}$$

Substituting Eq. (b) in Eq. (a), we have

$$R_A + 28 = 88$$
$$R_A = 60 \text{ kN} \qquad \text{... Eq. (c)}$$

Consider a section X-X at a distance x from end A and in the region DB as shown in **Fig. 8.29**.

Bending moment at X-X is

$$M_x = R_A \langle x \rangle - W_1 \langle x - 1000 \rangle - W_2 \langle x - 3000 \rangle$$

i.e.

$$EI \frac{d^2 y}{dx^2} = 60 \times 10^3 \langle x \rangle - 48 \times 10^3 \langle x - 1000 \rangle$$
$$- 40 \times 10^3 \langle x - 3000 \rangle$$

Integrating once we have

$$EI \frac{dy}{dx} = 30000 \langle x \rangle^2 + C_1 - 24000 \langle x - 1000 \rangle^2$$
$$- 20000 \langle x - 3000 \rangle^2 \qquad \text{... Eq. (i)}$$

Integrating again we have

$$EIy = 10000 \langle x \rangle^3 + C_1 \langle x \rangle + C_2 - 8000 \langle x - 1000 \rangle^3$$
$$- \frac{20000 \langle x - 3000 \rangle^3}{3} \qquad \text{... Eq. (ii)}$$

Boundary conditions:

At $x = 0, y = 0$:

Eq. (ii) yields...

$$0 = 0 + 0 + C_2 - 0 - 0$$

Ignore brackets containing negative value

$$C_2 = 0$$

At $x = L = 6000$ mm, $y = 0$:

Eq. (ii) yields...

$$0 = 10000 \langle 6000 \rangle^3 + C_1 \langle 6000 \rangle - 8000 \langle 6000 - 1000 \rangle^3$$
$$- \frac{20000 \langle 6000 - 3000 \rangle^3}{3}$$
$$C_1 = -1.\omega \times 10^{11}$$

Substituting C_1 in Eq. (i) we get

$$EI\frac{dy}{dx} = 30000\langle x\rangle^2 - 1.63 \times 10^{11} - 24000\langle x - 1000\rangle^2$$

$$- 20000\langle x - 3000\rangle^2 \ ... \ \text{Eq. (iii)}$$

Substituting C_1 and C_2 in Eq. (ii) we get

$$EIy = 10000\langle x\rangle^3 - 1.63 \times 10^{11}\langle x\rangle - 8000\langle x - 1000\rangle^3$$

$$- \frac{20000\langle x - 3000\rangle^3}{3} \qquad\qquad ... \ \text{Eq. (iv)}$$

a. *Deflection under each load*

At C, $x = 1000$ mm

Eq. (iv) yields... $\qquad EIy_C = 10000\langle 1000\rangle^3 - 1.63 \times 10^{11}\langle 1000\rangle - 0 - 0$

$$y_C = \frac{-1.53 \times 10^{14}}{(2 \times 10^5)(85 \times 10^6)} = -9.02 \text{ mm}$$

At D, $x = 3000$ mm

Eq. (iv) yields... $\qquad EIy_D = 10000\langle 1000\rangle^3 - 1.63 \times 10^{11}\langle 3000\rangle$

$$- 8000\langle 3000 - 1000\rangle^3$$

$$y_D = \frac{-2.83 \times 10^{14}}{(2 \times 10^5)(85 \times 10^6)} = -16.65 \text{ mm}$$

b. *The point at which maximum deflection occurs*

For maximum deflection $\qquad \dfrac{dy}{dx} = 0$

From Eq. (iii) we have $\qquad 0 = 30000\langle x\rangle^2 - 1.63 \times 10^{11} - 24000\langle x - 1000\rangle^2$

$$- 20000\langle x - 3000\rangle^2$$

$$0 = 1.5x^2 - 8.15 \times 10^6 - 1.2(x^2 + 1 \times 10^6 - 2000x)$$
$$- (x^2 + 9 \times 10^6 - 6000x)$$

$$0.7\,x^2 - 8400x + 18.35 \times 10^6 = 0$$
$$x = 2871.78 \text{ mm}$$

c. *Maximum deflection*

Eq. (iv) yields ... $\qquad EIy_{max} = 10000\langle 2871.78\rangle^3 - 1.63 \times 10^{11}\langle 2871.78\rangle$

$$- 8000\langle 2871.78 - 1000\rangle^3 - 0$$

$$y_{max} = \frac{-2.84 \times 10^{14}}{(2 \times 10^5)(85 \times 10^6)} = -16.71 \text{ mm}$$

Note: On the other hand if we assume that the maximum deflection will be in the region CD (based on maximum BM), then we have

$x = 2871.84$ mm $\quad$ and $\quad y_{max} = -16.75$ mm

28. A simply supported steel beam having uniform cross section is 14 m span and is simply supported at its ends. It carries concentrated loads of 120 kN and 80 kN at two points 3 m and 4.5 m from the left and right ends respectively. If $I = 160 \times 10^7$ mm^4 and $E = 210$ GPa, calculate the deflection of the beam at load points. Also find the maximum deflection.

VTU – Dec. 14/Jan. 15 – 10 Marks, June/July – 10 Marks,
Jan. 2013 – 10 Marks, June 2012 – 12 Marks;
[Civil: June/July 2017 – 14 Marks, Dec. 09/
Jan. 10 – 14 Marks, June/July 2013 – 10 Marks,
Dec. 13/Jan. 14 – 12 Marks]

Solution: $L = 14000$ mm, $W_1 = 120 \times 10^3$ N, $W_2 = 80 \times 10^3$ N, $x_1 = 3000$ mm, $x_2 = 9500$ mm, $E = 210 \times 10^3$ MPa, $I = 160 \times 10^7$ mm^4 a) y_A , y_B = ?, b) y_{max} = ?

Based on given data, the problem is as shown in **Fig. 8.30**.

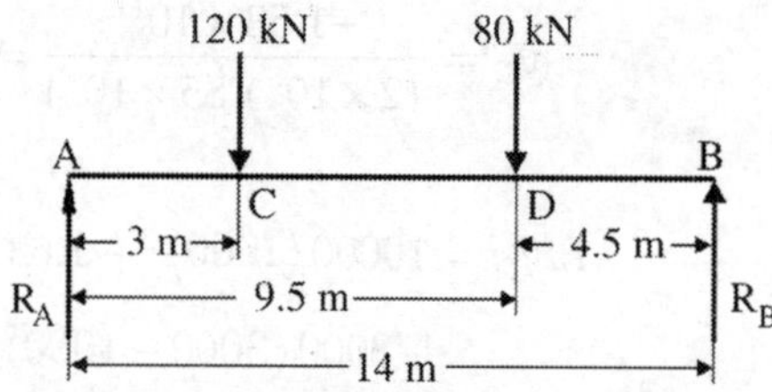

Fig. 8.30: Problem 28

Reactions at supports:
$$R_A + R_B = 120 + 80 = 200 \text{ kN} \qquad \text{... Eq. (a)}$$
Taking moments about A and equating to zero, we have
$$R_B \times 14 = (120 \times 3) + (80 \times 9.5)$$
$$R_B = 80 \text{ kN} \qquad \text{... Eq. (b)}$$
Substituting Eq. (b) in Eq. (a), we have
$$R_A + 80 = 200$$
$$R_A = 120 \text{ kN} \qquad \text{... Eq. (c)}$$
Consider a section X-X at a distance x from end A and in the region DB.

Bending moment at X-X is
$$M_x = R_A.\langle x \rangle - W_1 \langle x - 3000 \rangle - W_2 \langle x - 7000 \rangle$$

i.e.
$$EI \frac{d^2 y}{dx^2} = 120 \times 10^3 \langle x \rangle - 120 \times 10^3 \langle x - 3000 \rangle$$
$$- 80 \times 10^3 \langle x - 9500 \rangle$$

Integrating once we have
$$EI \frac{dy}{dx} = 60000 \langle x \rangle^2 + C_1 - 60000 \langle x - 3000 \rangle^2$$
$$- 40000 \langle x - 9500 \rangle^2 \qquad \text{... Eq. (i)}$$

Integrating again we have
$$EIy = 20000 \langle x \rangle^3 + C_1 \langle x \rangle + C_2 - 20000 \langle x - 3000 \rangle^3$$
$$- \frac{40000 \langle x - 9500 \rangle^3}{3} \qquad \text{... Eq. (ii)}$$

Boundary conditions:
At $x = 0$, $y = 0$:
Eq. (ii) yields...
$$0 = 0 + 0 + C_2 - 0 - 0$$

Ignore brackets containing negative value

$$C_2 = 0$$

At $x = L = 14000$ mm, $y = 0$:

Eq. (ii) yields... $\quad 0 = 20000\langle 14000\rangle^3 + C_1\langle 14000\rangle - 20000\langle 14000 - 3000\rangle^3$

$$-\frac{40000\langle x - 9500\rangle^3}{3}$$

$$C_1 = -1.93 \times 10^{12}$$

Substituting C_1 in Eq. (i) we get

$$EI\frac{dy}{dx} = 60000\langle x\rangle^2 - 1.93 \times 10^{12} - 60000\langle x - 3000\rangle^2 - 40000\langle x - 9500\rangle^2$$

$$\ldots \text{Eq. (iii)}$$

Substituting C_1 and C_2 in Eq. (ii) we get

$$EIy = 20000\langle x\rangle^3 - 1.93 \times 10^{12}\langle x\rangle - 20000\langle x - 3000\rangle^3 - \frac{40000\langle x - 9500\rangle^3}{3}$$

$$\ldots \text{Eq. (iv)}$$

a. *Deflection under each load*
   At C, $x = 3000$ mm

   Eq. (iv) yields... $\quad EIy_C = 20000\langle 3000\rangle^3 - 1.93 \times 10^{12}\langle 3000\rangle - 0 - 0$

   $$y_C = \frac{-5.25 \times 10^{15}}{(210 \times 10^3) \times (160 \times 10^7)} = -15.63 \text{ mm}$$

   At D, $x = 9500$ mm

   Eq. (iv) yields... $\quad EIy_D = 20000\langle 9500\rangle^3 - 1.93 \times 10^{12}\langle 9500\rangle$

   $$-20000\langle 9500 - 3000\rangle^3$$

   $$y_D = \frac{-6.68 \times 10^{15}}{(210 \times 10^3) \times (160 \times 10^7)} = -19.88 \text{ mm}$$

b. *Maximum deflection*

   For maximum deflection $\dfrac{dy}{dx} = 0$

   Eq. (iii) yields ... $\quad 0 = 60000\langle x\rangle^2 - 1.93 \times 10^{12} - 60000\langle x - 3000\rangle^2$

   $$-40000\langle x - 9500\rangle^2$$

   $$0 = 1.5x^2 - 48.25 \times 10^6 - 1.5(x^2 + 9 \times 10^6 - 6000x)$$
   $$-(x^2 + 90.25 \times 10^6 - 19000x)$$

   $$x^2 - 28000x + 152 \times 10^6 = 0$$
   $$x = 7366.75 \text{ mm}$$

   Eq. (iv) yields ... $\quad EIy_{max} = 20000\langle 7366.75\rangle^3 - 1.93 \times 10^{12}\langle 7366.75\rangle$

   $$-20000\langle 7366.75 - 3000\rangle^3 - 0$$

$$y_{max} = \frac{-7.88 \times 10^{15}}{(210 \times 10^3) \times (160 \times 10^7)} = -23.47 \text{ mm}$$

Note: On the other hand if we assume that the maximum deflection will be in the region CD (based on maximum BM), then we have

$x = 6866.07 \text{ mm}$ and $y_{max} = -23.65 \text{ mm}$

29. A simply supported beam carrying the point loads is as shown in Fig. 8.31. Determine:
   (a) Slope at supports
   (b) Deflection at points C and D.
   (c) Deflection at the mid span
   (d) The location and magnitude of the maximum deflection.
   Take $E = 200$ GPa, $I = 80 \times 10^{-5} \text{ m}^4$

VTU – (CV) June/July 2011 – 14 Marks;
[Similar: (CV) May/June 2010 – 10 Marks; (ME) Dec. 07/Jan. 08 – 10 Marks

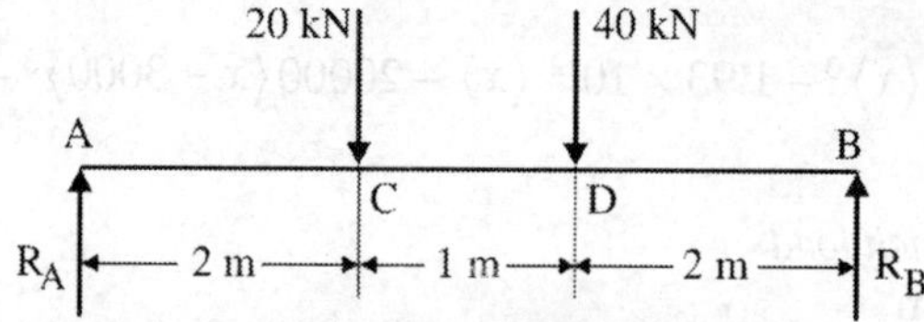

Fig. 8.31: Problem 29

Solution: $L = 5000$ mm, $W_1 = 20 \times 10^3$ N, $W_2 = 40 \times 10^3$ N, $x_1 = 2000$ mm, $x_2 = 3000$ mm, $E = 200 \times 10^3$ MPa, $I = 80 \times 10^{-5} \text{ m}^4 = 800 \times 10^6 \text{ mm}^4$. a) θ_A, $\theta_B = ?$, b) y_C, $y_D = ?$, c) $y_{L/2} = ?$, d) $x = ?$, $y_{max} = ?$

Based on given data, the problem is as shown in **Fig. 8.31**.

Reactions at supports:

$$R_A + R_B = 20 + 40 = 60 \text{ kN} \qquad \text{... Eq. (a)}$$

Taking moments about A and equating to zero, we have

$$R_B \times 5 = (20 \times 2) + (40 \times 3)$$
$$R_B = 32 \text{ kN} \qquad \text{... Eq. (b)}$$

Substituting Eq. (b) in Eq. (a), we have

$$R_A + 32 = 60$$
$$R_A = 28 \text{ kN} \qquad \text{... Eq. (c)}$$

Consider a section X-X at a distance x from end A and in the region DB.

Bending moment at X-X is $M_x = R_A.\langle x \rangle - W_1 \langle x - 2000 \rangle - W_2 \langle x - 3000 \rangle$

i.e. $$EI\frac{d^2y}{dx^2} = 28 \times 10^3 \langle x \rangle - 20 \times 10^3 \langle x - 2000 \rangle$$

$$- 40 \times 10^3 \langle x - 3000 \rangle$$

Integrating once we have $$EI\frac{dy}{dx} = 14000 \langle x \rangle^2 + C_1 - 10000 \langle x - 2000 \rangle^2$$

$$- 20000 \langle x - 3000 \rangle^2 \qquad \text{... Eq. (i)}$$

Integrating again we have

$$EIy = \frac{14000\langle x\rangle^3}{3} + C_1\langle x\rangle + C_2 - \frac{10000\langle x-2000\rangle^3}{3}$$

$$- \frac{20000\langle x-2000\rangle^3}{3} \qquad \text{... Eq. (ii)}$$

Boundary conditions:

At $x = 0, y = 0$:

Eq. (ii) yields... $\qquad 0 = 0 + 0 + C_2 - 0 - 0$

Ignore brackets containing negative value

$$C_2 = 0$$

At $x = L = 5000$ mm, $y = 0$:

Eq. (ii) yields... $\quad 0 = \dfrac{14000\langle 5000\rangle^3}{3} + C_1\langle 5000\rangle - \dfrac{10000\langle 5000-2000\rangle^3}{3}$

$$- \frac{20000\langle 5000-3000\rangle^3}{3}$$

$$C_1 = -8.8 \times 10^{10}$$

Substituting C_1 in Eq. (i) we get

$$EI\frac{dy}{dx} = 14000\langle x\rangle^2 - 8.8 \times 10^{10} - 10000\langle x-2000\rangle^2$$

$$- 20000\langle x-3000\rangle^2 \qquad \text{... Eq. (iii)}$$

Substituting C_1 and C_2 in Eq. (ii) we get

$$EIy = \frac{14000\langle x\rangle^3}{3} - 8.8 \times 10^{10}\langle x\rangle - \frac{10000\langle x-2000\rangle^3}{3}$$

$$- \frac{20000\langle x-3000\rangle^3}{3} \qquad \text{... Eq. (iv)}$$

a. *Slope at supports*

At A, $x = 0$

Eq. (iii) yields... $EI\theta_A = 0 - 8.8 \times 10^{10} - 0 - 0$

Ignore brackets containing negative value

$$\theta_A = \frac{-8.8 \times 10^{10}}{(200 \times 10^3) \times (800 \times 10^6)} = -0.00055 \text{ rad}$$

(Clockwise)

At B, $x = 5000$ mm

Eq. (iii) yields... $EI\theta_B = 14000\langle 5000\rangle^2 - 8.8 \times 10^{10} - 10000\langle 5000-2000\rangle^2$

$$- 20000\langle 5000-3000\rangle^2$$

$$\theta_B = \frac{9.2 \times 10^{10}}{(200 \times 10^3) \times (800 \times 10^6)} = 0.00057 \text{ rad}$$

(Counter clockwise)

b. *Deflection at points C and D*
   At C, $x = 2000$ mm

Eq. (iv) yields... $EIy_C = \dfrac{14000\,\langle 2000 \rangle^3}{3} - 8.8 \times 10^{10}\,\langle 2000 \rangle - 0 - 0$

$$y_C = \frac{-1.39 \times 10^{14}}{(200 \times 10^3) \times (800 \times 10^6)} = -0.867 \text{ mm}$$

At D, $x = 3000$ mm

Eq. (iv) yields... $EIy_D = \dfrac{14000\,\langle 3000 \rangle^3}{3} - 8.8 \times 10^{10}\,\langle 3000 \rangle$

$$- \frac{10000\,\langle 3000 - 2000 \rangle^3}{3} - 0$$

$$y_D = \frac{-1.41 \times 10^{14}}{(200 \times 10^3) \times (800 \times 10^6)} = -0.883 \text{ mm}$$

c. *Deflection at the mid span*
   At mid-span, $x = 2500$ mm

Eq. (iv) yields... $EIy_{L/2} = \dfrac{14000\,\langle 2500 \rangle^3}{3} - 8.8 \times 10^{10}\,\langle 2500 \rangle$

$$- \frac{10000\,\langle 2500 - 2000 \rangle^3}{3} - 0$$

$$y_{L/2} = \frac{-1.48 \times 10^{14}}{(200 \times 10^3) \times (800 \times 10^6)} = -0.922 \text{ mm}$$

d. *The location and magnitude of the maximum deflection.*

For maximum deflection $\dfrac{dy}{dx} = 0$

Eq. (iii) yields ... $0 = 14000\,\langle x \rangle^2 - 8.8 \times 10^{10} - 10000\,\langle x - 2000 \rangle^2$

$$- 20000\,\langle x - 3000 \rangle^2$$

$$0 = 0.7x^2 - 4.4 \times 10^6 - 0.5(x^2 + 4 \times 10^6 - 4000x)$$
$$- (x^2 + 9 \times 10^6 - 6000x)$$

$$0.8x^2 - 8000x + 15.4 \times 10^6 = 0$$

$$x = 2602.08 \text{ mm}$$

Eq. (iv) yields ... $EIy_{max} = \dfrac{14000\,\langle 2602.08 \rangle^3}{3} - 8.8 \times 10^{10}\,\langle 2602.08 \rangle$

$$- \frac{10000\,\langle 2602.08 - 2000 \rangle^3}{3} - 0$$

$$y_{max} = \frac{-1.47 \times 10^{15}}{(210 \times 10^3) \times (160 \times 10^7)} = -0.921 \text{ mm}$$

Note: On the other hand if we assume that the maximum deflection will be in the region CD (based on maximum BM), then we have

$$x = 2549.83 \text{ mm} \quad \text{and} \quad y_{max} = -0.922 \text{ mm}$$

30. A simply supported beam 8 m long carries two concentrated loads of 80 kN and 60 kN at distances of 3 m and 6m from left end support respectively. Calculate the slope and deflection under loads. Given E = 200 GPa and I = 300 $\times 10^6$ mm^4.

VTU – (CV): June/July 2016 – 14 Marks, June 2012 – 14 Marks

Solution: L = 8000 mm, W_1 = 80 $\times 10^3$ N, W_2 = 60 $\times 10^3$ N, x_1 = 3000 mm, x_2 = 6000 mm, E = 200 $\times 10^3$ MPa, I = 300 $\times 10^6$ mm^4. a) θ_C , θ_D = ?, b) y_C , y_D = ?
Based on given data, the problem is as shown in **Fig. 8.32**.

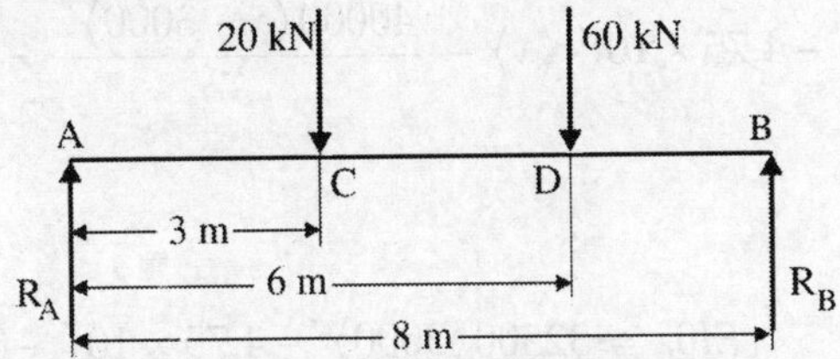

Fig. 8.32: Problem 30

Reactions at supports:

$$R_A + R_B = 80 + 60 = 140 \text{ kN} \qquad \text{... Eq. (a)}$$

Taking moments about A and equating to zero, we have

$$R_B \times 8 = (80 \times 3) + (60 \times 6)$$
$$R_B = 75 \text{ kN} \qquad \text{... Eq. (b)}$$

Substituting Eq. (b) in Eq. (a), we have

$$R_A + 75 = 140$$
$$R_A = 65 \text{ kN} \qquad \text{... Eq. (c)}$$

Consider a section X-X at a distance x from end A and in the region DB.

Bending moment at X-X is

$$M_x = R_A \langle x \rangle - W_1 \langle x - 3000 \rangle - W_2 \langle x - 6000 \rangle$$

i.e.

$$EI \frac{d^2y}{dx^2} = 65 \times 10^3 \langle x \rangle - 80 \times 10^3 \langle x - 3000 \rangle$$

$$- 60 \times 10^3 \langle x - 6000 \rangle$$

Integrating once we have

$$EI \frac{dy}{dx} = 32500 \langle x \rangle^2 + C_1 - 40000 \langle x - 3000 \rangle^2$$

$$- 30000 \langle x - 6000 \rangle^2 \qquad \text{... Eq. (i)}$$

Integrating again we have

$$EIy = \frac{32500 \langle x \rangle^3}{3} + C_1 \langle x \rangle + C_2 - \frac{40000 \langle x - 3000 \rangle^3}{3}$$

$$- 10000 \langle x - 6000 \rangle^3 \qquad \text{... Eq. (ii)}$$

Boundary conditions:
At $x = 0$, $y = 0$:
Eq. (ii) yields...

$$0 = 0 + 0 + C_2 - 0 - 0$$

Ignore brackets containing negative value

$$C_2 = 0$$

At $x = L = 8000$ mm, $y = 0$:

Eq. (ii) yields...
$$0 = \frac{32500 \langle 8000 \rangle^3}{3} + C_1 \langle 8000 \rangle - \frac{40000 \langle 8000 - 3000 \rangle^3}{3}$$
$$- 10000 \langle 8000 - 6000 \rangle^3$$
$$C_1 = -4.75 \times 10^{11}$$

Substituting C_1 in Eq. (i) we get

$$EI\frac{dy}{dx} = 32500 \langle x \rangle^2 - 4.75 \times 10^{11} - 40000 \langle x - 3000 \rangle^2 - 30000 \langle x - 6000 \rangle^2 \ldots \text{Eq. (iii)}$$

Substituting C_1 and C_2 in Eq. (ii) we get

$$EIy = \frac{32500 \langle x \rangle^3}{3} - 4.75 \times 10^{11} \langle x \rangle - \frac{40000 \langle x - 3000 \rangle^3}{3} - 10000 \langle x - 6000 \rangle^3$$

$$\ldots \text{Eq. (iv)}$$

a. *Slope at load points*
   At C, $x = 3000$

Eq. (iii) yields... $\qquad EI\theta_C = 32500 \langle 3000 \rangle^2 - 4.75 \times 10^{11} - 0 - 0$

Ignore brackets containing negative value

$$\theta_C = \frac{1.825 \times 10^{11}}{(200 \times 10^3) \times (300 \times 10^6)} = -0.00304 \text{ rad}$$

(Clockwise)

At D, $x = 6000$ mm

Eq. (iii) yields... $EI\theta_D = 32500 \langle 6000 \rangle^2 - 4.75 \times 10^{11} - 40000 \langle 6000 - 3000 \rangle^2 - 0$

$$\theta_D = \frac{3.39 \times 10^{11}}{(200 \times 10^3) \times (300 \times 10^6)} = 0.0056 \text{ rad}$$

(Counter clockwise)

b. *Deflection at load points*
   At C, $x = 3000$ mm

Eq. (iv) yields... $\qquad EIy_C = \frac{32500 \langle 3000 \rangle^3}{3} - 4.75 \times 10^{11} \langle 3000 \rangle - 0 - 0$

$$y_C = \frac{-1.133 \times 10^{15}}{(200 \times 10^3) \times (300 \times 10^6)} = -18.875 \text{ mm}$$

At D, $x = 6000$ mm

Eq. (iv) yields... $\qquad EIy_D = \frac{32500 \langle 6000 \rangle^3}{3} - 4.75 \times 10^{11} \langle 6000 \rangle$

$$- \frac{40000 \langle 6000 - 3000 \rangle^3}{3} - 0$$

$$y_D = \frac{-8.7 \times 10^{14}}{(200 \times 10^3) \times (300 \times 10^6)} = -14.50 \text{ mm}$$

31. A simply supported beam of span 7 m carries concentrated loads of 120 kN, 20 kN and 60 kN at 1 m, 4 m and 5 m respectively from left support. If $I = 400 \times 10^6$ mm^4 and $E = 210$ GPa, find the maximum deflection.

Solution: $L = 7000$ mm, $W_1 = 120 \times 10^3$ N, $W_2 = 20 \times 10^3$ N, $W_3 = 60 \times 10^3$ N, $x_1 = 1000$ mm, $x_2 = 4000$ mm, $x_3 = 5000$ mm, $E = 210 \times 10^3$ MPa, $I = 400 \times 10^6$ mm^4. $y_{max} = ?$

Based on given data, the problem is as shown in **Fig. 8.33**.

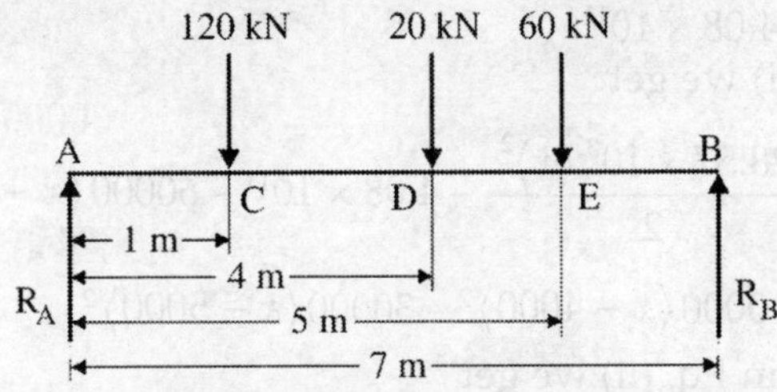

Fig. 8.33: Problem 31

Reactions at supports:

$$R_A + R_B = 120 + 20 + 60 = 200 \text{ kN} \qquad \text{... Eq. (a)}$$

Taking moments about A and equating to zero, we have

$$R_B \times 7 = (120 \times 1) + (20 \times 4) + (60 \times 5)$$
$$R_B = 71.43 \text{ kN} \qquad \text{... Eq. (b)}$$

Substituting Eq. (b) in Eq. (a), we have

$$R_A + 71.43 = 200$$
$$R_A = 128.57 \text{ kN} \qquad \text{... Eq. (c)}$$

Consider a section X-X at a distance x from end A and in the region EB.

Bending moment at X-X is $\quad M_x = R_A . \langle x \rangle - W_1 \langle x - 1000 \rangle - W_2 \langle x - 4000 \rangle$

$$- W_3 \langle x - 5000 \rangle$$

i.e. $\quad EI \dfrac{d^2y}{dx^2} = 128.57 \times 10^3 \langle x \rangle - 120 \times 10^3 \langle x - 1000 \rangle - 20 \times 10^3 \langle x - 4000 \rangle$

$$- 60 \times 10^3 \langle x - 5000 \rangle$$

Integrating once we have

$$EI \dfrac{dy}{dx} = \dfrac{128.57 \times 10^3 \langle x \rangle^2}{2} + C_1 - 60000 \langle x - 1000 \rangle^2 - 10000 \langle x - 4000 \rangle^2$$

$$- 30000 \langle x - 5000 \rangle \qquad \text{... Eq. (i)}$$

Integrating again we have

$$EIy = \dfrac{128.57 \times 10^3 \langle x \rangle^3}{6} + C_1 \langle x \rangle + C_2 - 20000 \langle x - 1000 \rangle^3$$

$$- \dfrac{10000 \langle x - 4000 \rangle^3}{3} - 10000 \langle x - 5000 \rangle^3 \qquad \text{... Eq. (ii)}$$

Boundary conditions:

At $x = 0, y = 0$:

Eq. (ii) yields... $\quad 0 = 0 + 0 + C_2 - 0 - 0 - 0$

Ignore brackets containing negative value

$$C_2 = 0$$

At $x = L = 7000$ mm, $y = 0$:

Eq. (ii) yields... $0 = \dfrac{128.57 \times 10^3 \langle 7000 \rangle^3}{6} + C_1 \langle 7000 \rangle - 20000 \langle 7000 - 1000 \rangle^3$

$$- \frac{10000 \langle 7000 - 4000 \rangle^3}{3} - 10000 \langle 7000 - 5000 \rangle^3$$

$$C_1 = -4.08 \times 10^{11}$$

Substituting C_1 in Eq. (i) we get

$$EI\frac{dy}{dx} = \frac{128.57 \times 10^3 \langle x \rangle^2}{2} - 4.08 \times 10^{11} - 60000 \langle x - 1000 \rangle^2$$

$$- 10000 \langle x - 4000 \rangle^2 - 30000 \langle x - 5000 \rangle^2 \qquad \dots \text{Eq. (iii)}$$

Substituting C_1 and C_2 in Eq. (ii) we get

$$EIy = \frac{128.57 \times 10^3 \langle x \rangle^3}{6} - 4.08 \times 10^{11} \langle x \rangle - 20000 \langle x - 1000 \rangle^3$$

$$- \frac{10000 \langle x - 4000 \rangle^3}{3} - 10000 \langle x - 5000 \rangle^3 \qquad \dots \text{Eq. (iv)}$$

For maximum deflection $\dfrac{dy}{dx} = 0$

Eq. (iii) yields ... $\qquad 0 = \dfrac{128.57 \times 10^3 \langle x \rangle^2}{2} - 4.08 \times 10^{11} - 60000 \langle x - 1000 \rangle^2$

$$-10000 \langle x - 4000 \rangle^2 - 30000 \langle x - 5000 \rangle^2$$

$$0 = 1.07 \langle x \rangle^2 - 6.8 \times 10^6 - \langle x - 1000 \rangle^2$$

$$- 0.167 \langle x - 4000 \rangle^2 - 0.5 \langle x - 5000 \rangle^2$$

$$0 = 1.07 x^2 - 6.8 \times 10^6 - (x^2 + 1 \times 10^6 - 2000x)$$

$$- 0.167(x^2 + 16 \times 10^6 - 8000x)$$

$$- 0.5(x^2 + 25 \times 10^6 - 10000x)$$

$$0.597 x^2 - 8336 x + 22.972 \times 10^6 = 0$$

$$x = 3777.93 \text{ mm}$$

Eq. (iv) yields ... $\qquad EIy_{max} = \dfrac{128.57 \times 10^3 \langle 3777.93 \rangle^3}{6} - 4.08 \times 10^{11} \langle 3777.93 \rangle$

$$- 20000 \langle 3777.93 - 1000 \rangle^3 - 0 - 0$$

$$y_{max} = \frac{-8.15 \times 10^{14}}{(210 \times 10^3) \times (400 \times 10^6)} = -9.70 \text{ mm}$$

Note: On the other hand if we assume that the maximum deflection will be in the region CD (based on maximum BM), then we have

$\qquad x = 3473.77$ mm $\quad$ and $\quad y_{max} = -9.81$ mm

32. **A simply supported beam carrying the point loads as shown in Fig. 8.34. If the maximum stress is 90 MPa and the beam is 300 mm deep. Determine:**
   (a) Slope at supports
   (b) slope at load points

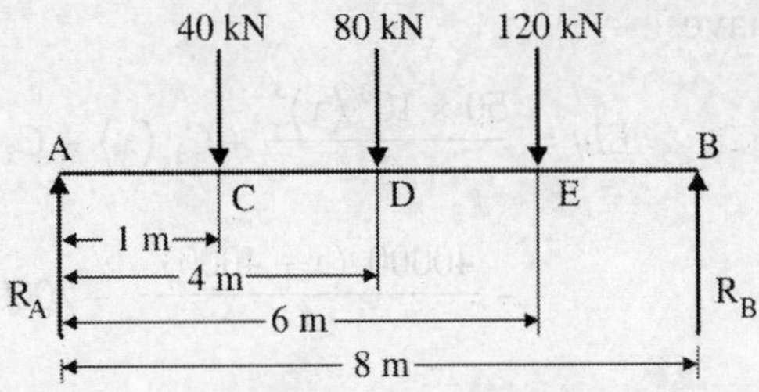

Fig. 8.34: Problem 32

(c) Deflection at load points

(d) The location and magnitude of the maximum deflection. Take E = 200 GPa

Solution: $L = 8000$ mm, $W_1 = 40 \times 10^3$ N, $W_2 = 80 \times 10^3$ N, $W_3 = 120 \times 10^3$ N, $x_1 = 2000$ mm, $x_2 = 4000$ mm, $x_3 = 6000$ mm, $E = 200 \times 10^3$ MPa. Bending stress $\sigma = 90$ MPa, Depth $h = 300$ mm a) $\theta_A, \theta_B = ?$, b) $\theta_C, \theta_D, \theta_E = ?$ c) $y_C, y_D, y_E = ?$, d) $x = ?$, $y_{max} = ?$

Reactions at supports:

$$R_A + R_B = 40 + 80 + 120 = 240 \text{ kN} \qquad \text{... Eq. (a)}$$

Taking moments about A and equating to zero, we have

$$R_B \times 8 = (40 \times 2) + (80 \times 4) + (120 \times 6)$$
$$R_B = 140 \text{ kN} \qquad \text{... Eq. (b)}$$

Substituting Eq. (b) in Eq. (a), we have

$$R_A + 140 = 240$$
$$R_A = 100 \text{ kN} \qquad \text{... Eq. (c)}$$

Bending moment calculations:

$$M_A = 0, M_B = 0$$
$$M_C = 100 \times 2 = 200 \text{ kN} - \text{m}$$
$$M_D = (100 \times 4) - (40 \times 2) = 320 \text{ kN} - \text{m}$$
$$M_E = 140 \times 2 = 280 \text{ kN} - \text{m} \quad \text{(from RHS)}$$

Thus the maximum BM occurs at D i.e. $M_D = 320$ kN $-$ m

To find I

$$\text{Bending stress } \sigma = \frac{M}{Z} = \frac{Mc}{I}$$

$$90 = \frac{320 \times 10^6 \times (300/2)}{I} \qquad \text{since } c = \frac{h}{2}$$

$$I = 533.33 \times 10^6 \text{ mm}^4$$

Consider a section X-X at a distance x from end A and in the region EB.

Bending moment at X-X is $\quad M_x = R_A.\langle x \rangle - W_1 \langle x - 2000 \rangle - W_2 \langle x - 4000 \rangle$

$$- W_3 \langle x - 6000 \rangle$$

i.e. $\qquad EI\dfrac{d^2y}{dx^2} = 100 \times 10^3 \langle x \rangle - 40 \times 10^3 \langle x - 4000 \rangle$

$$- 80 \times 10^3 \langle x - 6000 \rangle - 120 \times 10^3 \langle x - 6000 \rangle$$

Integrating once we have

$$EI\dfrac{dy}{dx} = 50 \times 10^3 \langle x \rangle^2 + C_1 - 20000 \langle x - 2000 \rangle^2$$

$$- 40000 \langle x - 4000 \rangle^2 - 60000 \langle x - 6000 \rangle^2 \qquad \text{... Eq. (i)}$$

Integrating again we have

$$EIy = \frac{50 \times 10^3 \langle x \rangle^3}{3} + C_1 \langle x \rangle + C_2 - \frac{20000 \langle x - 2000 \rangle^3}{3}$$

$$- \frac{40000 \langle x - 4000 \rangle^3}{3} - 20000 \langle x - 6000 \rangle^3 \dots \text{Eq. (ii)}$$

Boundary conditions:
At $x = 0$, $y = 0$:
Eq. (ii) yields... $\qquad 0 = 0 + 0 + C_2 - 0 - 0 - 0$

Ignore brackets containing negative value

$$C_2 = 0$$

At $x = L = 8000$ mm, $y = 0$:

Eq. (ii) yields... $\quad 0 = \dfrac{50 \times 10^3 \langle 8000 \rangle^3}{3} + C_1 \langle 8000 \rangle - \dfrac{20000 \langle 8000 - 2000 \rangle^3}{3}$

$$- \frac{40000 \langle 8000 - 4000 \rangle^3}{3} - 20000 \langle 8000 - 6000 \rangle^3$$

$$C_1 = -7.6 \times 10^{11}$$

Substituting C_1 in Eq. (i) we get

$$EI \frac{dy}{dx} = 50 \times 10^3 \langle x \rangle^2 - 7.6 \times 10^{11} - 20000 \langle x - 2000 \rangle^2$$

$$- 40000 \langle x - 4000 \rangle^2 - 60000 \langle x - 6000 \rangle^2 \qquad \dots \text{Eq. (iii)}$$

Substituting C_1 and C_2 in Eq. (ii) we get

$$EIy = \frac{50 \times 10^3 \langle x \rangle^3}{3} - 7.6 \times 10^{11} \langle x \rangle - \frac{20000 \langle x - 2000 \rangle^3}{3}$$

$$- \frac{40000 \langle x - 4000 \rangle^3}{3} - 20000 \langle x - 6000 \rangle^3 \qquad \dots \text{Eq. (iv)}$$

a. *Slope at supports*
At A, $x = 0$
Eq. (iii) yields... $EI\theta_A = 0 - 7.6 \times 10^{11} - 0 - 0 - 0$

Ignore brackets containing negative value

$$\theta_A = \frac{-7.6 \times 10^{11}}{(200 \times 10^3) \times (533.33 \times 10^6)} = -0.00713 \text{ rad(Clockwise)}$$

At B, $x = 8000$ mm

Eq. (iii) yields... $EI\theta_B = 50 \times 10^3 \langle 8000 \rangle^2 - 7.6 \times 10^{11} - 20000 \langle 8000 - 2000 \rangle^2$

$$- 40000 \langle 8000 - 4000 \rangle^2 - 60000 \langle 8000 - 6000 \rangle^2$$

$$\theta_B = \frac{8.4 \times 10^{11}}{(200 \times 10^3) \times (533.33 \times 10^6)} = 0.00788 \text{ rad}$$

(Counter clockwise)

b. *Slope at load points*
  At C, $x = 2000$ mm

Eq. (iii) yields... $EI\theta_C = 50 \times 10^3 \langle 2000 \rangle^2 - 7.6 \times 10^{11} - 0 - 0 - 0$

$$\theta_C = \frac{-5.6 \times 10^{11}}{(200 \times 10^3) \times (533.33 \times 10^6)} = -0.00525 \text{ rad}$$

(Clockwise)

At D, $x = 4000$ mm

Eq. (iii) yields... $EI\theta_D = 50 \times 10^3 \langle 4000 \rangle^2 - 7.6 \times 10^{11}$

$$- 20000 \langle 4000 - 2000 \rangle^2 - 0 - 0$$

$$\theta_D = \frac{-4 \times 10^{10}}{(200 \times 10^3) \times (533.33 \times 10^6)} = -0.00038 \text{ rad}$$

(Clockwise)

At E, $x = 6000$ mm

Eq. (iii) yields... $EI\theta_E = 50 \times 10^3 \langle 6000 \rangle^2 - 7.6 \times 10^{11} - 20000 \langle 6000 - 2000 \rangle^2$

$$- 40000 \langle 6000 - 4000 \rangle^2 - 0$$

$$\theta_E = \frac{5.6 \times 10^{11}}{(200 \times 10^3) \times (533.33 \times 10^6)} = 0.00525 \text{ rad}$$

(Counter clockwise)

c. *Deflection at load points*
  At C, $x = 2000$ mm

Eq. (iv) yields... $EIy_C = \dfrac{50 \times 10^3 \langle 2000 \rangle^3}{3} - 7.6 \times 10^{11} \langle 2000 \rangle - 0 - 0 - 0$

$$y_C = \frac{-1.386 \times 10^{15}}{(200 \times 10^3) \times (533.33 \times 10^6)} = -13 \text{ mm}$$

At D, $x = 4000$ mm

Eq. (iv) yields... $EIy_D = \dfrac{50 \times 10^3 \langle 4000 \rangle^3}{3} - 7.6 \times 10^{11} \langle 4000 \rangle$

$$- \frac{20000 \langle 4000 - 2000 \rangle^3}{3} - 0 - 0$$

$$y_D = \frac{-2.026 \times 10^{15}}{(200 \times 10^3) \times (533.33 \times 10^6)} = -19 \text{ mm}$$

At E, $x = 6000$ mm

Eq. (iv) yields... $EIy_E = \dfrac{50 \times 10^3 \langle 6000 \rangle^3}{3} - 7.6 \times 10^{11} \langle 6000 \rangle$

$$- \frac{20000 \langle 6000 - 2000 \rangle^3}{3} - \frac{40000 \langle 6000 - 4000 \rangle^3}{3} - 0$$

$$y_E = \frac{-1.493 \times 10^{15}}{(200 \times 10^3) \times (533.33 \times 10^6)} = -14 \text{ mm}$$

d. *The location and magnitude of the maximum deflection.*

For maximum deflection $\dfrac{dy}{dx} = 0$

Eq. (iii) yields ...

$$0 = 50 \times 10^3 \langle x \rangle^2 - 7.6 \times 10^{11} - 20000 \langle x - 2000 \rangle^2$$
$$- 40000 \langle x - 4000 \rangle^2 - 60000 \langle x - 6000 \rangle^2$$
$$0 = \langle x \rangle^2 - 15.2 \times 10^6 - 0.4 \langle x - 2000 \rangle^2 - 0.8 \langle x - 4000 \rangle^2$$
$$- 1.2 \langle x - 6000 \rangle^2$$
$$0 = x^2 - 15.2 \times 10^6 - 0.4(x^2 + 4 \times 10^6 - 4000x)$$
$$- 0.8(x^2 + 16\, x \, 10^6 - 8000x) - 1.2(x^2 + 36 \times 10^6 - 12000x)$$
$$1.4x^2 - 22400x + 72.8 \times 10^6 = 0$$
$$x = 4535.90 \text{ mm}$$

Eq. (iv) yields ...

$$EIy_{max} = \frac{50 \times 10^3 \langle 4535.90 \rangle^3}{3} - 7.6 \times 10^{11} \langle 4535.90 \rangle$$

$$- \frac{20000 \langle 4535.90 - 2000 \rangle^3}{3} - \frac{40000 \langle 4535.90 - 4000 \rangle^3}{3} - 0$$

$$y_{max} = \frac{-2.11 \times 10^{15}}{(200 \times 10^3) \times (533.33 \times 10^6)} = -18.78 \text{ mm}$$

Note: On the other hand if we assume that the maximum deflection will be in the region CD (based on maximum BM) then we have

$$x = 4125.5 \text{ mm} \quad \text{and} \quad y_{max} = -19.02 \text{ mm}$$

SSB WITH FULL UDL

33. **A beam of uniform rectangular section 250 mm wide and 350 mm deep is simply supported at its ends. It carries an UDL of 12 kN/m over the entire span of 6m. If $E = 1 \times 10^4$ N/mm^2, find**
    (a) Slope at the supports   **(b) maximum deflection**

Solution: $b = 250$ mm, $h = 350$ mm, $w = 12$ kN/m $= 12$ N/mm, $L = 6000$ mm, $E = 1 \times 10^4$ MPa, $\theta_{max} = ?$, $y_{max} = ?$.

Moment of inertia
$$I = \frac{bh^3}{12} = \frac{250 \times 350^3}{12} = 8.93 \times 10^8 \text{ mm}^4$$

Method 1: Using direct relations:

a. *Slope at both ends:*

Slope at A: Here $x = 0$
$$\theta_A = -\frac{wL^3}{24EI} = -\frac{12 \times 6000^3}{24 \times (1 \times 10^4) \times (8.93 \times 10^8)}$$
$$= -0.0121 \text{ rad (Clockwise)}$$

Slope at B: Here x = 6000 mm $\quad \theta_B = \dfrac{wL^3}{24EI} = \dfrac{12 \times 6000^3}{24 \times (1 \times 10^4) \times (8.93 \times 10^8)} = 0.0121$ rad

(Counter clockwise)

b. *Maximum deflection:*

Since the beam is uniformly loaded, maximum deflection occurs at mid-span where $x = \dfrac{L}{2}$

$$y_{max} = -\frac{5wL^4}{384EI} = -\frac{5 \times 12 \times 6000^4}{384 \times (1 \times 10^4) \times (8.93 \times 10^8)}$$

$$= -22.67 \text{ mm (Downward)}$$

Method 2: Using Macaulay's method

Reactions at supports:

$$R_A + R_B = (12 \times 6) = 72 \text{ kN} \qquad \qquad \dots \text{Eq. (a)}$$

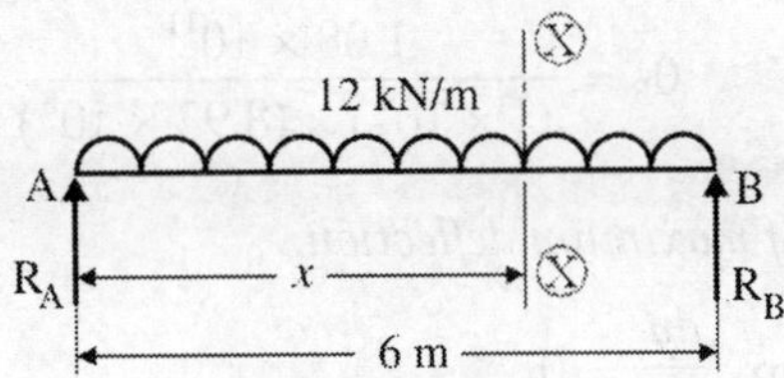

Fig. 8.35: Problem 33

Taking moments about A and equating to zero, we have

$$R_B \times 6 = (12 \times 6)\left(\frac{6}{2}\right)$$

$$R_B = 36 \text{ kN} \qquad \qquad \dots \text{Eq. (b)}$$

Substituting Eq. (b) in Eq. (a), we have

$$R_A + 72 = 36$$

$$R_A = 36 \text{ kN} \qquad \qquad \dots \text{Eq. (c)}$$

Consider a section X-X at a distance x from free end A as shown in **Fig. 8.35**

Bending moment at X-X is $\quad M_x = R_A \langle x \rangle - \left(\dfrac{w}{2}\right)\langle x \rangle^2$

i.e. $\qquad \qquad EI\dfrac{d^2y}{dx^2} = 36 \times 10^3 \langle x \rangle - \dfrac{12\langle x \rangle^2}{2}$

Integrating once we have $EI\dfrac{dy}{dx} = 18 \times 10^3 \langle x \rangle^2 + C_1 - 2\langle x \rangle^3 \qquad \dots \text{Eq. (i)}$

Integrating again we have $\quad EIy = 6 \times 10^3 \langle x \rangle^3 + C_1 \langle x \rangle + C_2 - 0.5\langle x \rangle^4 \qquad \dots \text{Eq. (ii)}$

Boundary conditions:

At x = 0, y = 0:

Eq. (ii) yields... $\qquad \qquad 0 = 0 + 0 + C_2 - 0$

$$C_2 = 0$$

At x = L = 6000, y = 0:

Eq. (ii) yields... $\qquad \qquad 0 = 6 \times 10^3 \langle 6000 \rangle^3 + C_1 \langle 6000 \rangle + 0 - 0.5\langle 6000 \rangle^4$

$$C_1 = -1.08 \times 10^{11}$$

Substituting C_1 in Eq. (i) we get

$$EI\frac{dy}{dx} = 18 \times 10^3 \langle x \rangle^2 - 1.08 \times 10^{11} - 2\langle x \rangle^3 \qquad \text{... Eq. (iii)}$$

Substituting C_1 and C_2 in Eq. (ii) we get

$$EIy = 6 \times 10^3 \langle x \rangle^3 - 1.08 \times 10^{11} \langle x \rangle - 0.5\langle x \rangle^4 \qquad \text{... Eq. (iv)}$$

a. *Slope at both ends:*

At A, $x = 0$

Eq. (iii) yields... $\qquad EI\theta_A = 0 - 1.08 \times 10^{11} - 0$

$$\theta_A = \frac{-1.08 \times 10^{11}}{(1 \times 10^4) \times (8.93 \times 10^8)} = -0.0121 \text{ rad}$$

(Clockwise)

At B, $x = 6000$ mm

Eq. (iii) yields... $\qquad EI\theta_B = 18 \times 10^3 \langle 6000 \rangle^2 - 1.08 \times 10^{11} - 2\langle 6000 \rangle^3$

$$\theta_B = \frac{1.08 \times 10^{11}}{(1 \times 10^4) \times (8.93 \times 10^8)} = 0.0121 \text{ rad}$$

(Counter clockwise)

b. *Position and magnitude of maximum deflection:*

For maximum deflection $\dfrac{dy}{dx} = 0$

Eq. (iii) yields ... $\qquad 0 = 18 \times 10^3 \langle x \rangle^2 - 1.08 \times 10^{11} - 2\langle x \rangle^3$

$$x = 3000 \text{ mm}$$

Eq. (iv) yields ... $\qquad EIy_{max} = 6 \times 10^3 \langle 3000 \rangle^3 - 1.08 \times 10^{11} \langle 3000 \rangle - 0.5\langle 3000 \rangle^4$

$$y_{max} = \frac{-2.025 \times 10^{14}}{(1 \times 10^4) \times (8.93 \times 10^8)} = -22.67 \text{ mm}$$

SSB WITH FULL UDL AND POINT LOADS

34. **A simply supported beam of span 6m is subjected to a concentrated load of 25 kN acting at 3m from left support and a uniformly distributed load of 10 kN/m over the entire span. If $E = 200 \times 10^3$ MPa, $I = 150 \times 10^6$ mm^4, determine:**
    (a) Slope at both ends
    (b) Deflection at load point
    (c) The position and magnitude of maximum deflection.

Solution: $L = 6000$ mm, $W = 25 \times 10^3$ N, $w = 10$ kN/m $= 10$ N/mm, $E = 200 \times 10^3$ MPa, $I = 150 \times 10^6$ mm^4.

a) $\theta_A, \theta_B = ?$, b) $y_C = ?$, c) $x = ?, y_{max} = ?$

Based on given data, the problem is as shown in **Fig. 8.36**.

Reactions at supports:

$$R_A + R_B = (10 \times 6) + 25 = 85 \text{ kN} \qquad \text{... Eq. (a)}$$

Taking moments about A and equating to zero, we have

$$R_B \times 6 = (25 \times 3) + (10 \times 6)(6/2)$$
$$R_B = 42.5 \text{ kN} \qquad \text{... Eq. (b)}$$

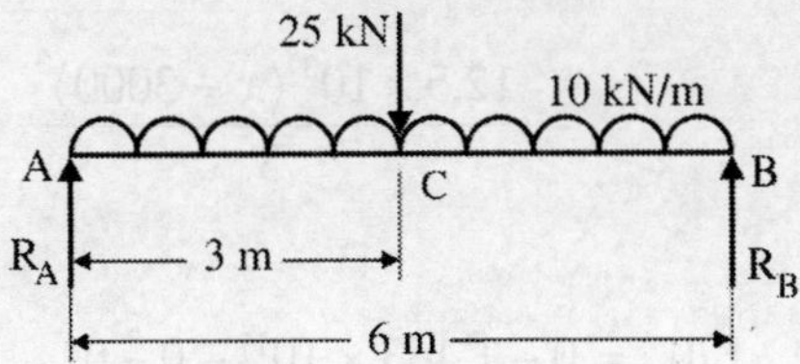

Fig. 8.36: Problem 34 (Problem 19 repeated)

Substituting Eq. (b) in Eq. (a), we have

$$R_A + 85 = 42.5$$

$$R_A = 42.5 \text{ kN} \qquad \qquad \text{... Eq. (c)}$$

Consider a section X-X at a distance x from free end A and in the region CB.

Bending moment at X-X is $\quad M_x = R_A \cdot \langle x \rangle - W \langle x - 3000 \rangle - \left(\dfrac{w}{2} \right) \langle x \rangle^2$

i.e. $\qquad \qquad EI \dfrac{d^2 y}{dx^2} = 42.5 \times 10^3 \langle x \rangle - 25 \times 10^3 \langle x - 3000 \rangle - \dfrac{10 \langle x \rangle^2}{2}$

Integrating once we have $EI \dfrac{dy}{dx} = 21.25 \times 10^3 \langle x \rangle^2 + C_1 - 12.5 \times 10^3 \langle x - 3000 \rangle^2$

$$- \dfrac{5 \langle x \rangle^3}{3} \qquad \qquad \text{... Eq. (i)}$$

Integrating again we have $\quad EIy = \dfrac{21.25 \times 10^3 \langle x \rangle^3}{3} + C_1 \langle x \rangle + C_2$

$$- \dfrac{12.5 \times 10^3 \langle x - 3000 \rangle^3}{3} - \dfrac{5 \langle x \rangle^4}{12} \qquad \text{... Eq. (ii)}$$

Boundary conditions:
At $x = 0$, $y = 0$:
Eq. (ii) yields... $\qquad \qquad 0 = 0 + 0 + C_2 - 0 - 0$

$$C_2 = 0$$

At $x = L = 6000$, $y = 0$:

Eq. (ii) yields... $\qquad 0 = \dfrac{21.25 \times 10^3 \langle 6000 \rangle^3}{3} + C_1 \langle 6000 \rangle$

$$- \dfrac{12.5 \times 10^3 \langle 6000 - 3000 \rangle^3}{3} - \dfrac{5 \langle 6000 \rangle^4}{12}$$

$$C_1 = -1.463 \times 10^{11}$$

Substituting C_1 in Eq. (i) we get

$$EI \dfrac{dy}{dx} = 21.25 \times 10^3 \langle x \rangle^2 - 1.463 \times 10^{11}$$

$$- 12.5 \times 10^3 \langle x - 3000 \rangle^2 - \dfrac{5 \langle x \rangle^3}{3} \qquad \text{... Eq. (iii)}$$

Substituting C_1 and C_2 in Eq. (ii) we get

$$EIy = \dfrac{21.25 \times 10^3 \langle x \rangle^3}{3} - 1.463 \times 10^{11} \langle x \rangle$$

$$-\frac{12.5\times10^3\,\langle x-3000\rangle^3}{3}-\frac{5\langle x\rangle^4}{12} \qquad\qquad \dots \text{Eq. (iv)}$$

a. *Slope at both ends*

At A, $x = 0$

Eq. (iii) yields...
$$EI\theta_A = 0 - 1.463\times10^{11} - 0 - 0$$

$$\theta_A = \frac{-1.463\times10^{11}}{(200\times10^3)\times(150\times10^6)} = -0.0048 \text{ rad}$$

$$\text{(Clockwise)}$$

At B, $x = 6000$ mm

Eq. (iii) yields...
$$EI\theta_B = 21.25\times10^3\,\langle6000\rangle^2 - 1.463\times10^{11}$$

$$-12.5\times10^3\,\langle6000-3000\rangle^2 - \frac{5\langle6000\rangle^3}{3}$$

$$\theta_B = \frac{1.462\times10^{11}}{(200\times10^3)\times(150\times10^6)} = 0.0048 \text{ rad}$$

$$\text{(Counter clockwise)}$$

b. *Deflection at load point*

At C, $x = 3000$ mm

Eq. (iv) yields...
$$EIy_C = \frac{21.25\times10^3\,\langle3000\rangle^3}{3} - 1.463\times10^{11}\,\langle3000\rangle$$

$$-0 - \frac{5\langle3000\rangle^4}{12}$$

$$y_C = \frac{-2.814\times10^{14}}{(200\times10^3)\times(150\times10^6)} = -9.38 \text{ mm}$$

c. *The position and magnitude of maximum deflection*

For maximum deflection $\dfrac{dy}{dx} = 0$

Eq. (iii) yields ...
$$0 = 21.25\times10^3\,\langle x\rangle^2 - 1.463\times10^{11}$$

$$-12.5\times10^3\,\langle x-3000\rangle^2 - \frac{5\langle x\rangle^3}{3}$$

$$0 = x^2 - 6.88\times10^6 - 0.59(x^2 + 9\times10^6 - 6000x)$$
$$- 78.43\times10^{-6}\,x^3$$

i.e. $\quad 78.43\times10^{-6}\,x^3 - 0.41x^2 - 3540x + 12.19\times10^6 = 0$

$$x = 3000 \text{ mm}$$

Eq. (iv) yields ...
$$EIy_{max} = \frac{21.25\times10^3\,\langle3000\rangle^3}{3} - 1.463\times10^{11}\,\langle3000\rangle$$

$$-0 - \frac{5\langle3000\rangle^4}{12}$$

$$y_{max} = \frac{-2.814 \times 10^{14}}{(200 \times 10^3) \times (150 \times 10^6)} = -9.38 \text{ mm}$$

Here case (b) and case (c) have same answer as the beam is symmetric.

35. **A simply supported beam of span 7 m is subjected to two concentrated loads of 100 N each acting at 2 m from either supports as shown in Fig. 8.37. It is also acted upon by a uniformly distributed load of 6 N/m over the entire span. If $E = 200 \times 10^3$ MPa, $I = 100 \times 10^6$ mm^4, determine:**

(a) Deflection at load points

(b) The position and magnitude of maximum deflection.

Solution: $L = 7000$ mm, $W_1 = W_2 = 100$ N, $w = 6$ N/m $= 0.006$ N/mm, $x_1 = 2000$ mm, $x_2 = 5000$ mm $E = 200 \times 10^3$ MPa, $I = 100 \times 10^6$ mm^4. a) $y_C, y_D = ?$, b) $x = ?, y_{max} = ?$

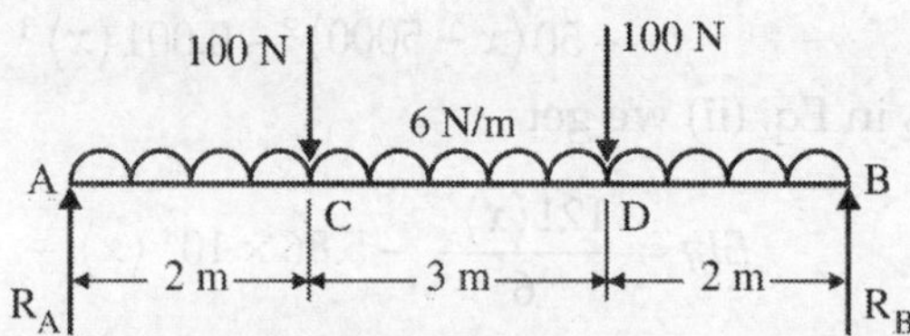

Fig. 8.37: Problem 35

Reactions at supports:

$$R_A + R_B = (6 \times 7) + 100 + 100 = 242 \text{ N} \qquad \text{... Eq. (a)}$$

Taking moments about A and equating to zero, we have

$$R_B \times 7 = (100 \times 2) + (100 \times 5) + (6 \times 7)\left(\frac{7}{2}\right)$$

$$R_B = 121 \text{ N} \qquad \text{... Eq. (b)}$$

Substituting Eq. (b) in Eq. (a), we have

$$R_A + 242 = 121$$

$$R_A = 121 \text{ N} \qquad \text{... Eq. (c)}$$

Consider a section X-X at a distance x from end A and in the region DB.

Bending moment at X-X is $M_x = R_A.\langle x \rangle - W_1 \langle x - 2000 \rangle - W_2 \langle x - 5000 \rangle - \left(\frac{w}{2}\right)\langle x \rangle^2$

i.e. $\qquad EI\dfrac{d^2y}{dx^2} = 121\langle x \rangle - 100\langle x - 2000 \rangle - 100\langle x - 5000 \rangle - \dfrac{0.006\langle x \rangle^2}{2}$

Integrating once we have $EI\dfrac{dy}{dx} = \dfrac{121\langle x \rangle^2}{2} + C_1 - 50\langle x - 2000 \rangle^2 - 50\langle x - 5000 \rangle^2$

$$- 0.001\langle x \rangle^3 \qquad \text{... Eq. (i)}$$

Integrating again we have $\quad EIy = \dfrac{121\langle x \rangle^3}{6} + C_1\langle x \rangle + C_2 - \dfrac{50\langle x - 2000 \rangle^3}{3}$

$$- \dfrac{50\langle x - 5000 \rangle^3}{3} - 2.5 \times 10^{-4}\langle x \rangle^4 \qquad \text{... Eq. (ii)}$$

Boundary conditions:

At $x = 0, y = 0$:

Eq. (ii) yields... $\qquad\qquad 0 = 0 + 0 + C_2 - 0 - 0$

Ignore brackets containing negative value

$$C_2 = 0$$

At $x = L = 7000$ mm, $y = 0$:

Eq. (ii) yields…

$$0 = \frac{121\langle 7000 \rangle^3}{6} + C_1 \langle 7000 \rangle - \frac{50\langle 7000 - 2000 \rangle^3}{3}$$

$$- \frac{50\langle 7000 - 5000 \rangle^3}{3} - 2.5 \times 10^{-4}\langle 7000 \rangle^4$$

$$C_1 = -5.86 \times 10^8$$

Substituting C_1 in Eq. (i) we get

$$EI\frac{dy}{dx} = \frac{121\langle x \rangle^2}{2} - 5.86 \times 10^8 - 50\langle x - 2000 \rangle^2$$

$$- 50\langle x - 5000 \rangle^2 - 0.001\langle x \rangle^3 \qquad \text{… Eq. (iii)}$$

Substituting C_1 and C_2 in Eq. (ii) we get

$$EIy = \frac{121\langle x \rangle^3}{6} - 5.86 \times 10^8 \langle x \rangle - \frac{50\langle x - 2000 \rangle^3}{3}$$

$$- \frac{50\langle x - 5000 \rangle^3}{3} - 2.5 \times 10^{-4}\langle x \rangle^4 \qquad \text{… Eq. (iv)}$$

a. *Deflection at load points*
   At C, $x = 2000$ mm

Eq. (iv) yields…

$$EIy_C = \frac{121\langle 2000 \rangle^3}{6} - 5.86 \times 10^8 \langle 2000 \rangle - 0 - 0$$

$$- 2.5 \times 10^{-4}\langle 2000 \rangle^4$$

$$y_C = \frac{-1.015 \times 10^{12}}{(200 \times 10^3) \times (100 \times 10^6)} = -0.0507 \text{ mm}$$

At D, $x = 5000$ mm

Eq. (iv) yields…

$$EIy_D = \frac{121\langle 5000 \rangle^3}{6} - 5.86 \times 10^8 \langle 5000 \rangle$$

$$- \frac{50\langle 5000 - 2000 \rangle^3}{3} - 0 - 2.5 \times 10^{-4}\langle 5000 \rangle^4$$

$$y_D = \frac{-1.015 \times 10^{12}}{(200 \times 10^3) \times (100 \times 10^6)} = -0.0507 \text{ mm}$$

Note: Here $y_C = y_D$, since the beam is symmetrically loaded.

b. *The position and magnitude of maximum deflection*

For maximum deflection $\frac{dy}{dx} = 0$

Eq. (iii) yields ...
$$0 = \frac{121\langle x\rangle^2}{2} - 5.86 \times 10^8 - 50\langle x - 2000\rangle^2$$
$$- 50\langle x - 5000\rangle^2 - 0.001\langle x\rangle^3$$
$$0 = 60.5x^2 - 5.86 \times 10^8 - 50(x^2 + 4 \times 10^6 - 4000x)$$
$$- 50(x^2 + 25 \times 10^6 - 10000x) - 0.001\langle x\rangle^3$$
$$0 = -0.001\langle x\rangle^3 - 39.5x^2 + 700.06 \times 10^3\, x - 2.036 \times 10^9$$
$$x = 3802.87 \text{ mm}$$

Eq. (iv) yields ...
$$EIy_{max} = \frac{121\langle 3802.87\rangle^3}{6} - 5.86 \times 10^8\,\langle 3802.87\rangle$$
$$- \frac{50\langle 3802.87 - 2000\rangle^3}{3} - 0 - 2.5 \times 10^{-4}\langle 3802.87\rangle^4$$
$$y_{max} = \frac{-1.269 \times 10^{14}}{(200 \times 10^3) \times (100 \times 10^6)} = -0.063 \text{ mm}$$

36. **A simply supported beam of span 7 m carries concentrated loads of 120 kN, 20 kN and 60 kN at 1 m, 4 m and 5 m respectively from left support, along with a UDL of 24 kN/m over the entire span. If $I = 400 \times 10^6$ mm^4 and $E = 210$ GPa, find**
    (a) Slope at supports   (b) Slope at load points   (c) Deflection at load points
    (d) The location and magnitude of the maximum deflection.

Solution: $L = 7000$ mm, $w = 24$ kN/m $= 24$ N/mm, $W_1 = 120 \times 10^3$ N, $W_2 = 20 \times 10^3$ N, $W_3 = 60 \times 10^3$ N, $x_1 = 1000$ mm, $x_2 = 4000$ mm, $x_3 = 5000$ mm, $E = 210 \times 10^3$ MPa, $I = 400 \times 10^6$ mm^4. a) θ_A, $\theta_B = ?$, b) θ_C, θ_D, $\theta_E = ?$, c) y_C, y_D, $y_E = ?$ d) $x = ?$, $y_{max} = ?$
Based on given data, the problem is as shown in **Fig. 8.38**.

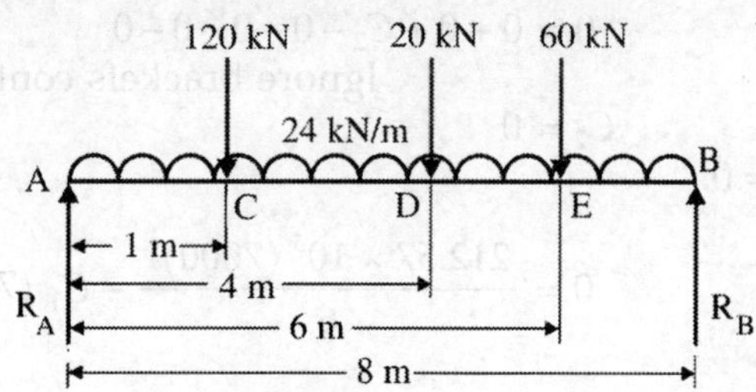

Fig. 8.38: Problem 36

Reactions at supports:
$$R_A + R_B = (24 \times 7) + 120 + 20 + 60 = 368 \text{ kN} \qquad \text{... Eq. (a)}$$
Taking moments about A and equating to zero, we have
$$R_B \times 7 = (120 \times 1) + (20 \times 4) + (60 \times 5) + (24 \times 7)\left(\frac{7}{2}\right)$$
$$R_B = 155.43 \text{ kN} \qquad \text{... Eq. (b)}$$
Substituting Eq. (b) in Eq. (a), we have
$$R_A + 155.43 = 368$$
$$R_A = 212.57 \text{ kN} \qquad \text{... Eq. (c)}$$

Consider a section X-X at a distance x from end A and in the region EB. Bending moment at X-X is

$$M_x = R_A \langle x \rangle - W_1 \langle x - 1000 \rangle - W_2 \langle x - 4000 \rangle$$

$$- W_3 \langle x - 5000 \rangle - \left(\frac{w}{2}\right)\langle x \rangle^2$$

i.e.
$$EI\frac{d^2y}{dx^2} = 212.57 \times 10^3 \langle x \rangle - 120 \times 10^3 \langle x - 1000 \rangle$$

$$- 20 \times 10^3 \langle x - 4000 \rangle - 60 \times 10^3 \langle x - 5000 \rangle$$

$$- \frac{24 \langle x \rangle^2}{2}$$

Integrating once we have

$$EI\frac{dy}{dx} = \frac{212.57 \times 10^3 \langle x \rangle^2}{2} + C_1 - 60000 \langle x - 1000 \rangle^2$$

$$- 10000 \langle x - 4000 \rangle^2 - 30000 \langle x - 5000 \rangle - 4 \langle x \rangle^3$$

$$\dots \text{Eq. (i)}$$

Integrating again we have

$$EIy = \frac{212.57 \times 10^3 \langle x \rangle^3}{6} + C_1 \langle x \rangle + C_2 - 20000 \langle x - 1000 \rangle^3$$

$$- \frac{10000 \langle x - 4000 \rangle^3}{3} - 10000 \langle x - 5000 \rangle^3 - \langle x \rangle^4$$

$$\dots \text{Eq. (ii)}$$

Boundary conditions:
At $x = 0, y = 0$:
Eq. (ii) yields...
$$0 = 0 + 0 + C_2 - 0 - 0 - 0 - 0$$

Ignore brackets containing negative value
$$C_2 = 0$$

At $x = L = 7000$ mm, $y = 0$:

Eq. (ii) yields...
$$0 = \frac{212.57 \times 10^3 \langle 7000 \rangle^3}{6} + C_1 \langle 7000 \rangle$$

$$- 20000 \langle 7000 - 1000 \rangle^3 - \frac{10000 \langle 7000 - 4000 \rangle^3}{3}$$

$$- 10000 \langle 7000 - 5000 \rangle^3 - \langle 7000 \rangle^4$$
$$C_1 = -7.52 \times 10^{11}$$

Substituting C_1 in Eq. (i) we get

$$EI\frac{dy}{dx} = \frac{212.57 \times 10^3 \langle x \rangle^2}{2} - 7.52 \times 10^{11} - 60000 \langle x - 1000 \rangle^2$$

$$- 10000 \langle x - 4000 \rangle^2 - 30000 \langle x - 5000 \rangle^2 - 4 \langle x \rangle^3$$

$$\dots \text{Eq. (iii)}$$

Substituting C_1 and C_2 in Eq. (ii) we get

$$EIy = \frac{212.57 \times 10^3 \, \langle x \rangle^3}{6} - 7.52 \times 10^{11} \, \langle x \rangle$$

$$- 20000 \, \langle x - 1000 \rangle^3 - \frac{10000 \, \langle x - 4000 \rangle^3}{3}$$

$$- 10000 \, \langle x - 5000 \rangle^3 - \langle x \rangle^4 \qquad \ldots \text{ Eq. (iv)}$$

a. *Slope at supports*

At A, $x = 0$

Eq. (iii) yields...
$$EI\theta_A = 0 - 7.52 \times 10^{11} - 0 - 0 - 0 - 0$$

Ignore brackets containing negative value

$$\theta_A = \frac{-7.52 \times 10^{11}}{(210 \times 10^3) \times (400 \times 10^6)} = -0.00895 \text{ rad}$$

(Clockwise)

At B, $x = 7000$ mm

Eq. (iii) yields...
$$EI\theta_B = \frac{212.57 \times 10^3 \, \langle 7000 \rangle^2}{2} - 7.52 \times 10^{11}$$

$$- 60000 \, \langle 7000 - 1000 \rangle^2 - 10000 \, \langle 7000 - 4000 \rangle^2$$

$$- 30000 \, \langle 7000 - 5000 \rangle^2 - 4 \, \langle 7000 \rangle^3$$

$$\theta_B = \frac{8.4 \times 10^{11}}{(210 \times 10^3) \times (400 \times 10^6)} = 0.0085 \text{ rad}$$

(Counter clockwise)

b. *Slope at load points*

At C, $x = 1000$ mm

Eq. (iii) yields...
$$EI\theta_C = \frac{212.57 \times 10^3 \, \langle 1000 \rangle^2}{2} - 7.52 \times 10^{11} - 0 - 0$$

$$- 0 - 4 \, \langle 1000 \rangle^3$$

$$\theta_C = \frac{-6.49 \times 10^{11}}{(210 \times 10^3) \times (400 \times 10^6)} = -0.0077 \text{ rad}$$

(Clockwise)

At D, $x = 4000$ mm

Eq. (iii) yields...
$$EI\theta_D = \frac{212.57 \times 10^3 \, \langle 4000 \rangle^2}{2} - 7.52 \times 10^{11}$$

$$- 60000 \, \langle 4000 - 1000 \rangle^2 - 0 - 0 - 4 \, \langle 4000 \rangle^3$$

$$\theta_D = \frac{1.53 \times 10^{11}}{(210 \times 10^3) \times (400 \times 10^6)} = 0.00182 \text{ rad}$$

(Clockwise)

At E, $x = 5000$ mm

Eq. (iii) yields...

$$EI\theta_E = \frac{212.57 \times 10^3 \langle 5000 \rangle^2}{2} - 7.52 \times 10^{11}$$

$$- 60000 \langle 5000 - 1000 \rangle^2 - 10000 \langle 5000 - 4000 \rangle^2$$

$$- 0 - 4 \langle 5000 \rangle^3$$

$$\theta_E = \frac{4.35 \times 10^{11}}{(210 \times 10^3) \times (400 \times 10^6)} = 0.00518 \text{ rad}$$

(Clockwise)

c. *Deflection at load points*
   At C, $x = 1000$ mm

Eq. (iv) yields...

$$EIy_C = \frac{212.57 \times 10^3 \langle 6000 \rangle^3}{6} - 7.52 \times 10^{11} \langle 1000 \rangle$$

$$- 0 - 0 - 0 - \langle 1000 \rangle^4$$

$$y_C = \frac{-7.176 \times 10^{14}}{(210 \times 10^3) \times (400 \times 10^6)} = -8.54 \text{ mm}$$

At D, $x = 4000$ mm

Eq. (iv) yields...

$$EIy_D = \frac{212.57 \times 10^3 \langle 4000 \rangle^3}{6} - 7.52 \times 10^{11} \langle 4000 \rangle$$

$$- 20000 \langle 4000 - 1000 \rangle^3 - 0 - 0 - \langle 4000 \rangle^4$$

$$y_D = \frac{-1.536 \times 10^{15}}{(210 \times 10^3) \times (400 \times 10^6)} = -18.29 \text{ mm}$$

At $x = 5000$ mm

Eq. (iv) yields...

$$EIy_E = \frac{212.57 \times 10^3 \langle 5000 \rangle^3}{6} - 7.52 \times 10^{11} \langle 5000 \rangle$$

$$- 20000 \langle 5000 - 1000 \rangle^3 - \frac{10000 \langle 5000 - 4000 \rangle^3}{3}$$

$$- 0 - \langle 5000 \rangle^4$$

$$y_E = \frac{-1.239 \times 10^{15}}{(210 \times 10^3) \times (400 \times 10^6)} = -14.75 \text{ mm}$$

d. *The location and magnitude of the maximum deflection.*

For maximum deflection $\dfrac{dy}{dx} = 0$

Eq. (iii) yields ...

$$0 = \frac{212.57 \times 10^3 \langle x \rangle^2}{2} - 7.52 \times 10^{11}$$

$$- 60000 \langle x - 1000 \rangle^2 - 10000 \langle x - 4000 \rangle^2$$

$$- 30000 \langle x - 5000 \rangle^2 - 4 \langle x \rangle^3$$

$$0 = 3.54\langle x\rangle^2 - 25.06 \times 10^6 - 2\langle x - 1000\rangle^2$$

$$- 0.334\langle x - 4000\rangle^2 - \langle x - 5000\rangle^2$$

$$- 1.334 \times 10^{-6}\langle x\rangle^3$$

$$0 = 3.54x^2 - 25.06 \times 10^6 - 2(x^2 + 1 \times 10^6 - 2000x)$$
$$- 0.334(x^2 + 16 \times 10^6 - 8000x)$$

$$- (x^2 + 25 \times 10^6 - 10000x) - 1.334 \times 10^{-4}\langle x\rangle^3$$

i.e.

$$1.334 \times 10^{-4}\langle x\rangle^3 - 0.206x^2 - 16672x + 57.404 \times 10^6 = 0$$

$$x = 3672.91 \text{ mm}$$

Eq. (iv) yields ...

$$EIy_{\max} = \frac{212.57 \times 10^3 \langle 3672.91\rangle^3}{6} - 7.52 \times 10^{11}\langle 3672.91\rangle$$

$$- 20000\langle 3672.91 - 1000\rangle^3 - 0 - 0 - \langle 3672.91\rangle^4$$

$$y_{\max} = \frac{-1.57 \times 10^{15}}{(210 \times 10^3) \times (400 \times 10^6)} = -18.69 \text{ mm}$$

8.9.3 Simply supported beams with partial UDL

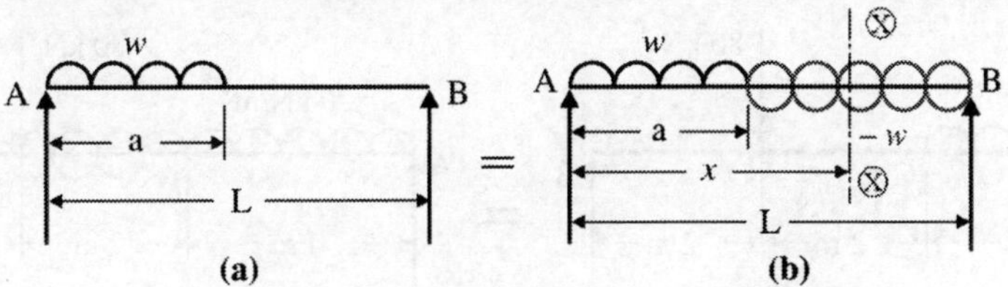

Fig. 8.39: Beam with partial UDL @ left end

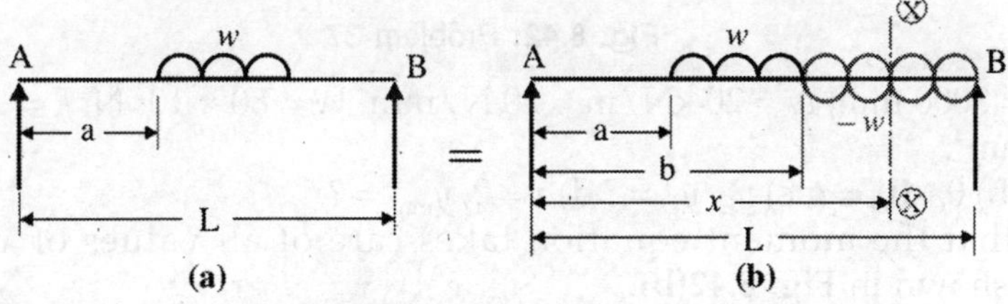

Fig. 8.40: Beam with intermediate partial UDL

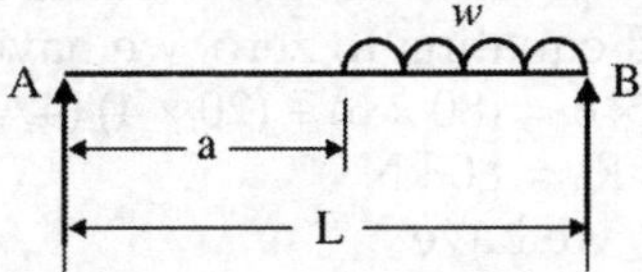

Fig. 8.41: Beam with partial UDL @ right end

Fig's 8.39, 8.40 and **8.41** represent different cases of simply supported beams subjected to partial loads.

Fig. 8.39(a) shows a beam with partial UDL at left end. In order that the moment equation takes care of all values of x, we extend the UDL up to the right end of the beam. Now an equal and opposite UDL is added for the extended portion of the beam to cancel the unwanted portion of the initial distributed load, as shown in **Fig. 8.39(b)**.

$$EI\frac{d^2y}{dx^2} = R_A \cdot \langle x \rangle - \frac{w\langle x \rangle^2}{2} + \frac{w\langle x-a \rangle^2}{2} \qquad \text{... (Eq. 8.57)}$$

Fig. 8.40(a) shows a beam with intermediate partial UDL. On similar lines as discussed above, we have

$$EI\frac{d^2y}{dx^2} = R_A \cdot \langle x \rangle - \frac{w\langle x-a \rangle^2}{2} + \frac{w\langle x-b \rangle^2}{2}$$

Fig. 8.41 shows a beam with partial UDL starting anywhere and extending up to the right end. The general equation for bending moment will hold good for the entire beam. In this case there is no extension and subtraction of the UDL.

$$EI\frac{d^2y}{dx^2} = R_A \cdot \langle x \rangle - \frac{w\langle x-a \rangle^2}{2}$$

SSB WITH DISTRIBUTED LOAD AT LEFT END

37. **A simply supported beam is loaded as shown in Fig. 8.42(a). If E = 200 GPa and $I = 60 \times 10^6$ mm^4, determine:**

   (a) **Slope at supports**   (b) **slope at load points**   (c) **Deflection at load points**

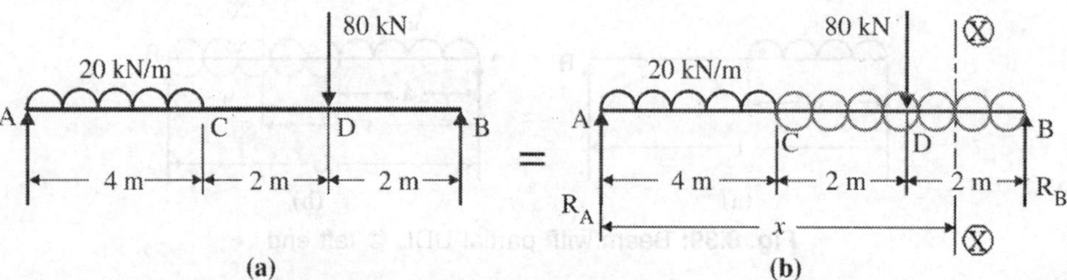

Fig. 8.42: Problem 37

Solution: L = 8000 mm, w = 20 kN/m = 20 N/mm, $W = 80 \times 10^3$ N, $E = 200 \times 10^3$ MPa, $I = 60 \times 10^6$ mm^4.

a) θ_A , θ_B = ?, b) θ_C ,θ_D = ?, c) y_C, y_D = ? d) x = ?, y_{max} = ?

In order that the moment equation takes care of all values of x, the beam is modified as shown in **Fig. 8.42(b)**.

Reactions at supports:

$$R_A + R_B = (20 \times 4) + 80 = 160 \text{ kN} \qquad \text{... Eq. (a)}$$

Taking moments about A and equating to zero, we have

$$R_B \times 8 = (80 \times 6) + (20 \times 4)(4/2)$$
$$R_B = 80 \text{ kN} \qquad \text{... Eq. (b)}$$

Substituting Eq. (b) in Eq. (a), we have

$$R_A + 80 = 160$$
$$R_A = 80 \text{ kN} \qquad \text{... Eq. (c)}$$

Consider a section X-X at a distance x from end A and in the region DB. Bending moment at X-X is

$$M_x = R_A \langle x \rangle - \frac{w\langle x \rangle^2}{2} - W\langle x-6000 \rangle + \frac{w\langle x-4000 \rangle^2}{2}$$

i.e. $$EI\frac{d^2y}{dx^2} = 80000\langle x \rangle - \frac{20\langle x \rangle^2}{2} - 80000\langle x-6000 \rangle + \frac{20\langle x-4000 \rangle^2}{2}$$

Integrating once we have

$$EI\frac{dy}{dx} = 40000\langle x\rangle^2 + C_1 - \frac{10\langle x\rangle^3}{3} - 40000\langle x - 6000\rangle^2 + \frac{10\langle x - 4000\rangle^3}{3}$$

$$\dots \text{Eq. (i)}$$

Integrating again we have

$$EIy = \frac{40000\langle x\rangle^3}{3} + C_1\langle x\rangle + C_2 - \frac{5\langle x\rangle^4}{6} - \frac{40000\langle x - 6000\rangle^3}{3}$$

$$+ \frac{5\langle x - 4000\rangle^4}{6} \qquad \dots \text{Eq. (ii)}$$

Boundary conditions:
At $x = 0, y = 0$:
Eq. (ii) yields... $\qquad 0 = 0 + 0 + C_2 - 0 - 0 + 0$

Ignore brackets containing negative value

$$C_2 = 0$$

At $x = L = 8000$ mm, $y = 0$:

Eq. (ii) yields... $\qquad 0 = \dfrac{40000\langle 8000\rangle^3}{3} + C_1\langle 8000\rangle - \dfrac{5\langle 8000\rangle^4}{6}$

$$- \frac{40000\langle 8000 - 6000\rangle^3}{3} + \frac{5\langle 8000 - 4000\rangle^4}{6}$$

$$C_1 = -4.4 \times 10^{11}$$

Substituting C_1 in Eq. (i) we get

$$EI\frac{dy}{dx} = 40000\langle x\rangle^2 - 4.4 \times 10^{11} - \frac{10\langle x\rangle^3}{3} - 40000\langle x - 6000\rangle^2$$

$$+ \frac{10\langle x - 4000\rangle^3}{3} \qquad \dots \text{Eq. (iii)}$$

Substituting C_1 and C_2 in Eq. (ii) we get

$$EIy = \frac{40000\langle x\rangle^3}{3} - 4.4 \times 10^{11}\langle x\rangle + C_2 - \frac{5\langle x\rangle^4}{6} - \frac{40000\langle x - 6000\rangle^3}{3}$$

$$+ \frac{5\langle x - 4000\rangle^4}{6} \qquad \dots \text{Eq. (iv)}$$

a. *Slope at supports*
   At A, $x = 0$
   Eq. (iii) yields...$EI\theta_A = 0 - 4.4 \times 10^{11} - 0 - 0 + 0$

Ignore brackets containing negative value

$$\theta_A = \frac{-4.4 \times 10^{11}}{(200 \times 10^3) \times (60 \times 10^6)} = -0.0366 \text{ rad} \qquad \text{(Clockwise)}$$

   At B, $x = 8000$ mm

Eq. (iii) yields...$EI\theta_B = 40000\langle 8000\rangle^2 - 4.4 \times 10^{11} - \dfrac{10\langle 8000\rangle^3}{3} - 40000\langle 8000 - 6000\rangle^2$

$$+ \frac{10\langle 8000 - 4000\rangle^3}{3}$$

$$\theta_B = \frac{4.67 \times 10^{11}}{(200 \times 10^3) \times (60 \times 10^6)} = 0.0388 \text{ rad} \qquad \text{(Counter clockwise)}$$

b. *Slope at load points*
   At C, $x = 4000$ mm

Eq. (iii) yields... $EI\theta_C = 40000\langle 4000\rangle^2 - 4.4 \times 10^{11} - \dfrac{10\langle 4000\rangle^3}{3} - 0 + 0$

$$\theta_C = \frac{-1.33 \times 10^{10}}{(200 \times 10^3) \times (60 \times 10^6)} = -0.0011 \text{ rad} \qquad \text{(Counter clockwise)}$$

   At D, $x = 6000$ mm

Eq. (iii) yields... $EI\theta_D = 40000\langle 6000\rangle^2 - 4.4 \times 10^{11} - \dfrac{10\langle 6000\rangle^3}{3} - 0$

$$+ \frac{10\langle 6000 - 4000\rangle^3}{3}$$

$$\theta_D = \frac{3.066 \times 10^{11}}{(200 \times 10^3) \times (60 \times 10^6)} = 0.0255 \text{ rad} \qquad \text{(Counter clockwise)}$$

c. *Deflection at load points*
   At C, $x = 4000$ mm

Eq. (iv) yields... $EIy_C = \dfrac{40000\langle 4000\rangle^3}{3} - 4.4 \times 10^{11}\langle 4000\rangle - \dfrac{5\langle 4000\rangle^4}{6} - 0 + 0$

$$y_C = \frac{-1.12 \times 10^{15}}{(200 \times 10^3) \times (60 \times 10^6)} = -93.33 \text{ mm}$$

   At D, $x = 6000$ mm

Eq. (iv) yields... $EIy_D = \dfrac{40000\langle 6000\rangle^3}{3} - 4.4 \times 10^{11}\langle 6000\rangle - \dfrac{5\langle 6000\rangle^4}{6} - 0$

$$+ \frac{5\langle 6000 - 4000\rangle^4}{6}$$

$$y_D = \frac{-8.266 \times 10^{14}}{(200 \times 10^3) \times (60 \times 10^6)} = -68.89 \text{ mm}$$

SSB WITH DISTRIBUTED INTERMEDIATE LOAD

38. A simply supported beam of span 8 m is loaded s shown in Fig. 8.43(a). If the moment of inertia of the section is 4.3×10^8 mm^4 and Young's modulus is 200 GPa, calculate

(a) The deflection at mid span   (b) Maximum deflection   (c) Slope at point D.

VTU – June/ July 2014 – 14 Marks; (CV) Dec. 13/ Jan. 14 – 14 Marks; [Similar: Dec. 2010 – 20 Marks]

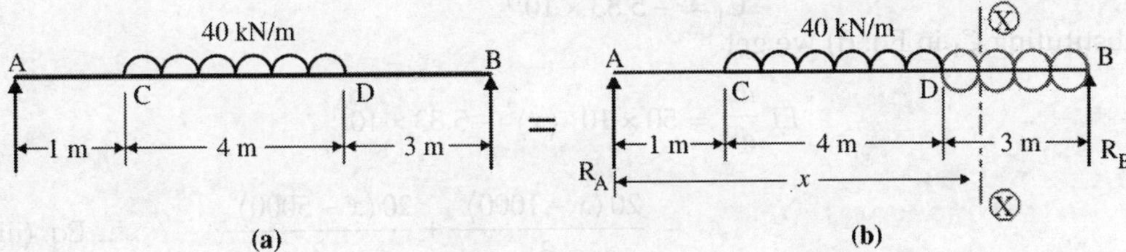

(a)   **(b)**

Fig. 8.43: Problem 38

Solution: $w = 40$ kN/m $= 40$ N/mm, $L = 8000$ mm, $I = 4.3 \times 10^8$ mm^4, $E = 200 \times 10^3$ MPa. a) $y_{L/2} = ?$, b) $y_{max} = ?$, c) $\theta_D = ?$

In order that the moment equation takes care of all values of x, the beam is modified as shown in **Fig. 8.43(b)**.

Reactions at supports:
$$R_A + R_B = WL = 40 \times 4 = 160 \text{ kN} \qquad \text{... Eq. (a)}$$
Taking moments about A and equating to zero, we have
$$R_B \times 8 = [40 \times 4 \times (4/2 + 1)]$$
$$R_B = 60 \text{ kN} \qquad \text{... Eq. (b)}$$
Substituting Eq. (ii) in Eq. (i), we have
$$R_A + 60 = 160$$
$$R_A = 100 \text{ kN} \qquad \text{... Eq. (c)}$$
Consider a section X-X at a distance x from end A and in the region DB. Bending moment at X-X is

$$M_x = R_A \langle x \rangle - \frac{w(x - 1000)^2}{2} + \frac{w(x - 5000)^2}{2}$$

i.e.
$$EI \frac{d^2y}{dx^2} = 100 \times 10^3 \langle x \rangle - \frac{40 \langle x - 1000 \rangle^2}{2} + \frac{40 \langle x - 5000 \rangle^2}{2}$$

Integrating once we have

$$EI \frac{dy}{dx} = 50 \times 10^3 \langle x \rangle^2 + C_1 - \frac{20 \langle x - 2000 \rangle^3}{3} + \frac{20 \langle x - 5000 \rangle^3}{3} \qquad \text{... Eq. (i)}$$

Integrating again we have

$$EIy = \frac{50 \times 10^3 \langle x \rangle^3}{3} + C_1 \langle x \rangle + C_2 - \frac{5 \langle x - 1000 \rangle^4}{3} + \frac{5 \langle x - 5000 \rangle^4}{3} \qquad \text{... Eq. (ii)}$$

Boundary conditions:
At $x = 0, y = 0$:
Eq. (ii) yields... $0 = 0 + 0 + C_2 - 0 + 0$

Ignore brackets containing negative value

$$C_2 = 0$$

At $x = L = 8000$ mm, $y = 0$:

Eq. (ii) yields...

$$0 = \frac{50 \times 10^3 \langle 8000 \rangle^3}{3} + C_1 \langle 8000 \rangle$$

$$- \frac{5 \langle 8000 - 1000 \rangle^4}{3} + \frac{5 \langle 8000 - 5000 \rangle^4}{3}$$

$$C_1 = -5.83 \times 10^{11}$$

Substituting C_1 in Eq. (i) we get

$$EI \frac{dy}{dx} = 50 \times 10^3 \langle x \rangle^2 - 5.83 \times 10^{11}$$

$$- \frac{20 \langle x - 1000 \rangle^3}{3} + \frac{20 \langle x - 5000 \rangle^3}{3} \qquad \text{... Eq. (iii)}$$

Substituting C_1 and C_2 in Eq. (ii) we get

$$EIy = \frac{50 \times 10^3 \langle x \rangle^3}{3} - 5.83 \times 10^{11} \langle x \rangle + C_2$$

$$- \frac{5 \langle x - 1000 \rangle^4}{3} + \frac{5 \langle x - 5000 \rangle^4}{3} \qquad \text{... Eq. (iv)}$$

a. *Deflection at mid span*
   At $L/2$, $x = 4000$ mm

Eq. (iv) yields...

$$EIy_{L/2} = \frac{50 \times 10^3 \langle 4000 \rangle^3}{3} - 5.83 \times 10^{11} \langle 4000 \rangle$$

$$- \frac{5 \langle 4000 - 1000 \rangle^4}{3} + 0$$

$$y_{L/2} = \frac{-1.40 \times 10^{15}}{(200 \times 10^3) \times (4.3 \times 10^8)} = -16.28 \text{ mm}$$

b. *Maximum deflection.*

For maximum deflection $\dfrac{dy}{dx} = 0$

Eq. (iii) yields ...

$$0 = 50 \times 10^3 \langle x \rangle^2 - 5.83 \times 10^{11} - \frac{20 \langle x - 1000 \rangle^3}{3} + \frac{20 \langle x - 5000 \rangle^3}{3}$$

$$0 = 50 \times 10^3 \langle x \rangle^2 - 5.83 \times 10^{11} - 6.67 \langle x - 1000 \rangle^3 + 6.67 \langle x - 5000 \rangle^3$$

Upon solving we get $x = 3875.88$ mm

Eq. (iv) yields ...

$$EIy_{max} = \frac{50 \times 10^3 \langle 3875.88 \rangle^3}{3} - 5.83 \times 10^{11} \langle 3875.88 \rangle$$

$$- \frac{5 \langle 3875.88 - 1000 \rangle^4}{3} + 0$$

$$y_{max} = \frac{-1.403 \times 10^{15}}{(200 \times 10^3) \times (4.3 \times 10^8)} = -16.32\,\text{mm}$$

c. *Slope at D*
   At D, $x = 5000$ mm,

Eq. (iii) yields...
$$EI\theta_D = 50 \times 10^3 \langle 5000 \rangle^2 - 5.83 \times 10^{11}$$

$$- \frac{20 \langle 5000 - 1000 \rangle^3}{3} + 0$$

$$\theta_D = \frac{3.066 \times 10^{11}}{(200 \times 10^3) \times (4.3 \times 10^8)} = 0.0028\,\text{rad}$$

(Counter clockwise)

39. Determine the deflection at points C, D and E for the beam shown in Fig. 8.44(a). Take $E = 200$ kN/mm^2 and $I = 60 \times 10^6$ mm^4.

VTU – Dec. 16/ Jan. 17 – 10 Marks, June/ July 15 – 10 Marks

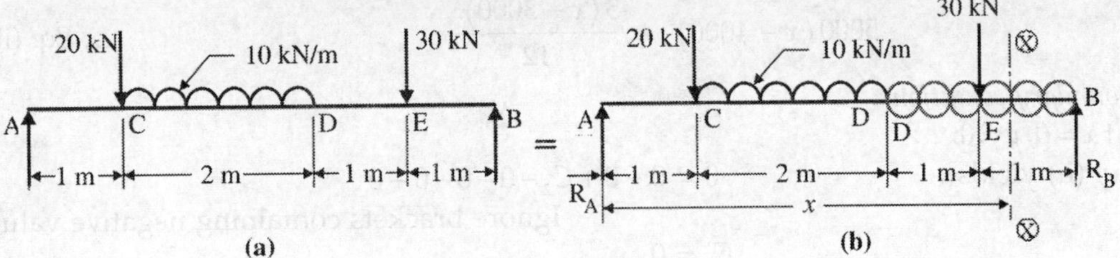

Fig. 8.44: Problem 39

Solution: $w = 10$ kN/m $= 10$ N/mm, $W_1 = 20 \times 10^3$ N, $W_2 = 30 \times 10^3$ N, $L = 5000$ mm, $E = 200 \times 10^3$ MPa, $I = 60 \times 10^6$ mm^4. $y_C, y_D, y_E = ?$

In order that the moment equation takes care of all values of x, the beam is modified as shown in **Fig. 8.44(b)**.

Reactions at supports:
$$R_A + R_B = 20 + 30 + (10 \times 2) = 70\,\text{kN} \qquad \text{... Eq. (a)}$$

Taking moments about A aand equating to zero, we have

$$R_B \times 5 = (30 \times 4) + \left[10 \times 2 \times \left(\frac{2}{2} + 1 \right) \right] + (20 + 1)$$

$$R_B = 36\,\text{kN} \qquad \text{... Eq. (b)}$$

Substituting eq. (ii) in Eq. (i), we have
$$R_A + 36 = 70$$
$$R_A = 34\,\text{kN} \qquad \text{... Eq. (c)}$$

Consider a section X-X at a distance x from end A and in the region EB. Bending moment at X-X is

$$M_x = R_A \langle x \rangle - W_1 \langle x - 1000 \rangle - \frac{w \langle x - 1000 \rangle^2}{2}$$

$$- W_2 \langle x - 4000 \rangle + \frac{w \langle x - 3000 \rangle^2}{2}$$

i.e.
$$EI\frac{d^2y}{dx^2} = 34000\langle x\rangle - 20000\langle x-1000\rangle - \frac{10(x-1000)^2}{2}$$

$$-30000\langle x-4000\rangle + \frac{10\langle x-3000\rangle^2}{2}$$

Integrating once we have

$$EI\frac{dy}{dx} = 17000\langle x\rangle^2 + C_1 - 10000\langle x-1000\rangle^2 - \frac{5\langle x-1000\rangle^3}{3}$$

$$-15000\langle x-4000\rangle^2 + \frac{5\langle x-3000\rangle^3}{3} \qquad \text{... Eq. (i)}$$

Integrating again we have

$$EIy = \frac{17000\langle x\rangle^3}{3} + C_1\langle x\rangle + C_2 - \frac{10000\langle x-1000\rangle^3}{3} - \frac{5\langle x-1000\rangle^4}{12}$$

$$-5000\langle x-4000\rangle^3 + \frac{5\langle x-3000\rangle^4}{12} \qquad \text{... Eq. (ii)}$$

Boundary conditions:
At $x = 0$, $y = 0$:
Eq. (ii) yields...
$$0 = 0+0+C_2-0-0-0+0$$

Ignore brackets containing negative value
$$C_2 = 0$$

At $x = L = 5000$ mm, $y = 0$:

Eq. (ii) yields...
$$0 = \frac{17000\langle 5000\rangle^3}{3} + C_1\langle 5000\rangle - \frac{10000\langle 5000-1000\rangle^3}{3}$$

$$- \frac{5\langle 5000-1000\rangle^4}{12} - 5000\langle 5000-4000\rangle^3 + \frac{5\langle 5000-3000\rangle^4}{12}$$

$$C_1 = -7.8 \times 10^{10}$$

Substituting C_1 in Eq. (i) we get

$$EI\frac{dy}{dx} = 17000\langle x\rangle^2 - 7.8 \times 10^{10} - 10000\langle x-1000\rangle^2 - \frac{5\langle x-1000\rangle^3}{3}$$

$$-15000\langle x-4000\rangle^2 + \frac{5\langle x-3000\rangle^3}{3} \qquad \text{... Eq. (iii)}$$

Substituting C_1 and C_2 in Eq. (ii) we get

$$EIy = \frac{17000\langle x\rangle^3}{3} - 7.8 \times 10^{10}\langle x\rangle - \frac{10000\langle x-1000\rangle^3}{3} - \frac{5\langle x-1000\rangle^4}{12}$$

$$-5000\langle x-4000\rangle^3 + \frac{5\langle x-3000\rangle^4}{12} \qquad \text{... Eq. (iv)}$$

Deflection

a. At C, $x = 1000$ mm

Eq. (iv) yields...

$$EIy_C = \frac{17000\langle 1000\rangle^3}{3} - 7.8 \times 10^{10}\langle 1000\rangle - 0 - 0 - 0 + 0$$

$$y_C = \frac{-7.23 \times 10^{13}}{(200 \times 10^3) \times (60 \times 10^6)} = -6.028 \text{ mm}$$

b. At D, $x = 3000$ mm

Eq. (iv) yields...

$$EIy_D = \frac{17000\langle 3000\rangle^3}{3} - 7.8 \times 10^{10}\langle 3000\rangle$$

$$- \frac{10000\langle 3000 - 1000\rangle^3}{3} - \frac{5\langle 3000 - 1000\rangle^4}{12} - 0 + 0$$

$$y_D = \frac{-1.143 \times 10^{14}}{(200 \times 10^3) \times (60 \times 10^6)} = -9.528 \text{ mm}$$

c. At E, $x = 4000$ mm

Eq. (iv) yields...

$$EIy_E = \frac{17000\langle 4000\rangle^3}{3} - 7.8 \times 10^{10}\langle 4000\rangle$$

$$- \frac{10000\langle 4000 - 1000\rangle^3}{3} - \frac{5\langle 4000 - 1000\rangle^4}{12} - 0$$

$$+ \frac{5\langle 4000 - 3000\rangle^4}{12}$$

$$y_E = \frac{-7.27 \times 10^{13}}{(200 \times 10^3) \times (60 \times 10^6)} = -6.056 \text{ mm}$$

SSB WITH DISTRIBUTED LOAD AT RIGHT END

40. A beam AB of span 6 m is simply supported at the ends and is loaded as shown in Fig. 8.45. Determine:

(a) Deflection at C   (b) maximum deflection and   (c) slope at the end A.

Take $E = 2 \times 10^5$ N/mm^2, $I = 2 \times 10^7$ mm^4.

VTU – June/ July 2008 – 15 Marks, May/ June 2010 – 14 Marks;
(CV) June/ July 2008 – 14 Marks

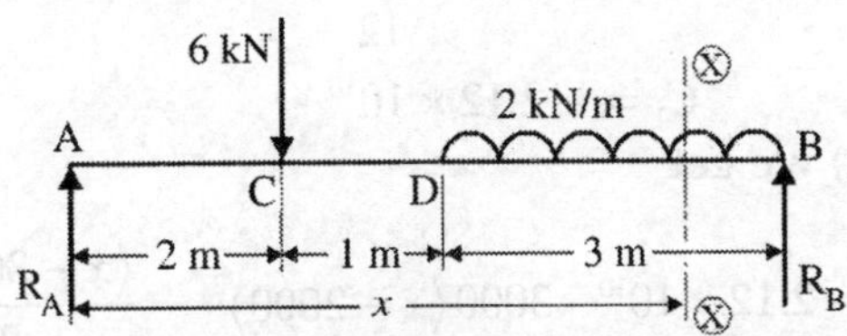

Fig. 8.45: Problem 40

Solution: $L = 6000$ mm, $W = 6000$ N, $w = 2$ kN/m $= 2$ N/mm, $E = 2 \times 10^5$ MPa, $I = 2 \times 10^7$ mm, a) $y_C = ?$, b) $y_{max} = ?$, c) $\theta_A = ?$.

Reactions at supports:

$$R_A + R_B = 6 + (2 \times 3) = 12 \text{ kN} \qquad \text{... Eq. (a)}$$

Taking moments about A and equating to zero, we have

$$R_B \times 6 = (6 \times 2) + (2 \times 3)\left[\frac{3}{2} + 3\right]$$

$$R_B = 6.5 \text{ kN} \qquad \text{... Eq. (b)}$$

Substituting Eq. (b) in Eq. (a), we have

$$R_A + 6.5 = 12$$

$$R_A = 5.5 \text{ kN} \qquad \text{... Eq. (c)}$$

Consider a section X-X at a distance x from end A and in the region DB. Bending moment at X-X is

$$M_x = R_A \langle x \rangle - W \langle x - 2000 \rangle - \frac{w \langle x - 3000 \rangle^2}{2}$$

i.e.

$$EI \frac{d^2 y}{dx^2} = 5500 \langle x \rangle - 6000 \langle x - 2000 \rangle - \frac{2 \langle x - 3000 \rangle^2}{2}$$

Integrating once we have

$$EI \frac{dy}{dx} = 2750 \langle x \rangle^2 + C_1 - 3000 \langle x - 2000 \rangle^2 - \frac{\langle x - 3000 \rangle^3}{3}$$

$$\text{... Eq. (i)}$$

Integrating again we have

$$EIy = \frac{2750 \langle x \rangle^3}{3} + C_1 \langle x \rangle + C_2 - 1000 \langle x - 2000 \rangle^3$$

$$- \frac{\langle x - 3000 \rangle^4}{12} \qquad \text{... Eq. (ii)}$$

Boundary conditions:

At $x = 0, y = 0$:

Eq. (ii) yields...
$$0 = 0 + 0 + C_2 - 0 - 0$$

Ignore brackets containing negative value

$$C_2 = 0$$

At $x = L = 6000$ mm, $y = 0$:

Eq. (ii) yields...
$$0 = \frac{2750 \langle 6000 \rangle^3}{3} + C_1 \langle 6000 \rangle - 1000 \langle 6000 - 2000 \rangle^3$$

$$- \frac{\langle 6000 - 3000 \rangle^4}{12}$$

$$C_1 = -2.12 \times 10^{10}$$

Substituting C_1 in Eq. (i) we get

$$EI \frac{dy}{dx} = 2750 \langle x \rangle^2 - 2.12 \times 10^{10} - 3000 \langle x - 2000 \rangle^2 - \frac{\langle x - 3000 \rangle^3}{3} \qquad \text{... Eq. (iii)}$$

Substituting C_1 and C_2 in Eq. (ii) we get

$$EIy = \frac{2750\langle x\rangle^3}{3} - 2.12 \times 10^{10}\langle x\rangle - 1000\langle x - 2000\rangle^3$$

$$- \frac{\langle x - 3000\rangle^4}{12} \qquad \text{... Eq. (iv)}$$

a. *Deflection at C*

At C, $x = 2000$ mm

Eq. (iv) yields... $EIy_C = \dfrac{2750\langle 2000\rangle^3}{3} - 2.12 \times 10^{10}\langle 2000\rangle - 0 - 0$

$$y_C = \frac{-3.51 \times 10^{13}}{(2 \times 10^5) \times (2 \times 10^7)} = -8.77 \text{ mm}$$

b. *Maximum deflection.*

For maximum deflection $\dfrac{dy}{dx} = 0$

Eq. (iii) yields ... $\qquad 0 = 2750\langle x\rangle^2 - 2.12 \times 10^{10} - 3000\langle x - 2000\rangle^2$

$$- \frac{\langle x - 3000\rangle^3}{3}$$

Assuming that the deflection to be maximum in portion CD, we have

$$0 = 2750\langle x\rangle^2 - 2.12 \times 10^{10} - 3000(x^2 + 4 \times 10^6 - 4000x)$$

$$0 = -250\langle x\rangle^2 + 12 \times 10^6 x - 3.32 \times 10^{10}$$

$$x = 2947.68 \text{ mm}$$

Eq. (iv) yields ... $\qquad EIy_{max} = \dfrac{2750\langle 2947.68\rangle^3}{3} - 2.12 \times 10^{10}\langle 2947.68\rangle$

$$- 1000\langle 2947.68 - 2000\rangle^3 - 0$$

$$y_{max} = \frac{-3.98 \times 10^{13}}{(2 \times 10^5) \times (2 \times 17^7)} = -9.966 \text{ mm}$$

c. *Slope at A*

At A, $x = 0$ mm

Eq. (iii) yields... $\qquad EI\theta_A = 0 - 2.12 \times 10^{10} - 0 - 0$

$$\theta_A = \frac{-2.12 \times 10^{10}}{(2 \times 10^5) \times (2 \times 10^7)} = -0.0053 \text{ rad(Clockwise)}$$

41. Find the maximum deflection and the maximum slope for the beam loaded as shown in Fig. 8.46. Take flexural rigidity $EI = 15 \times 10^9$ kN-mm^2.

VTU – Dec. 2011 – 12 Marks, June/ July 2011 – 12 Marks;
[Similar: (CV) Dec. 10 – 10 Marks]

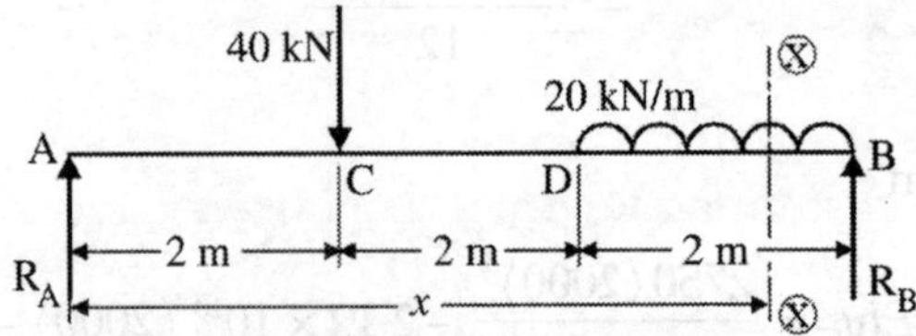

Fig. 8.46: Problem 41

Solution: $L = 6000$ mm, $W = 40 \times 10^3$ N, $w = 20$ kN/m $= 20$ N/mm, $EI = 15 \times 10^9$ kN-mm$^2 = 15 \times 10^{12}$ N-mm^2.

a) $y_{max} = ?$, c) $\theta_{max} = ?$.

Reactions at supports:

$$R_A + R_B = 40 + (20 \times 2) = 80 \text{ kN} \qquad \text{... Eq. (a)}$$

Taking moments about A and equating to zero, we have

$$R_B \times 6 = (40 \times 2) + (20 \times 2)\left(\frac{2}{2} + 4\right)$$

$$R_B = 46.67 \text{ kN} \qquad \text{... Eq. (b)}$$

Substituting Eq. (b) in Eq. (a), we have

$$R_A + 46.67 = 80$$

$$R_A = 33.33 \text{ kN} \qquad \text{... Eq. (c)}$$

Consider a section X-X at a distance x from end A and in the region DB. Bending moment at X-X is

$$M_x = R_A \langle x \rangle - W \langle x - 2000 \rangle - \frac{w \langle x - 4000 \rangle^2}{2}$$

i.e.

$$EI \frac{d^2y}{dx^2} = 33.33 \times 10^3 \langle x \rangle - 40 \times 10^3 \langle x - 2000 \rangle - \frac{20 \langle x - 4000 \rangle^2}{2}$$

Integrating once we have

$$EI \frac{dy}{dx} = \frac{33.33 \times 10^3 \langle x \rangle^2}{2} + C_1 - 20 \times 10^3 \langle x - 2000 \rangle^2 - \frac{10 \langle x - 4000 \rangle^3}{3}$$

$$\text{... Eq. (i)}$$

Integrating again we have

$$EIy = \frac{33.33 \times 10^3 \langle x \rangle^3}{6} + C_1 \langle x \rangle + C_2 - \frac{20 \times 10^3 \langle x - 2000 \rangle^3}{3}$$

$$- \frac{5(x - 4000)^4}{6} \qquad \text{... Eq. (ii)}$$

Boundary conditions:

At $x = 0$, $y = 0$:

Eq. (ii) yields... $\qquad 0 = 0 + 0 + C_2 - 0 - 0$

Ignore brackets containing negative value

$$C_2 = 0$$

At $x = L = 6000$ mm, $y = 0$:

Eq. (ii) yields... $\qquad 0 = \dfrac{33.33 \times 10^3 \langle 6000 \rangle^3}{6} + C_1 \langle 6000 \rangle$

$$- \frac{20^3 \times 10^3 \langle 6000 - 2000 \rangle^3}{3} - \frac{\langle 60000 - 4000 \rangle^4}{6}$$

$$C_1 = -1.26 \times 10^{11}$$

Substituting C_1 in Eq. (i) we get

$$EI \frac{dy}{dx} = \frac{33.33 \times 10^3 \langle x \rangle^2}{2} - 1.26 \times 10^{11}$$

$$- 20 \times 10^3 \langle x - 2000 \rangle^2 - \frac{10 \langle x - 4000 \rangle^3}{3} \quad \text{... Eq. (iii)}$$

Substituting C_1 and C_2 in Eq. (ii) we get

$$EIy = \frac{33.33 \times 10^3 \langle x \rangle^3}{6} - 1.26 \times 10^{11}$$

$$- \frac{20 \times 10^3 \langle x - 2000 \rangle^3}{3} - \frac{5 \langle x - 4000 \rangle^4}{4} \quad \text{... Eq. (iv)}$$

a. *Maximum deflection.*

For maximum deflection $\dfrac{dy}{dx} = 0$

Eq. (iii) yields ... $\qquad 0 = \dfrac{33.33 \times 10^3 \times \langle x \rangle^2}{2} - 1.26 \times 10^{11}$

$$- 20 \times 10^3 \langle x - 2000 \rangle^2 - \frac{10 \langle x - 4000 \rangle^3}{3}$$

Assuming that the deflection to be maximum in portion CD, we have

$$0 = \frac{33.33 \times 10^3 \langle x \rangle}{2} - 1.26 \times 10^{11} - 20 \times 10^3 (x^2 + 4 \times 10^6 - 4000x)$$

$$0 = -3335 \langle x \rangle^2 + 80 \times 10^6 x - 2.06 \times 10^{11}$$

$$x = 2933.82 \text{ mm}$$

Eq. (iv) yields ... $\qquad EIy_{max} = \dfrac{33.33 \times 10^3 \langle 2933.82 \rangle^3}{6} - 1.26 \times 10^{11} \langle 2933.82 \rangle$

$$- \frac{20 \times 10^3 \langle 2933.82 - 2000 \rangle^3}{3} - 0$$

$$y_{max} = \frac{-3.98 \times 10^{13}}{15 \times 10^{12}} = -15.65 \text{ mm}$$

b. *Maximum slope*

At A, $x = 0$ mm

Eq. (iii) yields... $EI\theta_A = 0 - 1.26 \times 10^{11} - 0 - 0$

$$\theta_A = \frac{-1.26 \times 10^{11}}{15 \times 10^{12}} = -0.0084 \text{ rad} \quad \text{(Clockwise)}$$

At B, $x = 6000$ mm

Eq. (iii) yields... $EI\theta_B = \dfrac{33.33 \times 10^3 \langle 6000 \rangle^2}{2} - 1.26 \times 10^{11}$

$$- 20 \times 10^3 \langle 6000 - 2000 \rangle^2 - \frac{10 \langle 6000 - 4000 \rangle^3}{3}$$

$$\theta_B = \frac{1.26 \times 10^{11}}{15 \times 10^{12}} = 0.0085 \text{ rad (Counter clockwise)}$$

42. **A simply supported is loaded as shown in Fig. 8.47. Determine**
    (a) Slope at load points
    (b) Deflection under load points.
    (c) The position and magnitude of the maximum deflection. Take E = 200 GPa,
    $I = 83 \times 10^6$ mm^4

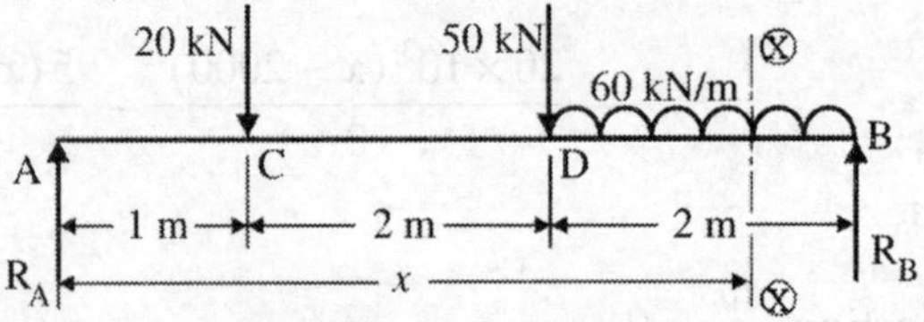

Fig. 8.47: Problem 42

Solution: L = 5000 mm, $W_1 = 20 \times 10^3$ N, $W_2 = 50 \times 10^3$ N, w = 60 kN/m = 60 N/mm, $E = 200 \times 10^3$ MPa, $I = 83 \times 10^6$ mm^4. a) θ_C, θ_D = ?, b) y_C, y_D = ?, c) y_{max} = ?

Reactions at supports:

$$R_A + R_B = 20 + 50 + (60 \times 2) = 190 \text{ kN} \qquad \text{... Eq. (a)}$$

Taking moments about A and equating to zero, we have

$$R_B \times 5 = (20 \times 1) + (50 \times 3) + (60 \times 2)\left(\frac{2}{2} + 3\right)$$

$$R_B = 130 \text{ kN} \qquad \text{... Eq. (b)}$$

Substituting Eq. (b) in Eq. (a), we have

$$R_A + 130 = 190$$

$$R_A = 60 \text{ kN} \qquad \text{... Eq. (c)}$$

Consider a section X-X at a distance x from end A and in the region DB. Bending moment at X-X is

$$M_x = R_A \langle x \rangle - W_1 \langle x - 1000 \rangle - W_2 \langle x - 3000 \rangle - \frac{w \langle x - 3000 \rangle^2}{2}$$

i.e. $EI\dfrac{d^2y}{dx^2} = 60 \times 10^3 \langle x \rangle - 20 \times 10^3 \langle x - 1000 \rangle - 50 \times 10^3 \langle x - 3000 \rangle$

$$- \frac{60 \langle x - 3000 \rangle^2}{2}$$

Integrating once we have

$$EI\frac{dy}{dx} = 30 \times 10^3 \langle x \rangle^2 + C_1 - 10 \times 10^3 \langle x - 1000 \rangle^2$$

$$- 25 \times 10^3 \langle x - 3000 \rangle^2 - 10 \langle x - 3000 \rangle^3 \quad \dots \text{Eq. (i)}$$

Integrating again we have

$$EIy = 10 \times 10^3 \langle x \rangle^3 + C_1 \langle x \rangle + C_2 - \frac{10 \times 10^3 \langle x - 1000 \rangle^3}{3}$$

$$- \frac{25 \times 10^3 \langle x - 3000 \rangle^3}{3} - 2.5 \langle x - 3000 \rangle^4 \quad \dots \text{Eq. (ii)}$$

Boundary conditions:

At $x = 0$, $y = 0$:

Eq. (ii) yields... $0 = 0 + 0 + C_2 - 0 - 0 - 0$

Ignore brackets containing negative value

$$C_2 = 0$$

At $x = L = 5000$ mm, $y = 0$:

Eq. (ii) yields... $\quad 0 = 10 \times 10^3 \langle 5000 \rangle^3 + C_1 \langle 5000 \rangle - \dfrac{10 \times 10^3 \langle 5000 - 1000 \rangle^3}{3}$

$$- \frac{25 \times 10^3 \langle 5000 - 3000 \rangle^3}{3} - 2.5 \langle 5000 - 3000 \rangle^4$$

$$C_1 = -1.86 \times 10^{11}$$

Substituting C_1 in Eq. (i) we get

$$EI\frac{dy}{dx} = 30 \times 10^3 \langle x \rangle^2 - 1.86 \times 10^{11} - 10 \times 10^3 \langle x - 1000 \rangle^2$$

$$- 25 \times 10^3 \langle x - 3000 \rangle^2 - 10 \langle x - 3000 \rangle^3 \quad \dots \text{Eq. (iii)}$$

Substituting C_1 and C_2 in Eq. (ii) we get

$$EIy = 10 \times 10^3 \langle x \rangle^3 - 1.86 \times 10^{11} \langle x \rangle + C_2 - \frac{10 \times 10^3 \langle x - 1000 \rangle^3}{3}$$

$$- \frac{25 \times 10^3 \langle x - 3000 \rangle^3}{3} - 2.5 \langle x - 3000 \rangle^4 \quad \dots \text{Eq. (iv)}$$

a. *Slope at load points*

   At C, $x = 1000$ mm

   Eq. (iii) yields... $\quad EI\theta_C = 30 \times 10^3 \langle 1000 \rangle^2 - 1.86 \times 10^{11} - 0 - 0 - 0$

$$\theta_C = \frac{-1.56 \times 10^{11}}{(200 \times 10^3)(83 \times 10^6)} = -0.0094 \text{ rad} \quad \text{(Clockwise)}$$

   At D, $x = 3000$ mm

Eq. (iii) yields... $\quad EI\theta_D = 30 \times 10^3 \langle 3000 \rangle^2 - 1.86 \times 10^{11} - 10 \times 10^3 \langle 3000 - 1000 \rangle^2 - 0 - 0$

$$\theta_D = \frac{3.066 \times 10^{11}}{(200 \times 10^3)(83 \times 10^6)} = 0.00265 \text{ rad} \quad (\text{Clockwise})$$

b. *Deflection at load points*

At C, $x = 1000$ mm

Eq. (iv) yields... $\quad EIy_C = 10 \times 10^3 \langle 1000 \rangle^3 - 1.86 \times 10^{11} \langle 1000 \rangle - 0 - 0 - 0$

$$y_C = \frac{-1.76 \times 10^{14}}{(200 \times 10^3)(83 \times 10^6)} = -10.60 \text{ mm}$$

At D, $x = 3000$ mm

Eq. (iv) yields... $\quad EIy_D = 10 \times 10^3 \langle 3000 \rangle^3 - 1.86 \times 10^{11} \langle 3000 \rangle$

$$- \frac{10 \times 10^3 \langle 3000 - 1000 \rangle^3}{3} - 0 - 0$$

$$y_D = \frac{-3.14 \times 10^{14}}{(200 \times 10^3)(83 \times 10^6)} = -18.96 \text{ mm}$$

c. *Maximum deflection.*

For maximum deflection $\dfrac{dy}{dx} = 0$

Eq. (iii) yields ... $\quad 0 = 30 \times 10^3 \langle x \rangle^2 - 1.86 \times 10^{11} - 10 \times 10^3 \langle x - 1000 \rangle^2$

$$- 25 \times 10^3 \langle x - 3000 \rangle^2 - 10 \langle x - 3000 \rangle^3$$

Assuming that the deflection to be maximum in portion CD, we have

$$0 = 30 \times 10^3 \langle x \rangle^2 - 1.86 \times 10^{11} - 10 \times 10^3 \langle x - 1000 \rangle^2 - 25 \times 10^3 \langle x - 3000 \rangle^2$$

$$0 = 1.2 \langle x \rangle^2 - 7.44 \times 10^6 - 0.4 \langle x - 1000 \rangle^2 - \langle x - 3000 \rangle^2$$

$$0 = 1.2 \langle x \rangle^2 - 7.44 \times 10^6 - 0.4(x^2 + 1 \times 10^6 - 2000x) - (x^2 + 9 \times 10^6 - 6000x)$$

$$0 = -0.2 \langle x \rangle^2 + 6800x - 16.84 \times 10^6$$

$$x = 2689.16 \text{ mm}$$

Eq. (iv) yields ... $\quad EIy_{\max} = 10 \times 10^3 \langle 2689.16 \rangle^3 - 1.86 \times 10^{11} \langle 2689.16 \rangle$

$$- \frac{10 \times 10^3 \langle 2689.16 - 1000 \rangle^3}{3} - 0 - 0$$

$$y_{\max} = \frac{-3.22 \times 10^{14}}{(200 \times 10^3) \times (83 \times 10^6)} = -19.38 \text{ mm}$$

43. A simply supported is loaded as shown in Fig. 8.48(a). Determine:
(a) Slope at supports   (b) Deflection at C and D   (c) Deflection at mid-span
Take $E = 200$ GPa, $I = 83 \times 10^6$ mm^4

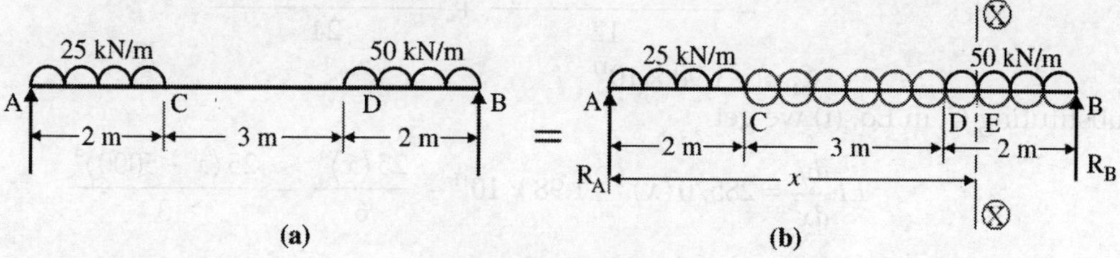

(a)   (b)

Fig. 8.48: Problem 43

Solution: $L = 7000$ mm, $w_1 = 25$ kN/m $= 25$ N/mm, $w_2 = 50 \times 10^3$ kN/m $= 50$ N/mm, $E = 200 \times 10^3$ MPa, $I = 83 \times 10^6$ mm^4. a) $\theta_A, \theta_B = ?$, b) $y_C, y_D = ?$, c) $y_{L/2} = ?$

Reactions at supports:

$$R_A + R_B = (25 \times 2) + (50 \times 2) = 150 \text{ kN} \qquad \text{... Eq. (a)}$$

Taking moments about A and equating to zero, we have

$$R_B \times 7 = (25 \times 2) \left(\frac{2}{2}\right) + (50 \times 2) \left(\frac{2}{2} + 5\right)$$

$$R_B = 92.86 \text{ kN} \qquad \text{... Eq. (b)}$$

Substituting Eq. (b) in Eq. (a), we have

$$R_A + 92.86 = 150$$

$$R_A = 57.14 \text{ kN} \qquad \text{... Eq. (c)}$$

Consider a section X-X at a distance x from end A and in the region DB as shown in **Fig. 8.48(b)**.

Bending moment at X-X is

$$M_x = R_A \langle x \rangle - \frac{w_1 \langle x \rangle^2}{2} - \frac{w_2 \langle x - 5000 \rangle^2}{2} + \frac{w_1 \langle x - 2000 \rangle^2}{2}$$

i.e.

$$EI \frac{d^2y}{dx^2} = 57140 \langle x \rangle - \frac{25 \langle x \rangle^2}{2} - \frac{50 \langle x - 5000 \rangle^2}{2} + \frac{25 \langle x - 2000 \rangle^2}{2}$$

Integrating once we have

$$EI \frac{dy}{dx} = 28570 \langle x \rangle^2 + C_1 - \frac{25 \langle x \rangle^3}{6} - \frac{25 \langle x - 5000 \rangle^3}{3} + \frac{25 \langle x - 2000 \rangle^3}{6}$$

$$\text{... Eq. (i)}$$

Integrating again we have

$$EIy = \frac{28570 \langle x \rangle^3}{3} + C_1 \langle x \rangle + C_2 - \frac{25 \langle x \rangle^4}{24} - \frac{25 \langle x - 5000 \rangle^4}{12} + \frac{25 \langle x - 2000 \rangle^4}{24}$$

$$\text{... Eq. (ii)}$$

Boundary conditions:

At $x = 0$, $y = 0$:

Eq. (ii) yields...
$$0 = 0 + 0 + C_2 - 0 - 0 - 0$$

Ignore brackets containing negative value

$$C_2 = 0$$

At $x = L = 7000$ mm, $y = 0$:

Eq. (ii) yields...
$$0 = \frac{28570 \langle 7000 \rangle^3}{3} + C_1 \langle 7000 \rangle - \frac{25 \langle 7000 \rangle^4}{24}$$

$$- \frac{25 \langle 7000 - 5000 \rangle^4}{12} + \frac{25 \langle 7000 - 2000 \rangle^4}{24}$$

$$C_1 = -1.98 \times 10^{11}$$

Substituting C_1 in Eq. (i) we get

$$EI \frac{dy}{dx} = 28570 \langle x \rangle^2 - 1.98 \times 10^{11} - \frac{25 \langle x \rangle^3}{6} - \frac{25 \langle x - 5000 \rangle^3}{3}$$

$$+ \frac{25 \langle x - 2000 \rangle^3}{6} \qquad \text{... Eq. (iii)}$$

Substituting C_1 and C_2 in Eq. (ii) we get

$$EIy = \frac{28570 \langle x \rangle^3}{3} - 1.98 \times 10^{11} \langle x \rangle - \frac{25 \langle x \rangle^4}{24}$$

$$- \frac{25 \langle x - 5000 \rangle^4}{12} + \frac{25 \langle x - 2000 \rangle^4}{24} \qquad \text{... Eq. (iv)}$$

a. *Slope at supports*

At A, $x = 0$

Eq. (iii) yields...$EI\theta_A = 0 - 1.98 \times 10^{11} - 0 - 0 + 0$

$$\theta_A = \frac{-1.98 \times 10^{11}}{(200 \times 10^3) \times (83 \times 10^6)} = -0.012 \text{ mm}$$

At B, $x = 7000$ mm

Eq. (iii) yields...
$$EI\theta_B = 28570 \langle 7000 \rangle^2 - 1.98 \times 10^{11} - \frac{25 \langle 7000 \rangle^3}{6}$$

$$- \frac{25 \langle 7000 - 5000 \rangle^3}{3} + \frac{25 \langle 7000 - 2000 \rangle^3}{6}$$

$$\theta_B = \frac{2.27 \times 10^{11}}{(200 \times 10^3) \times (83 \times 10^6)} = 0.0136 \text{ mm}$$

b. *Deflection*

At C, $x = 2000$ mm

Eq. (iv) yields...
$$EIy_C = \frac{28570 \langle 2000 \rangle^3}{3} - 1.98 \times 10^{11} \langle 2000 \rangle - \frac{25 \langle 2000 \rangle^4}{24} - 0 + 0$$

$$y_C = \frac{-3.36 \times 10^{14}}{(200 \times 10^3) \times (83 \times 10^6)} = -20.27 \text{ mm}$$

At D, $x = 5000$ mm

Eq. (iv) yields...
$$EIy_D = \frac{28570 \langle 5000 \rangle^3}{3} - 1.98 \times 10^{11} \langle 5000 \rangle - \frac{25 \langle 5000 \rangle^4}{24}$$

$$-0 + \frac{25\langle 5000 - 2000\rangle^4}{24}$$

$$y_D = \frac{-3.668 \times 10^{14}}{(200 \times 10^3) \times (83 \times 10^6)} = -22.06 \text{ mm}$$

c. *Deflection at mid-span*
   At $L/2$, $x = 3500$ mm

Eq. (iv) yields... $EIy_{L/2} = \dfrac{28570\langle 3500\rangle^3}{3} - 1.98 \times 10^{11}\langle 3500\rangle - \dfrac{25\langle 3500\rangle^4}{24}$

$$-0 + \frac{25\langle 3500 - 2000\rangle^4}{24}$$

$$y_{L/2} = \frac{-4.36 \times 10^{14}}{(200 \times 10^3) \times (83 \times 10^6)} = -26.25 \text{ mm}$$

8.9.4 SSB subjected to a couple

44. Obtain the expressions for slope and deflection for a simply supported beam subjected to a counter clock wise couple acting at a distance a from the left support.

Solution: Fig. 8.49(a) indicates a simply supported beam subjected to a CCW couple at a distance a from left support

Let M = couple
         L = Length of the beam

Reactions at supports:

    $R_A + R_B = 0$ kN since no load is acting on the beam
$$\qquad\qquad\qquad\qquad\qquad\qquad\qquad \dots \text{ Eq. (a)}$$

Taking moments about A and equating to zero, we have

$$R_B L + M = 0$$

$$R_B = -\frac{M}{L} \qquad\qquad \dots \text{ Eq. (b)}$$

Substituting Eq. (b) in Eq. (a), we have

$$R_A - \frac{M}{L} = 0$$

$$R_A = \frac{M}{L} \qquad\qquad\qquad\qquad\qquad \dots \text{ Eq. (c)}$$

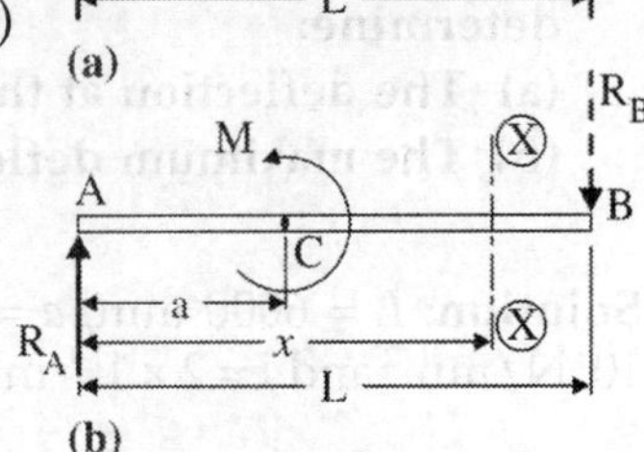

Fig. 8.49: Problem 44

Note: Since no other load is acting on the beam, reaction at the other support would be in the opposite sense to keep the system in equilibrium as shown in Fig. 8.49(b).

Consider a section X-X at a distance x from free end A and in the region CB. Bending moment at X-X is

$$M_x = R_A \cdot \langle x\rangle - M\langle x - a\rangle^0$$

i.e. $\qquad\qquad EI\dfrac{d^2y}{dx^2} = \dfrac{M\langle x\rangle}{L} - M\langle x - a\rangle^0$

Integrating once we have

$$EI\frac{dy}{dx} = \frac{M\langle x\rangle^2}{2L} + C_1 - M\langle x-a\rangle^1 \qquad \text{... Eq. (i)}$$

Integrating again we have

$$EIy = \frac{M\langle x\rangle^3}{6L} + C_1\langle x\rangle + C_2 - \frac{M\langle x-a\rangle^2}{2} \qquad \text{... Eq. (ii)}$$

Boundary conditions:

At $x = 0$, $y = 0$:

Eq. (ii) yields...
$$0 = 0 + 0 + C_2 - 0$$
$$C_2 = 0$$

At $x = L$, $y = 0$:

Eq. (ii) yields...
$$0 = \frac{ML^3}{6L} + C_1\langle L\rangle - \frac{M\langle L-a\rangle^2}{2}$$

$$C_1 = \frac{M\langle L-a\rangle^2}{2L} - \frac{ML}{6}$$

Substituting C_1 in Eq. (i) we get

$$EI\frac{dy}{dx} = \frac{M\langle x\rangle^2}{2L} + \frac{M\langle L-a\rangle^2}{2L} - \frac{ML}{6} - M\langle x-a\rangle^1 \qquad \text{... Eq. (iii)}$$

Substituting C_1 and C_2 in Eq. (ii) we get

$$EIy = \frac{M\langle x\rangle^3}{6L} + \left[\frac{M\langle L-a\rangle^2}{2L} - \frac{ML}{6}\right]\langle x\rangle - \frac{M\langle x-a\rangle^2}{2} \qquad \text{... Eq. (iv)}$$

45. **A horizontal beam AB is simply supported at A and B, 6m apart. The beam is subjected to a clockwise couple of 300 kN-m at a distance of 4m from the left end as shown in Fig. 8.50(a). If $E = 2.1 \times 10^5$ N/mm^2 and $I = 2 \times 10^8$ mm^4, determine:**

(a) The deflection at the point where the couple is acting

(b) The maximum deflection.

VTU – Dec. 13/ Jan. 14 – 16 Marks

Solution: $L = 6000$ mm, $a = 4000$ mm, $M = 300$ kN-m $= 300 \times 10^6$ N-mm, $E = 2.1 \times 10^5$ N/mm^2 and $I = 2 \times 10^8$ mm^4, a) $y_C = ?$, b) $y_{max} = ?$

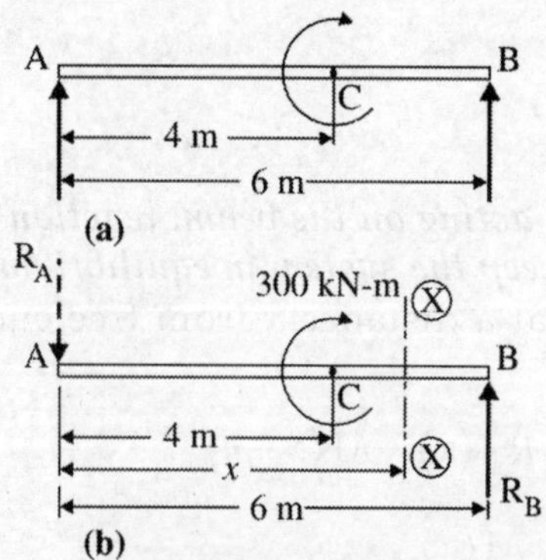

Fig. 8.50: Problem 45

Reactions at supports:

$$R_A + R_B = 0 \text{ kN since no load is acting on the beam} \qquad \ldots \text{Eq. (a)}$$

Taking moments about A and equating to zero, we have

$$R_B L = M$$
$$6R_B = 300$$
$$R_B = 50 \text{ kN} \qquad \ldots \text{Eq. (b)}$$

Substituting Eq. (b) in Eq. (a), we have

$$R_A + 50 = 0$$
$$R_A = -50 \text{ kN} \qquad \ldots \text{Eq. (c)}$$

Note: Since no other load is acting on the beam, reaction at the other support would be in the opposite sense to keep the system in equilibrium as shown in Fig. 8.50(b).

Consider a section X-X at a distance x from free end A and in the region CB as shown in **Fig. 8.50(b)**. Bending moment at X-X is

$$M_x = R_A.\langle x \rangle + M \langle x - a \rangle^0$$

i.e.

$$EI \frac{d^2y}{dx^2} = -50 \times 10^3 \langle x \rangle + 300 \times 10^6 \langle x - 4000 \rangle^0$$

Integrating once we have

$$EI \frac{dy}{dx} = -25 \times 10^3 \langle x \rangle^2 + C_1 + 300 \times 10^6 \langle x - 4000 \rangle^1 \qquad \ldots \text{Eq. (i)}$$

Integrating again we have

$$EIy = -\frac{25 \times 10^3}{3} \langle x \rangle^3 + C_1 \langle x \rangle + C_2 + 150 \times 10^6 \langle x - 4000 \rangle^2$$

$$\ldots \text{Eq. (ii)}$$

Boundary conditions:

At $x = 0, y = 0$:

Eq. (ii) yields…

$$0 = -0 + 0 + C_2 + 0$$
$$C_2 = 0$$

At $x = L = 6000$ mm, $y = 0$:

Eq. (ii) yields…

$$0 = -\frac{25 \times 10^3}{3} \langle 6000 \rangle^3 + C_1 \langle 6000 \rangle + 150 \times 10^6 \langle 6000 - 4000 \rangle^2$$

$$C_1 = 2 \times 10^{11}$$

Substituting C_1 in Eq. (i) we get

$$EI \frac{dy}{dx} = -25 \times 10^3 \langle x \rangle^2 + 2 \times 10^{11} + 300 \times 10^6 \langle x - 4000 \rangle^1 \qquad \ldots \text{Eq. (iii)}$$

Substituting C_1 and C_2 in Eq. (ii) we get

$$EIy = -\frac{25 \times 10^3}{3} \langle x \rangle^3 + 2 \times 10^{11} \langle x \rangle + 150 \times 10^6 \langle x - 4000 \rangle^2$$

$$\ldots \text{Eq. (iv)}$$

a. *Deflection at C*

At C, $x = 4000$ mm

Eq. (iv) yields... $EIy_C = -\dfrac{25 \times 10^3}{3} \langle 4000 \rangle^3 + 2 \times 10^{11} \langle 4000 \rangle + 0$

$$y_C = \frac{2.667 \times 10^{14}}{(2.1 \times 10^5) \times (2 \times 10^8)} = 6.35 \text{ mm}$$

b. *Maximum deflection.*

For maximum deflection $\dfrac{dy}{dx} = 0$

Eq. (iii) yields ... $0 = -25 \times 10^3 \langle x \rangle^2 + 2 \times 10^{11} + 300 \times 10^6 \langle x - 4000 \rangle^1$

Assuming that the deflection to be maximum in portion AC, we have

$$0 = -25 \times 10^3 \langle x \rangle^2 + 2 \times 10^{11}$$
$$x = 2828.43 \text{ mm}$$

Eq. (iv) yields... $EIy_{max} = -\dfrac{25 \times 10^3}{3} \langle 2828.43 \rangle^3 + 2 \times 10^{11} \langle 2828.43 \rangle + 0$

$$y_{max} = \frac{-3.77 \times 10^{14}}{(2.1 \times 10^5) \times (2 \times 10^8)} = -8.98 \text{ mm}$$

46. For the beam shown in Fig. 8.51(a), determine slope at the supports and mid span deflection.

VTU – (CV) June/ July 2009 – 14 Marks

Solution: $L = 9000$ mm, $M = 120$ kN–m$= 120 \times 10^6$ N-mm. a) $\theta_A, \theta_B = ?$, b) $y_{L/2} = ?$
Reactions at supports:

$$R_A + R_B = 80 \text{ kN} \qquad \qquad \text{... Eq. (a)}$$

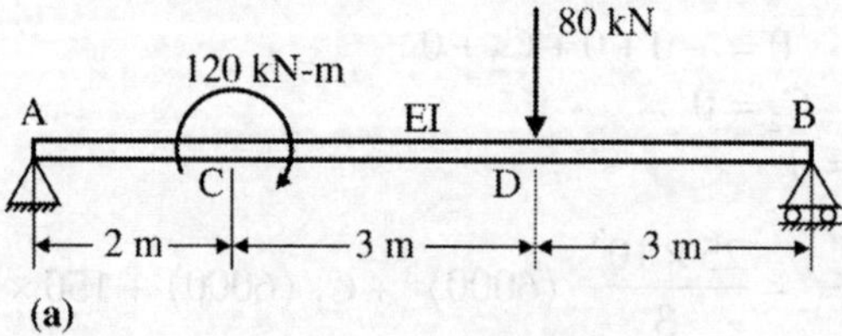

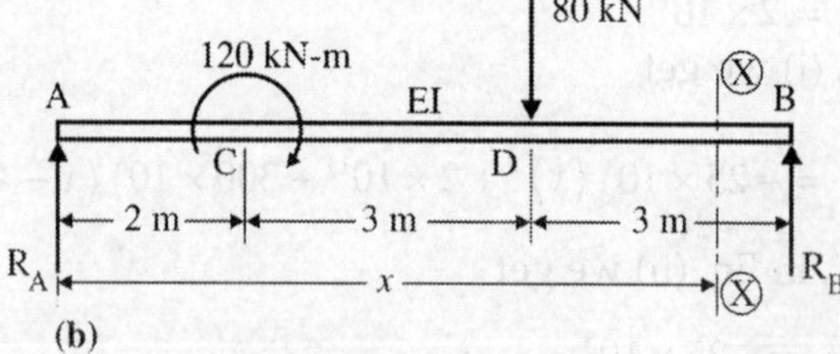

Fig. 8.51: Problem 46

Taking moments about A and equating to zero, we have
$$8R_B = 120 + (80 \times 5)$$
$$R_B = 65 \text{ kN} \qquad \qquad \text{... Eq. (b)}$$

Substituting Eq. (b) in Eq. (a), we have
$$R_A + 65 = 80$$
$$R_A = 15 \text{ kN} \qquad \qquad \text{... Eq. (c)}$$

Consider a section X-X at a distance x from free end A and in the region DB as shown in **Fig. 8.51(b)**. Bending moment at X-X is

$$M_x = R_A.\langle x \rangle + M\langle x - 2000 \rangle^0 - W\langle x - 5000 \rangle$$

i.e.
$$EI\frac{d^2y}{dx} = 15000\langle x \rangle + 120 \times 10^6 \langle x - 2000 \rangle^0 - 80000\langle x - 5000 \rangle$$

Integrating once we have

$$EI\frac{dy}{dx} = 7500\langle x \rangle^2 + C_1 + 120 \times 10^6 \langle x - 2000 \rangle^1 - 40000\langle x - 5000 \rangle^2$$
$$\text{... Eq. (i)}$$

Integrating again we have

$$EIy = 2500\langle x \rangle^3 + C_1\langle x \rangle + C_2 + 60 \times 10^6 \langle x - 2000 \rangle^2$$
$$- \frac{40000\langle x - 5000 \rangle^3}{3} \qquad \text{... Eq. (ii)}$$

Boundary conditions:
At $x = 0, y = 0$:
Eq. (ii) yields...
$$0 = 0 + 0 + C_2 + 0 - 0$$
$$C_2 = 0$$

At $x = L = 8000$ mm, $y = 0$:

Eq. (ii) yields...
$$0 = 2500\langle 8000 \rangle^3 + C_1\langle 8000 \rangle + 60 \times 10^6 \langle 8000 - 2000 \rangle^2$$
$$- \frac{40000\langle 8000 - 5000 \rangle^3}{3}$$
$$C_1 = -3.85 \times 10^{11}$$

Substituting C_1 in Eq. (i) we get

$$EI\frac{dy}{dx} = 7500\langle x \rangle^2 - 3.85 \times 10^{11} + 120 \times 10^6 \langle x - 2000 \rangle^1$$
$$- 40000\langle x - 5000 \rangle^2 \qquad \text{... Eq. (iii)}$$

Substituting C_1 and C_2 in Eq. (ii) we get

$$EIy = 2500\langle x \rangle^3 - 3.85 \times 10^{11}\langle x \rangle + C_2 + 60 \times 10^6 \langle x - 2000 \rangle^2$$
$$- \frac{40000\langle x - 5000 \rangle^3}{3} \qquad \text{... Eq. (iv)}$$

a. *Slope at supports*
   At A, $x = 0$
   Eq. (iii) yields... $EI\theta_A = 0 - 3.85 \times 10^{11} + 0 + 0$

$$\theta_A = \frac{-3.85 \times 10^{11}}{EI}$$

At B, $x = 8000$ mm

Eq. (iii) yields...
$$EI\theta_B = 7500\langle 8000\rangle^2 - 3.85\times 10^{11} + 120\times 10^6\langle 8000 - 2000\rangle^1$$
$$-40000\langle 8000 - 5000\rangle^2$$

$$\theta_B = \frac{4.55\times 10^{11}}{EI}$$

b. *Deflection at mid-span*
   At $L/2$, $x = 4000$ mm

Eq. (iv) yields... $EIy_{L/2} = 2500\langle 4000\rangle^3 - 3.85\times 10^{11}\langle 4000\rangle$
$$+ 60\times 10^6\langle 4000 - 2000\rangle^2 - 0$$

$$y_{L/2} = \frac{-1.14\times 10^{15}}{EI}$$

47. A simply supported is loaded as shown in Fig. 8.52(a). Determine:
(a) Slope at supports   (b) Deflection at C and D.
Take $E = 200$ GPa, $I = 2\times 10^8$ mm^4

Solution: $L = 6000$ mm, $w = 20$ kN/m $= 20$ N/mm, $W = 40\times 10^3$N, $M = 120\times 10^6$ N-mm, $E = 2\times 10^5$ MPa, $I = 2\times 10^8$ mm^4. a) θ_A, $\theta_B = ?$, b) y_C, $y_D = ?$

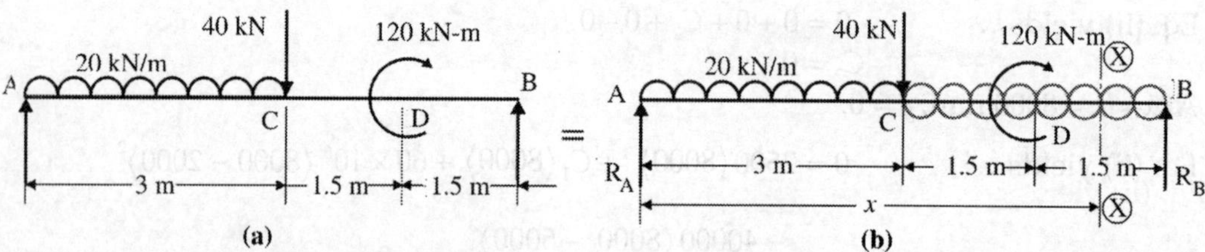

Fig. 8.52: Problem 47

Reactions at supports:
$$R_A + R_B = (20\times 3) + 40 = 100 \text{ kN} \quad\quad \text{... Eq. (a)}$$
Taking moments about A and equating to zero, we have
$$R_B \times 6 = 120 + (40\times 3) + [(20\times 3)\times (3/2)]$$
$$R_B = 55 \text{ kN} \quad\quad \text{... Eq. (b)}$$
Substituting Eq. (b) in Eq. (a), we have
$$R_A + 55 = 100$$
$$R_A = 45 \text{ kN} \quad\quad \text{... Eq. (c)}$$
Consider a section X-X at a distance x from free end A and in the region DB as shown in **Fig. 8.52(b)**.

Bending moment at X-X is $M_x = R_A.\langle x\rangle - \dfrac{w\langle x\rangle^2}{2} - W\langle x - 3000\rangle + M\langle x - 4500\rangle^0$
$$+ \frac{w\langle x - 3000\rangle^2}{2}$$

i.e.
$$EI\frac{d^2y}{dx^2} = 45000\langle x\rangle - \frac{20\langle x\rangle^2}{2} - 40000\langle x - 3000\rangle$$

$$+ 120 \times 10^6 \langle x - 4500\rangle^0 + \frac{20\langle x - 3000\rangle^2}{2}$$

Integrating once we have

$$EI\frac{dy}{dx} = 22500\langle x\rangle^2 + C_1 - \frac{10\langle x\rangle^3}{3} - 20000\langle x - 3000\rangle^2$$

$$+ 120 \times 10^6 \langle x - 4500\rangle^1 + \frac{10\langle x - 3000\rangle^3}{3} \qquad \dots \text{Eq. (i)}$$

Integrating again we have

$$EIy = 7500\langle x\rangle^3 + C_1\langle x\rangle + C_2 - \frac{5\langle x\rangle^4}{6} - \frac{20000\langle x - 3000\rangle^3}{3}$$

$$+ 60 \times 10^6 \langle x - 4500\rangle^2 + \frac{5\langle x - 3000\rangle^4}{6} \qquad \dots \text{Eq. (ii)}$$

Boundary conditions:
At $x = 0$, $y = 0$:

 Eq. (ii) yields… $0 = 0 + 0 + C_2 - 0 - 0 + 0 + 0$

        $C_2 = 0$

At $x = L = 6000$ mm, $y = 0$:

Eq. (ii) yields… $0 = 7500\langle 6000\rangle^3 + C_1\langle 6000\rangle - \frac{5\langle 6000\rangle^4}{6}$

$$- \frac{20000\langle 6000 - 3000\rangle^3}{3} + 60 \times 10^6 \langle 6000 - 4500\rangle^2$$

$$+ \frac{5\langle 6000 - 3000\rangle^4}{6}$$

      $C_1 = -9.375 \times 10^{10}$

Substituting C_1 in Eq. (i) we get

$$EI\frac{dy}{dx} = 22500\langle x\rangle^2 - 9.375 \times 10^{10} - \frac{10\langle x\rangle^3}{3} - 20000\langle x - 3000\rangle^2$$

$$+ 120 \times 10^6 \langle x - 4500\rangle^1 + \frac{10\langle x - 3000\rangle^3}{3} \qquad \dots \text{Eq. (iii)}$$

Substituting C_1 and C_2 in Eq. (ii) we get

$$EIy = 7500\langle x\rangle^3 - 9.375 \times 10^{10}\langle x\rangle - \frac{5\langle x\rangle^4}{6} - \frac{20000\langle x - 3000\rangle^3}{3}$$

$$+ 60 \times 10^6 \langle x - 4500\rangle^2 + \frac{5\langle x - 3000\rangle^4}{6} \qquad \dots \text{Eq. (iv)}$$

a. *Slope at supports*

At A, $x = 0$

Eq. (iii) yields... $EI\theta_A = 0 - 9.375 \times 10^{10} - 0 - 0 + 0 + 0$

$$\theta_A = \frac{-9.375 \times 10^{10}}{(2 \times 10^5) \times (2 \times 10^8)} = -0.0023 \text{ rad}$$

At B, $x = 6000$ mm

Eq. (iii) yields... $EI\theta_B = 22500\langle 6000 \rangle^2 - 9.375 \times 10^{10} - \dfrac{10\langle 6000 \rangle^3}{3}$

$$- 20000\langle 6000 - 3000 \rangle^2 + 120 \times 10^6 \langle 6000 - 4500 \rangle^1$$

$$+ \frac{10\langle 6000 - 3000 \rangle^3}{3}$$

$$\theta_B = \frac{8.625 \times 10^{10}}{(2 \times 10^5) \times (2 \times 10^8)} = 0.0022 \text{ rad}$$

b. *Deflection*

At C, $x = 3000$ mm

Eq. (iv) yields... $EIy_C = 7500\langle 3000 \rangle^3 - 9.375 \times 10^{10} \langle 3000 \rangle - \dfrac{5\langle 3000 \rangle^4}{6} - 0 + 0 + 0$

$$y_C = \frac{-1.463 \times 10^{14}}{(2 \times 10^5) \times (2 \times 10^8)} = -3.66 \text{ mm}$$

At D, $x = 4500$ mm

Eq. (iv) yields... $EIy_D = 7500\langle 4500 \rangle^3 - 9.375 \times 10^{10} \langle 4500 \rangle - \dfrac{5\langle 4500 \rangle^4}{6}$

$$- \frac{20000\langle 4500 - 3000 \rangle^3}{3} + 0 + \frac{5\langle 4500 - 3000 \rangle^4}{6}$$

$$y_D = \frac{-9.84 \times 10^{13}}{(2 \times 10^5) \times (2 \times 10^8)} = -2.46 \text{ mm}$$

48. A simply supported is loaded as shown in Fig. 8.53(a). Determine:
(a) Slope at supports   (b) Deflection at C, D and E.
Take $E = 200$ GPa, $I = 90 \times 10^6$ mm^4

Solution: $L = 7000$ mm, $W = 40 \times 10^3$ N, $w = 20$ kN/m $= 20$ N/mm, $M = 80 \times 10^6$ N-mm, $E = 2 \times 10^5$ MPa, $I = 90 \times 10^6$ mm^4. a) θ_A, $\theta_B = ?$, b) y_C, y_D, $y_E = ?$

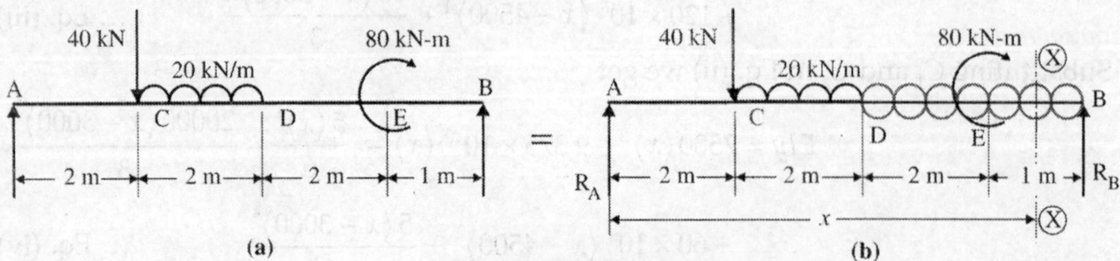

Fig. 8.53: Problem 48

Reactions at supports:

$$R_A + R_B = (20 \times 2) + 40 = 80 \text{ kN} \qquad \text{... Eq. (a)}$$

Taking moments about A and equating to zero, we have

$$R_B \times 7 = 80 + \left[(20 \times 2) \times \left(\frac{2}{2} + 2 \right) \right] + (40 \times 2)$$

$$R_B = 40 \text{ kN} \qquad \text{... Eq. (b)}$$

Substituting Eq. (b) in Eq. (a), we have

$$R_A + 40 = 80$$

$$R_A = 40 \text{ kN} \qquad \text{... Eq. (c)}$$

Consider a section X-X at a distance x from free end A and in the region DB as shown in **Fig. 8.53(b)**.

Bending moment at X-X is

$$M_x = R_A. \langle x \rangle - W \langle x - 2000 \rangle - \frac{w \langle x - 2000 \rangle^2}{2}$$

$$+ M \langle x - 6000 \rangle^0 + \frac{w \langle x - 4000 \rangle^2}{2}$$

i.e.

$$EI \frac{d^2y}{dx^2} = 40000 \langle x \rangle - 40000 \langle x - 2000 \rangle - \frac{20 \langle x - 2000 \rangle^2}{2}$$

$$+ 80 \times 10^6 \langle x - 6000 \rangle^0 + \frac{20 \langle x - 4000 \rangle^2}{2}$$

Integrating once we have

$$EI \frac{dy}{dx} = 20000 \langle x \rangle^2 + C_1 - 20000 \langle x - 2000 \rangle^2 - \frac{10 \langle x - 2000 \rangle^3}{3}$$

$$+ 80 \times 10^6 \langle x - 6000 \rangle^1 + \frac{10 \langle x - 4000 \rangle^3}{3} \qquad \text{... Eq. (i)}$$

Integrating again we have

$$EIy = \frac{20000 \langle x \rangle^3}{3} + C_1 \langle x \rangle + C_2 - \frac{20000 \langle x - 2000 \rangle^3}{3}$$

$$- \frac{5 \langle x - 2000 \rangle^4}{6} + 40 \times 10^6 \langle x - 6000 \rangle^2 + \frac{5 \langle x - 4000 \rangle^4}{6}$$

$$\text{... Eq. (ii)}$$

Boundary conditions:

At $x = 0$, $y = 0$:

Eq. (ii) yields...

$$0 = 0 + 0 + C_2 - 0 - 0 + 0 + 0$$

$$C_2 = 0$$

At $x = L = 7000$ mm, $y = 0$:

Eq. (ii) yields...

$$0 = \frac{20000 \langle 7000 \rangle^3}{3} + C_1 \langle 7000 \rangle - \frac{20000 \langle 7000 - 2000 \rangle^3}{3}$$

$$- \frac{5 \langle 7000 - 2000 \rangle^4}{6} + 40 \times 10^6 \langle 7000 - 6000 \rangle^2$$

$$+ \frac{5 \langle 7000 - 4000 \rangle^4}{6}$$

$$C_1 = -1.49 \times 10^{11}$$

Substituting C_1 in Eq. (i) we get

$$EI \frac{dy}{dx} = 20000 \langle x \rangle^2 - 1.49 \times 10^{11} - 20000 \langle x - 2000 \rangle^2$$

$$- \frac{10 \langle x - 2000 \rangle^3}{3} + 80 \times 10^6 \langle x - 6000 \rangle^1 + \frac{10 \langle x - 4000 \rangle^3}{3}$$

$$\dots \text{ Eq. (iii)}$$

Substituting C_1 and C_2 in Eq. (ii) we get

$$EIy = \frac{20000 \langle x \rangle^3}{3} - 1.49 \times 10^{11} \langle x \rangle - \frac{20000 \langle x - 2000 \rangle^3}{3}$$

$$- \frac{5 \langle x - 2000 \rangle^4}{6} + 40 \times 10^6 \langle x - 6000 \rangle^2 + \frac{5 \langle x - 4000 \rangle^4}{6}$$

$$\dots \text{ Eq. (iv)}$$

a. *Slope at supports*

At A, $x = 0$

Eq. (iii) yields...
$$EI\theta_A = 0 - 1.49 \times 10^{11} - 0 - 0 + 0 + 0$$

$$\theta_A = \frac{-1.49 \times 10^{11}}{(2 \times 10^5) \times (90 \times 10^6)} = -0.0083 \text{ rad}$$

At B, $x = 7000$ mm

Eq. (iii) yields...
$$EI\theta_B = 20000 \langle 7000 \rangle^2 - 1.49 \times 10^{11} - 20000 \langle 7000 - 2000 \rangle^2$$

$$- \frac{10 \langle 7000 - 2000 \rangle^3}{3} + 80 \times 10^6 \langle 7000 - 6000 \rangle^1$$

$$+ \frac{10 \langle 7000 - 4000 \rangle^3}{3}$$

$$\theta_B = \frac{8.48 \times 10^{10}}{(2 \times 10^5) \times (90 \times 10^6)} = 0.0047 \text{ rad}$$

b. *Deflection*

At C, $x = 2000$ mm

Eq. (iv) yields...
$$EIy_C = \frac{20000 \langle 2000 \rangle^3}{3} - 1.49 \times 10^{11} \langle 2000 \rangle - 0 - 0 + 0 + 0$$

$$y_C = \frac{-2.45 \times 10^{14}}{(2 \times 10^5) \times (90 \times 10^6)} = -13.59 \text{ mm}$$

At D, $x = 4000$ mm

Eq. (iv) yields... $\quad EIy_D = \frac{20000 \langle 4000 \rangle^3}{3} - 1.49 \times 10^{11} \langle 4000 \rangle$

$$- \frac{20000 \langle 4000 - 2000 \rangle^3}{3} - \frac{5 \langle 4000 - 2000 \rangle^4}{6} + 0 + 0$$

$$y_D = \frac{-2.36 \times 10^{14}}{(2 \times 10^5) \times (90 \times 10^6)} = -13.11 \text{ mm}$$

At E, $x = 6000$ mm

Eq. (iv) yields... $\quad EIy_E = \frac{20000 \langle 6000 \rangle^3}{3} - 1.49 \times 10^{11} \langle 6000 \rangle$

$$- \frac{20000 \langle 6000 - 2000 \rangle^3}{3} - \frac{5 \langle 6000 - 2000 \rangle^4}{6} + 0$$

$$+ \frac{5 \langle 6000 - 4000 \rangle^4}{6}$$

$$y_E = \frac{-8.06 \times 10^{13}}{(2 \times 10^5) \times (90 \times 10^6)} = -4.48 \text{ mm}$$

8.9.5 Overhanging beams

49. **Calculate the deflection at E for the overhanging beam loaded as shown in Fig. 8.54(a). Take $E = 200$ GPa, $I = 50 \times 10^6$ mm^4. Use Macaulay's method.**

VTU – (CV) Dec. 2011 – 14 Marks

Solution: $E = 2 \times 10^5$ MPa, $I = 50 \times 10^6$ mm^4. $y_E = ?$
Reactions at supports:

$$R_C + R_D = 40 + 20 = 60 \text{ kN} \qquad \ldots \text{Eq. (a)}$$

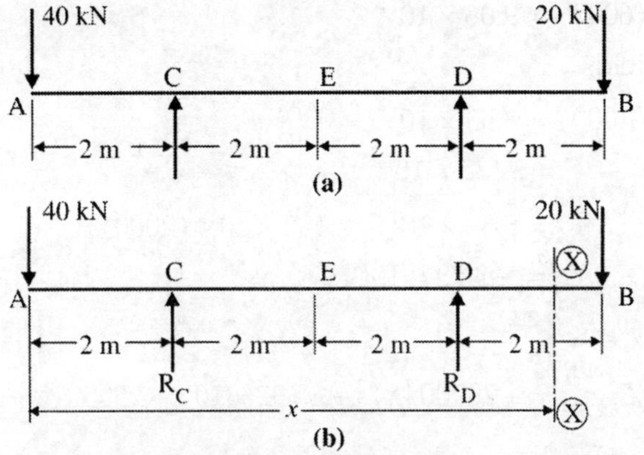

Fig. 8.54: Problem 49

Taking moments about A and equating to zero, we have

$$R_D \times 4 = (20 \times 6) - (40 \times 2)$$

$$R_D = 10 \text{ kN} \qquad \ldots \text{Eq. (b)}$$

Substituting Eq. (b) in Eq. (a), we have

$$R_C + 10 = 60$$

$$R_C = 50 \text{ kN} \qquad \ldots \text{Eq. (c)}$$

Consider a section X-X at a distance x from free end A and in the region DB as shown in **Fig. 8.54(b)**.

Bending moment at X-X is

$$M_x = -40000 \langle x \rangle + R_C \langle x - 2000 \rangle + R_D \langle x - 6000 \rangle$$

i.e. $\qquad EI \dfrac{d^2y}{dx^2} = -40000 \langle x \rangle + 50000 \langle x - 2000 \rangle + 10000 \langle x - 6000 \rangle$

Integrating once we have

$$EI \frac{dy}{dx} = -20000 \langle x \rangle^2 + C_1 + 25000 \langle x - 2000 \rangle^2 + 5000 \langle x - 6000 \rangle^2$$

$$\ldots \text{Eq. (i)}$$

Integrating again we have

$$EIy = \frac{-20000 \langle x \rangle^3}{3} + C_1 \langle x \rangle + C_2 + \frac{25000 \langle x - 2000 \rangle^3}{3}$$

$$+ \frac{5000 \langle x - 6000 \rangle^3}{3} \qquad \ldots \text{Eq. (ii)}$$

Boundary conditions:

At $x = 2000$ mm, $y = 0$:

Eq. (ii) yields... $\qquad 0 = \dfrac{-20000 \langle 2000 \rangle^3}{3} + C_1 \langle 2000 \rangle + C_2 + 0 + 0$

$$C_2 + C_1 \langle 2000 \rangle = 5.33 \times 10^{13} \qquad \ldots \text{Eq. (iii)}$$

At $x = 6000$ mm, $y = 0$:

Eq. (ii) yields... $\qquad 0 = \dfrac{-20000 \langle 6000 \rangle^3}{3} + C_1 \langle 6000 \rangle + C_2 + \dfrac{25000 \langle 6000 - 2000 \rangle^3}{3}$

$$C_2 + C_1 \langle 6000 \rangle = 9.06 \times 10^{14} \qquad \ldots \text{Eq. (iv)}$$

Eq. (iv) – Eq. (iii) yields...

$$C_1 \langle 4000 \rangle = 8.53 \times 10^{14}$$

$$C_1 = 2.132 \times 10^{11}$$

Eq. (iii) yields... $\qquad C_2 = 5.33 \times 10^{13} - 2.132 \times 10^{11} \langle 2000 \rangle$

$$C_2 = -3.73 \times 10^{14}$$

Substituting C_1 in Eq. (i) we get

$$EI \frac{dy}{dx} = -20000 \langle x \rangle^2 + 2.132 \times 10^{11} + 25000 \langle x - 2000 \rangle^2$$

$$+ 5000 \langle x - 6000 \rangle^2 \qquad \ldots \text{Eq. (v)}$$

Substituting C_1 and C_2 in Eq. (ii) we get

$$EIy = \frac{-20000 \langle x \rangle^3}{3} + 2.132 \times 10^{11} \langle x \rangle - 3.73 \times 10^{14}$$

$$+ \frac{25000 \langle x - 2000 \rangle^3}{3} + \frac{5000 \langle x - 6000 \rangle^3}{3} \qquad \dots \text{Eq. (vi)}$$

Deflection at E
At E, $x = 4000$ mm

Eq. (vi) yields... $\qquad EIy_E = \dfrac{-20000 \langle 4000 \rangle^3}{3} + 2.132 \times 10^{11} \langle 4000 \rangle - 3.73 \times 10^{14}$

$$+ \frac{25000 \langle 4000 - 2000 \rangle^3}{3} + 0$$

$$y_E = \frac{1.198 \times 10^{14}}{(2 \times 10^5) \times (50 \times 10^6)} = 11.98 \text{ mm}$$

50. Determine the deflections at free ends and also at center for the beam of uniform cross section shown in Fig. 8.55(a). Given $E = 210$ kN/mm^2, $I = 40 \times 10^6$ mm^4.

VTU – (CV) Dec. 15/ Jan. 16 – 14 Marks

Solution: $E = 210 \times 10^3$ MPa, $I = 40 \times 10^6$ mm^4. $y_C, y_D, y_E = ?$

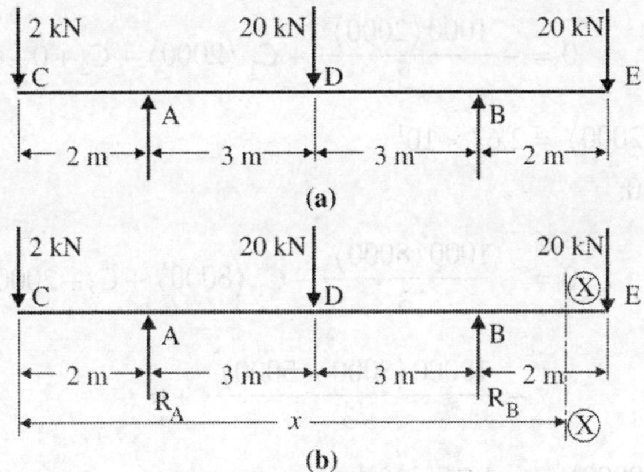

Fig. 8.55: Problem 49

Reactions at supports:

$$R_A + R_B = 2 + 20 + 2 = 24 \text{ kN} \qquad \dots \text{Eq. (a)}$$

Taking moments about A and equating to zero, we have

$$R_B \times 6 = (2 \times 8) + (20 \times 3) - (2 \times 2)$$

$$R_B = 12 \text{ kN} \qquad \dots \text{Eq. (b)}$$

Substituting Eq. (b) in Eq. (a), we have

$$R_A + 12 = 24$$

$$R_A = 12 \text{ kN} \qquad \dots \text{Eq. (c)}$$

Consider a section X-X at a distance x from free end A and in the region BE as shown in **Fig. 8.55(b)**. Bending moment at X-X is

$$M_x = -2000\langle x\rangle + R_A.\langle x - 2000\rangle - 20000\langle x - 5000\rangle$$

$$+ R_B\langle x - 8000\rangle$$

i.e.
$$EI\frac{d^2y}{dx^2} = -2000\langle x\rangle + 12000\langle x - 2000\rangle - 20000\langle x - 5000\rangle$$

$$+ 12000\langle x - 8000\rangle$$

Integrating once we have

$$EI\frac{dy}{dx} = -1000\langle x\rangle^2 + C_1 + 6000\langle x - 2000\rangle^2 - 10000\langle x - 5000\rangle^2$$

$$+ 6000\langle x - 8000\rangle^2 \qquad\qquad \text{... Eq. (i)}$$

Integrating again we have

$$EIy = -\frac{1000\langle x\rangle^3}{3} + C_1\langle x\rangle + C_2 + 2000\langle x - 2000\rangle^3$$

$$- \frac{10000\langle x - 5000\rangle^3}{3} + 2000\langle x - 8000\rangle^3 \qquad \text{... Eq. (ii)}$$

Boundary conditions:
At $x = 2000$ mm, $y = 0$:

Eq. (ii) yields...
$$0 = -\frac{1000\langle 2000\rangle^3}{3} + C_1\langle 2000\rangle + C_2 + 0 - 0 + 0$$

$$C_2 + C_1\langle 2000\rangle = 2.67 \times 10^{12} \qquad\qquad \text{... Eq. (iii)}$$

At $x = 8000$ mm, $y = 0$:

Eq. (ii) yields...
$$0 = -\frac{1000\langle 8000\rangle^3}{3} + C_1\langle 8000\rangle + C_2 + 2000\langle 8000 - 2000\rangle^3$$

$$- \frac{10000\langle 8000 - 5000\rangle^3}{3} + 0$$

$$C_2 + C_1\langle 8000\rangle = -1.71 \times 10^{14} \qquad\qquad \text{... Eq. (iv)}$$

Eq. (iv) – Eq. (iii) yields...
$$C_1\langle 6000\rangle = -1.737 \times 10^{14}$$

$$C_1 = -2.90 \times 10^{10}$$

Eq. (iii) yields...
$$C_2 = 2.67 \times 10^{12} + 2.90 \times 10^{10}\langle 2000\rangle$$

$$C_2 = 6.07 \times 10^{13}$$

Substituting C_1 in Eq. (i) we get

$$EI\frac{dy}{dx} = -1000\langle x\rangle^2 - 2.90 \times 10^{10} + 6000\langle x - 2000\rangle^2$$

$$- 10000\langle x - 5000\rangle^2 + 6000\langle x - 8000\rangle^2 \qquad \text{... Eq. (v)}$$

Substituting C_1 and C_2 in Eq. (ii) we get

$$EIy = -\frac{1000\langle x\rangle^3}{3} - 2.90 \times 10^{10}\,\langle x\rangle + 6.07 \times 10^{13}$$

$$+ 2000\langle x - 2000\rangle^3 - \frac{10000\langle x - 5000\rangle^3}{3} + 2000\langle x - 8000\rangle^3$$

$$\ldots \text{Eq. (vi)}$$

Deflection

At C, $x = 0$

Eq. (vi) yields... $\quad EIy_C = -0 - 0 + 6.07 \times 10^{13} + 0 - 0 + 0$

$$y_D = \frac{6.07 \times 10^{13}}{(210 \times 10^3) \times (40 \times 10^6)} = 7.23 \text{ mm}$$

At D, $x = 5000$ mm

Eq. (vi) yields... $\quad EIy_D = -\frac{1000\langle 5000\rangle^3}{3} - 2.90 \times 10^{10}\,\langle 5000\rangle + 6.07 \times 10^{13}$

$$+ 2000\langle 5000 - 2000\rangle^3 - 0 + 0$$

$$y_D = \frac{-7.20 \times 10^{13}}{(210 \times 10^3) \times (40 \times 10^6)} = -8.57 \text{ mm}$$

At E, $x = 10000$ mm

Eq. (vi) yields... $\quad EIy_E = -\frac{1000\langle 10000\rangle^3}{3} - 2.90 \times 10^{10}\,\langle 10000\rangle + 6.07 \times 10^{13}$

$$+ 2000\langle 10000 - 2000\rangle^3 - \frac{10000\langle 10000 - 5000\rangle^3}{3}$$

$$+ 2000\langle 10000 - 8000\rangle^3$$

$$y_E = \frac{6.07 \times 10^{13}}{(210 \times 10^3) \times (40 \times 10^6)} = 7.23 \text{ mm}$$

51. A beam AB shown in Fig. 8.56(a) is 6 m long and has flexural rigidity of $EI = 9 \times 10^{13}$ N-mm^2. Determine: (a) Slope at A   (b) Deflection at mid-span

VTU – Dec. 2010 – 20 Marks

Solution: $w = 10$ kN/m $= 10$ N/mm, $EI = 9 \times 10^{13}$ N-mm^2. a) $\theta = ?$ b) $y_{L/2} = ?$

Reactions at supports:

$$R_C + R_D = (10 \times 3) = 30 \text{ kN} \qquad \ldots \text{Eq. (a)}$$

Taking moments about A and equating to zero, we have

$$R_D \times 3 = (10 \times 3) \times \left(\frac{3}{2}\right)$$

$$R_D = 15 \text{ kN} \qquad \ldots \text{Eq. (b)}$$

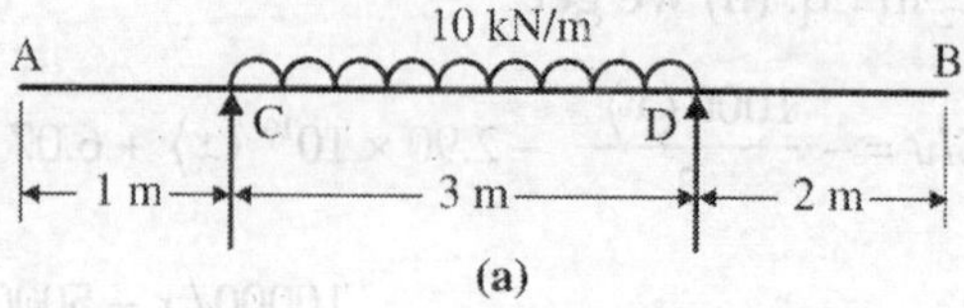

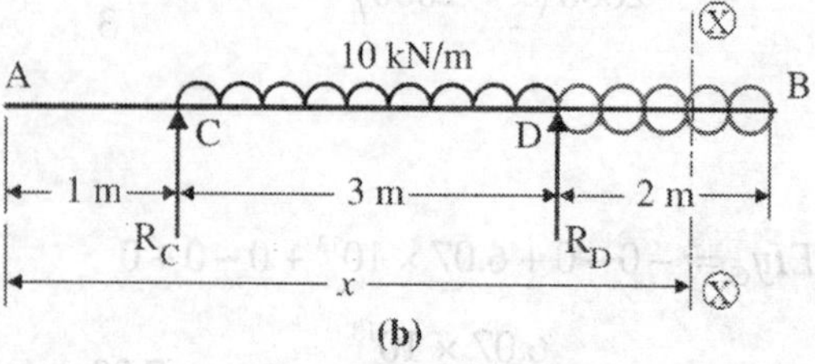

Fig. 8.56: Problem 51

Substituting Eq. (b) in Eq. (a), we have

$$R_C + 15 = 30$$

$$R_C = 15 \text{ kN} \qquad \qquad \text{... Eq. (c)}$$

Consider a section X-X at a distance x from free end A and in the region DB as shown in **Fig. 8.56(b)**. Bending moment at X-X is

$$M_x = R_C . \langle x - 1000 \rangle - \frac{w \langle x - 1000 \rangle^2}{2} + R_D \langle x - 4000 \rangle$$

$$+ \frac{w \langle x - 4000 \rangle^2}{2}$$

i.e.

$$EI \frac{d^2 y}{dx^2} = 15000 \langle x - 1000 \rangle - \frac{10 \langle x - 1000 \rangle^2}{2} + 15000 \langle x - 4000 \rangle$$

$$+ \frac{10 \langle x - 4000 \rangle^2}{2}$$

Integrating once we have

$$EI \frac{dy}{dx} = 7500 \langle x \rangle^2 + C_1 - \frac{5 \langle x - 1000 \rangle^3}{3} + 7500 \langle x - 4000 \rangle^2$$

$$+ \frac{5 \langle x - 4000 \rangle^3}{3} \qquad \qquad \text{... Eq. (i)}$$

Integrating again we have

$$EIy = 2500 \langle x \rangle^4 + C_1 \langle x \rangle + C_2 - \frac{5 \langle x - 1000 \rangle^4}{3}$$

$$+ 2500 \langle x - 4000 \rangle^3 + \frac{5 \langle x - 4000 \rangle^4}{12} \qquad \text{... Eq. (ii)}$$

Boundary conditions:

At x = 1000 mm, $y = 0$:

Eq. (ii) yields...
$$0 = 2500 \langle 1000 \rangle^3 + C_1 \langle 1000 \rangle + C_2 - 0 + 0 + 0$$

$$C_2 + C_1 \langle 1000 \rangle = -2.5 \times 10^{12} \qquad \text{... Eq. (iii)}$$

At $x = 4000$ mm, $y = 0$:

$$0 = 2500 \langle 4000 \rangle^3 + C_1 \langle 4000 \rangle + C_2 - \frac{5 \langle 4000 - 1000 \rangle^4}{12} + 0 + 0$$

$$C_2 + C_1 \langle 4000 \rangle = -1.263 \times 10^{14} \qquad \text{... Eq. (iv)}$$

Eq. (iv) – Eq. (iii) yields...

$$C_1 \langle 3000 \rangle = -1.238 \times 10^{14}$$

$$C_1 = -4.125 \times 10^{10}$$

Eq. (iii) yields... $\qquad C_2 = -2.5 \times 10^{12} + 4.125 \times 10^{10} \langle 1000 \rangle$

$$C_2 = 3.875 \times 10^{13}$$

Substituting C_1 in Eq. (i) we get

$$EI \frac{dy}{dx} = 7500 \langle x \rangle^2 - 4.125 \times 10^{10} - \frac{5 \langle x - 1000 \rangle^3}{3} + 7500 \langle x - 4000 \rangle^2$$

$$+ \frac{5 \langle x - 4000 \rangle^3}{3} \qquad \text{... Eq. (v)}$$

Substituting C_1 and C_2 in Eq. (ii) we get

$$EIy = 2500 \langle x \rangle^3 - 4.125 \times 10^{10} \langle x \rangle + 3.875 \times 10^{13} - \frac{5 \langle x - 1000 \rangle^4}{12}$$

$$+ 5000 \langle x - 4000 \rangle^3 + \frac{5 \langle x - 4000 \rangle^4}{12} \qquad \text{... Eq. (vi)}$$

a. *Slope at A*

At A, $x = 0$

Eq. (v) yields... $\qquad EI\theta_A = 0 - 4.125 \times 10^{10} - 0 + 0 + 0$

$$\theta_A = \frac{-4.125 \times 10^{10}}{9 \times 10^{13}} = -0.00046 \text{ rad}$$

b. *Deflection at mid-span*

At C, $x = L/2 = 3000$ mm

Eq. (vi) yields... $EIy_{3000} = 2500 \langle 3000 \rangle^3 - 4.125 \times 10^{10} \langle 3000 \rangle + 3.875 \times 10^{13}$

$$- \frac{5 \langle 3000 - 1000 \rangle^4}{12} + 0 + 0$$

$$y_{3000} = \frac{-2.417 \times 10^{13}}{9 \times 10^{13}} = -0.2685 \text{ mm}$$

52. An overhanging beam is loaded as shown in Fig. 8.57(a). If $EI = 9 \times 10^{13}$ N-mm^2. Determine:

  (a) Slope at all points   **(b) Deflection at C, D, E**

Solution: $w = 30$ kN/m $= 30$ N/mm, $EI = 9 \times 10^{13}$ N-mm^2.

(a) $\theta_C, \theta_A, \theta_D, \theta_E, \theta_B = ?$ (b) $y_C, y_D, y_E = ?$

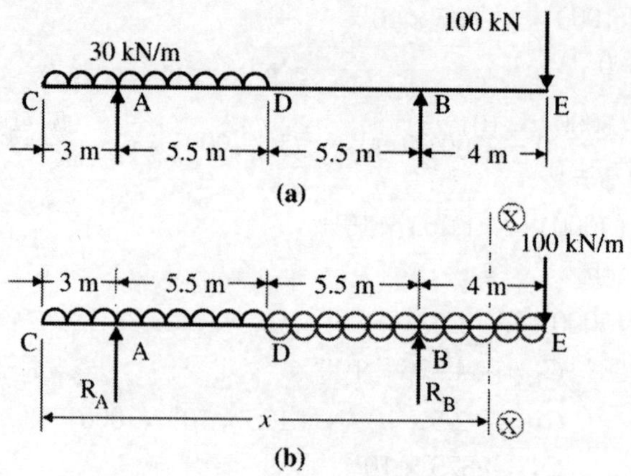

Fig. 8.57: Problem 52

Reactions at supports:

$$R_A + R_B = 100 + (30 \times 8.5) = 355 \text{ kN} \qquad \dots \text{Eq. (a)}$$

Taking moments about A and equating to zero, we have

$$R_B \times 11 = (100 \times 15) + (30 \times 5.5) \times \left(\frac{5.5}{2}\right) - (30 \times 3) \times \left(\frac{3}{2}\right)$$

$$R_B = 165.34 \text{ kN} \qquad \dots \text{Eq. (b)}$$

Substituting Eq. (b) in Eq. (a), we have

$$R_A + 165.34 = 190$$

$$R_A = 189.66 \text{ kN} \qquad \dots \text{Eq. (c)}$$

Consider a section X-X at a distance x from free end C and in the region BE as shown in **Fig. 8.57(b)**. Bending moment at X-X is

$$M_x = -\frac{w \langle x \rangle^2}{2} + R_A \cdot \langle x - 3000 \rangle + R_B \langle x - 14000 \rangle + \frac{w \langle x - 8500 \rangle^2}{2}$$

i.e.

$$EI\frac{d^2y}{dx^2} = -\frac{30 \langle x \rangle^2}{2} + 189.66 \times 10^3 \langle x - 3000 \rangle + 165.34 \times 10^3 \langle x - 14000 \rangle$$

$$+ \frac{30 \langle x - 8500 \rangle^2}{2}$$

Integrating once we have

$$EI\frac{dy}{dx} = -5 \langle x \rangle^3 + C_1 + 94.83 \times 10^3 \langle x - 3000 \rangle^2$$

$$+ 82.67 \times 10^3 \langle x - 14000 \rangle^2 + 5 \langle x - 8500 \rangle^3 \qquad \dots \text{Eq. (i)}$$

Integrating again we have

$$EIy = -\frac{5 \langle x \rangle^4}{4} + C_1 \langle x \rangle + C_2 + 31.61 \times 10^3 \langle x - 3000 \rangle^3$$

$$+ 27.56 \times 10^3 \langle x - 14000 \rangle^3 + \frac{5 \langle x - 8500 \rangle^4}{4} \qquad \dots \text{Eq. (ii)}$$

Boundary conditions:

At $x = 3000$ mm, $y = 0$:

Eq. (ii) yields...

$$0 = -\frac{5\langle 3000\rangle^4}{4} + C_1\langle 3000\rangle + C_2 + 0 + 0 + 0$$

$$C_2 + C_1\langle 3000\rangle = 101.25 \times 10^{12} \qquad \text{... Eq. (iii)}$$

At $x = 14000$ mm, $y = 0$:

$$0 = -\frac{5\langle 14000\rangle^4}{4} + C_1\langle 14000\rangle + C_2 + 31.61$$

$$\times 10^3\langle 14000 - 3000\rangle^3 + 0 + \frac{5\langle 14000 - 8500\rangle^4}{4}$$

$$C_2 + C_1\langle 14000\rangle = 4.81 \times 10^{15} \qquad \text{... Eq. (iv)}$$

Eq. (iv)-Eq. (iii) yields...

$$C_1\langle 11000\rangle = 4.71 \times 10^{15}$$

$$C_1 = 4.28 \times 10^{11}$$

Eq. (iii) yields...

$$C_2 = 101.25 \times 10^{12} - 4.28 \times 10^{11}\langle 3000\rangle$$

$$C_2 = -1.18 \times 10^{15}$$

Substituting C_1 in Eq. (i) we get

$$EI\frac{dy}{dx} = -5\langle x\rangle^3 + 4.28 \times 10^{11} + 94.83 \times 10^3\langle x - 3000\rangle^2$$

$$+ 82.67 \times 10^3\langle x - 14000\rangle^2 + 5\langle x - 8500\rangle^3 \qquad \text{... Eq. (v)}$$

Substituting C_1 and C_2 in Eq. (ii) we get

$$EIy = -\frac{5\langle x\rangle^4}{4} + 4.28 \times 10^{11}\langle x\rangle - 1.18 \times 10^{15}$$

$$+ 31.61 \times 10^3\langle x - 3000\rangle^3 + 27.56 \times 10^3\langle x - 14000\rangle^3$$

$$+ \frac{5\langle x - 8500\rangle^4}{4} \qquad \text{... Eq. (vi)}$$

a. *Slope at all points*
At C, $x = 0$
Eq. (v) yields...

$$EI\theta_C = 0 + 4.28 \times 10^{11} + 0 + 0 + 0$$

$$\theta_C = \frac{4.28 \times 10^{11}}{9 \times 10^{13}} = 0.00475 \text{ rad}$$

At A, $x = 3000$ mm

Eq. (v) yields...

$$EI\theta_A = -5\langle 3000\rangle^3 + 4.28 \times 10^{11} + 0 + 0 + 0$$

$$\theta_A = \frac{2.93 \times 10^{11}}{9 \times 10^{13}} = 0.00325 \text{ rad}$$

At D, $x = 8500$ mm

Eq. (v) yields...

$$EI\theta_D = -5\langle 8500\rangle^3 + 4.28 \times 10^{11} + 94.83 \times 10^3\langle 8500 - 3000\rangle^2$$

$$+ 0 + 0$$

$$\theta_D = \frac{2.26 \times 10^{11}}{9 \times 10^{13}} = 0.0025 \text{ rad}$$

At B, $x = 14000$ mm

Eq. (v) yields... $\quad EI\theta_B = -5\langle 14000 \rangle^3 + 4.28 \times 10^{11} + 94.83 \times 10^3 \langle 14000 - 3000 \rangle^2$

$$+ 0 + 5\langle 14000 - 8500 \rangle^3$$

$$\theta_B = \frac{-9.86 \times 10^{11}}{9 \times 10^{13}} = -0.0110 \text{ rad}$$

At E, $x = 18000$ mm

Eq. (v) yields... $\quad EI\theta_E = -5\langle 18000 \rangle^3 + 4.28 \times 10^{11} + 94.83 \times 10^3 \langle 18000 - 3000 \rangle^2$

$$+ 82.67 \times 10^3 \langle 18000 - 14000 \rangle^2 + 5\langle 18000 - 8500 \rangle^3$$

$$\theta_E = \frac{-1.78 \times 10^{12}}{9 \times 10^{13}} = -0.0198 \text{ rad}$$

b. *Deflection at C*

At C, $x = 0$ mm

Eq. (vi) yields... $\quad EIy_C = 0 + 0 - 1.18 \times 10^{15} + 0 + 0 + 0$

$$y_C = \frac{-1.18 \times 10^{15}}{9 \times 10^{13}} = -13.11 \text{ mm}$$

At D, $x = 8500$ mm

Eq. (vi) yields... $\quad EIy_D = -\frac{5\langle 8500 \rangle^4}{4} + 4.28 \times 10^{11} \langle 8500 \rangle - 1.18 \times 10^{15}$

$$+ 31.61 \times 10^3 \langle 8500 - 3000 \rangle^3 + 0 + 0$$

$$y_D = \frac{1.192 \times 10^{15}}{9 \times 10^{13}} = 13.24 \text{ mm}$$

At E, $x = 18000$ mm

Eq. (vi) yields... $\quad EIy_E = -\frac{5\langle 18000 \rangle^4}{4} + 4.28 \times 10^{11} \langle 18000 \rangle - 1.18 \times 10^{15}$

$$+ 31.61 \times 10^3 \langle 18000 - 3000 \rangle^3 + 27.56$$

$$\times 10^3 \langle 18000 - 14000 \rangle^3 + \frac{5\langle 18000 - 8500 \rangle^4}{4}$$

$$y_E = \frac{-60.67 \times 10^{15}}{9 \times 10^{13}} = -67.41 \text{ mm}$$

53. Determine the deflection under the loads in the beam shown in Fig. 8.58(a). Take flexural rigidity as *EI*, throughout.

VTU – June 2012 – 10 Marks, Dec. 08/ Jan. 09 – 10 Marks, Dec. 15/ Jan. 16 – 10 Marks

Solution: $W_1 = 40 \times 10^3$ N, $W_2 = 10 \times 10^3$ N, $a = 2000$ mm, $b = 4000$ mm, $EI = $ constant.
$y_C, y_D = ?$

Reactions at supports:

$$R_A + R_B = 40 + 10 = 50 \text{ kN} \qquad \qquad \text{... Eq. (a)}$$

Taking moments about A and equating to zero, we have

$$R_B \times 4 = (40 \times 2) + (10 \times 6)$$

$$R_B = 35 \text{ kN} \qquad \qquad \text{... Eq. (b)}$$

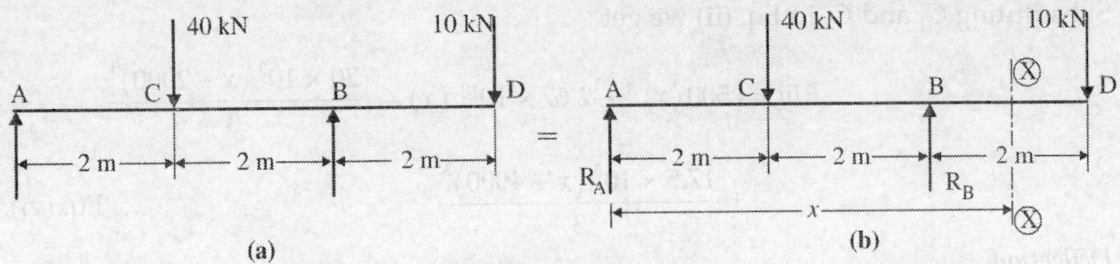

Fig. 8.58: Problem 53

Substituting Eq. (b) in Eq. (a), we have

$$R_A + 35 = 50$$

$$R_A = 15 \text{ kN} \qquad \qquad \text{... Eq. (c)}$$

Consider a section X-X at a distance x from free end A and in the region BD as shown in **Fig. 8.58(b)**. Bending moment at X-X is

$$M_x = R_A \langle x \rangle - W_1 \langle x - a \rangle + R_B \langle x - b \rangle$$

i.e. $\qquad EI\dfrac{d^2 y}{dx^2} = 15 \times 10^3 \langle x \rangle - 40 \times 10^3 \langle x - 2000 \rangle + 35 \times 10^3 \langle x - 4000 \rangle$

Integrating once we have

$$EI\dfrac{dy}{dx} = 7500 \langle x \rangle^2 + C_1 - 20 \times 10^3 \langle x - 2000 \rangle^2$$

$$+ 17.5 \times 10^3 \langle x - 4000 \rangle^2 \qquad \text{... Eq. (i)}$$

Integrating again we have

$$EIy = 2500 \langle x \rangle^3 + C_1 \langle x \rangle + C_2 - \dfrac{20 \times 10^3 \langle x - 2000 \rangle^3}{3}$$

$$+ \dfrac{17.5 \times 10^3 \langle x - 4000 \rangle^3}{3} \qquad \text{... Eq. (ii)}$$

Boundary conditions:

At $x = 0$, $y = 0$:

Eq. (ii) yields... $\qquad 0 = 0 + 0 + C_2 - 0 - 0$

Ignore brackets containing negative value

$$C_2 = 0 \qquad \qquad \text{... Eq. (iii)}$$

At $x = 4000$ mm, $y = 0$:

Eq. (ii) yields... $\qquad 0 = 2500 \langle 4000 \rangle^3 + C_1 \langle 4000 \rangle - \dfrac{20 \times 10^3 \langle 4000 - 2000 \rangle^3}{3} + 0$

$$C_1 = -2.67 \times 10^{10} \qquad \qquad \text{... Eq. (iv)}$$

Substituting C_1 in Eq. (i) we get

$$EI\dfrac{dy}{dx} = 7500 \langle x \rangle^2 - 2.67 \times 10^{10} - 20 \times 10^3 \langle x - 2000 \rangle^2$$

$$+ 17.5 \times 10^3 \langle x - 4000 \rangle^2 \qquad \text{... Eq. (v)}$$

Substituting C_1 and C_2 in Eq. (ii) we get

$$EIy = 2500 \langle x \rangle^3 - 2.67 \times 10^{10} \langle x \rangle - \frac{20 \times 10^3 \langle x - 2000 \rangle^3}{3}$$

$$+ \frac{17.5 \times 10^3 \langle x - 4000 \rangle^3}{3} \qquad \text{... Eq. (vi)}$$

Deflection

At C, $x = 2000$ mm

Eq. (vi) yields... $\quad EIy_C = 2500 \langle 2000 \rangle^3 - 2.67 \times 10^{10} \langle 2000 \rangle - 0 + 0$

$$y_C = \frac{3.33 \times 10^{13}}{EI}$$

At D, $x = 6000$ mm

Eq. (vi) yields... $\quad EIy_D = 2500 \langle 6000 \rangle^3 - 2.67 \times 10^{10} \langle 6000 \rangle$

$$- \frac{20 \times 10^3 \langle 6000 - 2000 \rangle^3}{3} + \frac{17.5 \times 10^3 \langle 6000 - 4000 \rangle^3}{3}$$

$$y_D = \frac{2 \times 10^{11}}{EI}$$

54. Determine slopes at supports at A and B, and deflections at D and E using Macaulay's method for the beam shown in Fig. 8.59(a).

VTU – (CV) Dec. 2011 – 14 Marks

Solution: $W_1 = W_3 = 40 \times 10^3$ N, $W_2 = 80 \times 10^3$ N, $a = 2000$ mm, $b = 7000$ mm, $c = 10000$ mm, $EI = $ constant.

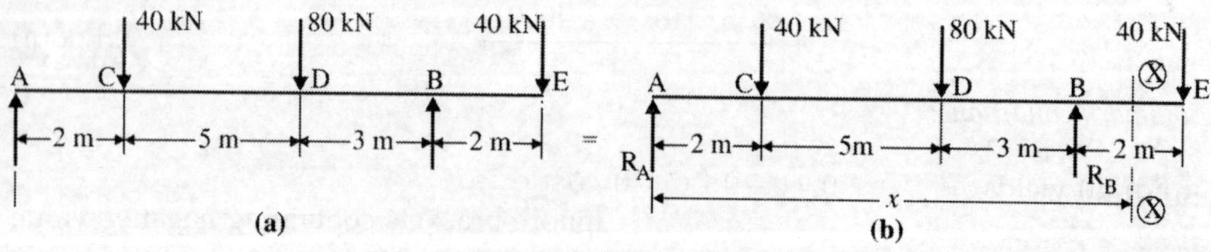

Fig. 8.59: Problem 54

(a) $\theta_A, \theta_B = ?$, (b) $y_D, y_E = ?$

Reactions at supports:

$$R_A + R_B = 40 + 80 + 40 = 160 \text{ kN} \qquad \text{... Eq. (a)}$$

Taking moments about A and equating to zero, we have

$$R_B \times 10 = (40 \times 2) + (80 \times 7) + (40 \times 12)$$

$$R_B = 112 \text{ kN} \qquad \text{... Eq. (b)}$$

Substituting Eq. (b) in Eq. (a), we have

$$R_A + 112 = 160$$

$$R_A = 48 \text{ kN} \qquad \text{... Eq. (c)}$$

Consider a section X-X at a distance x from free end A and in the region BE as shown in **Fig. 8.59(b)**. Bending moment at X-X is

$$M_x = R_A \langle x \rangle - W_1 \langle x - a \rangle - W_2 \langle x - b \rangle + R_B \langle x - c \rangle$$

i.e.
$$EI\frac{d^2y}{dx^2} = 48 \times 10^3 \langle x \rangle - 40 \times 10^3 \langle x - 2000 \rangle - 80 \times 10^3 \langle x - 7000 \rangle$$

$$+ 112 \times 10^3 \langle x - 10000 \rangle$$

Integrating once we have

$$EI\frac{dy}{dx} = 24000 \langle x \rangle^2 + C_1 - 20 \times 10^3 \langle x - 2000 \rangle^2$$

$$- 40 \times 10^3 \langle x - 7000 \rangle^2 + 56 \times 10^3 \langle x - 10000 \rangle^2 \quad \text{... Eq. (i)}$$

Integrating again we have

$$EIy = 8000 \langle x \rangle^3 + C_1 \langle x \rangle + C_2 - \frac{20 \times 10^3 \langle x - 2000 \rangle^3}{3}$$

$$- \frac{40 \times 10^3 \langle x - 7000 \rangle^3}{3} + \frac{56 \times 10^3 \langle x - 10000 \rangle^3}{3} \quad \text{... Eq. (ii)}$$

Boundary conditions:
At $x = 0, y = 0$:
Eq. (ii) yields...
$$0 = 0 + 0 + C_2 - 0 - 0 + 0$$

Ignore brackets containing negative value
$$C_2 = 0 \quad \text{... Eq. (iii)}$$

At $x = 10000$ mm, $y = 0$:

Eq. (ii) yields...
$$0 = 8000 \langle 10000 \rangle^3 + C_1 \langle 10000 \rangle - \frac{20 \times 10^3 \langle 10000 - 2000 \rangle^3}{3}$$

$$- \frac{40 \times 10^3 \langle 10000 - 7000 \rangle^3}{3}$$

$$C_1 = -4.23 \times 10^{11} \quad \text{... Eq. (iv)}$$

Substituting C_1 in Eq. (i) we get

$$EI\frac{dy}{dx} = 24000 \langle x \rangle^2 - 4.23 \times 10^{11} - 20 \times 10^3 \langle x - 2000 \rangle^2$$

$$- 40 \times 10^3 \langle x - 7000 \rangle^2 + 56 \times 10^3 \langle x - 10000 \rangle^2 \quad \text{... Eq. (v)}$$

Substituting C_1 and C_2 in Eq. (ii) we get

$$EIy = 8000 \langle x \rangle^3 - 4.23 \times 10^{11} \langle x \rangle - \frac{20 \times 10^3 \langle x - 2000 \rangle^3}{3}$$

$$- \frac{40 \times 10^3 \langle x - 7000 \rangle^3}{3} + \frac{56 \times 10^3 \langle x - 10000 \rangle^3}{3}$$

$$\text{... Eq. (vi)}$$

a. *Slope at supports*
   At A, $x = 0$

   Eq. (v) yields... $EI\theta_A = 0 - 4.23 \times 10^{11} - 0 - 0 + 0$

   $$\theta_A = \frac{-4.23 \times 10^{11}}{EI}$$

   At B, $x = 10000$ mm

   Eq. (v) yields... $EI\theta_B = 24000\langle 10000 \rangle^2 - 4.23 \times 10^{11} - 20 \times 10^3 \langle 10000 - 2000 \rangle^2$

   $$- 40 \times 10^3 \langle 10000 - 7000 \rangle^2 + 0$$

   $$\theta_B = \frac{3.37 \times 10^{11}}{EI}$$

b. *Deflection*
   At D, $x = 7000$ mm

   Eq. (vi) yields... $EIy_D = 8000\langle 7000 \rangle^3 - 4.23 \times 10^{11} \langle 7000 \rangle$

   $$- \frac{20 \times 10^3 \langle 7000 - 2000 \rangle^3}{3} - 0 + 0$$

   $$y_D = \frac{-1.05 \times 10^{15}}{EI}$$

   At E, $x = 12000$ mm

   Eq. (vi) yields... $EIy_E = 8000\langle 12000 \rangle^3 - 4.23 \times 10^{11} \langle 12000 \rangle$

   $$- \frac{20 \times 10^3 \langle 12000 - 2000 \rangle^3}{3} - \frac{40 \times 10^3 \langle 12000 - 7000 \rangle^3}{3}$$

   $$+ \frac{56 \times 10^3 \langle 12000 - 10000 \rangle^3}{3}$$

   $$y_E = \frac{5.64 \times 10^{14}}{EI}$$

55. Determine the deflection at B and D for the beam shown in Fig. 8.60(a). Take $E = 210$ GPa and $I = 1.6 \times 10^7$ mm^4.

VTU – (CV) Dec. 14/ Jan. 15 – 12 Marks

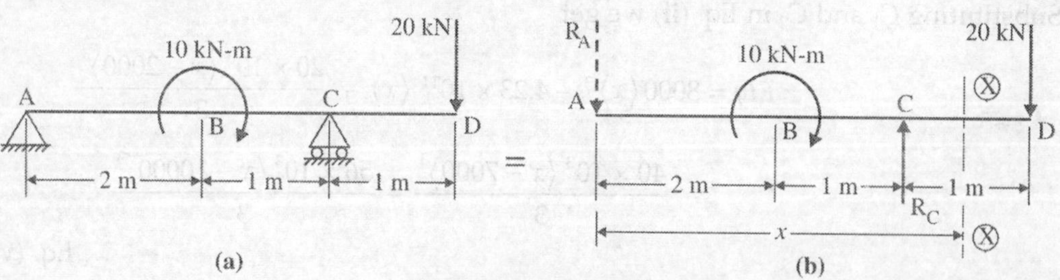

Fig. 8.60: Problem 55

Solution: $W = 20 \times 10^3$ N, $M = 10$ kN-m $= 10 \times 10^6$ N-mm, $a = 2000$ mm, $b = 3000$ mm, $E = 210 \times 10^3$ MPa, $I = 1.6 \times 10^7$ mm^4. $y_B = ?$

Reactions at supports:

$$R_A + R_C = 20 \text{ kN} \qquad \qquad \text{... Eq. (a)}$$

Taking moments about A and equating to zero, we have

$$R_C \times 3 = (20 \times 4) + 10$$
$$R_C = 30 \text{ kN} \qquad \qquad \text{... Eq. (b)}$$

Substituting Eq. (b) in Eq. (a), we have

$$R_A + 30 = 20$$
$$R_A = -10 \text{ kN} \qquad \qquad \text{... Eq. (c)}$$

Consider a section X-X at a distance x from free end A and in the region CD as shown in **Fig. 8.60(b)**. Bending moment at X-X is

$$M_x = R_A.\langle x \rangle + M\langle x - a \rangle^0 + R_C \langle x - b \rangle$$

i.e.

$$EI\frac{d^2y}{dx^2} = -10000\langle x \rangle + 10 \times 10^6 \langle x - 2000 \rangle^0 + 30000\langle x - 3000 \rangle$$

Integrating once we have

$$EI\frac{dy}{dx} = -5000\langle x \rangle^2 + C_1 + 10 \times 10^6 \langle x - 2000 \rangle^1 + 15000\langle x - 3000 \rangle^2$$
$$\text{... Eq. (i)}$$

Integrating again we have

$$EIy = -\frac{5000\langle x \rangle^3}{3} + C_1 \langle x \rangle + C_2 + 5 \times 10^6 \langle x - 2000 \rangle^2$$

$$+ 5000\langle x - 3000 \rangle^3 \qquad \qquad \text{... Eq. (ii)}$$

Boundary conditions:

At $x = 0$, $y = 0$:

Eq. (ii) yields...

$$0 = -0 + 0 + C_2 + 0 - 0$$

Ignore brackets containing negative value

$$C_2 = 0 \qquad \qquad \text{... Eq. (iii)}$$

At $x = 3000$ mm, $y = 0$:

Eq. (ii) yields...

$$0 = -\frac{5000\langle 3000 \rangle^3}{3} + C_1 \langle 3000 \rangle + 5 \times 10^6 \langle 3000 - 2000 \rangle^2 + 0$$

$$C_1 = 1.33 \times 10^{10} \qquad \qquad \text{... Eq. (iv)}$$

Substituting C_1 in Eq. (i) we get

$$EI\frac{dy}{dx} = -5000\langle x \rangle^2 + 1.33 \times 10^{10} + 10 \times 10^6 \langle x - 2000 \rangle^1$$

$$+ 15000\langle x - 3000 \rangle^2 \qquad \qquad \text{... Eq. (v)}$$

Substituting C_1 and C_2 in Eq. (ii) we get

$$EIy = -\frac{5000\langle x \rangle^3}{3} + 1.33 \times 10^{10} \langle x \rangle + 5 \times 10^6 \langle x - 2000 \rangle^2$$

$$+ 5000\langle x - 3000 \rangle^3 \qquad \qquad \text{... Eq. (vi)}$$

Deflection

At B, $x = 2000$ mm

Eq. (vi) yields... $EIy_B = -\dfrac{5000\langle 2000\rangle^3}{3} + 1.33 \times 10^{10}\langle 2000\rangle + 0 - 0$

$$y_B = \frac{1.326 \times 10^{13}}{(210 \times 10^3) \times (1.6 \times 10^7)} = 3.95 \text{ mm}$$

At D, $x = 4000$ mm

Eq. (vi) yields... $EIy_B = -\dfrac{5000\langle 4000\rangle^3}{3} + 1.33 \times 10^{10}\langle 4000\rangle$

$$+ 5 \times 10^6 \langle 4000 - 2000\rangle^2 + 5000\langle 4000 - 3000\rangle^3$$

$$y_B = \frac{-2.85 \times 10^{13}}{(210 \times 10^3) \times (1.6 \times 10^7)} = -8.47 \text{ mm}$$

56. A beam 25 m long is supported at A and B and is loaded as shown in Fig. 8.61(a). If $E = 200$ GPa, and $I = 160 \times 10^7$ mm^4, determine:

(a) Slope at all points   **(b) Deflection C, D & E**

Solution: $w = 10$ kN/m $= 10$ N/mm, $W_1 = 40 \times 10^3$ N, $W_2 = 30 \times 10^3$ N, $E = 200 \times 10^3$ MPa, $I = 160 \times 10^7$ mm^4. $a = 10000$ mm, $b = 15000$ mm, $c = 20000$ mm. a) $\theta_A, \theta_C, \theta_D, \theta_B, \theta_E = ?$, b) $y_C, y_D, y_E = ?$

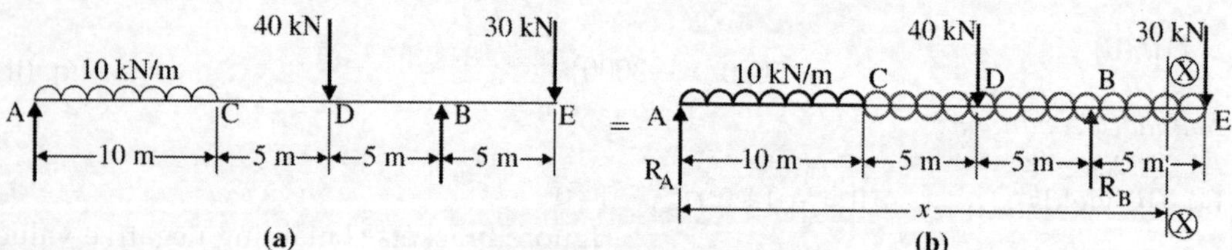

Fig. 8.61: Problem 56

Reactions at supports:

$$R_A + R_B = 30 + 40 + (10 \times 10) = 170 \text{ kN} \qquad \dots \text{Eq. (a)}$$

Taking moments about A and equating to zero, we have

$$R_B \times 20 = (30 \times 25) + (40 \times 15) + (10 \times 10) \times \left(\frac{10}{2}\right)$$

$$R_B = 92.50 \text{ kN} \qquad \dots \text{Eq. (b)}$$

Substituting Eq. (b) in Eq. (a), we have

$$R_A + 92.50 = 170$$

$$R_A = 77.50 \text{ kN} \qquad \dots \text{Eq. (c)}$$

Consider a section X-X at a distance x from free end A and in the region BE as shown in **Fig. 8.61(b)**. Bending moment at X-X is

$$M_x = R_A\langle x\rangle - \frac{w\langle x\rangle^2}{2} + \frac{w\langle x - a\rangle^2}{2} - W_1\langle x - b\rangle + R_B\langle x - c\rangle$$

i.e.
$$EI \frac{d^2y}{dx^2} = 77500\langle x \rangle - \frac{10\langle x \rangle^2}{2} + \frac{10\langle x - 10000 \rangle^2}{2} - 40000\langle x - 15000 \rangle$$
$$+ 92500\langle x - 20000 \rangle$$

Integrating once we have
$$EI \frac{dy}{dx} = 38750\langle x \rangle^2 + C_1 - \frac{5\langle x \rangle^3}{3} + \frac{5\langle x - 10000 \rangle^3}{3}$$
$$- 20000\langle x - 15000 \rangle^2 + 46250\langle x - 20000 \rangle^2 \qquad \ldots \text{Eq. (i)}$$

Integrating again we have
$$EIy = \frac{38750\langle x \rangle^3}{3} + C_1\langle x \rangle + C_2 - \frac{5\langle x \rangle^4}{12} + \frac{5\langle x - 10000 \rangle^4}{12}$$
$$- \frac{20000\langle x - 15000 \rangle^3}{3} + \frac{46250\langle x - 20000 \rangle^3}{3} \qquad \ldots \text{Eq. (ii)}$$

Boundary conditions:
At $x = 0, y = 0$:
Eq. (ii) yields... $\qquad 0 = 0 + 0 + C_2 - 0 + 0 - 0 + 0$

$\qquad\qquad\qquad\qquad\qquad\qquad$ Ignore brackets containing negative value
$$C_2 = 0 \qquad \ldots \text{Eq. (iii)}$$
At $x = 20000$ mm, $y = 0$:

Eq. (ii) yields... $\qquad 0 = \dfrac{38750\langle 20000 \rangle^3}{3} + C_1\langle 20000 \rangle - \dfrac{5\langle 20000 \rangle^4}{12}$
$$+ \frac{5\langle 20000 - 10000 \rangle^4}{12} - \frac{20000\langle 20000 - 15000 \rangle^3}{3} + 0$$
$$C_1 = -2 \times 10^{12} \qquad \ldots \text{Eq. (iv)}$$
Substituting C_1 in Eq. (i) we get
$$EI \frac{dy}{dx} = 38750\langle x \rangle^2 - 2 \times 10^{12} - \frac{5\langle x \rangle^3}{3} + \frac{5\langle x - 10000 \rangle^3}{3}$$
$$- 20000\langle x - 15000 \rangle^2 + 46250\langle x - 20000 \rangle^2 \qquad \ldots \text{Eq. (v)}$$

Substituting C_1 and C_2 in Eq. (ii) we get
$$EIy = \frac{38750\langle x \rangle^3}{3} - 2 \times 10^{12}\langle x \rangle - \frac{5\langle x \rangle^4}{12} + \frac{5\langle x - 10000 \rangle^4}{12}$$
$$- \frac{20000\langle x - 15000 \rangle^3}{3} + \frac{46250\langle x - 20000 \rangle^3}{3} \qquad \ldots \text{Eq. (vi)}$$

a. *Slope at all points*
   At A, $x = 0$
   Eq. (v) yields... $\qquad EI\theta_A = 0 - 2 \times 10^{12} - 0 + 0 - 0 + 0$
$$\theta_A = \frac{-2 \times 10^{12}}{(200 \times 10^3) \times (160 \times 10^7)} = -0.00625 \text{ rad}$$

At C, $x = 10000$ mm

Eq. (v) yields... $\quad EI\theta_C = 38750\langle 10000\rangle^2 - 2\times 10^{12} - \dfrac{5\langle 10000\rangle^3}{3} + 0$

$$\theta_C = \dfrac{2.083\times 10^{12}}{(200\times 10^3)\times(160\times 10^7)} = 0.00065 \text{ rad}$$

At D, $x = 15000$ mm

Eq. (v) yields... $\quad EI\theta_D = 38750\langle 15000\rangle^2 - 2\times 10^{12} - \dfrac{5\langle 15000\rangle^3}{3}$

$$+ \dfrac{5\langle 15000 - 10000\rangle^3}{3} - 0 + 0$$

$$\theta_D = \dfrac{1.302\times 10^{12}}{(200\times 10^3)\times(160\times 10^7)} = 0.00407 \text{ rad}$$

At B, $x = 20000$ mm

Eq. (v) yields... $\quad EI\theta_B = 38750\langle 20000\rangle^2 - 2\times 10^{12} - \dfrac{5\langle 20000\rangle^3}{3}$

$$+ \dfrac{5\langle 20000 - 10000\rangle^3}{3} - 20000\langle 20000 - 15000\rangle^2 + 0$$

$$\theta_B = \dfrac{1.33\times 10^{12}}{(200\times 10^3)\times(160\times 10^7)} = 0.00417 \text{ rad}$$

At E, $x = 25000$ mm

Eq. (v) yields... $\quad EI\theta_E = 38750\langle 25000\rangle^2 - 2\times 10^{12} - \dfrac{5\langle 25000\rangle^3}{3}$

$$+ \dfrac{5\langle 25000 - 10000\rangle^3}{3} - 20000\langle 25000 - 15000\rangle^2$$

$$+ 46250\langle 25000 - 20000\rangle^2$$

$$\theta_E = \dfrac{9.58\times 10^{11}}{(200\times 10^3)\times(160\times 10^7)} = 0.00299 \text{ rad}$$

b. *Deflection*

At C, $x = 10000$ mm

Eq. (vi) yields... $\quad EIy_C = \dfrac{38750\langle 10000\rangle^3}{3} - 2\times 10^{12}\langle 10000\rangle - \dfrac{5\langle 10000\rangle^4}{12}$

$$+ 0 - 0 + 0$$

$$y_C = \dfrac{-1.125\times 10^{16}}{(200\times 10^3)\times(160\times 10^7)} = -35.16 \text{ mm}$$

At D, $x = 15000$ mm

Eq. (vi) yields... $EIy_D = \dfrac{38750\langle 15000\rangle^3}{3} - 2\times 10^{12}\langle 15000\rangle - \dfrac{5\langle 15000\rangle^4}{12}$

$$+ \dfrac{5\langle 15000 - 10000\rangle^4}{12} - 0 + 0$$

$$y_D = \dfrac{-7.24\times 10^{15}}{(200\times 10^3)\times(160\times 10^7)} = -22.62 \text{ mm}$$

At E, $x = 25000$ mm

Eq. (vi) yields... $EIy_E = \dfrac{38750\langle 25000\rangle^3}{3} - 2\times 10^{12}\langle 25000\rangle - \dfrac{5\langle 25000\rangle^4}{12}$

$$+ \dfrac{5\langle 25000 - 10000\rangle^4}{12} - \dfrac{20000\langle 25000 - 15000\rangle^3}{3}$$

$$+ \dfrac{6250\langle 25000 - 20000\rangle^3}{3}$$

$$y_E = \dfrac{5.42\times 10^{15}}{(200\times 10^3)\times(160\times 10^7)} = 16.93 \text{ mm}$$

57. **An overhanging beam is loaded as shown in Fig. 8.62(a). If $E = 200$ GPa, and $I = 150\times 10^6$ mm^4, determine:**

(a) Slope at all points   (b) Deflection C, D & E

Solution: $W = 20\times 10^3$ N, $w = 3$ kN/m $= 3$ N/mm, $E = 200\times 10^3$ MPa, $I = 150\times 10^6$ mm^4.
$a = 2000$ mm, $b = 4000$ mm, $c = 8000$ mm. a) $\theta_A,\ \theta_C,\ \theta_D,\ \theta_B,\ \theta_E = ?$, b) $y_C,\ y_D,\ y_E = ?$

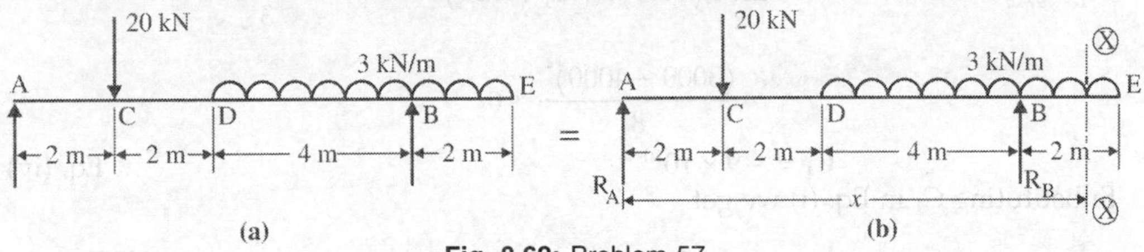

Fig. 8.62: Problem 57

Reactions at supports:

$$R_A + R_B = 20 + (3\times 6) = 38 \text{ kN} \qquad \text{... Eq. (a)}$$

Taking moments about A and equating to zero, we have

$$R_B\times 8 = (20\times 2) + (3\times 6)\times\left(\dfrac{6}{2} + 4\right)$$

$$R_B = 20.75 \text{ kN} \qquad \text{... Eq. (b)}$$

Substituting Eq. (b) in Eq. (a), we have
$$R_A + 20.75 = 38$$
$$R_A = 17.25 \text{ kN} \qquad \text{... Eq. (c)}$$

Consider a section X-X at a distance x from free end A and in the region BE as shown in **Fig. 8.62(b)**. Bending moment at X-X is

$$M_x = R_A \langle x \rangle - W \langle x - a \rangle - \frac{w \langle x - b \rangle^2}{2} + R_B \langle x - c \rangle$$

i.e.

$$EI \frac{d^2y}{dx^2} = 17250 \langle x \rangle - 20000 \langle x - 2000 \rangle - \frac{3 \langle x - 4000 \rangle^2}{2}$$
$$+ 20500 \langle x - 8000 \rangle$$

Integrating once we have

$$EI \frac{dy}{dx} = 8625 \langle x \rangle^2 + C_1 - 10000 \langle x - 2000 \rangle^2 - \frac{\langle x - 4000 \rangle^3}{2}$$
$$+ 10250 \langle x - 8000 \rangle^2 \qquad \ldots \text{Eq. (i)}$$

Integrating again we have

$$EIy = 2875 \langle x \rangle^3 + C_1 \langle x \rangle + C_2 - \frac{10000 \langle x - 2000 \rangle^3}{3}$$
$$- \frac{\langle x - 4000 \rangle^4}{8} + \frac{10250 \langle x - 8000 \rangle^3}{3} \qquad \ldots \text{Eq. (ii)}$$

Boundary conditions:
At $x = 0, y = 0$:
Eq. (ii) yields... $\qquad 0 = 0 + 0 + C_2 - 0 + 0 - 0 + 0$

Ignore brackets containing negative value
$$C_2 = 0 \qquad \ldots \text{Eq. (iii)}$$
At $x = 8000$ mm, $y = 0$:

Eq. (ii) yields... $\qquad 0 = 2875 \langle 8000 \rangle^3 + C_1 \langle 8000 \rangle - \frac{10000 \langle 8000 - 2000 \rangle^3}{3}$
$$- \frac{\langle 8000 - 4000 \rangle^4}{8} + 0$$
$$C_1 = -9 \times 10^{10} \qquad \ldots \text{Eq. (iv)}$$

Substituting C_1 in Eq. (i) we get

$$EI \frac{dy}{dx} = 8625 \langle x \rangle^2 - 9 \times 10^{10} - 10000 \langle x - 2000 \rangle^2 - \frac{\langle x - 4000 \rangle^3}{2}$$
$$+ 10250 \langle x - 8000 \rangle^2 \qquad \ldots \text{Eq. (v)}$$

Substituting C_1 and C_2 in Eq. (ii) we get

$$EIy = 2875 \langle x \rangle^3 - 9 \times 10^{10} \langle x \rangle - \frac{10000 \langle x - 2000 \rangle^3}{3}$$
$$- \frac{\langle x - 4000 \rangle^4}{8} + \frac{10250 \langle x - 8000 \rangle^3}{3} \qquad \ldots \text{Eq. (vi)}$$

a. *Slope at all points*
At A, $x = 0$

Eq. (v) yields... $EI\theta_A = 0 - 9 \times 10^{10} - 0 + 0 - 0 + 0$

$$\theta_A = \frac{-9 \times 10^{10}}{(200 \times 10^3) \times (150 \times 10^6)} = -0.003 \text{ rad}$$

At C, $x = 2000$ mm

Eq. (v) yields... $EI\theta_C = 8625\langle 2000 \rangle^2 - 9 \times 10^{10} - 0 - 0 + 0$

$$\theta_C = \frac{-3.45 \times 10^{10}}{(200 \times 10^3) \times (150 \times 10^6)} = -0.00185 \text{ rad}$$

At D, $x = 4000$ mm

Eq. (v) yields... $EI\theta_D = 8625\langle 4000 \rangle^2 - 9 \times 10^{10} - 10000\langle 4000 - 2000 \rangle^2 - 0 + 0$

$$\theta_D = \frac{8 \times 10^9}{(200 \times 10^3) \times (150 \times 10^6)} = 0.000275 \text{ rad}$$

At B, $x = 8000$ mm

Eq. (v) yields... $EI\theta_B = 8625\langle 8000 \rangle^2 - 9 \times 10^{10} - 10000\langle 8000 - 2000 \rangle^2$

$$- \frac{\langle 8000 - 4000 \rangle^3}{2} + 0$$

$$\theta_B = \frac{7 \times 10^{10}}{(200 \times 10^3) \times (150 \times 10^6)} = 0.0023 \text{ rad}$$

At E, $x = 10000$ mm

Eq. (v) yields... $EI\theta_E = 8625\langle 10000 \rangle^2 - 9 \times 10^{10} - 10000\langle 10000 - 2000 \rangle^2$

$$- \frac{\langle 10000 - 4000 \rangle^3}{2} + 10250\langle 10000 - 8000 \rangle^2$$

$$\theta_E = \frac{6.55 \times 10^{10}}{(200 \times 10^3) \times (150 \times 10^6)} = 0.00218 \text{ rad}$$

b. *Deflection*
At C, $x = 2000$ mm

Eq. (vi) yields... $EIy_C = 2875\langle 2000 \rangle^3 - 9 \times 10^{10}\langle 2000 \rangle - 0 - 0 + 0$

$$y_C = \frac{-1.57 \times 10^{14}}{(200 \times 10^3) \times (150 \times 10^6)} = -5.23 \text{ mm}$$

At D, $x = 4000$ mm

Eq. (vi) yields... $EIy_D = 2875\langle 4000 \rangle^3 - 9 \times 10^{10}\langle 4000 \rangle - \dfrac{10000\langle 4000 - 2000 \rangle^3}{3}$

$$- 0 + 0$$

$$y_D = \frac{-2.03 \times 10^{14}}{(200 \times 10^3) \times (150 \times 10^6)} = -6.76 \text{ mm}$$

At E, $x = 10000$ mm

Eq. (vi) yields... $EIy_E = 2875 \langle 10000 \rangle^3 - 9 \times 10^{10} \langle 10000 \rangle$

$$- \frac{10000 \langle 10000 - 2000 \rangle^3}{3} - \frac{\langle 10000 - 4000 \rangle^4}{8}$$

$$+ \frac{10250 \langle 10000 - 8000 \rangle^3}{3}$$

$$y_E = \frac{1.33 \times 10^{14}}{(200 \times 10^3) \times (150 \times 10^6)} = 4.45 \text{ mm}$$

58. **An overhanging beam is loaded as shown in Fig. 8.63(a). If $E = 200$ GPa, and $I = 150 \times 10^6$ mm^4, determine:**

(a) Slope at all points   (b) Deflection C, D & E

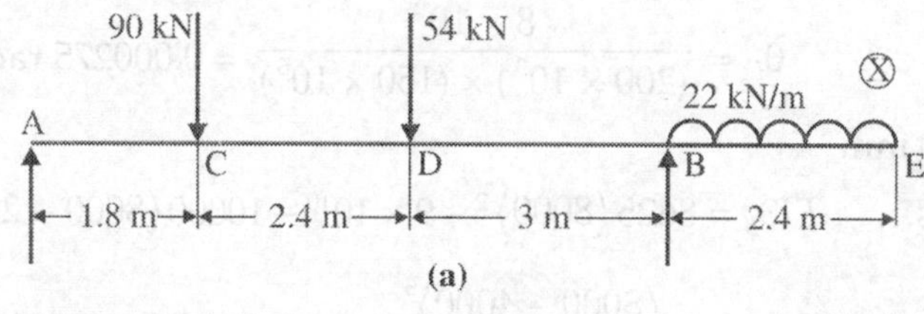

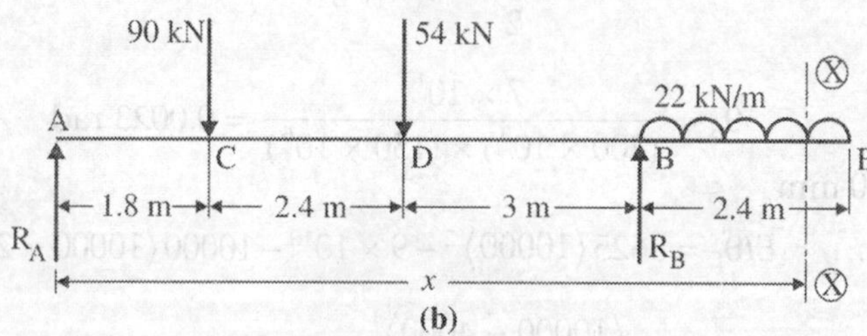

Fig. 8.63: Problem 58

Solution: $W_1 = 90 \times 10^3$ N, $W_2 = 54 \times 10^3$ N, $w = 22$ kN/m $= 22$ N/mm, $E = 200 \times 10^3$ MPa, $I = 150 \times 10^6$ mm^4. $a = 1800$ mm, $b = 4200$ mm, $c = 7200$ mm. a) θ_A, θ_C, θ_D, θ_B, $\theta_E = ?$, b) y_C, y_D, $y_E = ?$

Reactions at supports:

$$R_A + R_B = 90 + 54 + (22 \times 2.4) = 196.8 \text{ kN} \qquad \text{... Eq. (a)}$$

Taking moments about A and equating to zero, we have

$$R_B \times 7.2 = (90 \times 1.8) + (54 \times 4.2) + (22 \times 2.4) \times \left(\frac{2.4}{2} + 7.2 \right)$$

$$R_B = 115.60 \text{ kN} \qquad \text{... Eq. (b)}$$

Substituting Eq. (b) in Eq. (a), we have

$$R_A + 115.6 = 196.80$$

$$R_A = 81.20 \text{ kN} \qquad \text{... Eq. (c)}$$

Consider a section X-X at a distance x from free end A and in the region BE as shown in **Fig. 8.63(b)**. Bending moment at X-X is

$$M_x = R_A \langle x \rangle - W_1 \langle x - a \rangle - W_2 \langle x - b \rangle + R_B \langle x - c \rangle - \frac{w \langle x - c \rangle^2}{2}$$

i.e.
$$EI\frac{d^2y}{dx^2} = 81200\langle x\rangle - 90000\langle x - 1800\rangle - 54000\langle x - 4200\rangle$$

$$+ 115600\langle x - 7200\rangle - \frac{22\langle x - 7200\rangle^2}{2}$$

Integrating once we have

$$EI\frac{dy}{dx} = \frac{81200\langle x\rangle^2}{2} + C_1 - 45000\langle x - 1800\rangle^2 - 27000\langle x - 4200\rangle^2$$

$$+ 57800\langle x - 7200\rangle^2 - \frac{11\langle x - 7200\rangle^3}{3} \qquad \ldots \text{Eq. (i)}$$

Integrating again we have

$$EIy = \frac{40600\langle x\rangle^3}{3} + C_1\langle x\rangle + C_2 - 15000\langle x - 1800\rangle^3$$

$$- 9000\langle x - 4200\rangle^3 + \frac{57800\langle x - 7200\rangle^3}{3} - \frac{11\langle x - 7200\rangle^4}{12}$$

$$\ldots \text{Eq. (ii)}$$

Boundary conditions:

At $x = 0$, $y = 0$:

Eq. (ii) yields... $\qquad 0 = 0 + 0 + C_2 - 0 - 0 + 0 - 0$

Ignore brackets containing negative value

$$C_2 = 0 \qquad \ldots \text{Eq. (iii)}$$

At $x = 7200$ mm, $y = 0$:

Eq. (ii) yields... $\qquad 0 = \frac{40600\langle 7200\rangle^3}{3} + C_1\langle 7200\rangle - 15000\langle 7200 - 1800\rangle^3$

$$- 9000\langle 7200 - 4200\rangle^3 + 0 - 0$$

$$C_1 = -3.40 \times 10^{11} \qquad \ldots \text{Eq. (iv)}$$

Substituting C_1 in Eq. (i) we get

$$EI\frac{dy}{dx} = \frac{81200\langle x\rangle^2}{2} - 3.40 \times 10^{11} - 45000\langle x - 1800\rangle^2$$

$$- 27000\langle x - 4200\rangle^2 + 57800\langle x - 7200\rangle^2 - \frac{11\langle x - 7200\rangle^3}{3}$$

$$\ldots \text{Eq. (v)}$$

Substituting C_1 and C_2 in Eq. (ii) we get

$$EIy = \frac{40600\langle x\rangle^3}{3} - 3.40 \times 10^{11}\langle x\rangle - 15000\langle x - 1800\rangle^3$$

$$- 9000\langle x - 4200\rangle^3 + \frac{57800\langle x - 7200\rangle^3}{3} - \frac{11\langle x - 7200\rangle^4}{12}$$

$$\ldots \text{Eq. (vi)}$$

a. *Slope at all points*

At A, $x = 0$

Eq. (v) yields... $EI\theta_A = 0 - 3.40 \times 10^{11} - 0 - 0 + 0 - 0$

$$\theta_A = \frac{-3.40 \times 10^{11}}{(200 \times 10^3) \times (150 \times 10^6)} = -0.0113 \text{ rad}$$

At C, $x = 1800$ mm

Eq. (v) yields... $EI\theta_C = \dfrac{81200 \langle 1800 \rangle^2}{2} - 3.40 \times 10^{11} - 0 - 0 + 0 - 0$

$$\theta_C = \frac{-2.08 \times 10^{11}}{(200 \times 10^3) \times (150 \times 10^6)} = -0.0069 \text{ rad}$$

At D, $x = 4200$ mm

Eq. (v) yields... $EI\theta_D = \dfrac{81200 \langle 4200 \rangle^2}{2} - 3.40 \times 10^{11} - 45000 \langle 4200 - 1800 \rangle^2 - 0 + 0 - 0$

$$\theta_D = \frac{1.17 \times 10^{11}}{(200 \times 10^3) \times (150 \times 10^6)} = 0.00390 \text{ rad}$$

At B, $x = 7200$ mm

Eq. (v) yields... $EI\theta_B = \dfrac{81200 \langle 7200 \rangle^2}{2} - 3.40 \times 10^{11} - 45000 \langle 7200 - 1800 \rangle^2$

$$- 27000 \langle 7200 - 4200 \rangle^2 + 0 - 0$$

$$\theta_B = \frac{2.09 \times 10^{11}}{(200 \times 10^3) \times (150 \times 10^6)} = 0.00698 \text{ rad}$$

At E, $x = 9600$ mm

Eq. (v) yields... $EI\theta_E = \dfrac{81200 \langle 9600 \rangle^2}{2} - 3.40 \times 10^{11} - 45000 \langle 9600 - 1800 \rangle^2$

$$- 27000 \langle 9600 - 4200 \rangle^2 + 57800 \langle 9600 - 7200 \rangle^2$$

$$- \frac{11 \langle 9600 - 7200 \rangle^3}{3}$$

$$\theta_E = \frac{1.59 \times 10^{11}}{(200 \times 10^3) \times (150 \times 10^6)} = 0.0053 \text{ rad}$$

b. *Deflection*

At C, $x = 1800$ mm

Eq. (vi) yields... $EIy_C = \dfrac{40600 \langle 1800 \rangle^3}{3} - 3.40 \times 10^{11} \langle 1800 \rangle - 0 - 0 + 0 - 0$

$$y_C = \frac{-5.33 \times 10^{14}}{(200 \times 10^3) \times (150 \times 10^6)} = -17.77 \text{ mm}$$

At D, $x = 4200$ mm

Eq. (vi) yields... $\quad EIy_D = \dfrac{40600\langle 4200\rangle^3}{3} - 3.40 \times 10^{11}\langle 4200\rangle$

$$- 15000\langle 4200 - 1800\rangle^3 - 0 + 0 - 0$$

$$y_D = \frac{-6.33 \times 10^{14}}{(200 \times 10^3) \times (150 \times 10^6)} = -21.09 \text{ mm}$$

At E, $x = 9600$ mm

Eq. (vi) yields... $\quad EIy_E = \dfrac{40600\langle 9600\rangle^3}{3} - 3.40 \times 10^{11}\langle 9600\rangle$

$$- 15000\langle 9600 - 1800\rangle^3 - 9000\langle 9600 - 4200\rangle^3$$

$$+ \frac{57800\langle 9600 - 7200\rangle^3}{3} - \frac{11\langle 9600 - 7200\rangle^4}{12}$$

$$y_E = \frac{4.10 \times 10^{14}}{(200 \times 10^3) \times (150 \times 10^6)} = 13.66 \text{ mm}$$

59. An overhanging beam is loaded as shown in Fig. 8.64(a). If $E = 200$ GPa, and $I = 100 \times 10^6$ mm^4, determine:

(a) Slope at all points $\qquad$ (b) Deflection C, D & E

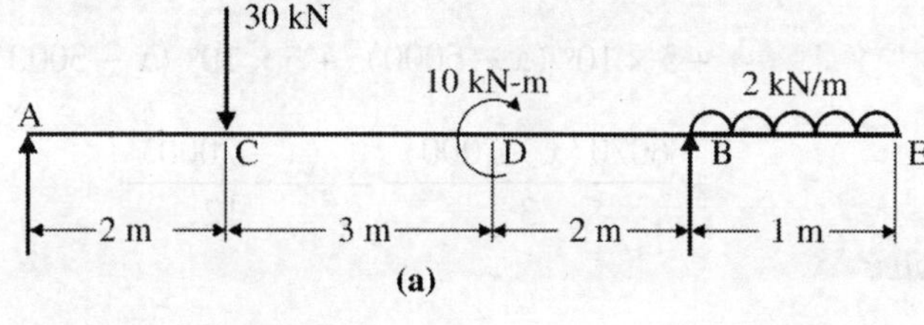

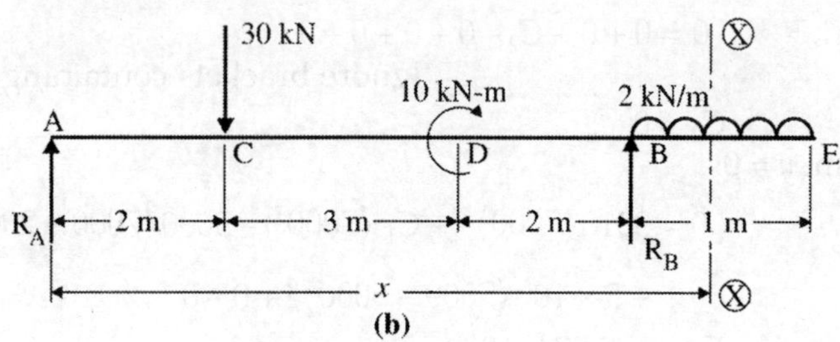

Fig. 8.64: Problem 59

Solution: $W = 30 \times 10^3$ N, $M = 10 \times 10^6$ N-mm, $w = 2$ kN/m $= 2$ N/mm, $E = 200 \times 10^3$ MPa, $I = 100 \times 10^6$ mm^4. $a = 2000$ mm, $b = 5000$ mm, $c = 7000$ mm. a) θ_A, θ_C, θ_D, θ_B, $\theta_E = ?$, b) y_C, y_D, $y_E = ?$

Reactions at supports:

$$R_A + R_B = 30 + (2 \times 1) = 32 \text{ kN} \qquad\qquad \text{... Eq. (a)}$$

Taking moments about A and equating to zero, we have

$$R_B \times 7 = (30 \times 2) + 10 + (2 \times 1) \times \left(\frac{1}{2} + 7\right)$$

$$R_B = 12.14 \text{ kN} \qquad \text{... Eq. (b)}$$

Substituting Eq. (b) in Eq. (a), we have

$$R_A + 12.14 = 32$$

$$R_A = 19.86 \text{ kN} \qquad \text{... Eq. (c)}$$

Consider a section X-X at a distance x from free end A and in the region BE as shown in **Fig. 8.64(b)**. Bending moment at X-X is

$$M_x = R_A.\langle x \rangle - W\langle x-a \rangle + M\langle x-b \rangle^0 + R_B \langle x-c \rangle - \frac{w\langle x-c \rangle^2}{2}$$

i.e.

$$EI\frac{d^2y}{dx^2} = 19860\langle x \rangle - 30000\langle x-2000 \rangle + 10 \times 10^6 \langle x-5000 \rangle^0$$

$$+ 12140\langle x-7000 \rangle - \frac{2\langle x-7000 \rangle^2}{2}$$

Integrating once we have

$$EI\frac{dy}{dx} = 9930\langle x \rangle^2 + C_1 - 15000\langle x-2000 \rangle^2 + 10 \times 10^6 \langle x-5000 \rangle^1$$

$$+ 6070\langle x-7000 \rangle^2 - \frac{\langle x-7000 \rangle^3}{3} \qquad \text{... Eq. (i)}$$

Integrating again we have

$$EIy = 3310\langle x \rangle^3 + C_1 \langle x \rangle + C_2 - 5000\langle x-2000 \rangle^3$$

$$+ 5 \times 10^6 \langle x-5000 \rangle^2 + 5 \times 10^6 \langle x-5000 \rangle^2$$

$$+ \frac{6070\langle x-7000 \rangle^3}{3} - \frac{\langle x-7000 \rangle^4}{12} \qquad \text{... Eq. (ii)}$$

Boundary conditions:

At $x = 0, y = 0$:

Eq. (ii) yields...

$$0 = 0 + 0 + C_2 - 0 + 0 + 0 - 0$$

Ignore brackets containing negative value

$$C_2 = 0 \qquad \text{... Eq. (iii)}$$

At $x = 7000$ mm, $y = 0$:

Eq. (ii) yields...

$$0 = 3310\langle 7000 \rangle^3 + C_1 \langle 7000 \rangle - 5000\langle 7000 - 2000 \rangle^3$$

$$+ 5 \times 10^6 \langle 7000 - 5000 \rangle^2 + 0 - 0$$

$$C_1 = -7.57 \times 10^{10} \qquad \text{... Eq. (iv)}$$

Substituting C_1 in Eq. (i) we get

$$EI\frac{dy}{dx} = 9930\langle x \rangle^2 - 7.57 \times 10^{10} - 15000\langle x-2000 \rangle^2$$

$$+ 10 \times 10^6 \langle x-5000 \rangle^1 + 6070\langle x-7000 \rangle^2 - \frac{\langle x-7000 \rangle^3}{3}$$

$$\text{... Eq. (v)}$$

Substituting C_1 and C_2 in Eq. (ii) we get

$$EIy = 3310\langle x \rangle^3 - 7.57 \times 10^{10} \langle x \rangle - 5000\langle x - 2000 \rangle^3$$

$$+ 5 \times 10^6 \langle x - 5000 \rangle^2 + \frac{6070\langle x - 7000 \rangle^3}{3} - \frac{\langle x - 7000 \rangle^4}{12}$$

$$\dots \text{Eq. (vi)}$$

a. *Slope at all points*

At A, $x = 0$

Eq. (v) yields... $\quad EI\theta_A = 0 - 7.57 \times 10^{10} - 0 + 0 + 0 - 0$

$$\theta_A = \frac{-7.57 \times 10^{10}}{(200 \times 10^3) \times (100 \times 10^6)} = -0.00379 \text{ rad}$$

At C, $x = 2000$ mm

Eq. (v) yields... $\quad EI\theta_C = 9930\langle 2000 \rangle^2 - 7.57 \times 10^{10} - 0 + 0 + 0 - 0$

$$\theta_C = \frac{-3.60 \times 10^{10}}{(200 \times 10^3) \times (100 \times 10^6)} = -0.00180 \text{ rad}$$

At D, $x = 5000$ mm

Eq. (v) yields... $\quad EI\theta_D = 9930\langle 5000 \rangle^2 - 7.57 \times 10^{10} - 15000\langle 5000 - 2000 \rangle^2 + 0 + 0 - 0$

$$\theta_D = \frac{3.78 \times 10^{10}}{(200 \times 10^3) \times (100 \times 10^6)} = 0.00187 \text{ rad}$$

At B, $x = 7000$ mm

Eq. (v) yields... $\quad EI\theta_B = 9930\langle 7000 \rangle^2 - 7.57 \times 10^{10} - 15000\langle 7000 - 2000 \rangle^2$

$$+ 10 \times 10^6 \langle 7000 - 5000 \rangle^1 + 0 - 0$$

$$\theta_B = \frac{5.59 \times 10^{10}}{(200 \times 10^3) \times (100 \times 10^6)} = 0.00279 \text{ rad}$$

At E, $x = 8000$ mm

Eq. (v) yields... $\quad EI\theta_E = 9930\langle 8000 \rangle^2 - 7.57 \times 10^{10} - 15000\langle 8000 - 2000 \rangle^2$

$$+ 10 \times 10^6 \langle 8000 - 5000 \rangle^1 + 6070\langle 8000 - 7000 \rangle^2$$

$$- \frac{\langle 8000 - 7000 \rangle^3}{3}$$

$$\theta_E = \frac{5.56 \times 10^{10}}{(200 \times 10^3) \times (100 \times 10^6)} = 0.00277 \text{ rad}$$

b. *Deflection*

At C, $x = 2000$ mm

Eq. (vi) yields... $\quad EIy_C = 3310\langle 2000 \rangle^3 - 7.57 \times 10^{10} \langle 2000 \rangle - 0 + 0 + 0 - 0$

$$y_C = \frac{-1.25 \times 10^{14}}{(200 \times 10^3) \times (100 \times 10^6)} = -6.25 \text{ mm}$$

At D, $x = 5000$ mm

Eq. (vi) yields... $EIy_D = 3310\langle 5000 \rangle^3 - 7.57 \times 10^{10} \langle 5000 \rangle - 5000 \langle 5000 - 2000 \rangle^3$
$$+ 0 + 0 - 0$$

$$y_D = \frac{-9.98 \times 10^{13}}{(200 \times 10^3) \times (100 \times 10^6)} = -4.99 \text{ mm}$$

At E, $x = 8000$ mm

Eq. (vi) yields... $EIy_E = 3310\langle 8000 \rangle^3 - 7.57 \times 10^{10} \langle 8000 \rangle - 5000 \langle 8000 - 2000 \rangle^3$

$$+ 5 \times 10^6 \langle 8000 - 5000 \rangle^2 + \frac{6070 \langle 8000 - 7000 \rangle^3}{3}$$

$$- \frac{\langle 8000 - 7000 \rangle^4}{12}$$

$$y_E = \frac{5.61 \times 10^{13}}{(200 \times 10^3) \times (100 \times 10^6)} = 2.81 \text{ mm}$$

60. An overhanging beam is loaded as shown in Fig. 8.65(a). If $E = 200$ GPa, and $I = 100 \times 10^6$ mm^4, determine: (a) Slope at all points (b) Deflection C, D, E & F

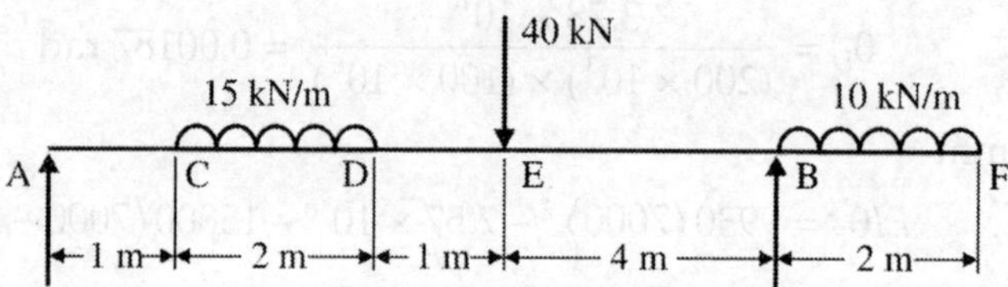

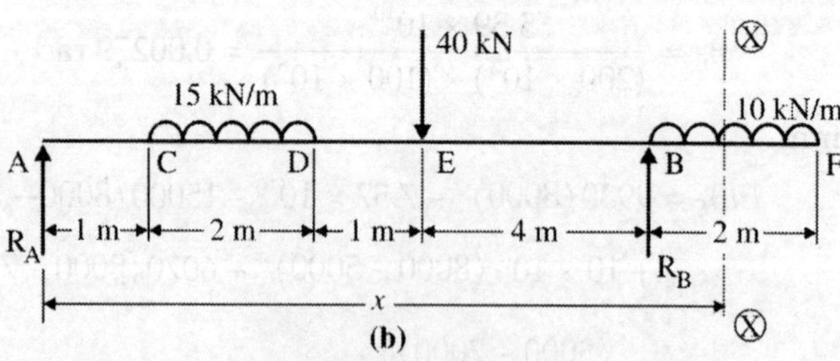

Fig. 8.65: Problem 60

Solution: $W = 40 \times 10^3$ N, $w_1 = 15$ kN/m $= 15$ N/mm, $w_2 = 10$ kN/m $= 10$ N/mm, $E = 200 \times 10^3$ MPa, $I = 100 \times 10^6$ mm^4. $a = 1000$ mm, $b = 3000$ mm, $c = 4000$ mm, $d = 8000$ mm.

a) $\theta_A, \theta_C, \theta_D, \theta_B, \theta_E, \theta_F = ?$, b) $y_C, y_D, y_E, y_F = ?$

Reactions at supports:

$$R_A + R_B = 40 + (15 \times 2) + (10 \times 2) = 90 \text{ kN} \qquad \text{... Eq. (a)}$$

Taking moments about A and equating to zero, we have

$$R_B \times 8 = (40 \times 4) + (15 \times 2) \times \left(\frac{2}{2} + 1 \right) + (10 \times 2) \times \left(\frac{2}{2} + 8 \right)$$

$$R_B = 50 \text{ kN} \qquad \text{... Eq. (b)}$$

Substituting Eq. (b) in Eq. (a), we have

$$R_A + 50 = 90$$
$$R_A = 40 \text{kN} \quad\quad \text{... Eq. (c)}$$

Consider a section X-X at a distance x from free end A and in the region BF as shown in **Fig. 8.65(b)**. Bending moment at X-X is

$$M_x = R_A \langle x \rangle - \frac{w_1 \langle x - a \rangle^2}{2} + \frac{w_1 \langle x - b \rangle^2}{2} - W \langle x - c \rangle$$

$$+ R_B \langle x - d \rangle - \frac{w_2 \langle x - d \rangle^2}{2}$$

i.e.

$$EI\frac{d^2y}{dx^2} = 40000 \langle x \rangle - \frac{15 \langle x - 1000 \rangle^2}{2} + \frac{15 \langle x - 3000 \rangle^2}{2}$$

$$- 40000 \langle x - 4000 \rangle + 50000 \langle x - 8000 \rangle - \frac{10 \langle x - 8000 \rangle^2}{2}$$

Integrating once we have

$$EI\frac{dy}{dx} = 20000 \langle x \rangle^2 + C_1 - \frac{5 \langle x - 1000 \rangle^3}{2} + \frac{5 \langle x - 1000 \rangle^3}{2}$$

$$- 20000 \langle x - 4000 \rangle^2 + 25000 \langle x - 8000 \rangle^2 - \frac{5 \langle x - 8000 \rangle^3}{3}$$

$$\text{... Eq. (i)}$$

Integrating again we have

$$EIy = \frac{20000 \langle x \rangle^3}{3} + C_1 \langle x \rangle + C_2 - \frac{5 \langle x - 1000 \rangle^4}{8}$$

$$+ \frac{5 \langle x - 3000 \rangle^4}{8} - \frac{20000 \langle x - 4000 \rangle^3}{3}$$

$$+ \frac{25000 \langle x - 8000 \rangle^3}{3} - \frac{5 \langle x - 8000 \rangle^4}{12} \quad\quad \text{... Eq. (ii)}$$

Boundary conditions:

At $x = 0, y = 0$:

Eq. (ii) yields... $\quad\quad 0 = 0 + 0 + C_2 - 0 + 0 - 0 + 0 - 0$

Ignore brackets containing negative value

$$C_2 = 0 \quad\quad \text{... Eq. (iii)}$$

At $x = 8000$ mm, $y = 0$:

Eq. (ii) yields... $\quad 0 = \dfrac{20000 \langle 8000 \rangle^3}{3} + C_1 \langle 8000 \rangle - \dfrac{5 \langle 8000 - 1000 \rangle^4}{8}$

$$+ \frac{5 \langle 8000 - 3000 \rangle^4}{8} - \frac{20000 \langle 8000 - 4000 \rangle^4}{3} + 0 - 0$$

$$C_1 = -2.35 \times 10^{11} \quad\quad \text{... Eq. (iv)}$$

Substituting C_1 in Eq. (i) we get

$$EI\frac{dy}{dx} = 20000\langle x\rangle^2 - 2.35\times 10^{11} - \frac{5\langle x-1000\rangle^3}{2} + \frac{5\langle x-3000\rangle^3}{2}$$

$$-20000\langle x-4000\rangle^2 + 25000\langle x-8000\rangle^2 - \frac{5\langle x-8000\rangle^3}{3}$$

$$\ldots \text{Eq. (v)}$$

Substituting C_1 and C_2 in Eq. (ii) we get

$$EIy = \frac{20000\langle x\rangle^3}{3} - 2.35\times 10^{11}\langle x\rangle - \frac{5\langle x-1000\rangle^4}{8}$$

$$+\frac{5\langle x-3000\rangle^4}{8} - \frac{20000\langle x-4000\rangle^3}{3}$$

$$+\frac{25000\langle x-8000\rangle^3}{3} - \frac{5\langle x-8000\rangle^4}{12} \qquad \ldots \text{Eq. (vi)}$$

a. *Slope at all points*

At A, $x = 0$

Eq. (v) yields... $\quad EI\theta_A = 0 - 2.35\times 10^{11} - 0 + 0 - 0 + 0 - 0$

$$\theta_A = \frac{-2.35\times 10^{11}}{(200\times 10^3)\times(100\times 10^6)} = -0.00117 \text{ rad}$$

At C, $x = 1000$ mm

Eq. (v) yields... $\quad EI\theta_C = 20000\langle 1000\rangle^2 - 2.35\times 10^{11} - 0 + 0 - 0 + 0 - 0$

$$\theta_C = \frac{-2.15\times 10^{11}}{(200\times 10^3)\times(100\times 10^6)} = -0.01075 \text{ rad}$$

At D, $x = 3000$ mm

Eq. (v) yields... $\quad EI\theta_D = 20000\langle 3000\rangle^2 - 2.35\times 10^{11} - \frac{5\langle 3000-1000\rangle^3}{2} + 0 - 0 + 0 - 0$

$$\theta_D = \frac{-7.5\times 10^{10}}{(200\times 10^3)\times(100\times 10^6)} = -0.00375 \text{ rad}$$

At E, $x = 4000$ mm

Eq. (v) yields... $\quad EI\theta_E = 20000\langle 4000\rangle^2 - 2.35\times 10^{11} - \frac{5\langle 4000-1000\rangle^3}{2}$

$$+\frac{5\langle 4000-3000\rangle^3}{2} - 0 + 0 - 0$$

$$\theta_E = \frac{2\times 10^{10}}{(200\times 10^3)\times(100\times 10^6)} = 0.001 \text{ rad}$$

At B, $x = 8000$ mm

Eq. (v) yields... $EI\theta_B = 20000\langle 8000\rangle^2 - 2.35 \times 10^{11} - \dfrac{5\langle 8000 - 1000\rangle^3}{2}$

$$+ \dfrac{5\langle 8000 - 3000\rangle^3}{2} - 20000\langle 8000 - 4000\rangle^2 + 0 - 0$$

$$\theta_B = \dfrac{1.8 \times 10^{11}}{(200 \times 10^3) \times (100 \times 10^6)} = 0.009 \text{ rad}$$

At F, $x = 10000$ mm

Eq. (v) yields... $EI\theta_F = 20000\langle 10000\rangle^2 - 2.35 \times 10^{11} - \dfrac{5\langle 10000 - 1000\rangle^3}{2}$

$$+ \dfrac{5\langle 10000 - 3000\rangle^3}{2} - 20000\langle 10000 - 4000\rangle^2$$

$$+ 25000\langle 10000 - 8000\rangle^2 - \dfrac{5\langle 10000 - 8000\rangle^3}{3}$$

$$\theta_F = \dfrac{1.67 \times 10^{11}}{(200 \times 10^3) \times (100 \times 10^6)} = 0.0083 \text{ rad}$$

b. *Deflection*

At C, $x = 1000$ mm

Eq. (vi) yields... $EIy_C = \dfrac{20000\langle 1000\rangle^3}{3} - 2.35 \times 10^{11}\langle 1000\rangle - 0 + 0 - 0 + 0 - 0$

$$y_C = \dfrac{-2.28 \times 10^{14}}{(200 \times 10^3) \times (100 \times 10^6)} = -11.42 \text{ mm}$$

At D, $x = 3000$ mm

Eq. (vi) yields... $EIy_D = \dfrac{20000\langle 3000\rangle^3}{3} - 2.35 \times 10^{11}\langle 3000\rangle - \dfrac{5\langle 3000 - 1000\rangle^4}{8}$

$$+ 0 - 0 + 0 - 0$$

$$y_D = \dfrac{-5.35 \times 10^{14}}{(200 \times 10^3) \times (100 \times 10^6)} = -26.75 \text{ mm}$$

At E, $x = 4000$ mm

Eq. (vi) yields... $EIy_E = \dfrac{20000\langle 4000\rangle^3}{3} - 2.35 \times 10^{11}\langle 4000\rangle - \dfrac{5\langle 4000 - 1000\rangle^4}{8}$

$$+ \dfrac{5\langle 4000 - 3000\rangle^4}{8} - 0 + 0 - 0$$

$$y_E = \dfrac{-5.63 \times 10^{14}}{(200 \times 10^3) \times (100 \times 10^6)} = -28.16 \text{ mm}$$

At F, $x = 10000$ mm

Eq. (vi) yields...

$$EIy_F = \frac{20000\langle 10000\rangle^3}{3} - 2.35\times 10^{11}\langle 10000\rangle - \frac{5\langle 10000-1000\rangle^4}{8}$$

$$+\frac{5\langle 10000-3000\rangle^4}{8} - \frac{20000\langle 10000-4000\rangle^3}{3}$$

$$+\frac{25000\langle 10000-8000\rangle^3}{3} - \frac{5\langle 10000-8000\rangle^4}{12}$$

$$y_F = \frac{3.367\times 10^{14}}{(200\times 10^3)\times(100\times 10^6)} = 16.83\text{ mm}$$

61. An overhanging beam is loaded as shown in Fig. 8.66(a). If $E = 200$ GPa, and $I = 100 \times 10^6$ mm^4, determine: (a) Slope at all points   (b) Deflection C, D & E

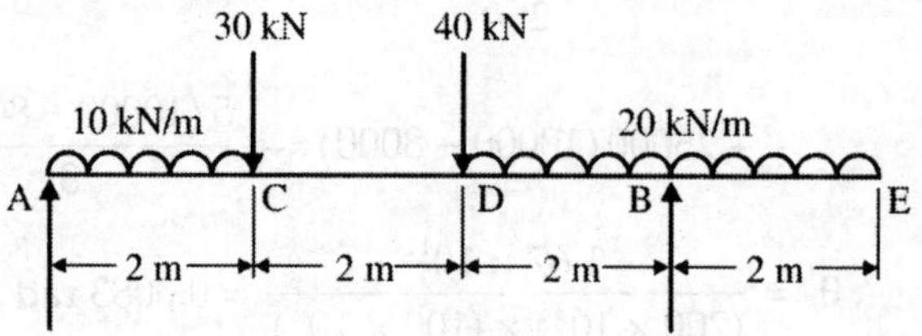

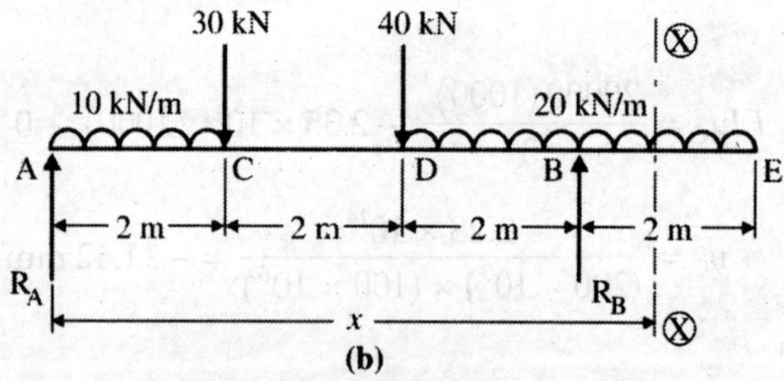

Fig. 8.66: Problem 61

Solution: $w_1 = 10$ kN/m $= 10$ N/mm, $w_2 = 20$ kN/m $= 20$ N/mm, $W_1 = 30\times 10^3$ N, $W_2 = 40\times 10^3$ N, $E = 200\times 10^3$ MPa, $I = 100\times 10^6$ mm^4. $a = 2000$ mm, $b = 4000$ mm, $c = 6000$ mm. a) $\theta_A, \theta_C, \theta_D, \theta_B, \theta_E = ?$, b) $y_C, y_D, y_E = ?$

Reactions at supports:

$$R_A + R_B = (10\times 2) + 30 + 40 + (20\times 4) = 170\text{ kN} \qquad \text{... Eq. (a)}$$

Taking moments about A and equating to zero, we have

$$R_B \times 6 = (20\times 4)\times\left(\frac{4}{2}+4\right) + (40\times 4) + (30\times 2) + (10\times 2)\times\left(\frac{2}{2}\right)$$

$$R_B = 120\text{ kN} \qquad \text{... Eq. (b)}$$

Substituting Eq. (b) in Eq. (a), we have

$$R_A + 120 = 70$$

$$R_A = 50\text{kN} \qquad \text{... Eq. (c)}$$

Consider a section X-X at a distance x from free end A and in the region BE as shown in **Fig. 8.66(b)**. Bending moment at X-X is

$$M_x = R_A\,\langle x\rangle - \frac{w_1\langle x\rangle^2}{2} + \frac{w_1\langle x-a\rangle^2}{2} - W_1\langle x-a\rangle$$

$$- W_2 \langle x - b \rangle - \frac{w_2 \langle x - b \rangle^2}{2} + R_B \langle x - c \rangle$$

i.e. $\qquad EI\dfrac{d^2y}{dx^2} = 50000 \langle x \rangle - \dfrac{10 \langle x \rangle^2}{2} + \dfrac{10 \langle x - 2000 \rangle^2}{2} - 30000 \langle x - 2000 \rangle$

$$- 40000 \langle x - 4000 \rangle - \frac{20 \langle x - 4000 \rangle^2}{2} + 120000 \langle x - 6000 \rangle$$

Integrating once we have

$$EI\frac{dy}{dx} = 25000 \langle x \rangle^2 + C_1 - \frac{5 \langle x \rangle^3}{3} + \frac{5 \langle x - 2000 \rangle^3}{3}$$

$$- 15000 \langle x - 2000 \rangle^2 - 20000 \langle x - 4000 \rangle^2$$

$$- \frac{10 \langle x - 4000 \rangle^3}{3} + 60000 \langle x - 6000 \rangle^2 \qquad \text{... Eq. (i)}$$

Integrating again we have

$$EIy = \frac{25000 \langle x \rangle^3}{3} + C_1 \langle x \rangle + C_2 - \frac{5 \langle x \rangle^4}{12} + \frac{5 \langle x - 2000 \rangle^4}{12}$$

$$- 5000 \langle x - 2000 \rangle^3 - \frac{20000 \langle x - 4000 \rangle^3}{3}$$

$$- \frac{5 \langle x - 4000 \rangle^4}{12} + 20000 \langle x - 6000 \rangle^3 \qquad \text{... Eq. (ii)}$$

Boundary conditions:
At $x = 0$, $y = 0$:

Eq. (ii) yields... $\qquad 0 = 0 + 0 + C_2 - 0 + 0 - 0 - 0 - 0 + 0$

$\qquad\qquad\qquad\qquad\qquad\qquad$ Ignore brackets containing negative value

$\qquad\qquad\qquad C_2 = 0 \qquad\qquad\qquad\qquad\qquad\qquad\qquad\qquad \text{... Eq. (iii)}$

At $x = 6000$ mm, $y = 0$:

Eq. (ii) yields... $\qquad 0 = \dfrac{25000 \langle 6000 \rangle^3}{3} + C_1 \langle 6000 \rangle - \dfrac{5 \langle 6000 \rangle^4}{12}$

$$+ \frac{5 \langle 6000 - 2000 \rangle^4}{12} - 5000 \langle 6000 - 2000 \rangle^3$$

$$- \frac{20000 \langle 6000 - 4000 \rangle^3}{3} - \frac{5 \langle 6000 - 4000 \rangle^4}{12} + 0$$

$$C_1 = -1.64 \times 10^{11} \qquad\qquad\qquad \text{... Eq. (iv)}$$

Substituting C_1 in Eq. (i) we get

$$EI\frac{dy}{dx} = 25000 \langle x \rangle^2 - 1.64 \times 10^{11} - \frac{5 \langle x \rangle^3}{3} + \frac{5 \langle x - 2000 \rangle^3}{3}$$

$$- 15000 \langle x - 2000 \rangle^2 - 20000 \langle x - 4000 \rangle^2$$

$$-\frac{10\langle x-4000\rangle^3}{3}+60000\langle x-6000\rangle^2 \qquad \dots \text{Eq. (v)}$$

Substituting C_1 and C_2 in Eq. (ii) we get

$$EIy=\frac{25000\langle x\rangle^3}{3}-1.64\times10^{11}\langle x\rangle-\frac{5\langle x\rangle^4}{12}+\frac{5\langle x-2000\rangle^4}{12}$$

$$-5000\langle x-2000\rangle^3-\frac{20000\langle x-4000\rangle^3}{3}$$

$$-\frac{5\langle x-4000\rangle^4}{6}+20000\langle x-6000\rangle^3 \qquad \dots \text{Eq. (vi)}$$

a. *Slope at all points*
   At A, $x=0$
   Eq. (v) yields... $\quad EI\theta_A=0-1.64\times10^{11}-0+0-0-0-0+0$

$$\theta_A=\frac{-1.64\times10^{11}}{(200\times10^3)\times(100\times10^6)}=-0.0082 \text{ rad}$$

At C, $x=2000$ mm

Eq. (v) yields... $\quad EI_C=25000\langle2000\rangle^2-1.64\times10^{11}-\frac{5\langle2000\rangle^3}{3}+0-0+0-0$

$$\theta_C=\frac{-7.73\times10^{10}}{(200\times10^3)\times(100\times10^6)}=-0.00386 \text{ rad}$$

At D, $x=4000$ mm

Eq. (v) yields... $\quad EI\theta_D=25000\langle4000\rangle^2-1.64\times10^{11}-\frac{5\langle4000\rangle^3}{3}$

$$+\frac{5\langle4000-2000\rangle^3}{3}-15000\langle4000-2000\rangle^2-0-0+0$$

$$\theta_D=\frac{8.27\times10^{10}}{(200\times10^3)\times(100\times10^6)}=0.00413 \text{ rad}$$

At B, $x=6000$ mm

Eq. (v) yields... $\quad EI\theta_B=25000\langle6000\rangle^2-1.64\times10^{11}-\frac{5\langle6000\rangle^3}{3}$

$$+\frac{5\langle6000-2000\rangle^3}{3}-15000\langle6000-2000\rangle^2$$

$$-20000\langle6000-4000\rangle^2-\frac{10\langle6000-4000\rangle^3}{3}$$

$$\theta_B=\frac{1.36\times10^{11}}{(200\times10^3)\times(100\times10^6)}=0.0068 \text{ rad}$$

At E, $x = 8000$ mm

Eq. (v) yields... $\quad EI\theta_E = 25000\langle 8000\rangle^2 - 1.64 \times 10^{11} - \dfrac{5\langle 8000\rangle^3}{3} + \dfrac{5\langle 8000-2000\rangle^3}{3}$

$$- 15000\langle 8000-2000\rangle^2 - 20000\langle 8000-4000\rangle^2$$

$$- \dfrac{10\langle 8000-4000\rangle^3}{3} + 60000\langle 8000-6000\rangle^2$$

$$\theta_E = \dfrac{1.043 \times 10^{12}}{(200 \times 10^3)\times(100 \times 10^6)} = 0.0521 \text{ rad}$$

b. *Deflection*

At C, $x = 2000$ mm

Eq. (vi) yields... $\quad EIy_C = \dfrac{25000\langle 2000\rangle^3}{3} - 1.64 \times 10^{11}\langle 2000\rangle - \dfrac{5\langle 2000\rangle^4}{12}$

$$+ 0 - 0 - 0 - 0 + 0$$

$$y_C = \dfrac{-2.68 \times 10^{14}}{(200 \times 10^3)\times(100 \times 10^6)} = -13.4 \text{ mm}$$

At D, $x = 4000$ mm

Eq. (vi) yields... $\quad EIy_D = \dfrac{25000\langle 4000\rangle^3}{3} - 1.64 \times 10^{11}\langle 4000\rangle - \dfrac{5\langle 4000\rangle^4}{12}$

$$+ \dfrac{5\langle 4000-2000\rangle^4}{12} - 5000\langle 4000-2000\rangle^3 - 0 - 0 + 0$$

$$y_D = \dfrac{-2.63 \times 10^{14}}{(200 \times 10^3)\times(100 \times 10^6)} = -13.13 \text{ mm}$$

At E, $x = 8000$ mm

Eq. (vi) yields... $\quad EIy_E = \dfrac{25000\langle 8000\rangle^3}{3} - 1.64 \times 10^{11}\langle 8000\rangle - \dfrac{5\langle 8000\rangle^4}{12}$

$$+ \dfrac{5\langle 8000-2000\rangle^4}{12} - 5000\langle 8000-2000\rangle^3$$

$$- \dfrac{20000\langle 8000-4000\rangle^3}{3} - \dfrac{5\langle 8000-4000\rangle^4}{6}$$

$$+ 20000\langle 8000-6000\rangle^3$$

$$y_E = \dfrac{-2.28 \times 10^{14}}{(200 \times 10^3)\times(100 \times 10^6)} = -11.4 \text{ mm}$$

62. Determine the deflection under the loads for an overhanging beam carrying loads as shown in Fig. 8.67(a). Take $E = 200$ GPa and $I = 45 \times 10^6$ mm^4.

VTU – Dec. 16/ Jan. 17 – 12 Marks

Solution: $W_1 = 30 \times 10^3$ N, $W_2 = 60 \times 10^3$ N, $E = 200 \times 10^3$ MPa, $I = 45 \times 10^6$ mm^4. $a = 2000$ mm, $b = 4000$ mm. $y_C, y_D = ?$

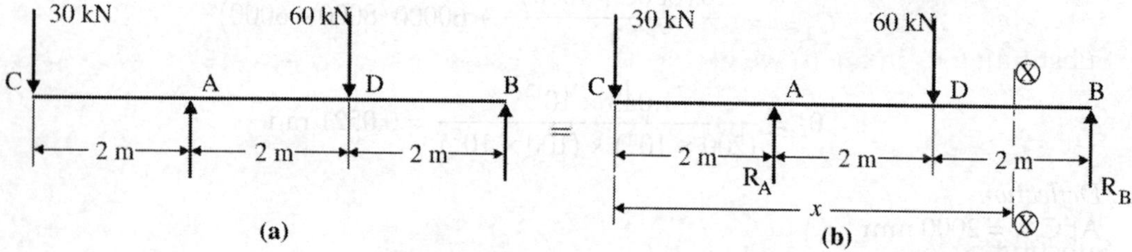

Fig. 8.67: Problem 62

Reactions at supports:
$$R_A + R_B = 30 + 60 = 90 \text{ kN} \qquad \text{... Eq. (a)}$$
Taking moments about A and equating to zero, we have
$$R_B \times 4 = (60 \times 2) - (30 \times 2)$$
$$R_B = 15 \text{ kN} \qquad \text{... Eq. (b)}$$
Substituting Eq. (b) in Eq. (a), we have
$$R_A + 15 = 90$$
$$R_A = 75 \text{ kN} \qquad \text{... Eq. (c)}$$
Consider a section X-X at a distance x from free end A and in the region DB as shown in **Fig. 8.67(b)**. Bending moment at X-X is

$$M_x = -W_1 \langle x \rangle + R_A \langle x - a \rangle - W_2 \langle x - b \rangle$$

i.e. $\qquad EI \dfrac{d^2 y}{dx^2} = -30000 \langle x \rangle + 75000 \langle x - 2000 \rangle - 60000 \langle x - 4000 \rangle$

Integrating once we have

$$EI \dfrac{dy}{dx} = -15000 \langle x \rangle^2 + C_1 + 37500 \langle x - 2000 \rangle^2 - 30000 \langle x - 4000 \rangle^2$$
$$\text{... Eq. (i)}$$

Integrating again we have

$$EIy = -5000 \langle x \rangle^3 + C_1 \langle x \rangle + C_2 + 12500 \langle x - 2000 \rangle^3$$
$$- 10000 \langle x - 4000 \rangle^3 \qquad \text{... Eq. (ii)}$$

Boundary conditions:
At $x = 2000$ mm, $y = 0$:

Eq. (ii) yields... $\qquad 0 = -5000 \langle 2000 \rangle^3 + C_1 \langle 2000 \rangle + C_2 + 0 - 0$

$$C_2 + C_1 \langle 2000 \rangle = 4 \times 10^{13} \qquad \text{... Eq. (iii)}$$

At $x = 6000$ mm, $y = 0$:

$$0 = -5000 \langle 6000 \rangle^3 + C_1 \langle 6000 \rangle + C_2 + 12500 \langle 6000 - 2000 \rangle^3$$
$$- 10000 \langle 6000 - 4000 \rangle^3$$

$$C_2 + C_1 \langle 6000 \rangle = 3.60 \times 10^{14} \qquad \text{... Eq. (iv)}$$

Eq. (iv) – Eq. (iii) yields...

$$C_1 \langle 4000 \rangle = 4.71 \times 10^{15}$$

$$C_1 = 8 \times 10^{10}$$

Eq. (iii) yields...
$$C_2 = 4 \times 10^{13} - 8 \times 10^{10} \langle 2000 \rangle$$

$$C_2 = -1.20 \times 10^{14}$$

Substituting C_1 in Eq. (i) we get

$$EI \frac{dy}{dx} = -15000 \langle x \rangle^2 + 8 \times 10^{10} + 37500 \langle x - 2000 \rangle^2$$

$$- 30000 \langle x - 4000 \rangle^2 \qquad \text{... Eq. (v)}$$

Substituting C_1 and C_2 in Eq. (ii) we get

$$EIy = -5000 \langle x \rangle^3 + 8 \times 10^{10} \langle x \rangle - 1.20 \times 10^{14} + 12500 \langle x - 2000 \rangle^3$$

$$- 10000 \langle x - 4000 \rangle^3 \qquad \text{... Eq. (vi)}$$

Deflection at load points

At C, $x = 0$ mm

Eq. (vi) yields...
$$EIy_C = 0 + 0 - 1.20 \times 10^{14} + 0 - 0$$

$$y_C = \frac{-1.20 \times 10^{14}}{(200 \times 10^3) \times (45 \times 10^6)} = -13.33 \text{ mm}$$

At D, $x = 4000$ mm

Eq. (vi) yields...
$$EIy_D = -5000 \langle 4000 \rangle^3 + 8 \times 10^{10} \langle 4000 \rangle - 1.20 \times 10^{14}$$

$$+ 12500 \langle 4000 - 2000 \rangle^3 - 0$$

$$y_D = \frac{-2 \times 10^{13}}{(200 \times 10^3) \times (45 \times 10^6)} = -2.22 \text{ mm}$$

63. An overhanging beam is loaded as shown in Fig. 8.68(a). If E = 200 GPa and I = 50 × 10⁶ mm⁴, determine: (a) Slope at all points   (b) Deflection C & D

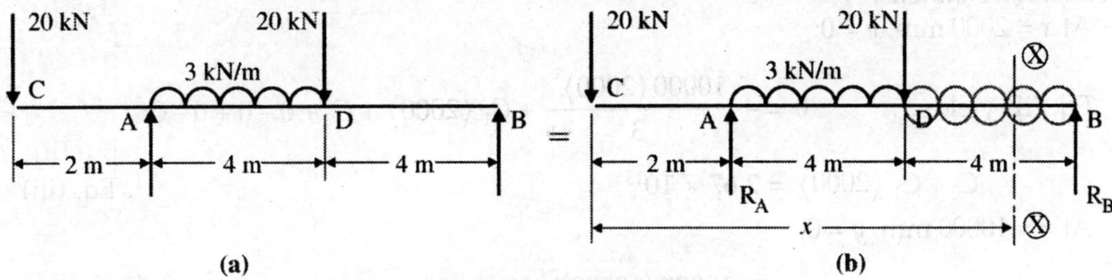

Fig. 8.68: Problem 63

Solution: $W_1 = 20 \times 10^3$ N, $W_2 = 20 \times 10^3$ N, $w = 3$ kN/m = 3 N/mm, $E = 200 \times 10^3$ MPa, $I = 50 \times 10^6$ mm⁴. $a = 2000$ mm, $b = 6000$ mm. a) θ_A, θ_C, θ_D, θ_B = ?   b) y_C, y_D = ?

Reactions at supports:

$$R_A + R_B = 20 + 20 + (3 \times 4) = 52 \text{ kN} \qquad \text{... Eq. (a)}$$

Taking moments about A and equating to zero, we have

$$R_B \times 8 = -(20 \times 2) + (20 \times 4) + (3 \times 4)\left(\frac{4}{2}\right)$$

$$R_B = 8 \text{ kN} \qquad\qquad \text{... Eq. (b)}$$

Substituting Eq. (b) in Eq. (a), we have

$$R_A + 8 = 52$$

$$R_A = 44 \text{ kN} \qquad\qquad \text{... Eq. (c)}$$

Consider a section X-X at a distance x from free end A and in the region DB as shown in **Fig. 8.68(b)**. Bending moment at X-X is

$$M_x = -W_1 \langle x \rangle + R_A \langle x - a \rangle - \frac{w \langle x - a \rangle^2}{2} + \frac{w \langle x - b \rangle^2}{2} - W_2 \langle x - b \rangle$$

i.e.

$$EI\frac{d^2y}{dx^2} = -20000\langle x \rangle + 44000\langle x - 2000 \rangle - \frac{3\langle x - 2000 \rangle^2}{2}$$

$$+ \frac{3\langle x - 6000 \rangle^2}{2} - 20000\langle x - 6000 \rangle$$

Integrating once we have

$$EI\frac{dy}{dx} = -10000\langle x \rangle^2 + C_1 + 22000\langle x - 2000 \rangle^2 - \frac{\langle x - 2000 \rangle^3}{2}$$

$$+ \frac{\langle x - 6000 \rangle^3}{2} - 10000\langle x - 6000 \rangle^2 \qquad \text{... Eq. (i)}$$

Integrating again we have

$$EIy = -\frac{10000\langle x \rangle^3}{3} + C_1\langle x \rangle + C_2 + \frac{22000\langle x - 2000 \rangle^3}{3}$$

$$- \frac{\langle x - 2000 \rangle^4}{8} + \frac{\langle x - 6000 \rangle^4}{8} - \frac{10000\langle x - 6000 \rangle^3}{3} \qquad \text{... Eq. (ii)}$$

Boundary conditions:

At $x = 2000$ mm, $y = 0$:

Eq. (ii) yields...

$$0 = -\frac{10000\langle 2000 \rangle^3}{3} + C_1\langle 2000 \rangle + C_2 + 0 - 0 + 0 - 0$$

$$C_2 + C_1\langle 2000 \rangle = 2.67 \times 10^{13} \qquad \text{... Eq. (iii)}$$

At $x = 10000$ mm, $y = 0$:

$$0 = -\frac{10000\langle 10000 \rangle^3}{3} + C_1\langle 10000 \rangle + C_2$$

$$+ \frac{22000\langle 10000 - 2000 \rangle^3}{3} - \frac{\langle 10000 - 2000 \rangle^4}{8}$$

$$+ \frac{\langle 10000 - 6000 \rangle^4}{8} - \frac{10000\langle 10000 - 6000 \rangle^3}{3}$$

$$C_2 + C_1 \langle 10000 \rangle = 2.72 \times 10^{14} \qquad \text{... Eq. (iv)}$$

Eq. (iv) – Eq. (iii) yields...

$$C_1 \langle 8000 \rangle = 4.71 \times 10^{15}$$

$$C_1 = 3.07 \times 10^{10}$$

Eq. (iii) yields... $\quad C_2 = 2.67 \times 10^{13} - 3.07 \times 10^{10} \langle 2000 \rangle$

$$C_2 = -3.47 \times 10^{13}$$

Substituting C_1 in Eq. (i) we get

$$EI \frac{dy}{dx} = -10000 \langle x \rangle^2 + 3.07 \times 10^{10} + 22000 \langle x - 2000 \rangle^2$$

$$- \frac{\langle x - 2000 \rangle^3}{2} + \frac{\langle x - 6000 \rangle^3}{2} - 10000 \langle x - 6000 \rangle^2 \text{... Eq. (v)}$$

Substituting C_1 and C_2 in Eq. (ii) we get

$$EIy = - \frac{10000 \langle x \rangle^3}{3} + 3.07 \times 10^{10} \langle x \rangle - 3.47 \times 10^{13}$$

$$+ \frac{22000 \langle x - 2000 \rangle^3}{3} - \frac{\langle x - 2000 \rangle^4}{8} + \frac{\langle x - 6000 \rangle^4}{8}$$

$$- \frac{10000 \langle x - 6000 \rangle^3}{3} \qquad \text{... Eq. (vi)}$$

a. *Slope at all points*

At C, $x = 0$

Eq. (v) yields... $\quad EI\theta_C = 0 + 3.07 \times 10^{10} + 0 - 0 + 0 - 0$

$$\theta_C = \frac{3.07 \times 10^{10}}{(200 \times 10^3) \times (50 \times 10^6)} = 0.0037 \text{ rad}$$

At A, $x = 2000$ mm

Eq. (v) yields... $\quad EI\theta_A = -10000 \langle 2000 \rangle^2 + 3.07 \times 10^{10} + 0 - 0 + 0 - 0$

$$\theta_A = \frac{-9.3 \times 10^9}{(200 \times 10^3) \times (50 \times 10^6)} = -0.00093 \text{ rad}$$

At D, $x = 6000$ mm

Eq. (v) yields... $\quad EI_D = -10000 \langle 6000 \rangle^2 + 3.07 \times 10^{10} + 22000 \langle 6000 - 2000 \rangle^2$

$$- \frac{\langle 6000 - 2000 \rangle^3}{2} + 0 - 0$$

$$\theta_D = \frac{-9.3 \times 10^9}{(200 \times 10^3) \times (50 \times 10^6)} = -0.00093 \text{ rad}$$

At B, $x = 10000$ mm

Eq. (v) yields... $EI\theta_B = -10000\langle10000\rangle^2 + 3.07 \times 10^{10} + 22000\langle10000 - 2000\rangle^2$

$$- \frac{\langle10000 - 2000\rangle^3}{2} + \frac{\langle10000 - 6000\rangle^3}{2}$$

$$- 10000\langle10000 - 6000\rangle^2$$

$$\theta_B = \frac{5.47 \times 10^{10}}{(200 \times 10^3) \times (50 \times 10^6)} = 0.00547 \text{ rad}$$

b. *Deflection*

At C, $x = 0$ mm

Eq. (vi) yields... $EIy_C = 0 + 0 - 3.47 \times 10^{13} + 0 - 0 + 0 - 0$

$$y_C = \frac{-3.47 \times 10^{13}}{(200 \times 10^3) \times (50 \times 10^6)} = -3.47 \text{ mm}$$

At D, $x = 6000$ mm

Eq. (vi) yields... $EIy_D = -\dfrac{10000\langle6000\rangle^3}{3} + 3.07 \times 10^{10}\langle6000\rangle - 3.47 \times 10^{13}$

$$+ \frac{22000\langle6000 - 2000\rangle^3}{3} - \frac{\langle6000 - 2000\rangle^4}{8} + 0 - 0$$

$$y_D = \frac{-1.33 \times 10^{14}}{(200 \times 10^3) \times (50 \times 10^6)} = -13.32 \text{ mm}$$

64. An overhanging beam is loaded as shown in Fig. 8.69(a). If $E = 200$ GPa and $I = 50 \times 10^6$ mm^4, determine: (a) Slope at all points (b) Deflection C & D

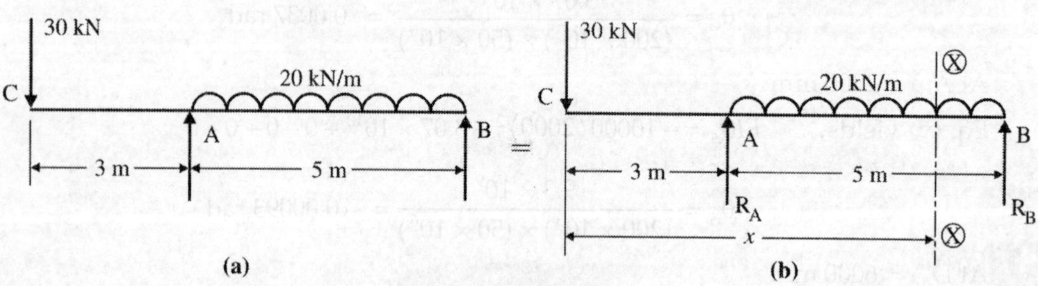

(a)   =   (b)

Fig. 8.69: Problem 64

Solution: $W = 30 \times 10^3$ N, $w = 20$ kN/m $= 20$ N/mm, $E = 200 \times 10^3$ MPa, $I = 50 \times 10^6$ mm^4. $a = 3000$ mm. a) $\theta_A, \theta_C, \theta_B = ?$ b) $y_C = ?$

Reactions at supports:

$$R_A + R_B = 30 + (20 \times 5) = 130 \text{ kN} \qquad \text{... Eq. (a)}$$

Taking moments about A and equating to zero, we have

$$R_B \times 5 = -(30 \times 3) + (20 \times 5) \times \left(\frac{5}{2}\right)$$

$$R_B = 32 \text{ kN} \qquad \text{... Eq. (b)}$$

Substituting Eq. (b) in Eq. (a), we have

$$R_A + 32 = 130$$
$$R_A = 98 \text{ kN} \qquad \qquad \text{... Eq. (c)}$$

Consider a section X-X at a distance x from free end A and in the region AB as shown in **Fig. 8.69(b)**. Bending moment at X-X is

$$M_x = -W\langle x \rangle + R_A \langle x - a \rangle - \frac{w\langle x - a \rangle^2}{2}$$

i.e.

$$EI\frac{d^2y}{dx^2} = -30000\langle x \rangle + 98000\langle x - 3000 \rangle - \frac{20\langle x - 3000 \rangle^2}{2}$$

Integrating once we have

$$EI\frac{dy}{dx} = -15000\langle x \rangle^2 + C_1 + 49000\langle x - 3000 \rangle^2 - \frac{10\langle x - 3000 \rangle^3}{3}$$

$$\text{... Eq. (i)}$$

Integrating again we have

$$EIy = -5000\langle x \rangle^3 + C_1\langle x \rangle + C_2 + \frac{49000\langle x - 3000 \rangle^3}{3}$$

$$- \frac{5\langle x - 3000 \rangle^4}{6} \qquad \qquad \text{... Eq. (ii)}$$

Boundary conditions:

At $x = 3000$ mm, $y = 0$:

Eq. (ii) yields...
$$0 = -5000\langle 3000 \rangle^3 + C_1\langle 3000 \rangle + C_2 + 0 - 0$$

$$C_2 + C_1\langle 3000 \rangle = 1.35 \times 10^{14} \qquad \qquad \text{... Eq. (iii)}$$

At $x = 8000$ mm, $y = 0$:

$$0 = -5000\langle 8000 \rangle^3 + C_1\langle 6000 \rangle + C_2 + \frac{49000\langle 8000 - 3000 \rangle^3}{3}$$

$$- \frac{5\langle 8000 - 3000 \rangle^4}{6}$$

$$C_2 + C_1\langle 8000 \rangle = 1.04 \times 10^{15} \qquad \qquad \text{... Eq. (iv)}$$

Eq. (iv) – Eq. (iii) yields...

$$C_1\langle 5000 \rangle = 9.05 \times 10^{14}$$
$$C_1 = 1.81 \times 10^{11}$$

Eq. (iii) yields...
$$C_2 = 1.35 \times 10^{14} - 1.81 \times 10^{11}\langle 3000 \rangle$$
$$C_2 = -4.08 \times 10^{14}$$

Substituting C_1 in Eq. (i) we get

$$EI\frac{dy}{dx} = -15000\langle x \rangle^2 + 1.81 \times 10^{11} + 49000\langle x - 3000 \rangle^2$$

$$- \frac{10\langle x - 3000 \rangle^3}{3} \qquad \qquad \text{... Eq. (v)}$$

Substituting C_1 and C_2 in Eq. (ii) we get

$$EIy = -5000\langle x\rangle^3 + 1.81 \times 10^{11}\langle x\rangle - 4.08 \times 10^{14}$$

$$+ \frac{49000\langle x - 3000\rangle^3}{3} - \frac{5\langle x - 3000\rangle^4}{6} \qquad \dots \text{Eq. (vi)}$$

a. *Slope at all points*

At C, $x = 0$

Eq. (v) yields… $\quad EI\theta_C = 0 + 1.81 \times 10^{11} + 0 - 0$

$$\theta_C = \frac{1.81 \times 10^{11}}{(200 \times 10^3) \times (50 \times 10^6)} = 0.0181 \text{ rad}$$

At A, $x = 3000$ mm

Eq. (v) yields… $\quad EI\theta_A = -15000\langle 3000\rangle^2 + 1.81 \times 10^{11} + 0 - 0$

$$\theta_A = \frac{4.6 \times 10^{11}}{(200 \times 10^3) \times (50 \times 10^6)} = 0.0046 \text{ rad}$$

At B, $x = 8000$ mm

Eq. (v) yields… $\quad EI\theta_B = -15000\langle 8000\rangle^2 + 1.81 \times 10^{11} + 49000\langle 8000 - 3000\rangle^2$

$$- \frac{10\langle 8000 - 3000\rangle^3}{3}$$

$$\theta_B = \frac{2.93 \times 10^{10}}{(200 \times 10^3) \times (50 \times 10^6)} = 0.00293 \text{ rad}$$

b. *Deflection*

At C, $x = 0$ mm

Eq. (vi) yields… $\quad EIy_C = 0 + 0 - 4.08 \times 10^{10} + 0 - 0$

$$y_C = \frac{-4.08 \times 10^{14}}{(200 \times 10^3) \times (50 \times 10^6)} = -40.8 \text{ mm}$$

VTU QUESTION PAPERS

Dec. 07/Jan. 08 (06ME34)

1. a. A beam of length 4 m is simply supported at the ends and carries two concentrated lads of 20 kN and 30 kN at a distance of 1.5 m and 2.5 m from the left end. Refer **Fig. U8.1**. Find the deflection at the mid span. Take $E = 200$ GPa and moment of inertia $I = 3 \times 10^8$ mm^4 of the cross section. **(10 Marks)**

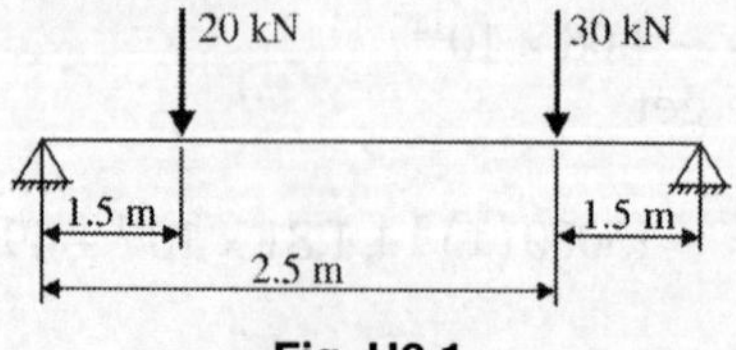

Fig. U8.1

b. Derive an expression relating slope, deflection and radius of curvature in a beam fro first principle in terms of E, I and M, with usual notations.

(07 Marks)

c. Explain how the deflection in beams can be reduced. **(03 Marks)**

June/July 2008 (06ME34)

2. a. For simply supported beam with uniformly distributed load over whole length show that the maximum deflection is equal to $\dfrac{-5wL^4}{384EI}$ **(05 Marks)**

b. A beam AB of span 6 m is simply supported at the ends and is loaded as shown in **Fig. U8.2**. Determine:
i. deflection at C   ii. maximum deflection an   iii. slope at the end A
Take $E = 2 \times 10^5\,\text{N/mm}^2$, $I = 2 \times 10^7\,\text{mm}^4$. **(15 Marks)**

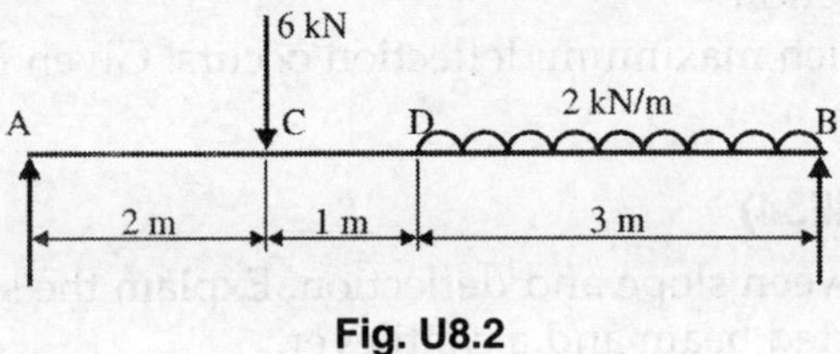

Fig. U8.2

Dec. 08/Jan. 09 (06ME34)

3. a. Derive the expression $E = \dfrac{d^2y}{dx^2} = M$, with usual notations. **(10 Marks)**

b. Determine the deflection under the loads in the beam shown in **Fig. U8.3**. Take flexural rigidity as EI throughout. **(10 Marks)**

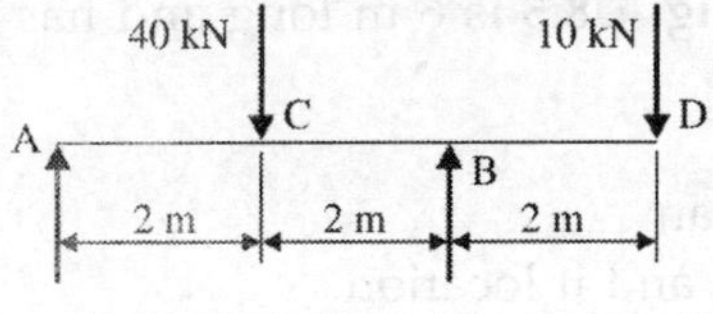

Fig. U8.3

June/July 2009 (06ME34)

4. a. Derive an expression with usual notations for the maximum deflection in a beam subjected to point load at mid span. **(08 Marks)**

b. A steel girder of length 6 m acting as a beam carries a udl w N/m run throughout its length as shown in **Fig. U8.4**. If $I = 30 \times 10^{-6}\,\text{mm}^4$ and depth 270 mm, calculate:
(i) Magnitude of w so that the maximum stress developed in the beam section does not exceed 72 MPa,
(ii) The slope and deflection in the beam at a distance of 1.8 m from one end. Take $E = 200\,\text{GPa}$. **(12 Marks)**

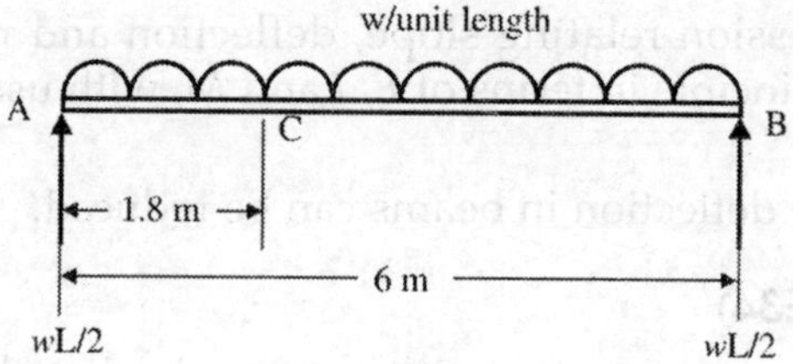

Fig. U8.4

Dec. 09/Jan. 10 (06ME34)

5. A beam of length 6 m is simply supported at its ends and carries two point loads of 40 kN at a distance of 1 m and 3 m respectively from the left support. By using Macaulay's method, determine:
   i. Deflection under each load
   ii. Maximum deflection
   iii. The point at which maximum deflection occurs. Given $E = 2 \times 10^5$ N/mm^2 and $I = 85 \times 10^6$ mm^4. **(20 Marks)**

May/June 2010 (06ME34)

6. a. Distinguish between slope and deflection. Explain the same with examples for a simply supported beam and a cantilever. **(06 Marks)**
   b. A beam AB of 6 m span is simply supported at the ends and is loaded with a point load of 6 kN at 2 m from the left support and uniformly distributed load of 2 kN/m for the second half of the beam. Find:
   i. Deflection at mid-span
   ii. Maximum deflection
   iii. Slope at left support. Take $E = 20$ GPa and $I = 2 \times 10^7$ mm^4. **(14 Marks)**

Dec. 2010 (06ME34)

7. A beam AB shown in **Fig. U8.5** is 6 m long and has flexural rigidity of $EI = 9 \times 10^{13}$ N-mm^2. Determine:
   i. Slope at A
   ii. Deflection at mid-span
   iii. maximum deflection and it location. **(20 Marks)**

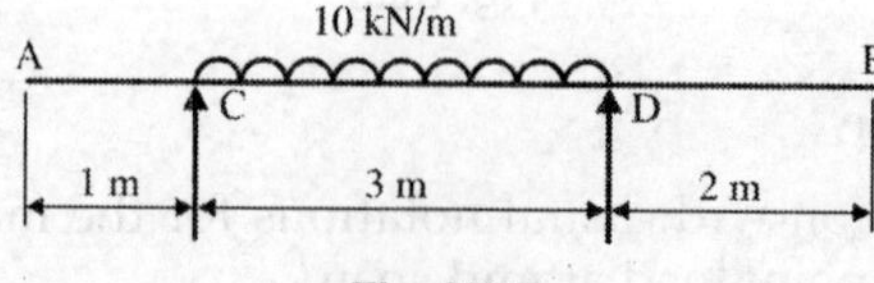

Fig. U8.5

June/July 2011 (06ME34)

8. a. Derive an expression with usual notations for the maximum deflection in a simply supported beam subjected to point load at mid span. **(08 Marks)**
   b. Find the maximum deflection and maximum slope for the beam loaded as shown in **Fig. U8.6**. Take flexural rigidity $EI = 15 \times 10^9$ kN-mm^2. **(12 Marks)**

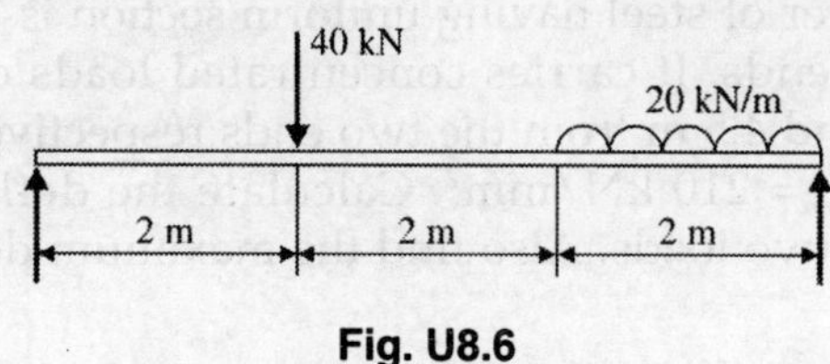

Fig. U8.6

Dec. 2011 (06ME34)

9. a. Derive an expression for the maximum deflection of a cantilever beam carrying a point load at its free end. **(08 Marks)**

b. Find the maximum deflection and the maximum slope for the beam loaded as shown in **Fig. U8.7**. Take flexural rigidity $EI = 15 \times 10^9$ kN-mm^2. **(12 Marks)**

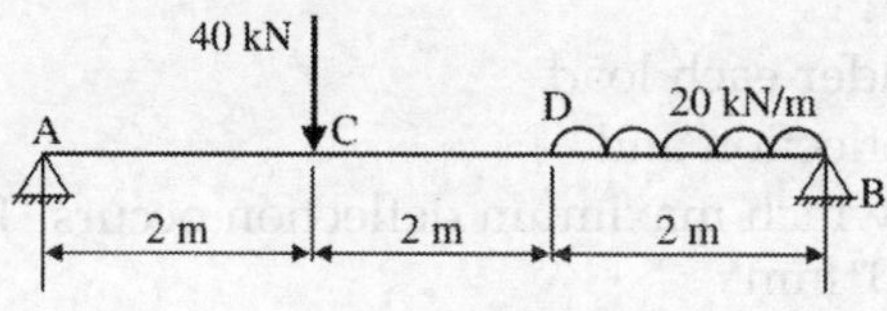

Fig. U8.7

Dec. 2011 (10ME34)

10. a. Using standard notations derive an expression for deflection, slope and maximum deflection of a simply supported beam of span L subjected to concentrated load W at its mid span. **(10 Marks)**

b. A simply supported beam of span 20 m carries two concentrated loads 4 kN at 8 m and 10 kN at 12 m from the left end support. Calculate:

i. The deflection under each load ii. The maximum deflection.

Take $E = 2 \times 10^5$ N/mm^2, and $I = 1 \times 10^9$ mm^4. **(10 Marks)**

June 2012 (06ME34)

11. a. Derive an expression $EI = \dfrac{d^2y}{dx^2} = M$, with usual notations. **(10 Marks)**

b. Determine the deflection under the loads in the beam as shown in **Fig. U8.8**. Take flexural rigidity as EI throughout. **(10 Marks)**

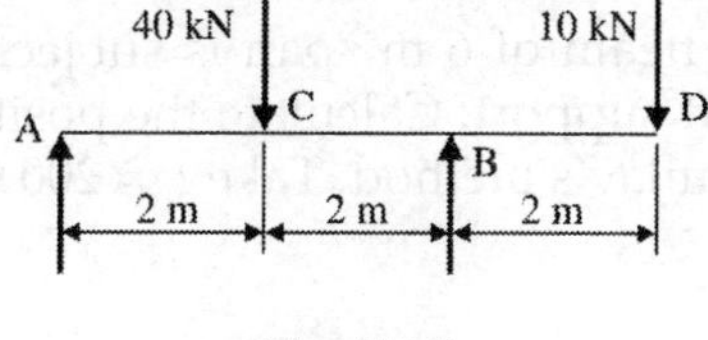

Fig. U8.8

June 2012 (10ME34)

12. a. Find the expressions for the slope and deflection of a cantilever beam of length L carrying uniformly distributed load over the whole length. **(08 Marks)**

b. A horizontal girder of steel having uniform section is 14 m long and is simply supported at its ends. It carries concentrated loads of 120 kN and 80 kN at two points 3 m and 4.5 m from the two ends respectively. $I = 16 \times 10^8$ mm^4 for the girder and $E_s = 210$ kN/mm^2. Calculate the deflections of the girder at points under the two loads. Also find the maximum deflection. **(12 Marks)**

Dec. 2012 (10ME34)

13. a. A cantilever of length 2.5 m carries a uniformly distributed load of 16.4 kN/m over the entire length. If the moment of inertia of the beam is 7.95×10^7 mm^4 and $E = 2 \times 10^5$ N/mm^2, determine the deflection at the free end. Derive the equation used. **(10 Marks)**

b. A beam of length 6 m is simply supported at its ends and caries two point loads of 48 kN and 40 kN at a distance of 1 m and 3 m respectively from the left support. Find:
   i. Deflection under each load
   ii. Maximum deflection and
   iii. The point at which maximum deflection occurs. Take $E = 2 \times 10^5$ N/mm^2, and $I = 85 \times 10^6$ mm^4 **(10 Marks)**

Jan. 2013 (06ME34)

14. a. Prove that the slope and deflection at the free end of a cantilever of length L, which carries a gradually varying load from zero at the free end to w/m run at the fixed end are given by

$$\theta = \frac{WL^3}{24EI} \quad \text{and} \quad y = \frac{WL^4}{30EI} \qquad \text{where } EI = \text{flexural rigidity} \qquad \textbf{(10 Marks)}$$

b. A horizontal girder of steel having uniform section is 14 m long and is simply supported at its ends. It carries concentrated loads of 120 kN and 80 kN at two points 3 m and 4.5 m from the two ends respectively. $I = 16 \times 10^8$ mm^4 for the girder and $E_s = 210$ kN/mm^2. Calculate the deflections of the girder at points under the two loads. Also find the maximum deflection. **(10 Marks)**

June/July 2013 (06ME34)

15. a. Derive an expression for maximum deflection of a simply supported beam by double integration method. The beam is subjected to uniformly distributed load of w/unit length, L being the length of the beam, E the Young's modulus and I moment of inertia of the cross section. **(10 Marks)**

b. A simply supported beam of 6 m span is subjected to concentrated load of 18 kN at 4 m from left support. Calculate the position and value of maximum deflection using Macaulay's method. Take $E = 200$ GPa & $I = 15 \times 10^6$ mm^4.

(10 Marks)

June/July 2013 (10ME34)

16. a. Show that for a simply supported beam of length l carrying a concentrated load W at its mid-span, the maximum deflection is Wl^3/48EI. **(10 Marks)**

b. A simply supported steel beam having uniform cross section is 14 m span and is simply supported at its ends. It carries concentrated loads of 120 kN and 80 kN at two points 3 m and 4.5 m from the left and right ends respectively.

If $I = 160 \times 10^7$ mm^4 and $E = 210$ GPa, calculate the deflection of the beam at load points. **(10 Marks)**

DEC. 13/JAN. 14 (06ME34)

17. a. Derive an expression $M = EI \dfrac{d^2y}{dx^2}$ with usual notations. **(05 Marks)**

b. A simply supported beam of 6m is subjected to a concentrated load of 18 kN at 4m from left hand support as shown in **Fig. U8.9**. Calculate the position and magnitude of maximum deflection if $E = 200$ GPa and $I = 30 \times 10^6$ mm^4. **(10 Marks)**

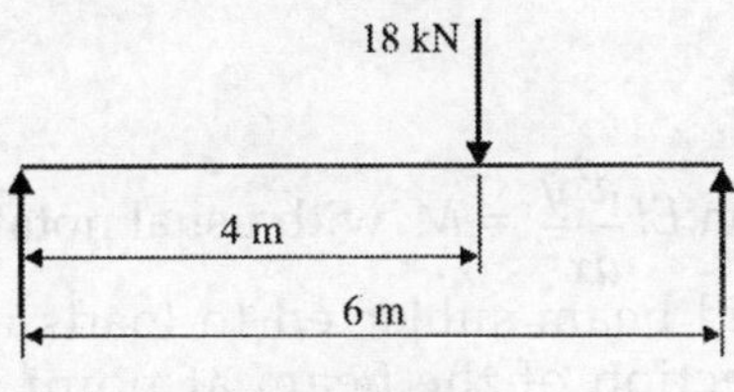

Fig. U8.9

Dec. 13/Jan. 14 (10ME34)

18. a. A cantilever 120 mm wide and 200 mm deep is 2.5 m long. What is the uniformly distributed load which the beam can carry in order to a deflection of 5 mm at the free end? Take $E = 200$ GPa. **(04 Marks)**

b. A horizontal beam AB is simply supported at A and B, 6m apart. The beam is subjected to a clockwise couple of 300 kN-m at a distance of 4m from the left end as shown in **Fig. U8.10**. If $E = 2.1 \times 10^5$ N/mm^2 and $I = 2 \times 10^8$ mm^4, determine: i) the deflection at the point where the couple is acting ii) the maximum deflection. **(16 Marks)**

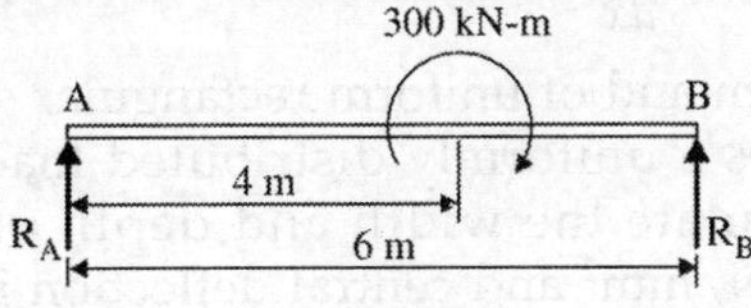

Fig. U8.10

June/July 2014 (06ME34)

19. a. Prove that the slope and deflection of a simply supported beam of length L and carrying a uniformly distributed load of W per unit length over the entire span is given as

Slope at supports $= \dfrac{WL^2}{24EI}$ and deflection at center $= \dfrac{5WL^3}{384EI}$ **(10 Marks)**

b. A beam of length 5 m and of uniform rectangular cross section is simply supported at its ends. It carries a uniformly distributed load of 9 kN/m run over the entire length. Calculate the width and depth of the beam if permissible bending stress is 7 N/mm^2 and central deflection is not to exceed 1 cm. **(10 Marks)**

June/July 2014 (10ME34)

20. a. Derive the deflection equation for the beam in standard form $EI\dfrac{d^2y}{dx^2} = M(x)$

   (06 Marks)

   b. For the beam loaded as shown in **Fig. U8.11**, find the position and magnitude of maximum deflection. Take $I = 4.3 \times 10^8$ and $E = 200$ kN/mm^2.   **(14 Marks)**

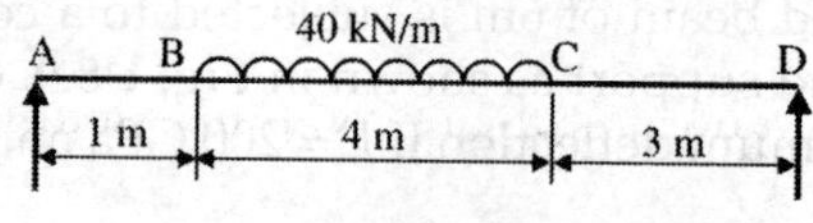

Fig. U8.11

Dec. 14/Jan. 15 (06ME34)

21. a. Derive the expression $EI\dfrac{d^2y}{dx^2} = M$, with usual notations.   **(10 Marks)**

   b. A simply supported beam subjected to loads is as shown in **Fig. U8.12**. Calculate the deflection of the beam at point of application of load by Macaulay's method. Take $E = 200$ GPa, $I = 200 \times 10^6$ mm^4.   **(10 Marks)**

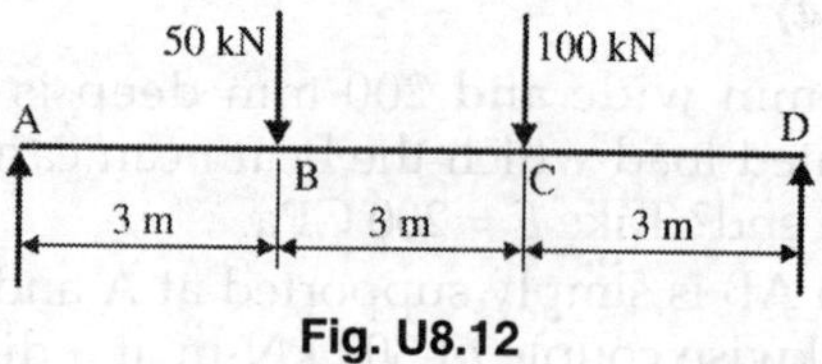

Fig. U8.12

Dec. 14/Jan. 15 (10ME34)

22. a. Derive an expression $EI\dfrac{d^2y}{dx^2} = M$ with usual notations.   **(10 Marks)**

   b. A beam of length 5 m and of uniform rectangular section is simply supported at its ends. It carries a uniformly distributed load of 9 kN/m run over the entire length. Calculate the width and depth of the beam if permissible bending stress is 7 N/mm^2 and central deflection is not to exceed 1 cm. Take $E = 1 \times 10^4$ N/mm^2.   **(10 Marks)**

June/July 15 (10ME34)

23. a. Derive the expression $EI\dfrac{d^2y}{dx^2} = M$, with usual notations.   **(10 Marks)**

   b. Determine he deflections at points C, D and E in the beam shown in **Fig. U8.13**. Take $E = 200$ kN/mm^2 and $I = 60 \times 10^6$ mm^4.   **(10 Marks)**

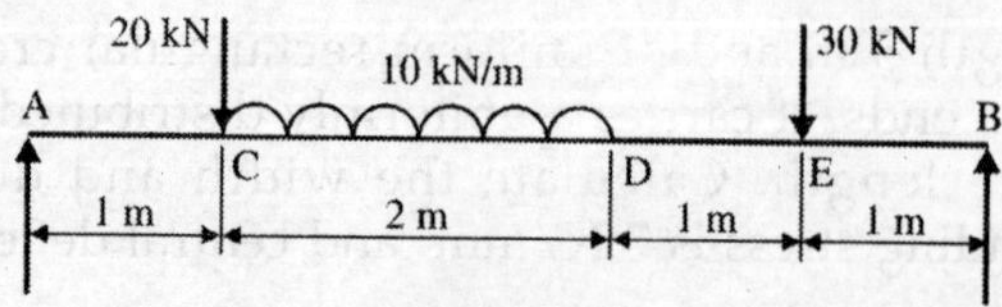

Fig. U8.13

Dec. 15/Jan. 16 (10ME/AU34)

24. a. Derive an expression $EI\dfrac{d^2y}{dx^2} = M$, with usual notations. **(10 Marks)**

   b. Determine the deflection under the loads in the beam shown in **Fig. U8.14**. Take flexural rigidity as EI, throughout. **(10 Marks)**

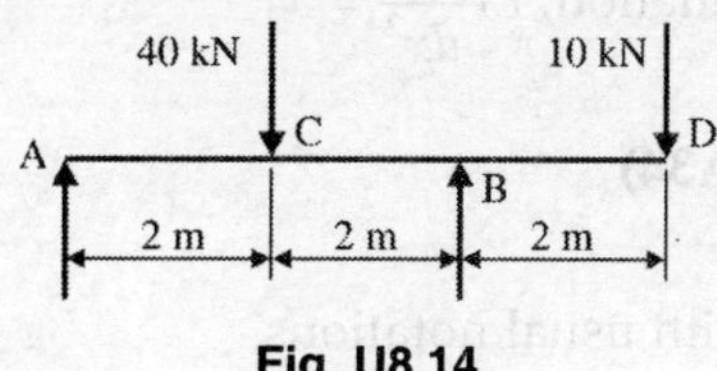

Fig. U8.14

June/July 2016 (10ME/AU34)

25. a. Find the expression for the slope and deflection of a cantilever of length L carrying a udl over the whole length. **(10 Marks)**

   b. A beam of length 6 m is simply supported at its ends and carries two point loads of 48 kN and 40 kN at a distance of 1m and 3 m respectively from the left support. Find:
   - i. Deflection under each load
   - ii. Maximum deflection and
   - iii. Point at which maximum deflection occurs. Take $E = 2 \times 10^5$ MPa and $I = 85 \times 10^6$ mm^4. **(10 Marks)**

Dec. 16/Jan. 17 (10ME/AU34)

26. a. Derive deflection equation for a simply supported beam subjected to uniformly distributed load. **(10 Marks)**

   b. Determine the deflection at points C, D and E for the beam shown in **Fig. U8.15**. Take $E = 200$ kN/mm^2 and $I = 60 \times 10^6$ mm^4. **(10 Marks)**

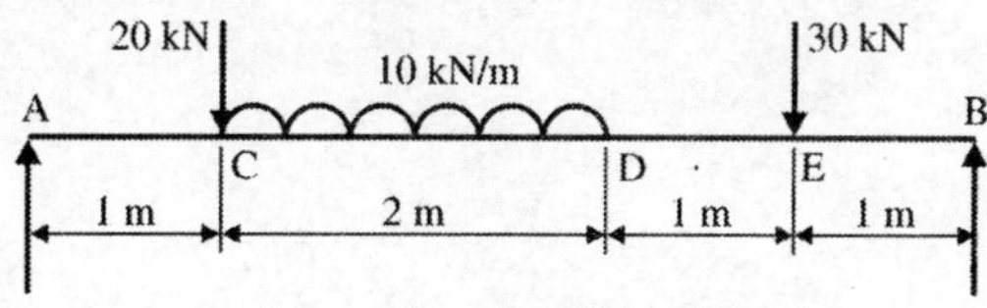

Fig. U8.15

Dec. 16/Jan. 17 (15ME/MA34)

27. Using Double Integration method, determine the slope and deflection for a cantilever beam subjected to concentrated load at free end.

(08 Marks)

June/July 2017 (15ME/MA34)

28. a. Derive an equation for deflection. **(10 Marks)**

   b. What is Macaulay's method? Where is it used? **(04 Marks)**

   c. A 2 m long cantilever is subjected to a UDL of 10 kN/m throughout its length and has a vertically downward point load of 20 kN at its free end. Taking

E = 200 GPa and minimum deflection as 0.3 mm, determine the width and depth of the rectangular section. Depth of the section is twice the width.

(06 Marks)

Dec. 17/Jan. 18 (10ME/AU34)

29. Derive the deflection equation, $EI\dfrac{d^2y}{dx^2} = M$

(08 Marks)

Dec. 17/Jan. 18 (15ME/MA34)

30. a. Derive $EI\dfrac{d^2y}{dx^2} = M$, with usual notations.

(08 Marks)

b. A cantilever of length 3 m and cross section 150 mm width and 300 mm depth is loaded as shown in **Fig. U8.16**. Take E = 210 GPa. Calculate the maximum slope and maximum deflection.

(12 Marks)

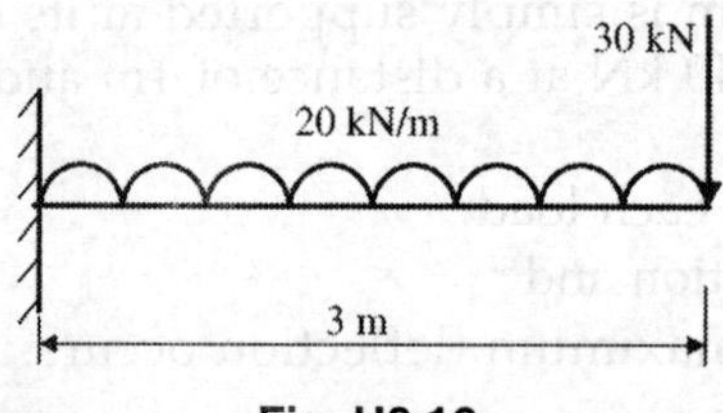

Fig. U8.16

9

Torsion of Circular Shafts

Chapter Outline

9.1 INTRODUCTION

The term shaft usually refers to a relatively long member of circular cross-section that rotates and transmits power. Various members such as gears, bearings, pulleys, sprockets, cams, flywheels, cranks, etc. are mounted on the shaft for power transmission. These members are secured to the shaft by means pins, keys, splines, snap rings and other devices.

However, a shaft can have a noncircular cross section and need not be rotating, such as axles and spindles.

- *Axle* is a non-rotating member used for supporting rotating wheels, pulleys, etc. and do not transmit any torque.
- *Spindle* is simply defined as a short shaft. Examples: Lathe spindles, drill press spindle, etc.

9.2 TYPES OF SHAFTS

Shafts are divided into two main groups:
- *Transmission shafts:* Shafts used to transmit power between the source and the machines absorbing power are called transmission shafts. These shafts carry machine parts or members such as pulleys, gears etc., and therefore are subjected to bending in addition to twisting.
  Examples: Counter shafts, line shafts, over head shafts and all factory shafts.
- *Machine shafts:* These shafts form an integral part of the machine itself.
  Examples: Crank shaft

9.3 ASSUMPTIONS IN THEORY OF PURE TORSION

- The material of the shaft is uniform throughout.
- The twist along the shaft is uniform.
- The shaft is circular in section remains circular after loading.
- The plane section of the shaft normal to its axis before loading remains plane after the torque is applied.
- The distance between any two normal cross-sections remains the same after the application of torque.
- The maximum shear stress induced in the shaft due to application of torque does not exceed its elastic limit value.

9.4 DERIVATION OF TORSIONAL EQUATION

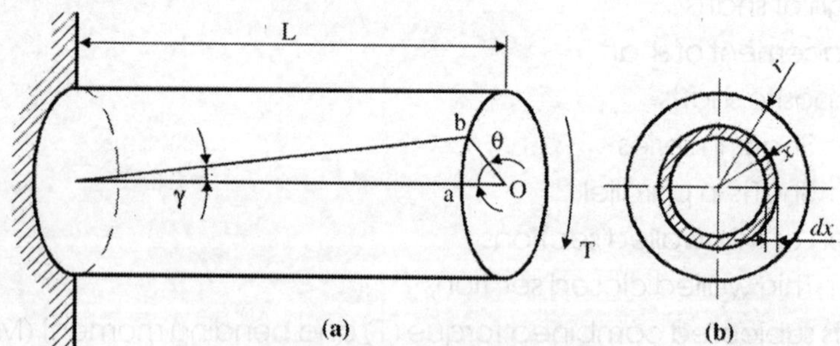

Fig. 9.1: Shaft subjected to torque

Let, r = Radius of the shaft
   τ = Shear stress
   T = Torque
   J = Polar moment of inertia
   G = Modulus of rigidity
   θ = Angle of twist
   L = Length of the shaft
   γ = shear strain

Consider a shaft fixed at one end and subjected to torque at the other end as shown in **Fig. 9.1(a)**. If oa is the initial position before twist, then the final position after twist is ob, i.e. the cross-section will be twisted through an angle θ and the surface by an angle γ. This is then the angle of distortion (shear strain) of the shaft.

From **Fig. 9.1(a)**, $arc\,ab = r\theta = L\gamma$

$$\gamma = \frac{r\theta}{L} \qquad\qquad \text{... Eq. (i)}$$

But Modulus of rigidity, $\qquad G = \dfrac{\tau}{\gamma}$

$$\therefore \qquad \gamma = \dfrac{\tau}{G} \qquad\qquad \dots \text{Eq. (ii)}$$

From Eqs (i) and (ii), we have

$$\dfrac{r\theta}{L} = \dfrac{\tau}{G}$$

$$\therefore \qquad \dfrac{\tau}{r} = \dfrac{G\theta}{L} = \left(\dfrac{\tau_x}{x}\right) \qquad\qquad \dots \text{(Eq. 9.1)}$$

Where τ_x is the shear stress at any radius x.

Consider an elementary ring of thickness dx at a radius x as shown in **Fig. 9.1(b)**. Let τ' be the shear stress developed in the element.

Turning force on the ring $= \tau_x.A = \tau_x\,(2\pi x.dx)$

Turning moment of the ring, $\ dT = \text{force} \times \text{distance} = \tau_x\,(2\pi x.dx).x$

$$dT = 2\pi\tau_x\, x^2.dx$$

Thus the total torque may be obtained by integrating the above equation.

i.e. $\qquad\qquad \displaystyle\int dT = \int_{0}^{r} 2\pi\tau_x x^2 \cdot dx \qquad\qquad \dots \text{(Eq. 9.2)}$

but $\qquad\qquad\qquad \tau_x = \dfrac{\tau x}{r} \qquad\qquad\qquad \dots \text{using (Eq. 9.1)}$

$$\int dT = \int_{0}^{r}\left(\dfrac{\tau x}{r}\right) 2\pi x^2 \cdot dx = \left(\dfrac{2\pi\tau}{r}\right) = \int_{0}^{r} x^3 \cdot dx$$

$$T = \left(\dfrac{2\pi\tau}{r}\right)\left[\dfrac{x^4}{4}\right]_{0}^{r}$$

$$= \left(\dfrac{2\pi\tau}{4r}\right) r^4 = \left(\dfrac{\pi\tau}{2}\right) r^3$$

$$= \left(\dfrac{\pi\tau}{2}\right)\left(\dfrac{d}{2}\right)^3 \qquad\qquad (\because\ r = d/2)$$

$$\therefore \qquad T = \left(\dfrac{\pi d^3}{16}\right)\tau, \text{ is known as strength of a solid shaft} \qquad \dots \text{(Eq. 9.3)}$$

But for a circular cross-section, polar second moment of inertia

$$J = \dfrac{\pi d^4}{32}$$

i.e. $\qquad\qquad\qquad \dfrac{2J}{d} = \dfrac{\pi d^3}{16} \qquad\qquad\qquad \dots \text{(Eq. 9.4)}$

Substituting (Eq. 9.4) in (Eq. 9.3), we have

$$T = \left(\dfrac{2J}{d}\right)\tau = \left(\dfrac{2J}{2r}\right)\tau$$

$$\therefore \qquad \frac{T}{J} = \frac{\tau}{r} \qquad \qquad \text{... (Eq. 9.5)}$$

Combining Eqns. (9.1) and (9.5), we have

$$\frac{\tau}{r} = \frac{G\theta}{L} = \frac{T}{J}$$

Or

$$\frac{T}{J} = \frac{G\theta}{L} = \frac{\tau}{r} \qquad \qquad \text{... (Eq. 9.6)}$$

(Eq. 9.6) is called the **torsional equation** for a solid circular shaft

Note:
- The term $J/r = Z_p$ is known as *torsional or polar section modulus.*
- The term GJ is known as *torsional rigidity* or *stiffness of the shaft.*

9.5 EFFECTS OF TORSION

The effects of a torsional load applied to a bar or shaft are:
- To impart an angular displacement of one end cross section with respect to the other end.
- To setup shear stresses on any cross section of the bar perpendicular to its axis.

9.6 SOME DEFINITIONS

- *Line shaft:* refers to a shaft which transmits power to several machines by means of belts.
- *Counter shaft:* A shaft that connects a prime mover to a line shaft of a machine is referred to as counter shaft.
- *Flexible shaft:* A flexible shaft transmits motion between two points (say motor and machine), where the rotational axes are at an angle with respect to one another.
- *Torsional moment of resistance or torque or twisting moment(T):* The twisting moment for any section along the bar or shaft is defined as the algebraic sum of moments of the applied couples that lie to one side of the section under consideration.

For a solid shaft,
$$T = \left(\frac{\pi d^3}{16}\right)\tau \qquad \text{... strength of a solid shaft ... (Eq. 9.7)}$$

For a hollow shaft,
$$T = \left[\frac{\pi}{16}\left(\frac{d_o^4 - d_i^4}{d_o}\right)\right]\tau = \frac{\pi}{16}d_o^3\left(1 - K^4\right)\tau$$

$$\text{... strength of a hollow shaft ... (Eq. 9.8)}$$

Where
$$d = \text{Diameter of solid shaft}$$
$$d_o = \text{Outer diameter of hollow shaft}$$
$$d_i = \text{Inner diameter of hollow shaft}$$

$$K = \frac{d_i}{d_o} = \text{Ratio of inner diameter to outer diameter}$$

$$\text{of hollow shaft}$$

- *Angle of Twist (θ):* If a shaft of length L is subjected to a constant twisting moment T along its length, then the angle θ through which one end of the shaft will twist relative to the other is known is the angle of twist.

$$\theta = \frac{TL}{GJ} \text{ radians per unit length} \qquad \text{... (Eq. 9.9)}$$

In the above equation G and J are constants for a given shaft, therefore the angle of twist is directly proportional to the twisting moment.

Note: The standard and widely used relation is that the deflection should not exceed $1°$ in a length equal to twenty times the diameter of the shaft ($L = 20d$).

- *Torsional rigidity or stiffness of shaft:* It is defined as the torque produced per unit twist of the shaft for a unit length.

We know that, $$\frac{T}{J} = \frac{G\theta}{L}$$

$$GJ = \frac{TL}{\theta} \qquad \text{... (Eq. 9.10)}$$

The term GJ is called as **torsional rigidity or torsional stiffness** of the shaft. Since GJ is a constant for a given shaft, a graph between torque T and the angle of twist per unit length will be a straight line.

A shaft is said to be *torsionally rigid*, if it does not twist too much under the action of external torque.

Examples: Cam shaft, machine tool spindles, etc.

A shaft is said to be *laterally rigid*, if it does not deflect too much under the action of external forces and bending moment.

- *Polar moment of inertia (J):* The Moment of inertia (MI) of a plane about an axis perpendicular to the plane of the area is called polar moment of inertia of the area with respect to the point at which the axis intersects the plane.

For a solid shaft, $$J = \frac{\pi d^4}{32} \qquad \text{... (Eq. 9.11)}$$

For a hollow shaft, $$J = \frac{\pi}{32}\left(d_o^4 - d_i^4\right) = \frac{\pi}{32} d_o^4(1 - K^4) \qquad \text{... (Eq. 9.12)}$$

- *Polar section modulus (Z_p):* It is defined as the ratio of polar moment of inertia to the extreme distance of the fibre from the center.

i.e. $$Z_P = J/r$$

For a solid shaft, polar modulus $$Z_P = \frac{\pi d^4/32}{d/2} = \frac{\pi d^3}{16} \qquad \text{... (Eq. 9.13)}$$

For a hollow shaft, polar modulus $$Z_P = \frac{\pi d_o^4(1 - K^4)/32}{d_o/2} = \frac{\pi}{16} d_o^3(1 - K^4)$$

$$\text{... (Eq. 9.14)}$$

- *Power transmitted (P):* The power transmitted by a shaft is given as

$$P = \frac{2\pi NT}{60} \quad (Watts) \qquad \text{... (Eq. 9.15)}$$

BASIC PROBLEMS ON SOLID SHAFT

1. What must be the length of a 5 mm diameter wire so that it can be twisted through one complete revolution without exceeding a shear stress of 42 N/mm^2. Take $G = 27$ GN/m^2.

VTU – (CV) Dec. 13/ Jan. 14 – 04 Marks

Solution: $L = ?, d = 5$ mm, $\theta = 360° = 2\pi$ rads, $\tau = 42$ N/mm^2, $G = 27 \times 10^3$ N/mm^2

We know that
$$\frac{T}{J} = \frac{G\theta}{L} = \frac{\pi}{r}$$

$$L = \frac{G\theta r}{\tau} = \frac{(27 \times 10^3) \times 2\pi(5/2)}{42} = 10098 \text{ mm} \ \Box \ 10.10 \text{ m}$$

2. Determine the diameter of a solid steel shaft which will transmit 90 kW at 160 rpm. Also determine the length of the shaft if the twist must not exceed 1° over the entire length. The maximum shear stress is limited to 60 N/mm^2. Take the value of rigidity as 8×10^4 N/mm^2.

VTU – Dec. 2012 – 10 Marks

Solution: $d = ?, L = ?, P = 90$ kW $= 90 \times 10^3$ W, $N = 160$ rpm, $\theta = 1° = 0.0175$ rad, $\tau = 60$ N/mm^2, $G = 8 \times 10^4$ N/mm^2

Torque transmitted:

We know that
$$P = \frac{2\pi NT}{60}$$

$$90 \times 10^3 = \frac{2\pi \times 160 \times T}{60}$$

$$T = 5371.48 \text{ N-m} = 5371.48 \times 10^3 \text{ N-mm}$$

Diameter of shaft:

Strength of a solid shaft,
$$T = \left(\frac{\pi d^3}{16}\right)\tau$$

$$5371.48 \times 10^3 = \left(\frac{\pi d^3}{16}\right) \times 60$$

$$d = 76.97 \text{ mm} \approx 78 \text{ mm}$$

Length of the shaft:

We know that
$$\frac{T}{J} = \frac{G\theta}{L} = \frac{\tau}{r}$$

$$L = \frac{G\theta J}{T}$$

Here
$$T = \left(\frac{\pi d^3}{16}\right)\tau = \left(\frac{\pi \times 78^3}{16}\right) \times 60 = 5.59 \times 10^6 \text{ N-mm}$$

$$J = \left(\frac{\pi d^4}{32}\right) = \left(\frac{\pi \times 78^4}{32}\right) = 3.63 \times 10^6 \text{ mm}^4$$

$$\therefore \quad L = \frac{(8 \times 10^4) \times 0.0175 \times 3.63 \times 10^6}{5.59 \times 10^6} = 909.12 \text{ mm} \approx 0.910 \text{ m}$$

Or $$L = \frac{G\theta r}{\tau} = \frac{(8 \times 10^4) \times 0.0175 \times (78/2)}{60} = 910 \text{ mm} = 0.910 \text{ m}$$

3. **A solid steel shaft transmits 100 kW at 150 rpm. Determine suitable diameter of the shaft, if the shear stress in the shaft is not to exceed 60 MPa. Also find the maximum angle of twist, of the shaft length is 4 m. Take modulus of rigidity as 80 GPa.**

VTU – June/ July 2013 – 10 Marks

Solution: $P = 100 \text{ kW} = 100 \times 10^3 \text{ W}$, $N = 150 \text{ rpm}$, $d = ?$, $\tau = 60 \text{ MPa}$, $\theta = ?$, $L = 4000 \text{ mm}$, $G = 80 \times 10^3 \text{ MPa}$

Torque transmitted:

We know that $$P = \frac{2\pi NT}{60}$$

$$100 \times 10^3 = \frac{2\pi \times 150 \times T}{60}$$

$$T = 6366.20 \text{ N-m} = 6366.20 \times 10^3 \text{ N-mm}$$

Diameter of shaft:

Strength of a solid shaft, $$T = \left(\frac{\pi d^3}{16}\right)\tau$$

$$6366.20 \times 10^3 = \left(\frac{\pi d^3}{16}\right) \times 60$$

$$d = 81.45 \text{ mm} \approx 82 \text{ mm}$$

Angle of twist:

We know that $$\frac{T}{J} = \frac{G\theta}{L} = \frac{\tau}{r}$$

$$\theta = \frac{TL}{GJ}$$

Here $$T = \left(\frac{\pi d^3}{16}\right)\tau = \left(\frac{\pi \times 82^3}{16}\right) \times 60 = 6.50 \times 10^6 \text{ N-mm}$$

$$J = \left(\frac{\pi d^4}{32}\right) = \left(\frac{\pi \times 82^4}{32}\right) = 4.44 \times 10^6 \text{ mm}^4$$

$$\therefore \quad \theta = \frac{(6.50 \times 10^6) \times 4000}{(80 \times 10^3) \times (4.44 \times 10^6)} = 0.073 \text{ rad.} = 4.19°$$

Or $\qquad \theta = \dfrac{L\tau}{Gr} = \dfrac{4000 \times 60}{(80 \times 10^3) \times (82/2)} = 0.073 \text{ rad} = 4.19°$

4. Find the diameter of the shaft required to transmit 60 kW at 150 rpm if the maximum torque is 25% more than the mean torque for a maximum shear stress of 60 MPa. Find also the angle of twist in a length of 4 m. Take $G = 80$ GPa.

VTU – June/ July 2014 – 10 Marks; Dec. 07/ Jan. 08 – 10 Marks

Solution: $d = ?$, $P = 60$ kW $= 60 \times 10^3$ W, $N = 150$ rpm, $T_{max} = 1.25 \, T$, $\tau = 60$ MPa, $\theta = ?$, $L = 4000$ mm, $G = 80 \times 10^3$ MPa

Torque transmitted:

Given $\qquad\qquad\qquad T_{max} = 1.25 \, T \qquad\qquad\qquad\qquad …$ Eq. (i)

But $\qquad\qquad\qquad P = \dfrac{2\pi N T}{60}$

$$60 \times 10^3 = \dfrac{2\pi \times 150 \times T}{60}$$

$$T = 3819.72 \text{ N-m} = 3819.72 \times 10^3 \text{ N-mm}$$

Eq. (i) yields… $\qquad T_{max} = 1.25 \times (3819.72 \times 10^3) = 4774.65 \times 10^3 \text{ N-mm}$

Diameter of shaft:

Strength of a solid shaft, $T_{max} = \left(\dfrac{\pi d^3}{16}\right)\tau$

$$4774.65 \times 10^3 = \left(\dfrac{\pi d^3}{16}\right) \times 60$$

$$d = 74 \text{ mm}$$

Angle of twist:

We know that $\qquad\qquad \dfrac{T_{max}}{J} = \dfrac{G\theta}{L} = \dfrac{\tau}{r}$

$$\theta = \dfrac{T_{max} L}{GJ}$$

Here $\qquad T_{max} = \left(\dfrac{\pi d^3}{16}\right)\tau = \left(\dfrac{\pi \times 74^3}{16}\right) \times 60 = 4.77 \times 10^6 \text{ N-mm}$

$$J = \left(\dfrac{\pi d^4}{32}\right) = \left(\dfrac{\pi \times 74^4}{32}\right) = 2.94 \times 10^6 \text{ mm}^4$$

$\therefore \quad \theta = \dfrac{(4.77 \times 10^6) \times 4000}{(80 \times 10^3) \times (2.94 \times 10^6)} = 0.081 \text{ rad} = 4.65°$

Or $\qquad \theta = \dfrac{L\tau}{Gr} = \dfrac{4000 \times 60}{(80 \times 10^3) \times (74/2)} = 0.081 \text{ rad} = 4.65°$

5. **A solid shaft of 60 mm diameter runs at 160 rpm. Find the power that can be transmitted if permissible shear stress is 80 N/mm^2 and the maximum torque is likely to exceed 30% over the average torque. Also find the angle of twist in degrees for a length of 8000 mm. Take $G = 80$ GPa.**

VTU – (CV) Dec. 09/ Jan. 10 – 08 Marks

Solution: $d = 60$ mm, $N = 160$ rpm, $P = ?$, $\tau = 80$ N/mm^2, $T_{max} = 1.30$ T, $\theta = ?$, $L = 8000$ mm, $G = 80 \times 10^3$ MPa

$$\text{Given} \qquad T_{max} = 1.30 \ T \qquad\qquad \text{... Eq. (i)}$$

$$\text{But} \qquad T = \left(\frac{\pi d^3}{16}\right)\tau = \left(\frac{\pi \times 60^3}{16}\right) \times 80 = 3.40 \times 10^6 \text{ N-mm}$$

$$\text{Eq. (i) yields...} \qquad T_{max} = 1.30 \times (3.40 \times 10^6)$$
$$T_{max} = 4.42 \times 10^6 \text{ N-mm} = 4.42 \times 10^3 \text{ N-m}$$

$$\text{Power transmitted} \qquad P = \frac{2\pi N T_{max}}{60} = \frac{2\pi \times 160 \times (4.42 \times 10^3)}{60} = 74.05 \times 10^3 \text{ W}$$
$$P = 74.05 \text{ kW}$$

6. **A 150 mm diameter solid steel shaft is transmitting 450 kW power at 90 rpm. Compute the maximum shearing stress. Find the change that would occur in the shearing stress, if the speed was increased to 360 rpm.**

VTU – (CV) June/ July 2014 –10 Marks

Solution: $d = 150$ mm, $P = 450 \times 10^3$ W, $N = 90$ rpm. $\tau = ?$, $\tau_1 = ?$, if $N_1 = 360$ rpm

$$\text{We know that} \qquad P = \frac{2\pi N T}{60} \qquad\qquad \text{... Eq. (i)}$$

$$450 \times 10^3 = \frac{2\pi \times 90 \times T}{60}$$

$$T = 47746.48 \text{ N-m} = 47746.48 \times 10^3 \text{ N-mm}$$

$$\text{Strength of a solid shaft, } T_{max} = \left(\frac{\pi d^3}{16}\right)\tau \qquad\qquad \text{... Eq. (ii)}$$

$$47746.48 \times 10^3 = \left(\frac{\pi \times 150^3}{16}\right) \times \tau$$

$$\tau = 72.05 \text{ MPa}$$

$$\text{For } N_1 = 360 \text{ rpm, Eq. (i) yields... } 450 \times 10^3 = \frac{(2\pi \times 360 \times T_1)}{60}$$

$$T_1 = 11936.62 \text{ N-m}$$
$$T_1 = 11936.62 \times 10^3 \text{ N-mm}$$

$$\text{Eq. (ii) yields...} \qquad T_1 = \left(\frac{\pi d^3}{16}\right)\tau_1$$

$$11936.62 \times 10^3 = \frac{(\pi \times 150^3)}{16} \times \tau_1$$

$$\tau_1 = 18.01 \text{ MPa}$$

Change in shear stress $= \tau - \tau_1 = 72.05 - 18.01 = 54.04$ MPa

BASIC PROBLEMS ON HOLLOW SHAFT

7. **A shaft transmits 300 kW power at 120 rpm. Determine:**
   (a) The necessary diameter of the solid circular shaft.
   (b) The necessary outer diameter of the hollow circular section such that inner diameter being 2/3 of the outer diameter. Take allowable shear stress as 70 MPa.

VTU – (CV) June/ July 2013 – 10 Marks

Solution: $P = 300 \times 10^3$ W, $N = 120$ rpm, $\tau = 70$ MPa. a) $d = ?$. b) $d_o = ?$, if $d_i = (2/3)d_o$
$\Rightarrow K = 2/3 = d_i/d_o$

Torque transmitted:

We know that
$$P = \frac{2\pi NT}{60} \qquad \text{... Eq. (i)}$$

$$300 \times 10^3 = \frac{2\pi \times 120 \times T}{60}$$

$$T = 23873.24 \text{ N-m} = 23873.24 \times 10^3 \text{ N-mm}$$

a. *Diameter of solid shaft:*

Strength of a solid shaft, $\quad T = \left(\frac{\pi d^3}{16}\right)\tau$

$$23873.24 \times 10^3 = \left(\frac{\pi d^3}{16}\right) \times 70$$

$$d = 120.21 \text{ mm} \approx 122 \text{ mm}$$

b. *Diameter of hollow shaft:*

Strength of a hollow shaft, $\quad T = \left[\frac{\pi}{16}\left(\frac{d_o^4 - d_i^4}{d_o}\right)\right]\tau = \frac{\pi}{16}d_o^3(1 - K^4)\tau$

$$23873.24 \times 10^3 = \left(\frac{\pi}{16}\right)d_o^3 \times \left[(1 - (2/3)^4)\right] \times 70$$

$$d_o = 129.36 \text{ mm} \approx 130 \text{ mm}$$

and $\qquad d_i = \left(\frac{2}{3}\right) \times 130 = 86.67$ mm

8. **A hollow circular steel shaft has to transmit 60 kW at 210 rpm such that the shear stress does not exceed 60 MPa. If the ratio of internal to external diameter is 3/4 and the value of rigidity modulus is 84 GPa, find the dimensions of the shaft and angle of twist in a length of 3 m.**

VTU – Dec. 15/ Jan. 16 – 08 Marks; June/ July 2013 – 10 Marks

Solution: $P = 60 \times 10^3$ W, $N = 210$ rpm, $\tau = 60$ MPa, $K = \dfrac{d_i}{d_o} = \dfrac{3}{4}$, $G = 84 \times 10^3$ MPa,

$L = 3000$ mm. a) $d_o, d_i = ?$, b) $\theta = ?$

Torque transmitted:

We know that
$$P = \frac{2\pi N T}{60} \qquad \text{... Eq. (i)}$$

$$60 \times 10^3 = \frac{2\pi \times 210 \times T}{60}$$

$$T = 2728.37 \text{ N-m} = 2728.37 \times 10^3 \text{ N-mm}$$

a. *Diameter of solid shaft:*

Strength of a hollow shaft, $\quad T = \dfrac{\pi}{10} d_o^3 (1 - K^4)\tau$

$$2728.37 \times 10^3 = \left(\frac{\pi}{16}\right) d_o^3 \times \left[(1 - (3/4)^4)\right] \times 60$$

$$d_o = 69.71 \text{ mm} \approx 70 \text{ mm}$$

and
$$d_i = \left(\frac{3}{4}\right) \times 70 = 52.5 \text{ mm}$$

b. *Angle of twist:*

We know that
$$\frac{T}{J} = \frac{G\theta}{L} = \frac{\tau}{r}$$

$$\theta = \frac{TL}{GJ}$$

Here
$$J = \frac{\pi}{32} d_o^4 (1 - K^4) = \frac{\pi}{32} \times 70^4 \times [1 - (3/4)^4]$$

$$= 1.62 \times 10^6 \text{ mm}^4$$

$$\therefore \quad \theta = \frac{(2728.37 \times 10^3) \times 3000}{(84 \times 10^3) \times (1.62 \times 10^6)} = 0.0601 \text{ rad} = 3.45°$$

9. A hollow circular shaft is to transmit 300 kW power at 80 rpm. If the shear stress is not to exceed 60 N/mm² and the internal diameter is 0.6 times the outer diameter, find the external and internal diameters assuming that the maximum torque is 1.4 times the mean.

VTU – (CV) June/ July 2013 – 10 Marks

Solution: $P = 300 \times 10^3$ W, $N = 80$ rpm, $\tau = 60$ MPa, $K = 0.6 = \dfrac{d_i}{d_o}$, $T_{max} = 1.4$ T. $d_o, d_i = ?$

Torque transmitted:

Given $\qquad\qquad T_{max} = 1.40\ T \qquad\qquad\qquad$ ... Eq. (i)

But $\qquad\qquad P = \dfrac{2\pi NT}{60}$

$$300 \times 10^3 = \frac{2\pi \times 80 \times T}{60}$$

$$T = 35809.86\ \text{N-m} = 35809.86 \times 10^3\ \text{N-mm}$$

Eq. (i) yields... $\qquad T_{max} = 1.4 \times (35809.86 \times 10^3) = 50133.81 \times 10^3\ \text{N-mm}$

Diameter of hollow shaft:

Strength of a hollow shaft, $\quad T = \dfrac{\pi}{16} d_o^3 (1 - K^4)\tau$

$$50133.81 \times 10^3 = \left(\frac{\pi}{16}\right) d_o^3 \times \left[(1 - 0.6^4)\right] \times 60$$

$$d_o = 169.72\ \text{mm} \approx 170\ \text{mm}$$

and $\qquad\qquad\qquad d_i = 0.6 \times 170 = 102\ \text{mm}$

10. A hollow shaft of external diameter 120 mm transmits 300 kW power at 200 rpm. Determine the maximum internal diameter, if the maximum stress is not to exceed 60 N/mm².

VTU – (CV) June 2012 – 10 Marks

Solution: $d_o = 120$ mm, $P = 300 \times 10^3$ W, $N = 200$ rpm, $d_i = ?$, $\tau = 60$ MPa.

Torque transmitted:

We know that $\qquad\qquad P = \dfrac{2\pi NT}{60}$

$$300 \times 10^3 = \frac{2\pi \times 200 \times T}{60}$$

$$T = 14323.94\ \text{N-m} = 14323.94 \times 10^3\ \text{N-mm}$$

Diameter of hollow shaft:

Strength of a hollow shaft, $\quad T = \dfrac{\pi}{16} d_o^3 (1 - K^4)\tau$

$$14323.94 \times 10^3 = \left(\frac{\pi}{16}\right) \times 120^3 \times (1 - K^4) \times 60$$

$$1 - K^4 = 0.7036$$
$$K^4 = 0.2964$$

i.e. $\qquad\qquad\qquad \dfrac{d_i}{d_o} = 0.7378$

$$d_i = 120 \times 0.7378 = 88.54\ \text{mm}$$

11. A hollow shaft of internal diameter 400 mm and external diameter 460 mm is required to transmit power at 180 rpm. Determine the power it can transmit if the shear stress is not to exceed 60 MPa and the maximum torque exceeds the mean by 30%.

VTU – (CV) June/ July 2016 – 06 Marks

Solution: $d_i = 400$ mm, $d_o = 460$ mm, $N = 180$ rpm, $P = ?$, $\tau = 60$ MPa. $T_{max} = 1.30\,T$

Power transmitted:

Given
$$T_{max} = 1.30\,T \qquad \text{... Eq. (i)}$$

But
$$T = \frac{\pi}{16} d_o^3 (1 - K^4)\tau$$

Also
$$K = \frac{d_i}{d_o} = \frac{400}{460} = 0.870$$

$$\therefore \quad T = \left(\frac{\pi \times 460^3}{16}\right) \times 60[(1 - (0.870)^4)]$$

$$T = 490 \times 10^6 \text{ N-mm}$$

Eq. (i) yields...
$$T_{max} = 1.30 \times (490 \times 10^6) = 637 \times 10^6 \text{ N-mm}$$
$$= 637 \times 10^3 \text{ N-m}$$

Power transmitted
$$P = \frac{2\pi N T_{max}}{60} = \frac{2\pi \times 180 \times (637 \times 10^3)}{60} = 12.007 \times 10^6 \text{W}$$

$$P = 12.007 \times 10^3 \text{ kW}$$

9.7 DESIGN OF SHAFTS

In designing a shaft, two approaches are used given as follows:

1. *Based on strength or shear stress:*

Strength of a solid shaft, $\quad T = \left(\frac{\pi d^3}{16}\right)\tau$

Strength of a hollow shaft, $\quad T = \frac{\pi}{16} d_o^3 (1 - K^4)\tau \qquad \text{... Eq. (a)}$

2. *Based on rigidity or stiffness:*

We know that
$$\frac{T}{J} = \frac{G\theta}{L} = \frac{\tau}{r}$$

$$\theta = \frac{TL}{GJ} \qquad \text{... Eq. (b)}$$

Where
$$J = \frac{\pi d^4}{32}, \text{ for a solid shaft,}$$

$$J = \frac{\pi}{32} d_o^4 (1 - K^4), \text{ for a hollow shaft,}$$

and
$$K = \frac{d_i}{d_o}$$

Based on Eqs (a) and (b), select:
- Maximum value of diameter for design
- Minimum value of torque for design

DESIGN PROBLEMS ON SOLID SHAFT

12. Compute the maximum permissible torque to which the solid circular shaft, 3m long and 100 mm in diameter can be subjected when specification require that shearing stress must not exceed 50 N/mm^2 and twist must not exceed 3.5° in this length. Take $G = 7 \times 10^4$ N/mm^2

VTU – (CV) Dec. 10 – 10 Marks

Solution: T = ?, L = 3000 mm, d = 100 mm, τ = 50 N/mm^2, θ = 3.5° = 0.0611 rad, $G = 7 \times 10^4$ MPa

i. *Based on strength:*

Strength of a solid shaft, $\quad T = \left(\dfrac{\pi d^3}{16}\right)\tau = \left(\dfrac{\pi \times 100^3}{16}\right) \times 50 = 9.82 \times 10^6$ N-mm

$$\text{... Eq. (a)}$$

ii. *Based on rigidity or stiffness:*

We know that $\quad T = \dfrac{G\theta J}{L}$

But $\quad\quad J = \dfrac{\pi d^4}{32} = \dfrac{\pi \times 100^4}{32} = 9.82 \times 10^6$ mm^4

$$T = \frac{(7 \times 10^4) \times 0.0611 \times 9.82 \times 10^6}{3000} = 14 \times 10^6 \text{ N-mm}$$

$$\text{... Eq. (b)}$$

Based on Eqs (a) and (b), select minimum value of torque for design
i.e. $\quad\quad\quad T = 9.82 \times 10^6$ N-mm

13. Determine the diameter of a solid shaft which will transmit 440 kW at 280 rpm. The angle of twist must not exceed one degree per meter length and the maximum torsional stress is to be limited to 40 N/mm^2. Assume $G = 84$ kN/mm^2.

VTU – June/ July 2016 – 10 Marks; Dec. 2011 – 08 Marks;
[Similar: (CV) Dec. 13/ Jan. 14 – 12 Marks]

Solution: d = ?, $P = 440 \times 10^3$ W, N = 280 rpm, θ = 1° = 0.0175 rad, L = 1000 mm, τ = 40 N/mm^2, $G = 84 \times 10^3$ N/mm^2
Torque transmitted:

We know that $\quad\quad\quad P = \dfrac{2\pi NT}{60}$

$$400 \times 10^3 = \frac{2\pi \times 280 \times T}{60}$$

$$T = 15 \times 10^3 \text{ N-m} = 15 \times 10^6 \text{ N-mm}$$

Diameter of shaft:

i. Based on strength: $\quad\quad T = \left(\dfrac{\pi d^3}{16}\right)\tau$

$$15 \times 10^6 = \left(\frac{\pi d^3}{16}\right) \times 40$$

$$d = 124.07 \text{ mm} \qquad \qquad \ldots \text{ Eq. (a)}$$

ii. Based on rigidity: $\quad J = \dfrac{TL}{G\theta} = \dfrac{(15 \times 10^6) \times 1000}{(84 \times 10^3) \times 0.0175} = 10.20 \times 10^6 \text{ mm}^4$

But $\qquad \qquad \qquad J = \dfrac{\pi d^4}{32}$

$$10.20 \times 10^6 = \dfrac{\pi d^4}{32}$$

$$d = 100.96 \text{ mm} \qquad \qquad \ldots \text{ Eq. (b)}$$

Based on Eqs (a) and (b), select maximum value of diameter for design

i.e. $\qquad \qquad \qquad d = 124.07 \text{ mm} \approx 124 \text{ mm}$

14. A solid shaft has to transmit 120 kW of power at 160 rpm. If the shear stress is not to exceed 60 MPa and the twist in a length of 3 m must not exceed 1°, find the suitable diameter of the shaft. Take G = 80 GPa.

VTU – (CV) Dec.07/ Jan.08 – 10 Marks; [Similar: (CV) Dec. 2011 – 08 Marks]

Solution: $P = 120 \times 10^3$ W, $N = 160$ rpm, $\tau = 60$ MPa, $\theta = 1° = 0.0175$ rad, $L = 3000$ mm, $G = 80 \times 10^3$ MPa, $d = ?$

Torque transmitted:

We know that $\qquad \qquad P = \dfrac{2\pi NT}{60}$

$$120 \times 10^3 = \dfrac{2\pi \times 160 \times T}{60}$$

$$T = 7162 \text{ N-m} = 7162 \times 10^3 \text{ N-mm}$$

Diameter of shaft:

i. *Based on strength:* $\qquad T = \left(\dfrac{\pi d^3}{16}\right)\tau$

$$7162 \times 10^3 = \left(\dfrac{\pi d^3}{16}\right) \times 60$$

$$d = 84.71 \text{ mm} \qquad \qquad \ldots \text{ Eq. (a)}$$

ii. *Based on rigidity:* $\quad J = \dfrac{TL}{G\theta} = \dfrac{(7162 \times 10^3) \times 3000}{(80 \times 10^3) \times 0.0175} = 15.35 \times 10^6 \text{ mm}^4$

But $\qquad \qquad \qquad J = \dfrac{\pi d^4}{32}$

$$15.35 \times 10^6 = \dfrac{\pi d^4}{32}$$

$$d = 111.82 \text{ mm} \qquad \qquad \ldots \text{ Eq. (b)}$$

Based on Eqs (a) and (b), select maximum value of diameter for design

i.e. $\qquad \qquad \qquad d = 111.82 \text{ mm} \approx 112 \text{ mm}$

15. Determine a suitable diameter for a solid circular shaft to transmit 112.5 kW of power at 200 rpm. The allowable shear stress is 75 N/mm^2 and the allowable twist is 1° in a length of 3 m. Take modulus of rigidity as 82 × 10^3 N/mm^2.

VTU – (CV) Dec.08/ Jan.09 – 12 Marks

Solution: d = ?, P = 112.5 × 10^3 W, N = 200 rpm, τ = 75 N/mm^2, θ = 1° = 0.0175 rad, L = 3000 mm, G = 82 × 10^3 N/mm^2

Torque transmitted:

We know that
$$P = \frac{2\pi NT}{60}$$

$$112.5 \times 10^3 = \frac{2\pi \times 200 \times T}{60}$$

$$T = 5371.48 \text{ N-m} = 5371.48 \times 10^3 \text{ N-mm}$$

Diameter of shaft:

i. *Based on strength:*
$$T = \left(\frac{\pi d^3}{16}\right)\tau$$

$$5371.48 \times 10^3 = \left(\frac{\pi d^3}{16}\right) \times 75$$

$$d = 71.45 \text{ mm} \qquad \qquad \text{... Eq. (a)}$$

ii. *Based on rigidity:*
$$J = \frac{TL}{G\theta} = \frac{(5371.48 \times 10^3) \times 3000}{(82 \times 10^3) \times 0.0175} = 11.23 \times 10^6 \text{ mm}^4$$

But
$$J = \frac{\pi d^4}{32}$$

$$11.23 \times 10^6 = \frac{\pi d^4}{32}$$

$$d = 103.42 \text{ mm} \qquad \qquad \text{... Eq. (b)}$$

Based on Eqs (a) and (b), select maximum value of diameter for design
i.e. $\quad\quad d$ = 103.42 mm ≈ 104 mm

16. A solid shaft rotating at 500 rpm transmits 30 kW. Maximum torque is 20% more than the mean torque. Allowable shear stress is 65 MPa and modulus of rigidity is 81 GPa, angle of twist in the shaft should not exceed 1° in a length of 1m. Determine suitable diameter.

VTU – June 2012 – 12 Marks; Dec. 08/ Jan. 09 – 10 Marks

Solution: N = 500 rpm, P = 30 × 10^3 W, T_{max} = 1.2 T, τ = 65 MPa, G = 81 × 10^3 MPa, θ = 1° = 0.0175 rad, L = 1000 mm, d = ?

Torque transmitted:

Given
$$T_{max} = 1.2\, T \qquad\qquad \text{... Eq. (i)}$$

But
$$P = \frac{2\pi NT}{60}$$

$$30 \times 10^3 = \frac{2\pi \times 500 \times T}{60}$$

$$T = 572.96 \text{ N-m} = 572.96 \times 10^3 \text{ N-mm}$$

Eq. (i) yields ... $T_{max} = 1.2 \times (572.96 \times 10^3) = 687.55 \times 10^3 \text{ N-mm}$

Diameter of shaft:

i. *Based on strength:* $T_{max} = \left(\frac{\pi d^3}{16}\right)\tau$

$$687.55 \times 10^3 = \left(\frac{\pi d^3}{16}\right) \times 65$$

$$d = 37.76 \text{ mm} \qquad\qquad \text{... Eq. (a)}$$

ii. *Based on rigidity:* $J = \dfrac{T_{max}L}{G\theta} = \dfrac{(687.55 \times 10^3) \times 1000}{(81 \times 10^3) \times 0.0175} = 485.05 \times 10^3 \text{ mm}^4$

But $$J = \frac{\pi d^4}{32}$$

$$485.05 \times 10^3 = \frac{\pi d^4}{32}$$

$$d = 47.15 \text{ mm} \qquad\qquad \text{... Eq. (b)}$$

Based on Eqs (a) and (b), select maximum value of diameter for design
i.e. $d = 47.15 \text{ mm} \approx 48 \text{ mm}$

17. **A mild steel shaft has to transmit 75 kW at 200 rev/min. The allowable stress in the shaft material is limited to 40 MPa and the angle of twist is not to exceed 1° in a length of 20 diameters. Calculate the suitable diameter of the shaft. Take $G = 78.5 \times 10^3$ MPa**

Solution: $P = 75 \times 10^3$ W, $N = 200$ rpm, $\tau = 40$ MPa, $\theta = 1° = 0.0175$ rad, $L = 20d$, $d = ?$, $G = 78.5 \times 10^3$ MPa.

Torque transmitted:

We know that $$P = \frac{2\pi NT}{60}$$

$$75 \times 10^3 = \frac{2\pi \times 200 \times T}{60}$$

$$T = 3580.98 \text{ N-m} = 3580.98 \times 10^3 \text{ N-mm}$$

Diameter of shaft:

i. *Based on strength:* $T = \left(\frac{\pi d^3}{16}\right)\tau$

$$3580.98 \times 10^3 = \left(\frac{\pi d^3}{16}\right) \times 40$$

$$d = 76.97 \text{ mm} \qquad\qquad \text{... Eq. (a)}$$

ii. *Based on rigidity:* $\quad J = \dfrac{TL}{G\theta} = \dfrac{(3580.98 \times 10^3) \times (20d)}{(78.5 \times 10^3) \times 0.0175} = (52.13 \times 10^3)d$

But $\qquad\qquad\qquad\qquad J = \dfrac{\pi d^4}{32}$

$$(52.13 \times 10^3)d = \dfrac{\pi d^4}{32}$$

$$d = 80.98 \text{ mm} \qquad\qquad \text{... Eq. (b)}$$

Based on Eqs (a) and (b), select maximum value of diameter for design
i.e. $\qquad\qquad\qquad d = 80.98 \text{ mm} \approx 81 \text{ mm}$

**18. A solid shaft is subjected to a torque of 40 kN-m. If the angle of twist is 0.6°
per meter length of shaft and the shear stress is not to exceed 80 MPa, find:**
(a) Suitable diameter of the shaft
(b) Maximum shear stress
(c) Maximum shear strain. Take G = 80 GPa.

Solution: $T = 40 \times 10^6$ N-mm, $\theta = 0.6° = 0.01047$ rad, $L = 1000$ mm, $\tau = 80$ MPa, $G = 80 \times 10^3$ MPa. a) $d = ?$ b) $\tau_{max} = ?$ c) $\gamma = ?$

a. *Diameter of shaft:*

i. *Based on strength:* $\qquad\qquad T = \left(\dfrac{\pi d^3}{16}\right)\tau$

$$40 \times 10^6 = \left(\dfrac{\pi d^3}{16}\right) \times 80$$

$$d = 136.56 \text{ mm} \qquad\qquad \text{... Eq. (a)}$$

ii. *Based on rigidity:* $\qquad J = \dfrac{TL}{G\theta} = \dfrac{(40 \times 10^6) \times 1000}{(80 \times 10^3) \times 0.01047} = 47.76 \times 10^6 \text{ mm}^4$

But $\qquad\qquad\qquad\qquad J = \dfrac{\pi d^4}{32}$

$$47.76 \times 10^6 = \dfrac{\pi d^4}{32}$$

$$d = 148.51 \text{ mm} \qquad\qquad \text{... Eq. (b)}$$

Based on Eqs (a) and (b), select maximum value of diameter for design
i.e. $d = 148.51 \text{ mm} \approx 150 \text{ mm}$

b. *Maximum shear stress:*

We know that $\qquad\qquad\qquad T = \left(\dfrac{\pi d^3}{16}\right)\tau_{max}$

$$40 \times 10^6 = \left(\dfrac{\pi \times 150^3}{16}\right) \times \tau_{max}$$

$$\tau_{max} = 60.36 \text{ MPa}$$

c. *Maximum shear strain:*

We know that
$$G = \frac{\tau}{\gamma} = \frac{\tau_{max}}{\gamma}$$

$$80 \times 10^3 = \frac{60.36}{\gamma}$$

$$\theta = 7.55 \times 10^{-4}$$

DESIGN PROBLEMS ON HOLLOW SHAFT

19. A hollow shaft with inner diameter to outer diameter ratio 0.75 is to transmit a torque of 2500 N-m. Taking allowable shear stress for the shaft material as 50 N/mm² and limiting the angle of twist as 1.5° in a length of 2 meters, determine the inner and outer diameters. Take $G = 80$ kN/mm².

VTU – June/ July 2011 – 12 Marks

Solution: $K = 0.75$, $T = 2500 \times 10^3$ N-mm, $\tau = 50$ N/mm², $\theta = 1.5° = 0.02617$ rad, $L = 2000$ mm, $G = 80 \times 10^3$ N/mm², $d_o = ?$, $d_i = ?$.

Diameter of hollow shaft:

i. *Based on strength:*
$$T = \frac{\pi}{16} d_o^3 (1 - K^4)\tau$$

$$2500 \times 10^3 = \frac{\pi}{16} d_o^3 \times (1 - 0.6^4) \times 50$$

$$d_o = 66.39 \text{ mm} \qquad \qquad \text{... Eq. (a)}$$

ii. *Based on rigidity:*
$$J = \frac{TL}{G\theta} = \frac{(2500 \times 10^3) \times 2000}{(80 \times 10^3) \times 0.02617} = 2.39 \times 10^6 \text{ mm}^4$$

But
$$J = \frac{\pi}{32} d_o^4 (1 - K^4)$$

$$2.39 \times 10^6 = \frac{\pi}{32} d_o^4 \times [1 - 0.6^4]$$

$$d_o = 72.72 \text{ mm} \qquad \qquad \text{... Eq. (b)}$$

Based on Eqs (a) and (b), select maximum value of diameter for design

i.e. $\qquad d_o = 72.72$ mm ≈ 75 mm and $\quad d_i = 0.6 \times 75 = 45$ mm

20. A hollow shaft of diameter ratio 3/8 is required to transmit 588 kW at 110 rpm, the torque being 20% of the mean. Shear stress is not to exceed 63 N/mm² and twist in a length of 3 m not to exceed 1.4 degrees. Calculate the external diameter of the shaft which would satisfy these conditions. Take $G = 84$ GPa.

VTU – June/ July 15 – 12 Marks

Solution: $K = 3/8$, $P = 588 \times 10^3$ W, $N = 110$ rpm, $T_{max} = 1.2$ T, $\tau = 63$ N/mm², $\theta = 1.4° = 0.0244$ rad, $L = 3000$ mm, $G = 84 \times 10^3$ N/mm², $d_o = ?$.

Torque transmitted:

Given
$$T_{max} = 1.2 \text{ T} \qquad \qquad \text{... Eq. (i)}$$

But
$$P = \frac{2\pi NT}{60}$$

$$588 \times 10^3 = \frac{2\pi \times 110 \times T}{60}$$

$$T = 51.05 \times 10^3 \text{ N-}M = 51.05 \times 10^6 \text{ N-mm}$$

Eq. (i) yields ...
$$T_{max} = 1.2 \times (51.05 \times 10^6) = 61.26 \times 10^6 \text{ N-mm}$$

Diameter of hollow shaft:

i. *Based on strength:*
$$T_{max} = \frac{\pi}{16} d_o^3 \, (1 - K^4)\tau$$

$$61.26 \times 10^6 = \frac{\pi}{16} d_o^3 \times [(1 - (3/8)^4)] \times 63$$

$$d_o = 171.60 \text{ mm} \qquad \text{... Eq. (a)}$$

ii. *Based on rigidity:*
$$J = \frac{T_{max} L}{G\theta} = \frac{(61.26 \times 10^6) \times 3000}{(84 \times 10^3) \times 0.0244} = 89.67 \times 10^6 \text{ mm}^4$$

But
$$J = \frac{\pi}{32} d_o^4 (1 - K^4)$$

$$89.66 \times 10^6 = \frac{\pi}{32} d_o^4 \times [(1 - (3/8)^4)]$$

$$d_o = 174.72 \text{ mm} \qquad \text{... Eq. (b)}$$

Based on Eqs (a) and (b), select maximum value of diameter for design

i.e.
$$d_o = 174.72 \text{ mm} \approx 175 \text{ mm} \qquad \text{or } 176 \text{ mm}$$

and
$$d_i = 175 \times (3/8) = 65.63 \text{ mm} \qquad \text{or } 66 \text{ mm}$$

21. A hollow shaft having internal diameter 40% of external diameter, transmits 562.5 kW power at 100 rpm. Determine the cross-sectional dimensions of the shaft if shear stress is not to exceed 60 MPa and twist in a length of 2.5 m should not exceed 1.3°. Maximum torque transmitted is 25% higher than average torque. Rigidity modulus is 90 GPa.

Solution: $d_i = 0.4 \, d_o \Rightarrow K = 0.4$, $P = 562.5 \times 10^3$ W, $N = 100$ rpm, $d_o = ?$, $d_i = ?$, $\tau = 60$ MPa, $L = 2500$ mm, $\theta = 1.3° = 0.0227$ rad, $T_{max} = 1.25$ T, $G = 90 \times 10^3$ MPa.

Torque transmitted:

Given
$$T_{max} = 1.25 \text{ T} \qquad \text{... Eq. (i)}$$

But
$$P = \frac{2\pi NT}{60}$$

$$562.5 \times 10^3 = \frac{2\pi \times 110 \times T}{60}$$

$$T = 53.715 \times 10^3 \text{ N-m} = 53.715 \times 10^6 \text{ N-mm}$$

Eq. (i) yields ...
$$T_{max} = 1.25 \times (53.715 \times 10^6) = 67.14 \times 10^6 \text{ N-mm}$$

Diameter of hollow shaft:

i. *Based on strength:*
$$T_{max} = \frac{\pi}{16} d_o^3 \, (1 - K^4)\tau$$

$$67.14 \times 10^6 = \frac{\pi}{16} d_o^3 \times (1 - 0.4^4) \times 60$$

$$d_o = 180.17 \text{ mm} \qquad \qquad \dots \text{Eq. (a)}$$

ii. *Based on rigidity:* $\quad J = \dfrac{T_{max}L}{G\theta} = \dfrac{(67.14 \times 10^6) \times 2500}{(90 \times 10^3) \times 0.0227} = 82.16 \times 10^6 \text{ mm}^4$

But $\qquad \qquad \qquad J = \dfrac{\pi}{32} d_o^4 (1 - K^4)$

$$82.16 \times 10^6 = \frac{\pi}{32} d_o^4 \times (1 - 0.4^4)$$

$$d_o = 171.19 \text{ mm} \qquad \qquad \dots \text{Eq. (b)}$$

Based on Eqs (a) and (b), select maximum value of diameter for design

i.e. $\qquad \qquad \qquad d_o = 180.17 \text{ mm} \approx 182 \text{ mm}$

and $\qquad \qquad \qquad d_i = 182 \times 0.4 = 72.8 \text{ mm}$

22. A shaft required to transmit 245 kW at 240 rpm. The maximum torque may be 1.5 times the mean torque. The shear stress in the shaft should not exceed 40 N/mm² and twist 1° per meter length. Determine the diameter required if:

(a) The shaft is solid

(b) The shaft is hollow with external diameter twice the internal diameter. Take $G = 80$ kN/mm².

VTU – Dec. 14/ Jan. 15 – 12 Marks

Solution: $P = 245 \times 10^3$ W, $N = 240$ rpm, $T_{max} = 1.5$ T, $\tau = 40$ N/mm², $\theta = 1° = 0.0175$ rad, $L = 1000$ mm, $G = 80 \times 10^3$ N/mm². a) $d = ?$ b) $d_o = ?$, $d_i = ?$, if $d_o = 2d_i \Rightarrow K = 0.5$

Torque transmitted:

Given $\qquad \qquad \qquad T_{max} = 1.5 \text{ T} \qquad \qquad \dots \text{Eq. (i)}$

But $\qquad \qquad \qquad P = \dfrac{2\pi NT}{60}$

$$245 \times 10^3 = \frac{2\pi \times 240 \times T}{60}$$

$$T = 9748.24 \text{ N-m} = 9748.24 \times 10^3 \text{ N-mm}$$

Eq. (i) yields ... $\qquad T_{max} = 1.5 \times (9748.24 \times 10^3) = 14.62 \times 10^6 \text{ N-mm}$

a. *Solid shaft:*

i. *Based on strength:* $\quad T_{max} = \left(\dfrac{\pi d^3}{16}\right)\tau$

$$14.62 \times 10^6 = \frac{\pi d^3}{16} \times 40$$

$$d = 123.01 \text{ mm} \qquad \qquad \dots \text{Eq. (a)}$$

ii. *Based on rigidity:* $\quad J = \dfrac{T_{max}L}{G\theta} = \dfrac{(14.62 \times 10^6) \times 1000}{(80 \times 10^3) \times 0.0175} = 10.44 \times 10^6 \text{ mm}^4$

But
$$J = \frac{\pi d^4}{32}$$

$$10.44 \times 10^6 = \frac{\pi d^4}{32}$$

$$d = 101.56 \text{ mm} \qquad \qquad \dots \text{Eq. (b)}$$

Based on Eqs (a) and (b), select maximum value of diameter for design

i.e. $\qquad \qquad d = 123.01 \text{ mm} \simeq 123 \text{ mm}$

b. Hollow shaft:

i. *Based on strength:* $\qquad T_{\max} = \frac{\pi}{16} d_o^3 (1 - K^4)\tau$

$$14.62 \times 10^6 = \frac{\pi}{16} d_o^3 \times (1 - 0.5^4) \times 40$$

$$d_o = 125.68 \text{ mm} \qquad \qquad \dots \text{Eq. (c)}$$

ii. *Based on rigidity:* $\qquad J = \frac{T_{\max} L}{G\theta} = \frac{(14.62 \times 10^6) \times 1000}{(80 \times 10^3) \times 0.0175} = 10.44 \times 10^6 \text{ mm}^4$

But
$$J = \frac{\pi}{32} d_o^4 (1 - K^4)$$

$$10.44 \times 10^6 = \frac{\pi}{32} d_o^4 \times (1 - 0.5^4)$$

$$d_o = 103.20 \text{ mm} \qquad \qquad \dots \text{Eq. (d)}$$

Based on Eqs (c) and (d), select maximum value of diameter for design

i.e. $\qquad \qquad d_o = 125.68 \text{ mm} \approx 126 \text{ mm}$

and $\qquad \qquad d_i = 0.5 \times 126 = 63 \text{ mm}$

23. **A hollow circular shaft is to transmit a torque of 4.05 kN-m.**
    (a) Determine the shaft dimensions for the following data:
        Ratio of inside to outside diameter = 0.8, Allowable shear stress = 40 N/mm²,
        Limiting angle of twist = 1°/20 dia length, Modulus of rigidity = 80 GPa.
    (b) For the above dimensions, calculate the maximum shear stress.

VTU – May/ June 2010 – 08 Marks

Solution: $T = 4.05 \times 10^6$ N-mm, $K = 0.8$, $\tau = 40$ N/mm², $\theta = 1° = 0.0175$ rad, $L = 20d_o$, $G = 80 \times 10^3$ N/mm². a) $d_o = ?, d_i = ?$. b) $\tau_{\max} = ?$

a. *Diameter of hollow shaft:*

i. *Based on strength:* $\qquad T = \frac{\pi}{16} d_o^3 (1 - K^4)\tau$

$$4.05 \times 10^6 = \frac{\pi}{16} d_o^3 \times (1 - 0.8^4) \times 40$$

$$d_o = 95.59 \text{ mm} \qquad \qquad \dots \text{Eq. (a)}$$

ii. *Based on rigidity:* $\qquad J = \dfrac{T_{max}L}{G\theta} = \dfrac{(4.05 \times 10^6) \times (20d_o)}{(80 \times 10^3) \times 0.0175} = (57.86 \times 10^3)\, d_o$

But $\qquad\qquad\qquad J = \dfrac{\pi}{32} d_o^4 \,(1 - K^4)$

$$(57.86 \times 10^3)\, d_o = \dfrac{\pi}{32} d_o^4 \times (1 - 0.8^4)$$

$$d_o = 99.94 \text{ mm} \qquad\qquad \text{... Eq. (b)}$$

Based on Eqs (a) and (b), select maximum value of diameter for design

$$\text{i.e. } d_o = 99.94 \text{ mm} \approx 100 \text{ mm}$$
$$\text{and } d_i = 0.8 \times 100 = 80 \text{ mm}$$

b. *Maximum shear stress:*

We know that $\qquad\qquad T = \dfrac{\pi}{16} d_o^3 \,(1 - K^4) T_{max}$

$$4.05 \times 10^6 = \dfrac{\pi}{16} \times 100^3 \times (1 - 0.8^4) \times T_{max}$$

$$T_{max} = 34.94 \text{ N/mm}^2$$

24. A hollow shaft 3 m long transmits a torque of 25 kN-m. The total angle of twist in this length is not to exceed 2.5° and allowable shear stress is 90 MPa. Determine the inside and outside diameters of the shaft, if $G = 85$ GPa.

VTU – June/ July 2009 – 10 Marks

Solution: $L = 3000$ mm, $T = 25 \times 10^6$ N-mm, $\theta = 2.5° = 0.0436$ rad, $\tau = 90$ MPa, $G = 85 \times 10^3$ MPa, $d_o, d_i = ?$

Diameter of hollow shaft:

i. *Based on strength:* $\qquad T = \dfrac{\pi}{16} d_o^3 \,(1 - K^4)\tau$

$$25 \times 10^6 = \dfrac{\pi}{16} d_o^3 \,(1 - K^4) \times 90$$

$$d_o^3 \,(1 - K^4) = 1.412 \times 10^6 \qquad\qquad \text{... Eq. (a)}$$

ii. *Based on rigidity:* $\qquad J = \dfrac{TL}{G\theta} = \dfrac{(25 \times 10^6) \times 3000}{(85 \times 10^3) \times 0.0436} = 20.22 \times 10^6 \text{ mm}^4$

But $\qquad\qquad\qquad J = \dfrac{\pi}{32} d_o^4 \,(1 - K^4)$

$$20.22 \times 10^6 = \dfrac{\pi}{32} d_o^4 \,(1 - K^4)$$

$$d_o^4 \,(1 - K^4) = 206 \times 10^6$$

$$d_o^3 \,(1 - K^4) = \dfrac{206 \times 10^6}{d_o} \qquad\qquad \text{... Eq. (b)}$$

Equating Eqs (a) and (b), we have

$$1.412 \times 10^6 = \frac{206 \times 10^6}{d_o}$$

$$d_o = 145.89 \text{ mm} \approx 146 \text{ mm}$$

Eq. (a) yields... $146^3 \times (1 - K^4) = 1.412 \times 10^6$

$$1 - K^4 = 0.4537$$

$$K = 0.8597$$

Also

$$K = \frac{d_i}{d_o}$$

$$0.8957 = \frac{d_i}{146}$$

$$d_i = 0.8597 \times 146 = 125.52 \text{ mm}$$

25. A hollow steel shaft transmits 200 kW of power at 150 rpm. The total angle of twist in a length of 5 m of shaft is 3°. Find the inner and outer diameters of the shaft if the permissible shear stress is 60 MPa. Take $G = 80$ GPa.

VTU – Dec. 2011 – 10 Marks

Solution: $P = 200 \times 10^3$ W, $N = 150$ rpm, $\theta = 3° = 0.0524$ rad, $L = 5000$ mm, $\tau = 60$ MPa, $G = 80 \times 10^3$ MPa, d_o, $d_i = ?$

Torque transmitted:

We know that
$$P = \frac{2\pi NT}{60}$$

$$200 \times 10^3 = \frac{2\pi \times 150 \times T}{60}$$

$$T = 12.73 \times 10^3 \text{ N-m} = 12.73 \times 10^6 \text{ N-mm}$$

Diameter of hollow shaft:

i. *Based on strength:*
$$T = \frac{\pi}{16} d_o^3 (1 - K^4)\tau$$

$$12.73 \times 10^6 = \frac{\pi}{16} d_o^3 (1 - K^4) \times 60$$

$$d_o^3 (1 - K^4) = 1.08 \times 10^6 \qquad \text{... Eq. (a)}$$

ii. *Based on rigidity:*
$$J = \frac{TL}{G\theta} = \frac{(12.73 \times 10^6) \times 5000}{(80 \times 10^3) \times 0.0524} = 15.18 \times 10^6 \text{ mm}^4$$

But
$$J = \frac{\pi}{32} d_o^4 (1 - K^4)$$

$$15.18 \times 10^6 = \frac{\pi}{32} d_o^4 (1 - K^4)$$

$$d_o^4 (1 - K^4) = 154.66 \times 10^6$$

$$d_o^3 (1 - K^4) = \frac{154.66 \times 10^6}{d_o} \qquad \text{... Eq. (b)}$$

Equating Eqs (a) and (b), we have

$$1.08 \times 10^6 = \frac{154.66 \times 10^6}{d_o}$$

$$d_o = 143.2 \text{ mm} \approx 144 \text{ mm}$$

Eq. (a) yields... $144^3 \times (1 - K^4) = 1.08 \times 10^6$

$$1 - K^4 = 0.3617$$

$$K = 0.8938$$

Also

$$K = \frac{d_i}{d_o}$$

$$0.8938 = \frac{d_i}{144}$$

$$d_i = 0.6383 \times 144 = 128.70 \text{ mm}$$

26. **A hollow steel shaft 3 m long transmits 41 kW power at 100 rpm. Maximum torque is 25% more than the mean torque. The total angle of twist is not to exceed 3° and allowable shear stress of the materials is 100 MPa. Determine the dimensions of the shaft. The rigidity modulus of the shaft material is 85 GPa.**

VTU – June/ July 2014 – 10 Marks

Solution: $L = 3000$ mm, $P = 41 \times 10^3$ W, $N = 100$ rpm, $T_{max} = 1.25\ T$, $\theta = 3° = 0.0524$ rad, $\tau = 100$ MPa, $G = 85 \times 10^3$ MPa, d_o, $d_i = ?$

Torque transmitted:
Given

$$T_{max} = 1.25\ T \qquad \qquad \text{... Eq. (i)}$$

But

$$P = \frac{2\pi NT}{60}$$

$$41 \times 10^3 = \frac{2\pi \times 100 \times T}{60}$$

$$T = 3915.21 \text{ N-m} = 3915.21 \times 10^3 \text{ N-mm}$$

Eq. (i) yields...

$$T_{max} = 1.25 \times (3915.21 \times 10^3) = 4.89 \times 10^6 \text{ N-mm}$$

Diameter of hollow shaft:

i. *Based on strength:*

$$T_{max} = \frac{\pi}{16} d_o^3 (1 - K^4)\tau$$

$$4.89 \times 10^6 = \frac{\pi}{16} d_o^3 (1 - K^4) \times 100$$

$$d_o^3 (1 - K^4) = 0.249 \times 10^6 \qquad \qquad \text{... Eq. (a)}$$

ii. *Based on rigidity:*

$$J = \frac{T_{max} L}{G\theta} = \frac{(4.89 \times 10^6) \times 3000}{(85 \times 10^3) \times 0.0524} = 3.29 \times 10^6 \text{ mm}^4$$

But

$$J = \frac{\pi}{32} d_o^4 (1 - K^4)$$

$$3.29 \times 10^6 = \frac{\pi}{32} d_o^4 (1 - K^4)$$

$$d_o^4 \left(1 - K^4\right) = 33.51 \times 10^6$$

$$d_o^3 \left(1 - K^4\right) = \frac{33.51 \times 10^6}{d_o} \qquad \text{... Eq. (b)}$$

Equating Eqs (a) and (b), we have

$$0.249 \times 10^6 = \frac{33.51 \times 10^6}{d_o}$$

$$d_o = 134.58 \text{ mm} \approx 135 \text{ mm}$$

Eq. (a) yields... $135^3 \times \left(1 - K^4\right) = 0.249 \times 10^6$

$$1 - K^4 = 0.1012$$

$$K = 0.9737$$

Also

$$K = \frac{d_i}{d_o}$$

$$0.9737 = \frac{d_i}{135}$$

$$d_i = 0.9737 \times 135 = 131.45 \text{ mm}$$

9.8 COMPARISON OF SOLID AND HOLLOW SHAFTS OR REPLACEMENT OF SHAFTS

Until unless specified, when a shaft is replaced by another, the following data or parameters are assumed to be common for both the shafts:
- Length of the shaft
- Power transmitted
- Torque transmitted
- Speed

On the other hand if both the shafts are made of same material, then in addition to the above parameters, the following parameters may also be assumed to be common for both the shafts:
- Material properties (shear stress and modulus of rigidity)
- Weight per unit volume

REPLACEMENT OF SOLID SHAFT WITH HOLLOW SHAFT

27. Compare the weight, strength and stiffness of a hollow shaft with that of a solid shaft having same material and length.

Solution:

Let, d = Diameter of solid shaft

d_o = Outer diameter of hollow shaft

d_i = Inner diameter of hollow shaft

$K = \dfrac{d_i}{d_o}$ = Ratio of inner diameter to outer diameter of hollow shaft

$L = L_s = L_H$ = Length of the shaft

$\tau = \tau_s = T_H$ = Shear stress of shaft material   (material is same)

ρ = Density of shaft material

W_H, W_s = Weight of hollow shaft and solid shaft respectively

T_H, T_s = Torque transmitted by hollow shaft and solid shaft respectively
S_H, S_s = Stiffness of hollow shaft and solid shaft respectively

a. Comparison of weight:

We know that $\qquad$ Weight = density × volume = density × (area × length)

$$W = \rho AL$$

Thus for a solid shaft, $\quad W_s = \rho A_s L = \rho L \left(\dfrac{\pi d^2}{4}\right)$ $\qquad$ ... Eq. (i)

and for a hollow shaft, $\quad W_H = \rho A_H L = \rho L \left[\dfrac{\pi\left(d_o^2 - d_i^2\right)}{4}\right]$ $\qquad$ ... Eq. (ii)

Dividing Eq. (ii) by Eq. (i) yields

$$\frac{W_H}{W_s} = \frac{\rho L\left[\pi\left(d_o^2 - d_i^2\right)/4\right]}{\rho L(\pi d^2/4} = \frac{d_o^2 - d_i^2}{d^2}$$

$$\therefore \qquad \frac{W_H}{W_s} = \frac{d_o^2(1 - K^2)}{d^2} \qquad \text{... Eq. (iii)}$$

b. Comparison of strength:

For a hollow shaft, $\qquad T_H = \dfrac{\pi}{16} d_o^3 (1 - K^4)\tau$ $\qquad$ ... Eq. (iv)

For a solid shaft substituting $\quad K = 0$ and $d_o = d$, in Eq. (iv), we have

$$T_s = \left(\frac{\pi}{16}\right) d^3\tau \qquad \text{... Eq. (v)}$$

Dividing Eq. (iv) by Eq. (v) yields

$$\frac{T_H}{T_s} = \frac{(\pi/16)\, d_o^3(1 - K^4)\tau}{(\pi/16)d^3\tau}$$

$$\therefore \qquad \frac{T_H}{T_s} = \frac{d_o^3(1 - K^4)}{d^3} \qquad \text{... Eq. (vi)}$$

Since the material is same, Equating Eqs (i) and (ii), we have

$$\rho L\left[\pi\left(d_o^2 - d_i^2\right)/4\right] = \rho L\left(\pi d^2/4\right)$$

$$d_o^2(1 - K^2) = d^2$$

$$d_o\sqrt{(1 - K^2)} = d \qquad \text{... Eq. (iii-a)}$$

Substituting Eq. (iii-a) in Eq. (vi), we have

$$\frac{T_H}{T_s} = \frac{d_o^3(1 - K^4)}{\left[d_o\sqrt{(1 - K^2)}\right]^3} = \frac{(1 - K^4)}{\left[\sqrt{(1 - K^2)}\right]^3} = \frac{(1 + K^2)(1 - K^2)}{(1 - K^2)\sqrt{(1 - K^2)}}$$

$$\therefore \quad \frac{T_H}{T_s} = \frac{(1+K^2)}{\sqrt{(1-K^2)}} \qquad \text{... Eq. (vi-a)}$$

c. Comparison of stiffness:

Stiffness is defined as $\quad S = \dfrac{T}{\theta}$ $\qquad$ ... Eq. (vii)

We know that $\qquad \dfrac{T}{J} = \dfrac{G\theta}{L} = \dfrac{\tau}{r}$

$$S = \frac{T}{\theta} = \frac{GJ}{L}$$

For a solid shaft, $J = \left[\dfrac{\pi d^4}{32}\right]$ and for a hollow shaft $J = \left[\dfrac{\pi\left(d_o^4 - d_i^4\right)}{32}\right]$

For a hollow shaft, $\quad S_H = \dfrac{G}{L}\left[\dfrac{\pi\left(d_o^4 - d_i^4\right)}{32}\right] = \dfrac{G}{L}\left[\dfrac{\pi\, d_o^4(1-K^4)}{32}\right]$

$$\text{... Eq. (viii)}$$

For a solid shaft substituting $K = 0$ and $d_o = d$, in Eq. (viii), we have

For a solid shaft, $\quad S_s = \dfrac{G}{L}\left[\dfrac{\pi d^4}{32}\right]$ $\qquad$ ... Eq. (ix)

Dividing Eq. (viii) by Eq. (ix) yields

$$\frac{S_H}{S_s} = \frac{(G/L)\times\left[\pi d_o^4(1-K^4)/32\right]}{(G/L)\times(\pi d^4/32)}$$

$$\therefore \quad \frac{S_H}{S_s} = \frac{d_o^4(1-K^4)}{d^4} \qquad \text{... Eq. (x)}$$

Substituting Eq. (iii-a) in Eq. (x), we have

$$\frac{S_H}{S_s} = \frac{d_o^4(1-K^4)}{\left[d_o\sqrt{(1-K^2)}\right]^4} = \frac{(1-K^4)}{\left[\sqrt{(1-K^2)}\right]^4} = \frac{(1+K^2)(1-K^2)}{(1-K^2)^2}$$

$$\therefore \quad \frac{S_H}{S_s} = \frac{(1+K^2)}{(1-K^2)} \qquad \text{... Eq. (x-a)}$$

28. **Prove that a hollow shaft is stronger and stiffer than the solid shaft of the same material, length and weight.**

VTU – Dec. 15/ Jan. 16 – 08 Marks; Dec. 2011 – 08 Marks;
June/ July 2008 – 08 Marks

Solution: Refer to Problem 27 Case (b) and (c)

29. Compare the weight, strength and stiffness of a hollow shaft of same outside diameter as that of a solid shaft.

Proceeding on similar lines to problem 27, we have:

a. *Comparison of strength:*

$$\frac{T_H}{T_s} = \frac{d_o^3(1-K^4)}{d^3} \qquad \text{... using Eq. (vi)}$$

Since $d_o = d$, we have

$$\frac{T_H}{T_s} = \frac{d^3(1-K^4)}{d^3} = (1-K^4) \qquad \text{... Eq. (vi-a)}$$

b. *Comparison of stiffness:*

$$\frac{S_H}{S_s} = \frac{d_o^4(1-K^4)}{d^4} \qquad \text{... using Eq. (x)}$$

Since $d_o = d$, we have

$$\frac{S_H}{S_s} = \frac{d_o^4(1-K^4)}{d^4} = (1-K^4) \qquad \text{... Eq. (x-a)}$$

30. Compare the weight, strength and stiffness of a hollow shaft with that of a solid shaft having same material and length. The external diameter of hollow shaft is same as that of solid shaft, while the internal diameter of hollow shaft is half the external diameter hollow shaft. OR

Compare the torsional strength and angle of twist of two shafts of same material, length and weight having same maximum shear stress. One is solid and the other is hollow with a ratio of diameters = 0.5 (d/D = 0.5). Take same rigidity modulus.

VTU – June 2012 – 14 Marks; Dec. 09/ Jan. 10 – 12 Marks

Solution: $T_s = T_H$, $L_s = L_H$, $d_o = d$, $d_i = d_o/2$, $K = \dfrac{d_i}{d_o} = 0.5$,

Let, L = Length of the shaft

d = Diameter of solid shaft

d_o = Outer diameter of hollow shaft

d_i = Inner diameter of hollow shaft

$K = \dfrac{d_i}{d_o}$ = Ratio of inner diameter to outer diameter of hollow shaft

$\tau = \tau_s = \tau_H$ = Shear stress of shaft material (material is same)

ρ = Density of shaft material

W_H, W_s = Weight of hollow shaft and solid shaft respectively

T_H, T_s = Torque transmitted by hollow shaft and solid shaft respectively

S_H, S_s = Stiffness of hollow shaft and solid shaft respectively

a. *Comparison of weight:*

We know that   Weight = density × volume = density × (area × length)

$$W = \rho A L$$

Thus for a solid shaft, $W_s = \rho A_s L = \rho L \left(\dfrac{\pi d^2}{4}\right) \qquad \text{... Eq. (i)}$

and for a hollow shaft, $W_H = \rho A_H L = \rho L \left[\dfrac{\pi\left(d_o^2 - d_i^2\right)}{4}\right] \qquad \text{... Eq. (ii)}$

Dividing Eq. (ii) by Eq. (i) yields

$$\frac{W_H}{W_s} = \frac{\rho L\left[\pi\left(d_o^2 - d_i^2\right)/4\right]}{\rho L(\pi d^2/4)} = \frac{d_o^2 - d_i^2}{d^2}$$

$$\therefore \quad \frac{W_H}{W_s} = \frac{d_o^2(1 - K^2)}{d^2}$$

Since $d_o = d$, we have

$$\frac{W_H}{W_s} = (1 - K^2) = (1 - 0.5^2)$$

$$\therefore \quad \frac{W_H}{W_s} = 0.75 \qquad \qquad \text{... Eq. (iv)}$$

b. *Comparison of strength:*

For a hollow shaft,
$$T_H = \frac{\pi}{16} d_o^3\,(1 - K^4)\tau \qquad \qquad \text{... Eq. (v)}$$

For a solid shaft substituting $K = 0$ and $d_o = d$, in Eq. (iv), we have

$$T_s = \left(\frac{\pi}{16}\right) d^3 \tau \qquad \qquad \text{... Eq. (vi)}$$

Dividing Eq. (vi) by Eq. (v) yields

$$\frac{T_H}{T_s} = \frac{(\pi/16)\, d_o^3(1 - K^4)\tau}{(\pi/16)d^3\tau}$$

$$\therefore \quad \frac{T_H}{T_s} = \frac{d_o^3(1 - K^4)}{d^3} \qquad \qquad \text{... Eq. (vii)}$$

Since $d_o = d$, we have

$$\frac{T_H}{T_s} = (1 - K^4) = (1 - 0.5^4)$$

$$\therefore \quad \frac{T_H}{T_s} = 0.9375 \qquad \qquad \text{... Eq. (viii)}$$

c. *Comparison of stiffness:*

Stiffness is defined as
$$S = \frac{T}{\theta} \qquad \qquad \text{... Eq. (ix)}$$

We know that
$$\frac{T}{J} = \frac{G\theta}{L} = \frac{\tau}{r}$$

$$S = \frac{T}{\theta} = \frac{GJ}{L}$$

For a solid shaft, $J = \left[\dfrac{\pi d^4}{32}\right]$ and for a hollow shaft $J = \left[\dfrac{\pi\left(d_o^4 - d_i^4\right)}{32}\right]$

For a hollow shaft,
$$S_H = \frac{G}{L}\left[\frac{\pi\left(d_o^4 - d_i^4\right)}{32}\right] = \frac{G}{L}\left[\frac{\pi\, d_o^4(1 - K^4)}{32}\right]$$

$$\text{... Eq. (x)}$$

For a solid shaft, $\qquad S_s = \dfrac{G}{L}\left[\dfrac{\pi d^4}{32}\right]$ $\hspace{2cm}$ ... Eq. (xi)

Dividing Eq. (x) by Eq. (xi) yields

$$\dfrac{S_H}{S_s} = \dfrac{(G/L)\times\left[\pi d_o^4(1-K^4)/32\right]}{(G/L)\times(\pi d^4/32)}$$

$\therefore \qquad \dfrac{S_H}{S_s} = \dfrac{\pi d_o^4(1-K^4)}{d^4}$ $\hspace{2cm}$ ... Eq. (xii)

Since $d_o = d$, we have

$$\dfrac{S_H}{S_s} = (1-K^4) = (1-0.5^4)$$

$\therefore \qquad \dfrac{S_H}{S_s} = 0.9375$ $\hspace{2cm}$ ... Eq. (xiii)

31. Compare the strength of a hollow shaft with that of a solid shaft for the same diameter and material. The diameter ratio of hollow shaft is 0.75.

Solution: $K = 0.75 = \dfrac{d_i}{d_o}$, $d_o = $ d, $\tau_s = \tau_H$

Let, $\qquad d$ = Diameter of solid shaft

$\qquad\qquad d_o$ = Outer diameter of hollow shaft

$\qquad\qquad d_i$ = Inner diameter of hollow shaft

$\qquad K = \dfrac{d_i}{d_o}$ = Ratio of inner diameter to outer diameter of hollow shaft

From case (b) of Problem 30, we have $\dfrac{T_H}{T_s} = \dfrac{d_o^3(1-K^4)}{d^3}$ $\hspace{1cm}$ ... using Eq. (vii)

Since $d_o = d$, we have $\qquad\qquad \dfrac{T_H}{T_s} = (1-K^4) = (1-0.75^4) = 0.6836$

32. Two shafts of same material and of same lengths are subjected to the same torque. If the first shaft is a solid circular section and the second shaft is of hollow circular section, whose internal diameter is 2/3 of the outside diameter and the maximum shear stress developed in each shaft is the same, compare the weights of the shafts.

VTU – Dec. 09/ Jan. 10 – 10 Marks

Solution: $\tau_s = \tau_H, L_s = L_H, T_s = T_H, d_i = 2d_o/3 \Rightarrow K = \dfrac{d_i}{d_o} = \dfrac{2}{3}, \dfrac{W_H}{W_s} = ?$

Let, $\qquad d$ = Diameter of solid shaft

$\qquad\qquad d_o$ = Outer diameter of hollow shaft

$\qquad\qquad d_i$ = Inner diameter of hollow shaft

$\qquad K = \dfrac{d_i}{d_o}$ = Ratio of inner diameter to outer diameter of hollow shaft

$\qquad L$ = Length of the shaft

$\qquad \tau = \tau_s = \tau_H$ = Shear stress of shaft material $\hspace{2cm}$ (material is same)

$\qquad \rho$ = Density of shaft material

T_H, T_s = Torque transmitted by hollow shaft and solid shaft respectively
W_H, W_s = Weight of hollow shaft and solid shaft respectively

For a hollow shaft, $\qquad T_H = \left(\dfrac{\pi}{16}\right) d_o^3 \tau (1 - K^4)$ $\qquad\qquad$ ... Eq. (i)

For a solid shaft substituting $K = 0$ and $d_o = d$, in Eq. (i), we have

$$T_s = \left(\dfrac{\pi}{16}\right) d^3 \tau \qquad\qquad \text{... Eq. (ii)}$$

Since the material is same, equating Eq. (ii) and Eq. (i) yields
$$T_H = T_s$$

$$\left(\dfrac{\pi}{16}\right) d_o^3 \tau (1 - K^4) = \left(\dfrac{\pi}{16}\right) d^3 \tau$$

$$d_o^3 (1 - K^4) = d^3$$

$$d_o^3 \left[1 - \left(\dfrac{2}{3}\right)^4\right] = d^3$$

$$(0.8025)\ d_o^3 = d^3$$

$$\therefore \quad d = 0.9293 d_o \qquad\qquad \text{... Eq. (iii)}$$

Comparison of weight:

For a hollow shaft, $\qquad W_H = \rho A_H L = \rho L \left[\dfrac{\pi\left(d_o^2 - d_i^2\right)}{4}\right]$ $\qquad$ ... Eq. (iv)

For a solid shaft substituting $d_i = 0$ and $d_o = d$, in Eq. (iv), we have

$$W_s = \rho A_s L = \rho L \left(\dfrac{\pi d^2}{4}\right) \qquad\qquad \text{... Eq. (v)}$$

Dividing Eq. (iv) by Eq. (v) yields

$$\dfrac{W_H}{W_s} = \dfrac{\rho L \left[\pi\left(d_o^2 - d_i^2\right)/4\right]}{\rho L (\pi d^2 / 4)} = \dfrac{d_o^2 - d_i^2}{d^2} = \dfrac{d_o^2 (1 - K^2)}{d^2}$$

$$\therefore \quad \dfrac{W_H}{W_s} = \dfrac{d_o^2 \left[1 - (2/3)^2\right]}{(0.9293 d_o)^2} = 0.6433$$

33. A hollow shaft having an inside diameter 60% of its outer diameter, is to replace a solid shaft transmitting the same power at the same speed. Calculate the percentage saving in material, if the material to be used is also the same.

VTU – Dec. 14/ Jan. 15 – 10 Marks

Solution: $d_i = 0.6 d_o \Rightarrow K = \dfrac{d_i}{d_o} = 0.6$, $P_s = P_H$, $N_s = N_H$, $\tau_s = \tau_H$, percentage saving in

material = ?

Let, d = Diameter of solid shaft

d_o = Outer diameter of hollow shaft

d_i = Inner diameter of hollow shaft

$K = \dfrac{d_i}{d_o}$ = Ratio of inner diameter to outer diameter of hollow shaft

L = Length of the shaft

$\tau = \tau_s = \tau_H$ = Shear stress of shaft material   (material is same)

ρ = Density of shaft material

T_H, T_s = Torque transmitted by hollow shaft and solid shaft respectively

W_H, W_s = Weight of hollow shaft and solid shaft respectively

For a hollow shaft, $\quad\quad W_H = \rho A_H L = \rho L \left[\dfrac{\pi\left(d_o^2 - d_i^2\right)}{4} \right]$ ... Eq. (i)

For a solid shaft substituting $d_i = 0$ and $d_o = d$, in Eq. (i), we have

$$W_s = \rho A_s L = \rho L \left(\dfrac{\pi d^2}{4} \right) \quad\quad\quad\quad \text{... Eq. (ii)}$$

Dividing Eq. (ii) by Eq. (i) yields

$$\dfrac{W_H}{W_s} = \dfrac{\rho L \left[\pi\left(d_o^2 - d_i^2\right)/4 \right]}{\rho L (\pi d^2 / 4)} = \dfrac{d_o^2 - d_i^2}{d^2} = \dfrac{d_o^2(1 - K^2)}{d^2}$$

$$\text{Percentage saving in material} = \left[1 - \dfrac{W_H}{W_s} \right] \times 100$$

$$= \left[1 - \dfrac{d_o^2(1 - K^2)}{d^2} \right] \times 100$$

$$= \left[1 - \dfrac{d_o^2(1 - 0.6^2)}{d^2} \right] \times 100$$

$$\text{Percentage saving in material} = \left[1 - 0.64 \left(\dfrac{d_o}{d} \right)^2 \right] \times 100 \quad\quad \text{... Eq. (iii)}$$

Since power transmitted by both shafts is same, we have

$$P_H = P_s$$

$$\dfrac{2\pi N T_H}{60} = \dfrac{2\pi N T s}{60}$$

$$T_H = T_s$$

$$\left(\dfrac{\pi}{16} \right) d_o^3 \tau \, (1 - K^4) = \left(\dfrac{\pi}{16} \right) d^3 \tau$$

$$d_o^3 \, (1 - K^4) = d^3$$

$$d_o^3 \, [1 - (0.6)^4] = d^3$$

$$\frac{d_o}{d} = 1.047 \qquad \text{... Eq. (iv)}$$

Substituting Eq. (iv) in Eq. (iii), we have

Percentage saving in material = $[1 - 0.64 (1.047)^2] \times 100 = 29.84\%$

34. A solid shaft and a hollow shaft are made of same material and have equal strength in torsion. The outside diameter of hollow shaft is 25% larger than the solid shaft. What will be the ratio weight of hollow shaft to solid shaft?

Solution: $d_o = 1.25d$, $T_H = T_s$, $W_H/W_s = ?$

Let, d = Diameter of solid shaft

      d_o = Outer diameter of hollow shaft

      d_i = Inner diameter of hollow shaft

$$K = \frac{d_i}{d_o} = \text{Ratio of inner diameter to outer diameter of hollow shaft}$$

$\tau = \tau_s = \tau_H$ = Shear stress of shaft material   (material is same)

For a hollow shaft, $T_H = \left(\dfrac{\pi}{16}\right) d_o^3 \tau (1 - K^4)$ ... Eq. (i)

For a solid shaft substituting $K = 0$ and $d_o = d$, in Eq. (i), we have

$$T_s = \left(\frac{\pi}{16}\right) d^3 \tau \qquad \text{... Eq. (ii)}$$

Since the material is same, Equating Eqs (i) and (ii), we have

$$\left(\frac{\pi}{16}\right) d_o^3 \tau (1 - K^4) = \left(\frac{\pi}{16}\right) d^3 \tau$$

$$d_o^3 (1 - K^4) = d^3$$
$$(1.25 d)^3 (1 - K^4) = d^3$$
$$(1 - K^4) = 0.512$$
$$\therefore \quad K = 0.8358$$

Comparison of weight:

For a hollow shaft, $W_H = \rho A_H L = \rho L \left[\dfrac{\pi \left(d_o^2 - d_i^2 \right)}{4} \right]$ ... Eq. (iii)

For a solid shaft substituting $d_i = 0$ and $d_o = d$, in Eq. (iii), we have

$$W_s = \rho A_s L = \rho L \left(\frac{\pi d^2}{4} \right) \qquad \text{... Eq. (iv)}$$

Dividing Eq. (iii) by Eq. (iv) yields

$$\frac{W_H}{W_s} = \frac{\rho L \left[\pi \left(d_o^2 - d_i^2 \right)/4 \right]}{\rho L (\pi d^2/4)} = \frac{d_o^2 - d_i^2}{d^2} = \frac{d_o^2 (1 - K^2)}{d^2}$$

$$\therefore \quad \frac{W_H}{W_s} = \frac{(1.25d)^2 (1 - 0.8358^2)}{d^2} = 0.4709$$

35. **A solid shaft of diameter *d* is used in power transmission. Due to modification of existing transmission system, it is required to replace the solid shaft by a hollow shaft of the same material and equally strong in torsion. Further, the weight of the hollow shaft per meter length should be half of solid shaft. Determine the outer diameter of hollow shaft in terms of *d*.**

Solution: $T_H = T_s$, $\tau_s = \tau_H$, $W_H = W_s/2$

Let, $\quad d$ = Diameter of solid shaft

$\qquad d_o$ = Outer diameter of hollow shaft

$\qquad d_i$ = Inner diameter of hollow shaft

$$K = \frac{d_i}{d_o} = \text{Ratio of inner diameter to outer diameter of hollow shaft}$$

$\qquad L$ = Length of the shaft

$\qquad \tau = \tau_s = \tau_H$ = Shear stress of shaft material $\qquad\qquad$ (material is same)

$\qquad \rho$ = Density of shaft material

$\quad T_H, T_s$ = Torque transmitted by hollow shaft and solid shaft respectively

$\quad W_H, W_s$ = Weight of hollow shaft and solid shaft respectively

For a hollow shaft, $\qquad\qquad T_H = \left(\dfrac{\pi}{16}\right) d_o^3 \tau (1 - K^4)$ $\qquad\qquad\qquad$ ... Eq. (i)

For a solid shaft substituting $K = 0$ and $d_o = d$, in Eq. (i), we have

$$T_s = \left(\dfrac{\pi}{16}\right) d^3 \tau \qquad\qquad\qquad \text{... Eq. (ii)}$$

Since the material is equally strong in torsion, equating Eq. (ii) and Eq. (i) yields

$$T_H = T_s$$

$$\left(\dfrac{\pi}{16}\right) d_o^3 \tau (1 - K^4) = \left(\dfrac{\pi}{16}\right) d^3 \tau$$

$$d_o^3 (1 - K^4) = d^3$$

$$d_o^3 \left(1 - \dfrac{d_i^4}{d_o^4}\right) = d^3$$

$$\left(d_o^3 - \dfrac{d_i^4}{d_o}\right) = d^3$$

$$\dfrac{d_o^4 - d_i^4}{d_o} = d^3$$

$$\therefore \quad d_i^4 = d_o^4 - d^3 d_o \qquad\qquad\qquad \text{... Eq. (iii)}$$

Also, $\qquad\qquad\qquad W_H = W_s/2$

$$\rho A_H L = \rho A_s L/2$$

$$A_H = A_s/2$$

$$\dfrac{\pi\left(d_o^2 - d_i^2\right)}{4} = \dfrac{1}{2}\left(\dfrac{\pi d^2}{4}\right)$$

$$\left(d_o^2 - d_i^2\right) = \frac{d^2}{2}$$

$$\left(d_o^2 - d_i^2\right) = 0.5d^2$$

$$d_i^2 = d_o^2 - 0.5d^2$$

Squaring both sides, we have

$$\therefore \quad d_i^4 = \left(d_o^2 - 0.5d^2\right)^2 \qquad \qquad \text{... Eq. (iv)}$$

Equating Eqs (iii) and (iv), we have

$$d_o^4 - d^3 d_o = \left(d_o^2 - 0.5d^2\right)^2$$

$$= d_o^4 + 0.25d^4 - d_o^2 d^2$$

$$(d^2)\, d_o^2 - (d^3)\, d_o - 0.25d^4 = 0 \qquad \qquad \text{... Eq. (v)}$$

This is a quadratic equation, having $a = d^2$, $b = -d^3$ and $c = -0.25d^4$

$$d_o = \frac{-(-d^3) \pm \sqrt{d^6 - [4d^2(-0.25d^4)]}}{2d^2} = \frac{d^3 \pm \sqrt{d^6 + d^6}}{2d^2} = \frac{d^3 \pm \sqrt{2d^6}}{2d^2}$$

$$d_o = \frac{d^2\left(d \pm \sqrt{2d^2}\right)}{2d^2} = \frac{\left(d \pm \sqrt{2}d\right)}{2}$$

Thus the roots are $d_o = \dfrac{\left(d \pm \sqrt{2}d\right)}{2}$ and $d_o = \dfrac{\left(d - \sqrt{2}d\right)}{2}$

36. A 250 mm diameter solid shaft is used to drive the propeller of a marine vessel. It is necessary to replace the weight of the shaft by 70%. What would be the dimensions of the hollow shaft made of same material as that of solid shaft?

Solution: $d = 250$ mm, $W_H/W_s = 0.7$, $\Rightarrow W_H = 0.7W_s$, $\tau_s = \tau_H$

Let, $\quad d$ = Diameter of solid shaft

$\quad d_o$ = Outer diameter of hollow shaft

$\quad d_i$ = Inner diameter of hollow shaft

$$K = \frac{d_i}{d_o} = \text{Ratio of inner diameter to outer diameter of hollow shaft}$$

$\quad L$ = Length of the shaft

$\quad \tau = \tau_s = \tau_H$ = Shear stress of shaft material $\qquad \qquad$ (material is same)

$\quad \rho$ = Density of shaft material

$\quad T_H, T_s$ = Torque transmitted by hollow shaft and solid shaft respectively

$\quad W_H, W_s$ = Weight of hollow shaft and solid shaft respectively

For a hollow shaft, $\qquad T_H = \left(\dfrac{\pi}{16}\right) d_o^3 \tau (1 - K^4) \qquad \qquad \text{... Eq. (i)}$

For a solid shaft substituting $K = 0$ and $d_o = d$, in Eq. (i), we have

$$T_s = \left(\frac{\pi}{16}\right) d^3 \tau \qquad \qquad \text{... Eq. (ii)}$$

Since the material is equally strong in torsion, equating Eq. (ii) and Eq. (i) yields

$$T_H = T_s$$

$$\left(\frac{\pi}{16}\right) d_o^3 \tau (1 - K^4) = \left(\frac{\pi}{16}\right) d^3 \tau$$

$$d_o^3 (1 - K^4) = d^3$$

$$d_o^3 \left(1 - \frac{d_i^4}{d_o^4}\right) = d^3$$

$$\left(d_o^3 - \frac{d_i^4}{d_o}\right) = d^3$$

$$\frac{d_o^4 - d_i^4}{d_o} = d^3$$

$$\therefore \quad d_i^4 = d_o^4 - d^3 d_o \qquad \qquad \text{... Eq. (iii)}$$

Also,

$$W_H = 0.7 \, W_s$$
$$\rho A_H L = 0.7 \, \rho A_s L$$
$$A_H = 0.7 A_s$$

$$\frac{\pi\left(d_o^2 - d_i^2\right)}{4} = 0.7\left(\frac{\pi d^2}{4}\right)$$

$$\left(d_o^2 - d_i^2\right) = 0.7 d^2$$

$$d_i^2 = d_o^2 - 0.7 d^2$$

Squaring both sides, we have

$$\therefore \quad d_i^4 = \left(d_o^2 - 0.7 d^2\right)^2 \qquad \qquad \text{... Eq. (iv)}$$

Equating Eqs (iii) and (iv), we have

$$d_o^4 - d^3 d_o = \left(d_o^2 - 0.7 d^2\right)^2$$

$$= d_o^4 + 0.49 d^4 - 1.4 d_o^2 d^2$$

i.e. $$(1.4 d^2)\, d_o^2 - (d^3)\, d_o - 0.49 d^4 = 0$$

$$(1.4 \times 250^2)\, d_o^2 - 250^3 d_o - (0.49 \times 250^4) = 0$$

$$87500 \, d_o^2 - (15.625 \times 10^6) d_o - 1.914 \times 10^9 = 0$$

This is a quadratic equation, having $a = 87500$, $b = -15.625 \times 10^6$ and $c = -1.914 \times 10^9$
Thus the roots are $d_o = 262$ mm, -83.48 mm
$\therefore$ Standard size of shaft, $\quad d_o = 262$ mm

Eq. (iii) yields... $\quad d_i^4 = 262^4 - (250^3 \times 262)$

$$\therefore \quad d_i = 157.68 \text{ mm}$$

37. **Determine the diameter of a solid circular shaft to transmit a power of 50 kW at a rated speed of 1000 rpm. The maximum allowable shear stress for the material is 75 MPa. Replace this solid shaft by a hollow circular shaft assuming the value of 0.6 for the ratio of diameters. As the consequences of this replacement, determine:**

   (a) Percentage of reduction in weight assuming same length for the shafts.

   (b) The ratio of torsional strengths of the hollow shaft to that of the solid shaft.

Solution: $P = 50$ kW, $N = 1000$ rpm, $\tau = 75$ MPa, $K = 0.6$. a) $d = ?$, b) $d_o, d_i = ?$ c) Percentage saving in weight = ? d) $T_H/T_s = ?$

Torque transmitted:

We know that
$$P = \frac{2\pi NT}{60}$$

$$50 \times 10^3 = \frac{2\pi \times 1000 \times T}{60}$$

$$T = 477.46 \text{ N-m} = 477.46 \times 10^3 \text{ N-mm}$$

a. *Diameter of solid shaft:*

Strength of a solid shaft, $\quad T = \left(\dfrac{\pi d^3}{16}\right)\tau$

$$477.46 \times 10^3 = \left(\frac{\pi d^3}{16}\right) \times 75$$

$$d = 31.88 \text{ mm} \approx 32 \text{ mm}$$

b. *Diameter of hollow shaft:*

Strength of a hollow shaft, $\quad T = \left[\dfrac{\pi}{16}\left(\dfrac{d_o^4 - d_i^4}{d_o}\right)\right]\tau = \dfrac{\pi}{16}d_o^3(1 - K^4)\tau$

$$477.46 \times 10^3 = \left(\frac{\pi}{16}\right)d_o^3 \times [(1 - 0.6^4)] \times 75$$

$$d_o = 33.40 \text{ mm} \approx 34 \text{ mm}$$

and
$$d_i = 0.6 \times 34 = 20.04 \text{ mm}$$

c. *Percentage saving in weight:*

Percentage saving in weight $= \left(1 - \dfrac{W_H}{W_s}\right) \times 100 \qquad\qquad$ (where $W = \rho AL$)

Since the material is same, cancelling the common terms, we have

$$= \left(1 - \frac{A_H}{A_s}\right) \times 100$$

$$= \left(1 - \frac{d_o^2(1 - K^2)}{d^2}\right) \times 100$$

$$= \left(1 - \frac{34^2(1 - 0.6^2)}{32^2}\right) \times 100$$

$\therefore$ Percentage saving in weight = 27.75 %

d. *The ratio of torsional strengths of the hollow shaft to that of the solid shaft*

We know that
$$\frac{T_H}{T_s} = \frac{d_o^3(1-K^4)}{d^3}$$

$$= \frac{34^2(1-0.6^2)}{32^2}$$

$$\therefore \quad \frac{T_H}{T_s} = 0.7225$$

38. **A solid shaft is of 50 mm diameter. Determine the diameters of a hollow shaft such that its area of cross section is same as that of solid shaft. The inner diameter of hollow one is 0.6 times outer diameter. Compare the torsional strengths and torsional stiffness of the hollow and solid shafts, the length material being same in both cases.**

VTU – Dec. 13/ Jan. 14 – 08 Marks

Solution: $d = 50$ mm, $A_H = A_s$, $d_i = 0.6\, d_o \Rightarrow K = \dfrac{d_i}{d_o} = 0.6$. a) $T_H/T_s = ?$ b) $S_H/S_s = ?$

Given
$$A_H = A_s$$
$$d_o^2 - d_i^2 = d^2$$
$$d_o^2 (1 - K^2) = d^2$$
$$d_o^2 (1 - 0.6^2) = 50^2$$
$$d_o^2 = 3906.25$$
$$\therefore \quad d_o = 62.5 \text{ mm} \approx 64 \text{ mm}$$

a. *Comparison of torsional strength:*

$$\frac{T_H}{T_s} = \frac{d_o^4(1-K^4)}{d^3} = \frac{64^3(1-0.6^4)}{50^3} = 1.8254$$

b. *Comparison of torsional stiffness:*

$$\frac{S_H}{S_s} = \frac{d_o^4(1-K^4)}{d^4} = \frac{64^3(1-0.6^4)}{50^4} = 2.3365$$

39. **A hollow shaft of 250 mm outer diameter has the same area as that of solid shaft of 150 mm diameter. Compare:**
   (a) Power transmitted by the above shafts for the same speed.
   (b) Compare angle of twist of them for the same length and same material.

VTU – Dec. 13/ Jan. 14 – 10 Marks

Solution: $d_o = 250$ mm, $A_H = A_s$, $d = 150$ mm. a) $P_H/P_s = ?$, if $N_s = N_H$, b) $\theta_H/\theta_s = ?$, if $\tau_s = \tau_H$, $L_s = L_H$

Given
$$A_H = A_s$$
$$d_o^2 - d_i^2 = d^2$$
$$250^2 - d_i^2 = 150^2$$
$$d_i = 200 \text{ mm}$$

And
$$K = \frac{d_i}{d_o} = \frac{200}{250} = 0.8$$

a. *Ratio of power transmitted:*

$$\frac{P_H}{P_s} = \frac{(2\pi NT/60)_H}{(2\pi NT/60)s} = \frac{T_H}{T_s}$$

$$\frac{T_H}{T_s} = \frac{d_o^3(1-K^4)}{d^3} = \frac{250^3(1-0.8^4)}{150^3} = 2.7333$$

b. *Comparison of angle of twist:*

We know that
$$\frac{T}{J} = \frac{G\theta}{L} = \frac{\tau}{r}$$

$$\frac{G\theta}{L} = \frac{\tau}{r}$$

Since τ, G and L are constants, we have $\theta = \dfrac{1}{r}$

$$\frac{\theta_H}{\theta_s} = \frac{r_s}{r_H} = \frac{150}{250} = 0.6$$

Or
$$\frac{\theta_s}{\theta_H} = \frac{r_H}{r_s} = \frac{250}{150} = 1.667$$

Note: $\theta = \dfrac{TL}{GJ}$ can not be used, since $T_H \neq T_s$

40. A solid shaft is to transmit 192 kW at 450 rpm. Taking allowable stress for the shaft material as 70 MPa, find the diameter of the solid shaft. What percentage of saving in weight would be obtained, if this shaft were to be replaced by a hollow shaft, whose internal diameter is 0.8 times its external diameter? The length of the shaft, power to be transmitted and speed are equal in both cases.

VTU – June/ July 2011 – 10 Marks

Solution: $P = 192 \times 10^3$ W, $N = 450$ rpm, $\tau = 70$ MPa, $K = 0.8$. a) $d = ?$, b) Percentage saving in weight = ?, if $P_H = P_s$, $L_H = L_s$, $N_H = N_s$
Torque transmitted:

We know that
$$P = \frac{2\pi NT}{60}$$

$$192 \times 10^3 = \frac{2\pi \times 450 \times T}{60}$$

$$T = 4074.37 \text{ N-m} = 4074.37 \times 10^3 \text{ N-mm}$$

a. *Diameter of solid shaft:*

Strength of a solid shaft,
$$T = \left(\frac{\pi d^3}{16}\right)\tau$$

$$4074.37 \times 10^3 = \left(\frac{\pi d^3}{16}\right) \times 70$$

$$d = 66.67 \text{ mm} \approx 68 \text{ mm}$$

b. *Percentage saving in weight:*

$$\text{Percentage saving in weight} = \left(1 - \frac{W_H}{A_s}\right) \times 100 \qquad \text{(where } W = \rho AL\text{)}$$

Since the material is same, cancelling the common terms, we have

$$= \left(1 - \frac{A_H}{A_s}\right) \times 100$$

$$\text{Percentage saving in weight} = \left[1 - \frac{d_o^2(1 - K^2)}{d^2}\right] \times 100 \qquad \ldots \text{Eq. (i)}$$

But
$$P_H = P_s$$
$$(2\pi NT/60)_H = (2\pi NT/60)_s$$
$$\therefore \qquad T_H = T_s$$
$$d_o^3 (1 - K^4) = d^3$$
$$d_o^3 (1 - 0.8^4) = 68^3$$
$$d_o = 81.05 \text{ mm} \simeq 81 \text{ mm}$$

$\therefore$ Eq. (i) yields...

$$\text{Percentage saving in weight} = \left[\frac{1 - 81^2 \times (1 - 0.8^2)}{68^2}\right] \times 100 = 48.92\,\%$$

41. **A solid circular shaft is to transmit 300 kW at 100 rpm. If the shear stress is not to exceed 80 MPa, find the diameter of the shaft. What percentage saving in weight would be obtained, if this shaft is replaced by a hollow one, whose internal diameter is equal to 0.8 of external diameter, the length, material and allowable maximum shear stress being same?**

Solution: $P = 300 \times 10^3$ W, $N = 100$ rpm, $\tau = 80$ MPa, $K = 0.8$. a) $d = ?$, b) Percentage saving in weight = ?, if $L_H = L_s$, $T_H = T_s$.
Torque transmitted:

We know that
$$P = \frac{2\pi NT}{60}$$

$$300 \times 10^3 = \frac{2\pi \times 100 \times T}{60}$$

$$T = 28647.89 \text{ N-m} = 28647.89 \times 10^3 \text{ N-mm}$$

a. *Diameter of solid shaft:*

Strength of a solid shaft,
$$T = \left(\frac{\pi d^3}{16}\right)\tau$$

$$28647.89 \times 10^3 = \left(\frac{\pi d^3}{16}\right) \times 80$$

$$d = 122.18 \text{ mm} \approx 125 \text{ mm}$$

b. *Percentage saving in weight:*

$$\text{Percentage saving in weight} = \left(1 - \frac{W_H}{A_s}\right) \times 100 \qquad (\text{where } W = \rho AL)$$

Since the material is same, cancelling the common terms, we have

$$= \left(1 - \frac{A_H}{A_s}\right) \times 100$$

$$\text{Percentage saving in weight} = \left[1 - \frac{d_o^2(1 - K^2)}{d^2}\right] \qquad \dots \text{Eq. (i)}$$

But
$$T_H = T_s$$

$$d_o^3(1 - K^4) = d^3$$

$$d_o^3(1 - 0.8^4) = 125^3$$

$$d_o = 149 \text{ mm} \approx 150 \text{ mm}$$

$\therefore$ Eq. (i) yields…

$$\text{Percentage saving in weight} = \left[\frac{1 - 150^2 \times (1 - 0.8^2)}{125^2}\right] \times 100 = 48.16\,\%$$

42. A solid shaft transmits 250 kW at 100 rpm. If the shear stress is not to exceed 75 MPa, what should be the diameter of the shaft? If this shaft is replaced by a hollow shaft, whose diameter ratio is 0.6, determine the size and percentage saving in weight, the maximum shear stress being the same.

VTU – May/ June 2010 – 14 Marks; [Civil: June/ July 2016 – 10 Marks; Dec. 2012 – 10 Marks; June/ July 2008 – 12 Marks]

Solution: $P = 250 \times 10^3$ W, $N = 100$ rpm, $\tau = 75$ MPa, $K = 0.6$. a) $d = ?$, b) Percentage saving in weight = ?, $T_H = T_s$.
Torque transmitted:

We know that
$$P = \frac{2\pi NT}{60}$$

$$250 \times 10^3 = \frac{2\pi \times 100 \times T}{60}$$

$$T = 23873.24 \text{ N-m} = 23873.24 \times 10^3 \text{ N-mm}$$

a. *Diameter of solid shaft:*

Strength of a solid shaft,
$$T = \left(\frac{\pi d^3}{16}\right)\tau$$

$$23873.24 \times 10^3 = \left(\frac{\pi d^3}{16}\right) \times 75$$

$$d = 117.47 \text{ mm} \approx 118 \text{ mm}$$

b. *Percentage saving in weight:*

$$\text{Percentage saving in weight} = \left(1 - \frac{W_H}{A_s}\right) \times 100 \qquad \text{(where } W = \rho AL)$$

Since the material is same, cancelling the common terms, we have

$$= \left(1 - \frac{A_H}{A_s}\right) \times 100$$

$$\text{Percentage saving in weight} = \left[1 - \frac{d_o^2(1 - K^2)}{d^2}\right] \times 100 \qquad \qquad \dots \text{Eq. (i)}$$

But $\qquad\qquad\qquad T_H = T_s \qquad\qquad\qquad$ (Since the material is same)

$$d_o^3(1 - K^4) = d^3$$

$$d_o^3(1 - 0.6^4) = 118^3$$

$$d_o = 123.58 \text{ mm} \approx 124 \text{ mm}$$

$\therefore \quad$ Eq. (i) yields ...

$$\text{Percentage saving in weight} = \left[\frac{1 - 124^2 \times (1 - 0.6)^2}{118^2}\right] \times 100 = 29.33\,\%$$

43. **A solid shaft is to transmit 340 kN-m at 120 rpm. If the shear stress of the material should not exceed 80 MPa, find the diameter required. What percentage saving in weight would be obtained if this shaft is to be replaced by a hollow one whose $d_i = 0.6d_o$, the length, material and shear stress remaining same.**

VTU – June - July 2015 – 10 Marks

Solution: $T = 340 \times 10^6$ N-mm, $N = 120$ rpm, $\tau = 80$ MPa, $d_i = 0.6d_o \Rightarrow K = \dfrac{d_i}{d_o} = 0.6$.

a) $d = ?$, b) Percentage saving in weight $= ?$, $T_H = T_s$.

a. *Diameter of solid shaft:*

Strength of a solid shaft, $\qquad T = \left(\dfrac{\pi d^3}{16}\right)\tau$

$$340 \times 10^6 = \left(\frac{\pi d^3}{16}\right) \times 80$$

$$d = 278.69 \text{ mm} \approx 280 \text{ mm}$$

b. *Percentage saving in weight:*

$$\text{Percentage saving in weight} \left(1 - \frac{W_H}{A_s}\right) \times 100 \qquad \text{(where } W = \rho AL)$$

Since the material is same, cancelling the common terms, we have

$$= \left(1 - \frac{A_H}{A_s}\right) \times 100$$

$$\text{Percentage saving in weight} = \left[1 - \frac{d_o^2(1 - K^2)}{d^2}\right] \times 100 \qquad \qquad \text{... Eq. (i)}$$

$$\text{But} \qquad \qquad T_H = T_s \qquad \qquad \text{(Since the material is same)}$$

$$d_o^3(1 - K^4) = d^3$$

$$d_o^3(1 - 0.6^4) = 280^3$$

$$d_o = 293.26 \text{ mm} \approx 295 \text{ mm}$$

$\therefore$ Eq. (i) yields...

$$\text{Percentage saving in weight} = \left[\frac{1 - 295^2 \times (1 - 0.6^2)}{118^2}\right] \times 100 = 28.96\,\%$$

44. **A solid circular shaft has to transmit power of 1000 kW at 120 rpm. Find the diameter of the shaft if the shear stress must not exceed 80 MPa. Maximum torque is 1.25 times the mean, what percentage in material could be obtained if the shaft is replaced by a hollow shaft, whose inner diameter is 0.6 times the external diameter. The length of the material and maximum shear stress being same.**

> *VTU – Dec. 14/ Jan. 15 – 12 Marks; [Similar: (CV) Jan. 2013 – 12 Marks]*

Solution: $P = 1000 \times 10^3$ W, $N = 120$ rpm, $\tau = 80$ MPa, $T_{max} = 1.25\,T$, $K = 0.6$. a) $d = ?$, b) Percentage saving in weight = ?, $L_H = L_s$, $T_H = T_s$
Torque transmitted:

$$\text{Given} \qquad \qquad T_{max} = 1.25\,T \qquad \qquad \text{... Eq. (i)}$$

$$\text{But} \qquad \qquad P = \frac{2\pi NT}{60}$$

$$1000 \times 10^3 = \frac{2\pi \times 120 \times T}{60}$$

$$T = 79.58 \times 10^3 \text{ N-m} = 79.58 \times 10^6 \text{ N-mm}$$

Eq. (i) yields... $\qquad T_{max} = 1.25 \times (79.58 \times 10^6) = 99.48 \times 10^6$ N-mm

a. *Diameter of shaft:*

Strength of a solid shaft, $T_{max} = \left(\dfrac{\pi d^3}{16}\right)\tau$

$$99.48 \times 10^6 = \left(\frac{\pi d^3}{16}\right) \times 80$$

$$d = 185.01 \text{ mm} \approx 185 \text{ mm}$$

b. *Percentage saving in weight:*

$$\text{Percentage saving in weight} = \left(1 - \frac{W_H}{A_s}\right) \times 100 \qquad \qquad \text{(where } W = \rho AL)$$

Since the material is same, cancelling the common terms, we have

$$= \left(1 - \frac{A_H}{A_s}\right) \times 100$$

$$\text{Percentage saving in weight} = \left[1 - \frac{d_o^2(1 - K^2)}{d^2}\right] \times 100 \qquad \qquad \text{... Eq. (i)}$$

But
$$T_H = T_s \qquad\qquad \text{(Since the material is same)}$$

$$d_o^3\,(1 - K^4) = d^3$$

$$d_o^3\,(1 - 0.6^4) = 185^3$$

$$d_o = 193.76 \text{ mm} \approx 195 \text{ mm}$$

$\therefore$ Eq. (i) yields ...

$$\text{Percentage saving in weight} = \left[\frac{1 - 195^2 \times (1 - 0.6^2)}{185^2}\right] \times 100 = 28.89\ \%$$

9.9 COMPOSITE OR STEPPED SHAFTS OR SHAFTS OF VARYING DIAMETERS

If two or more shafts are connected together, they form a composite shaft. The shafts connected together may be of different materials and of different cross sections. Shafts can be joined in two ways:
   a. Shafts in series
   b. Shafts in parallel.

9.9.1 Shafts in series (common torque)

Shafts are said to be connected in series if the driving torque is applied at one end and the resisting torque at the other end, as shown in **Fig. 9.2**. Here each shaft transmits the same torque and the total angle of twist is the sum of angle of twists of individual shafts connected together.

i.e. $T = T_1 = T_2$ and $\theta = \theta_1 + \theta_2$ $\qquad\qquad$ ... (Eq. 9.16)

Here the composite shaft is analyzed by applying torsion theory to each of the component shafts.

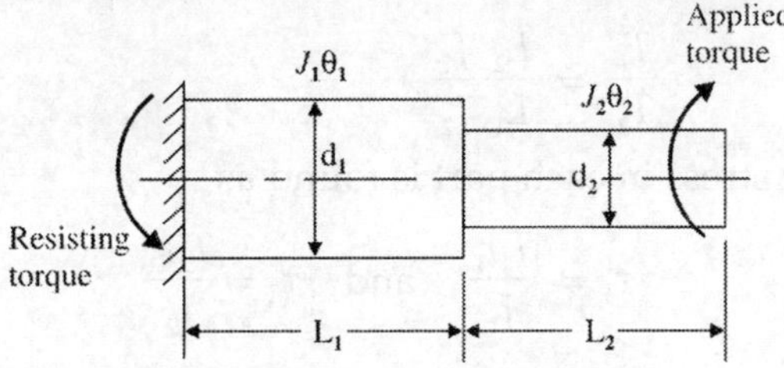

Fig. 9.2: Shafts in series

From torsional equation, we have

$$\theta = \frac{TL}{GJ}$$

Total angle of twist,

$$\theta = \theta_1 + \theta_2 = \frac{TL_1}{G_1J_1} + \frac{TL_2}{G_2J_2}$$

$$\theta = T\left[\frac{L_1}{G_1J_1} + \frac{L_2}{G_2J_2}\right] \qquad\qquad \text{... (Eq. 9.17a)}$$

If both shafts are made of same material, then $G_1 = G_2 = G$

$$\theta = \frac{T}{G}\left[\frac{L_1}{J_1} + \frac{L_2}{J_2}\right] \qquad \text{... (Eq. 9.17b)}$$

9.9.2 Shafts in parallel (shared torque)

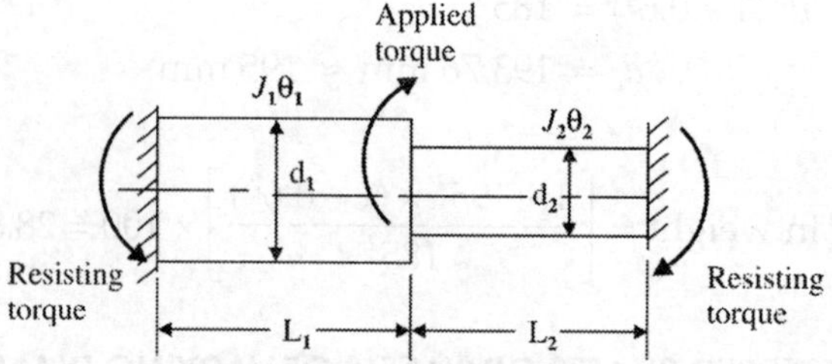

Fig. 9.3: Shafts in parallel

Shafts are said to be connected in parallel if the driving torque is applied at the junction of the two shafts connected together and the resisting torques at the other ends of the two shafts, as shown in **Fig. 9.3**. Here the angle of twist is same for each shaft but the torque applied is divided between the two shafts.

i.e. $\qquad\qquad T = T_1 + T_2 \quad$ and $\quad \theta = \theta_1 = \theta_2$ or $\Sigma\theta = 0$ ... (Eq. 9.18)

For parallel shafts, $\theta_1 = \theta_2$

$$\frac{T_1 L_1}{G_1 J_1} = \frac{T_2 L_2}{G_2 J_2} \qquad \text{... (Eq. 9.19a)}$$

If both shafts are made of same material, then $G_1 = G_2 = G$

$$\frac{T_1 L_1}{J_1} = \frac{T_2 L_2}{J_2} \qquad \text{... (Eq. 9.19b)}$$

Or

$$\frac{T_1}{T_2} = \frac{L_2}{L_1}\frac{J_1}{J_2} \qquad \text{... (Eq. 9.19c)}$$

The maximum shear stress in each part is found as

$$\tau_1 = \frac{T_1 r_1}{J_1} \quad \text{and} \quad \tau_2 = \frac{T_2 r_2}{J_2} \qquad \text{... (Eq. 9.19d)}$$

PROBLEMS ON SERIES SHAFTS – KNOWN TORQUE

45. Determine the angle of twist at free end for the stepped shaft shown in Fig. 9.4(a). The modulus of rigidity is 80 GPa.

Solution: $d_{AB} = 30$ mm, $d_{BC} = 60$ mm, $L_{AB} = 400$ mm, $L_{BC} = 800$ mm, $T_1 = 250$ N-m, $T_2 = 1000$ N-m, $G = 80 \times 10^3$ MPa. $\theta = ?$

The free-body diagram of the system is shown in **Fig. 9.4(b)**.

Assume that clockwise torques/moments are negative and counterclockwise torques/moments are positive.

Shaft AB: $\Sigma M = 0: T_{AB} - 250 = 0 \qquad \Rightarrow T_{AB} = 250$ N-m $= 250 \times 10^3$ N-mm

Shaft BC: $\Sigma M = 0: T_{BC} - 1000 - 250 = 0 \qquad \Rightarrow T_{BC} = 1250$ N-m $= 1250 \times 10^3$ N-mm

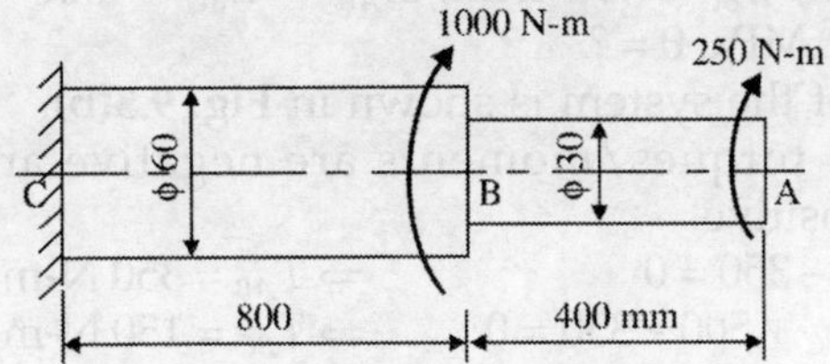

Fig. 9.4(a): Problem 45

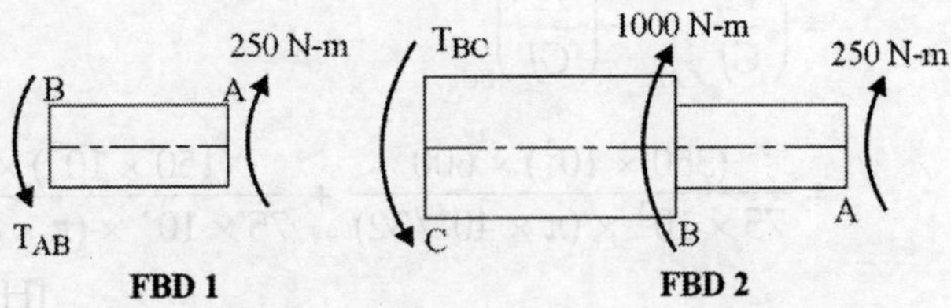

Fig. 9.4(b): Problem 45: Free body diagrams

Total angle of twist:

$$\theta = \theta_{AB} + \theta_{BC}$$

$$= \left(\frac{TL}{GJ}\right)_{AB} + \left(\frac{TL}{GJ}\right)_{BC}$$

$$= \frac{(250 \times 10^3) \times 400}{80 \times 10^3 \times (\pi \times 30^4/32)} + \frac{(1250 \times 10^3) \times 800}{80 \times 10^3 \times (\pi \times 60^4/32)}$$

$$= 0.0157 + 0.0098$$

$$\theta = 0.0255 \text{ rad} = 1.464°$$

46. Determine the angle of twist at the free end for the stepped shaft shown in Fig. 9.5(a). The modulus of rigidity is 75 GPa.

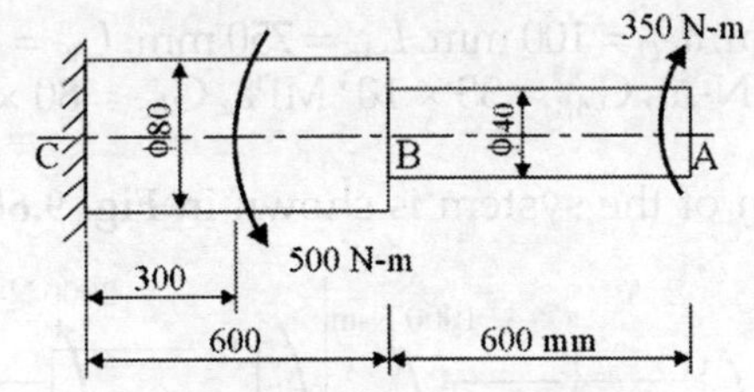

Fig. 9.5(a): Problem 46

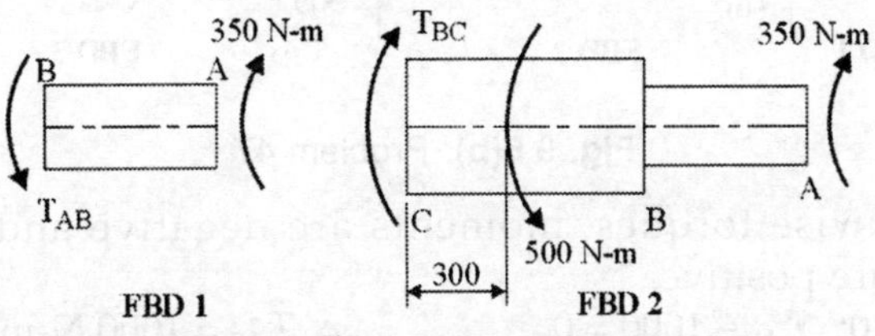

Fig. 9.5(b): Problem 46: Free body diagrams

Solution: $d_{AB} = 40$ mm, $d_{BC} = 80$ mm, $L_{AB} = L_{BC} = 600$ mm, $T_1 = 350$ N-m, $T_2 = 500$ N-m, $G = 75 \times 10^3$ MPa. $\theta = ?$

The free-body diagram of the system is shown in **Fig. 9.5(b)**.

Assume that clockwise torques/moments are negative and counterclockwise torques/moments are positive.

Shaft AB: $\Sigma M = 0$: $T_{AB} - 350 = 0$ $\Rightarrow T_{AB} = 350$ N-m $= 350 \times 10^3$ N-mm

Shaft BC: $\Sigma M = 0$: $-T_{BC} + 500 - 350 = 0$ $\Rightarrow T_{BC} = 150$ N-m $= 150 \times 10^3$ N-mm

Total angle of twist:

$$\theta = \theta_{AB} + \theta_{BC}$$

$$= \left(\frac{TL}{GJ}\right)_{AB} + \left(\frac{TL}{GJ}\right)_{BC}$$

$$= \frac{(350 \times 10^3) \times 600}{75 \times 10^3 \times (\pi \times 40^4/32)} + \frac{(150 \times 10^3) \times 300}{75 \times 10^3 \times (\pi \times 80^4/32)}$$

[Here $L_{BC} = 300$ mm]

$$= 0.0111 + 0.0001$$
$$\theta = 0.0112 \text{ rad} = 0.642°$$

47. **Fig. 9.6(a) represents a compound shaft made of three different materials. The modulus of rigidity is 28 GPa for aluminum, 80 GPa for steel, and 35 GPa for bronze. Find the angle of rotation at the free end of the shaft. Also calculate the maximum shear stress in each material.**

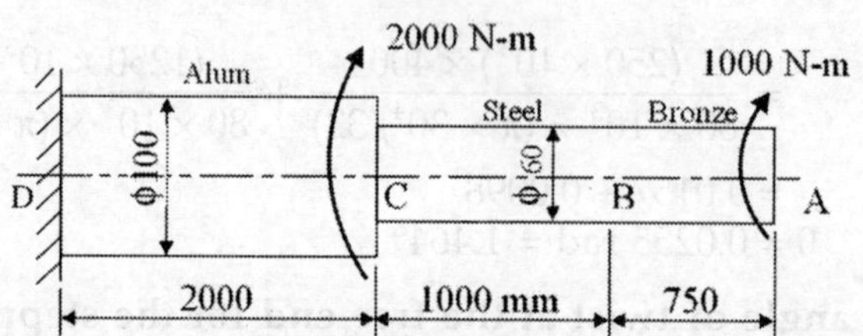

Fig. 9.6(a): Problem 47

Solution: $d_{AB} = d_{BC} = 60$ mm, $d_{CD} = 100$ mm, $L_{AB} = 750$ mm, $L_{BC} = 1000$ mm, $L_{CD} = 2000$ mm, $T_1 = 1000$ N-m, $T_2 = 2000$ N-m, $G_{AB} = 35 \times 10^3$ MPa, $G_{BC} = 80 \times 10^3$ MPa, $G_{CD} = 28 \times 10^3$ MPa. a) $\theta = ?$ b) $\tau = ?$

The free-body diagram of the system is shown in **Fig. 9.6(b)**.

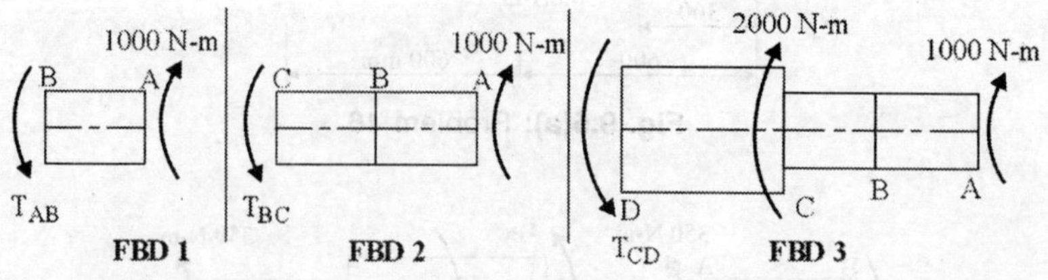

Fig. 9.6(b): Problem 47

Assume that clockwise torques/moments are negative and counterclockwise torques/moments are positive.

Shaft AB: $\Sigma M = 0$: $T_{AB} - 1000 = 0$ $\Rightarrow T_{AB} = 1000$ N-m $= 1000 \times 10^3$ N-mm

Shaft BC: $\Sigma M = 0$: $T_{BC} - 1000 = 0$ $\Rightarrow T_{BC} = 1000$ N-m $= 1000 \times 10^3$ N-mm

Shaft CD: $\Sigma M = 0$: $T_{CD} - 2000 - 1000 = 0$ $\Rightarrow T_{CD} = 3000$ N-m $= 3000 \times 10^3$ N-mm

a. *Total angle of twist:*

$$\theta = \sum\left(\frac{TL}{GJ}\right) = \left(\frac{TL}{GJ}\right)_{AB} + \left(\frac{TL}{GJ}\right)_{BC} + \left(\frac{TL}{GJ}\right)_{CD}$$

$$= \frac{(1000 \times 10^3) \times 750}{35 \times 10^3 \times (\pi \times 60^4/32)} + \frac{(1000 \times 10^3) \times 1000}{80 \times 10^3 \times (\pi \times 60^4/32)}$$

$$+ \frac{(3000 \times 10^3) \times 2000}{28 \times 10^3 \times (\pi \times 100^4/32)}$$

$$= 0.0168 + 0.0098 + 0.0218$$
$$\theta = 0.04842 \text{ rad} = 2.773°$$

b. *Shear stress:*

For a solid shaft, $\tau = \dfrac{16T}{\pi d^3}$

$$\tau_{AB} = \left(\frac{16T}{\pi d^3}\right)_{AB} = \left(\frac{16 \times 1000 \times 10^3}{\pi \times 60^3}\right) = 23.57 \text{ MPa}$$

$$\tau_{BC} = \left(\frac{16T}{\pi d^3}\right)_{BC} = \left(\frac{16 \times 1000 \times 10^3}{\pi \times 60^3}\right) = 23.57 \text{ MPa}$$

$$\tau_{CD} = \left(\frac{16T}{\pi d^3}\right)_{CD} = \left(\frac{16 \times 3000 \times 10^3}{\pi \times 100^3}\right) = 15.28 \text{ MPa}$$

48. Determine the angle of rotation at free end of a stepped shaft shown in Fig. 9.7(a).
   Take $G = 80$ GPa

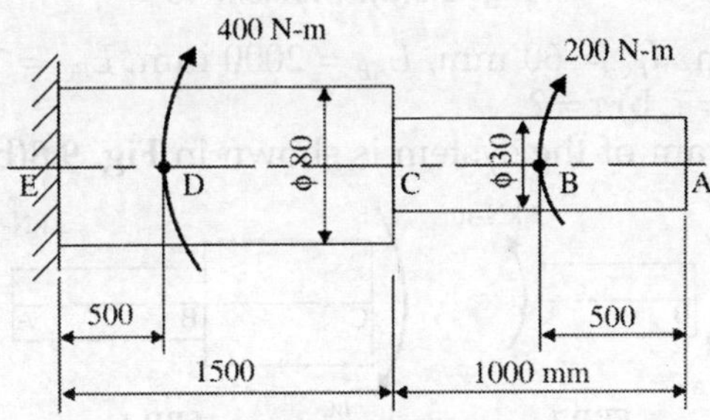

Fig. 9.7(a): Problem 48

Solution: $d_{AB} = d_{BC} = 30$ mm, $d_{CD} = d_{DE} = 80$ mm, $L_{AB} = 500$ mm, $L_{BC} = 500$ mm, $L_{CD} = 1000$ mm, $L_{DE} = 500$ mm, $T_1 = 200$ N-m, $T_2 = 400$ N-m, $G = 80 \times 10^3$ MPa. $\theta = ?$
The free-body diagram of the system is shown in **Fig. 9.7(b)**.

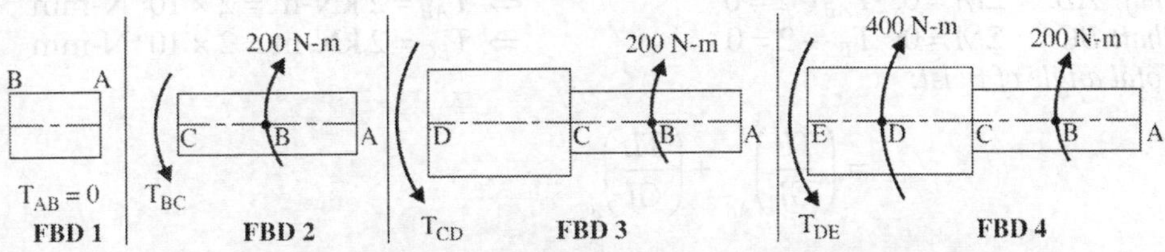

Fig. 9.7(b): Problem 48: Free body diagrams

Assume that clockwise torques/moments are negative and counterclockwise torques/moments are positive.

Shaft AB: $\Sigma M = 0$: $T_{AB} = 0$

Shaft BC: $\Sigma M = 0$: $T_{BC} - 200 = 0$ $\Rightarrow T_{BC} = 200$ N-m $= 200 \times 10^3$ N-mm

Shaft CD: $\Sigma M = 0$: $T_{CD} - 200 = 0$ $\Rightarrow T_{CD} = 200$ N-m $= 200 \times 10^3$ N-mm

Shaft DE: $\Sigma M = 0$: $T_{DE} - 400 - 200 = 0$ $\Rightarrow T_{DE} = 600$ N-m $= 600 \times 10^3$ N-mm

Total angle of twist:

$$\theta = \sum \left(\frac{TL}{GJ}\right) = \left(\frac{TL}{GJ}\right)_{AB} + \left(\frac{TL}{GJ}\right)_{BC} + \left(\frac{TL}{GJ}\right)_{CD} + \left(\frac{TL}{GJ}\right)_{DE}$$

$$= \frac{(200 \times 10^3) \times 500}{80 \times 10^3 \times (\pi \times 30^4/32)} + \frac{(200 \times 10^3) \times 1000}{80 \times 10^3 \times (\pi \times 80^4/32)}$$

$$+ \frac{(600 \times 10^3) \times 500}{80 \times 10^3 \times (\pi \times 80^4/32)}$$

$$= 0.0157 + 0.0006 + 0.0009$$

$$\theta = 0.0172 \text{ rad} = 0.985°$$

49. Two shafts are connected in series as shown in Fig. 9.8(a). Determine the total angle of twist and the shear stress induced in each shaft. Take $G = 85$ GPa

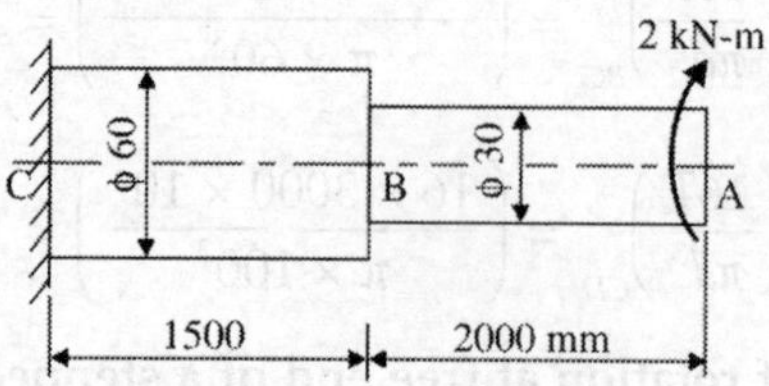

Fig. 9.8(a): Problem 49

Solution: $d_{AB} = 30$ mm, $d_{BC} = 60$ mm, $L_{AB} = 2000$ mm, $L_{BC} = 1500$ mm, $T = 2$ kN-m, $G = 85 \times 10^3$ MPa. a) $\theta = ?$, b) $\tau = ?$

The free-body diagram of the system is shown in **Fig. 9.8(b)**.

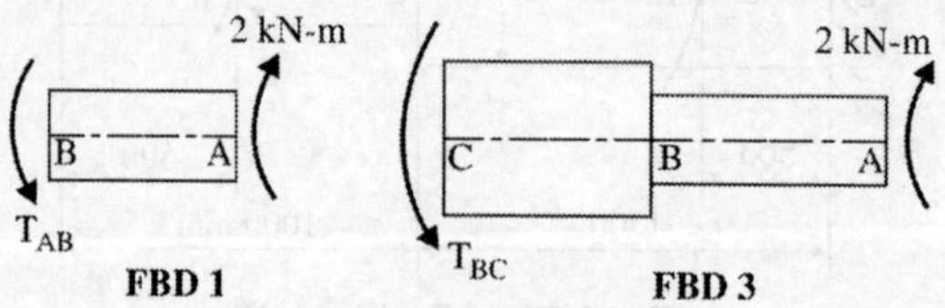

Fig. 9.8(b): Problem 49: Free body diagrams

Assume that clockwise torques/moments are negative and counterclockwise torques/moments are positive.

Shaft AB: $\Sigma M = 0$: $T_{AB} - 2 = 0$ $\Rightarrow T_{AB} = 2$ kN-m $= 2 \times 10^6$ N-mm

Shaft BC: $\Sigma M = 0$: $T_{BC} - 2 = 0$ $\Rightarrow T_{BC} = 2$ kN-m $= 2 \times 10^6$ N-mm

a. *Total angle of twist:*

$$= \left(\frac{TL}{GJ}\right)_{AB} + \left(\frac{TL}{GJ}\right)_{BC}$$

$$= \frac{(2 \times 10^6) \times 2000}{85 \times 10^3 \times (\pi \times 30^4/32)} + \frac{(2 \times 10^6) \times 1500}{85 \times 10^3 \times (\pi \times 60^4/32)}$$

$$= 0.5918 + 0.0277$$

$$\theta = 0.6195 \text{ rad} = 35.5°$$

b. *Shear stress:*

For a solid shaft, $\qquad \tau_{AB} = \left(\dfrac{16T}{\pi d^3}\right)_{AB} = \left(\dfrac{16 \times 2 \times 10^6}{\pi \times 30^3}\right) = 377.26 \text{ MPa}$

$$\tau_{BC} = \left(\frac{16T}{\pi d^3}\right)_{BC} = \left(\frac{16 \times 2 \times 10^6}{\pi \times 30^3}\right) = 47.16 \text{ MPa}$$

50. A stepped shaft ABCD is subjected to torques, as shown in Fig. 9.9(a). AB is made of aluminium having modulus of rigidity of 28 GPa while BD is made of steel having modulus of rigidity of 80 GPa. Find the angle of rotation at the free end of the shaft. Also calculate the maximum shear stress in each material.

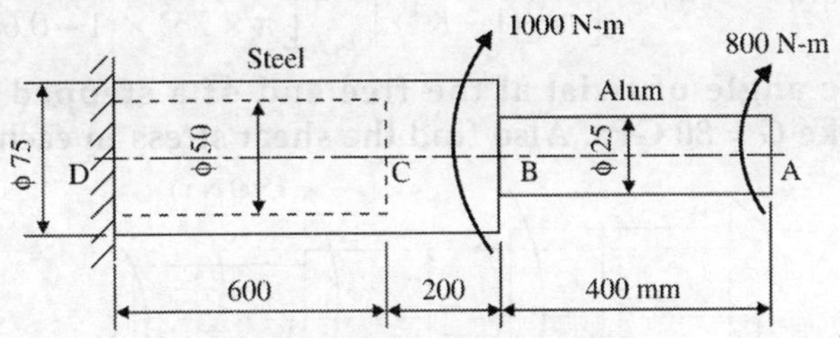

Fig. 9.9(a): Problem 50

Solution: $d_{AB} = 25$ mm, $d_{BC} = 75$ mm, $d_{CD} = 50$ mm, $\Rightarrow K = \dfrac{d_i}{d_o} = \dfrac{50}{75} = 0.667$, $L_{AB} = 400$ mm,

$L_{BC} = 200$ mm, $L_{CD} = 600$ mm, $T_1 = 800$ N-m, $T_2 = 1000$ N-m, $G_{AB} = 28 \times 10^3$ MPa, $G_{BC} = G_{CD} = 80 \times 10^3$ MPa. a) $\theta = ?$, b) $\tau = ?$

The free-body diagram of the system is shown in **Fig. 9.9(b)**.

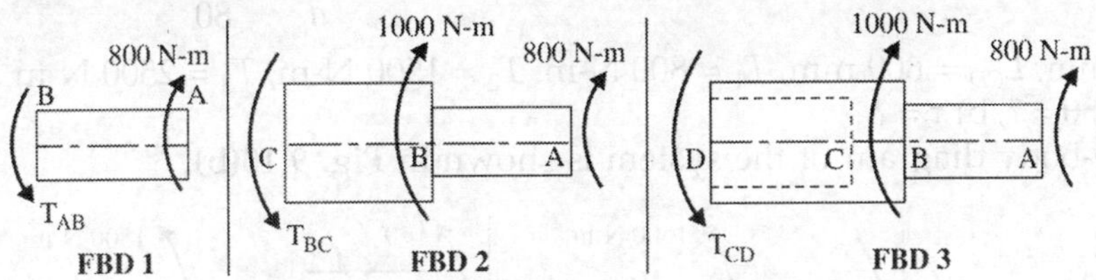

Fig. 9.9(b): Problem 49: Free body diagrams

Assume that clockwise torques/moments are negative and counterclockwise torques/moments are positive.

Shaft AB: $\quad \Sigma M = 0$: $T_{AB} - 800 = 0 \qquad\qquad \Rightarrow T_{AB} = 800$ N-m $= 800 \times 10^3$ N-mm

Shaft BC: $\quad \Sigma M = 0$: $T_{BC} - 1000 - 800 = 0 \qquad \Rightarrow T_{BC} = 1800$ N-m $= 1800 \times 10^3$ N-mm

Shaft CD: $\quad \Sigma M = 0$: $T_{CD} - 1000 - 800 = 0 \qquad \Rightarrow T_{CD} = 1800$ N-m $= 1800 \times 10^3$ N-mm

a. *Total angle of twist:*

$$\theta = \sum \left(\frac{TL}{GJ}\right) = \left(\frac{TL}{GJ}\right)_{AB} + \left(\frac{TL}{GJ}\right)_{BC} + \left(\frac{TL}{GJ}\right)_{CD}$$

$$= \frac{(800 \times 10^3) \times 400}{28 \times 10^3 \times (\pi \times 25^4/32)} + \frac{(1800 \times 10^3) \times 200}{80 \times 10^3 \times (\pi \times 75^4/32)}$$

$$+ \frac{(1800 \times 10^3) \times 600}{28 \times 10^3 \times \left[\pi \times 75^4 \times (1 - 0.667^4)/32)\right]}$$

$$= 0.2980 + 0.0014 + 0.0054$$
$$\theta = 0.3048 \text{ rad} = 17.46°$$

b. *Shear stress:*

For a solid shaft, $\qquad \tau_{AB} = \left(\dfrac{16T}{\pi d^3}\right)_{AB} = \left(\dfrac{16 \times 800 \times 10^3}{\pi \times 25^3}\right) = 260.76 \text{ MPa}$

$$\tau_{BC} = \left(\frac{16T}{\pi d^3}\right)_{BC} = \left[\frac{16 \times 1800 \times 10^3}{\pi \times 25^3}\right] = 21.73 \text{ MPa}$$

For a hollow shaft, $\qquad \tau_{CD} = \left[\dfrac{16T}{\pi d_o^3(1-K^4)}\right]_{CD} = \left[\dfrac{16 \times 1800 \times 10^3}{\pi \times 75^3 \times (1 - 0.6674)}\right] = 27.09 \text{ MPa}$

51. Determine the angle of twist at the free end of a stepped shaft shown in Fig. 9.10(a). Take $G = 80$ GPa. Also find the shear stress in each shaft.

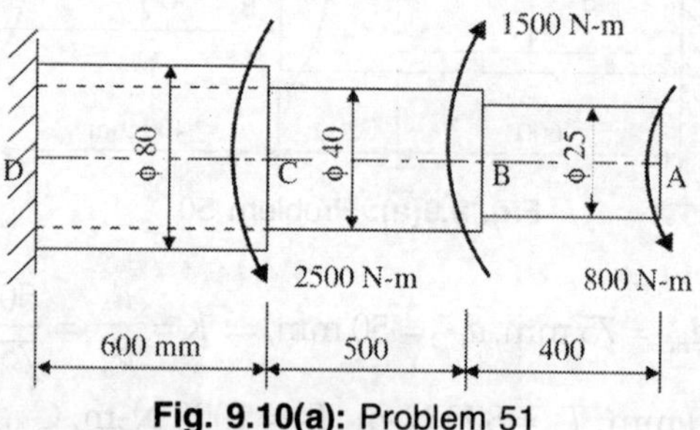

Fig. 9.10(a): Problem 51

Solution: $d_{AB} = 25$ mm, $d_{BC} = 40$ mm, $d_{CD} = 80$ mm, $\Rightarrow K = \dfrac{d_i}{d_o} = \dfrac{40}{80} = 0.5$, $L_{AB} = 400$ mm,

$L_{BC} = 500$ mm, $L_{CD} = 600$ mm, $T_1 = 800$ N-m, $T_2 = 1500$ N-m, $T_3 = 2500$ N-m, $G = 80 \times 10^3$ MPa. a) $\theta = ?$, b) $\tau = ?$

The free-body diagram of the system is shown in **Fig. 9.10(b)**.

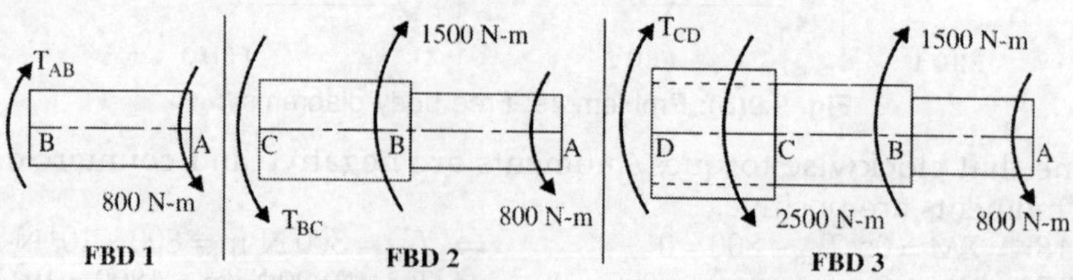

Fig. 9.10(b): Problem 51: Free body diagrams

Assume that clockwise torques/moments are negative and counterclockwise torques/moments are positive.

Shaft AB: $\quad \Sigma M = 0$: $\ -T_{AB} + 800 = 0 \qquad \Rightarrow T_{AB} = 800 \text{ N-m} = 800 \times 10^3 \text{ N-mm}$

Shaft BC: $\quad \Sigma M = 0$: $\ T_{BC} - 1500 + 800 = 0 \qquad \Rightarrow T_{BC} = 700 \text{ N-m} = 700 \times 10^3 \text{ N-mm}$

$$(CW, \textit{hence negative})$$

$$\text{Or} \qquad T_{BC} = -1500 + 800 \qquad \Rightarrow T_{BC} = -700 \text{ N-m} = -700 \times 10^3 \text{ N-mm}$$

Shaft CD: $\qquad \Sigma M = 0: \quad -T_{CD} + 2500 \qquad \Rightarrow T_{CD} = 1800 \text{ N-m} = 1800 \times 10^3 \text{ N-mm}$

$$-1500 + 800 = 0$$

a. *Total angle of twist:*

$$\theta = \sum \left(\frac{TL}{GJ} \right) = \left(\frac{TL}{GJ} \right)_{AB} + \left(\frac{TL}{GJ} \right)_{BC} + \left(\frac{TL}{GJ} \right)_{CD}$$

$$= \frac{(800 \times 10^3) \times 400}{80 \times 10^3 \times (\pi \times 25^4/32)} + \frac{(-700 \times 10^3) \times 500}{80 \times 10^3 \times (\pi \times 40^4/32)}$$

$$+ \frac{(1800 \times 10^3) \times 600}{80 \times 10^3 \times \left[\pi \times 80^4 \times (1 - 0.5^4)/32 \right]}$$

$$= 0.1043 - 0.0174 + 0.0036$$

$$\theta = 0.0905 \text{ rad} = 5.18°$$

b. *Shear stress:*

For a solid shaft, $\qquad \tau_{AB} = \left(\frac{16T}{\pi d^3} \right)_{AB} = \left(\frac{16 \times 800 \times 10^3}{\pi \times 25^3} \right) = 260.76 \text{ MPa}$

$$\tau_{BC} = \left(\frac{16T}{\pi d^3} \right)_{BC} = \left[\frac{16 \times (-700) \times 10^3}{\pi \times 25^3} \right] = 21.73 \text{ MPa}$$

For a hollow shaft, $\qquad \tau_{CD} = \left[\frac{16T}{\pi d_o^3 (1 - K^4)} \right]_{CD} = \left[\frac{16 \times 1800 \times 10^3}{\pi \times 80^3 \times (1 - 0.5^4)} \right] = 19.09 \text{ MPa}$

52. A stepped shaft is subjected to a torque as shown in Fig. 9.11(a). The compound shaft is made of steel having a modulus of rigidity of 80 GPa. Find the angle of rotation at the free end of the shaft. Also calculate the maximum shear stress in each shaft.

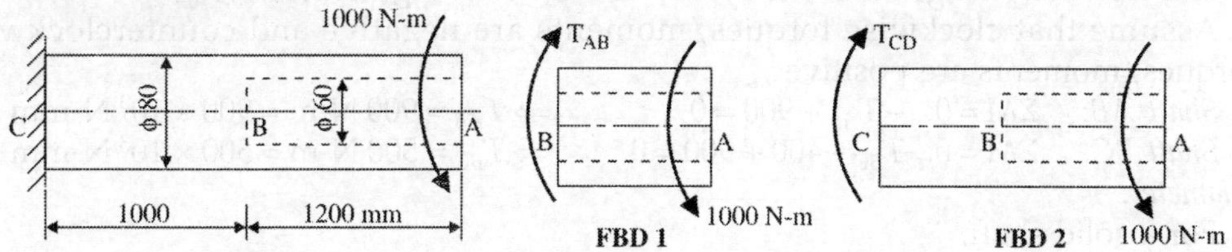

Fig. 9.11(a): Problem 52 $\qquad\qquad$ **Fig. 9.11(b):** Problem 52: Free body diagrams

Solution: $d_{AB})_i = 60 \text{ mm}, d_{AB})_o = 80 \text{ mm } K = \dfrac{d_i}{d_o} = \dfrac{60}{80} = 0.75, d_{BC} = 80 \text{ mm}, L_{AB} = 1200 \text{ mm},$

$L_{BC} = 1000 \text{ mm}, T = 1000 \text{ N-m}, G = 80 \times 10^3 \text{ MPa. a) } \theta = ?, \text{b) } \tau = ?$

The free-body diagram of the system is shown in **Fig. 9.11(b)**.

Assume that clockwise torques/moments are negative and counterclockwise torques/moments are positive.

Shaft AB: $\qquad \Sigma M = 0 \quad -T_{AB} + 1000 = 0 \qquad \Rightarrow T_{AB} = 1000 \text{ N-m} = 1000 \times 10^3 \text{ N-mm}$

Shaft BC: $\qquad \Sigma M = 0: \quad -T_{BC} + 1000 = 0 \qquad \Rightarrow T_{BC} = 1000 \text{ N-m} = 1000 \times 10^3 \text{ N-mm}$

a. *Total angle of twist:*

$$\theta = \sum\left(\frac{TL}{GJ}\right) = \left(\frac{TL}{GJ}\right)_{AB} + \left(\frac{TL}{GJ}\right)_{BC}$$

$$= \frac{(1000 \times 10^3) \times 1200}{80 \times 10^3 \times \left[\pi \times 80^4 \times (1 - 0.75^4)/32\right]} + \frac{(1000 \times 10^3) \times 1000}{80 \times 10^3 \times (\pi \times 80^4/32)}$$

$$= 0.0055 + 0.0031$$

$$\theta = 0.0086 \text{ rad} = 0.49°$$

b. *Shear stress:*

For a solid shaft, $\quad \tau_{AB} = \left[\dfrac{16T}{\pi d_o^3 (1 - K^4)}\right]_{AB} = \left[\dfrac{16 \times 1000 \times 10^3}{\pi \times 80^3 \times (1 - 0.75^4)}\right] = 14.55 \text{ MPa}$

$$\tau_{BC} = \left(\frac{16T}{\pi d^3}\right)_{CD} = \left[\frac{16 \times 1000 \times 10^3}{\pi \times 80^3}\right] = 9.95 \text{ MPa}$$

53. A uniform solid shaft carries two torques as shown in Fig. 9.12(a). Determine the diameter of the shaft if the angle of twist is limited to 3°. Take G = 78 GPa.

Solution: $T_1 = 900$ N-m, $T_2 = 400$ N-m, $L_{AB} = 1200$ mm, $L_{BC} = 1000$ mm, $\theta = 3° = 0.0524$ rad, $G = 78 \times 10^3$ MPa. $d = ?$

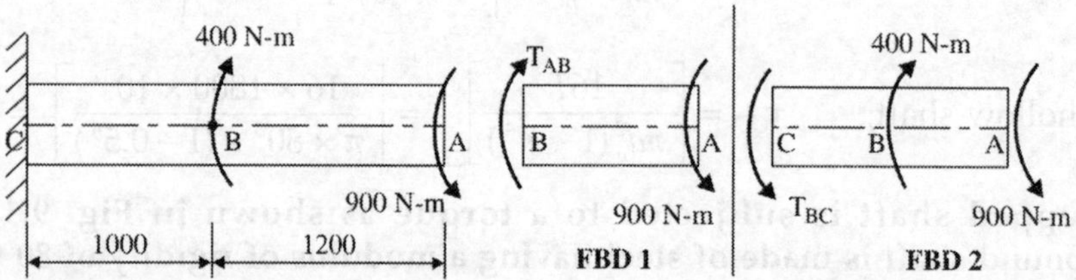

Fig. 9.12(a): Problem 53   **Fig. 9.12(b):** Problem 53: Free body diagrams

The free-body diagram of the system is shown in **Fig. 9.12(b)**.

Assume that clockwise torques/moments are negative and counterclockwise torques/moments are positive.

Shaft AB: $\quad \Sigma M = 0$: $\quad -T_{AB} + 900 = 0 \qquad \Rightarrow T_{AB} = 900$ N-m $= 900 \times 10^3$ N-mm

Shaft BC: $\quad \Sigma M = 0$: $\quad T_{BC} - 400 + 900 = 0 \qquad \Rightarrow T_{BC} = 500$ N-m $= 500 \times 10^3$ N-mm

Diameter:

For a solid shaft,

$$\theta = \sum\left(\frac{TL}{GJ}\right) = \left(\frac{TL}{GJ}\right)_{AB} + \left(\frac{TL}{GJ}\right)_{BC}$$

$$0.0524 = \frac{(900 \times 10^3) \times 1200}{78 \times 10^3 \times (\pi d^4/32)} + \frac{(500 \times 10^3) \times 1000}{78 \times 10^3 \times (\pi d^4/32)}$$

$$0.0524 = \frac{206.33 \times 10^3}{d^4}$$

$$d = 44.55 \text{ mm} \approx 45 \text{ mm}$$

54. Determine the diameter of the shaft shown in Fig. 9.13(a). Take $G = 80$ GPa. The angle of twist is limited to 4°. Also find the shear stress induced in the shaft.

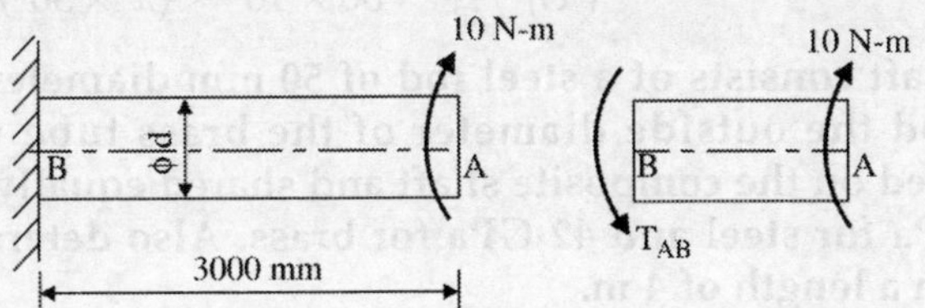

Fig. 9.13(a): Problem 54   **Fig. 9.13(b): Problem 54: Free body diagram**

Solution: $T = 10$ kN-m, $L = 3000$ mm, $\theta = 4° = 0.0698$ rad, $G = 80 \times 10^3$ MPa. a) $d = ?$ b) $\tau = ?$

The free-body diagram of the system is shown in **Fig. 9.13(b)**.

Assume that clockwise torques/moments are negative and counterclockwise torques/moments are positive.

Shaft AB: $\Sigma M = 0$: $T_{AB} - 100 = 0$ $\qquad\qquad \Rightarrow T_{AB} = 10$ kN-m $= 10 \times 10^6$ N-mm

a. *Diameter:*

For a solid shaft, $\qquad\qquad \theta = \left(\dfrac{TL}{GJ}\right)_{AB}$

$$0.0698 = \frac{(10 \times 10^6) \times 3000}{80 \times 10^3 \times (\pi \, d^4/32)}$$

$$d = 86 \, \text{mm}$$

b. *Shear stress:*

For a solid shaft $\qquad\qquad \tau_{AB} = \left(\dfrac{16T}{\pi d^3}\right)_{AB} = \left(\dfrac{16 \times 10 \times 10^6}{\pi \times 86^3}\right) = 80 \, \text{MPa}$

55. Determine the angle of twist at A, for the steel shaft shown in Fig. 9.14(a). Take $G = 80$ GPa.

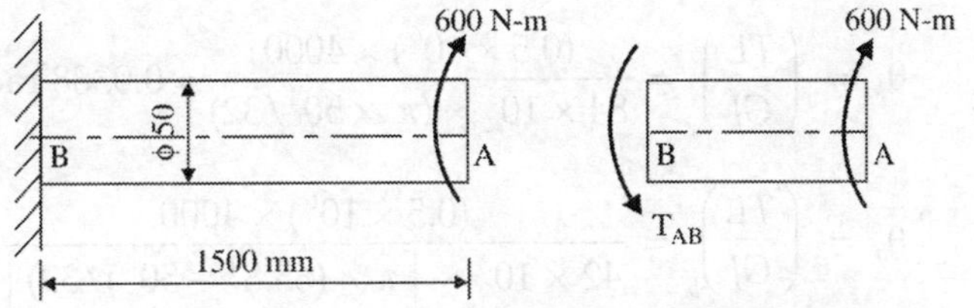

Fig. 9.14(a): Problem 54   **Fig. 9.14(b): Problem 54: Free body diagrams**

Solution: $d = 50$ mm, $L = 1500$ mm, $T = 600$ N-m, $G = 80 \times 10^3$ MPa, $\theta = ?$

The free-body diagram of the system is shown in **Fig. 9.14(b)**.

Assume that clockwise torques/moments are negative and counterclockwise torques/moments are positive.

Shaft AB: $\Sigma M = 0$: $T_{AB} - 600 = 0$ $\qquad\qquad \Rightarrow T_{AB} = 600$ N-m $= 600 \times 10^3$ N-mm

Total angle of twist:

$$\theta = \left(\frac{TL}{GJ}\right)_{AB} = \frac{(600 \times 10^3) \times 1500}{80 \times 10^3 \times (\pi \times 50^4/32)}$$

56. A composite shaft consists of a steel rod of 50 mm diameter surrounded by a brass tube. Find the outside diameter of the brass tube when a torque of 1 kN-m is applied on the composite shaft and shared equally by two materials. Take G = 84 GPa for steel and 42 GPa for brass. Also determine the common angle of twist in a length of 4 m.

Solution: $d_s = d_i)_b = 50$ mm, $T = 1$ kN-m $\Rightarrow T_s = T_b = 0.5$ kN-m (equally shared), $G_s = 84 \times 10^3$ MPa, $G_b = 42 \times 10^3$ MPa. a) $d_o)_b = ?$, for equal torques b) Common angle of twist $\theta_s = \theta_b = ?$

a. *Outside diameter:*

We know that
$$\theta = \frac{TL}{GJ}$$

$$\left(\frac{TL}{GJ}\right)_s = \left(\frac{TL}{GJ}\right)_b$$

Since T and L are equal, we have
$$(GJ)_b = (GJ)_s$$

$$J_b = J_s\left(\frac{G_s}{G_b}\right)$$

$$\frac{\pi}{32}\left(d_o^4 - d_i^4\right) = \frac{\pi}{32}d^4\left(\frac{G_s}{G_b}\right)$$

$$\left(d_o^4 - 50^4\right) = 50^4\left(\frac{84 \times 10^3}{42 \times 10^3}\right)$$

$$d_o = d_o)_b = 65.80 \text{ mm}$$

Fig. 9.15: Problem 56

b. *Common angle of twist:*

$$\theta_s = \left(\frac{TL}{GJ}\right)_s = \frac{(0.5 \times 10^6) \times 4000}{84 \times 10^3 \times (\pi \times 50^4/32)} = 0.0388 \text{ rad} = 2.223°$$

$$\theta_b = \left(\frac{TL}{GJ}\right)_b = \frac{(0.5 \times 10^6) \times 4000}{42 \times 10^3 \times \left[\pi \times (65.8^4 - 50^4)/32\right]} = 0.0388 \text{ rad}$$

$$= 2.223°$$

PROBLEMS ON SERIES SHAFTS – UNKNOWN TORQUE

57. A stepped shaft is subjected to torques T and 2T as shown in Fig. 9.16(a). What is the total angle of twist at the free end, if the maximum shear stress is limited to 70 MPa. Take G = 84 GPa

Solution: $d_{AB} = 50$ mm, $d_{BC} = 100$ mm, $L_{AB} = 1800$ mm, $L_{BC} = 1200$ mm, $\tau = 70$ MPa, $G = 84 \times 10^3$ MPa, $T_1 = T$, $T_1 = 2T$. $\theta = ?$

The free-body diagram of the system is shown in **Fig. 9.16(b)**.

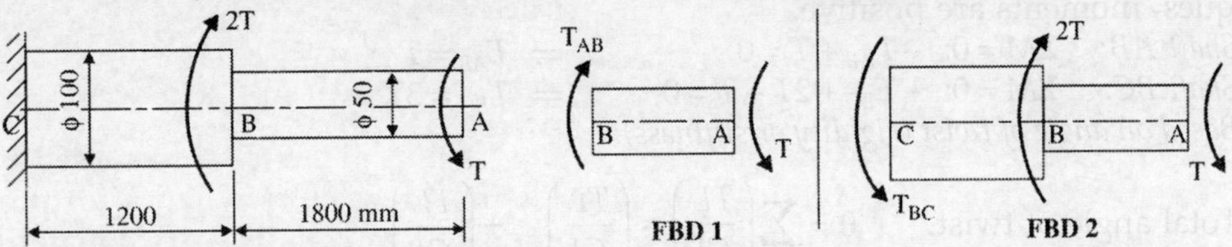

Fig. 9.16(a): Problem 57   **Fig. 9.16(b):** Problem 57: Free body diagrams

Assume that clockwise torques/moments are negative and counterclockwise torques/moments are positive.

Shaft AB: $\Sigma M = 0$: $-T_{AB} + T = 0$ $\Rightarrow T_{AB} = T$

Shaft BC: $\Sigma M = 0$: $T_{BC} - 2T + T = 0$ $\Rightarrow T_{BC} = T$ (CW, hence negative)

      Or $T_{BC} = -2T + T$ $\Rightarrow T_{BC} = -T$

Total angle of twist:

$$\theta = \sum\left(\frac{TL}{GJ}\right) = \left(\frac{TL}{GJ}\right)_{AB} + \left(\frac{TL}{GJ}\right)_{BC} \qquad \text{... Eq. (i)}$$

For a solid shaft, $T = \left(\dfrac{\pi d^3}{16}\right)\tau$

For shaft AB, $T = \left(\dfrac{\pi \times 50^3}{16}\right) \times 70 = 1.72 \times 10^6\,\text{N-mm}$ ... Eq. (a)

For shaft BC, $T = \left(\dfrac{\pi \times 100^3}{16}\right) \times 70 = 1.37 \times 10^7\,\text{N-mm}$ ... Eq. (b)

Based on Eqs (a) and (b), select minimum value of torque for design

   i.e. $T = 1.72 \times 10^6\,\text{N-mm}$

Eq. (i) yields... $\theta = \dfrac{1.72 \times 10^6 \times 1800}{84 \times 10^3 \times (\pi \times 50^4/32)} + \dfrac{-(1.72 \times 10^6) \times 1200}{84 \times 10^3 \times (\pi \times 100^4/32)}$

      $\theta = 0.0576\,\text{rad} = 3.29°$

58. **A compound shaft is acted upon by two torques as shown in Fig. 9.17(a). Determine the maximum permissible value of T subject to the following conditions: $\tau_s = 83$ MPa, $\tau_{al} = 55$ MPa, and the angle of rotation of the free end is limited to 6°. Talk $G = 83$ GPa for steel and $G = 28$ MPa for aluminum.**

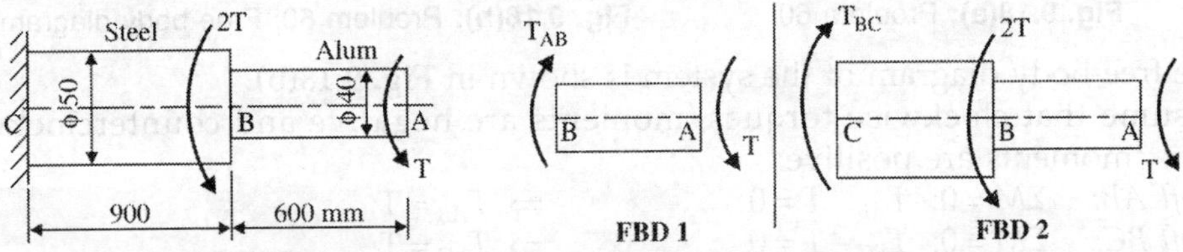

Fig. 9.17(a): Problem 58   **Fig. 9.17(b):** Problem 58: Free body diagrams

Solution: $d_{AB} = 40$ mm, $d_{BC} = 50$ mm, $L_{AB} = 600$ mm, $L_{BC} = 900$ mm, $\tau_{al} = \tau_{AB} = 55$ MPa, $\tau_s = \tau_{BC} = 83$ MPa, $\theta = 6° = 0.1047$ rad, $T_1 = T$, $T_2 = 2T$, $G_{AB} = G_{al} = 28 \times 10^3$ MPa, $G_{BC} = G_s = 83 \times 10^3$ MPa. $T = ?$

The free-body diagram of the system is shown in **Fig. 9.17(b)**.

Assume that clockwise torques/moments are negative and counterclockwise torques/moments are positive.

Shaft AB: $\Sigma M = 0$: $-T_{AB} + T = 0$ $\Rightarrow$ $T_{AB} = T$
Shaft BC: $\Sigma M = 0$: $-T_{BC} + 2T + T = 0$ $\Rightarrow$ $T_{BC} = 3T$

a. *Based on angle of twist (rigidity or stiffness):*

Total angle of twist, $\theta = \sum \left(\dfrac{TL}{GJ}\right) = \left(\dfrac{TL}{GJ}\right)_{AB} + \left(\dfrac{TL}{GJ}\right)_{BC}$

$$0.1047 = \frac{T \times 600}{28 \times 10^3 \times (\pi \times 40^4/32)} + \frac{(3T) \times 900}{83 \times 10^3 \times (\pi \times 50^4/32)}$$

$$T = 0.757 \times 10^6 \text{ N-mm} \qquad \qquad \text{... Eq. (a)}$$

b. *Based on strength:*

For a solid shaft, $T = \left(\dfrac{\pi d^3}{16}\right) \tau$

For shaft AB, $T = \left(\dfrac{\pi \times 40^3}{16}\right) \times 55 = 0.691 \times 10^6 \text{ N-mm}$ ... Eq. (b)

For shaft BC, $3T = \left(\dfrac{\pi \times 50^3}{16}\right) \times 83 = 0.679 \times 10^6 \text{ N-mm}$ ... Eq. (c)

Based on Eqs (a), (b) and (c), select minimum value of torque for design
    i.e. $T = 0.679 \times 10^6 \text{ N-mm} = 679 \text{ N-m}$

59. A stepped steel shaft carries a torque T as shown in Fig. 9.18(a). Determine the maximum allowable magnitude of T if the working shear stress is 12 MPa and the rotation of the free end is limited to 4°. Take G = 83 GPa for steel.

Solution: d_{AB} = 60 mm, d_{BC} = 80 mm, L_{AB} = 4000 mm, L_{BC} = 3000 mm, τ = 12 MPa, $\theta = 4° = 0.0698$ rad, $G = 83 \times 10^3$ MPa. $T = \theta$

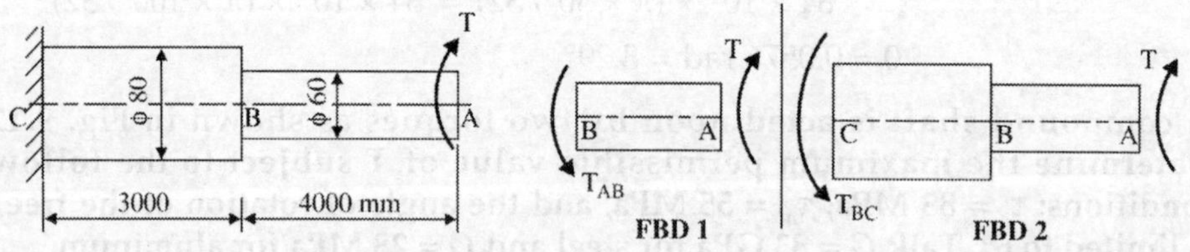

Fig. 9.18(a): Problem 60   Fig. 9.18(b): Problem 60: Free body diagrams

The free-body diagram of the system is shown in **Fig. 9.18(b)**.

Assume that clockwise torques/moments are negative and counterclockwise torques/moments are positive.

Shaft AB: $\Sigma M = 0$: $T_{AB} - T = 0$ $\Rightarrow$ $T_{AB} = T$
Shaft BC: $\Sigma M = 0$: $T_{BC} - T = 0$ $\Rightarrow$ $T_{BC} = T$

a. *Based on angle of twist (rigidity or stiffness):*

Total angle of twist, $\theta = \sum \left(\dfrac{TL}{GJ}\right) = \left(\dfrac{TL}{GJ}\right)_{AB} + \left(\dfrac{TL}{GJ}\right)_{BC}$

$$0.0698 = \frac{T \times 4000}{83 \times 10^3 \times (\pi \times 60^4/32)} + \frac{T \times 3000}{83 \times 10^3 \times (\pi \times 80^4/32)}$$

$$T = 1.48 \times 10^6 \text{ N-mm} \qquad \text{... Eq. (a)}$$

b. *Based on strength:*

Strength of a solid shaft, $T = \left(\dfrac{\pi d^3}{16}\right)\tau$

For shaft AB, $\qquad\qquad T = \left(\dfrac{\pi \times 60^3}{16}\right) \times 12 = 0.509 \times 10^6 \text{ N-mm} \qquad \text{... Eq. (b)}$

For shaft BC, $\qquad\qquad T = \left(\dfrac{\pi \times 80^3}{16}\right) \times 12 = 1.21 \times 10^6 \text{ N-mm} \qquad \text{... Eq. (c)}$

Based on Eqs (a), (b) and (c), select minimum value of torque for design
i.e. $\qquad\qquad T = 0.509 \times 10^6 \text{ N-mm} = 509 \text{ N-m}$

60. Determine the maximum torque T that can be applied to the ends of the shaft shown in Fig. 9.19(a) without exceeding a shear stress of 70 MPa. The angle of twist is limited to 2.5°. Use G = 83 GPa for steel.

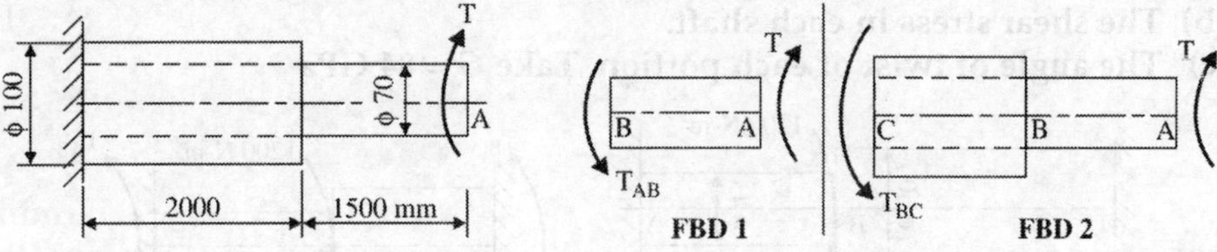

Fig. 9.19(a): Problem 60 $\qquad\qquad$ **Fig. 9.19(b):** Problem 60: Free body diagrams

Solution: $d_{AB} = d_{BC})_i = 70$ mm, $d_{BC})_o = 100$ mm, $K = \dfrac{d_i}{d_o} = \dfrac{70}{100} = 0.70$, $L_{AB} = 1500$ mm,

$L_{BC} = 2000$ mm, $\tau = 70$ MPa, $\theta = 2.5° = 0.0436$ rad, $G = 83 \times 10^3$ MPa. $T = ?$
The free-body diagram of the system is shown in **Fig. 9.19(b)**.

Assume that clockwise torques/moments are negative and counterclockwise torques/moments are positive.

Shaft AB: $\quad \Sigma M = 0$: $\ T_{AB} - T = 0 \qquad\qquad \Rightarrow T_{AB} = \text{T}$
Shaft BC: $\quad \Sigma M = 0$: $\ T_{BC} - T = 0 \qquad\qquad \Rightarrow T_{BC} = \text{T}$

a. *Based on angle of twist (rigidity or stiffness):*

Total angle of twist, $\qquad \theta = \Sigma\left(\dfrac{TL}{GJ}\right) = \left(\dfrac{TL}{GJ}\right)_{AB} + \left(\dfrac{TL}{GJ}\right)_{BC}$

$$0.0436 = \frac{T \times 1500}{83 \times 10^3 \times (\pi \times 70^4/32)}$$

$$+ \frac{T \times 2000}{83 \times 10^3 \times [\pi \times 100^4 \times (1 - 0.7^4)/32]}$$

$$T = 4.0 \times 10^6 \text{ N-mm} \qquad \text{... Eq. (a)}$$

b. *Based on strength:*

Strength of a solid shaft, $T = \left(\dfrac{\pi d^3}{16}\right)\tau$

For shaft AB, $\qquad T = \left(\dfrac{\pi \times 70^3}{16}\right) \times 70 = 4.71 \times 10^6$ N-mm $\qquad$ ... Eq. (b)

For a hollow shaft, $\qquad T = \left[\dfrac{\pi d_o^3 (1 - K^4)}{16}\right]\tau$

For shaft BC, $\qquad T = \left[\dfrac{\pi \times 100^3 \times (1 - 0.7^4)}{16}\right] \times 70 = 10.44 \times 10^6$ N-mm

$\qquad\qquad\qquad\qquad\qquad\qquad\qquad\qquad\qquad\qquad\qquad\qquad\qquad$ ... Eq. (c)

Based on Eqs (a), (b) and (c), select minimum value of torque for design
i.e. $\qquad\qquad\qquad T = 4 \times 10^6$ N-mm $= 4$ kN-m

PROBLEMS ON PARALLEL SHAFTS – KNOWN TORQUE

61. **Two shafts of same material are connected to fixed supports as shown in Fig. 9.20(a). For the loading shown, determine:**
   (a) The reaction at each support,
   (b) The shear stress in each shaft.
   (c) The angle of twist of each portion. Take $G = 84$ GPa

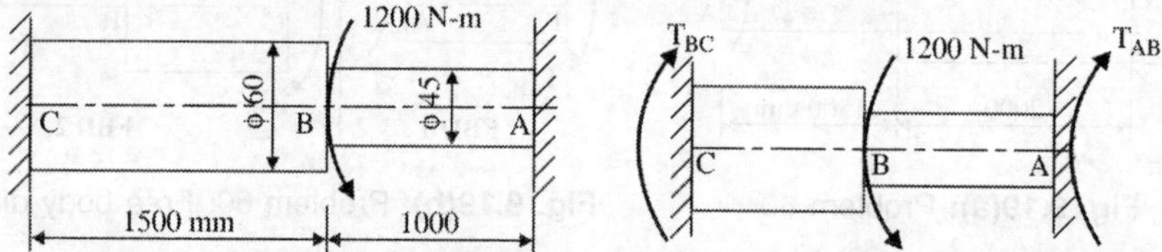

Fig. 9.20(a): Problem 61 $\qquad$ **Fig. 9.20(b):** Problem 61: Free body diagram

Solution: $d_{AB} = 45$ mm, $d_{BC} = 60$ mm, $L_{AB} = 1000$ mm, $L_{BC} = 1500$ mm, $T = 1200 \times 10^3$ N-mm, $G = 84 \times 10^3$ MPa. $T_{AB} = ?, T_{BC} = ?, \tau_{AB} = ?, \tau_{BC} = ?,$
The free-body diagram of the system is shown in **Fig. 9.20(b)**.
Assume that clockwise torques/moments are negative and counterclockwise torques/moments are positive.
For equilibrium,
$\qquad \Sigma M = 0: \ -T_{BC} + (1200 \times 10^3) - T_{AB} = 0 \qquad \Rightarrow \ T_{AB} + T_{BC} = 1200 \times 10^3$ N-mm
$\qquad\qquad\qquad\qquad\qquad\qquad\qquad\qquad\qquad\qquad\qquad\qquad\qquad\qquad\qquad$ ... Eq. (i)

Since the shafts are connected in parallel, we have
$$\theta_{AB} = \theta_{BC}$$
$$\left(\frac{TL}{GJ}\right)_{AB} = \left(\frac{TL}{GJ}\right)_{BC}$$

Since the material is same
$$\left(\frac{TL}{J}\right)_{AB} = \left(\frac{TL}{J}\right)_{BC}$$

$$\left[\frac{T_{AB} \times 1000}{(\pi \times 45^4/32)}\right] = \left[\frac{T_{BC} \times 1500}{(\pi \times 60^4/32)}\right]$$

$$T_{AB} = (0.4746)T_{BC} \qquad \text{... Eq. (ii)}$$

Substituting Eq. (ii) in Eq. (i), we have

$$1200 \times 10^3 = (0.4746)\,T_{BC} + T_{BC}$$
$$T_{BC} = 813.78 \times 10^3 \text{ N-mm}$$

Eq. (ii) yields... $\qquad T_{AB} = (0.4746) \times (813.78 \times 10^3) = 386.22 \times 10^3$ N-mm

a. *Reactions:* $\qquad T_{AB} = 386.22 \times 10^3$ N-mm and $T_{BC} = 813.78 \times 10^3$ N-mm

b. *Shear stress:*

For a solid shaft, $\qquad \tau_{AB} = \left(\dfrac{16T}{\pi d^3}\right)_{AB} = \left(\dfrac{16 \times 386.22 \times 10^3}{\pi \times 45^3}\right) = 21.58$ MPa

(maximum shear stress)

$$\tau_{BC} = \left(\frac{16T}{\pi d^3}\right)_{AB} = \left(\frac{16 \times 813.78 \times 10^3}{\pi \times 60^3}\right) = 19.18 \text{ MPa}$$

c. *Angle of twist for each portion:*

$$\theta_{AB} = \theta_{BC} = \left(\frac{TL}{GJ}\right)_{AB} = \left[\frac{386.22 \times 10^3 \times 1000}{84 \times 10^3 \times (\pi \times 45^4/32)}\right]$$
$$= 0.01142 \text{ rad} = 0.654°$$

62. Two shafts are connected to a coupling disk B and to fixed supports at A and C. Determine:

(a) The reaction at each support,

(b) The shear stress in each shaft.

(c) The angle of twist of each portion. Take $G = 84$ GPa for steel and 28 GPa for aluminium.

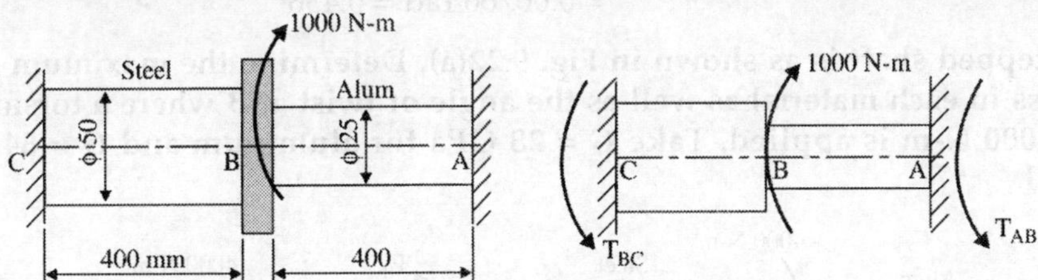

Fig. 9.21(a): Problem 62   Fig. 9.21(b): Problem 62: Free body diagram

Solution: $d_{AB} = 25$ mm, $d_{BC} = 50$ mm, $L_{AB} = L_{BC} = 400$ mm, $T = 1000 \times 10^3$ N-mm, $G_{AB} = 28 \times 10^3$ MPa, $G_{BC} = 84 \times 10^3$ MPa. $T_{AB} = ?, T_{BC} = ?, \tau_{AB} = ?, \tau_{BC} = ?, \theta = ?$.

The free-body diagram of the system is shown in **Fig. 9.21(b)**.

Assume that clockwise torques/moments are negative and counterclockwise torques/moments are positive.

For equilibrium,

$$\Sigma M = 0: T_{BC} - 1000 \times 10^3 + T_{AB} = 0 \Rightarrow T_{AB} + T_{BC} = 1000 \times 10^3 \text{ N-mm} \qquad \text{... Eq. (i)}$$

Since the shafts are connected in parallel, we have

$$\theta_{AB} = \theta_{BC}$$

$$\left(\frac{TL}{GJ}\right)_{AB} = \left(\frac{TL}{GJ}\right)_{BC}$$

$$\left[\frac{T_{AB} \times 400}{28 \times 10^3 \times (\pi \times 25^4/32)}\right] = \left[\frac{T_{BC} \times 400}{84 \times 10^3 \times (\pi \times 50^4/32)}\right]$$

$$T_{AB} = (0.0208)\, T_{BC} \qquad\qquad \ldots \text{Eq. (ii)}$$

Substituting Eq. (ii) in Eq. (i), we have

$$1000 \times 10^3 = (0.0208)\, T_{BC} + T_{BC}$$
$$T_{BC} = 979.62 \times 10^3 \text{ N-mm}$$

Eq. (ii) yields... $\quad T_{AB} = (0.0208) \times (813.78 \times 10^3) = 20.38 \times 10^3$ N-mm

a. *Reactions:* $\quad T_{AB} = 20.38 \times 10^3$ N-mm and $T_{BC} = 979.62 \times 10^3$ N-mm

b. *Shear stress:*

For a solid shaft, $\quad \tau_{AB} = \left(\frac{16T}{\pi d^3}\right)_{AB} = \left(\frac{16 \times 20.38 \times 10^3}{\pi \times 25^3}\right) = 6.64$ MPa

$$\tau_{BC} = \left(\frac{16T}{\pi d^3}\right)_{BC} = \left(\frac{16 \times 979.62 \times 10^3}{\pi \times 50^3}\right) = 39.91 \text{ MPa}$$

(maximum shear stress)

c. *Angle of twist for each portion:*

$$\theta_{AB} = \theta_{BC} = \left(\frac{TL}{GJ}\right)_{AB} = \left[\frac{20.83 \times 10^3 \times 400}{28 \times 10^3 \times (\pi \times 25^4/32)}\right]$$
$$= 0.00760 \text{ rad} = 0.436°$$

Check: $\quad \theta_{AB} = \theta_{BC} = \left(\frac{TL}{GJ}\right)_{BC} = \left[\frac{979.62 \times 10^3 \times 400}{84 \times 10^3 \times (\pi \times 50^4/32)}\right]$
$$= 0.00760 \text{ rad} = 0.436°$$

63. **A stepped shaft is as shown in Fig. 9.22(a). Determine the maximum shearing stress in each material as well as the angle of twist at B where a torsional load of 4000 N-m is applied. Take $G = 28$ GPa for aluminum and $G = 84$ GPa for steel.**

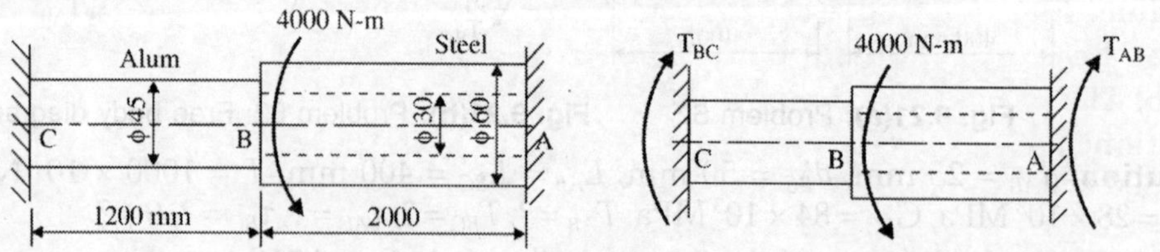

Fig. 9.22(a): Problem 63   **Fig. 9.22(b):** Problem 63: Free body diagram

Solution: $d_{AB})_i = 30$ mm, $d_{AB})_o = 60$ mm, $K = \dfrac{d_i}{d_o} = \dfrac{30}{60} = 0.5$, $d_{BC} = 45$ mm, $L_{AB} = 2000$ mm,

$L_{BC} = 1200$ mm, $T = 4000 \times 10^3$ N-mm, $G_{AB} = 84 \times 10^3$ MPa, $G_{BC} = 28 \times 10^3$ MPa. $\tau_{AB} = ?$, $\tau_{BC} = ?$, $\theta = ?$.

The free-body diagram of the system is shown in **Fig. 9.22(b)**.
Assume that clockwise torques/moments are negative and counterclockwise torques/moments are positive.

For equilibrium,
$\Sigma M = 0: - T_{BC} + 4000 \times 10^3 - T_{AB} = 0 \implies T_{AB} + T_{BC} = 4000 \times 10^3$ N-mm   ... Eq. (i)

Since the shafts are connected in parallel, we have
$$\theta_{AB} = \theta_{BC}$$

$$\left(\frac{TL}{GJ}\right)_{AB} = \left(\frac{TL}{GJ}\right)_{BC}$$

$$\left[\frac{T_{AB} \times 2000}{84 \times 10^3 \times [\pi \times 60^4 \times (1 - 0.5^4)/32]}\right] = \left[\frac{T_{BC} \times 1200}{28 \times 10^3 \times (\pi \times 45^4/32)}\right]$$

$$T_{AB} = (5.333)\, T_{BC} \qquad \text{... Eq. (ii)}$$

Substituting Eq. (ii) in Eq. (i), we have
$$4000 \times 10^3 = (5.333)\, T_{BC} + T_{BC}$$
$$T_{BC} = 631.61 \times 10^3 \text{ N-mm}$$

Eq. (ii) yields... $T_{AB} = (5.333) \times (631.61 \times 10^3) = 3.37 \times 10^6$ N-mm

a. *Shear stress:*

For a solid shaft, $\tau_{AB} = \left[\dfrac{16T}{\pi d_o^3 (1 - K^4)}\right]_{AB} = \left(\dfrac{16 \times 3.37 \times 10^6}{\pi \times 60^3 \times (1 - 0.5^4)}\right) = 84.75$ MPa

(maximum shear stress)

For a solid shaft, $\tau_{BC} = \left(\dfrac{16T}{\pi d^3}\right)_{BC} = \left(\dfrac{16 \times 631.61 \times 10^3}{\pi \times 45^3}\right) = 35.30$ MPa

b. *Angle of twist for each portion:*

$$\theta_{AB} = \theta_{BC} = \left(\frac{TL}{GJ}\right)_{AB} = \left[\frac{3.37 \times 10^6 \times 2000}{84 \times 10^3 \times [\pi \times 60^4 \times (1 - 0.5^4)/32]}\right]$$
$$= 0.0673 \text{ rad} = 3.86°$$

64. A compound shaft, composed of steel, aluminum, and bronze segments, carries the two torques as shown in Fig. 9.23(a). The modulus of rigidity for steel, aluminum and bronze are 83 GPa, 28 GPa and 35 GPa respectively. Determine:

(a) Reactions at the supports

(b) The absolute maximum shear stress in the shaft

Solution: $d_{AB} = d_{CD} = 25$ mm, $d_{BC} = 50$ mm, $L_{AB} = L_{BC} = 2000$ mm, $L_{CD} = 2500$ mm, $T_1 = 300 \times 10^3$ N-mm, $T_2 = 700 \times 10^3$ N-mm, $G_{AB} = 35 \times 10^3$ MPa, $G_{BC} = 28 \times 10^3$ MPa, $G_{CD} = 83 \times 10^3$ MPa a) $T_{AB} = ?$, $T_{CD} = ?$, b) Maximum shear stress

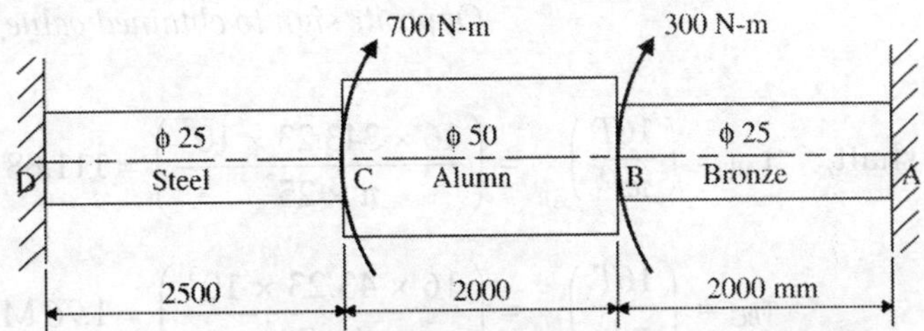

Fig. 9.23(a): Problem 64

The free-body diagram of the system is shown in **Fig. 9.23(b)**.

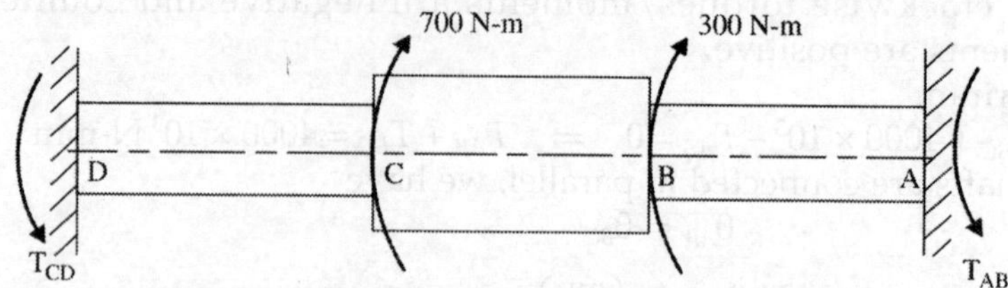

Fig. 9.23(b): Problem 64: Free body diagram

Assume that clockwise torques/moments are negative and counterclockwise torques/moments are positive.

For equilibrium,

$$\Sigma M = 0: \; T_{CD} - T_2 - T_1 + T_{AB} = 0$$
$$T_{AB} + T_{CD} = T_1 + T_2 = (300 \times 10^3) + (700 \times 10^3)$$
$$T_{AB} + T_{CD} = 1000 \times 10^3 \text{ N-mm} \qquad \qquad \text{... Eq. (i)}$$

Since the shafts are connected in parallel, we have

$$\theta_{AB} = \theta_{BC} = \theta_{CD} \quad \text{or} \quad \Sigma\theta = 0$$

i.e.

$$\left(\frac{TL}{GJ}\right)_{AB} + \left(\frac{TL}{GJ}\right)_{BC} + \left(\frac{TL}{GJ}\right)_{CD} = 0$$

Here $T_{AB} = T_{AB}$; $T_{BC} = (T_{AB} - T_1)$; $T_{CD} = [T_{AB} - (T_1 + T_2)]$

$$\left[\frac{T_{AB} \times 2000}{35 \times 10^3 \times (\pi \times 25^4 / 32)}\right] + \left[\frac{\left[T_{AB} - (300 \times 10^3)\right] \times 2000}{28 \times 10^3 \times (\pi \times 50^4 / 32)}\right]$$

$$+ \left[\frac{\left[T_{AB} - (1000 \times 10^3)\right] \times 2500}{83 \times 10^3 \times (\pi \times 25^4 / 32)}\right]$$

$$(1.49 \times 10^{-6})\, T_{AB} + [T_{AB} - (300 \times 10^3)](1.164 \times 10^{-7})$$
$$+ [T_{AB} - (1000 \times 10^3)](7.854 \times 10^{-7}) = 0$$
$$(2.39 \times 10^{-6})\, T_{AB} - 0.03492 - 0.7854 = 0$$
$$(2.39 \times 10^{-6})\, T_{AB} = 0.82032$$
$$T_{AB} = 343.23 \times 10^3 \text{ N-mm}$$

Eq. (i) yields...
$$T_{CD} = 1000 \times 10^3 - 343.23 \times 10^3 = 656.77 \times 10^3 \text{ N-mm}$$

a. *Reactions at the supports:*

$$T_{AB} = 343.23 \times 10^3 \text{ N-mm}$$
$$T_{BC} = [T_{AB} - T_1] = [343.23 \times 10^3 - 300 \times 10^3] = 43.23 \times 10^3 \text{ N-mm}$$
$$T_{CD} = 656.77 \times 10^3 \text{ N-mm}$$

Check for equilibrium:

$$T_{CD} = [T_{AB} - (T_1 + T_2)] = (343.23 \times 10^3) - (300 \times 10^3 + 700 \times 10^3)$$
$$= -656.77 \times 10^3 \text{ N-mm}$$

Opposite sign to obtained value, hence balanced

b. *Shear stress:*

For a solid shaft,
$$\tau_{AB} = \left(\frac{16T}{\pi d^3}\right)_{AB} = \left(\frac{16 \times 343.23 \times 10^3}{\pi \times 25^3}\right) = 111.88 \text{ MPa}$$

$$\tau_{BC} = \left(\frac{16T}{\pi d^3}\right)_{BC} = \left(\frac{16 \times 43.23 \times 10^3}{\pi \times 50^3}\right) = 1.76 \text{ MPa}$$

$$\tau_{CD} = \left(\frac{16T}{\pi d^3}\right)_{CD} = \left(\frac{16 \times 656.77 \times 10^3}{\pi \times 25^3}\right) = 214.07 \text{ MPa}$$

Maximum shear stress occurs in shaft CD

65. A steel shaft having rigidity modulus of 84 GPa is fixed at its ends. If it is subjected to the torques as shown in Fig. 9.24(a), determine:

(a) Reactions at the supports

(b) The absolute maximum shear stress in the shaft

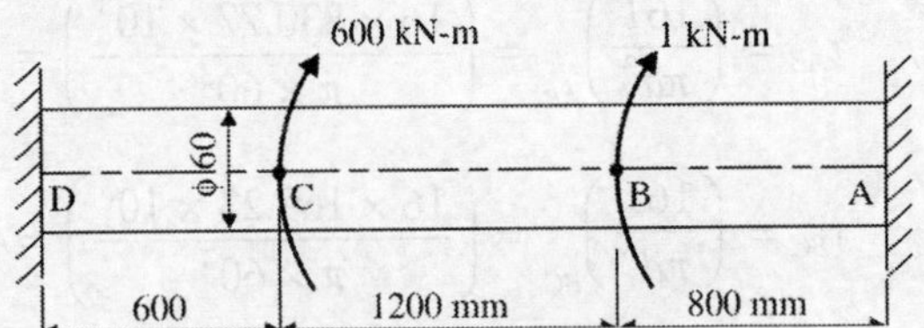

Fig. 9.24(a): Problem 65

Solution: $d = 60$ mm, $L_{AB} = 800$ mm, $L_{BC} = 1200$ mm, $L_{CD} = 600$ mm, $T_1 = 1$ kN-m, $T_2 = 600$ kN-m, $G = 84 \times 10^3$ MPa. a) $T_{AB} = ?$, $T_{CD} = ?$, b) Maximum shear stress

The free-body diagram of the system is shown in **Fig. 9.24(b)**.

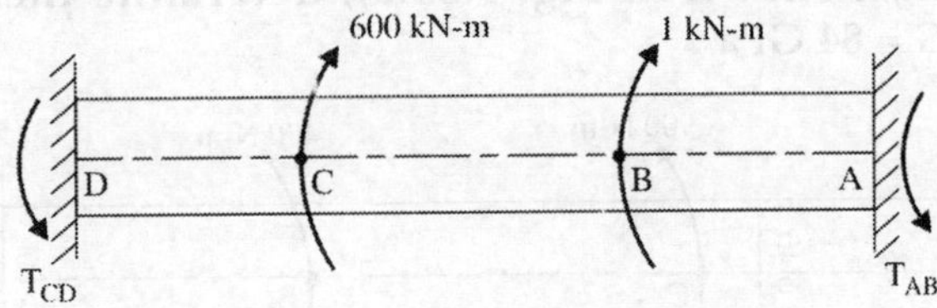

Fig. 9.24(b): Problem 65: Free body diagram

Assume that clockwise torques/moments are negative and counterclockwise torques/moments are positive.

For equilibrium, $\Sigma M = 0$: $T_{CD} - T_2 - T_1 + T_{AB} = 0$

$$T_{AB} + T_{CD} = T_1 + T_2 = (1 \times 10^6) + (600 \times 10^3)$$
$$T_{AB} + T_{CD} = 1600 \times 10^3 \text{ N-mm} \qquad \text{... Eq. (i)}$$

Since the shafts are connected in parallel, we have

$$\theta_{AB} = \theta_{BC} = \theta_{CD} \quad \text{or} \quad \Sigma\theta = 0$$

i.e. $\left(\dfrac{TL}{GJ}\right)_{AB} + \left(\dfrac{TL}{GJ}\right)_{BC} + \left(\dfrac{TL}{GJ}\right)_{CD} = 0$

Here $T_{AB} = T_{AB}$; $T_{BC} = (T_{AB} - T_1)$; $T_{CD} = [T_{AB} - (T_1 + T_2)]$

Since J and G remain same, we have

$$[T_{AB} \times 800] + [T_{AB} - (1 \times 10^6)] \times 1200$$
$$+ [T_{AB} - (1600 \times 10^3)] \times 600 = 0$$
$$(2600)\,T_{AB} - 1.2 \times 10^9 - 0.96 \times 10^9 = 0$$
$$(2600)\,T_{AB} = 2.16 \times 10^9$$

$$T_{AB} = 830.77 \times 10^3 \text{ N-mm}$$

Eq. (i) yields... $T_{CD} = 1600 \times 10^3 - 830.77 \times 10^3 = 769.23 \times 10^3 \text{ N-mm}$

a. *Reactions at the supports:*

$$T_{AB} = 830.77 \times 10^3 \text{ N-mm}$$
$$T_{BC} = [T_{AB} - T_1] = [830.77 \times 10^3 - 1 \times 10^6] = -169.23 \times 10^3 \text{ N-mm}$$
$$T_{CD} = 769.23 \times 10^3 \text{ N-mm}$$

Check for equilibrium:

$$T_{CD} = [T_{AB} - (T_1 + T_2)] = (830.77 \times 10^3) - (1000 \times 10^3 + 600 \times 10^3)$$
$$= -769.23 \times 10^3 \text{ N-mm}$$

Opposite sign to obtained value, hence balanced

b. *Shear stress:*

For a solid shaft,
$$\tau_{AB} = \left(\frac{16T}{\pi d^3}\right)_{AB} = \left(\frac{16 \times 830.77 \times 10^3}{\pi \times 60^3}\right) = 19.58 \text{ MPa}$$

$$\tau_{BC} = \left(\frac{16T}{\pi d^3}\right)_{BC} = \left(\frac{16 \times 169.23 \times 10^3}{\pi \times 60^3}\right) = 4.0 \text{ MPa}$$

$$\tau_{CD} = \left(\frac{16T}{\pi d^3}\right)_{CD} = \left(\frac{16 \times 769.23 \times 10^3}{\pi \times 60^3}\right) = 18.13 \text{ MPa}$$

Maximum shear stress occurs in shaft AB

66. For the steel shaft shown in Fig. 9.25(a), determine the reactions at the supports. Take G = 84 GPa.

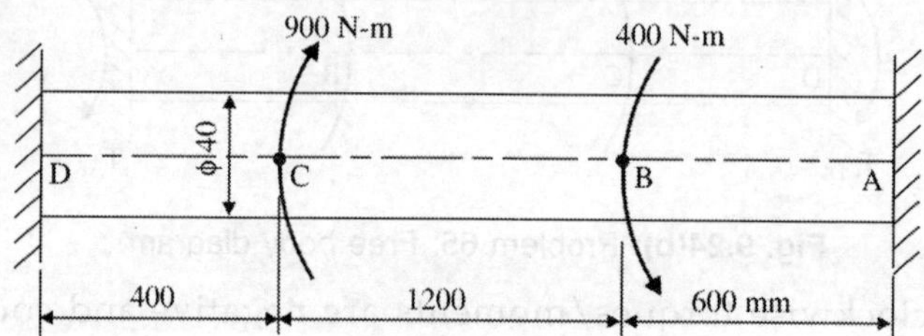

Fig. 9.25(a): Problem 66

Solution: d = 40 mm, L_{AB} = 600 mm, L_{BC} = 1200 mm, L_{CD} = 400 mm, T_1 = 400 N-m, T_2 = 900 N-m, G = 84 × 10³ MPa. T_{AB} = ?, T_{CD} = ?

The free-body diagram of the system is shown in **Fig. 9.25(b)**.

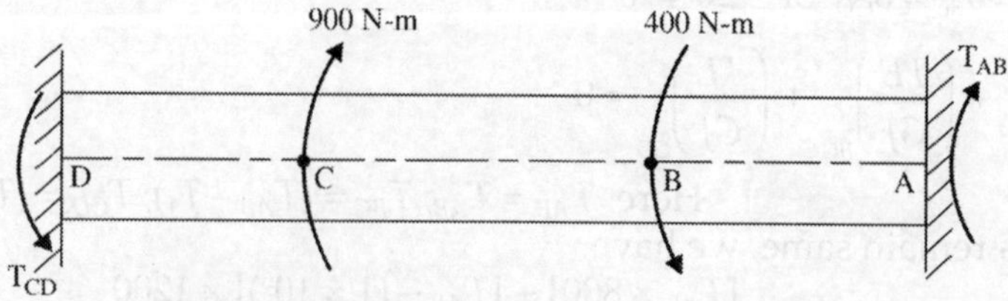

Fig. 9.25(b): Problem 66: Free body diagram

Assume that clockwise torques/moments are negative and counterclockwise torques/moments are positive.

For equilibrium, $\Sigma M = 0$: $T_{CD} - T_2 - T_1 + T_{AB} = 0$

$$T_{CD} - T_{AB} = T_2 - T_1 = (900 \times 10^3) - (400 \times 10^3)$$
$$T_{CD} - T_{AB} = 500 \times 10^3 \text{ N-mm} \qquad \text{... Eq. (i)}$$

Since the shafts are connected in parallel, we have
$$\theta_{AB} = \theta_{BC} = \theta_{CD} \quad \text{or} \quad \Sigma\theta = 0$$

i.e. $\left(\dfrac{TL}{GJ}\right)_{AB} + \left(\dfrac{TL}{GJ}\right)_{BC} + \left(\dfrac{TL}{GJ}\right)_{CD} = 0$

Here $T_{AB} = T_{AB}$; $T_{BC} = (T_{AB} - T_1)$; $T_{CD} = [T_{AB} - (T_1 + T_2)]$

Since J and G remain same , we have
$$[T_{AB} \times 600] + [T_{AB} - (400 \times 10^3)] \times 1200 + [T_{AB} - (-500 \times 10^3)] \times 400 = 0$$
$$(2200)\, T_{AB} - 480 \times 10^6 + 200 \times 10^6 = 0$$
$$(2200)\, T_{AB} = 280 \times 10^6$$
$$T_{AB} = 127.27 \times 10^3 \text{ N-mm}$$

Eq. (i) yields... $T_{CD} = 500 \times 10^3 + 127.27 \times 10^3 = 627.23 \times 10^3 \text{ N-mm}$

Reactions at the supports:
$$T_{AB} = 127.27 \times 10^3 \text{ N-mm}$$
$$T_{BC} = [T_{AB} - T_1] = [127.27 \times 10^3 - 400 \times 10^3] = -272.73 \times 10^3 \text{ N-mm}$$
$$T_{CD} = 627.23 \times 10^3 \text{ N-mm}$$

67. A steel shaft 1m long, 30 mm diameter is rigidly fixed at its ends. A torque of 600 N-m is applied at a distance of 250 mm from the left end in CCW direction. Calculate:

(a) Reactions at the supports

(b) Maximum shear stress

(c) Angle of twist at the point of application of torque. Take G = 84 GPa

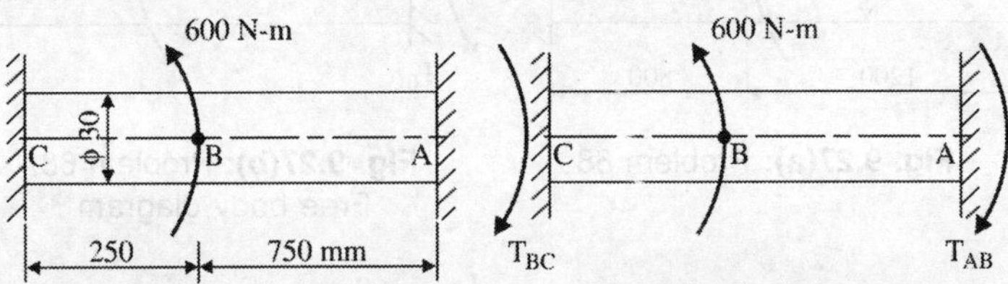

Fig. 9.26(a): Problem 67   **Fig. 9.26(b):** Problem 67:
                                        Free body diagram

Solution: d = 30 mm, L_{AB} = 750 mm, L_{BC} = 250 mm, T = 600 N-m, G = 84 × 10³ MPa.
a) T_{AB} = ?, T_{CD} = ? b) T_{AB} = ?, T_{CD} = ? c) θ = ?

The free-body diagram of the system is shown in **Fig. 9.26(b)**.

Assume that clockwise torques/moments are negative and counterclockwise torques/moments are positive.

For equilibrium,
$\Sigma M = 0: -T_{BC} + 600 \times 10^3 - T_{AB} = 0 \Rightarrow T_{AB} + T_{BC} = 600 \times 10^3 \text{ N-mm}$ ... Eq. (i)

Since the shafts are connected in parallel, we have
$$\theta_{AB} = \theta_{BC}$$

$$\left(\frac{TL}{GJ}\right)_{AB} = \left(\frac{TL}{GJ}\right)_{BC}$$

Since J and G remain same, we have
$$T_{AB} \times 750 = T_{BC} \times 250$$
$$T_{BC} = 3\, T_{AB}$$ ... Eq. (ii)

Substituting Eq. (ii) in Eq. (i), we have
$$600 \times 10^3 = T_{AB} + 3 T_{AB}$$

$$T_{AB} = 150 \times 10^3 \, \text{N-mm}$$

Eq. (ii) yields... $\quad T_{BC} = 3 \times (150 \times 10^3) = 450 \times 10^3 \, \text{N-mm}$

a. *Reactions:* $\quad T_{AB} = 150 \times 10^3 \, \text{N-mm} \;$ and $\; T_{BC} = 450 \times 10^3 \, \text{N-mm}$

b. *Shear stress:*

For a solid shaft, $\quad \tau_{AB} = \left(\dfrac{16T}{\pi d^3}\right)_{AB} = \left(\dfrac{16 \times 150 \times 10^3}{\pi \times 30^3}\right) = 28.29 \, \text{MPa}$

$$\tau_{BC} = \left(\dfrac{16T}{\pi d^3}\right)_{BC} = \left(\dfrac{16 \times 450 \times 10^3}{\pi \times 30^3}\right) = 84.88 \, \text{MPa}$$

(maximum shear stress)

c. *Angle of twist for each portion:*

$$\tau_{CD} = \left(\dfrac{TL}{GJ}\right)_{AB} = \left[\dfrac{150 \times 10^3 \times 750}{84 \times 10^3 \times (\pi \times 30^4/32)}\right] = 0.0168 \, \text{rad}$$

$$= 0.965°$$

68. For the shaft shown in Fig. 9.27(a), determine:

(a) Reactions at the supports

(b) Maximum shear stress. Take $G = 84$ GPa

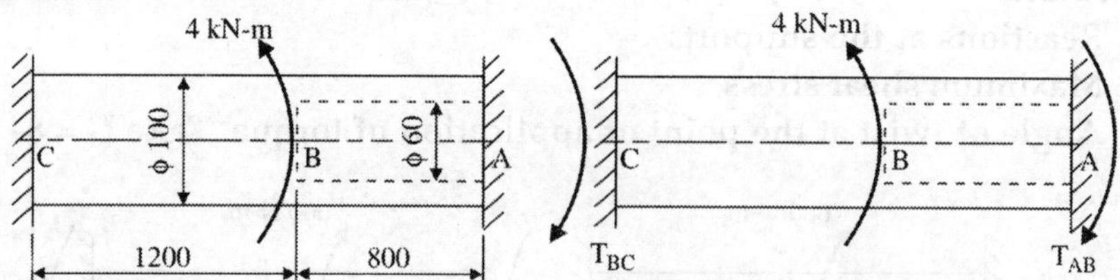

Fig. 9.27(a): Problem 68   **Fig. 9.27(b):** Problem 68:
Free body diagram

Solution: $d_{AB})_i = 60$ mm, $d_{AB})_o = 100$ mm, $K = \dfrac{d_i}{d_o} = \dfrac{60}{100} = 0.6$, $d_{BC} = 100$ mm, $L_{AB} = 800$ mm,

$L_{BC} = 1200$ mm, $T = 4000 \times 10^3$ N-mm, $G = 84 \times 10^3$ MPa. a) $T_{AB} = ?$, $T_{CD} = ?$ b) $\tau_{AB} = ?$, $\tau_{CD} = ?$ c) $\theta = ?$

The free-body diagram of the system is shown in **Fig. 9.27(b)**.

Assume that clockwise torques/moments are negative and counterclockwise torques/moments are positive.

For equilibrium,

$\Sigma M = 0$: $\quad -T_{BC} + 4000 \times 10^3 - T_{AB} = 0 \qquad \Rightarrow \; T_{AB} + T_{BC} = 4000 \times 10^3$ N-mm $\quad$ ... Eq. (i)

Since the shafts are connected in parallel, we have

$$\theta_{AB} = \theta_{BC}$$

$$\left(\dfrac{TL}{GJ}\right)_{AB} = \left(\dfrac{TL}{GJ}\right)_{BC}$$

$$\left[\dfrac{T_{AB} \times 800}{84 \times 10^3 \times [\pi \times 100^4 \times (1 - 0.6^4)/32]}\right] = \left[\dfrac{T_{BC} \times 1200}{84 \times 10^3 \times (\pi \times 100^4/32)}\right]$$

$$T_{AB} = 1.3056 \, T_{BC} \qquad \qquad \text{... Eq. (ii)}$$

Substituting Eq. (ii) in Eq. (i), we have
$$4000 \times 10^3 = 1.3056\, T_{BC} + T_{BC}$$
$$T_{BC} = 1735 \times 10^3 \text{ N-mm}$$

Eq. (ii) yields...
$$T_{AB} = 1.3056 \times (1735 \times 10^3) = 2265.22 \times 10^3 \text{ N-mm}$$

a. *Reactions:* $\quad T_{AB} = 2265.22 \times 10^3$ N-mm and $T_{BC} = 1735 \times 10^3$ N-mm

b. *Shear stress:*

For a solid shaft, $\quad \tau_{AB} = \left[\dfrac{16T}{\pi d_o^3 (1 - K^4)} \right]_{AB} = \left[\dfrac{16 \times 2265.22 \times 10^3}{\pi \times 100^3 \times (1 - 0.6^4)} \right] = 13.25$ MPa

(maximum shear stress)

$$\tau_{BC} = \left(\dfrac{16T}{\pi d^3} \right)_{BC} = \left(\dfrac{16 \times 1735 \times 10^3}{\pi \times 100^3} \right) = 8.84 \text{ MPa}$$

PROBLEMS ON PARALLEL SHAFTS – UNKNOWN TORQUE

69. **A stepped shaft of same material with two different diameters is held against rotation as shown in Fig. 9.28(a). If the allowable shear stress in the shaft is 43 MPa, what is the maximum torque that can be applied? Take G = 84 GPa.**

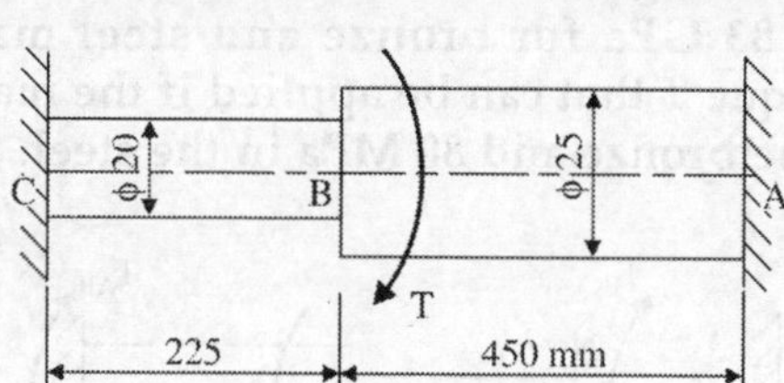

Fig. 9.28(a): Problem 69

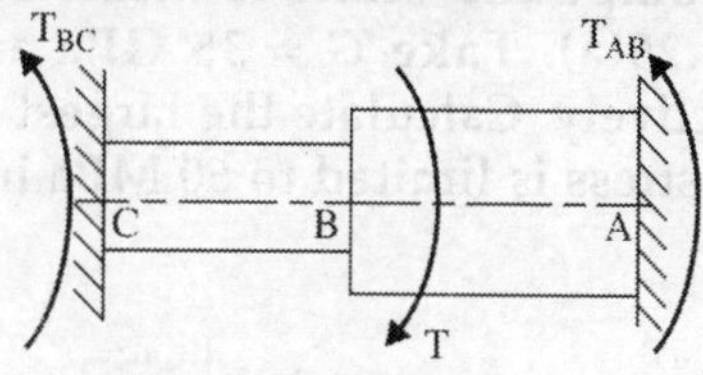

Fig. 9.28(b): Problem 69:
Free body diagrams

Solution: $d_{AB} = 25$ mm, $d_{BC} = 20$ mm, $L_{AB} = 450$ mm, $L_{BC} = 225$ mm, $\tau = 43$ MPa, $G = 84 \times 10^3$ MPa. $T = ?$.

The free-body diagram of the system is shown in **Fig. 9.28(b)**.

Assume that clockwise torques/moments are negative and counterclockwise torques/moments are positive.

For equilibrium, $\quad \Sigma M = 0$: $\quad T_{BC} - T + T_{AB} = 0 \quad \Rightarrow \quad T_{AB} + T_{BC} = T \qquad$ ... Eq. (i)

Since the shafts are connected in parallel, we have
$$\theta_{AB} = \theta_{BC}$$

$$\left(\frac{TL}{GJ} \right)_{AB} = \left(\frac{TL}{GJ} \right)_{BC}$$

$$\left[\frac{T_{AB} \times 450}{84 \times 10^3 \times [\pi \times 25^4/32)} \right] = \left[\frac{T_{BC} \times 225}{84 \times 10^3 \times (\pi \times 20^4/32)} \right]$$

$$T_{AB} = 1.2207\, T_{BC} \qquad \text{... Eq. (ii)}$$

To find T:

a. *Based on Shaft AB:*

For a solid shaft, $\qquad \tau_{AB} = \left(\dfrac{16T}{\pi d^3} \right)_{AB}$

$$43 = \left(\frac{16 \times T_{AB}}{\pi \times 25^3}\right)$$

$$T_{AB} = 131.92 \times 10^3 \text{ N-mm} = 131.92 \text{ N-m} \qquad \text{... Eq. (iii)}$$

Eq. (ii) yields... $\qquad 131.92 = 1.2207\, T_{BC}$

$$T_{BC} = 108.07 \text{ N-m} \qquad \text{... Eq. (iv)}$$

b. *Based on Shaft BC:*

For a solid shaft, $\qquad T_{BC} = \left(\frac{16T}{\pi d^3}\right)_{BC}$

$$43 = \left(\frac{16 \times T_{BC}}{\pi \times 20^3}\right)$$

$$T_{BC} = 67.54 \times 10^3 \text{ N-mm} = 67.54 \text{ N-m} \qquad \text{... Eq. (v)}$$

Eq. (ii) yields... $\qquad T_{AB} = 1.2207 \times 67.54$

$$T_{AB} = 82.45 \text{ N-m} \qquad \text{... Eq. (vi)}$$

Permissible torque is the minimum of Eqs (iii) to (vi)

$$T_{AB} = 82.45 \text{ N-m and } T_{BC} = 67.54 \text{ N-m}$$

Eq. (i) yields... $\qquad T = 82.45 + 67.54 = 149.99 \simeq 150 \text{ N-m}$

70. The compound shaft is attached to a rigid wall at each end as shown in Fig. 9.29(a). Take $G = 35$ GPa and 83 GPa for bronze and steel materials respectively. Calculate the largest torque T that can be applied if the maximum shear stress is limited to 60 MPa in the bronze and 80 MPa in the steel.

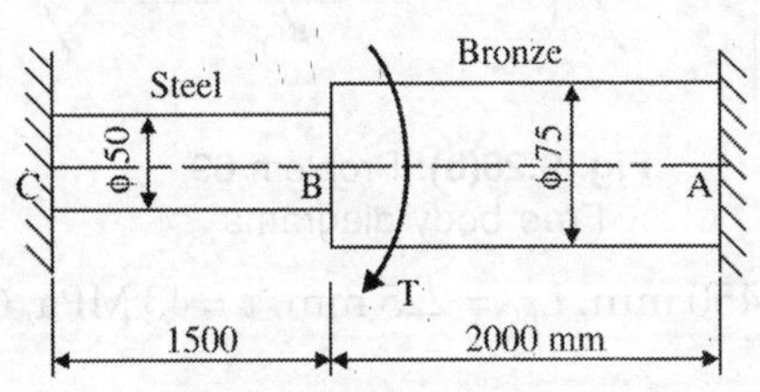

Fig. 9.29(a): Problem 70

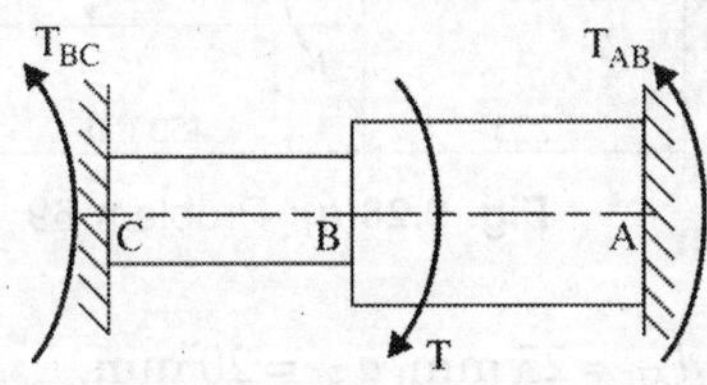

Fig. 9.29(b): Problem 70: Free body diagram

Solution: $d_{AB} = 75$ mm, $d_{BC} = 50$ mm, $L_{AB} = 2000$ mm, $L_{BC} = 1500$ mm, $\tau_{AB} = 60$ MPa, $\tau_{BC} = 80$ MPa, $G_{AB} = 35 \times 10^3$ MPa, $G_{BC} = 83 \times 10^3$ MPa. $T = ?$.

The free-body diagram of the system is shown in **Fig. 9.29(b)**.

Assume that clockwise torques/moments are negative and counterclockwise torques/moments are positive.

For equilibrium, $\qquad \Sigma M = 0$: $\quad T_{BC} - T + T_{AB} = 0 \implies T_{AB} + T_{BC} = T \qquad \text{... Eq. (i)}$

Since the shafts are connected in parallel, we have

$$\theta_{AB} = \theta_{BC}$$

$$\left(\frac{TL}{GJ}\right)_{AB} = \left(\frac{TL}{GJ}\right)_{BC}$$

$$\left[\frac{T_{AB} \times 2000}{35 \times 10^3 \times [\pi \times 75^4 / 32]}\right] = \frac{T_{BC} \times 1500}{83 \times 10^3 \times (\pi \times 50^4 / 32)}$$

$$T_{AB} = 1.6011\, T_{BC} \qquad \text{... Eq. (ii)}$$

To find T:
a. *Based on Shaft AB:*

For a solid shaft,
$$T_{AB} = \left(\frac{16T}{\pi d^3}\right)_{AB}$$

$$43 = \left(\frac{16 \times T_{AB}}{\pi \times 75^3}\right)$$

$$T_{AB} = 4970.1 \times 10^3 \text{ N-mm} = 4970.1 \text{ N-m} \qquad \text{... Eq. (iii)}$$

Eq. (ii) yields...
$$4970.1 = 1.6011\, T_{BC}$$
$$T_{BC} = 3104.18 \text{ N-m} \qquad \text{... Eq. (iv)}$$

b. *Based on Shaft BC:*

For a solid shaft,
$$T_{AB} = \left(\frac{16T}{\pi d^3}\right)_{BC}$$

$$80 = \left(\frac{16 \times T_{BC}}{\pi \times 50^3}\right)$$

$$T_{BC} = 1963.50 \times 10^3 \text{ N-mm} = 1963.50 \text{ N-m} \qquad \text{... Eq. (v)}$$

Eq. (ii) yields...
$$T_{AB} = 1.6011 \times 1963.50$$
$$T_{AB} = 3143.76 \text{ N-m} \qquad \text{... Eq. (vi)}$$

Permissible torque is the minimum of Eqs (iii) to (vi)
$$T_{AB} = 3143.76 \text{ N-m and } T_{BC} = 1963.50 \text{ N-m}$$

Eq. (i) yields...
$$T = 3143.76 + 1963.50 = 5107.26 \text{ N-m}$$

71. **A stepped shaft is as shown in Fig. 9.30(a). The material of the bar is the same throughout both segments. Obtain:**
    (a) The reactive torques at the supports.
    (b) The maximum shear stresses in each segment of the shaft, and
    (c) The angle of rotation at the cross section where *T* is applied.

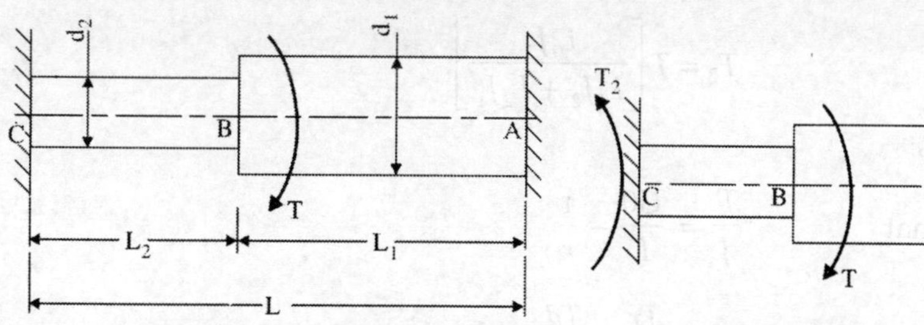

Fig. 9.30(a): Problem 71   **Fig. 9.30(b):** Problem 71:
Free body diagram

Solution: $d_{AB} = d_1$, $d_{BC} = d_2$, $L_{AB} = L_1$, $L_{BC} = L_2$, $G = G_{AB} = G_{BC}$
Let $T_{AB} = T_1$, be the reactive torque at support A
        $T_{BC} = T_2$, be the reactive torque at support C
        $J_{AB} = J_1$, be the polar modulus of portion AB
        $J_{BC} = J_2$, be the polar modulus of portion BC

The free-body diagram of the system is shown in **Fig. 9.30(b)**.

Assume that clockwise torques/moments are negative and counterclockwise torques/moments are positive.

For equilibrium,
$$\Sigma M = 0: \quad T_{BC} - T + T_{AB} = 0 \Rightarrow T_{AB} + T_{BC} = T \quad \text{i.e.} \quad T_1 + T_2 = T \qquad \text{... Eq. (i)}$$

Since the shafts are connected in parallel, we have
$$\theta_{AB} = \theta_{BC} \quad \text{or} \quad \Sigma\theta = 0$$

$$\left(\frac{TL}{GJ}\right)_{AB} = \left(\frac{TL}{GJ}\right)_{BC}$$

$$\left[\frac{T_1 L_1}{GJ_1}\right] = \left[\frac{T_2 L_2}{GJ_2}\right]$$

$$T_1 = T_2 \left(\frac{L_2}{L_1}\right)\left(\frac{J_1}{J_2}\right) \qquad \text{... Eq. (ii)}$$

Or
$$T_2 = T_1 \left(\frac{L_1}{L_2}\right)\left(\frac{J_2}{J_1}\right) \qquad \text{... Eq. (iii)}$$

Substituting Eq. (iii) in Eq. (i) yields...

$$T = T_1 + T_1 \left(\frac{L_1}{L_2}\right)\left(\frac{J_2}{J_1}\right)$$

$$= \frac{T_1 L_2 J_1 + T_1 L_1 J_2}{L_2 J_1} = T_1\left[\frac{L_2 J_1 + L_1 J_2}{L_2 J_1}\right]$$

$$T_1 = T\left[\frac{L_2 J_1}{L_1 J_2 + L_2 J_1}\right] \qquad \text{... Eq. (iv)}$$

On similar lines, we have

$$T_2 = T\left[\frac{L_1 J_2}{L_1 J_2 + L_2 J_1}\right] \qquad \text{... Eq. (v)}$$

Shear stresses:

We know that
$$\frac{T}{J} = \frac{G\theta}{L} = \frac{\tau}{r}$$

$$\tau = \frac{Tr}{J} = \frac{Td}{2J}$$

Thus
$$\tau_{AB} = \left(\frac{Td}{2J}\right)_{AB} = \frac{T_1 d_1}{2J_1} = \left(\frac{Td_1}{2J_1}\right)\left[\frac{L_2 J_1}{L_1 J_2 + L_2 J_1}\right]$$

$$\tau_1 = \left[\frac{TL_2 d_1}{2(L_1 J_2 + L_2 J_1)}\right]$$

$$\tau_{BC} = \left(\frac{Td}{2J}\right)_{AB} = \frac{T_2 d_2}{2J_2} = \left(\frac{Td_2}{2J_2}\right)\left[\frac{L_1 J_2}{L_1 J_2 + L_2 J_1}\right]$$

$$\tau_2 = \left[\frac{TL_1 d_2}{2(L_1 J_2 + L_2 J_1)}\right]$$

Angle of twist:

$$\theta_{AB} = \theta_{BC} = \left(\frac{TL}{GL}\right)_{AB} = \frac{T_1 L_1}{GJ_1} = \left(\frac{L_1}{GJ_1}\right)\left[\frac{TL_2 J_1}{L_1 J_2 + L_2 J_1}\right]$$

$$\theta_1 = \theta_2 = \left[\frac{TL_1 L_2}{G(L_1 J_2 + L_2 J_1)}\right]$$

72. A uniform shaft is as shown in Fig. 9.31(a). The material of the bar is the same throughout Obtain:

   (a) The reactive torques at the supports.

   (b) The maximum shear stresses in each segment of the shaft, and

   (c) The angle of rotation at the cross section where T is applied.

Solution: $L_{AB} = L_1$, $L_{BC} = L_2$, $G = G_{AB} = G_{BC}$

   Let d = diameter of the shaft

   $T_{AB} = T_1$, be the reactive torque at support A

   $T_{BC} = T_2$, be the reactive torque at support C

   $J_{AB} = J_1$, be the polar modulus of portion AB

   $J_{BC} = J_2$, be the polar modulus of portion BC

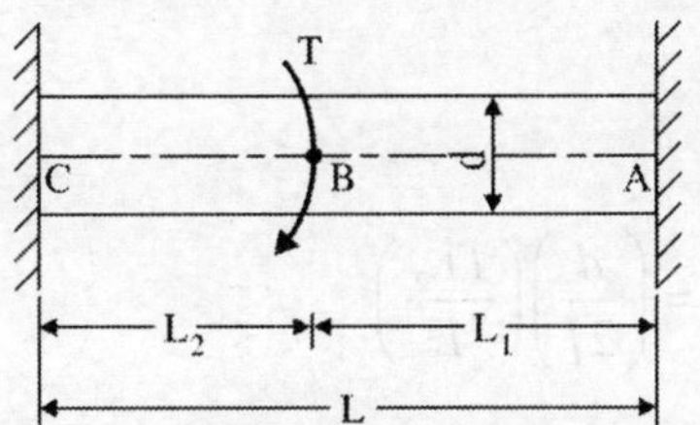

Fig. 9.31(a): Problem 72   **Fig. 9.31(b):** Problem 72:
Free body diagrams

The free-body diagram of the system is shown in **Fig. 9.31(b)**.

Assume that clockwise torques/moments are negative and counterclockwise torques/moments are positive.

For equilibrium, $\Sigma M = 0$: $T_{BC} - T + T_{AB} = 0 \Rightarrow T_{AB} + T_{BC} = T$

   i.e. $T_1 + T_2 = T$ ... Eq. (i)

Since the shafts are connected in parallel, we have

$$\theta_{AB} = \theta_{BC} \quad \text{or} \quad \Sigma\theta = 0$$

$$\left(\frac{TL}{GJ}\right)_{AB} = \left(\frac{TL}{GJ}\right)_{BC}$$

$$\left[\frac{T_1 L_1}{GJ_1}\right] = \left[\frac{T_2 L_2}{GJ_2}\right]$$

Since the diameter is uniform, $J_1 = J_2$

$$T_1 = T_2 \left(\frac{L_2}{L_1}\right) \qquad \text{... Eq. (ii)}$$

Or

$$T_2 = T_1 \left(\frac{L_1}{L_2} \right) \qquad \text{... Eq. (iii)}$$

Substituting Eq. (iii) in Eq. (i) yields...

$$T = T_1 + T_1 \left(\frac{L_1}{L_2} \right)$$

$$= \frac{T_1 L_2 + T_1 L_1}{L_2} = T_1 \left[\frac{L_2 + L_1}{L_2} \right] = \left(\frac{T_1 L}{L_2} \right) \qquad (\because L = L_1 + L_2)$$

$$T_1 = \left(\frac{T L_2}{L} \right) \qquad \text{... Eq. (iv)}$$

On similar lines, we have

$$T_2 = \left(\frac{T L_1}{L} \right) \qquad \text{... Eq. (v)}$$

Shear stresses:

We know that

$$\frac{T}{J} = \frac{G\theta}{L} = \frac{\tau}{r}$$

$$\tau = \frac{Tr}{J} = \frac{Td}{2J}$$

Thus

$$\tau_{AB} = \left(\frac{Td}{2J} \right)_{AB} = \frac{T_1 d}{2J} = \left(\frac{d}{2J} \right) \left(\frac{T L_2}{L} \right)$$

$$\tau_1 = \left[\frac{Td L_2}{2LJ} \right]$$

$$\tau_{BC} = \left(\frac{Td}{2J} \right)_{AB} = \frac{T_2 d}{2J} = \left(\frac{d}{2J} \right) \left(\frac{T L_1}{L} \right)$$

$$\tau_2 = \left[\frac{Td L_1}{2LJ} \right]$$

Angle of twist:

$$\theta_{AB} = \theta_{BC} = \left(\frac{TL}{GJ} \right)_{AB} = \frac{T_1 L_1}{GJ} = \left(\frac{L_1}{GJ} \right) \left(\frac{T L_2}{L} \right)$$

$$\theta_1 = \theta_2 = \left[\frac{T L_1 L_2}{GJL} \right]$$

9.10 TORSION OF THIN WALLED SECTIONS

Thin walled sections are common where light weight is of primary importance. These can be analyzed for torsion using similar assumptions as for circular sections;

i.e., plane sections remain plane, shear strains are small. However, since the thickness of the section is very small, the shear stresses remain almost constant across the thickness instead of varying linearly from the center of rotation.

The thin walled members or sections are divided into two groups:
1. Thin walled closed profiles
2. Thin walled open profiles

Some examples of closed thin wall sections include tube, box, aircraft fuselage, aircraft wings and tail, etc. These are more effective in resisting torque than open thin wall sections. Closed thin walled sections are further classified into single cell or multi-cellular, depending on whether there is only one shear flow circuit or several flow circuits.

9.10.1 Thin walled closed sections

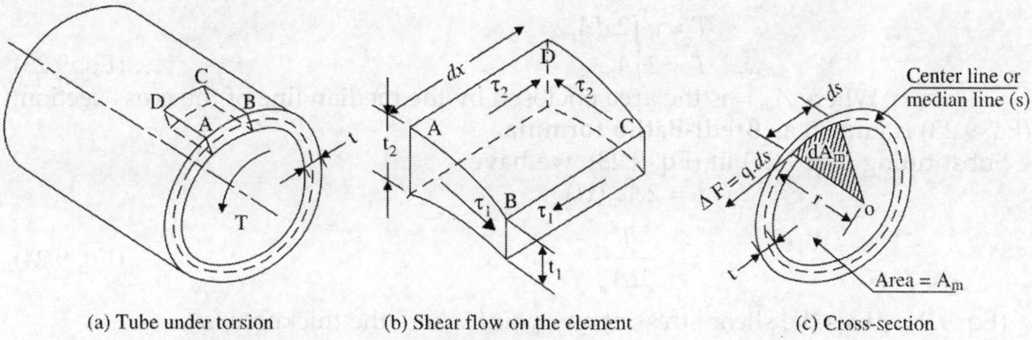

Fig. 9.32: Torison of thin walled closed tube of any cross-section

Limitations in analysis of thin walled closed tubes:
- The material is homogeneous and isotropic.
- The cross-section must be thin-walled, but not necessarily of constant thickness.
- Variations in thickness must not be abrupt except at re-entrant corners.
- No buckling occurs.
- The shear stress does not exceed the shearing proportional limit and is proportional to the shear strain.

Consider the thin-walled closed tube shown in **Fig. 9.32(a)** subjected to a torque T. The thickness t of the wall is not necessarily constant but may vary around the cross section. However, the thickness must be small in comparison with the total width of the tube. For the purpose of analysis, it is assumed that the thickness does not vary along the length of the tube.

Consider a small element of the tube as shown in **Fig. 9.32(b)**. At one end, the element has a thickness t_1 while at the other end, the thickness is t_2. If τ_1 is the shear stress at B and τ_2 is the shear stress at A then, from the equilibrium of the complementary shears on the sides CB and AD, it follows that

$$\tau_1 \, t \, dx = \tau_2 \, t \, dx$$

$$\tau_1 \, dx = \tau_2 \, dx \qquad \qquad \text{... (Eq. 9.20)}$$

i..e. the product of the shear stress and the thickness is constant at all points on the periphery of the tube. This constant is termed the shear flow and denoted by the symbol q and has the units of a load per unit length of the circumference of the tube.

Thus $\qquad\qquad\qquad q = \tau \, t = \text{constant} \qquad\qquad \text{... (Eq. 9.21)}$

The quantity q is termed the shear flow because q is analogous to water flowing through a tube of rectangular cross section having a constant depth and variable width w Although the water's velocity v at each point along the tube will be different, the flow $q = vw$ will be constant.

Torque:

Force acting on elementary length ds of tube, $\Delta F = q.ds$

The moment of this force about an arbitrary point O, $\Delta T = r.\Delta F = rq.ds$

Thus the moment or torque for the whole section,

$$T = \int \Delta T = \int rq.ds = q \int r.ds \qquad \text{... (Eq. 9.22)}$$

Area of shaded triangle **[Fig. 9.32(c)]** $dA_m = \dfrac{1}{2}\, r.ds$

$$\text{i.e. } r.ds = 2\, dA_m$$

$$T = q \int 2.dA_m$$

$$\therefore \quad T = 2qA_m \qquad \text{... (Eq. 9.23)}$$

Where $A_m = $ is the area enclosed by the median line of the cross-section. (Eq. 9.23) is known as **Bredt-Batho formula**.

Substituting (Eq. 9.21) in (Eq. 9.23), we have

$$T = 2A_m\,(\tau t)$$

$$\tau = \frac{T}{2tA_m} \qquad \text{... (Eq. 9.24)}$$

(Eq. 9.24) gives the shear stress at any point where the thickness is t

Angle of twist:

To find the angle of twist of the tube we consider the strain energy stored in the tube, and equate this to the work done by the torque T in twisting the tube.

Strain energy stored per unit volume $= \displaystyle\int \frac{\tau^2 V}{2G}$

Here

$$V = area \times length = (t.ds)L$$
$$ds = \text{Width}$$
$$t = \text{thickness}$$
$$L = \text{Length of the element}$$

$$= \int \frac{\tau^2}{2G}\,(t.L.ds) = \int \left(\frac{T^2}{4A_m^2 t^2} \right)\left(\frac{tL}{2G} \right) ds \ \text{ ... using (Eq. 9.24)}$$

$$= \frac{T^2 L}{8GA_m^2} \int \frac{ds}{t} \qquad \text{... (Eq. 9.25)}$$

Work done by torque $\quad = \dfrac{1}{2} T\theta \qquad \text{... (Eq. 9.26)}$

Equating Eqs (9.25) and (9.26), we have

$$\frac{1}{2} T\theta = \frac{T^2 L}{8GA_m^2} \int \frac{ds}{t}$$

$$\theta = \frac{TL}{4GA_m^2} \int \frac{ds}{t} \qquad \text{... (Eq. 9.27)}$$

For tube of constant thickness, (Eq. 9.27) reduces to the form,

$$\theta = \frac{TLs}{4GA_m^2 t} = \frac{\tau Ls}{2GA_m} \qquad \text{... (Eq. 9.28a) using (Eq.9.24)}$$

Where s = length or perimeter of median line

For closed sections which have constant thickness over specified lengths but varying from one part of the perimeter to another:

$$\frac{\theta}{L} = \left[\frac{s_1}{t_1} + \frac{s_2}{t_2} + \frac{s_2}{t_2} + \cdots \right] \qquad \text{... (Eq. 9.28b)}$$

Torsion constant: For a thin-walled tube, the torsion constant (J) is defined as:

$$J = \frac{4A_m^2}{\int \dfrac{ds}{t}} \qquad \text{... (Eq. 9.29)}$$

For tube of constant thickness, (Eq. 9.29) reduces to the form,

$$J = \frac{4A_m^2}{s} \qquad \text{... (Eq. 9.30)}$$

73. For a thin cylindrical tube of mean radius r_m, constant thickness t, and length L, prove that the polar moment of inertia of the cross-sectional area can be approximated by $J = 2\pi r_m^3 t$. Also find the angle of twist.

Solution: Consider a thin cylindrical tube as shown in **Fig. 9.33**.

Let r_m = mean radius of tube

$A_m = \pi r_m^2$ = mean area of tube or area enclosed by the median line

L = Length of the tube

t = thickness of the tube

d_o = outer diameter of the tube

d_i = inner diameter of the tube

J = Polar moment of inertia

s = length or perimeter of median line

a. *To find J:*

Shear stress at any point $\tau = \dfrac{T}{2A_m t} = \dfrac{T}{2\pi t r_m^2}$

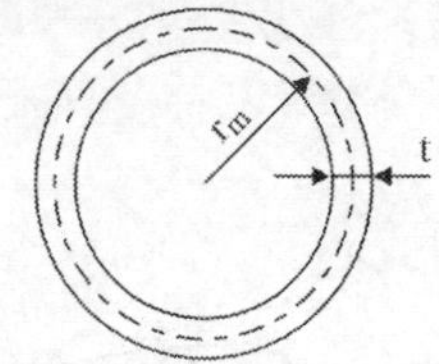

Fig. 9.33: Problem 73

For a hollow shaft $\quad J = \dfrac{\pi}{32}\left(d_o^4 - d_i^4 \right) = \dfrac{\pi}{2}\left(r_o^4 - r_i^4 \right)$

$$= \frac{\pi}{2}\left(r_o^2 + r_i^2 \right)\left(r_o^2 - r_i^2 \right)$$

$$= \frac{\pi}{2}\left(r_o^2 + r_i^2 \right)\left[(r_o + r_i)(r_o - r_i) \right]$$

Since $r_m \approx r_o \approx r_i$ and $t = (r_o - r_i)$, we have

$$J = \frac{\pi}{2}\left(2r_m^2\right)\left(2r_m\right)t$$

$$\therefore \quad J = \left(2\pi r_m^3 t\right) \qquad \qquad \text{... (Eq. 9.31)}$$

b. *Angle of twist:*

We know that $\qquad \theta = \dfrac{TL}{4GA_m^2}\displaystyle\int \dfrac{ds}{t} \qquad\qquad$ ... using (Eq. 9.27)

For tube of constant thickness, Eq. (9.27) reduces to the form,

$$\theta = \frac{TLs}{4GA_m^2 t} \qquad\qquad \text{... using (Eq. 9.28a)}$$

$$\theta = \frac{TL(2\pi r_m)}{4G(\pi r_m^2)^2 t} \qquad\qquad [\text{Here perimeter, } s = \pi d_m = 2\pi r_m]$$

$$\theta = \frac{TL}{2\pi r_m^3 Gt} = \frac{TL}{GJ} \qquad\qquad \text{... (Eq. 9.32)}$$

74. A circular tube and a square tube are constructed of the same material and subjected to the same torque. Both tubes have the same length, same wall thickness, and same cross-sectional area. What are the ratios of their shear stresses and angles of twist?. Neglect stress concentration

Solution: $A_c = A_s, L_c = L_s , T_c = T_s = T.$ a) $\tau_c/\tau_s = ?$ b) $\theta_c/\theta_s = ?$

Based on data, the problem is as shown in **Fig. 9.34**

Let *suffix 'c' denote circular tube and 's' denote square tube.*

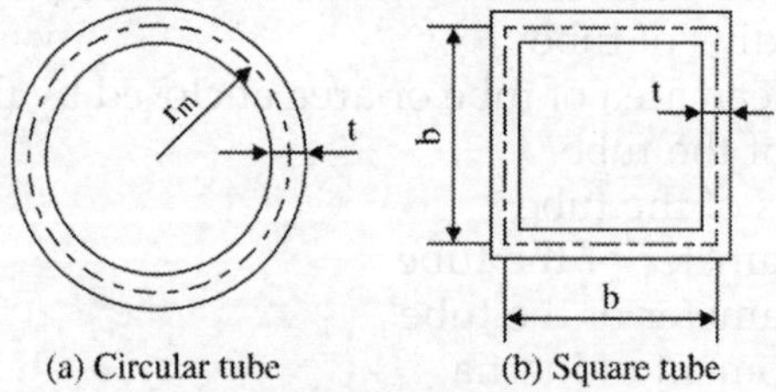

(a) Circular tube   (b) Square tube

Fig. 9.34: Problem 74

A_c = Cross-sectional area of circular tube
A_s = Cross-sectional area of square tube
L_c = Length of circular tube
L_s = Length of square tube
T_c = Torque transmitted by circular tube
T_s = Torque transmitted by square tube
τ_c = Shear stress in circular tube
τ_s = Shear stress in square tube
J_c = Torsion constant for circular tube
J_s = Torsion constant of square tube
t = Thickness of the tube.
A_{mc} = Area enclosed by the median line of the cross-section in circular tube.
A_{ms} = Area enclosed by the median line of the cross-section in square tube

Cross-sectional area of circular tube, $A_c = 2\pi r_m t$ ... Eq. (i)

Cross-sectional area of square tube, $A_s = 4bt$ ... Eq. (ii)

Since $A_c = A_s$, we have

$$2\pi r_m t = 4bt$$

$$b = \frac{\pi r_m}{2}$$ ... Eq. (iii)

Thus the area enclosed by median line of respective tubes are

$$A_{mc} = \pi r_m^2$$ ... Eq. (iv)

$$A_{ms} = b^2 = \left(\frac{\pi r_m}{2}\right)^2 = \frac{\pi^2 r_m^2}{4}$$ ... Eq. (v)

But torsion constant, $$J = \frac{4 A_m^2}{\displaystyle\int \frac{ds}{t}}$$ ... using (Eq. 9.29)

For a circular tube, $$J_c = \left(2\pi r_m^2 t\right)$$ ... Eq. (vi) using (Eq. 9.31)

For a square tube, $$\int \frac{ds}{t} = \left[\frac{s_1}{t_1} + \frac{s_2}{t_2} + \frac{s_2}{t_2} + \cdots\right] = \left[\frac{b}{t} + \frac{b}{t} + \frac{b}{t} + \frac{b}{t}\right] = \frac{4b}{t}$$

$$J_s = \frac{4 A_{ms}^2}{\displaystyle\int \frac{ds}{t}} = \frac{4(b^2)^2}{4b/t} = b^3 t = \left(\frac{\pi r_m}{2}\right)^3 t$$

$$J_s = \left(\frac{\pi^3 r_m^3}{8}\right) t$$ ... Eq. (vii)

a. *Ratio of shear stresses:*

Shear stress at any point $\tau = \dfrac{T}{2t A_m}$

$$\frac{\tau_c}{\tau_s} = \frac{A_{ms}}{A_{mc}}$$ (since other terms cancel out)

$$= \frac{\pi^2 r_m^2 / 4}{\pi r_m^2}$$ ... using Eqs (iv) and (v)

$$\frac{\tau_c}{\tau_s} = \frac{\pi}{4} = 0.7854$$

b. *Ratio of angle of twist:*

Angle of twist, $\theta = \dfrac{TL}{GJ}$

$$\frac{\theta_c}{\theta_s} = \frac{J_s}{J_c}$$ (since other terms cancel out)

$$= \frac{\pi^3 r_m^3 t / 8}{2\pi r_m^3 t} \qquad \text{... using Eqs (vi) and (vii)}$$

$$\frac{\theta_c}{\theta_s} = \frac{\pi^2}{16} = 0.6169$$

75. A thin walled box section having dimensions $2a \times a \times t$ is to be compared with a solid circular rod as shown in Fig. 9.35. Determine the thickness so that the two sections have:

(a) The same maximum shear stress for the same torque

(b) Same stiffness.

Solution: $t = ?$ a) based on shear stress, b) based on stiffness.

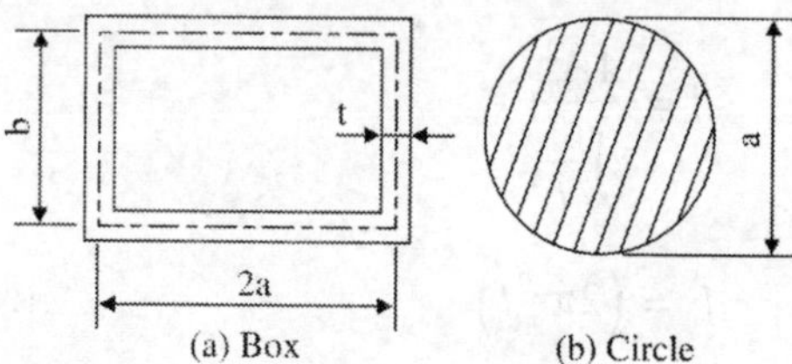

(a) Box   (b) Circle

Fig. 9.35: Problem 75

For a box or thin walled tubes:

Shear stress at any point $\tau = \dfrac{T}{2tA_m}$

$$\text{Here } A_m = 2a.a = 2a^2$$

$$\tau = \frac{T}{2(2a^2)t} = \frac{T}{4a^2 t} \qquad \text{... Eq. (i)}$$

For a Circular rod:

We know that $\dfrac{T}{J} = \dfrac{G\theta}{L} = \dfrac{\tau}{r}$

From which we have $\quad \tau = \dfrac{16T}{\pi d^3} = \dfrac{16T}{\pi a^3} \quad$ [since diameter is a] $\qquad$ ... Eq. (ii)

a. *Based on shear stress*

Equating Eqs (i) and (ii), we have

$$\frac{T}{4a^2 t} = \frac{16T}{\pi a^3}$$

$$t = \frac{\pi a}{64} \qquad \text{... Eq. (iii)}$$

b. *Based on torsional stiffness:*

   i. For a box or thin walled tubes:

Angle of twist $\qquad \theta = \dfrac{TL}{4GA_m^2} \displaystyle\int \dfrac{ds}{t}$

$$= \frac{TL}{4GA_m^2} \left[\frac{s_1}{t_1} + \frac{s_2}{t_2} + \frac{s_2}{t_2} + \cdots \right]$$

$$= \frac{TL}{4GA_m^2} \left[\frac{a}{t} + \frac{2a}{t} + \frac{a}{t} + \frac{2a}{t} \right]$$

$$= \frac{6aTL}{4GA_m^2 t} = \frac{6aTL}{4(2a^2)^2 Gt}$$

$$\theta = \frac{6TL}{16a^3 Gt}$$

Stiffness $\qquad \dfrac{\theta}{L} = \dfrac{6T}{16a^3 Gt}$ ... Eq. (iii)

ii. For a Circular rod:

$$\theta = \frac{TL}{GJ} = \frac{TL}{G(\pi a^4 / 32)}$$

Stiffness $\qquad \dfrac{\theta}{L} = \dfrac{32T}{G\pi a^4}$ ... Eq. (iv)

Equating Eqs (iii) and (iv), we have

$$\frac{6T}{16a^3 Gt} = \frac{32T}{G\pi a^4}$$

$$\frac{3}{8t} = \frac{32}{\pi a}$$

$$t = \frac{3\pi a}{256} = \left(\frac{3}{4} \right)\left(\frac{\pi a}{64} \right)$$

76. A thin-walled steel tube of rectangular cross section has a constant thickness as shown in Fig. 9.36. Determine:
   (a) The shear stress in the tube due to a torque T = 1.2 kN-m.
   (b) The angle of twist, if the length L of the tube is 1.5 m. Take G = 84 GPa.

Solution: $b = 120$ mm, $h = 100$ mm, $t = 5$ mm, $T = 1.2 \times 10^6$ N-mm, $L = 1500$ mm, $G = 84 \times 10^3$ MPa. a) $\tau = ?$ b) $\theta = ?$

a. *Shear stress:*

Shear stress at any point $\tau = \dfrac{T}{2tA_m}$

$\qquad$ Here $A_m = bh$

$\qquad A_m = 120 \times 100 = 12000$ mm^2

$$\tau = \frac{1.2 \times 10^6}{2 \times 12000 \times 5} = 10 \, \text{MPa}$$

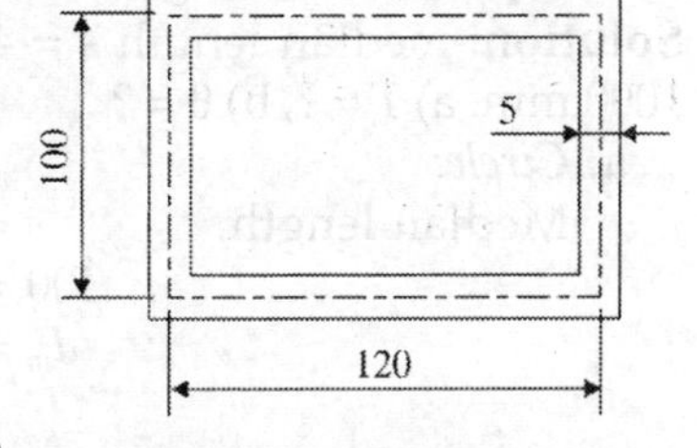

Fig. 9.36: Problems 76

b. *Angle of twist:* $\qquad \theta = \dfrac{TL}{4GA_m^2} \displaystyle\int \frac{ds}{t}$

$$\text{Here } \int \frac{ds}{t} = \frac{120}{5} + \frac{100}{5} + \frac{120}{5} + \frac{100}{5} = 88$$

$$\theta = \frac{(1.2 \times 10^6) \times 1500 \times 88}{4 \times (84 \times 10^3) \times (12000)^2}$$

$$\theta = 0.00327 \text{ rad} = 0.1875°$$

77. A rectangular tube has ouside dimensions of 80 mm × 60 mm and has a wall thicknes of 4 mm as shown in Fig. 9.37. Calculate the maximum shear stress when a torque of 1.5 kN-m is applied. Also find the angle of twist in a length of 1 m. Take G = 75 GPa.

Solution: $t = 4$ mm, $b = (80 - 4) = 76$ mm, $h = (60 - 4) = 56$ mm, $T = 1.5 \times 10^6$ N-m, $L = 1000$ mm, $G = 75 \times 10^3$ MPa. a) $\tau = ?$ b) $\theta = ?$

a. *Shear stress:*

$$\tau = \frac{T}{2tA_m}$$

$$\text{Here } A_m = bh = 76 \times 56 = 4256 \text{ mm}^2$$

$$\tau = \frac{1.5 \times 10^6}{2 \times 4256 \times 4} = 44.06 \text{ MPa}$$

Fig. 9.37: Problems 77

b. *Angle of twist:*

$$\theta = \frac{TL}{4GA_m^2} \int \frac{ds}{t}$$

$$\text{Here } \int \frac{ds}{t} = \frac{76}{4} + \frac{56}{4} + \frac{76}{4} + \frac{56}{4} = 66$$

$$\theta = \frac{(1.5 \times 10^6) \times 1000 \times 66}{4 \times (75 \times 10^3) \times (4256)^2}$$

$$\theta = 0.0182 \text{ rad} = 1.0438°$$

78. A steel sheet, 400 mm wide by 2 mm thick, is to be formed into a hollow section by bending through 360° and butt-welding the long edges together. The shape may be (a) circular, (b) square, (c) a rectangle 140 mm × 60 mm. Assume a median length of 400 mm in each case (i.e. no stretching) and square corners for non-circular sections. The allowable shearing stress is 90 MPa. For each of the shapes listed determine the magnitude of the maximum permissible torque and the angles of twist per metre length if G = 80 GPa.

Solution: median length $s = 400$ mm, $t = 2$ mm, $\tau = 90$ MPa, $G = 80 \times 10^3$ MPa, $L = 1000$ mm. a) $T = ?$, b) $\theta = ?$

a. *Circle:*

Median length, $s = \pi d_m$

$$400 = \pi d_m$$

$$\therefore \quad d_m = 127.32 \text{ mm}$$

$$\Rightarrow A_m = \frac{\pi d_m^2}{4} = \frac{\pi \times 127.32^2}{4} = 12731.60 \text{ mm}^2$$

i. Torque:

$$\tau = \frac{T}{2tA_m}$$

$$90 = \frac{T}{2 \times 2 \times 12732.60}$$

$$T = 4.58 \times 10^6 \text{ N-mm}$$

ii. Angle of twist: $\theta = \dfrac{TL}{4GA_m^2} \displaystyle\int \dfrac{ds}{t}$ or $\qquad \theta = \dfrac{TL}{GJ}$

Here $\displaystyle\int \dfrac{ds}{t} = \dfrac{s}{t} = \dfrac{400}{2} = 200$ $\qquad$ here $J = 2\pi t r_m^3$ ... using (Eq. 9.31)

$$\theta = \frac{(4.58 \times 10^6) \times 1000 \times 200}{4 \times (80 \times 10^3) \times (12732.60)^2} \qquad \theta = \left[\frac{(4.58 \times 10^6) \times 1000}{(80 \times 10^3) \times [2\pi \times 2 \times (127.32/2)^3]}\right]$$

$$\theta = 0.0176 \text{ rad} = 1.0117° \qquad\qquad \theta = 0.0176 \text{ rad} = 1.0117°$$

b. *Square:*

Median length, $\qquad s = 4b$

$$400 = 4b$$

$$\therefore \quad b = 100 \text{ mm} \qquad\qquad \therefore \quad A_m = b^2 = 100^2 = 10000 \text{ mm}^2$$

i. Torque: $\qquad\qquad \tau = \dfrac{T}{2tA_m}$

$$90 = \frac{T}{2 \times 2 \times 10000}$$

$$T = 3.6 \times 10^6 \text{ N-mm}$$

ii. Angle of twist: $\qquad \theta = \dfrac{TL}{4GA_m^2} \displaystyle\int \dfrac{ds}{t}$

Here $\displaystyle\int \dfrac{ds}{t} = \dfrac{4b}{t} = 4\left(\dfrac{100}{2}\right) = 200$

$$\theta = \frac{(3.6 \times 10^6) \times 1000 \times 200}{4 \times (80 \times 10^3) \times (10000)^2}$$

$$\theta = 0.0225 \text{ rad} = 1.289°$$

c. *Rectangle:* From data $b = 140$ mm, $h = 60$ mm $\Rightarrow A_m = bh = 140 \times 60 = 8400 \text{ mm}^2$

i. Torque: $\qquad\qquad t = \dfrac{T}{2tA_m}$

$$90 = \frac{T}{2 \times 2 \times 8400}$$

$$T = 3.024 \times 10^6 \text{ N-mm}$$

ii. Angle of twist: $\quad \theta = \dfrac{TL}{4GA_m^2} \displaystyle\int \dfrac{ds}{t}$

Here $\displaystyle\int \dfrac{ds}{t} = \dfrac{2b}{t} + \dfrac{2h}{t} = \left(\dfrac{2 \times 140}{2}\right) + \left(\dfrac{2 \times 60}{2}\right) = 200$

$$\theta = \frac{(3.024 \times 10^6) \times 1000 \times 200}{4 \times (80 \times 10^3) \times (8400)^2}$$

$$\theta = 0.0268 \text{ rad} = 1.535°$$

79. A tubular shaft having an inside diameter of 50 mm and a wall thickness of 5 mm is subjected to a torque of 1.5 kN-m. Determine the maximum shear stress in the tube using:

(a) The (approximate) thin-wall torsion theory, and

(b) The (exact theory) torsion of circular shafts

Solution: $d_i = 50$, $t = 5$ mm, $d_o = d_i + 2t = 50 + 10 = 60$ mm, $K = d_i/d_o = 50/60 = 0.8334$, $T = 1.5 \times 10^6$ N-mm. $\tau = ?$

a. *Based on thin wall theory (approxiamte theory):*

Shear stress at any point $\tau = \dfrac{T}{2tA_m}$

$$\text{Here } \quad d_m = \frac{d_o + d_i}{2} = \frac{60 + 50}{2} = 55 \text{ mm}$$

$$A_m = \frac{\pi d_m^2}{4} = \frac{\pi \times 55^2}{4} = 2375.83 \text{ mm}^2$$

$$\tau = \frac{1.5 \times 10^6}{2 \times 2375.83 \times 5} = 63.14 \text{ MPa}$$

b. *Based on torsion of shafts (exact theory):*

Shear stress $\qquad \tau = \dfrac{16T}{\pi d_o^3 (1 - K^4)} = \dfrac{16 \times 1.5 \times 10^6}{\pi \times 60^3 \times (1 - 0.8334^4)} = 68.33 \text{ MPa}$

80. A tubular shaft having an inside diameter of 60 mm is subjected to a torque of 2 kN-m. If the allowable shear stress is 45 MPa, Determine the required wall thickness using:

(a) the (approximate) thin-wall torsion theory, and

(b) the (exact theory) torsion of circular shafts

Solution: $d_i = 60$, $T = 2 \times 10^6$ N-mm, $\tau = 45$ MPa, $t = ?$

$$d_o = d_i + 2t = (60 + 2t) \qquad d_m = \frac{d_o + d_i}{2} = \frac{(60 + 2t) + 60}{2} = 60 + t$$

a. *Based on thin wall theory (approxiamte theory):*

Shear stress at any point $\tau = \dfrac{T}{2tA_m}$

$$\text{Here } A_m = \frac{\pi d_m^2}{4} = \frac{\pi \times (60 + 2t)^2}{4}$$

$$45 = \frac{2 \times 10^6}{2t[\pi \times (60 + t)^2 / 4]}$$

$$t(60 + t)^2 = 28294.21$$
$$t(3600 + t^2 + 120t) = 28294.21$$
$$t^3 + 120t^2 + 3600t - 28294.21 = 0$$
$$t = 6.41 \text{ mm}$$

b. *Based on torsion of shafts (exact theory):*

We know that
$$\frac{T}{J} = \frac{G\theta}{L} = \frac{\tau}{r}$$

Shear stress
$$\tau = \frac{Tr_o}{J} = \frac{Td_o}{2J} = \frac{Td_o}{2\pi(d_o^4 - d_i^4)/32}$$

$$45 = \frac{16 \times (2 \times 10^6)d_o}{\pi(d_o^4 - d_i^4)}$$

$$\frac{(d_o^4 - d_i^4)}{d_o} = 226353.69$$

$$\frac{(60 + 2t)^4 - 60^4}{(60 + 2t)} = 226353.69$$

Using $(a^4 - b^4) = (a - b)(a + b)(a^2 + b^2)$
$$(60 + 2t - 60)(60 + 2t + 60)[(60 + 2t)^2 + 60^2] = (60 + 2t) \times 226353.69$$
$$(120 + 2t) \times 2t \times [3600 + 4t^2 + 240t + 3600] = (60 + 2t) \times 226353.69$$
$$(240t + 4t^2)[4t^2 + 240t + 7200] = (60 + 2t) \times 226353.69$$

Upon solving, we have $t = 6.90$ mm

9.11 SHAFTS SUBJECTED TO COMBINED TORQUE (T) AND BENDING MOMENT (M)

A shaft transmitting torque or power is not only subjected to shear stresses but also to bending moment due to self-weight of the shaft, pulleys and couplings and due to the pulls exerted by belts and rope drives. Hence the shafts must be designed on the basis of two moments viz. torque and bending moment simultaneously. Thus, at any point in the shaft, the components of stresses are:

i. Shear stress τ due to torsion,
ii. Bending stress σ_b (tensile or compressive), and
iii. Shear stress τ' due to bending forces.

Of the three stress components t and s_b are maximum at the surface and τ' is zero

As per torsional equation $\dfrac{T}{J} = \dfrac{\tau}{r}$, from which we have

Strength of a solid shaft, $T = \left(\dfrac{\pi d^3}{16}\right)$

$$\tau = \frac{16T}{\pi d^3} \qquad\qquad \dots \text{(Eq. 9.33) using (Eq. 9.3)}$$

The bending equation is given as

$$\frac{M}{I} = \frac{E}{R} = \frac{\sigma_b}{c}, \text{ from which we have}$$

$$\sigma_b = \frac{M}{Z} = \frac{32M}{\pi d^3}$$

where $Z = \pi d^3/32$ for a solid shaft   ... (Eq. 9.34)

Thus, the principal stresses may be obtained as

$$\sigma_{1,2} = \left(\frac{\sigma_x + \sigma_y}{2}\right) \pm \sqrt{\left(\frac{\sigma_x - \sigma_y}{2}\right)^2 + \tau_{xy}^2}$$

Here $\sigma_x = \sigma_b = \dfrac{32M}{\pi d^3}$, $\sigma_y = 0$; $\tau_{xy} = \tau = \dfrac{16T}{\pi d^3}$

$$\sigma_{1,2} = \frac{32M}{2 \times \pi d^3} \pm \sqrt{\left(\frac{32M}{2 \times \pi d^3}\right)^2 + \left(\frac{16T}{\pi d^3}\right)^2}$$

$$= \frac{16M}{\pi d^3} \pm \sqrt{\left(\frac{16M}{\pi d^3}\right)^2 + \left(\frac{16T}{\pi d^3}\right)^2}$$

$$= \frac{16M}{\pi d^3} \pm \frac{16}{\pi d^3}\sqrt{M^2 + T^2}$$

$$\sigma_{1,2} = \frac{16}{\pi d^3}\left(M + \sqrt{M^2 + T^2}\right)$$ ... (Eq. 9.34)

Thus the maximum principal stress,

$$\sigma_1 = \frac{16}{\pi d^3}\left(M + \sqrt{M^2 + T^2}\right)$$ ... (Eq. 9.35)

And minimum principal stress

$$\sigma_2 = \frac{16}{\pi d^3}\left(M - \sqrt{M^2 - T^2}\right)$$ ... (Eq. 9.36)

Maximum shear stress, $\tau_{max} = \sqrt{\left(\dfrac{\sigma_x - \sigma_y}{2}\right)^2 + \tau_{xy}^2} = \left(\dfrac{\sigma_1 - \sigma_2}{2}\right)$

$$\tau_{max} = \frac{16}{\pi d^3}\sqrt{M^2 + T^2}$$ ... (Eq. 9.37)

The principal planes are given as

$$\tan 2\phi = \left(\frac{2\tau_{xy}}{\sigma_x - \sigma_y}\right) = \frac{2 \times (16T / \pi d^3)}{(32 / \pi d^3)}$$

$$\tan 2\phi = \frac{T}{M}$$ ... (Eq. 9.38)

81. **A 60 mm shaft is subjected to a torque of 200 N-m and a bending moment of 600 N-m. Calculate:**

(a) Principal stresses

(b) Maximum shear stress and

(c) Plane position on which they act.

Solution: $d = 60$ mm, $T = 200 \times 10^3$ N-mm, $M = 600 \times 10^3$ N-m. a) $\sigma_1 = ?$, $\sigma_2 = ?$, b) $\tau_{max} = ?$ c) $\theta = ?$

Method 1: As per formulae

a. *Principal stresses:*

Maximum principal stress $\sigma_1 = \dfrac{16}{\pi d^3}\left(M + \sqrt{M^2 + T^2}\right)$

$$= \frac{16}{\pi \times 60^3}\left[6000 \times 10^3 + \sqrt{(600 \times 10^3)^2 + (200 \times 10^3)^2}\right]$$

$$\sigma_1 = 29.06 \text{ MPa}$$

Minimum principal stress $\sigma_2 = \dfrac{16}{\pi d^3}\left(M - \sqrt{M^2 + T^2}\right)$

$$= \frac{16}{\pi \times 60^3}\left[6000 \times 10^3 - \sqrt{(600 \times 10^3)^2 + (200 \times 10^3)^2}\right]$$

$$\sigma_1 = -0.77 \text{ MPa}$$

b. *Maximum shear stress:*

Maximum shear stress $\tau_{max} = \dfrac{16}{\pi d^3}\left(\sqrt{M^2 + T^2}\right)$

$$= \frac{16}{\pi \times 60^3}\left[\sqrt{(600 \times 10^3)^2 + (200 \times 10^3)^2}\right]$$

$$\tau_{max} = 14.91 \text{ MPa}$$

c. *Plane position:* $\quad \tan 2\phi = \dfrac{T}{M} = \dfrac{200 \times 10^3}{600 \times 10^3} = 0.667$

$$\phi = 9.22°$$

Method 2: Based on principal stresses:

• Bending stress $\quad \sigma_b = \dfrac{M}{Z} = \dfrac{M}{\pi d^3/32} = \dfrac{600 \times 10^3}{\pi \times 60^3/32} = 28.29 \text{ MPa}$

• Shear stress $\quad \tau = \dfrac{16}{\pi d^3} = \dfrac{16 \times (200 \times 10^3)}{\pi \times 60^3} = 4.72 \text{ MPa}$

a. *Principal stresses:* $\quad$ Here $\sigma_x = \sigma_b = 28.29$ MPa; $\sigma_y = 0$; $\tau = \sigma_{xy} = 35.37$ MPa

Maximum principal stress $\sigma_1 = \left(\dfrac{\sigma_x + \sigma_y}{2}\right) + \sqrt{\left(\dfrac{\sigma_x - \sigma_y}{2}\right)^2 + \tau_{xy}^2}$

$$= \left(\frac{28.29 + 0}{2}\right) + \sqrt{\left(\frac{28.29 - 0}{2}\right)^2 + 4.72^2}$$

$$\therefore \quad \sigma_1 = 29.06 \text{ MPa}$$

Minimum principal stress $\sigma_2 = \left(\frac{\sigma_x + \sigma_y}{2}\right) - \sqrt{\left(\frac{\sigma_x - \sigma_y}{2}\right)^2 + \tau_{xy}^2}$

$$= \left(\frac{28.29 + 0}{2}\right) - \sqrt{\left(\frac{28.29 - 0}{2}\right)^2 + 4.72^2}$$

$$\therefore \quad \sigma_2 = -0.77 \text{ MPa}$$

b. *Maximum shear stress:*

Maximum shear stress $\quad \tau_{max} = \sqrt{\left(\frac{\sigma_x - \sigma_y}{2}\right)^2 + \tau_{xy}^2}$

$$\tau_{max} = \sqrt{\left(\frac{28.29 - 0}{2}\right)^2 + 4.72^2} = 14.91 \text{ MPa}$$

c. *Plane position: Same as in method 1.*

82. A hollow shaft of 40 mm external diameter and 25 mm inner diameter is subjected to a twisting moment of 118 N-m and a bending moment of 79 N-m. Calculate the principal stresses and maximum shear stresses.

Solution: $d_o = 40$ mm, $d_i = 25$ mm, $K = d_i/d_o = 25/40 = 0.625$, $M = 79 \times 10^3$ N-mm, $T = 118 \times 10^3$ N-mm. a) $\sigma_1 = ?$, $\sigma_2 = ?$, b) $\tau_{max} = ?$

Method 1: As per formulae

a. *Principal stresses:*

Maximum principal stress $\sigma_1 = \dfrac{16}{\pi d_o^3 (1 - K^4)} \left(M + \sqrt{M^2 + T^2}\right)$

$$= \frac{16}{\pi \times 40^3 (1 - 0.625^4)} \left[79 \times 10^3 + \sqrt{(79 \times 10^3)^2 + (118 \times 10^3)^2}\right]$$

$$\sigma_1 = 20.75 \text{ MPa}$$

Minimum principal stress $\sigma_2 = \dfrac{16}{\pi d_o^3 (1 - K^4)} \left(M - \sqrt{M^2 + T^2}\right)$

$$= \frac{16}{\pi \times 40^3 (1 - 0.625^4)} \left[79 \times 10^3 - \sqrt{(79 \times 10^3)^2 + (118 \times 10^3)^2}\right]$$

$$\sigma_1 = -5.92 \text{ MPa}$$

b. *Maximum shear stress:*

Maximum shear stress $\quad \tau_{max} = \dfrac{16}{\pi d_o^3 (1 - K^4)} \sqrt{M^2 + T^2}$

$$= \frac{16}{\pi \times 40^3 (1 - 0.625^4)} \left[\sqrt{(79 \times 10^3)^2 + (118 \times 10^3)^2}\right]$$

$$\tau_{max} = 13.34 \text{ MPa}$$

Method 2: Based on principal stresses:

- Bending stress $\quad \sigma_b = \dfrac{M}{Z} = \dfrac{M}{\pi d_o^3 (1 - K^4)/32} = \dfrac{79 \times 10^3}{\pi \times 40^3 (1 - 0.625^4)/32}$

$$= 14.84 \text{ MPa}$$

- Shear stress $\quad \tau = \dfrac{16T}{\pi d_o^3 (1 - K^4)} = \dfrac{16 \times 118 \times 10^3}{\pi \times 40^3 (1 - 0.625^4)}$

$$= 11.08 \text{ MPa}$$

a. *Principal stresses:* $\quad$ Here $\sigma_x = \sigma_b = 14.84$ MPa; $\sigma_y = 0$; $\tau = \sigma_{xy} = 11.08$ MPa

$$\text{Maximum principal stress } \sigma_1 = \left(\frac{\sigma_x + \sigma_y}{2} \right) + \sqrt{\left(\frac{\sigma_x - \sigma_y}{2} \right)^2 + \tau_{xy}^2}$$

$$= \left(\frac{14.84 + 0}{2} \right) + \sqrt{\left(\frac{14.84 - 0}{2} \right)^2 + 11.08^2}$$

$$\therefore \quad \sigma_1 = 20.75 \text{ MPa}$$

$$\text{Minimum principal stress } \sigma_2 = \left(\frac{\sigma_x + \sigma_y}{2} \right) - \sqrt{\left(\frac{\sigma_x - \sigma_y}{2} \right)^2 + \tau_{xy}^2}$$

$$= \left(\frac{14.84 + 0}{2} \right) - \sqrt{\left(\frac{14.84 - 0}{2} \right)^2 + 11.08^2}$$

$$\therefore \quad \sigma_2 = -5.92 \text{ MPa}$$

b. *Maximum shear stress:*

$$\text{Maximum shear stress } T_{\max} = \sqrt{\left(\frac{\sigma_x - \sigma_y}{2} \right)^2 + \tau_{xy}^2}$$

$$= \sqrt{\left(\frac{14.84 - 0}{2} \right) + 11.08^2}$$

$$T_{\max} = 13.33 \text{ MPa}$$

83. A shaft carries a torque of 75 N-m and a bending moment of 100 N-m. The allowable tensile stress is 60 MPa and the allowable shear stress is 50 MPa. What size should the shaft be?

Solution: $T = 75 \times 10^3$ N-mm, $M = 100 \times 10^3$ N-m, $\sigma_1 = 60$ MPa, $\tau_{\max} = 50$ MPa. $d = ?$

Method 1: As per formulae

Based on maximum principal stress:

$$\text{Maximum principal stress } \sigma_1 = \frac{16}{\pi d^3} \left(M + \sqrt{M^2 + T^2} \right)$$

$$60 = \frac{16}{\pi d^3}\left[100 \times 10^3 + \sqrt{(100 \times 10^3)^2 + (75 \times 10^3)^2}\right]$$

$$d = 26.74 \text{ MPa} \qquad\qquad \ldots \text{Eq. (a)}$$

Based on maximum shear stress:

Maximum shear stress $\quad \tau_{\max} = \dfrac{16}{\pi d^3}\sqrt{M^2 + T^2}$

$$50 = \frac{16}{\pi d^3}\left[\sqrt{(100 \times 10^3)^2 + (75 \times 10^3)^2}\right]$$

$$d = 23.35 \text{ MPa} \qquad\qquad \ldots \text{Eq. (b)}$$

Based on Eqs (a) and (b), select maximum value of diameter for design

i.e. $\qquad\qquad d = 26.74 \text{ mm} \approx 27 \text{ mm}$

Method 2: Based on principal stresses:

- Bending stress $\quad \sigma_b = \dfrac{M}{Z} = \dfrac{M}{\pi d^3/32} = \dfrac{32 \times (100 \times 10^3)}{\pi \times d^3} = \dfrac{1.02 \times 10^6}{d^3}$

- Shear stress $\quad \tau = \dfrac{16T}{\pi d^3} = \dfrac{16 \times (75 \times 10^3)}{\pi \times d^3} = \dfrac{3.82 \times 10^5}{d^3}$

Here $\quad \sigma_x = \sigma_b = \dfrac{1.02 \times 10^6}{d^3}; \sigma_y = 0; \tau = \tau_{xy} = \dfrac{3.82 \times 10^5}{d^3}$

Based on maximum principal stress:

Maximum principal stress $\sigma_1 = \left(\dfrac{\sigma_x + \sigma_y}{2}\right) + \sqrt{\left(\dfrac{\sigma_x - \sigma_y}{2}\right)^2 + \tau_{xy}^2}$

$$60 = \left(\frac{1.02 \times 10^6 + 0}{2d^3}\right) + \sqrt{\left(\frac{1.02 \times 10^6 - 0}{2d^3}\right)^2 + \left(\frac{3.82 \times 10^5}{d^3}\right)^2}$$

$$60 = \left(\frac{1.15 \times 10^6}{d^3}\right)$$

$$d = 26.74 \text{ mm} \qquad\qquad \ldots \text{Eq. (c)}$$

Based on maximum shear stress:

Maximum shear stress $\quad T_{\max} = \sqrt{\left(\dfrac{\sigma_x - \sigma_y}{2}\right)^2 + \tau_{xy}^2}$

$$50 = \sqrt{\left(\frac{1.02 \times 10^6 - 0}{2d^3}\right) + \left(\frac{3.82 \times 10^5}{d^3}\right)^2}$$

$$50 = \frac{6.37 \times 10^5}{d^3}$$

$$d = 23.35 \text{ mm} \qquad\qquad \ldots \text{Eq. (d)}$$

Based on Eqs (c) and (d), select maximum value of diameter for design

i.e. $d = 26.74 \text{ mm} \approx 27 \text{ mm}$

84. A solid shaft 1.2 m long and supported at ends is subjected to a torque of 10 kN-m. Find the necessary diameter of the shaft when a central load of 2000 N is applied. The allowable tensile stress in the shaft material is 120 MPa and the shear stress is 60 MPa.

Solution: $L = 1200 \text{ mm}$, $T = 10 \times 10^6$ N-mm, $F = 2000$ N, $\sigma_1 = 120$ MPa, $\tau_{max} = 60$ MPa. $d = ?$

Method 1: As per formulae

Based on maximum principal stress:

Maximum principal stress $\sigma_1 = \dfrac{16}{\pi d^3}\left(M + \sqrt{M^2 + T^2} \right)$

For a SS beam with central load, $M = \dfrac{FL}{4}$

$$= \frac{2000 \times 1200}{4}$$

$$M = 600 \times 10^3 \text{ N-mm}$$

$$120 = \frac{16}{\pi d^3}\left[600 \times 10^3 + \sqrt{(600 \times 10^3)^2 + (10 \times 10^6)^2} \right]$$

$$d = 76.67 \text{ MPa} \qquad \text{... Eq. (a)}$$

Based on maximum shear stress:

Maximum shear stress $\tau_{max} = \dfrac{16}{\pi d^3}\sqrt{M^2 + T^2}$

$$60 = \frac{16}{\pi d^3}\left[\sqrt{(600 \times 10^3)^2 + (10 \times 10^6)^2} \right]$$

$$d = 94.74 \text{ MPa} \qquad \text{... Eq. (b)}$$

Based on Eqs (a) and (b), select maximum value of diameter for design

i.e. $d = 94.74 \text{ mm} \approx 95 \text{ mm}$

Method 2: Based on principal stresses:

- Bending stress $\quad \sigma_b = \dfrac{M}{Z} = \dfrac{M}{\pi d^3/32} = \dfrac{32 \times (600 \times 10^3)}{\pi \times d^3} = \dfrac{6.11 \times 10^6}{d^3}$

- Shear stress $\quad \tau = \dfrac{16T}{\pi d^3} = \dfrac{16 \times (10 \times 10^6)}{\pi \times d^3} = \dfrac{50.9 \times 10^6}{d^3}$

Here $\quad \sigma_x = \sigma_b = \dfrac{6.11 \times 10^6}{d^3}$; $\sigma_y = 0$; $\tau = \tau_{xy} = \dfrac{50.9 \times 10^6}{d^3}$

Based on maximum principal stress:

Maximum principal stress $\sigma_1 = \left(\dfrac{\sigma_x + \sigma_y}{2} \right) + \sqrt{\left(\dfrac{\sigma_x - \sigma_y}{2} \right)^2 + \tau_{xy}^2}$

$$120 = \left(\frac{6.11\times10^6 + 0}{2d^3}\right) + \sqrt{\left(\frac{6.11\times10^6 - 0}{2d^3}\right)^2 + \left(\frac{50.9\times10^6}{d^3}\right)^2}$$

$$120 = \left(\frac{54.05\times10^6}{d^3}\right)$$

$$d = 76.65 \text{ mm} \qquad\qquad \text{Eq. (c)}$$

Based on maximum shear stress:

Maximum shear stress $\quad \tau_{max} = \sqrt{\left(\frac{\sigma_x - \sigma_y}{2}\right)^2 + \tau_{xy}^2}$

$$60 = \sqrt{\left(\frac{6.11\times10^6 - 0}{2d^3}\right)^2 + \left(\frac{50.9\times10^6}{d^3}\right)^2}$$

$$60 = \frac{51\times10^6}{d^3}$$

$$d = 94.72 \text{ mm} \qquad\qquad \text{... Eq. (d)}$$

Based on Eqs (c) and (d), select maximum value of diameter for design
i.e. $\qquad\qquad d = 94.72 \text{ mm} \approx 95 \text{ mm}$

VTU QUESTION PAPERS

Dec. 07/Jan. 08 (06ME34)

1. Find the diameter of the shaft required to transmit 60 kW at 150 rpm if the maximum torque is 25% of the mean torque for a maximum permissible shear stress of 60 MN/m². Also find the angle of twist in a length of 4 m. Take $G = 80$ GPa **(10 Marks)**

June/July 2008 (06ME34)

2. Derive the torsional formula in the standard form $\dfrac{T}{J} = \dfrac{G\theta}{L} = \dfrac{\tau}{R}$ and list the assumptions made while deriving the same. **(08 Marks)**

Dec. 08/Jan. 09 (06ME34)

3. A solid shaft rotating at 500 rpm transmits 30 kW. Maximum torque is 20% more than the mean torque. Allowable shear stress is 65 MPa and modulus of rigidity is 81 GPa, angle of twist in the shaft should not exceed 1° per meter length. Determine suitable diameter. **(10 Marks)**

June/July 2009 (06ME34)

4. A hollow shaft 3 m long transmits a torque of 25 kN-m. The total angle of twist in this length is not to exceed 2.5° and allowable shear stress is 90 MPa. Determine the inside and outside diameters of the shaft, if $G = 85$ GPa. **(10 Marks)**

Dec. 09/Jan. 10 (06ME34)

5. Two shafts of same material and of same lengths are subjected to the same torque. If the first shaft is a solid circular section and the second shaft is of hollow circular section, whose internal diameter is 2/3 of the outside diameter and the maximum shear stress developed in each shaft is the same, compare the weights of the shafts. **(10 Marks)**

May/June 2010 (06ME34)

6. A solid shaft transmits 250 kW at 100 rpm. If the shear stress is not to exceed 75 MPa, what should be the diameter of the shaft? If this shaft is replaced by a hollow shaft, whose diameter ratio is 0.6, determine the size and percentage saving in weight, the maximum shear stress being the same. **(14 Marks)**

Dec. 2010 (06ME34)

7. State the assumptions made in pure torsion theory and derive $\dfrac{T}{I_p} = \dfrac{G\theta}{L}$, where

    T = torsional moment
    I_p = polar moment of inertia
    G = modulus of rigidity
    θ = angle of twist
    L = length of the shaft. **(08 Marks)**

June/July 2011 (06ME34)

8. A solid shaft is to transmit 192 kW at 450 rpm. Taking allowable stress for the shaft material as 70 MPa, find the diameter of the solid shaft. What percentage of saving in weight would be obtained, if this shaft were to be replaced by a hollow shaft, whose internal diameter is 0.8 times its external diameter? The length of the shaft, power to be transmitted and speed are equal in both cases. **(10 Marks)**

Dec. 2011 (06ME34)

9. a. State the assumptions made in theory of pure torsion. **(04 Marks)**
   b. Determine the diameter of a solid shaft which will transmit 440 kW at 280 rpm. The angle of twist must not exceed one degree per meter length and the maximum torsional stress is to be limited to 40 N/mm². Assume $G = 84$ kN/mm². **(08 Marks)**

Dec. 2011 (10ME34)

10. A hollow steel shaft transmits 200 kW of power at 150 rpm. The total angle of twist in a length of 5 m of shaft is 3°. Find the inner and outer diameters of the shaft if the permissible shear stress is 60 MPa. Take $G = 80$ GPa. **(10 Marks)**

June 2012 (06ME34)

11. A solid shaft rotating at 500 rpm transmits 30 kW. Maximum torque is 20% more than the mean torque. Allowable shear stress is 65 MPa and modulus of rigidity is 81 GPa, angle of twist in the shaft should not exceed 1° in a length of 1m. Determine suitable diameter. **(12 Marks)**

June 2012 (10ME34)

12. Derive the torsion equation with usual notations. State the assumptions made in the derivation. **(10 Marks)**

Dec. 2012 (10ME34)

13. Determine the diameter of a solid steel shaft which will transmit 90 kW at 160 rpm. Also determine the length of the shaft if the twist must not exceed 1° over the entire length. The maximum shear stress is limited to 60 N/mm². Take the value of rigidity as 8×10^4 N/mm². **(10 Marks)**

Jan. 2013 (06ME34)

14. Derive the equation derive $\dfrac{T}{J} = \dfrac{G\theta}{L} = \dfrac{\tau}{R}$ with usual notations and state the assumptions made in the derivation. **(10 Marks)**

June/July 2013 (06ME34)

15. A solid steel shaft transmits 100 kW at 150 rpm. Determine suitable diameter of the shaft, if the shear stress in the shaft is not to exceed 60 MPa. Also find the maximum angle of twist, of the shaft length is 4 m. Take modulus of rigidity as 80 GPa. **(10 Marks)**

June/July 2013 (10ME34)

16. A hollow circular steel shaft has to transmit 60 kW at 210 rpm such that the maximum shear stress does not exceed 60 MPa. If the ratio of internal to external diameter is equal to 3/4 and the value of rigidity modulus is 84 GPa, find the dimensions of the shaft and angle of twist in a length of 3 m. **(10 Marks)**

Dec. 13/Jan. 14 (06ME34)

17. A hollow shaft of 250 mm outer diameter has the same area as that of sold shaft of 150 mm diameter. Compare:
i. Power transmitted by the above shafts for the same speed.
ii. Compare angle of twists of them for the same length and same material.
(10 Marks)

Dec. 13/Jan. 14 (10ME34)

18. Derive torsion equation with usual notations. State the assumptions made in the theory of pure torsion. **(10 Marks)**

June/July 2014 (06ME34)

19. A solid circular shaft is to transmit 300 kW at 100 rpm. If the shear stress is not to exceed 80 N/mm², find the diameter of the shaft. What percentage saving in weight would be obtained, if this shaft is replaced by a hollow one, whose internal diameter is equal to 0.8 of external diameter, the length, material and allowable maximum shear stress being same? **(10 Marks)**

June/July 2014 (10ME34)

20. Find the diameter of the shaft required to transmit 60 kW at 150 rpm if the maximum torque is 25% more than the mean torque for a maximum shear stress of 60 MPa. Find also the angle of twist in a length of 4m. Take $G = 80$ GPa. **(10 Marks)**

Dec. 14/Jan. 15 (06ME34)

21. A shaft is required to transmit 245 kW at 240 rpm. The maximum torque may be 1.5 times the mean torque. The shear stress in the shaft should not exceed 40 N/mm^2 and twist is 1° per meter length. Determine the diameter required if:
    i.   The shaft is solid
    ii. The shaft is hollow with external diameter twice the internal diameter. Take $G = 80$ kN/mm^2. **(12 Marks)**

Dec. 14/Jan. 15 (10ME34)

22. A hollow shaft having an inside diameter 60% of its outer diameter, is to replace a solid shaft transmitting the same power at the same speed. Calculate the percentage saving in material, if the material to be used is also the same. **(10 Marks)**

June/July 15 (10ME34) – QP ME-23

23. A hollow shaft of diameter ratio 3/8 is required to transmit 588 kW at 110 rpm, the torque being 20% of the mean. Shear stress is not to exceed 63 N/mm^2 and twist in a length of 3m not to exceed 1.4 degrees. Calculate the external diameter of the shaft which would satisfy these conditions. Take $G = 84$ GPa. **(12 Marks)**

Dec. 15/Jan. 16 (10ME/AU34)

24. A hollow circular steel shaft has to transmit 60 kW at 210 rpm such that the shear stress does not exceed 60 MPa. If the ratio of internal to external diameter is 3/4 and the value of rigidity modulus is 84 GPa, find the dimensions of the shaft and angle of twist in a length of 3 m. **(08 Marks)**

June/July 2016 (10ME/AU34)

25. Determine the diameter of the shaft which will transmit 440 kW at 280 rpm, if maximum torsional shear stress is to be limited to 40 MPa. Assume $G = 84$ kN/mm^2. **(10 Marks)**

Dec. 16/Jan. 17 (10ME/AU34)

26. Determine the diameter of a solid shaft which will transmit 440 kW at 280 rpm. The angle of twist must not exceed one degree per meter length and the maximum torsional shear stress is limited to 40 MPa. Take $G = 84$ kN/mm^2. **(10 Marks)**

Dec. 16/Jan. 17 (15ME/MA34) – QP ME-27

27. A shaft is required to transmit 245 kW at 240 rpm. The maximum torque may be 1.5 times the mean torque. The shear stress in the shaft should not exceed 40 MPa and the twist is 1° per meter length. Determine the diameter, if:
    i. The shaft is solid.
    ii. The shaft is hollow with external diameter twice the internal diameter. Take modulus of rigidity as 80 kN/mm^2 **(12 Marks)**
28. State the assumptions made in pure torsion theory. **(06 Marks)**

June/July 2017 (15ME/MA34) – QP ME-28

29. Derive the relation for a circular shaft when subjected to torsion as given by $\dfrac{T}{J} = \dfrac{G\theta}{L} = \dfrac{\tau}{R}$. Also list out the assumptions made while deriving the relation.

(10 Marks)

June/July 2017 (15ME/MA34) – QP ME-29

30. a. State the assumptions made in theory of pure torsion. **(04 Marks)**
   b. A solid circular shaft has to transmit a power of 1000 kW at 120 rpm. Find the diameter of the shaft, if the shear stress of the material must not exceed 80 MPa. The maximum torque is 1.25 times of its mean. What percentage of saving in the material would be obtained if the shaft is replaced by a hollow one whose internal diameter is 0.6 times its external diameter, the length, material and maximum shear stress being same? **(12 Marks)**

Dec. 17/Jan. 18 (10ME/AU34) – QP ME-30

31. A hollow shaft of diameter ratio 3/5 is required to transit 700 kW at 110 rpm. The maximum torque being 12% greater than the mean. The shear stress is not to exceed 60 MPa and twist in a length of 3 m not to exceed 1°. Calculate the minimum external diameter. Take $G = 0.8 \times 10^5$ MPa. **(10 Marks)**

Dec. 17/Jan. 18 (15ME/MA34)

32. a. State the assumptions made in pure torsion. And derive $\dfrac{T}{J} = \dfrac{G\theta}{L} = \dfrac{\tau}{R}$ with usual meanings. **(08 Marks)**
   b. A 1.5 m long column has circular cross-section of 50 mm diameter. One end of the column is fixed in position and the other end is free. Taking FOS as 3, calculate:
   i. Safe load according to Rankine's formula taking $\sigma_c = 560$ MPa and $\sigma = 1/1600$.
   ii. Safe load according to Euler's formula taking $E = 120$ GPa. **(08 Marks)**
33. A solid circular shaft has to transmit a power of 1000 kW at 120 rpm. Find the diameter of the shaft if the shear stress of the material must not exceed 80 MPa. The maximum torque is 1.25 times the mean torque. If this solid shaft is replaced by a hollow shaft whose diameter is 0.6 times the external diameter, find the diameter of hollow shaft. **(08 Marks)**

Columns and Struts

Chapter Outline

10.1 INTRODUCTION

In the previous chapters (external loading on beams, pressure vessels, and torsion of shafts) we have had two primary concerns: the stiffness and the strength of the structure.

1. The *strength* of the structure is its ability to support the required loads without experiencing excessive stress.
2. The *stiffness* of the structure is its ability to support the required loads without undergoing excessive deformations.

In practice, we have a third concern: the stability of the structure, i.e. the ability of the structure to support the required loads without experiencing a sudden change in configuration.

The instability known as buckling occurs when forces much lower than those necessary to exceed material yield stresses are applied to beams. Buckling can occur whenever a slender structural member is subjected to compression. The most common occurrence of this kind of loading, and of buckling instability, is in columns.

Columns are essentially vertical members responsible for supporting compressive loads from roofs and floors and transmitting the vertical forces to the foundations and sub- soil. The structural work performed by the column is simpler than that of the beam, because the applied loads are in the same vertical orientation. Columns are used as major elements in trusses, building frames, and substructure supports for bridges. The loads are applied at the member ends, thereby producing axial compressive stresses. Common terms used to identify column elements include *struts, posts, piers, piles, and shafts.*

Column or Pillar or Stanchion: A long slender (long in relation to their lateral dimension) bar subjected to axial compression is called a column. The term "column" is frequently used to describe a vertical member.

Or   A vertical member subjected to axial compressive forces is referred to as column.

Many aircraft structural components, structural connections between stages of boosters for space vehicles, members in bridge trusses, and structural frameworks of buildings are common examples of columns. Columns are major structural components that significantly affect the building's overall performance and stability and, thus, are designed with larger safety factors than other structural components.

Failure of a column occurs by buckling, i.e. by lateral deflection of the bar. In comparison it is to be noted that failure of a short compression member occurs by yielding of the material. Buckling, and hence failure, of a column may occur even though the maximum stress in the bar is much less than the yield point of the material. Linkages in oscillating or reciprocating machines may also fail by buckling.

10.2 CLASSIFICATION OF COLUMNS

1. *Short columns:* Columns whose lengths are less than 8 times their diameter or whose slenderness ratio is less than 32 are called as short columns. (Ex: Footing piers)

   i.e. $L < 8d$ or $\dfrac{L}{k} < 32$

   Short columns are subjected to direct compressive stresses only and fail by crushing.

2. *Medium size columns:* Columns whose lengths vary from 8 times their diameter to 30 times their diameter or whose slenderness ratio lies between 32 to 120 are called medium columns.

   i.e. $L = 8d$ to $30d$ or $\dfrac{L}{k} = 32$ to 120

   Medium columns are subjected to both direct compressive stress and buckling stress.

3. *Long columns:* Columns whose lengths are more than 30 times their diameter or whose slenderness ratio is more than 120 are called as long columns.(Ex: Bridge and freeway piers)

   $L > 30d$ or $\dfrac{L}{k} > 120$

   Long columns are subjected to buckling only, which are far less than crushing load.

Difference between short and long column:

Sl No.	Short column	Long column
1.	It is subjected to direct compressive stresses only	It is subjected to buckling stress only.
2.	Failure occurs purely due to crushing only	Failure occurs purely due to bucking only.
3.	Slenderness ratio is less than 80	Slenderness ratio is more than 120.
4.	Its length to least lateral dimension is less than 8, i.e. $\left(\dfrac{L}{d} < 8\right)$	Its length to least lateral dimension is more than 30, i.e. $\left(\dfrac{L}{d} > 30\right)$

10.3 FAILURE OF A COLUMN

a. *Crushing failure:* The column will reach a stage, when it will be subjected to the ultimate crushing stress; beyond this the column will fail by crushing. The load corresponding to the crushing stress is called crushing load. This type of failure occurs in short column.

b. *Buckling failure:* This is due to lateral deflection of the column. The load at which the column just buckles is called buckling load or crippling load or critical load. This type of failure occurs in long column.

10.4 DEFINITIONS

- *Strut:* is a structural member subjected to axial compressive forces. A strut can be horizontal or inclined. "Strut" is occasionally used in regard to inclined bars, while horizontal members are referred to as beams.

- *Critical load or buckling load or crippling load:* The critical load of a slender bar subjected to axial compression is that value of the axial force that is just sufficient to keep the bar in a slightly deflected configuration.

   OR

The maximum limiting load at which the column tends to have lateral displacement or tends to buckle is called buckling or crippling load. Buckling takes place about the axis having minimum radius of gyration, or least moment of inertia.

As per Euler, the critical load of a column/strut is given as,

$$F_{cr} = \frac{\pi^2 EI}{L^2} \qquad \text{... (Eq. 10.1)}$$

F_{cr} = Crippling or buckling load,

E = Young's modulus,

I = Least moment of inertia

L = equivalent length of the column

- *Equivalent or effective length of column (L):* For a given column with given end conditions, the effective length of column is defined as the length of an equivalent column of same material and cross section with both ends hinged and having the value of crippling load equal to that of given column.

   OR

The distance between adjacent points of inflection is called equivalent length of the column. A point of inflection is found at every column end, that is free to rotate and every point where there is a change of the axis, i.e. there is no moment in the inflection points.

End conditions:

1. Both ends hinged or pinned : $L = l$

2. Both ends fixed or clamped : $L = \dfrac{l}{2}$

3. One end fixed, other end hinged : $L = \dfrac{l}{\sqrt{2}}$

4. One end fixed, other end free : $L = 2l$ ... (Eq. 10.2)

- *Safe load:* It is the load to which a column is actually subjected to and is well below the buckling load. It is obtained by dividing the buckling load by a suitable factor of safety (n).

$$\text{Safe load} = \frac{\text{Buckling load}}{\text{Factor of safety}}$$

$$F_s = \frac{F_{cr}}{n} \qquad \text{... (Eq. 10.3)}$$

- *Slenderness ratio (Buckling factor):* is defined as the ratio of the effective length of the column to the minimum radius of gyration of the cross-sectional end of the column.

$$\text{Slenderness ratio} = \frac{L}{k} \qquad \text{... (Eq. 10.4)}$$

Where L = effective length of column, k = least radius of gyration

- *Radius of gyration (k):* The radius of gyration expresses the relationship between the area of a cross-section and a centroidal moment of inertia. It is a shape factor that measures a column's resistance to buckling about an axis.

The radius of gyration of a cross-section (area) is defined as that distance from its moment of inertia axis at which the entire area could be considered as being concentrated without changing its moment of inertia.

$$k = \sqrt{\frac{I}{A}} \qquad \text{... (Eq. 10.5)}$$

Note: Factors affecting the strength column include Slenderness ratio and end conditions

10.5 EULER' THEORY

Assumptions in Euler's theory:

- The column is initially straight and is of uniform lateral dimension.
- The compressive load is axial and passes through the centroid of the column section.
- The material of the column is perfectly homogeneous and isotropic.
- Pin joints are frictionless and fixed ends are perfectly rigid.
- The self-weight of the column is neglected.
- The column fails by buckling alone.
- The limit of proportionality is not exceeded.

10.6 EULER'S EQUATION FOR VARIOUS END CONDITIONS

The end conditions of a column affect the way a column resists the load. The support conditions of a column can be of four types..
1. Both ends hinged
2. Both ends fixed
3. One end fixed, other end hinged
4. One end fixed, other end free

A long column with both ends hinged is taken as a standard case for analysis

Sign conventions used in columns
A moment which tends to bend the column with its convexity towards its initial center line is taken as positive, as shown in **Fig. 10.1(a)**.

A moment which tends to bend the column with its concavity towards its initial center line is taken as negative, as shown in **Fig. 10.1(b)**.

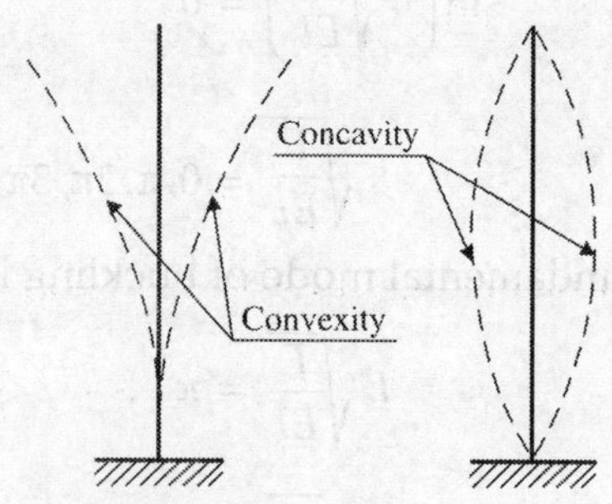

Fig. 10.1: Bending moment

10.6.1 Both ends of the column are hinged or pinned

Consider a column AB of length l and cross sectional area A hinged at both ends as shown in **Fig. 10.2**.

Let $\quad$ F = crippling load at which the column buckles.

$\qquad$ y = Lateral displacement of the section considered.

Consider a section X-X at a distance x from end B.

The bending moment at this section is

$$EI\left(\frac{d^2y}{dx^2}\right) = -Fy$$

i.e. $\qquad EI\left(\frac{d^2y}{dx^2}\right) + Fy = 0$

$$\left(\frac{d^2y}{dx^2}\right) + \left(\frac{F}{EI}\right)y = 0 \qquad \dots \text{(Eq. 10.6)}$$

The solution for the above differential equation is given as

Fig. 10.2: Both ends of the column are hinged

$$y = C_1 \cos\left(x.\sqrt{\frac{F}{EI}}\right) + C_2 \sin\left(x.\sqrt{\frac{F}{EI}}\right) \qquad \dots \text{(Eq. 10.7)}$$

$\qquad C_1$ and C_2 are constants which are to be evaluated from boundary conditions.
End B: At $x = 0, y = 0$
(Eq. 10.7) yields... $\qquad 0 = C_1 \cos(0) + C_2 \sin(0)$
$$\qquad\qquad C_1 = 0 \qquad \dots \text{(Eq. 10.8)}$$
End A: At $x = l, y = 0$

(Eq. 10.7) yields... $\qquad 0 = 0 + C_2 \sin\left(l.\sqrt{\dfrac{F}{EI}} \right)$ $\qquad$ ... using (Eq. 10.8)

Since $C_2 \neq 0$, we have

$$\sin\left(l.\sqrt{\dfrac{F}{EI}} \right) = 0$$

$$l.\sqrt{\dfrac{F}{EI}} = 0, \pi, 2\pi, 3\pi, 4\pi, \ldots$$

The fundamental mode of buckling in this case is the first value. Thus we have

$$l.\sqrt{\dfrac{F}{EI}} = \pi$$

$$\sqrt{\dfrac{F}{EI}} = \dfrac{\pi}{l}$$

$$F_{cr} = \dfrac{\pi^2 EI}{l^2} \qquad \ldots \text{(Eq. 10.9)}$$

Note: Column with hinged ends is taken as a standard for all practical purposes.

10.6.2 One end of the column is fixed and the other end is free

Consider a column AB of length l and cross sectional area A as shown in **Fig. 10.3**, with end B fixed while the upper end A is free.

$\qquad$ Let $\qquad$ F = crippling load at which the column buckles.

$\qquad\qquad\qquad$ y = Lateral displacement of the section considered.

$\qquad\qquad\qquad$ δ = Deflection at free end

Now consider a section X-X at a distance x from fixed end. The bending moment at this section is

$$EI\left(\dfrac{d^2y}{dx^2} \right) = F(\delta - y)$$

i.e. $\qquad$ $EI\left(\dfrac{d^2y}{dx^2} \right) - F(\delta - y) = 0$

$$EI\left(\dfrac{d^2y}{dx^2} \right) + Fy = F\delta$$

$$\left(\dfrac{d^2y}{dx^2} \right) + \left(\dfrac{F}{EI} \right)y = \dfrac{F\delta}{EI} \qquad \ldots \text{(Eq. 10.10)}$$

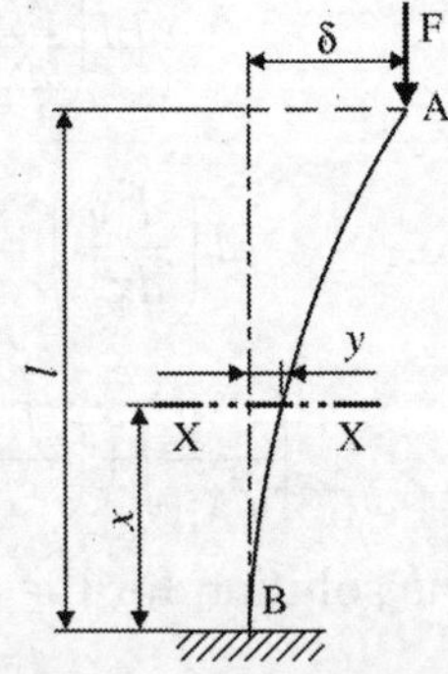

Fig. 10.3: One end of the column is fixed, while other end is free

The solution for the above differential equation is given as

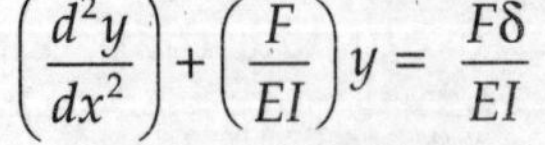

$$y = C_1 \cos\left(x.\sqrt{\dfrac{F}{EI}} \right) + C_2 \sin\left(x.\sqrt{\dfrac{F}{EI}} \right) + \delta \qquad \ldots \text{(Eq. 10.11)}$$

The slope at any section is obtained by differentiating (Eq. 10.11) as

$$\frac{dy}{dx} = C_1 \left[-\sin\left(x.\sqrt{\frac{F}{EI}} \right) \right]\left(\sqrt{\frac{F}{EI}} \right) + C_2 \left[\cos\left(x.\sqrt{\frac{F}{EI}} \right) \right]\left(\sqrt{\frac{F}{EI}} \right)$$

$$\dots \text{ (Eq. 10.12)}$$

C_1 and C_2 are constants which are to be evaluated from boundary conditions.

End B: At $x = 0$, $y = 0$

(Eq. 10.11) yields... $\quad 0 = C_1 \cos(0) + C_2 \sin(0) + \delta$
$$0 = C_1 + \delta$$
$$C_1 = -\delta \qquad\qquad\qquad \dots \text{ (Eq. 10.13)}$$

At $x = 0$, $\dfrac{dy}{dx} = 0$

(Eq. 10.12) yields... $\quad 0 = C_1 \left[-\sin(0)\right]\left(\sqrt{\frac{F}{EI}} \right) + C_2 \left[\cos(0)\right]\left(\sqrt{\frac{F}{EI}} \right)$

$$0 = C_2 \left(\sqrt{\frac{F}{EI}} \right)$$

$$C_2 = 0 \qquad\qquad \text{since } \sqrt{\frac{F}{EI}} \neq 0 \qquad \dots \text{ (Eq. 10.14)}$$

End A: At $x = l$, $y = d$

(Eq. 10.11) yields... $\quad \delta = C_1 \cos\left(l.\sqrt{\frac{F}{EI}} \right) + C_2 \sin\left(l.\sqrt{\frac{F}{EI}} \right) + \delta$

$$\delta = -\delta \cos\left(l.\sqrt{\frac{F}{EI}} \right) + 0 + \delta \quad \dots \text{ using Eqs (10.13) and (10.14)}$$

$$\cos\left(l.\sqrt{\frac{F}{EI}} \right) = 0$$

$$\left(l.\sqrt{\frac{F}{EI}} \right) = \frac{\pi}{2}, \frac{3\pi}{2}, \frac{5\pi}{2}, \dots$$

The fundamental mode of buckling in this case is the first value, we have

$$l.\sqrt{\frac{F}{EI}} = \frac{\pi}{2}$$

$$F_{cr} = \frac{\pi^2 EI}{4l^2} \qquad\qquad \dots \text{ (Eq. 10.15)}$$

10.6.3 One end of the column is fixed and the other end is hinged

Consider a column AB of length l and cross sectional area A as shown in **Fig. 10.4**, with end B fixed while the upper end A is hinged. Since B is fixed, a bending moment M is induced. In this case, there will be a horizontal reaction H at the hinge to keep the top end of the strut on the vertical axis; the product ($F.l$) balances the fixing (restraint) moment M at the base.

Let F = crippling load at which the column buckles.

         y = Lateral displacement of the section considered.

         H = Horizontal force at A

         M = Moment at fixed end B

Now consider a section X-X at a distance x from fixed end.

The bending moment at this section is

$$EI\left(\frac{d^2y}{dx^2}\right) = -Fy + H(l-x)$$

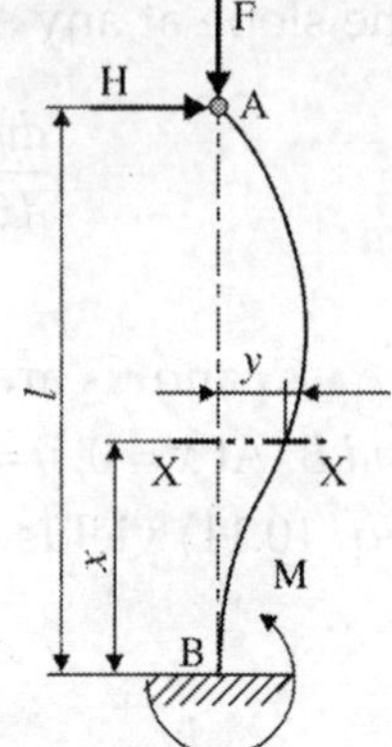

Fig. 10.4: One end of the column is fixed, while other end is hinged

$$EI\left(\frac{d^2y}{dx^2}\right) + Fy = H(l-x)$$

$$\left(\frac{d^2y}{dx^2}\right) + \left(\frac{F}{EI}\right)y = \frac{H(l-x)}{EI} \qquad \dots \text{(Eq. 10.16)}$$

The solution for the above differential equation is given as

$$y = C_1 \cos\left(x.\sqrt{\frac{F}{EI}}\right) + C_2 \sin\left(x.\sqrt{\frac{F}{EI}}\right) + \frac{H(l-x)}{F} \qquad \dots \text{(Eq. 10.17)}$$

The slope at any section is obtained by differentiating (Eq. 10.17) as

$$\frac{dy}{dx} = C_1\left[-\sin\left(x.\sqrt{\frac{F}{EI}}\right)\right]\left(\sqrt{\frac{F}{EI}}\right) + C_2\left[\cos\left(x.\sqrt{\frac{F}{EI}}\right)\right]\left(\sqrt{\frac{F}{EI}}\right) - \frac{H}{F}$$

$$\dots \text{(Eq. 10.18)}$$

C_1 and C_2 are constants which are to be evaluated from boundary conditions.

End B: At $x = 0$, $y = 0$

(Eq. 10.17) yields... $0 = C_1 \cos(0) + C_2 \sin(0) + \dfrac{Hl}{F}$

$$0 = C_1 + \frac{Hl}{F}$$

$$C_1 = -\frac{Hl}{F} \qquad \dots \text{(Eq. 10.19)}$$

At $x = 0$, $\dfrac{dy}{dx} = 0$

(Eq. 10.18) yields... $0 = C_1\left[-\sin(0)\right]\left(\sqrt{\dfrac{F}{EI}}\right) + C_2\left[\cos(0)\right]\left(\sqrt{\dfrac{F}{EI}}\right) - \dfrac{H}{F}$

$$0 = C_2\left(\sqrt{\frac{F}{EI}}\right) - \frac{H}{F}$$

$$C_2 = \frac{H}{F}\left(\sqrt{\frac{EI}{F}}\right) \qquad \qquad \text{... (Eq. 10.20)}$$

End A: At $x = l, y = 0$

(Eq. 10.17) yields... $0 = C_1 \cos\left(l.\sqrt{\frac{F}{EI}}\right) + C_2 \sin\left(l.\sqrt{\frac{F}{EI}}\right) + 0$

$$0 = -\frac{Hl}{F}\cos\left(l.\sqrt{\frac{F}{EI}}\right) + \frac{H}{F}\left(\sqrt{\frac{EI}{F}}\right)\sin\left(l.\sqrt{\frac{F}{EI}}\right)$$

... using Eqs (10.19) and (10.20)

$$\frac{Hl}{F}\cos\left(l.\sqrt{\frac{F}{EI}}\right) = \frac{H}{F}\left(\sqrt{\frac{EI}{F}}\right)\sin\left(l.\sqrt{\frac{F}{EI}}\right)$$

$$\tan\left(l.\sqrt{\frac{F}{EI}}\right) = \left(l\sqrt{\frac{F}{EI}}\right) \qquad \qquad \text{... (Eq. 10.21)}$$

The lowest value of $\left(l\sqrt{\frac{F}{EI}}\right)$ (neglecting zero) which satisfies this condition and

thereby produces the fundamental buckling condition is $\left(l\sqrt{\frac{F}{EI}}\right) = 4.5$ radians.

Thus $\left(l\sqrt{\frac{F}{EI}}\right) = 4.5$ radians.

$$\frac{l^2 F}{EI} = (4.5)^2 = 20.25$$

$$F_{cr} = 20.25\left(\frac{EI}{l^2}\right) \approx \frac{2\pi^2 EI}{l^2} \qquad \qquad \text{... (Eq. 10.22)}$$

10.6.4 Both ends of the column are fixed or clamped

Consider a column AB of length l and cross sectional area A as shown in **Fig. 10.5**, with both ends fixed. Since both ends are fixed, there will be fixing (restraint) moment M at the each end.

Let F = Crippling load at which the column buckles.

y = Lateral displacement of the section considered.

M = Moment at each end B

Now consider a section X-X at a distance x from fixed end.

The bending moment at this section is

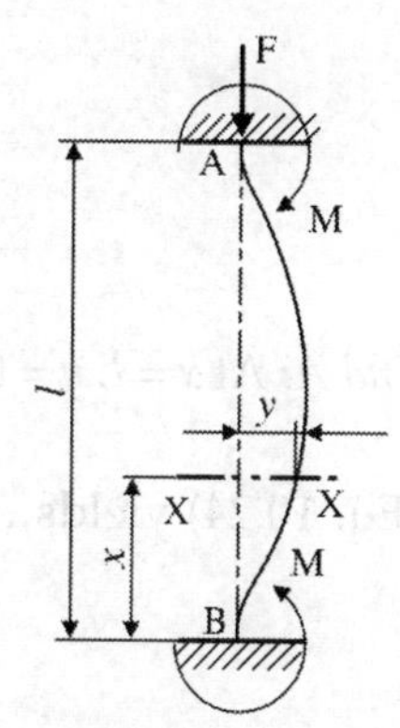

Fig. 10.5: Both ends fixed

$$EI\left(\frac{d^2 y}{dx^2}\right) = M - Fy$$

$$EI\left(\frac{d^2y}{dx^2}\right) + Fy = M$$

$$\left(\frac{d^2y}{dx^2}\right) + \left(\frac{F}{EI}\right)y = \frac{M}{EI} \qquad \qquad \dots \text{(Eq. 10.23)}$$

The solution for the above differential equation is given as

$$y = C_1 \cos\left(x.\sqrt{\frac{F}{EI}}\right) + C_2 \sin\left(x.\sqrt{\frac{F}{EI}}\right) + \frac{M}{F} \qquad \dots \text{(Eq. 10.24)}$$

The slope at any section is obtained by differentiating (Eq. 10.24) as

$$\frac{dy}{dx} = C_1\left[-\sin\left(x.\sqrt{\frac{F}{EI}}\right)\right]\left(\sqrt{\frac{F}{EI}}\right) + C_2\left[\cos\left(x.\sqrt{\frac{F}{EI}}\right)\right]\left(\sqrt{\frac{F}{EI}}\right)$$

$$\dots \text{(Eq. 10.25)}$$

C_1 and C_2 are constants which are to be evaluated from boundary conditions.
End B: At $x = 0$, $y = 0$

(Eq. 10.24) yields... $\quad 0 = C_1 \cos(0) + C_2 \sin(0) + \dfrac{M}{F}$

$$0 = C_1 + \frac{M}{F}$$

$$C_1 = -\frac{M}{F} \qquad \qquad \dots \text{(Eq. 10.26)}$$

At $x = 0$, $\dfrac{dy}{dx} = 0$

(Eq. 10.25) yields... $\quad 0 = C_1\,[-\sin(0)]\left(\sqrt{\frac{F}{EI}}\right) + C_2\,[\cos(0)]\left(\sqrt{\frac{F}{EI}}\right)$

$$0 = C_2\left(\sqrt{\frac{F}{EI}}\right) - \frac{H}{F}$$

$$C_2 = 0 \qquad \qquad \text{since } \sqrt{\frac{F}{EI}} \neq 0 \qquad \dots \text{(Eq. 10.27)}$$

End A: At $x = l$, $y = 0$

(Eq. 10.24) yields... $\quad 0 = C_1 \cos\left(l.\sqrt{\frac{F}{EI}}\right) + C_2 \sin\left(l.\sqrt{\frac{F}{EI}}\right) + \frac{M}{F}$

$$0 = -\frac{M}{F}\cos\left(l.\sqrt{\frac{F}{EI}}\right) + \frac{M}{F}$$

$$\dots \text{using Eqs (10.26) and (10.27)}$$

$$0 = \frac{M}{F}\left[1 - \cos\left(l.\sqrt{\frac{F}{EI}}\right)\right]$$

$$\left[1 - \cos\left(l.\sqrt{\frac{F}{EI}}\right)\right] = 0$$

$$\cos\left(l.\sqrt{\frac{F}{EI}}\right) = 1$$

$$\left(l.\sqrt{\frac{F}{EI}}\right) = 0, 2\pi, 4\pi, 6\pi \ldots$$

The fundamental mode of buckling in this case is the second value. Thus we have

$$\left(l.\sqrt{\frac{F}{EI}}\right) = 2\pi$$

$$F_{cr} = \frac{4\pi^2 EI}{l^2} \qquad \ldots \text{(Eq. 10.28)}$$

The comparison of various conditions is given in **Table 10.1**.

Table 10.1

Sl. No	End condition	Effective length (L)	Crippling or Buckling load (F_{cr})
1.	Both ends hinged or pinned	$L = l$	$\pi^2 EI/l^2$
2.	One end fixed, other end free	$L = 2l$	$\pi^2 EI/4l^2$
3.	One end fixed, other end hinged	$L = l/\sqrt{2}$	$2\pi^2 EI/l^2$
4.	Both ends fixed	$L = l/2$	$4\pi^2 EI/l^2$

Note: The moment of inertia in the relations should be the least value of I_{XX} and I_{YY}.

1. **A solid round bar of 60 mm diameter and 2.5 m long is used as a strut. Find the safe compressive load for the strut if:**

   (a) Both ends are hinged

   (b) Both ends are fixed.   Take $E = 2 \times 10^5$ MPa and factor of safety = 3.

VTU – June/ July 2016 – 10 Marks; Dec. 13/ Jan. 14 – 10 Marks

Solution: $d = 60$ mm, $l = 2500$ mm, safe load $F_s = ?$, $E = 2 \times 10^5$ MPa, $n = 3$

We know that $\qquad F_s = \dfrac{F_{cr}}{n}$ $\qquad\qquad \ldots$ Eq. (i)

But $\qquad\qquad F_{cr} = \dfrac{\pi^2 EI}{L^2}$ $\qquad\qquad \ldots$ Eq. (ii)

Also $\qquad\qquad I_{XX} = I_{YY} = \dfrac{\pi d^4}{64} = \dfrac{\pi \times 60^4}{64} = 6.36 \times 10^5 \text{ mm}^4$

Case a: Both ends are hinged:

Here effective length, $L = l = 2500$ mm

Eq. (ii) yields... $\qquad F_{cr} = \dfrac{\pi^2 \times 2 \times 10^5 \times (6.36 \times 10^5)}{2500^2} = 200.87 \times 10^3 \text{ N}$

Eq. (i) yields... $\qquad F_s = \dfrac{200.87 \times 10^3}{3} = 66.96 \times 10^3 \text{ N}$

Case b: Both ends fixed:

Here effective length, $L = \dfrac{l}{2} = \dfrac{2500}{2} = 1250 \text{ mm}$

Eq. (ii) yields... $\qquad F_{cr} = \dfrac{\pi^2 \times 2 \times 10^5 \times (6.36 \times 10^5)}{1250^2} = 803.46 \times 10^3 \text{ N}$

Eq. (i) yields... $\qquad F_s = \dfrac{803.46 \times 10^3}{3} = 267.82 \times 10^3 \text{ N}$

2. **A circular compression member is of 25 mm diameter and 950 mm long. Calculate the maximum buckling load. What will be the value of allowable load if a factor of safety of 3 is expected? Take for material of column σ_y = 441 MPa $E = 2.07 \times 10^5$ N/mm^2**

VTU – Dec. 2011 – 10 Marks

Solution: $d = 25$ mm, $l = 950$ mm, buckling load $F_{cr} = ?$, $n = 3$, safe load $F_s = ?$, $\sigma_y = 441$ MPa, $E = 2.07 \times 10^5$ N/mm^2

a. *Buckling load:*

We know that $\qquad F_{cr} = \dfrac{\pi^2 EI}{L^2}$ $\qquad\qquad\qquad$ ... Eq. (i)

But $\qquad I_{XX} = I_{YY} = \dfrac{\pi d^4}{64} = \dfrac{\pi \times 25^4}{64} = 19.17 \times 10^3 \text{ mm}^4$

Assume that both ends are hinged, we have effective length, $L = l = 950$ mm

Eq. (ii) yields... $\qquad F_{cr} = \dfrac{\pi^2 \times 2.07 \times 10^5 \times (19.17 \times 10^3)}{950^2} = 43.40 \times 10^3 \text{ N}$

b. *Safe or allowable load:*

We know that $\qquad F_s = \dfrac{F_{cr}}{L^2} = \dfrac{43.40 \times 10^3}{3} = 14.47 \times 10^3 \text{ N}$

3. **A column 6 m long has both of its ends fixed and has a timber section of 150 mm × 200 mm. Determine the crippling load on the column. Take $E = 17.5 \times 10^3$ MPa.**

VTU – (CV) Dec. 2016/ Jan. 2017 – 08 Marks;
(CV) Dec. 2008/ Jan. 2009 – 10 Marks

Solution: $l = 6000$ mm, $B = 150$ mm, $H = 200$ mm, $F_{cr} = ?$, $E = 17.5 \times 10^3$ MPa

We know that $\qquad F_{cr} = \dfrac{\pi^2 EI}{L^2}$ $\qquad\qquad\qquad$ ... Eq. (i)

But
$$I_{XX} = \frac{bh^3}{12} = \frac{150 \times 200^3}{12} = 100 \times 10^6 \text{ mm}^4$$

$$I_{YY} = \frac{bh^3}{12} = \frac{200 \times 150^3}{12} = 56.25 \times 10^6 \text{ mm}^4$$

Thus $\qquad I = I_{YY} = 56.25 \times 10^6 \text{ mm}^4 \qquad$ (minimum value)

For both ends fixed, effective length, $L = l/2 = 6000/2 = 3000$ mm

Eq. (i) yields... $\qquad F_{cr} = \dfrac{\pi^2 \times 17.5 \times 10^3 \times (56.25 \times 10^6)}{3000^2} = 1.08 \times 10^6 \text{ N}$

4. **A solid round bar 4 m long and 50 mm in diameter was found to extend 4.6 mm long under a tensile load of 50 kN. This bar is used as a strut with both ends hinged (pinned). Determine Euler's crippling load for the bar and also the safe load taking factor of safety as 4.**

VTU – (CV) Dec. 2012– 10 Marks; (CV) Dec. 2007/ Jan. 2008 – 10 Marks

Solution: $l = 4000$ mm, $d = 50$ mm, $\delta = 4.6$ mm, $F = 50 \times 10^3$ N, $F_{cr} = ?$, $n = 4$.

We know that $\qquad F_{cr} = \dfrac{F_{cr}}{n} \qquad\qquad\qquad$ ... Eq. (i)

But $\qquad\qquad F_{cr} = \dfrac{\pi^2 EI}{L^2} \qquad\qquad\qquad$ ... Eq. (ii)

$$I_{XX} = I_{YY} = \frac{\pi d^4}{64} = \frac{\pi \times 50^4}{64} = 3.07 \times 10^5 \text{ mm}^4$$

Also $\qquad\qquad \delta = \dfrac{Fl}{AE}$

$$4.6 = \frac{50 \times 10^3 \times 4000}{(\pi \times 50^2/4)E}$$

$$E = 22143.30 \text{ MPa}$$

For both ends hinged, effective length, $L = L = 4000$ mm

Eq. (ii) yields... $\qquad F_{cr} = \dfrac{\pi^2 \times 22143.30 \times (3.07 \times 10^5)}{4000^2} = 4193.34 \text{ N}$

Eq. (i) yields... $\qquad F_s = \dfrac{4193.34}{4} = 1048.34 \text{ N}$

5. **A hollow tube 6 m long and having diameters of 50 mm and 30 mm was found to extend by 6.4 mm under a tensile load of 80 kN. Find the safe load the tube can carry if it is used as a strut with both ends pinned? Take factor of safety as 4.**

Solution: $l = 6000$ mm, $d_o = 50$ mm, $d_i = 30$ mm, $\delta = 6.4$ mm, $F = 80 \times 10^3$ N, $F_{cr} = ?$, $n = 4$.

We know that $\qquad F_{cr} = \dfrac{F_{cr}}{n} \qquad\qquad\qquad$ ... Eq. (i)

$$\text{But} \qquad F_{cr} = \frac{\pi^2 EI}{L^2} \qquad \qquad \text{... Eq. (ii)}$$

$$I_{XX} = I_{YY} = \frac{\pi\left(d_o^4 - d_i^4\right)}{64} = \frac{\pi(50^4 - 30^4)}{64} = 267.04 \times 10^3 \text{ mm}^4$$

$$\text{Also} \qquad \delta = \frac{Fl}{AE}$$

$$6.4 = \frac{80 \times 10^3 \times 6000}{[\pi \times (50^2 - 30^2)/4]E}$$

$$E = 59.68 \times 10^3 \text{ MPa}$$

For both ends hinged or pinned, effective length, $L = l = 6000$ mm

Eq. (ii) yields... $\qquad F_{cr} = \dfrac{\pi^2 \times 59.68 \times 10^3 \times (267.04 \times 10^3)}{6000^2} = 4369.27 \text{ N}$

Eq. (i) yields... $\qquad F_s = \dfrac{4369.27}{4} = 1092.32 \text{ N}$

6. A simply supported beam of length 4 m is subjected to a udl of 30 kN/m over the entire span and deflects 15 mm at the center. Determine the crippling load when the beam is used as a column with both ends hinged.

VTU – (CV) June/ July 2013 – 10 Marks

Solution: $l = 4000$ mm, $w = 30$ kN/m $= 30$ N/mm, $\delta = 15$ mm, $F_{cr} = ?$.

We know that $\qquad F_{cr} = \dfrac{\pi^2 EI}{L^2} \qquad \qquad$ ... Eq. (i)

For a simply supported beam with udl over entire span,

$$\delta = \frac{5wl^4}{384EI}$$

$$15 = \frac{5 \times 30 \times 4000^4}{384EI}$$

$$EI = 6.67 \times 10^{12} \text{ N-mm}^2$$

For both ends hinged, effective length, $L = l = 4000$ mm

Eq. (i) yields... $\qquad F_{cr} = \dfrac{\pi^2 \times 6.67 \times 10^{12}}{4000^2} = 4114.40 \times 10^3 \text{ N}$

7. Repeat Problem 6 if the beam is a simply supported with point load of 120 N at mid-span.

Solution: $l = 4000$ mm, $W = 120$ N, $\delta = 15$ mm, $F_{cr} = ?$.

We know that $\qquad F_{cr} = \dfrac{\pi^2 EI}{L^2} \qquad \qquad$ ... Eq. (i)

For a simply supported beam with udl over entire span,

$$\delta = \frac{Wl^3}{48EI}$$

$$15 = \frac{120 \times 4000^3}{48EI}$$

$$EI = 1.07 \times 10^{10} \text{ N-mm}^2$$

For both ends hinged, effective length, $L = l = 4000$ mm

Eq. (i) yields... $\qquad F_{cr} = \dfrac{\pi^2 \times 1.07 \times 10^{10}}{4000^2} = 6579.74$ N

8. A circular rod is 50 mm in diameter and 3 m is used as a strut with both ends hinged. Calculate the maximum buckling load and slenderness ratio Take $E = 200$ GPa

Solution: $d = 50$ mm, $l = 3000$ mm, a) $F_{cr} = ?$, b) slenderness ratio $(L/k) = ?$

a. *To find F_{cr}:*

We know that $\qquad F_{cr} = \dfrac{\pi^2 EI}{L^2}$ $\qquad\qquad\qquad\qquad$ ... Eq. (i)

But $\qquad I_{XX} = I_{YY} = \dfrac{\pi d^4}{64} = \dfrac{\pi \times 50^4}{64} = 3.07 \times 10^5 \text{ mm}^4$

For both ends hinged, effective length, $L = l = 3000$ mm

Eq. (i) yields... $\quad F_{cr} = \dfrac{\pi^2 \times 200 \times 10^3 \times (3.07 \times 10^5)}{3000^2} = 67.33 \times 10^3$ N

b. *To find (L/k):*

We know that $\qquad F_{cr} = \dfrac{\pi^2 EI}{L^2}$

$$= \frac{\pi^2 E(Ak^2)}{L^2} = \frac{\pi^2 EA}{(L/k)^2} \qquad\qquad \text{since } I = Ak^2$$

$$67.33 \times 10^3 = \frac{\pi^2 \times 200 \times 10^3 \times (\pi \times 50^2/4)}{(L/k)^2}$$

$$(L/k)^2 = 57564$$
$$L/k = 239.93$$

9. A steel bar 2 m long and 40 mm × 50 mm in section with both ends hinged is subjected to axial compression. Determine the crippling load and the corresponding axial stress.

Also find the slenderness ratio if $E = 200$ GPa and the limit of proportionality for the material is 230 MPa.

Solution: $l = 2000$ mm, $b = 40$ mm, $h = 50$ mm, a) $F_{cr} = ?$, b) $\sigma_{cr} = ?$, c) $L/k = ?$, $E = 200 \times 10^3$ MPa, $\sigma_\alpha = 230$ MPa

a. *To find F_{cr}:*

We know that $\qquad F_{cr} = \dfrac{\pi^2 EI}{L^2}$ $\qquad\qquad\qquad\qquad$ ... Eq. (i)

But $\qquad I_{XX} = \dfrac{bh^3}{12} = \dfrac{40 \times 50^3}{12} = 416.67 \times 10^3 \text{ mm}^4$

$$I_{YY} = \frac{hb^3}{12} = \frac{50 \times 40^3}{12} = 266.67 \times 10^3 \text{ mm}^4$$

Thus $\qquad I = I_{YY} = 266.67 \times 10^3 \text{ mm}^4 \qquad$ (minimum value)

For both ends hinged, effective length, $L = l = 2000$ mm

Eq. (i) yields... $\quad F_{cr} = \dfrac{\pi^2 \times 200 \times 10^3 \times (266.67 \times 10^3)}{2000^2} = 131.59 \times 10^3 \text{ N}$

b. *To find* σ_{cr}:

We know that $\quad \sigma_{cr} = \dfrac{F_{cr}}{A} = \dfrac{131.59 \times 10^3}{40 \times 50} = 65.80 \text{ MPa}$

c. *To find* (L/k):

We know that $\quad F_{cr} = \dfrac{\pi^2 EI}{L^2} = \dfrac{\pi^2 E(Ak^2)}{L^2} \qquad\qquad$ since $I = Ak^2$

$$\frac{F_{cr}}{A} = \frac{\pi^2 E}{(L/k)^2}$$

$$230 = \frac{\pi^2 \times 200 \times 10^3}{(L/k)^2}$$

$\qquad\qquad\qquad\qquad$ [In this case $\dfrac{F_{cr}}{A} = \sigma_\alpha = 230$ MPa] as $\sigma_{cr} < \sigma_\alpha$

$$(L/k)^2 = 8582.26$$
$$L/k = 92.64$$

10. A hollow aluminium tube with both ends pinned has diameters of 50 mm and 30 mm. If the buckling load is 5 kN, estimate the length of the bar and calculate the slenderness ratio. Take $E = 70$ GPa

Solution: $d_o = 50$ mm, $d_i = 30$ mm, $F_{cr} = 5 \times 10^3$ N, a) slenderness ratio $(L/k) = ?$, b) $L = ?$,

a. *To find* (L/k):

We know that $\quad F_{cr} = \dfrac{\pi^2 EI}{L^2} = \dfrac{\pi^2 E(Ak^2)}{L^2} \qquad\qquad$ since $I = Ak^2$

$$\frac{F_{cr}}{A} = \frac{\pi^2 E}{(L/k)^2} \qquad\qquad \text{... Eq. (i)}$$

But $\quad A = \dfrac{\pi(d_o^2 - d_i^2)}{4} = \dfrac{\pi \times (50^2 - 30^2)}{4} = 1256.64 \text{ mm}^2$

$$I_{XX} = I_{YY} = \frac{\pi(d_o^4 - d_i^4)}{64} = \frac{\pi \times (50^4 - 30^4)}{64} = 267.04 \times 10^3 \text{ mm}^4$$

$$k = \sqrt{\frac{I}{A}} = \sqrt{\frac{267.04 \times 10^3}{1256.64}} = 14.58 \text{ mm}$$

Eq. (i) yields...

$$\frac{5000}{1256.64} = \frac{\pi^2 \times 70 \times 10^3}{(L/k)^2}$$

$$(L/k)^2 = 173635.56$$
$$L/k = 416.70$$

b. *To find L:*

Now
$$L/k = 416.70$$
$$L = 416.70 \times 14.58 = 6075.48 \text{ mm}$$

11. **A steel bar of solid circular cross-section is 50 mm in diameter. The bar is pinned at each end and subject to axial compression. If the proportional limit of the material is 210 MPa and $E = 200$ GPa, determine the minimum length for which Euler's formula is valid.**

Also, determine the value of the Euler buckling load if the column has this minimum length.

Solution: $d = 50$ mm, $\sigma_\alpha = 210$ MPa, $E = 200 \times 10^3$ MPa, , a) $L = $?, b) $F_{cr} = $?

a. *To find L:*

We know that
$$F_{cr} = \frac{\pi^2 EI}{L^2} = \frac{\pi^2 E(Ak^2)}{L^2} \qquad \text{since } I = Ak^2$$

$$\frac{F_{cr}}{A} = \frac{\pi^2 E}{(L/k)^2} \qquad \qquad \text{... Eq. (i)}$$

But
$$A = \frac{\pi d^2}{4} = \frac{\pi \times 50^2}{4} = 1963.50 \text{ mm}^2$$

$$I_{XX} = I_{YY} = \frac{\pi d^4}{64} = \frac{\pi \times 50^4}{64} = 306.80 \times 10^3 \text{ mm}^4$$

$$k = \sqrt{\frac{I}{A}} = \sqrt{\frac{306.80 \times 10^3}{1963.50}} = 12.50 \text{ mm}$$

Eq. (i) yields...
$$210 = \frac{\pi^2 \times 200 \times 10^3}{(L/k)^2}$$

$$(L/k)^2 = 9399.62$$
$$L/k = 96.95$$
$$L = 96.95 \times 12.50 = 1211.88 \text{ mm}$$

b. *To find F_{cr}:*

We know that
$$F_{cr} = \frac{\pi^2 EI}{L^2} = \frac{\pi^2 \times 200 \times 10^3 \times (306.80 \times 10^3)}{1211.88^2} = 412.35 \times 10^3 \text{ N}$$

12. **A steel bar 1.5 m long and 20 mm × 5 mm section with both ends hinged is compressed longitudinally until it buckles. Determine maximum central deflection before the steel passes the yield point at 320 MPa. Take $E = 210$ GPa.**

VTU – (CV) Jan. 2013 – 10 Marks

Solution: $l = 1500$ mm, $b = 5$ mm, $h = 20$ mm, $\delta = $?, $E = 210 \times 10^3$ MPa, $\sigma_y = 320$ MPa

Here the resultant stress is given as $\sigma_R = \sigma_D + \sigma_b$ ... Eq. (i)

Direct stress $\qquad \sigma_D = \sigma_{cr} = \dfrac{F_{cr}}{A}$ (tensile/compressive) $\qquad$ ... Eq. (ii)

Crippling load, $\qquad F_{cr} = \dfrac{\pi^2 EI}{L^2}$ $\qquad$ ... Eq. (iii)

But $\qquad I_{XX} = \dfrac{bh^3}{12} = \dfrac{5 \times 20^3}{12} = 3333.33 \text{ mm}^4$

$$I_{YY} = \dfrac{hb^3}{12} = \dfrac{20^3 \times 5}{12} = 208.33 \text{ mm}^4$$

Thus $\qquad I = I_{YY} = 208.33 \text{ mm}^4$ (minimum value)

For both ends hinged, effective length, $L = l = 2000$ mm

Eq. (iii) yields... $\qquad F_{cr} = \dfrac{\pi^2 \times 210 \times 10^3 \times 208.33}{1500^2} = 191.91 \text{ N}$

Eq. (ii) yields... $\qquad \sigma_D = \dfrac{191.91}{5 \times 20} = 1.92 \text{ MPa}$

Bending stress $\qquad \sigma_B = \dfrac{M}{Z} = \dfrac{F_{cr}.\delta}{Z_{yy}} = \dfrac{191.91 \times \delta}{25 \times 5^2/6} = (2.303)\delta$

Eq. (i) yields... $\qquad 320 = 1.92 + (2.303)\delta$

$$\delta = 138.12 \text{ mm}$$

13. A circular rod 25 mm in diameter and 2 m long is used as a strut with both ends hinged. Calculate the maximum buckling load and determine maximum lateral deflection . Take yield stress as 300 MPa and $E = 200$ GPa

Solution: $d = 25$ mm, $l = 2000$ mm, $F_{cr} = ?$, $\delta = ?$, $E = 200 \times 10^3$ MPa, $\sigma_y = 300$ MPa

Here the resultant stress is given as $\sigma_R = \sigma_D + \sigma_b$ $\qquad$ ... Eq. (i)

Direct stress $\qquad \sigma_D = \sigma_{cr} = \dfrac{F_{cr}}{A}$ (tensile/compressive) $\qquad$ ... Eq. (ii)

Crippling load, $\qquad F_{cr} = \dfrac{\pi^2 EI}{L^2}$ $\qquad$ ... Eq. (iii)

But $\qquad A = \dfrac{\pi d^2}{4} = \dfrac{\pi \times 25^2}{4} = 490.87 \text{ mm}^2$

$$I_{XX} = I_{YY} = \dfrac{\pi d^4}{64} = \dfrac{\pi \times 25^4}{64} = 19.17 \times 10^3 \text{ mm}^4$$

For both ends hinged, effective length, $L = l = 2000$ mm

Eq. (iii) yields... $\qquad F_{cr} = \dfrac{\pi^2 \times 200 \times 10^3 \times (19.17 \times 10^3)}{2000^2} = 9462.36 \text{ N}$

Eq. (ii) yields... $\qquad \sigma_D = \dfrac{9462.36}{490.87} = 19.28 \text{ MPa}$

Bending stress $\qquad \sigma_B = \dfrac{M}{Z} = \dfrac{F_{cr}.\delta}{Z_{yy}} = \dfrac{9462.36 \times \delta}{\pi \times 25^2/32} = (6.168)\delta$

Eq. (i) yields... $\qquad 300 = 19.28 + (6.168)\delta$

$\qquad\qquad\qquad \delta = 45.51$ mm

14. A 2 m long pin ended column of square section is made of a material with $E = 12 \times 10^3$ MPa and allowable stress of 12 MPa. Determine the dimension of the column using Euler's equation for the loads:

a) 95 kN $\qquad\qquad$ **b) 200 kN.** $\qquad$ **Use a factor of safety of 3.**

VTU – June/ July 2013 –12 Marks; Dec. 2011 – 08 Marks

Solution: $l = 2000$ mm, $E = 12 \times 10^3$ MPa, $\sigma_{allw} = 12$ MPa, $n = 3$, $b = ?$, a) $F_s = 95 \times 10^3$ N,
b) $F_s = 200 \times 10^3$ N

$\qquad$ Let $\qquad\qquad\qquad b = $ side of the square

Case a: $F_s = 95 \times 10^3$ N

$\qquad$ We know that $\qquad F_s = \dfrac{F_{cr}}{n}$

$\qquad\qquad\qquad\qquad F_{cr} = (95 \times 10^3) \times 3 = 285 \times 10^3$ N

Based on F_{cr}:

$\qquad$ We know that $\qquad F_{cr} = \dfrac{\pi^2 E I}{L^2}$

$\qquad\qquad\qquad\qquad I_{XX} = I_{YY} = \dfrac{bh^3}{12} = \dfrac{b^4}{12} \qquad\qquad$ [$b = h$, for square cross-section]

$\qquad\qquad$ For both ends hinged, effective length, $L = l = 2000$ mm

$\qquad\qquad 285 \times 10^3 = \dfrac{\pi^2 \times 12 \times 10^3 \times (b^4/12)}{2000^2}$

$\qquad\qquad\qquad\qquad b = 103.67$ mm $\qquad\qquad\qquad\qquad\qquad$ ... Eq. (a)

Based on σ_{allw}:

$\qquad\qquad \sigma_{allw} = \dfrac{F_s}{A} \qquad\qquad$ OR $\qquad \sigma_{cr} = n\sigma_{allw} = 3 \times 12 = 36$ MPa

$\qquad\qquad 12 = \dfrac{95 \times 10^3}{b^2} \qquad\qquad\qquad \sigma_{cr} = \dfrac{F_{cr}}{A} \Rightarrow 36 = \dfrac{285 \times 10^3}{b^2}$

$\qquad\qquad\quad b = 88.98$ mm $\qquad\qquad\qquad b = 88.98$ mm $\qquad$ ... Eq. (b)

Based on Eqs (a) and (b), select higher value for design.
Thus the dimensions of the column are 103.67×103.67 mm^2

Case b: $F_s = 200 \times 10^3$ N

$\qquad$ We know that $\quad F_s = \dfrac{F_{cr}}{n}$

$\qquad\qquad\qquad F_{cr} = (200 \times 10^3) \times 3 = 600 \times 10^3$ N

Based on F_{cr}:

$\qquad$ We know that $\qquad F_{cr} = \dfrac{\pi^2 E I}{L^2}$

$$600 \times 10^3 = \frac{\pi^2 \times 12 \times 10^3 \times (b^4/12)}{2000^2}$$

$$b = 124.88 \text{ mm} \qquad \qquad \text{... Eq. (c)}$$

Based on σ_{allw}:

$$\sigma_{allw} = \frac{F_s}{A} \qquad \text{OR} \qquad \sigma_{cr} = n\sigma_{allw} = 3 \times 12 = 36 \text{ MPa}$$

$$12 = \frac{200 \times 10^3}{b^2} \qquad \qquad \sigma_{cr} = \frac{F_{cr}}{A} \Rightarrow 36 = \frac{600 \times 10^3}{b^2}$$

$$b = 129.10 \text{ mm} \qquad \qquad b = 129.10 \text{ mm} \qquad \text{... Eq. (d)}$$

Based on Eqs (c) and (d), select higher value for design.

Thus the dimensions of the column are 129.10×129.10 mm^2

15. **An aluminum tube of length 4 m is used as a simply supported column carrying a 1500 N axial load. If the outer diameter of the tube is 50 mm, compute the inner diameter that would provide a factor of safety of 2 against buckling. Use $E = 75$ GPa.**

Solution: $l = 4000$ mm, $F_s = 1500$ N, $d_o = 50$ mm, $d_i = ?$, $n = 2$, $E = 75 \times 10^3$ MPa

We know that $\qquad F_s = \dfrac{F_{cr}}{n}$

$$F_{cr} = 1500 \times 2 = 3000 \text{ N}$$

Also $\qquad F_{cr} = \dfrac{\pi^2 EI}{L^2}$

But $\qquad I_{XX} = I_{YY} = \dfrac{\pi\left(d_o^4 - d_o^4\right)}{64}$

For both ends hinged, effective length, $L = l = 4000$ mm

$$3000 = \frac{\pi^2 \times 75 \times 10^3 \times [\pi(50^4 - d_i^4)/64]}{4000^2}$$

$$d_i = 47.12 \text{ mm}$$

16. **Determine the buckling load for a T-section shown in Fig. 10.6. The column is 3 m long and is hinged at both ends. Take $E = 200$ GPa.**

VTU – Dec. 16/ Jan. 17 – 10 Marks

Solution: $F_{cr} = ?$, $l = 3000$ mm, $E = 75 \times 10^3$ MPa

a. *To find $\bar{y}$:*

$a_1 = 10 \times 70 = 700$ mm^2, $\qquad\qquad a_2 = 100 \times 10 = 1000$ mm^2

$y_1 = 70/2 = 35$ mm, $\qquad\qquad\qquad y_2 = (10/2) + 70 = 75$ mm

$A = \Sigma A = a_1 + a_2 = 1700$ mm^2

$$\bar{y} = \frac{\Sigma ay}{\Sigma a} = \frac{(700 \times 35) + (1000 \times 75)}{1700} = 58.53 \text{ mm (w.r.t base)}$$

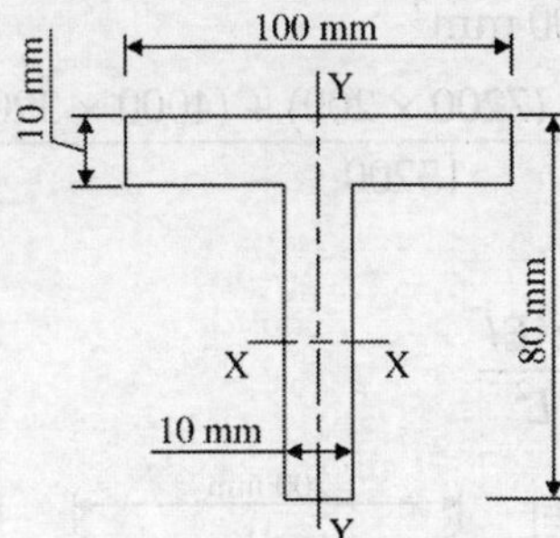

Fig. 10.6: Problems 16

We know that
$$F_{cr} = \frac{\pi^2 EI}{L^2} \qquad\qquad \text{... Eq. (i)}$$

But
$$I_{XX} = \Sigma I_{XX} = \sum\left[\frac{bh^3}{12} + a\left(\bar{y} \sim y_n\right)^2\right]$$

$$= \left\{\frac{10 \times 70^3}{12} + \left[700 \times (58.53 - 35)^2\right]\right\}$$

$$+ \left\{\frac{100 \times 10^3}{12} + \left[1000 \times (58.53 - 75)^2\right]\right\}$$

$$I_{XX} = 953 \times 10^3 \text{ mm}^4$$

$$I_{YY} = \Sigma I_{YY} = \sum\left[\frac{hb^3}{12} + a\left(x \sim x_n\right)^2\right]$$

$$= \sum\left(\frac{hb^3}{12}\right) \text{ since the given Fig. is symmetry about Y-Y axis}$$

$$= \frac{70 \times 10^3}{12} + \frac{10 \times 100^3}{12}$$

$$I_{YY} = 839.17 \times 10^3 \text{ mm}^4$$

Thus $\qquad I = I_{YY} = 839.17 \times 10^3 \text{ mm}^4 \qquad\qquad$ (minimum value)

For both ends hinged, effective length, $L = l = 3000$ mm

Eq. (i) yields... $\qquad F_{cr} = \dfrac{\pi^2 \times 200 \times 10^3 \times (839.17 \times 10^3)}{3000^2}$

$$F_{cr} = 184.05 \times 10^3 \text{ N} = 184.05 \text{ kN}$$

17. Determine the buckling load for a I-section shown in Fig. 10.7. The column is 6 m long and is fixed at both ends. Take $E = 200$ GPa.

Solution: $F_{cr} = ?$, $l = 6000$ mm, $E = 200 \times 10^3$ MPa

To find $\bar{y}$:

$a_1 = 200 \times 20 = 4000 \text{ mm}^2$, $\quad y_1 = 20/2 = 10$ mm,

$a_2 = 20 \times 360 = 7200 \text{ mm}^2 \quad y_2 = (360/2) + 20 = 200$ mm

$a_3 = 200 \times 20 = 4000 \text{ mm}^2 \quad y_3 = (20/2) + 360 + 20 = 390$ mm

$$A = \Sigma a = a_1 + a_2 + a_3 = 15200 \text{ mm}^2$$

$$\bar{y} = \frac{\Sigma ay}{\Sigma a} = \frac{(4000 \times 10) + (7200 \times 200) + (4000 \times 390)}{15200} = 200 \text{ mm (w.r.t base)}$$

To find F_{cr}:

We know that $\qquad F_{cr} = \dfrac{\pi^2 EI}{L^2}$ $\qquad\qquad\qquad\qquad$ ... Eq. (i)

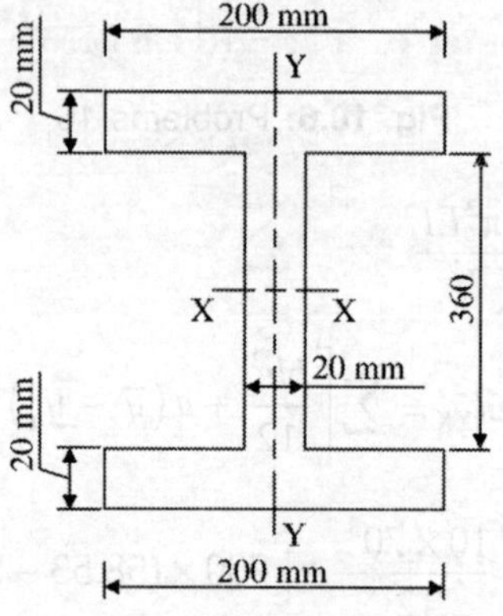

Fig. 10.7: Problems 17

But $\qquad I_{XX} = \Sigma I_{XX} = \sum \left[\dfrac{bh^3}{12} + a\left(\bar{y} \sim y_n\right)^2 \right]$

$$= \left\{ \frac{200 \times 20^3}{12} + \left[4000 \times (200 - 10)^2 \right] \right\}$$

$$+ \left\{ \frac{20 \times 360^3}{12} + \left[7200 \times (200 - 200)^2 \right] \right\}$$

$$+ \left\{ \frac{200 \times 20^3}{12} + \left[4000 \times (390 - 200)^2 \right] \right\}$$

$$I_{XX} = 236.87 \times 10^6 \text{ mm}^4$$

$$I_{YY} = \Sigma I_{YY} = \sum \left[\frac{hb^3}{12} + a\left(x \sim x_n\right)^2 \right]$$

$$= \sum \left(\frac{hb^3}{12} \right) \text{ since the given Fig. is symmetry about Y-Y axis}$$

$$= \frac{20 \times 200^3}{12} + \frac{360 \times 20^3}{12} + \frac{20 \times 200^3}{12}$$

$$I_{YY} = 26.91 \times 10^6 \text{ mm}^4$$

Thus $\qquad\qquad I = I_{YY} = 26.91 \times 10^6 \text{ mm}^4 \qquad\qquad$ (minimum value)

For both ends fixed, effective length, $l = l/2 = 6000/2 = 3000$ mm

Eq. (i) yields...
$$F_{cr} = \frac{\pi^2 \times 200 \times 10^3 \times (26.91 \times 10^6)}{3000^2}$$

$$F_{cr} = 5.90 \times 10^6 \text{ N} = 5.9 \text{ MN}$$

18. Determine the ratio of buckling strength of two columns of circular cross section, one hollow and the other solid when both are made of same material, same length and same cross-sectional area and end conditions. Assume that the inner diameter of hollow column is half the external diameter.

Solution: $d_i = 0.5 d_o \Rightarrow K = 0.5 = \dfrac{d_i}{d_o}$, $A_s = A_H,\, L_s = L_H$

Let, d = Diameter of solid rod

d_o = Outer diameter of hollow rod

d_i = Inner diameter of hollow rod

$K = \dfrac{d_i}{d_o}$ = Ratio of inner diameter to outer diameter of hollow rod

$L = L_s = L_H$ = Effective length of the column

$A = A_s = A_H$ = Area of the rod

$E = E_s = E_H$ = Young's modulus of the material

$F_{cr})_s$ = Crippling load of solid rod

$F_{cr})_H$ = Crippling load of hollow rod

Given $A_s = A_H$

$$\left(\frac{\pi d^2}{4}\right) = \left[\frac{\pi\left(d_o^2 - d_i^2\right)}{4}\right]$$

$$d^2 = \left(d_o^2 - d_i^2\right) = d_o^2\,(1 - K^2)$$

$$d^2 = d_o^2\,(1 - 0.5^2)$$

$$d^2 = 0.75\,d_o^2$$

$$d = 0.866\,d_o \qquad\qquad\qquad \text{... Eq. (i)}$$

Ratio of buckling strength:

$$\frac{F_{cr})_H}{F_{cr})_s} = \frac{(\pi^2 EI/L^2)_H}{(\pi^2 EI/L^2)_s}$$

$$= \frac{I_H}{I_s} = \frac{\pi\left(d_o^4 - d_i^4\right)/64}{\pi d^4/64}$$

$$= \frac{d_o^4 - d_i^4}{d^4} = \frac{d_o^4(1 - K^4)}{d^4}$$

$$= \frac{d_o^4(1 - 0.5^4)}{(0.866 d_o)^4} \qquad\qquad \text{... using Eq. (i)}$$

$$\frac{F_{cr})_H}{F_{cr})_s} = 1.667$$

19. Repeat the above problem if the ratio of diameters is 3/4.

Solution: $K = \dfrac{3}{4} = \dfrac{d_i}{d_o}$, $A_s = A_H$, $L_s = L_H$

Proceeding on similar lines to problem 18, we have
$$d = 0.6614\, d_o \qquad\qquad \text{... Eq. (i)}$$

$$\frac{F_{cr})_H}{F_{cr})_s} = \frac{d_o^4\left[1-(3/4)^4\right]}{\left(0.6614\, d_o\right)^4} = 3.572$$

20. There are two columns, one is a solid C.I column 150 mm in diameter and another hollow circular C.I column of the same cross-sectional area with a wall thickness of 25 mm. Both columns have same length and are pinned at the ends. Show that the hollow column can withstand 4.55 times greater than the solid column.

VTU – (CV) Dec. 2009/ Jan. 2010 – 10 Marks; (CV) June/ July 2009 – 08 Marks

Solution: $d = 150$ mm, $t = 25$ mm

Let, $\quad d = $ Diameter of solid rod

$d_o = $ Outer diameter of hollow rod

$d_i = $ Inner diameter of hollow rod

$K = \dfrac{d_i}{d_o} = $ Ratio of inner diameter to outer diameter of hollow rod

$L = L_s = L_H = $ Effective length of the column

$A = A_s = A_H = $ Area of the rod

$E = E_s = E_H = $ Young's modulus of the material

$F_{cr})_s = $ Crippling load of solid rod

$F_{cr})_H = $ Crippling load of hollow rod

Given $\qquad A_s = A_H$

$$\left(\frac{\pi d^2}{4}\right) = \left[\frac{\pi\left(d_o^2 - d_i^2\right)}{4}\right]$$

$$d^2 = \left(d_o^2 - d_i^2\right)$$

$$= d_o^2 - (d_o - 2t)^2 \qquad\qquad (\because\ \ d_o = d_i + 2t)$$

$$150^2 = d_o^2 - (d_o - 50)^2$$

$$22500 = d_o^2 - d_o^2 - 2500 + 100 d_o$$

$$100 d_o = 22500 + 2500$$

$$d_o = 250\,\text{mm}$$

And $\qquad\qquad d_i = 250 - (2 \times 25) = 200\,\text{mm}$

Ratio of buckling strength:

$$\frac{F_{cr})_H}{F_{cr})_s} = \frac{(\pi^2 EI/L^2)_H}{(\pi^2 EI/L^2)_s}$$

$$= \frac{I_H}{I_s} = \frac{\pi\left(d_o^4 - d_i^4\right)/64}{\pi d^4/64}$$

$$= \frac{d_o^4 - d_i^4}{d^4}$$

$$\frac{F_{cr})_H}{F_{cr})_s} = \frac{(250^4 - 200^4)}{150^4} = 4.555. \quad \text{Hence proved.}$$

21. **Calculate the value of slenderness ratio of a mild steel column for which the Euler's formula is valid. Take $E = 210$ GPa and compressive yield stress as 325 MPa.**

    OR   Explain the validity limit of Euler's formula

    OR   Write a note of limitations of Euler's theory.

Solution: $E = 210 \times 10^3$ MPa, $\sigma_c)_y = 325$ MPa

We know that $\qquad \sigma_{cr} = \dfrac{F_{cr}}{A}$

$$= \frac{\pi^2 EI}{AL^2} = \frac{\pi^2 E(Ak^2)}{AL^2}$$

$$\sigma_{cr} = \frac{\pi^2 E}{(L/k)^2} \qquad\qquad \text{... Eq. (i)}$$

Since a long column buckle at a stress far below the compressive yield stress of the material, for safe design, we have

$$\sigma_{cr} \leq \sigma_c)_y$$

$$\frac{\pi^2 E}{(L/k)^2} \leq \sigma_c)_y$$

$$\frac{\pi^2 \times (210 \times 10^3)}{(L/k)^2} \leq 325$$

$$(L/k)^2 \geq 6377.28$$
$$L/k \geq 79.86 \approx 80$$

It would therefore be impossible to use Euler's theory for such a strut of slenderness ratio less than this value i.e. Euler's equation is valid for $L/k \geq 80$.

22. **A both ends hinged cast iron hollow cylindrical column 3 m in length has a critical buckling load of F kN. When the column is fixed at both the ends, its critical buckling load raise by 400 kN more. If ratio of diameters is 0.75 and $E = 200$ GPa determine the external diameter of column.**

    Solution: $l = 3000$ mm, case 1: load = F kN, for both ends hinged; case 2: load = F = 400 kN, for both ends fixed, $K = 0.75$, $E = 200 \times 10^3$ MPa, $d_o = ?$

We know that

$$F_{cr} = \frac{\pi^2 EI}{L^2} \qquad \dots \text{Eq. (i)}$$

Case 1: Here $\quad F_{cr} = F$ and $L = l = 3000$ mm $\qquad \dots$ Eq. (ii)

Case 2: Here $\quad F_{cr} = (F + 400)$ and $L = l/2 = 1500$ mm $\qquad \dots$ Eq. (iii)

Dividing Eq. (iii) with Eq. (ii) as per Eq. (i), we have

$$\frac{(F + 400)}{F} = \frac{\pi^2 EI/l^2}{\pi^2 EI/(l/2)^2} = 4$$

$$F + 400 = 4F$$

$$F = 133.34 \text{ kN} = 133.34 \times 10^3 \text{ N}$$

Eq. (i) yields...

$$133.34 \times 10^3 = \frac{\pi^2 \times (200 \times 10^3) \times I}{3000^2}$$

$$I = 6.08 \times 10^5 \text{ mm}^4$$

Also

$$I_{XX} = I_{YY} = \frac{\pi \left(d_o^4 - d_i^4\right)}{64} = \frac{\pi d_o^4 \left(1 - K^4\right)}{64}$$

$$6.08 \times 10^5 = \frac{\pi d_o^4 (1 - 0.75^4)}{64}$$

$$d_o = 65.24 \text{ mm}$$

10.7 RANKINE–GORDON'S FORMULA FOR COLUMNS

Short columns fail by crushing while long columns fail by buckling. The struts we come across are neither too short nor too long (i.e. intermediate columns) which may not fail by crushing alone, and for which Euler's formulae are not applicable. Such columns may fail by a combination of crushing and buckling.

Rankine suggested an empirical relationship, taking into account the direct compressive stress and bending stress which is applicable to all columns (short, intermediate or long).

According to Rankine

$$\frac{1}{F_R} = \frac{1}{F_c} + \frac{1}{F_E} \qquad \dots \text{(Eq. 10.29)}$$

Where $\quad F_c = \sigma_c A = $ crushing load

$$F_{cr} = F_E = \frac{\pi^2 EI}{L^2} = \text{Buckling load}$$

$$\sigma_c = \text{crushing stress}$$

$$\frac{1}{F_R} = \frac{F_c + F_E}{F_c \cdot F_E}$$

$$F_R = \frac{F_c \cdot F_E}{F_c + F_E}$$

$$= \frac{F_c}{1 + \dfrac{F_c}{F_E}}$$

$$= \frac{\sigma_c A}{1 + \dfrac{\sigma_c A}{\pi^2 EI/L^2}}$$

$$= \frac{\sigma_c A}{1 + \dfrac{\sigma_c A L^2}{\pi^2 E A k^2}} \qquad \text{since } I = (Ak^2)$$

$$= \frac{\sigma_c A}{1 + \dfrac{\sigma_c}{\pi^2 E}\left(\dfrac{L}{k}\right)^2}$$

$$\therefore \quad F_R = \frac{\sigma_c A}{1 + a\left(\dfrac{L}{k}\right)^2} = \frac{F_c}{1 + a\left(\dfrac{L}{k}\right)^2} \qquad \dots \text{(Eq. 10.30)}$$

Where $\quad a = \dfrac{\sigma_c}{\pi^2 E}$ is a constant for a given material and is called the Rankine's constant.

Factor $1 + a\left(\dfrac{L}{k}\right)^2$ takes care of buckling effect.

Table 10.2 shows the values of σ_c and a for different materials

Table 10.2

Material	σ_c (MPa)	$a = \dfrac{\sigma_c}{\pi^2 E}$
Cast Iron (CI)	550	1/1600
Wrought iron (WI)	250	1/9000
Mild steel (MS)	320	1/7500
Timber	50	1/750

23. **Find the length of a column which gives the same value of buckling load by Euler and Rankine's formulae.**

Solution: $F_E = F_R$, $L = ?$

Given $\qquad F_E = F_R$

$$\frac{\pi^2 EI}{L^2} = \frac{\sigma_c A}{1 + a\left(\dfrac{L}{k}\right)^2}$$

$$\pi^2 EI\left[1 + a\left(\frac{L}{k}\right)^2\right] = \sigma_c A L^2$$

$$\pi^2 EI = \sigma_c AL^2 - \pi^2 EIa\left(\frac{L}{k}\right)^2$$

$$= L^2\left[\sigma_c A - \frac{\pi^2 EIa}{k^2}\right]$$

$$\pi^2 E(Ak^2) = L^2\left[\sigma_c A - \frac{\pi^2 Ea(Ak)^2}{k^2}\right]$$

$$L^2 = \frac{\pi^2 Ek^2}{\sigma_c - \pi^2 Ea}$$

$$L = \sqrt{\frac{\pi^2 Ek^2}{\sigma_c - \pi^2 Ea}} \qquad \qquad \text{... (Eq. 10.31)}$$

(Eq. 10.31) holds good for columns having both ends hinged.

24. **Using Rankine's formula, determine the crippling load for a mild steel strut 500 mm long, with a rectangular section 50 mm × 12.5 mm having:**
   a) hinged ends and   b) fixed ends.
   Take $a = 1/6500$, and $\sigma_c = 330$ N/mm².

VTU – (CV) June/ July 2009 – 08 Marks

Solution: $F_R = ?$, $l = 500$ mm, $b = 12.5$ mm, $h = 50$ mm, $\sigma_c = 330$ N/mm², $a = 1/6500$.

We know that
$$F_R = \frac{\sigma_c A}{1 + a\left(\dfrac{L}{K}\right)^2} \qquad \qquad \text{... Eq. (i)}$$

$$A = b.h = 12.5 \times 50 = 625 \text{ mm}^2$$

$$I_{XX} = \frac{bh^3}{12} = \frac{12.5 \times 50^3}{12} = 130.21 \times 10^3 \text{ mm}^4$$

$$I_{YY} = \frac{hb^3}{12} = \frac{50 \times 12.5^3}{12} = 8.13 \times 10^3 \text{ mm}^4$$

Thus $I = I_{YY} = 8.14 \times 10^3$ mm⁴   (minimum value)

$$k = \sqrt{\frac{I}{A}} = \sqrt{\frac{8.14 \times 10^3}{625}} = 3.61$$

Case a: For both ends hinged: Effective length, $L = l = 500$ mm

Eq. (i) yields...
$$F_R = \frac{330 \times 625}{1 + \left(\dfrac{1}{6500}\right) \times \left(\dfrac{500}{3.61}\right)^2} = 52.20 \times 10^3 \text{ N}$$

Case b: For both ends fixed: Effective length, $L = l/2 = 500/2 = 250$ mm

Eq. (i) yields...
$$F_R = \frac{330 \times 625}{1 + \left(\dfrac{1}{6500}\right) \times \left(\dfrac{250}{3.61}\right)^2} = 118.68 \times 10^3 \text{ N}$$

25. **Using Rankine's formula, determine the safe load for a cast iron column 7 m long, with both ends fixed. The circular column has an external diameter of 200 mm and internal diameter of 150 mm. It is subjected to an axial compressive load. Take factor of safety = 6, σ_c = 567 N/mm^2, and a = 1/1600.**

VTU – (CV) June 2012 – 10 Marks

Solution: F_s = ?, l = 7000 mm, d_o = 200 mm, d_i = 150 mm, n = 6, σ_c = 567 N/mm^2, a = 1/1600.

We know that
$$F_s = \frac{F_R}{n} \qquad \dots \text{Eq. (i)}$$

But
$$F_R = \frac{\sigma_c A}{1 + a\left(\dfrac{L}{k}\right)^2} \qquad \dots \text{Eq. (ii)}$$

$$A = \frac{\pi\left(d_o^2 - d_i^2\right)}{4} = \frac{\pi(200^2 - 150^2)}{4} = 13744.47 \text{ mm}^2$$

$$I_{XX} = I_{YY} = \frac{\pi\left(d_o^4 - d_i^4\right)}{64} = \frac{\pi(200^4 - 150^4)}{64} = 53.69 \times 10^6 \text{ mm}^4$$

$$k = \sqrt{\frac{I}{A}} = \sqrt{\frac{53.69 \times 10^6}{13744.47}} = 62.50$$

For both ends fixed, effective length, $L = l/2 = 7000/2 = 3500$ mm

Eq. (ii) yields...
$$F_R = \frac{567 \times 13744.47}{1 + \left(\dfrac{1}{1600}\right) \times \left(\dfrac{3500}{62.50}\right)^2} = 2632.81 \times 10^3 \text{ N}$$

Eq. (i) yields...
$$F_s = \frac{2632.81 \times 10^3}{6} = 438.80 \times 10^3 \text{ N}$$

26. **A 1.5 m long column has a circular cross section of 50 mm diameter. One end of the column is fixed in direction and position and the other end is free. Taking the factor of safety as 3, calculate the safe load using:**
   (a) Rankine's formula taking yield stress 560 N/mm^2 and a = 1/1600
   (b) Euler's formulas taking E = 1.2 × 10^5 N/mm^2.

VTU – June/ July 2013 – 10 Marks; Dec. 09/ Jan. 10 – 10 Marks;
[Similar: (CV) June 2012 – 10 Marks; (CV) Dec. 2010 – 10 Marks]

Solution: l = 1500 mm, d = 50 mm, n = 3, σ_c = 560 MPa, a = 1/1600, E = 1.2 × 10^5 N/mm^2, safe load F_s = ?

a. *According to Rankine's:*

We know that
$$F_s = \frac{F_R}{n} \qquad \dots \text{Eq. (i)}$$

But
$$F_R = \frac{\sigma_c A}{1 + a\left(\dfrac{L}{k}\right)^2} \qquad \dots \text{Eq. (ii)}$$

Also
$$A = \frac{\pi d^2}{4} = \frac{\pi \times 50^2}{4} = 1963.50 \text{ mm}^2$$

$$I_{XX} = I_{YY} = \frac{\pi d^4}{4} = \frac{\pi \times 50^4}{4} = 306.80 \times 10^3 \text{ mm}^4$$

$$k = \sqrt{\frac{I}{A}} = \sqrt{\frac{306.80 \times 10^3}{1963.50}} = 12.5$$

For a column with one end fixed in direction and position and the other end free.
Effective length, $L = 2l = 2 \times 1500 = 3000$ mm

Eq. (ii) yields... $F_R = \dfrac{560 \times 1963.50}{1 + \left(\dfrac{1}{1600}\right) \times \left(\dfrac{3000}{12.5}\right)} = 29.72 \times 10^3 \text{ N}$

Eq. (i) yields... $F_s = \dfrac{29.72 \times 10^3}{3} = 9906.67 \text{ N}$

b. *According to Euler:*

We know that $F_s = \dfrac{F_{cr}}{n}$ ... Eq. (iii)

But $F_{cr} = \dfrac{\pi^2 EI}{L^2}$

$$F_{cr} = \frac{\pi^2 \times 1.2 \times 10^5 \times (306.80 \times 10^3)}{3000^2} = 40.37 \times 10^3 \text{ N}$$

Eq. (i) yields... $F_s = \dfrac{40.37 \times 10^3}{3} = 13.46 \times 10^3 \text{ N}$

27. A hollow C.I column whose outer diameter is 200 mm has a thickness of 20 mm. It is 4.5m long and fixed at both ends. Calculate the safe load by Rankine's formula using a factor of safety of 4. Calculate the slenderness ratio and the ratio of Euler's and Rankine's critical loads. Take $\sigma_c = 550$ N/mm^2 and $a = 1/1600$ in Rankine's formula and $E = 9.4 \times 10^4$ N/mm^2.

VTU – Dec. 14/ Jan. 15 – 10 Marks; June/ July 2008 – 12 Marks;
(CV) Dec. 2016/ Jan. 2017 – 12 Marks

Solution: $d_o = 200$ mm, $t = 20$ mm, $d_i = d_o - 2t = 200 - 40 = 160$ mm, $l = 4500$ mm, $\sigma_c = 550$ N/mm^2 and $a = 1/1600$, $E = 9.4 \times 10^4$ N/mm^2. a) $F_s = ?$, b) $L/k = ?$ c) $F_E/F_R = ?$

a. *According to Rankine's:*

We know that $F_s = \dfrac{F_R}{n}$ ... Eq. (i)

But $F_R = \dfrac{\sigma_c A}{1 + a\left(\dfrac{L}{k}\right)^2}$ ... Eq. (ii)

$$A = \frac{\pi\left(d_o^2 - d_i^2\right)}{4} = \frac{\pi(200^2 - 160^2)}{4} = 11309.73 \text{ mm}^2$$

$$I_{XX} = I_{YY} = \frac{\pi\left(d_o^4 - d_i^4\right)}{64} = \frac{\pi(200^4 - 160^4)}{64} = 46.37 \times 10^6 \text{ mm}^4$$

$$k = \sqrt{\frac{I}{A}} = \sqrt{\frac{46.37 \times 10^6}{11309.73}} = 64.03$$

For both ends fixed, effective length, $L = l/2 = 4500/2 = 2250$ mm

Eq. (ii) yields... $\qquad F_R = \dfrac{550 \times 11309.73}{1 + \left(\dfrac{1}{1600}\right) \times \left(\dfrac{2250}{64.03}\right)^2} = 3.51 \times 10^6 \text{ N}$

Eq. (i) yields... $\qquad F_s = \dfrac{3.51 \times 10^6}{4} = 877.71 \times 10^3 \text{ N}$

b. *Slenderness ratio:*

Slenderness ratio $\dfrac{L}{k} = \dfrac{2250}{64.03} = 35.14$

c. *Ratio of Euler to Rankine's:*

We know that $\qquad F_{cr} = \dfrac{\pi^2 EI}{L^2} = \dfrac{\pi^2 \times 9.4 \times 10^4 \times (46.37 \times 10^6)}{2250^2} = 8.50 \times 10^6 \text{ N}$

Thus $\qquad \dfrac{F_E}{F_R} = \dfrac{8.50 \times 10^6}{3.51 \times 10^6} = 2.42$

28. **Find the Euler's crippling load for a hollow cylindrical steel column of 38 mm external diameter and 2.5 mm thick. Take the length of column as 2.3 m hinged at its both ends. Take $E = 2.05 \times 10^5$ N/mm^2. Also determine the crippling load by Rankine's formula using constants as 335 N/mm^2 and 1/7500.**

VTU – June/ July 2009 – 10 Marks; [similar (CV):
June/ July 2008 – 10 Marks; June/ July 2014 – 10 Marks; June/ July 2015 – 14
Marks; June/ July 2014 – 08 Marks; Dec. 2011– 10 Marks]

Solution: $d_o = 38$ mm, $t = 2.5$ mm, $d_i = d_o - 2t = 38 - 5 = 33$ mm, $l = 2300$ mm, $\sigma_c = 335$ N/mm^2 and $a = 1/7500$, $E = 2.05 \times 10^5$ N/mm^2. a) $F_{cr} = ?$, b) $F_R = ?$

a. *According to Euler:*

We know that $\qquad F_{cr} = \dfrac{\pi^2 EI}{L^2}$ $\hfill$ ... Eq. (i)

Here $\qquad I_{XX} = I_{YY} = \dfrac{\pi\left(d_o^4 - d_i^4\right)}{64} = \dfrac{\pi(38^4 - 33^4)}{64} = 44.14 \times 10^3 \text{ mm}^4$

For both ends hinged, effective length, $L = l = 2300$ mm

$$F_{cr} = \frac{\pi^2 \times 2.05 \times 10^5 \times (44.14 \times 10^3)}{2300^2} = 16.88 \times 10^3 \text{ N}$$

b. *According to Rankine's:*

We know that
$$F_R = \frac{\sigma_c A}{1 + a\left(\dfrac{L}{k}\right)^2}$$

But
$$A = \frac{\pi\left(d_o^2 - d_i^2\right)}{4} = \frac{\pi(38^2 - 33^2)}{4} = 278.82 \text{ mm}^2$$

$$k = \sqrt{\frac{I}{A}} = \sqrt{\frac{44.14 \times 10^3}{278.82}} = 12.58$$

$$F_R = \frac{335 \times 278.82}{1 + \left(\dfrac{1}{7500}\right) \times \left(\dfrac{2300}{12.58}\right)^2} = 17.12 \times 10^3 \text{ N}$$

29. **The cross-section of a column is a hollow rectangular section with its external dimensions 200 mm × 150 mm. The internal dimensions are 150 mm × 100 mm. The column is 5 m long and fixed at both ends. If E = 120 GPa, calculate the critical load using Euler's formula. Compare the above load with the value obtained from Rankine's formula. The permissible compressive stress is 500 N/mm^2. The Rankine's constant is 1/1600.**

VTU – Dec. 2013/ Jan. 2014 – 14 Marks

Solution: Outer dimensions: B = 150 mm, H = 200 mm; inner dimensions: b = 100 mm, h = 150 mm, l = 5000 mm, E = 120 × 10^3 MPa, σ_c = 500 N/mm^2, a = 1/1600. a) F_{cr} = ? b) F_R = ?

a. *According to Euler:*

We know that
$$F_{cr} = \frac{\pi^2 EI}{L^2}$$

Here
$$I_{YY} = \frac{BH^3 - bh^3}{12} = \frac{150 \times 200^3 - 100 \times 150^3}{12} = 71.88 \times 10^6 \text{ mm}^4$$

$$I_{XX} = \frac{HB^3 - hb^3}{12} = \frac{200 \times 150^3 - 150 \times 100^3}{12} = 43.75 \times 10^6 \text{ mm}^4$$

Thus
$$I = I_{YY} = 43.75 \times 10^6 \text{ mm}^4 \quad \text{(minimum value)}$$

For both ends fixed, effective length, $L = l/2 = 5000/2 = 2500$ mm

$$F_{cr} = \frac{\pi^2 \times 120 \times 10^3 \times (43.75 \times 10^3)}{2500^2} = 8.24 \times 10^6 \text{ N}$$

b. *According to Rankine's:*

We know that
$$F_R = \frac{\sigma_c A}{1 + a\left(\dfrac{L}{k}\right)^2}$$

But
$$A = (BH - bh) = (150 \times 200 - 100 \times 150) = 15000 \text{ mm}^2$$

$$k = \sqrt{\frac{I}{A}} = \sqrt{\frac{43.75 \times 10^6}{15000}} = 54.01$$

$$F_R = \frac{500 \times 15000}{1 + \left(\dfrac{1}{1600}\right) \times \left(\dfrac{2500}{54.01}\right)^2} = 3.21 \times 10^6 \text{ N}$$

30. Solve problem 17 using Rankine's formula. Take σ = 500 MPa, a = 1/1600

Solution: $F_R = ?$, $l = 6000$ mm, $E = 200 \times 10^3$ MPa, σ = 500 MPa, $a = 1/1600$

We know that $\qquad F_R = \dfrac{\sigma_c A}{1 + a\left(\dfrac{L}{k}\right)^2}$ $\qquad\qquad$ ... Eq. (i)

From problem 17, *we have*
$$A = 15200 \text{ mm}^2$$
$$I_{XX} = 236.87 \times 10^6 \text{ mm}^4$$
$$I_{YY} = 26.91 \times 10^6 \text{ mm}^4$$

Thus $\qquad I = I_{YY} = 26.91 \times 10^6 \text{ mm}^4$ $\qquad\qquad$ (minimum value)

$$k = \sqrt{\frac{I}{A}} = \sqrt{\frac{26.91 \times 10^6}{15200}} = 42.08$$

For both ends fixed, effective length, $L = l/2 = 6000/2 = 3000$ mm

Eq. (i) yields... $\qquad F_R = \dfrac{500 \times 15200}{1 + \left(\dfrac{1}{1600}\right) \times \left(\dfrac{3000}{42.08}\right)^2} = 1819.63 \times 10^3 \text{ N}$

31. A hollow square column of 120 mm outside dimensions and 5 mm thick is 8 m long and is fixed at both ends. Determine the buckling load using Rankine's formula assuming σ = 500 MPa, a = 1/1600. What is the equivalent solid square section?

VTU – (CV) May/ June 2010 – 08 Marks

Solution: $l = 8000$ mm, σ = σ_c = 500 MPa, $a = 1/1600$.
 a) $F_R = ?$, for hollow square section b) Size of equivalent solid square section $B = H = ?$
Given: Outer dimensions: $B = H = 120$ mm, $t = 5$ mm
$\qquad\quad$ Inner dimensions: $b = h = B - 2t = 120 - (2 \times 5) = 110$ mm
a. *Hollow square section:*

We know that $\qquad F_R = \dfrac{\sigma_c A}{1 + a\left(\dfrac{L}{k}\right)^2}$ $\qquad\qquad$ ... Eq. (i)

But $\qquad A = (BH - bh) = (B^2 - b^2) = (120^2 - 110^2) = 2300 \text{ mm}^2$

$$I_{XX} = I_{YY} = \frac{BH^3 - bh^3}{12} = \frac{B^4 - b^4}{12} = \frac{120^4 - 110^4}{12} = 5.08 \times 10^6 \text{ mm}^4$$

$$k = \sqrt{\frac{I}{A}} = \sqrt{\frac{5.09 \times 10^6}{2300}} = 47$$

For both ends fixed, effective length, $L = l/2 = 8000/2 = 4000$ mm

Eq. (i) yields...
$$F_R = \frac{500 \times 2300}{1 + \left(\dfrac{1}{1600}\right) \times \left(\dfrac{4000}{47}\right)^2} = 208.07 \times 10^3 \text{ N}$$

b. *Equivalent solid square section:*

Here
$$A = B.H = B^2$$

$$I_{XX} = I_{YY} = \frac{BH^3}{12} = \frac{B^4}{12}$$

$$k = \sqrt{\frac{I}{A}} = \sqrt{\frac{B^4/12}{B^2}} = 0.289\,B$$

For both ends fixed, effective length, $L = l/2 = 8000/2 = 4000$ mm
Eq. (i) yields...

$$208.07 \times 10^3 = \frac{500 \times B^2}{1 + \left(\dfrac{1}{1600}\right) \times \left(\dfrac{4000}{0.289B}\right)^2}$$

$$1 + \left(\frac{119.73 \times 10^3}{B^2}\right) = (2.40 \times 10^{-3})B^2$$

$$B^2 + 119.73 \times 10^3 = (2.40 \times 10^{-3})B^4$$
$$0 = B^4 - (416.67)B^2 - 49.88 \times 10^6$$
$$B = H = 85.29 \text{ mm} \approx 85.5 \text{ mm}$$

32. A 3 m long hollow circular column with inner to outer diameter ratio 0.8, carries a load of 140 kN. One end of the column is fixed and the other is hinged. Determine the diameters of other column. Take allowable stress as 320 MPa, Rankine's constant = 1/7500, and FOS = 2.

VTU – June/ July 2011 – 12 Marks

Solution: $l = 3000$ mm, $K = d_i/d_o = 0.8$, $F_s = 140 \times 10^3$ N, $\sigma_c = 320$ MPa, $a = 1/7500$, $n = 2$, $d_o, d_i = ?$.

We know that
$$F_s = \frac{F_R}{n}$$
$$F_R = 2 \times 140 \times 10^3 = 280 \times 10^3 \text{ N} \qquad \ldots \text{Eq. (i)}$$

Also
$$F_R = \frac{\sigma_c A}{1 + a\left(\dfrac{L}{k}\right)^2} \qquad \ldots \text{Eq. (ii)}$$

But
$$A = \frac{\pi(d_o^2 - d_i^2)}{4} = \frac{\pi d_o^2(1 - K^2)}{4} = \frac{\pi d_o^2(1 - 0.8^2)}{4} = (0.2827)d_o^2$$

$$I_{XX} = I_{YY} = \frac{\pi(d_o^4 - d_i^4)}{64} = \frac{\pi d_o^4(1 - K^4)}{64} = \frac{\pi d_o^4(1 - 0.8^4)}{64}$$

$$= (0.0289)d_o^4$$

$$k = \sqrt{\frac{I}{A}} = \sqrt{\frac{(0.0289)d_o^4}{(0.2827)d_o^2}} = (0.32)d_o$$

For one end fixed and the other hinged,

effective length, $L = l/\sqrt{2} = 3000/\sqrt{2} = 2121.32$ mm

From Eqs (i) and (ii) we have

$$280 \times 10^3 = \frac{320 \times (0.2827)d_o^2}{1 + \left(\dfrac{1}{7500}\right) \times \left(\dfrac{2121.32}{0.32d_o}\right)^2}$$

$$1 + \frac{5.86 \times 10^3}{d_o^2} = (3.23 \times 10^{-4})\, d_o^2$$

$$d_o^2 + 5.86 \times 10^3 = (3.23 \times 10^{-4})\, d_o^4$$

$$0 = d_o^4 - (3096)\, d_o^2 - 18.14 \times 10^6$$

$$d_o = 78 \text{ mm}$$

$$d_i = 0.8 \times 78 = 62.4 \text{ mm}$$

33. **A piston rod of steam engine 80 cm long in subjected to a maximum load of 60 kN. Determine the diameter of the rod using Rankine's formula with permissible compressive stress of 100 N/mm². Take constant in Rankine's formula as 1/7500 for hinged ends. The rod may be assumed to be fixed at both ends.**

Solution: $l = 800$ mm, $F_R = 60 \times 10^3$ N, $\sigma_c = 100$ MPa, $a = 1/7500$, $d = ?$.

We know that
$$F_R = \frac{\sigma_c A}{1 + a\left(\dfrac{L}{k}\right)^2}$$

But
$$A = \frac{\pi d^2}{4} = (0.7854)\, d^2$$

$$I_{XX} = I_{YY} = \frac{\pi d^4}{64} = (0.0491)\, d^4$$

$$k = \sqrt{\frac{I}{A}} = \sqrt{\frac{(0.0491)\, d^4}{(0.7854)d^2}} = (0.25)d$$

For both ends fixed, effective length, $L = l/2 = 800/2 = 400$ mm

From Eqs (i) and (ii) we have

$$60 \times 10^3 = \frac{100 \times (0.7854)d^2}{1 + \left(\dfrac{1}{7500}\right) \times \left(\dfrac{400}{0.25d}\right)^2}$$

$$1 + \left(\frac{341.33}{d^2}\right) = (1.31 \times 10^{-3})d^2$$

$$d^2 + 341.33 = (1.31 \times 10^{-3})d^4$$

$$0 = d^4 - (764)\,d^2 - 260.76 \times 10^3$$

$$d = 31.93 \text{ mm} \approx 32 \text{ mm}$$

34. Two 80 mm × 160 mm solid rectangular columns are 4 m long with ends hinged. They share equally the load carried by them. Find by Rankine's formula, the diameter of a single cast iron circular cross section column of the same length and end conditions to replace both of them. $a = 1/1600$ and $\sigma_c = 500$ N/mm^2.

VTU – Dec. 2013/ Jan. 2014 – 08 Marks

Solution: $b = 80$ mm, $h = 160$ mm, no. of columns $n' = 2$, $l = 4000$ mm, $d = ?$, $a = 1/1600$, and $\sigma_c = 500$ N/mm^2.

We know that

$$F_R = \frac{\sigma_c A}{1 + a\left(\dfrac{L}{k}\right)^2}$$

Since there are two columns, the above formula is modified as

$$F_R = \frac{\sigma_c A}{1 + a'\left(\dfrac{L}{k}\right)^2} \qquad \text{... Eq. (i)}$$

Here

$$a' = \frac{a}{n'} = \frac{1}{1600 \times 2} = \frac{1}{3200}$$

$$A = b.h = 80 \times 160 = 12800 \text{ mm}^2$$

$$I_{XX} = \frac{bh^3}{12} = \frac{80 \times 160^3}{12} = 27.31 \times 10^6 \text{ mm}^4$$

$$I_{YY} = \frac{hb^3}{12} = \frac{160 \times 80^3}{12} = 6.83 \times 10^6 \text{ mm}^4$$

Thus

$$I = I_{YY} = 6.83 \times 10^6 \text{ mm}^4 \qquad \text{(minimum value)}$$

$$k = \sqrt{\frac{I}{A}} = \sqrt{\frac{6.83 \times 10^6}{12800}} = 23.10$$

For both ends hinged, effective length, $L = l = 4000$ mm

Eq. (i) yields...

$$F_R = \frac{500 \times 12800}{1 + \left(\dfrac{1}{3200}\right) \times \left(\dfrac{4000}{23.10}\right)^2} = 617.16 \times 10^3 \text{ N}$$

Thus load taken by two columns $= n' F_R = 2 \times 617.16 \times 10^3 = 1.23 \times 10^6$ N

... Eq. (ii)

Equivalent solid circular section:

Here

$$A = \frac{\pi d^2}{4} = (0.7854)\,d^2 \text{ mm}^2$$

$$I_{XX} = I_{YY} = \frac{\pi d^4}{64} = (0.0491)\, d^4 \text{ mm}^4$$

$$k = \sqrt{\frac{I}{A}} = \sqrt{\frac{(0.0491)\, d^4}{(0.7854)d^2}} = (0.25)d$$

From Eqs (i) and (ii) we have

$$1.23 \times 10^6 = \frac{500 \times (0.7854)d^2}{1 + \left(\dfrac{1}{3200}\right) \times \left(\dfrac{4000}{0.25d}\right)^2}$$

$$1 + \left(\frac{80000}{d^2}\right) = (3.19 \times 10^{-4})\, d^2$$

$$d^2 + 80000 = (3.19 \times 10^{-4})\, d^4$$

$$0 = d^4 - (3134.80)\, d^2 - 250.78 \times 10^6$$

$$d = 132.8 \text{ mm} \approx 133 \text{ mm}$$

35. **A connecting rod of length 400 mm may be considered as a strut hinged at both ends and subjected to a maximum load of 150 kN. Find the suitable thickness for the proportions shown in Fig. 10.8. Take $a = 1/7500$ and $\sigma_c = 300$ N/mm^2. Assume that the connecting rod is equally strong in both planes of buckling.**

Solution: $l = 400$ mm, $F_R = 150 \times 10^3$ N, $\sigma_c = 300$ MPa, $a = 1/7500$, $t = ?$.

Consider an I-section of the connecting rod, as shown in **Fig. 10.8.**

Let $t =$ thickness of the flange and web

        $B =$ Width of the section $(= 4t)$

  D or $H =$ depth of the section $(= 5t)$

       $I_{XX} =$ Moment of inertia of the section about X-axis

       $I_{YY} =$ Moment of inertia of the section about Y-axis

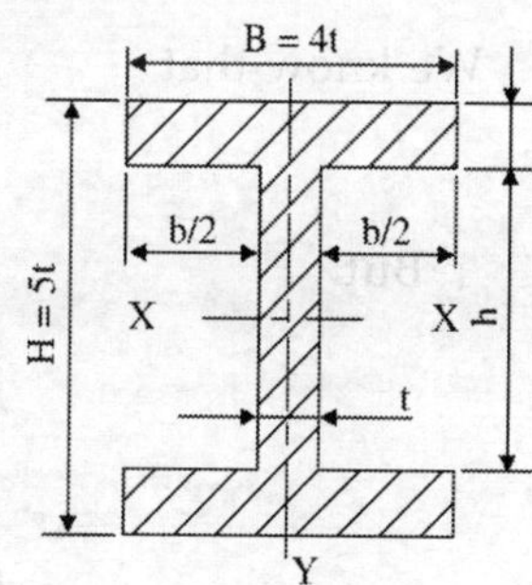

Fig. 10.8: Problem 35

We know that $F_R = \dfrac{\sigma_c A}{1 + a\left(\dfrac{L}{k}\right)^2}$ ... Eq. (i)

But $A = 2[(4t)t] + (t)(3t) = 11t^2$

$$I_{XX} = \frac{BH^3 - bh^3}{12} = \frac{(4t)(5t)^3 - (3t)(3t)^3}{12} = \frac{419t^4}{12}$$

$$I_{YY} = 2I_{yy\,flanges} + I_{yy\,web} = 2\left[\frac{(t)(4t)^3}{12}\right] + \left[\frac{(3t)(t)^3}{12}\right] = \frac{131t^4}{12}$$

$$k_{XX}^2 = \frac{I_{XX}}{A} = \frac{419t^4/12}{11t^2} = 3.1742\, t^2 \Rightarrow k_{XX} = 1.782t$$

$$k_{YY}^2 = \frac{I_{YY}}{A} = \frac{131t^4/12}{11t^2} = 0.9924\, t^2 \Rightarrow k_{YY} = 0.9962t$$

Here larger value of k governs the design. Hence $k = k_{XX} = 1.782t$

For both ends hinged, effective length, $L = l = 400$ mm

Eq. (i) yields...

$$150 \times 10^3 = \frac{300 \times (11)t^2}{1 + \left(\dfrac{1}{7500}\right) \times \left(\dfrac{400}{1.782t}\right)^2}$$

$$1 + \left(\frac{6.72}{t^2}\right) = (0.022)t^2$$

$$t^2 + 6.72 = (0.022)t^4$$
$$0 = t^4 - (45.45)\, t^2 - 305.45$$
$$t = 7.17 \text{ mm}$$

Note: If factor of safety is given, then $F_s = \dfrac{F_R}{n} \Rightarrow F_R = nF_s$ ... *(as in problem 31)*

36. A rectangular link 1 m long has width twice the thickness. It is subjected to a maximum load of 8 kN. Find the thickness of the link assuming both ends to be fixed. Take $a = 1/7500$ and $\sigma_c = 300$ N/mm^2.

Solution: $l = 1000$ mm, $b = t$, $h = 2t$, $F_R = 8000$ N, $\sigma_c = 300$ MPa, $a = 1/7500$, $t = ?$.

We know that $F_R = \dfrac{\sigma_c A}{1 + a\left(\dfrac{L}{k}\right)^2}$ ... Eq. (i)

But $A = b.h = t(2t) = 2t^2$

$$I_{XX} = \frac{bh^3}{12} = \frac{t(2t)^3}{12} = (0.667)t^4$$

$$I_{YY} = \frac{hb^3}{12} = \frac{2t(t)^3}{12} = (0.1667)t^4$$

Thus $I = I_{YY} = (0.1667)t^4$ (minimum value)

$$k = \sqrt{\frac{I}{A}} = \sqrt{\frac{(0.1667)t^4}{2t^2}} = (0.289)t^2$$

For both ends fixed, effective length, $L = l/2 = 1000/2 = 500$ mm

Eq. (i) yields...

$$8000 = \frac{300 \times 2t^2}{1 + \left(\dfrac{1}{7500}\right) \times \left(\dfrac{500}{0.289t}\right)^2}$$

$$1 + \left(\frac{399.10}{t^2}\right) = (0.075)t^2$$

$$t^2 + 399.10 = (0.075)t^4$$
$$0 = t^4 - (13.33)\, t^2 - 5321.33$$
$$t = 8.94 \text{ mm}$$

37. **A hollow cylindrical column with both ends hinged is 6m long and has an outer diameter of 120 mm and an inner diameter of 80 mm. Compare the crippling load by Euler's and Rankine's formulae. What is the length of the column if both crippling loads are equal?** E = 80,000 N/mm^2, σ_y = 550 N/mm^2, **Rankine's constant = 1/1600.**

VTU – (CV) Dec. 2015/ Jan. 2016 – 10 Marks

Solution: l = 6000 mm, d_o = 120 mm, d_i = 80 mm, E = 80000 N/mm^2, σ_y = 550 N/mm^2, a = 1/1600, F_{cr} = ?, F_R = ?, L = ?

a. *According to Euler:*

We know that
$$F_{cr} = \frac{\pi^2 EI}{L^2}$$

Here
$$I_{XX} = I_{YY} = \frac{\pi(d_o^4 - d_i^4)}{64} = \frac{\pi(120^4 - 80^4)}{64} = 8.17 \times 10^6 \text{ mm}^4$$

For both ends hinged, effective length, $L = l = 6000$ mm

$$F_{cr} = \frac{\pi^2 \times 80000 \times (8.17 \times 10^6)}{6000^2} = 179.19 \times 10^3 \text{ N}$$

b. *According to Rankine's:*

We know that
$$F_R = \frac{\sigma_c A}{1 + a\left(\dfrac{L}{k}\right)^2}$$

But
$$A = \frac{\pi(d_o^2 - d_i^2)}{4} = \frac{\pi(120^2 - 80^2)}{4} = 6283.19 \text{ mm}^2$$

$$k = \sqrt{\frac{I}{A}} = \sqrt{\frac{8.17 \times 10^6}{6283.19}} = 36.06$$

$$F_R = \frac{550 \times 6283.19}{1 + \left(\dfrac{1}{1600}\right) \times \left(\dfrac{600}{36.06}\right)^2} = 188.80 \times 10^3 \text{ N}$$

c. *To find L:*

Since both crippling loads are equal, we have
$$F_{cr} = F_R$$

$$\frac{\pi^2 EI}{L^2} = \frac{\sigma_c A}{1 + a\left(\dfrac{L}{k}\right)^2}$$

$$\frac{\pi^2 \times 80000 \times (8.17 \times 10^6)}{L^2} = \frac{550 \times 6283.19}{1 + \left(\dfrac{1}{1600}\right) \times \left(\dfrac{L}{36.06}\right)^2}$$

$$\frac{(6.45 \times 10^{12})}{L^2} = \frac{3.46 \times 10^6}{1 + (4.81 \times 10^{-7})L^2}$$

$$1 + (4.81 \times 10^{-7})\, L^2 = (5.36 \times 10^{-7})\, L^2$$
$$1 = (5.5 \times 10^{-8})\, L^2$$
$$L = 4264 \text{ mm} = 4.26 \text{ m}$$

38. **Compare the crippling loads given by Euler's and Rankine's formula for a tubular steel column 2.5 m long having outer and inner diameters as 40 mm and 30 mm respectively loaded through pin jointed ends. Take yield stress = 320 N/mm², a = 1/7500 and E = 210 GPa. For what length of the column of this cross section the Euler's formula cease to apply?**

VTU (CV) – Dec. 2014/ Jan. 2015 – 12 Marks; June/ July 2013 – 10 Marks; Dec. 2011 – 10 Marks; [similar: (CV) June/ July 2016 – 12 Marks]

Solution: l = 2500 mm, d_o = 40 mm, d_i = 30 mm, $\sigma_y = \sigma_c$ = 320 N/mm², a = 1/7500, $E = 210 \times 10^3$ N/mm², F_{cr} = ?, F_R = ?, L = ?

a. *According to Euler:*

We know that
$$F_{cr} = \frac{\pi^2 EI}{L^2}$$

Here
$$I_{XX} = I_{YY} = \frac{\pi(d_o^4 - d_i^4)}{64} = \frac{\pi(40^4 - 30^4)}{64} = 85.90 \times 10^3 \text{ mm}^4$$

For both ends hinged, effective length, $L = l = 2500$ mm

$$F_{cr} = \frac{\pi^2 \times 210 \times 10^3 \times (85.90 \times 10^3)}{2500^2} = 28.48 \times 10^3 \text{ N}$$

b. *According to Rankine's:*

We know that
$$F_R = \frac{\sigma_c A}{1 + a\left(\dfrac{L}{k}\right)^2}$$

But
$$A = \frac{\pi(d_o^2 - d_i^2)}{4} = \frac{\pi(40^2 - 30^2)}{4} = 549.78 \text{ mm}^2$$

$$k = \sqrt{\frac{I}{A}} = \sqrt{\frac{85.90 \times 10^3}{549.78}} = 12.50$$

$$F_R = \frac{320 \times 549.78}{1 + \left(\dfrac{1}{7500}\right) \times \left(\dfrac{2500}{12.50}\right)^2} = 27.78 \times 10^3 \text{ N}$$

c. *To find L, for Euler's to cease:*

Since both crippling loads are equal, we have

$$\frac{F_{cr}}{A} = \sigma_y$$

$$\frac{\pi^2 EI}{AL^2} = \sigma_y$$

$$\frac{\pi^2 E}{\left(L/k\right)^2} = \sigma_y$$

$$\frac{\pi^2 \times 210 \times 10^3}{\left(L/k\right)^2} = 320$$

$$(L/k) = 80.48$$
$$L = 80.48 \times 12.5 = 1006 \text{ mm}$$

39. **From tests on steel columns with hinged ends, following results were obtained:**

Test No	1	2
Slenderness ratio	70	170
Average failure stress (N/mm²)	200	70

If a steel bar of rectangular section 60 mm × 20 mm and length 1.25 m is to be used as a column with both ends fixed, determine the crippling load.

VTU – (CV) Dec. 2013/ Jan. 2014 – 08 Marks

Solution: $l = 1250$ mm, $b = 20$ mm, $h = 60$ mm, $F_R = ?$,
a. *To find a and σ_c*

We know that
$$F_R = \frac{\sigma_c A}{1 + a\left(\dfrac{L}{k}\right)^2} \qquad \text{... Eq. (i)}$$

$$\frac{F_R}{A} = \frac{\sigma_c}{1 + a\left(\dfrac{L}{k}\right)^2} \qquad \text{... Eq. (ii)}$$

For test 1: Eq. (ii) yields...

$$200 = \frac{\sigma_c}{1 + a(70)^2}$$

$$200 + (980000)a = \sigma_c \qquad \text{... Eq. (iii)}$$

For test 2: Eq. (ii) yields...

$$70 = \frac{\sigma_c}{1 + a(170)^2}$$

$$70 + (2023000)a = \sigma_c \qquad \text{... Eq. (iv)}$$

Eq. (iii) – Eq. (iv) yields...
$$130 - (1043000)a = 0$$

$$a = 1.246 \times 10^{-4} = \frac{1}{8023.08}$$

Substituting a in Eq.(iii), we have
$$\sigma_c = 200 + (980000) \times 1.246 \times 10^{-4} = 322.11 \text{ MPa}$$

b. *To find F_R*

Here
$$A = b.h = 20 \times 60 = 1200 \text{ mm}^2$$

$$I_{XX} = \frac{bh^3}{12} = \frac{20 \times 60^3}{12} = 360000 \text{ mm}^4$$

$$I_{YY} = \frac{hb^3}{12} = \frac{60 \times 20^3}{12} = 40000 \text{ mm}^4$$

Thus
$$I = I_{YY} = 40000 \text{ mm}^4 \quad \text{(minimum value)}$$

$$k = \sqrt{\frac{I}{A}} = \sqrt{\frac{40000}{1200}} = 5.77$$

For both ends fixed, effective length, $L = l/2 = 1250/2 = 625$ mm

Eq. (i) yields...
$$F_R = \frac{322.11 \times 1200}{1 + \left[1.246 \times 10^{-4} \times \left(\frac{625}{5.77} \right)^2 \right]} = 157 \times 10^3 \text{ N}$$

10.8 SECANT FORMULA FOR COLUMNS

In *section 10.5*, the Euler's formula was derived based on the assumption that column is perfectly straight; and that the load is always applied through the centroid of the cross-section of the member. In reality columns are never perfectly straight. Columns never buckle and commence to bend immediately upon application of the load; and the deflection at any point is directly related to the load.

Consider a column AB of length l and cross sectional area A as shown in **Fig. 10.9**, subjected to eccentric load.

Let
$$F = \text{Eccentric load.}$$
$$E = \text{Eccentricity}$$
$$y = \text{Lateral deflection of the section considered.}$$

Now consider a section X-X at a distance x from end B.

The bending moment at this section is

$$EI\left(\frac{d^2y}{dx^2}\right) = -F(y + e)$$

$$EI\left(\frac{d^2y}{dx^2}\right) + Fy = -Fe$$

$$\left(\frac{d^2y}{dx^2}\right) + \left(\frac{F}{EI}\right)y = -\frac{Fe}{EI} \quad \text{... (Eq. 10.32)}$$

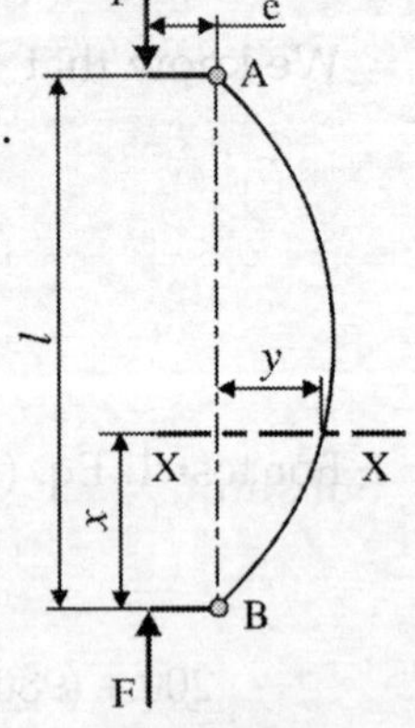

Fig. 10.9: Column with eccentric load

The solution for the above differential equation is given as

$$y = C_1 \cos\left(x.\sqrt{\frac{F}{EI}} \right) + C_2 \sin\left(x.\sqrt{\frac{F}{EI}} \right) - e \quad \text{... (Eq. 10.33)}$$

C_1 and C_2 are constants which are to be evaluated from boundary conditions.

End B: At $x = 0, y = 0$

(Eq. 10.33) yields...

$$0 = C_1 \cos(0) + C_2 \sin(0) - e$$
$$0 = C_1 - e$$
$$C_1 = e \qquad \text{... (Eq. 10.34)}$$

End A: At $x = l, y = 0$

(Eq. 10.33) yields...

$$0 = C_1 \cos\left(l.\sqrt{\frac{F}{EI}}\right) + C_2 \sin\left(l.\sqrt{\frac{F}{EI}}\right) - e \qquad \text{... (Eq. 10.35)}$$

$$0 = e \cos\left(l.\sqrt{\frac{F}{EI}}\right) + C_2 \sin\left(l.\sqrt{\frac{F}{EI}}\right) - e \quad \text{... using (Eq. 10.34)}$$

$$0 = e\left[\cos\left(l.\sqrt{\frac{F}{EI}}\right) - 1\right] + C_2 \sin\left(l.\sqrt{\frac{F}{EI}}\right)$$

$$C_2 \sin\left(l.\sqrt{\frac{F}{EI}}\right) = e\left[1 - \cos\left(l.\sqrt{\frac{F}{EI}}\right)\right]$$

$$C_2 = \frac{\left[1 - \cos\left(l.\sqrt{\frac{F}{EI}}\right)\right]}{C_2 \sin\left(l.\sqrt{\frac{F}{EI}}\right)} \qquad \text{... (Eq. 10.36)}$$

Since $1 - \cos\theta = 2\sin^2(\theta/2)$ and $\sin\theta = 2\sin(\theta/2)\cos(\theta/2)$, we have

$$C_2 = \frac{e\left[2\sin^2\left(\frac{l}{2}.\sqrt{\frac{F}{EI}}\right)\right]}{C_2\left[2\sin\left(\frac{l}{2}.\sqrt{\frac{F}{EI}}\right)\cos\left(\frac{l}{2}.\sqrt{\frac{F}{EI}}\right)\right]}$$

$$C_2 = e\tan\left(\frac{l}{2}.\sqrt{\frac{F}{EI}}\right) \qquad \text{... (Eq. 10.37)}$$

Substituting C_1 and C_2 in (Eq. 10.33), we have

$$y = e\left(x.\sqrt{\frac{F}{EI}}\right) + e\tan\left(\frac{l}{2}.\sqrt{\frac{F}{EI}}\right)\sin\left(x.\sqrt{\frac{F}{EI}}\right) - e$$

$$y = e\left[\cos\left(x.\sqrt{\frac{F}{EI}}\right) + \tan\left(\frac{l}{2}.\sqrt{\frac{F}{EI}}\right)\sin\left(x.\sqrt{\frac{F}{EI}}\right) - 1\right]$$

$$\text{... (Eq. 10.38)}$$

Maximum deflection: Due to symmetry of loading, both the maximum deflection and maximum stress occurs at the column's midpoint. i.e .at $x = l/2, y = y_{max}$

Eq. (10.38) yields... $y_{max} = e\left[\cos\left(\dfrac{l}{2}\cdot\sqrt{\dfrac{F}{EI}}\right) + \tan\left(\dfrac{l}{2}\cdot\sqrt{\dfrac{F}{EI}}\right)\sin\left(\dfrac{l}{2}\cdot\sqrt{\dfrac{F}{EI}}\right) - 1\right]$

$$= e\left[\frac{\cos^2\left(\dfrac{l}{2}\cdot\sqrt{\dfrac{F}{EI}}\right) + \sin^2\left(\dfrac{l}{2}\cdot\sqrt{\dfrac{F}{EI}}\right)}{\cos\left(\dfrac{l}{2}\cdot\sqrt{\dfrac{F}{EI}}\right)} - 1\right]$$

$$= e\left[\frac{1}{\cos\left(\dfrac{l}{2}\cdot\sqrt{\dfrac{F}{EI}}\right)} - 1\right]$$

$$y_{max} = e\left[\sec\left(\dfrac{l}{2}\cdot\sqrt{\dfrac{F}{EI}}\right) - 1\right] \qquad \text{... (Eq. 10.39)}$$

y_{max} becomes infinite, when

$$\frac{l}{2}\sqrt{\frac{E}{EI}} = \frac{\pi}{2} \qquad \text{... (Eq. 10.40)}$$

i.e. for critical load

$$\left[\sec\left(\frac{l}{2}\cdot\sqrt{\frac{F_{cr}}{EI}}\right)\right] = \infty$$

$$\frac{l}{2}\cdot\sqrt{\frac{F_{cr}}{EI}} = \frac{\pi}{2}$$

$$F_{cr} = \frac{\pi^2 EI}{l^2} \qquad \text{... (Eq. 10.41)}$$

(Eq. 10.41) is the same result as found from the Euler formula.

Solving (Eq. 10.41) for EI and substituting into (Eq. 10.39) the maximum deflection can be expressed in alternative form as

$$y_{max} = e\left[\sec\left(\frac{\pi}{2}\cdot\sqrt{\frac{F}{F_{cr}}}\right) - 1\right] \qquad \text{... (Eq. 10.42)}$$

Maximum bending moment: Maximum moment occurs at the column's midpoint i.e.

$$x = \frac{l}{2}$$

$$M_{max} = F(y_{max} + e)$$

$$= F\left\{e\left[\sec\left(\frac{l}{2}\cdot\sqrt{\frac{F}{EI}}\right)-1\right]+e\right\}$$

$$M_{max} = Fe\left[\sec\left(\frac{l}{2}\cdot\sqrt{\frac{F}{EI}}\right)\right] \quad \text{... using (Eq. 10.39) ... (Eq. 10.43a)}$$

OR $$M_{max} = Fe\left[\sec\left(\frac{\pi}{2}\cdot\sqrt{\frac{F}{F_{cr}}}\right)\right] \quad \text{... using (Eq. 10.42) ... (Eq. 10.43b)}$$

Maximum stress: The maximum stress in the column occurs at mid-span which is the combined effect of axial stress due to compressive load and bending stress due to moment.

$$\sigma_{max} = \frac{F}{A} + \frac{M_{max}}{Z} = \frac{F}{A} + \frac{M_{max}.c}{I}$$

Where c is the distance of extreme fiber from neutral axis.

$$\sigma_{max} = \frac{F}{A} + \frac{Fec}{I}\sec\left(\frac{l}{2}\cdot\sqrt{\frac{F}{EI}}\right) \quad \text{... (Eq. 10.44)}$$

(Eq. 10.44) is called the **secant formula**.

since $I = \sqrt{Ak^2}$, (Eq. 10.44) can be written as

$$\sigma_{max} = \frac{F}{A}\left[1+\frac{ec}{k^2}\sec\left(\frac{l}{2k}\cdot\sqrt{\frac{F}{EA}}\right)\right] \quad \text{... (Eq. 10.45a)}$$

OR $$\sigma_{max} = \frac{F}{A}\left[1+\frac{ec}{k^2}\sec\left(\frac{\pi}{2k}\cdot\sqrt{\frac{F}{EA}}\right)\right]$$

$$\text{... using (Eq. 10.42)} \qquad \text{... (Eq. 10.45b)}$$

The term (ec/k^2) is known as the eccentricity ratio, and $\left(\frac{l}{2k}\cdot\sqrt{\frac{F}{EA}}\right)$ called the **Euler angle.**

Note: Eqs (10.45a) and (10.45b) can be used with any end condition if we replace l with effective length L as in **Table 10.1.**

40. A steel rod of length 1.5 m and 40 mm in diameter, pin joined at ends is subjected to an axial load of 25 kN at an eccentricity of 5 mm. Determine:
   (a) the maximum deflection of the rod,
   (b) the maximum stress in the rod. Take $E = 210$ GPa.

Solution: $l = 1500$ mm, $d = 40$ mm, $F = 25 \times 10^3$ N, $e = 5$ mm, $E = 210 \times 10^3$ MPa.
a) $y_{max} = ?$ b) $\sigma_{max} = ?$

   a. *To find y_{max}:* Maximum deflection occurs at mid-span of the rod.

We know that $$y_{max} = e\left[\sec\left(\frac{l}{2}\cdot\sqrt{\frac{F}{EI}}\right)-1\right] \quad \text{... Eq. (i)}$$

But
$$A = \frac{\pi d^2}{64} = \frac{\pi \times 40^2}{4} = 1256.64 \text{ mm}^2$$

$$I_{XX} = I_{YY} = \frac{\pi d^4}{64} = \frac{\pi \times 40^4}{64} = 125.66 \times 10^3 \text{ mm}^4$$

$$k = \sqrt{\frac{I}{A}} = \sqrt{\frac{125.66 \times 10^3}{1256.64}} = 10$$

$$c = \frac{d}{2} = \frac{40}{2} = 20 \text{ mm}$$

Eq. (i) yields...
$$y_{max} = \left[\sec\left(\frac{1500}{2} \times \sqrt{\frac{25 \times 10^3}{210 \times 10^3 \times (125.66 \times 10^3)}} \right) - 1 \right]$$

$$= 1.71 \text{ mm}$$

b. *To find* σ_{max}: Maximum stress occurs at mid-span of the rod.

We know that $\sigma_{max} = \dfrac{F}{A}\left[1 + \dfrac{ec}{k^2} \sec\left(\dfrac{l}{2k} \cdot \sqrt{\dfrac{F}{EA}} \right) \right]$

$$= \frac{25 \times 10^3}{1256.64}\left[1 + \frac{5 \times 20}{10^2} \times \sec\left(\frac{1500}{2 \times 10} \times \sqrt{\frac{25 \times 10^3}{210 \times 10^3 \times 1256.64}} \right) \right]$$

$$\sigma_{max} = 46.59 \text{ MPa}$$

41. **A strut 2 m long and pin-joined at ends carries a load of 50 kN at an eccentricity of 4 mm. it is constructed of steel tube 70 mm outside diameter and 4 mm thick. Find**
    (a) the maximum deflection at mid-span.
    (b) the maximum and minimum stresses. Take E = 200 GPa.

Solution: l = 2000 mm, F = 50 × 10^3 N, e = 4 mm, d_o = 70 mm, t = 4 mm $\Rightarrow d_i = d_o - 2t$ = 62 mm, E = 200 × 10^3 MPa. a) y_{max} = ?, b) σ_{max} = ? , σ_{min} = ?

a. *To find* y_{max}: Maximum deflection occurs at mid-span of the rod.

We know that $\quad y_{max} = e\left[\sec\left(\dfrac{l}{2} \cdot \sqrt{\dfrac{F}{EI}} \right) - 1 \right]$ $\qquad$ ... Eq. (i)

But
$$A = \frac{\pi\left(d_o^2 - d_i^2\right)}{4} = \frac{\pi \times (70^2 - 62^2)}{4} = 829.39 \text{ mm}^2$$

$$I_{XX} = I_{YY} = \frac{\pi\left(d_o^4 - d_i^4\right)}{64} = \frac{\pi \times (70^4 - 62^4)}{64} = 4.53 \times 10^5 \text{ mm}^4$$

$$k = \sqrt{\frac{I}{A}} = \sqrt{\frac{4.53 \times 10^6}{829.39}} = 23.38$$

$$c = \frac{d_o}{2} = \frac{70}{2} = 35\,\text{mm}$$

Eq. (i) yields... $\quad y_{max} = \left[\sec\left(\frac{2000}{2} \times \sqrt{\frac{50 \times 10^3}{200 \times 10^3 \times (4.53 \times 10^5)}}\right) - 1\right]$

$$= 1.43\,\text{mm}$$

b. *To find stresses:*

We know that $\sigma_{max,min} = \dfrac{F}{A}\left[1 \pm \dfrac{ec}{k^2}\sec\left(\dfrac{l}{2k}\cdot\sqrt{\dfrac{F}{EA}}\right)\right]$

$$= \frac{50 \times 10^3}{829.39}\left[1 \pm \frac{4 \times 35}{23.28^2} \times \sec\left(\frac{2000}{2 \times 23.38} \times \sqrt{\frac{50 \times 10^3}{200 \times 10^3 \times 829.39}}\right)\right]$$

$$\sigma_{max,min} = 81.42\,,\,39.15\,\text{MPa}$$
$$\sigma_{max} = 81.42\,\text{MPa},\ \sigma_{min} = 39.15\,\text{MPa}$$

42. **A steel rod of length 1.2 m and 50 mm in diameter is pin joined at ends. When an axial load of 100 kN was applied the deflection at mid-span was observed to be 1.5 mm. Determine:**
    (a) the eccentricity of the rod,
    (b) the maximum stress in the rod. Take E = 210 GPa.

Solution: $l = 1200$ mm, $d = 50$ mm, $F = 100 \times 10^3$ N, $y_{max} = 1.5$ mm, $E = 200 \times 10^3$ MPa. a) $e = ?$ b) $\sigma_{max} = ?$

a. *To find e:*

We know that $\quad y_{max} = e\left[\sec\left(\dfrac{l}{2}\cdot\sqrt{\dfrac{F}{EI}}\right) - 1\right]$ $\qquad\qquad$ ... Eq. (i)

But $\qquad A = \dfrac{\pi d^2}{64} = \dfrac{\pi \times 50^2}{4} = 1963.50\,\text{mm}^2$

$$I_{XX} = I_{YY} = \frac{\pi d^2}{64} = \frac{\pi \times 50^2}{4} = 306.80 \times 10^3\,\text{mm}^4$$

$$k = \sqrt{\frac{I}{A}} = \sqrt{\frac{306.80 \times 10^6}{1963.50}} = 12.50$$

$$c = \frac{d}{2} = \frac{50}{2} = 25\,\text{mm}$$

Eq. (i) yields... $\quad 1.5 = e\left[\sec\left(\dfrac{1200}{2} \times \sqrt{\dfrac{100 \times 10^3}{200 \times 10^3 \times (306.80 \times 10^3)}}\right) - 1\right]$

$$e = 3.87\,\text{mm}$$

b. *To find* σ_{max}: Maximum stress occurs at mid-span of the rod.

We know that $\sigma_{max} = \dfrac{F}{A}\left[1 + \dfrac{ec}{k^2}\sec\left(\dfrac{l}{2k}\cdot\sqrt{\dfrac{F}{EA}}\right)\right]$

$$= \dfrac{100\times10^3}{1963.50}\left[1 + \dfrac{3.87\times25}{12.50^2}\times\sec\left(\dfrac{1200}{2\times12.50}\times\sqrt{\dfrac{100\times10^3}{200\times10^3\times1963.50}}\right)\right]$$

$$\sigma_{max} = 94.68\,\text{MPa}$$

VTU QUESTION PAPERS

Dec. 07/Jan. 08 (06ME34)

1. Derive an expression for the critical load in a column subjected to compressive load, when one end is fixed and the other end is free. **(10 Marks)**

June/July 2008 (06ME34)

2. A hollow column of C.I whose outside diameter is 200 mm has a thickness of 20 mm. It is 4.5 m long and is fixed at both ends. Calculate the safe load by Rankine's formula using a factor of safety of 4. Calculate slenderness ration and the ratio of Euler's and Rankine's critical loads.
Take $\sigma_c = 550\,\text{N/mm}^2$, $\alpha = 1/1600$ and $E = 8\times10^4\,\text{N/mm}^2$. **(12 Marks)**

Dec. 08/Jan. 09 (06ME34)

3. Define Slenderness ratio and derive Euler's expression for buckling load for column with both ends hinged. **(10 Marks)**

June/July 2009 (06ME34)

4. Find the Euler's crippling load for a hollow cylindrical steel column of 38 mm external diameter and 2.5 mm thick. Take the length of column as 2.3 m hinged at its both ends. Take $E = 2.05\times10^5\,\text{N/mm}^2$. Also determine the crippling load by Rankine's formula using constants as 335 N/mm^2 and 1/7500. **(10 Marks)**

Dec. 09/Jan. 10 (06ME34)

5. A 1.5 m long column has a circular cross section of 50 mm diameter. One of the ends of the column is fixed in direction and position and the other end is free. Take factor of safety as 3. Calculate the safe load using:
   i. Rankine's formula. Take yield stress as 560 N/mm^2 and $a = 1/1500$ for pinned ends.
   ii. Euler's formula. Young's modulus for CI as $1.2\times10^5\,\text{N/mm}^2$. **(10 Marks)**

May/June 2010 (06ME34)

6. Derive the expression for Euler's buckling load for a column with its one end fixed and the other end free. **(06 Marks)**

Dec. 2010 (06ME34)

7. Show the variation of Euler's critical load with slenderness ratio. Using the same, explain the limitations of Euler's theory. How the Rankine's formula overcomes theses limitations? **(12 Marks)**

June/July 2011 (06ME34)

8. Derive an expression for the critical load on a column subjected to compressive load, when both the ends are hinged. Also mention the assumptions made in the derivation. **(10 Marks)**

Dec. 2011 (06ME34)

9. A 2 m long pin ended column of square cross section is to be made of wood. Assuming $E = 12$ GPa and the allowable stress being limited to 12 MPa, determine the size of the column to support a load of 95 kN. Use a factor of safety of 3 and Euler's crippling load for buckling. **(08 Marks)**

Dec. 2011 (10ME34)

10. A circular compression member is of 25 mm diameter and 950 mm long. Calculate the maximum buckling load. What will be the value of allowable load if a factor of safety of 3 is expected? Take for material of column $\sigma_y = 441$ MPa $E = 2.07 \times 10^5$ N/mm^2 **(10 Marks)**

June 2012 (06ME34)

11. a. Derive an expression for the critical load in a column subjected to compressive load, when one end is fixed and the other end is free. **(08 Marks)**

June 2012 (10ME34)

12. Derive an expression for the Euler's buckling load for a long column having one end fixed and other end hinged. State the assumptions made in the derivation. **(10 Marks)**

Dec. 2012 (10ME34)

13. State the assumptions made in the theory of Euler's equation. Derive the Euler's expression for a column subjected to an axial compressive load. Consider both ends of the column as hinged. **(10 Marks)**

Jan. 2013 (06ME34)

14. State the assumptions made in Euler's theory for axially loaded elastic long columns. Prove that the crippling load by Euler's formula for a column having one end fixed and the other end free is given by

$$P = \frac{\pi^2 EI}{4l^2}$$ where l = actual length of the column, I = moment of inertia,

E = Young's modulus. **(10 Marks)**

June/July 2013 (06ME34)

15. A 2 m long pin ended column of square section is made of a material with $E = 12 \times 10^3$ MPa and allowable stress of 12 N/mm^2. Determine the dimension of the column using Euler's equation for the loads:
i. 95 kN   ii. 200 kN. Use a factor of safety of 3. **(12 Marks)**

June/July 2013 (10ME34)

16. A 1.5 m long column has a circular cross section of 50 mm diameter. One end of the column is fixed in direction and position and the other end is free. Taking the factor of safety as 3, calculate the safe load using:

   i. Rankine's formula taking yield stress 560 N/mm^2 and $a = 1/1600$

   ii. Euler's formulas taking $E = 1.2 \times 10^5$ N/mm^2.   **(10 Marks)**

Dec. 13/Jan. 14 (06ME34)

17. A solid round bar has 60 mm diameter and length 2.5 m. Find the safe compressive load for the column, if :

   i. both ends are hinged

   ii. if both ends are fixed. $E = 2 \times 10^5$ N/mm^2 and factor of safety $= 3$.   **(10 Marks)**

Dec. 13/Jan. 14 (10ME34)

18. Derive an expression for Euler's buckling load in a column when both ends are fixed.   **(10 Marks)**

June/July 2014 (06ME34)

19. i. What are the assumptions made in Euler's theory?   **(03 Marks)**

   ii. Derive an expression for Euler's buckling load for a column with both ends fixed condition.   **(07 Marks)**

June/July 2014 (10ME34)

20. i. What are the assumptions made in the theory of columns?   **(03 Marks)**

   ii. Derive an expression for the critical load in a column subjected to compressive load, when one end is fixed and other end is free.   **(07 Marks)**

Dec. 14/Jan. 15 (06ME34)

21. Define slenderness ratio and derive Euler's expression for buckling load for column with both ends hinged.   **(08 Marks)**

Dec. 14/Jan. 15 (10ME34)

22. A hollow C.I column whose outer diameter is 200 mm has a thickness of 20 mm. It is 4.5 m long and fixed at both ends. Calculate the safe load by Rankine's formula using a factor of safety of 4. Calculate the slenderness ratio and the ratio of Euler's and Rankine's critical loads. Take $\sigma_c = 550$ N/mm^2 and $a = 1/1600$ in Rankine's formula and $E = 9.4 \times 10^4$ N/mm^2.   **(10 Marks)**

June/July 15 (10ME34)

23. Define slenderness ratio and derive Euler's expression for buckling load for column with both ends hinged.   **(08 Marks)**

Dec. 15/Jan. 16 (10ME/AU34)

24. Derive an expression for the critical load in a column subjected to compressive load, when both ends are fixed.   **(10 Marks)**

June/uly 2016 (10ME/AU34)

25. A solid round bar of 60 mm diameter and 2.5 m long is used as a strut. Find the safe compressive load for the strut if:

   i. Both ends are hinged

   ii. Bothe ends are fixed.

Take $E = 2 \times 10^5$ MPa and factor of safety $= 3$.   **(10 Marks)**

Dec. 16/Jan. 17 (10ME/AU34)

26. Derive Euler's equation for a column with both ends hinged. **(10 Marks)**

Dec. 16/Jan. 17 (15ME/MA34)

27. i. Explain Slenderness ratio. **(04 Marks)**

    ii. Determine the buckling load for a T-section shown in **Fig. U10.1**. The column is 3 m long and is hinged at both ends. Take $E = 200$ GPa. **(10 Marks)**

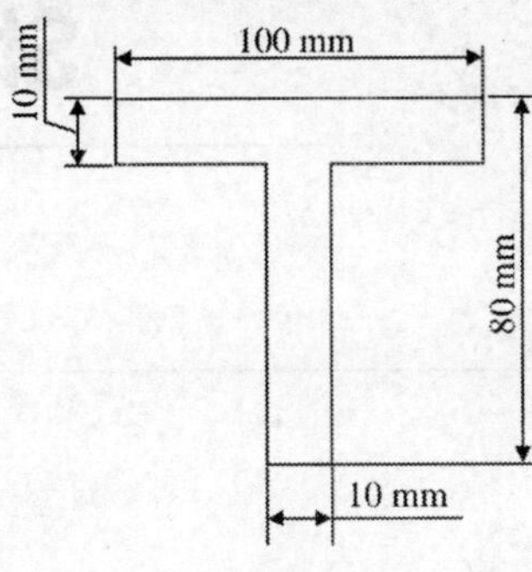

Fig. U10.1

June/July 2017 (15ME/MA34)

28. Derive an expression for the Euler's crippling load for a long column when both ends of the column are hinged. **(10 Marks)**

June/July 2017 (15ME/MA34)

29. i. Derive a Euler's crippling load for a column when both of its ends are hinged. **(08 Marks)**

    ii. A 1.5 m long column has a circular cross section of 50 mm diameter. One end of the column is fixed in direction and position and the other end is free. Taking the factor of safety as 3, calculate the safe load using Euler's formulae. Take $E = 2.1$ GPa. **(08 Marks)**

Dec. 17/Jan. 18 (10ME/AU34)

30. State at least 4 assumptions made in Euler's theory of columns, and derive an expression for Euler's formula for a column when both ends are fixed. **(10 Marks)**

Dec. 17/Jan. 18 (15ME/MA34)

31. A 1.5 m long column has circular cross-section of 50 mm diameter. One end of the column is fixed in position and the other end is free. Taking FOS as 3, calculate:
    i. Safe load according to Rankine's formula taking $\sigma_c = 560$ MPa and $a = 1/1600$.
    ii. Safe load according to Euler's formula taking $E = 120$ GPa. **(08 Marks)**
32. State the assumptions made while deriving Euler's column formula. Also derive Euler's expression for buckling load for a column with both ends hinged. **(08 Marks)**

11.1 INTRODUCTION

Whenever a body is subjected to a load within the elastic limit, the body undergoes deformation and work is done on it. This work done on an elastic member during loading is stored in the member as *strain energy*, and is recoverable upon unloading provided that the material remains elastic. This energy is caused by the action of either normal stress or shear stress.

For an elastic body, the work done (W) on the body by the applied force is stored as elastic strain energy (U).

11.2 WORK AND ENERGY

Work done on a body is defined as the product of force and displacement of the body in the direction of force.

Energy is defined as the capacity to do work and it may exist in many forms. Ex: Potential energy, kinetic energy, thermal energy, etc.

11.3 CONCEPT OF STRAIN ENERGY

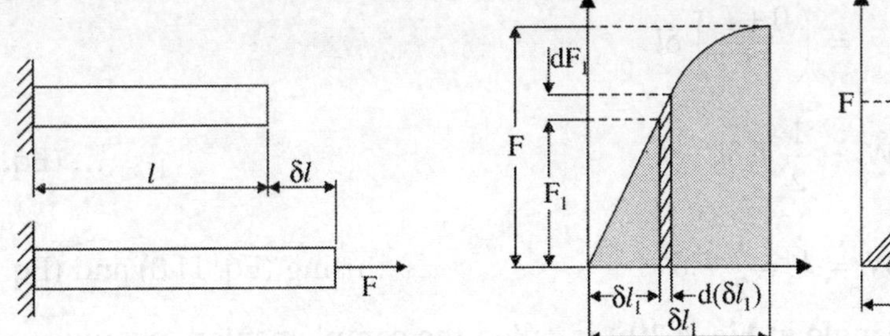

Fig. 11.1: Axially loaded rod   **Fig. 11.2:** Load-deformation diagram

Consider a rod fixed at one end as shown in **Fig. 11.1**

Let l = Length of the rod

  A = Cross-sectional area of the rod

  δl = Total deformation of the rod

  F = Gradually applied load

Fig. 11.2(a) represents a typical load-deformation diagram. Let F_1 be the load that varies between zero and the maximum value F, and the corresponding elongation of the rod as δl_1. Now as the load increases gradually from δF_1, then there will be a corresponding increment in elongation as $d(\delta l_1)$.

The work done by the load during this incremental elongation is equal to the product of the load and small elongation. i.e. $F_1\, d(\delta l_1)$ as represented by the area of the hatched strip, in **Fig. 11.2(a)**. The total work done by the load as it increases from zero to the maximum value F is the summation of all such elemental strips.

i.e.
$$W = \int_0^{\delta l} F_1 \left[d(\delta l_1) \right]$$
... (Eq. 11.1)

(Eq. 11.1) indicates that the work done by the load is equal to the area below the load-deformation curve between $\delta l = 0$ and $l = \delta l$. The work done by the load F_1 must result in the increase of energy associated with the deformation of the rod. This energy is referred to as the **strain energy**.

According to definition, strain energy is equal to the work done by a gradual increasing load applied to the member.

i.e. Strain energy $= U = \int_0^{\delta l} F_1 \left[d(\delta l_1) \right]$
... (Eq. 11.2)

(Eq. 11.2) holds for both linear elastic and non-linear elastic materials. If the material is linear elastic, then the load-deformation diagram can be represented by a straight line as shown in **Fig. 11.2(b)**.

The elastic strain energy stored in the material is determined from the area of triangle (hatched) as

$$U = \frac{1}{2} F.\delta l$$
... (Eq. 11.3)

Thus, as the force is gradually applied to the rod, its magnitude increases from zero to some value F, and consequently, the work done is equal to the average force magnitude $(F/2)$ times the total displacement (δl).

i.e. $\qquad W = $ *average force* $\times$ *deformation* $=$ *area of hatched triangle*

$$= \left(\frac{0 + F}{2} \right) \delta l$$

$$W = \frac{1}{2} F.\delta l$$
... (Eq. 11.4)

Thus $\qquad W = U = \frac{1}{2} F.\delta l$ $\qquad$ ... using (Eq. 11.3) and (Eq. 11.4)

The unshaded triangle in **Fig. 4.2(b)** is called the complementary energy.

Note: Unless otherwise stated, the load is assumed to be a gradually applied load.

11.4 STRAIN ENERGY DUE TO NORMAL STRESS: TENSION OR COMPRESSION

Work done on an elastic member during loading is stored in the member as strain energy, and is recoverable upon unloading provided that the material remains elastic. This energy is caused by the action of either normal stress or shear stress.

11.4.1 Neglecting the weight of the rod

Consider a rod or bar of uniform cross-section fixed at one end as shown in **Fig. 11.1**

Let $\qquad l \;\; =$ Length of the rod

$\qquad\quad A \;\; =$ Cross-sectional area of the rod

$\qquad\quad \delta l \;\; =$ Total deformation of the rod

$$F = \text{Gradually applied load}$$
$$\sigma = \text{Nominal stress (tensile or compressive)}$$
$$e = \text{Normal strain}$$
$$E = \text{Young's modulus}$$

For a linear elastic material, the load-deformation diagram is as shown in **Fig. 11.2(b)**. The shaded area under the graph gives the work done and hence the strain energy

i.e. $\qquad U = \dfrac{1}{2}\, F.\delta l$ $\hfill$ ... using (Eq. 11.3)

$$\text{Since} \quad \delta l = \frac{Fl}{AE}$$

$$U = \frac{1}{2} F\left(\frac{Fl}{AE}\right)$$

$$U = \frac{F^2 l}{2AE} \hspace{4cm} \text{... (Eq. 11.5a)}$$

In generalized terms, if the axial force varies along the length of the rod as dx, then the above equation can be written as

$$U = \int_0^l \frac{F^2 dx}{2AE} \hspace{3cm} \text{... (Eq. 11.5b)}$$

Since $\sigma = \dfrac{F}{A}$, substituting $F = \sigma A$ in (Eq. 11.5) yields...

$$U = \frac{(\sigma A)^2 l}{2AE} = \frac{\sigma^2 Al}{2E}$$

$$\therefore \quad U = \frac{\sigma^2 V}{2E} \hspace{4cm} \text{... (Eq. 11.6)}$$

$$\text{Where} \qquad V = Al = \text{volume of the rod}$$

In terms of stress and strain, (Eq. 11.6) can be written as

$$U = \frac{\sigma \varepsilon V}{2E} \hspace{4cm} \text{... (Eq. 11.7)}$$

The strain energy stored per unit volume is termed as ***resilience or strain energy density***.

i.e. $\qquad u = \dfrac{U}{V} = \dfrac{\sigma^2}{2E}$ $\hfill$ ... (Eq. 11.8), using (Eq. 11.6)

or $\qquad u = \dfrac{\sigma \varepsilon}{2}$ $\hfill$ ... (Eq. 11.9), using (Eq. 11.7)

The maximum energy per unit volume that the body can store up to the elastic limit (σ_y) is known as *Proof resilience or Modulus of resilience, as* shown in **Fig. 11.3**. Proof resilience is a mechanical property and indicates the capacity of the material to bear shocks.

$$\text{Proof resilience } u_p = \frac{\sigma_y^2}{2E} = \frac{E\varepsilon^2}{2} \hspace{3cm} \text{... (Eq. 11.10)}$$

Modulus of rupture is defined as the energy per unit volume required to cause the material to rupture.

$$\text{Modulus of rupture} = \frac{\sigma_R^2}{2E} = \frac{E\varepsilon_R^2}{2} \qquad \qquad \text{... (Eq. 11.11)}$$

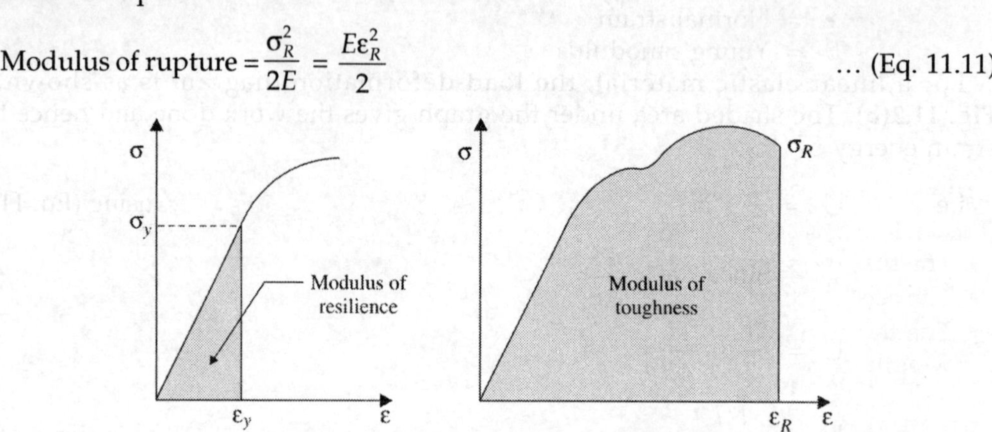

Fig. 11.3: Modulus of resilience and toughness

11.4.2 Including the weight of the rod

Consider a rod or bar of uniform cross-section, hanging freely under its own weight and subjected to axial load as shown in **Fig. 11.4.**

Let
- l = Length of the rod
- A = Cross-sectional area of the rod
- δl = Total deformation of the rod
- F = Gradually applied load
- σ = Nominal stress (tensile or compressive)
- ε = Normal strain
- E = Young's modulus
- w = Specific weight of the bar material ($= \rho g$)
- ρ = Specific mass or density of the material

Fig. 11.4: Self weight with axial load

Consider an elementary strip of length dy at a distance y from the free end. At any section, total load on the section will be the sum of external load and the weight of the rod below the strip.

i.e. Load below the section is $F_y = F \pm wAy$ ... (Eq. 11.12)

Positive sign for tensile load and negative sign for compressive load.

For the element
$$dU = \frac{1}{2}\left(\frac{F_y^2}{AE}\right)\delta y \qquad \qquad \text{... using (Eq. 11.5a)}$$

$$= \frac{\delta y}{2AE}\left(F \pm wAy\right)^2$$

$$= \frac{\delta y}{2AE}\left(F^2 \pm w^2 A^2 y^2 + 2FwAy\right)$$

$$\therefore \quad dU = \left[\left(\frac{F^2}{2AE}\right) + \left(\frac{w^2 Ay^2}{2E}\right) + \left(\frac{Fwy}{E}\right)\right]\delta y \qquad \text{... (Eq. 11.13)}$$

Thus the total stain energy is obtained by integrating the above equation in the limits from 0 to l.

i.e.
$$\int dU = \int_0^l \left[\left(\frac{F^2}{2AE} \right) + \left(\frac{w^2 Ay^2}{2E} \right) + \left(\frac{Fwy}{E} \right) \right] \delta y$$

$$\therefore \quad U = \frac{F^2 l}{2AE} + \frac{w^2 A l^3}{6E} + \frac{Fwl^2}{2E} \qquad \qquad \text{... (Eq. 11.14)}$$

(Eq. 11.14) consists of three componenets:
- The first term is the strain energy due to axial load
- The second term is the strain energy due to the self weight of the rod
- The third term is the strain energy due to combined effect of axial load and self weight.

11.5 STRAIN ENERGY DUE TO SHEAR STRESS

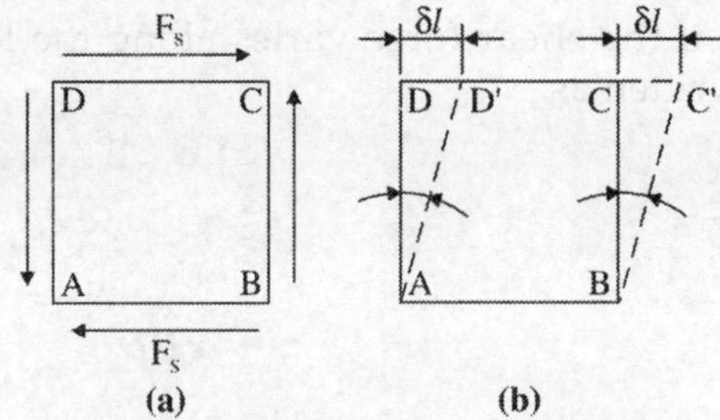

Fig. 11.5: Strain energy in shear

Consider an element ABCD of thickness t as shown in **Fig. 11.5(a)**.

Let
F_s = Shear load
τ = Shear stress
γ = Shear strain
G = Modulus of rigidity
t = thickmess

The shear force (F_s) applied on top face CD cause the element to deform to CC'. Work done by shear force is

W = average force × deformation

$$= \left(\frac{0 + F_s}{2} \right) \times CC'$$

$$W = \left(\frac{F_s}{2} \right) \times CC' \qquad \qquad \text{... (Eq. 11.15)}$$

Shear force, $F_s = \tau \times (DC \times t)$ \qquad where (area $= DC \times t$)

$$\tan \gamma = \frac{CC'}{BC} \approx \gamma \Rightarrow CC' = BC \times \gamma$$

$$W = \left(\frac{1}{2} \right) (\tau \times DC \times t) \times (BC \times \gamma)$$

Also \qquad Modulus of rigidity $G = \dfrac{\tau}{\gamma} \Rightarrow \gamma = \dfrac{\tau}{G}$

$$\therefore \quad U = W = \left(\frac{1}{2}\right)\frac{\tau^2}{G}(DC \times BC \times t)$$

$$U = \left(\frac{\tau^2 V}{2G}\right) \qquad\qquad \dots \text{(Eq. 11.16)}$$

Where $V = (DC \times BC \times t) = $ volume of the element.

Since $\tau = \dfrac{F_s}{A}$, (Eq. 11.16) yields…

$$U = \left(\frac{F_s^2}{A^2}\right)\left(\frac{Al}{2G}\right)$$

$$\therefore \quad U = \frac{F_s^2 l}{2AG} \qquad\qquad \dots \text{(Eq. 11.17)}$$

In generalized terms, if the shear force varies along the length of the rod as dx, then (Eq. 11.17) can be written as

$$U = \int_0^l \frac{F_s^2 dx}{2AG} \qquad\qquad \dots \text{(Eq. 11.17a)}$$

Strain energy density

$$u = \frac{U}{V}$$

$$u = \frac{\tau^2}{2G} \qquad\qquad \dots \text{(Eq. 11.18), using (Eq. 11.16)}$$

11.6 STRAIN ENERGY DUE TO TORSION

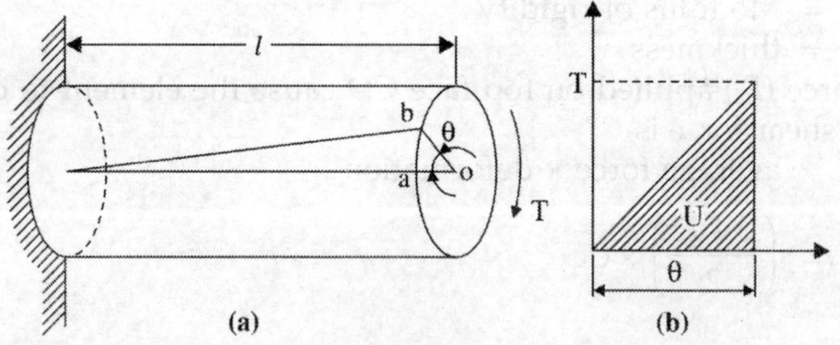

Fig. 11.6: Strain energy in torsion

Consider a shaft fixed at one end and subjected to torque at the other end as shown in **Fig. 11.6(a)**.

Let,
r = Radius of the shaft
τ = Shear stress
T = Torque
J = Polar moment of inertia
G = Modulus of rigidity
θ = Angle of twist
l = Length of the shaft

If *oa* is the initial position before twist, then the final position after twist is *ob*, i.e. the cross-section will be twisted through an angle θ. As long as the elastic limits are not exceeded, the relation between the angle of twist and the applied torque is linear as shown in **Fig. 11.6(b)**. The work done or strain energy, is the average torque multiplied by the angle through which it turns.

i.e. $\qquad W = U = \dfrac{1}{2}T\theta$ $\qquad\qquad$ ... (Eq. 11.19), using (Eq. 11.4)

But torsional equation is given as

$$\frac{T}{J} = \frac{G\theta}{l} = \frac{\tau}{r}$$

$$\theta = \left(\frac{Tl}{GJ}\right) \qquad\qquad\qquad \text{... (Eq. 11.20)}$$

Substituting (Eq. 11.20) in (Eq. 11.19), we have

$$U = \frac{T}{2}\left(\frac{Tl}{GJ}\right)$$

$$U = \frac{T^2 l}{2GJ} \qquad\qquad\qquad \text{... (Eq. 11.21)}$$

(Eq. 11.21) is applicable only to circular shafts as well as hollow circular shafts. In generalized terms, if the torque varies along the length of the rod as *dx*, then (Eq. 11.21) can be written as

$$U = \int_0^l \frac{T^2 dx}{2GJ} \qquad\qquad\qquad \text{... (Eq. 11.22)}$$

For solid shafts:

Since $T = \dfrac{\tau J}{r}$; $r = d/2$ and $J = \dfrac{\pi d^4}{32}$ in (Eq. 11.21) yields...

$$U = \frac{l}{2G}\left[\frac{\tau^2 J^2}{(d/2)^2}\right]\left(\frac{1}{J}\right)$$

$$= \frac{l}{2G}\left(\frac{4\tau^2 J}{d^2}\right)$$

$$= \frac{2\tau^2 l}{G}\left(\frac{\pi d^4/32}{d^2}\right)$$

$$= \frac{\pi d^2 \tau^2 l}{16G}$$

$$= \frac{\tau^2}{4G}\left[\left(\frac{\pi d^2}{4}\right)l\right]$$

$$U = \frac{\tau^2 V}{4G} \qquad \qquad \text{... (Eq. 11.23)}$$

$$\text{Where volume } V = A.l = \left(\frac{\pi d^2}{4}\right) l$$

Strain energy density or torsional resilience

$$u = \frac{U}{V} = \frac{\tau^2}{4G} \qquad \qquad \text{... (Eq. 11.24)}$$

For hollow shafts:

Substituting $\quad T = \dfrac{\tau J}{r}, r = \dfrac{d_o}{2}$ and $J = \dfrac{\pi}{32} d_o^4 (1 - K^4)$ in (Eq. 11.21) yields...

$$U = \frac{l}{2G}\left[\frac{\tau^2 J^2}{(d_o/2)^2}\right]\left(\frac{1}{J}\right)$$

$$= \frac{l}{2G}\left(\frac{4\tau^2 J}{d_o^2}\right)$$

$$= \frac{2\tau^2 l}{G}\left[\frac{\pi d_o^4 (1 - K^4)/32}{d_o^2}\right]$$

$$= \frac{\pi d_o^2 \tau^2 l (1 - K^4)}{16G}$$

$$= \frac{\pi d_o^2 \tau^2 (1 - K^2)(1 + K^2) l}{16G}$$

$$= \frac{\tau^2 (1 + K^2)}{4G}\left[\left(\frac{\pi d_o^2 (1 - K^2)}{4}\right) l\right]$$

$$\therefore \quad U = \frac{\tau^2 V}{4G}(1 + K^2) = \frac{\tau^2 V}{4G}\left(1 + \frac{d_i^2}{d_o^2}\right) \qquad \qquad \text{... (Eq. 11.25)}$$

$$\text{Where} \quad \text{volume} \quad V = A.l$$

$$\text{Area} \qquad A = \frac{\pi}{4}\left(d_o^2 - d_i^2\right) = \frac{\pi}{4} d_o^2 (1 - K^2)$$

$$K = \frac{d_i}{d_o}$$

Strain energy density or torsional resilience

$$u = \frac{U}{V} = \frac{\tau^2 (1 + K^2)}{4G} = \frac{\tau^2}{4G}\left(1 + \frac{d_i^2}{d_o^2}\right) \qquad \qquad \text{... (Eq. 11.26)}$$

As $d_i \rightarrow d_o \Rightarrow K = 1$
Then (Eq. 11.25) yields ...

$$U = \frac{\tau^2 V}{2G} \qquad \qquad \text{... (Eq. 11.27), same as (Eq. 11.16)}$$

And (Eq. 11.26) yields ...

$$u = \frac{\tau^2}{2G}$$ ... (Eq. 11.28), same as (Eq. 11.18)

11.7 STRAIN ENERGY DUE TO BENDING

Consider a beam initially straight, subjected to pure bending moment. Due to this moment, the beam bends into an arc of radius R, subtending an angle θ at the center as shown in **Fig. 11.7(a)**.

Let, M = Bending moment

              I = Moment of inertia about neutral axis

              E = Young's modulus

              R = Radius of curvature of the beam

              σ = Bending stress

              y = distance from neutral axis to extreme fibre

              θ = Angle of twist

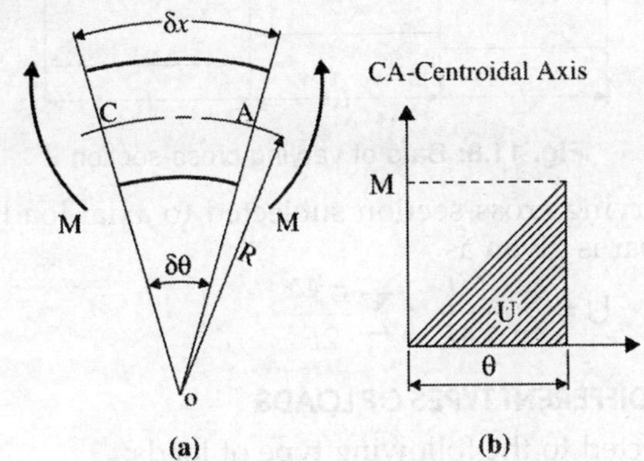

Fig. 11.7: Strain energy in bending

As long as the elastic limits are not exceeded, the relation between the angle of twist and the applied moment is linear as shown in **Fig. 11.7(b)**. The work done or strain energy, is the average moment multiplied by the angle through which it turns.

i.e. $W = \dfrac{1}{2} M\,\delta\theta = U$ ... (Eq. 11.29), using (Eq. 11.4)

But bending equation is given as

$$\frac{M}{I} = \frac{\sigma}{y} = \frac{E}{R}$$

$$M = \frac{EI}{R}$$ ... (Eq. 11.30)

From **Fig. 11.7(a)**, arc length $\delta x = R.\delta\theta$

$$R = \frac{\delta x}{\delta\theta}$$

(Eq. 11.30) yields...

$$M = \frac{EI}{\delta x / \delta\theta} = \frac{EI.\delta\theta}{\delta x}$$

$$\delta\theta = \frac{M.\delta x}{EI}$$ ... (Eq. 11.31)

Substituting (Eq. 11.31) in (Eq. 11.29), we have

$$U = \frac{M}{2}\left(\frac{M.\delta x}{EI}\right)$$

$$U = \frac{M^2 \delta x}{2EI} \qquad \text{... (Eq. 11.32a)}$$

In generalized terms, if the moment varies along the length of the rod as dx, then (Eq. 11.32a) can be written as

$$U = \int_0^l \frac{M^2 dx}{2EI} \qquad \text{... (Eq. 11.32b)}$$

11.8 STRAIN ENERGY IN BARS OF VARYING CROSS-SECTIONS

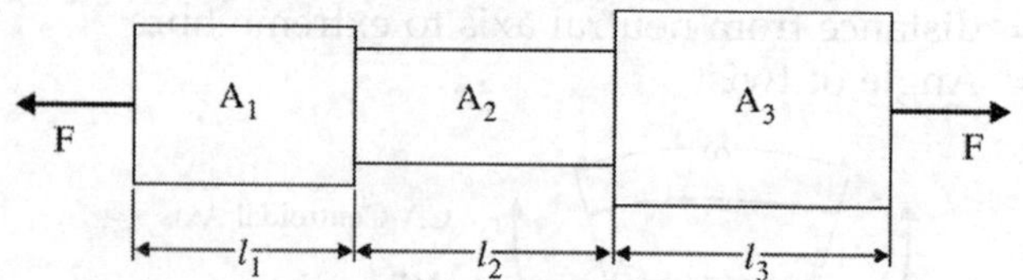
Fig. 11.8: Bars of varying cross-section

In case of bars of varying cross-section subjected to axial load **(Fig. 11.8)** the total strain energy of the bar is given as

Total strain energy, $\quad U = \sum \dfrac{F^2 l}{2AE} = \sum \dfrac{\sigma^2 V}{2E}$ $\qquad$ ... (Eq. 11.33)

11.9 STESSES DUE TO DIFFERENT TYPES OF LOADS

A body may be subjected to the following type of loads:
1. Gradually applied load
2. Suddenly applied load
3. Impact load

11.9.1 Gradually applied load

A load is said to be gradully applied if the load increases from zero to a maximum value gradually. Consider a rod or bar of uniform cross-section fixed at one end as shown in **Fig. 11.9(a)** (repeated)

Let $\quad l \;=\;$ Length of the rod

$\qquad A \;=\;$ Cross-sectional area of the rod

$\qquad \delta l \;=\;$ Total deformation of the rod

$\qquad F \;=\;$ Gradually applied load

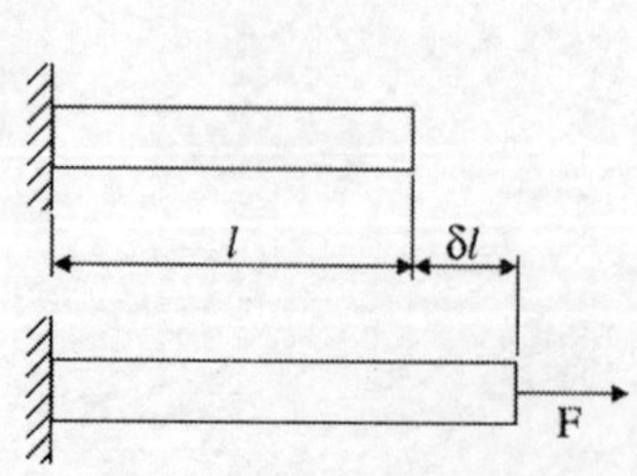
Fig. 11.9(a): Axially loaded rod

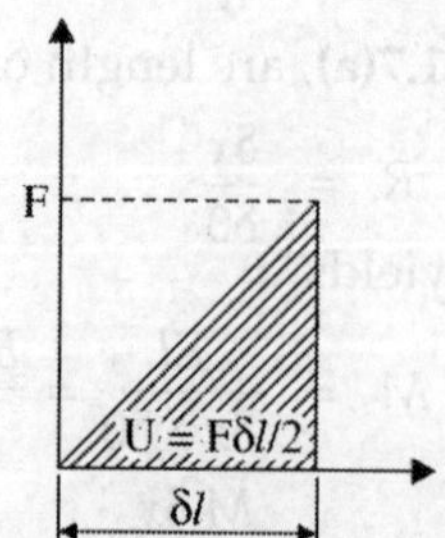
Fig. 11.9(b): Axially loaded rod

$$\sigma = \text{Nominal stress (tensile or compressive)}$$
$$\varepsilon = \text{Normal strain}$$
$$E = \text{Young's modulus}$$

As long as the load is within the elastic limit, the load-deformation diagram will be linear as shown in **Fig. 11.9(b)**.

Work done by external load,

$$W = \text{average force} \times \text{deformation} = \text{area of hatched triangle}$$

$$= \left(\frac{0+F}{2}\right)\delta l$$

$$W = \frac{1}{2}F.dl \qquad \qquad \text{... using (Eq. 11.3)}$$

Energy stored in the body,

$$U = \frac{\sigma^2 V}{2E} = \frac{\sigma^2 Al}{2E} \qquad \qquad \text{... using (Eq. 11.6)}$$

Since strain energy stored = work done on the body, equating the above two equations, we have

$$\frac{\sigma^2 Al}{2E} = \frac{1}{2}F.\delta l$$

Since $\quad \delta l = \dfrac{Fl}{AE} = \dfrac{\sigma l}{E}$

$$\frac{\sigma^2 Al}{2E} = \frac{1}{2}F\left(\frac{\sigma l}{E}\right)$$

$$\sigma = \frac{F}{A} \qquad \qquad \text{... (Eq. 11.34)}$$

11.9.2 Suddenly applied load

If the load is applied suddenly instead of being gradually applied, the value of load F remains constant throughout the deformation process, as shown in **Fig. 11.10**.

Work done by external load,

$$W = F.\delta l$$

Energy stored in the body,

$$U = \frac{\sigma^2 V}{2E} = \frac{\sigma^2 Al}{2E} \qquad \qquad \text{... using (Eq. 11.6)}$$

Since strain energy stored = work done on the body

$$\frac{\sigma^2 Al}{2E} = F.\delta l$$

Since $\delta l = \dfrac{Fl}{AE} = \dfrac{\sigma l}{E}$

$$\frac{\sigma^2 Al}{2E} = F\left(\frac{\sigma l}{E}\right)$$

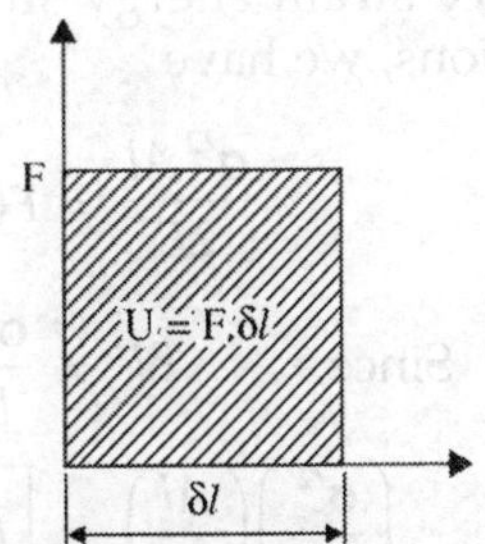

Fig. 11.10: Suddenly applied load

$$\sigma = \frac{2F}{A} \qquad \qquad \text{... (Eq. 11.35)}$$

(Eq. 11.35) indicates that the stress due to suddenly applied load is twice as that of gradually applied load.

11.9.3 Strain energy due to impact load (axial load or falling weight)

A load is said to be an impact load, if it is applied with some initial velocity. In general impact load is an external force applied to a structure or a part if the time of application is less than one-third its lowest natural period of vibration. It can occur in the following ways:

- A direct impact by another member or an external body moving with considerable velocity.
  Example: Punch press, two cars colliding.
- Sudden application of forces without a blow being involved
- Sudden creation of force on a member. Example: Power stroke in I.C. engines.
- Sudden moving of force on to a member. Example: Heavily loaded train or truck moving rapidly over the floor of the bridge.
- The inertia of the member resisting high acceleration and retardation. Example: Reciprocating levers.

Consider a bar shown in **Fig. 11.11** with a rigid collar firmly attached at the end. The load F is free to slide vertically and is suspended by some means at a distance h above the collar.

Let
F = Load applied with impact
h = Height through which the load falls
A = Cross sectional area of the bar
l = Length of the bar
σ = Static stress
δl = Deformation of bar due to static action
σ' = Impact stress
$\delta l'$ = Deformation due to impact action
E = Young's modulus of the bar material

When the load is dropped it will produce a maximum instantaneous extension $\delta l'$ of the bar, and thus

Work done = Force × distance moved
$$= F.(h + \delta l') \qquad \text{... (Eq. 11.36)}$$

Fig. 11.11: Impact stress due to axial load

Also strain energy $\cup = \dfrac{\sigma'^2 V}{2E} = \dfrac{\sigma'^2 Al}{2E} \qquad \text{... (Eq. 11.37)}$

Since strain energy stored = work done on the body, equating the above two equations, we have

$$\frac{\sigma'^2 Al}{2E} = F(h + \delta l')$$

Since $\delta l' = \dfrac{\sigma' l}{E}$, we have

$$\left(\frac{\sigma'^2}{2}\right)\left(\frac{Al}{E}\right) = \left[h + \frac{\sigma' l}{E}\right] F$$

$$\left(\frac{\sigma'^2}{2}\right)\left(\frac{Al}{E}\right) = Fh + \frac{F\sigma'l}{E}$$

$$\left(\frac{\sigma'^2}{2}\right)\left(\frac{Al}{E}\right) - \left(\frac{Fl}{E}\right)\sigma' - Fh = 0 \qquad \ldots (Eq.\ 11.38)$$

Multiplying with $\left(\dfrac{E}{Al}\right)$ on both sides of (Eq. 11.38), we have

$$\left(\frac{\sigma'^2}{2}\right) - \left(\frac{F}{A}\right)\sigma' - Fh\left(\frac{E}{Al}\right) = 0 \qquad \ldots (Eq.\ 11.39)$$

(Eq. 11.39) is a quadratic equation, the roots of which are found as

$$\sigma' = \frac{\dfrac{-(-F)}{A} \pm \sqrt{\dfrac{-(-F)}{A} - \left[4 \times \left(\dfrac{1}{2}\right) \times \left(\dfrac{-FEh}{Al}\right)\right]}}{2 \times \left(\dfrac{1}{2}\right)}$$

$$= \left(\frac{F}{A}\right) \pm \sqrt{\left(\frac{F}{A}\right)^2 + \left[\frac{2FEh}{Al}\right]}$$

$$= \left(\frac{F}{A}\right) \pm \left(\frac{F}{A}\right)\sqrt{1 + \left(\frac{2Eh}{l}\right)^2\left(\frac{A}{F}\right)}$$

$$\sigma' = \left(\frac{F}{A}\right)\left[1 + \sqrt{1 + \left(\frac{2AEh}{Fl}\right)}\right] \quad \text{(neglecting negative sign)} \ldots (Eq.\ 11.40)$$

OR

$$\sigma' = \sigma\left[1 + \sqrt{1 + \left(\frac{2AEh}{Fl}\right)}\right] = \sigma\left[1 + \sqrt{1 + \left(\frac{2h}{\delta l}\right)}\right] \qquad \ldots (Eq.\ 11.41)$$

The term $\quad \dfrac{\sigma'}{\sigma} = \left[1 + \sqrt{1 + \left(\dfrac{2h}{Fl}\right)}\right]$ is called the *"Impact/shock factor"* for stress.

$$\ldots (Eq.\ 11.42)$$

(Eq. 11.41) indicates that an impact load produces much larger effects than when the same load is applied statically.

But static deflection, $\delta l = \dfrac{Fl}{AE}$

Multiplying with $\left(\dfrac{l}{E}\right)$ on both sides of (Eq. 11.40), we have

$$\sigma'\left(\frac{l}{E}\right) = \left(\frac{F}{A}\right)\left(\frac{l}{E}\right)\left[1 \pm \sqrt{1 + \left(\frac{2AEh}{Fl}\right)}\right]$$

$$\delta l' = \delta l \left[1 + \sqrt{1 + \left(\frac{2h}{\delta l} \right)} \right] \qquad \text{... (Eq. 11.43)}$$

The term $\dfrac{\delta l'}{\delta l} = \left[1 + \sqrt{1 + \left(\dfrac{2h}{\delta l} \right)} \right]$ is called the *"Impact/ shock factor"* for deformation.

$$\text{... (Eq. 11.44)}$$

Impact factor is defined as the ratio of the dynamic response of a structure to the static response. This factor represents the amount by which the static elongation is amplified due to the dynamic effects of the impact.

11.9.4 Impact stresses due to bending

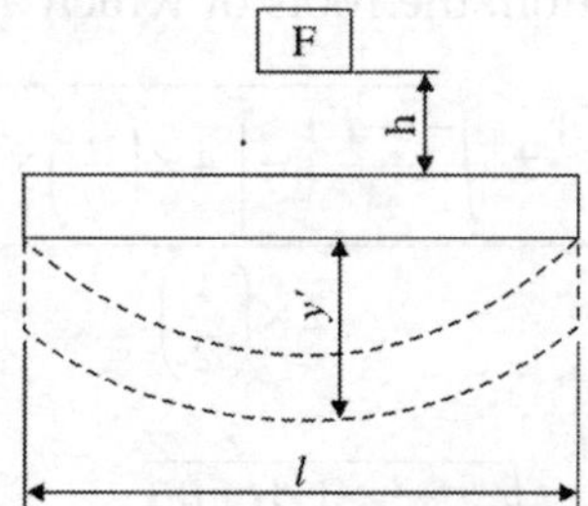

Fig. 11.12: Impact stress due to bending load

Consider a simply supported beam as shown in **Fig. 11.12**.

Let F = Weight of falling body

         h = Height through which the weight falls

         l = Length of the beam

         A = Cross sectional area of the beam ($= b.d$)

         y = Static deflection of the beam due to weight F

         y' = Deflection of the beam due to impact

         σ_b = Bending stress due to static weight

         σ_b' = Impact stress due to bending

         M = Bending moment of the beam

Work done = Force × distance moved

               $= F.(h + y')$ ... (Eq. 11.45)

Also strain energy, $U = \dfrac{1}{2} F_E y'$ ... (Eq. 11.46)

         F_E = Equivalent static load

Since strain energy stored = work done on the body, equating the above two equations, we have

$$\frac{1}{2} F_E y' = F \times (h + y')$$

$$F_E = \frac{2F(h + y')}{y'} \qquad \text{... (Eq. 11.47)}$$

For a static beam, deflection $y = \dfrac{Fl^3}{48EI}$ ... (Eq. 11.48)

On similar lines for F_E, $y' = \dfrac{F_E l^3}{48EI}$ ... (Eq. 11.49)

Substituting (Eq. 11.47) in (Eq. 11.49), we have

$$y' = \frac{2F(h + y')}{y'}\left(\frac{l^3}{48EI}\right)$$

$$y' = \frac{2(h + y')}{y'} \times y$$ ... using (Eq. 11.48)

i.e. $\quad y'^2 - 2yy' - 2hy = 0$ ... (Eq. 11.50)

(Eq. 11.50) is a quadratic equation, the roots of which are found as

$$y' = \frac{-(-2y) \pm \sqrt{(-2y)^2 - \left[4 \times (1) \times (-2hy)\right]}}{2 \times (1)} = \frac{2y \pm \sqrt{4y^2 + 8hy}}{2}$$

$$= \frac{2y + \sqrt{4y^2 + 8hy}}{2} \qquad \textit{(neglecting negative sign)}$$

$$= \frac{2y + 2y\sqrt{1 + \left(\dfrac{2h}{y}\right)}}{2} = \frac{2y\left[1 + \sqrt{1 + \left(\dfrac{2h}{y}\right)}\right]}{2}$$

$$y' = y\left[1 + \sqrt{1 + \left(\frac{2h}{y}\right)}\right] \qquad \text{... (Eq. 11.51)}$$

The term $\dfrac{y'}{y} = \left[1 + \sqrt{1 + \left(\dfrac{2h}{y}\right)}\right]$ is called the *"Impact/ shock factor"* for deflection.

... (Eq. 11.52)

In terms of bending stress, we have

$$\sigma_b' = \sigma_b\left[1 + \sqrt{1 + \left(\frac{2h}{y}\right)}\right] \qquad \text{... (Eq. 11.53)}$$

The term $\dfrac{\sigma_b'}{\sigma_b} = \left[1 + \sqrt{1 + \left(\dfrac{2h}{y}\right)}\right]$ is called the *"Impact/ shock factor"* for bending stress

... (Eq. 11.54)

Note:
- Impact stress due to sudden load, $\sigma' = 2\sigma, \sigma_b' = 2\sigma_b$ and $\tau' = 2\tau$
- Deformation under the action of sudden load, $\delta' = 2d$, $y' = 2y$ and $\theta' = 2\delta$

- Kinetic energy, $E_K = \dfrac{Wv^2}{2g} = \dfrac{1}{2}mv^2$ (F or W)

- Impact energy of a body falling from a height h (potential energy) is
$$E_k = Wh = (mg)h$$

11.10 PROBLEMS ON AXIAL LOAD

11.10.1 Problems on axial load: Basic

1. Calculate the strain energy and strain energy density stored in a circular rod of 200 mm diameter and 3 m long under the following cases:
   (a) When subjected to a tensile load of 25 kN.
   (b) When subjected to a shear force of 15 kN.
   (c) When subjected to a torque of 10 kN-m.
   (d) When subjected to a uniform bending moment of 20 kN-m.

Take $E = 200$ GPa and $G = 84$ GPa.

Solution: $d = 200$ mm, $l = 3000$ mm, $E = 200 \times 10^3$ MPa, $G = 84 \times 10^3$ MPa, $U = ?$, $u = ?$, if
a) $F = 25 \times 10^3$ N, b) $F_s = 15 \times 10^3$ N, c) $T = 10 \times 10^6$ N-mm, d) $M = 20 \times 10^6$ N-mm

Area $\qquad A = (\pi \times 200^2/4) = 31415.93$ mm^2

Volume $\qquad V = Al = 31415.93 \times 3000 = 94.25 \times 10^6$ mm$^3 = 94.25 \times 10^{-3}$ m^3

a. *Axial load:*

Strain energy $\qquad U = \dfrac{F^2 l}{2AE} = \dfrac{(25 \times 10^3)^2 \times 3000}{2 \times 31415.93 \times 200 \times 10^3} = 149.21$ N-mm

$$= 0.14291 \text{ N-m or J}$$

Strain energy density $\quad u = \dfrac{U}{V} = \dfrac{0.14291}{94.25 \times 10^{-3}} = 1.58$ N-m/m^3 or J/m^3

b. *Shear load:*

Strain energy $\qquad U = \dfrac{F^2 l}{2AG} = \dfrac{(15 \times 10^3)^2 \times 3000}{2 \times 31415.93 \times 84 \times 10^3} = 127.90$ N-mm

$$= 0.1279 \text{ N-m or J}$$

Strain energy density $\quad u = \dfrac{U}{V} = \dfrac{0.1279}{94.25 \times 10^{-3}} = 1.36$ N-m/m^3 or J/m^3

c. *Torque:*

Strain energy $\qquad U = \dfrac{T^2 l}{2GJ} = \dfrac{(10 \times 10^6)^2 \times 3000}{2 \times 84 \times 10^3 \times (\pi \times 200^4/32)}$

$$= 11.37 \times 10^3 \text{ N-mm} = 11.37 \text{ N-m or J}$$

Strain energy density $\quad u = \dfrac{U}{V} = \dfrac{11.37}{94.25 \times 10^{-3}} = 120.64$ N-m/m^3 or J/m^3

d. *Moment:*

Strain energy $\qquad U = \dfrac{M^2 l}{2EI} = \dfrac{(20 \times 10^6)^2 \times 3000}{2 \times 200 \times 10^3 \times (\pi \times 200^4/64)}$

$$= 38.20 \times 10^3 \text{ N-mm} = 38.20 \text{ N-m or J}$$

Strain energy density $\quad u = \dfrac{U}{V} = \dfrac{38.20}{94.25 \times 10^{-3}} = 405.31$ N-m/m^3 or J/m^3

2. **A cantilever circular rod has a diameter of 50 mm and 300 mm length. Calculate the strain energy under the following cases:**
   (a) **Appling an axial load of 20 kN.**
   (b) **Applying 4 kN load at an end, acting downwards creating a bending moment.**
   (c) **Applying a torque of 1.5 kN-m. Take E = 200 GPa and G = 84 GPa.**

Solution: l = 300 mm, d = 50 mm, U = ?, if a) F = 20 × 10³ N, b) F_b = 4000 N, c) T = 1.5 × 10⁶ N-mm

    Area $A = (\pi \times 50^2/4) = 1963.50 \text{ mm}^2$

    Volume $V = Al = 1963.50 \times 300 = 589050 \text{ mm}^3$

Based on the given data, the loading is as shown in **Figs 11.13(a) to 11.13(c)**

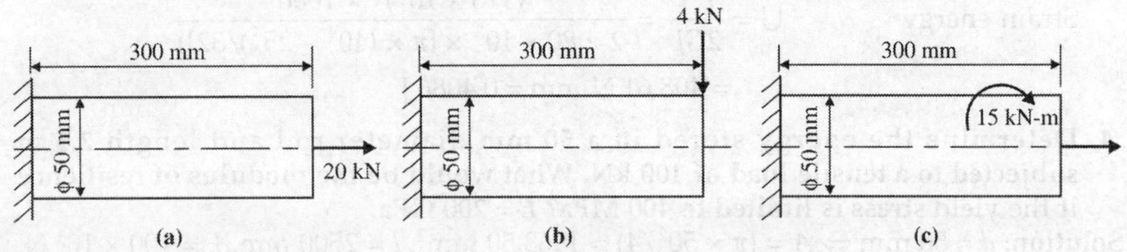

Fig. 11.13: Problem 2

a. Axial load [**Fig. 11.12(a)**]:

    Strain energy $\mathsf{U} = \dfrac{F^2 l}{2AE} = \dfrac{(20 \times 10^3)^2 \times 300}{2 \times 1963.50 \times 200 \times 10^3} = 152.78 \text{ N-mm}$

                                            = 0.1528 J

b. Moment [**Fig. 11.12(b)**]:

    From **Fig. 11.12(b)**, for a cantilever beam, $M = F_b.l = 4000 \times 300 = 1.2 \times 10^6$ N-mm

    Strain energy $\mathsf{U} = \dfrac{M^2 L}{2EI} = \dfrac{(1.2 \times 10^6)^2 \times 300}{2 \times 200 \times 10^3 \times (\pi \times 50^4/64)} = 3520.25 \text{ N-mm}$

                                            = 3.52 N-m

c. Torque [**Fig. 11.12(c)**]:

    Strain energy $\mathsf{U} = \dfrac{T^2 l}{2GJ} = \dfrac{(1.5 \times 10^6)^2 \times 300}{2 \times 84 \times 10^3 \times (\pi \times 50^4/32)} = 6548.08 \text{ N-mm}$

                                            = 6.55 N-m

3. **A hollow cantilever shaft 1 m long has an external diameter of 40 mm and internal diameter of 25 mm inner diameter. Calculate the strain energy under the following cases:**
   (a) **When subjected to an axial thrust of 9806 N.**
   (b) **When subjected to a bending moment of 79 N-m.**
   (c) **When subjected to a twisting moment of 118 N-m.**
       Take E = 210 GPa and G = 80 GPa

Solution: d_o = 40 mm, d_i = 25 mm, l = 1000 mm, U = ? if a) F = 9806 N, b) M = 79 × 10³ N-mm, c) T = 118 N-m = 118 × 10³ N-mm,

a. *Axial load:*

Strain energy
$$U = \frac{F^2 l}{2AE} = \frac{(9806)^2 \times 1000}{2 \times [\pi \times (40^2 - 25^2)/4] \times 210 \times 10^3}$$
$$= 298.98 \text{ N-mm} = 0.2989 \text{ J}$$

b. *Moment:*

Strain energy
$$U = \frac{M^2 L}{2EI} = \frac{(79 \times 10^3)^2 \times 1000}{2 \times 210 \times 10^3 \times [\pi \times (40^4 - 25^4)/64]}$$
$$= 139.54 \text{ N-mm} = 0.1395 \text{ J}$$

c. *Torque:*

Strain energy
$$U = \frac{T^2 l}{2GJ} = \frac{(118 \times 10^3)^2 \times 1000}{2 \times 80 \times 10^3 \times [\pi \times (40^4 - 25^4)/32])}$$
$$= 408.61 \text{ N-mm} = 0.4086 \text{ J}$$

4. **Determine the energy stored in a 50 mm diameter rod and length 2.5 m subjected to a tensile load of 100 kN. What would be the modulus of resilience if the yield stress is limited to 400 MPa? E = 200 GPa.**

Solution: $d = 50$ mm $\Rightarrow A = (\pi \times 50^2/4) = 1963.50$ mm^2, $l = 2500$ mm, $F = 100 \times 10^3$ N, $E = 200 \times 10^3$ MPa, $\sigma_y = 400$ MPa, $U = ?$, modulus of resilience = ?

a. Strain energy:
$$U = \frac{F^2 l}{2AE} = \frac{(100 \times 10^3)^2 \times 2500}{2 \times 1963.50 \times 200 \times 10^3} = 31.83 \times 10^3 \text{ N-mm}$$
$$= 31.83 \text{ J}$$

b. Modulus of resilience: $u_p = \dfrac{\sigma_y^2}{2E} = \dfrac{400^2}{2 \times 200 \times 10^3} = 0.4 \text{ N/mm}^2$

5. **Calculate the strain energy stored in a square bar of size 300 mm and 1m long under the following cases:**
   (a) When subjected to a tensile load of 25 kN.
   (b) When subjected to a uniform bending moment of 20 kN-m.
   Take E = 200 GPa and G = 84 GPa.

Solution: $A = 300 \times 300 = 90000$ mm^2, $l = 1000$ mm, $E = 200 \times 10^3$ MPa, $G = 84 \times 10^3$ MPa, $U = ?$ a) $F = 25 \times 10^3$ N, b) $M = 20 \times 10^6$ N-mm

a. *Axial load:*
$$U = \frac{F^2 l}{2AE} = \frac{(25 \times 10^3)^2 \times 1000}{2 \times 90000 \times 200 \times 10^3} = 17.36 \text{ N-mm}$$

b. *Moment:*
$$U = \frac{M^2 l}{2EI} = \frac{(20 \times 10^6)^2 \times 1000}{2 \times 200 \times 10^3 \times (300^4/12)} = 1.48 \times 10^3 \text{ N-mm}$$

6. **A steel rod 15mm in diameter and gauge length 80 mm stretches 0.04 mm under an axial load of 50 kN. Calculate the strain energy stored in the specimen at this point.**
   If the load at elastic limit for the specimen is 80 kN, calculate the elongation at elastic limit and resilience.

Solution: $d = 15$ mm, $l = 80$ mm, $\delta l = 0.04$ mm, $F = 50 \times 10^3$ N, $U = ?$, $F_y = 80 \times 10^3$ N, $U_p = ?$.

a. *To find* $\cup$:

We know that $\qquad \cup = \dfrac{1}{2} F.\delta l = \dfrac{1}{2} \times (50 \times 10^3) \times 0.04 = 1000 \text{ N-mm} = 1 \text{ J}$

b. *To find* $\cup_p$:

At elastic limit, $\qquad \cup_p = \dfrac{1}{2} F_y.\delta l_y$

But $\qquad F.\delta l = F_y.\delta l_y$ up to elastic limit

$$\delta l_y = \dfrac{F.\delta l}{F_y} = \dfrac{80 \times 10^3 \times 0.04}{50 \times 10^3} = 0.064 \text{ mm}$$

$$\cup_p = \dfrac{1}{2} \times (80 \times 10^3) \times 0.064 = 2560 \text{ N-mm} = 2.56 \text{ J}$$

7. **A cantilever rod 2 m long is subjected to an axial energy input of 15 N-m. Determine the diameter of the rod for a factor of safety of 6. The rod is made of steel having yield strength of 300 MPa and modulus of elasticity as 200 GPa.**

Solution: $l = 2000$ mm, $\cup = 15$ N-m $= 15 \times 10^3$ N-mm, $n = 6$, $\sigma_y = 300$ MPa, $E = 200 \times 10^3$ MPa, $d = ?$

Note: Since energy loads are not linearly related to the stresses they produce, factors of safety associated with energy loads should be applied to the energy loads and not to the stresses.

At yield point, $\qquad \cup = \dfrac{\sigma_y^2 V}{2E}$

Since factor of safety is given, the above relation takes the form

$$\cup.n = \dfrac{\sigma_y^2 Al}{2E}$$

$$(15 \times 10^3) \times 6 = \dfrac{300^2 \times A \times 2000}{2 \times (2 \times 10^5)}$$

$$A = 200 \text{ mm}^2$$

But $\qquad A = \dfrac{\pi d^2}{4}$

$$200 = \dfrac{\pi d^2}{4}$$

$$d = 15.96 \text{ mm} \ \square \ 16 \text{ mm}$$

8. **A rectangular copper bar 50 mm × 75 mm in cross-section is subjected to an axial energy input of 200 N-m. Determine the minimum length of the bar to limit the axial stress in the bar to 80 MPa. The modulus of elasticity of the bar is 1.15×10^5 N/mm².**

VTU – Dec. 2011 – 06 Marks

Solution: $b = 50$ mm, $h = 75$ mm, $\cup = 200 \times 10^3$ N-mm, $l = ?$, $\sigma = 80$ MPa, $E = 1.15 \times 10^5$ N/mm².

For axial load
$$U = \frac{\sigma^2 V}{2E} = \frac{\sigma^2 Al}{2E}$$

$$200 \times 10^3 = \frac{80^2 \times (50 \times 75) \times l}{2 \times (1.15 \times 10^5)} \qquad \Rightarrow \quad l = 1916.67 \text{ mm}$$

11.10.2 Problems on axial load: Stepped bars

9. For the rod shown in Fig. 11.14. Determine:
   (a) Strain Energy stored in each part and total strain energy.
   (b) Strain energy density in each part.
      Take $E = 75$ GPa

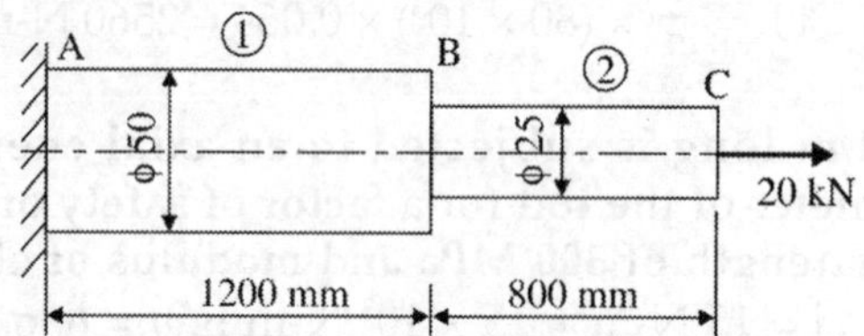

Fig. 11.14: Problem 9

Solution: *Let suffix '1' refers to rod AB and '2' refers to rod BC*
$d_1 = 50$ mm, $l_1 = 1200$ mm, $d_2 = 25$ mm, $l_2 = 800$ mm, $F = 10 \times 10^3$ N, $E = 75 \times 10^3$ MPa.
a) $U = ?$, b) $u = ?$

a. *To find* U:

For rod AB
$$U_1 = \frac{F_1^2 l_1}{2A_1 E} = \frac{(20 \times 10^3)^2 \times 1200}{2 \times (\pi \times 50^2/4) \times 75 \times 10^3} = 1629.75 \text{ N-mm}$$
$$= 1.630 \text{ J} \qquad \text{(here } F \text{ and } E \text{ are constants)}$$

For rod BC
$$U_2 = \frac{F_1^2 l_1}{2A_1 E} = \frac{(20 \times 10^3)^2 \times 800}{2 \times (\pi \times 25^2/4) \times 75 \times 10^3} = 4346 \text{ N-mm}$$
$$= 4.346 \text{ J}$$

Total strain energy for rod ABC

$$U = \sum \frac{F^2 l}{2AE} = U_1 + U_2 = 1629.75 + 4346$$
$$= 5975.75 \text{ N-mm} = 5.975 \text{ J}$$

b. *To find* u:

For rod AB
$$u_1 = \frac{U_1}{V_1} = \frac{U_1}{A_1 l_1} = \frac{1.63}{(\pi \times 50^2/4) \times 1200} = 6.92 \times 10^{-7} \text{ J/mm}^3$$
$$= 691.80 \text{ J/m}^3$$

For rod BC
$$u_2 = \frac{U_2}{V_2} = \frac{U_2}{A_2 l_2} = \frac{4.364}{(\pi \times 25^2/4) \times 800} = 1.11 \times 10^{-5} \text{ J/mm}^3$$
$$= 11.06 \times 10^3 \text{ J/m}^3$$

10. A bar with circular cross-section as shown in Fig. 11.15 is subjected to a load of 10 kN. Determine the strain energy stored in it. Take $E = 2.1 \times 10^5$ MPa.

VTU – June/ July 2013 – 07 Marks

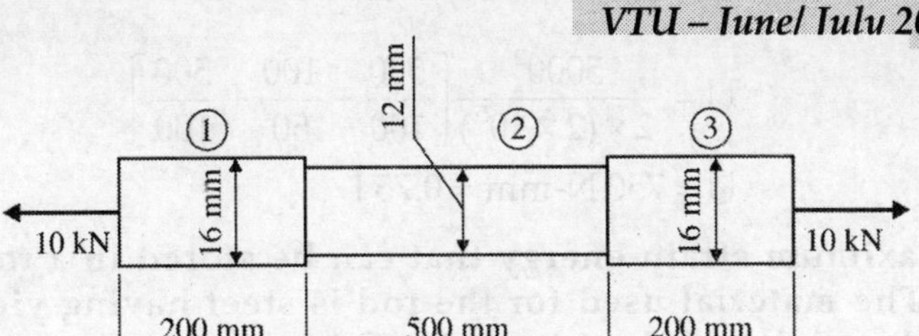

Fig. 11.15: Problem 10

Solution: $d_1 = d_3 = 16$ mm, $l_1 = l_3 = 200$ mm, $d_2 = 12$ mm, $l_2 = 500$ mm, $F = 10 \times 10^3$ N, $E = 2.1 \times 10^5$ MPa, $U = ?$

For bars of varying cross-section, we have

$$U = \sum \frac{F^2 l}{2AE} = \frac{F^2}{2E} \sum \frac{l}{A}$$

$$= \frac{4F^2}{2\pi E}\left[\frac{l_1}{d_1^2} + \frac{l_2}{d_2^2} + \frac{l_3}{d_3^2}\right] = \frac{2F^2}{\pi E}\left[\frac{l_1}{d_1^2} + \frac{l_2}{d_2^2} + \frac{l_3}{d_3^2}\right]$$

$$= \frac{2 \times (10 \times 10^3)^2}{\pi \times (2.1 \times 10^5)}\left[\frac{200}{16^2} + \frac{500}{12^2} + \frac{200}{16^2}\right]$$

$$U = 1526.29 \text{ N-mm} = 1.526 \text{ J}$$

11. The maximum stress produced by a pull in a bar of length 100 mm is 100 N/mm². The area of cross section and length are as shown in Fig. 11.16. Calculate the strain energy stored in the bar if $E = 2 \times 105$ N/mm².

VTU – Dec. 14/ Jan. 15 – 10 Marks

Solution: $A_1 = A_3 = 100$ mm², $l_1 = l_3 = 500$ mm, $A_2 = 50$ mm², $l_2 = 100$ mm, $\sigma_{max} = \sigma_2 = 100$ MPa, $E = 2 \times 10^5$ MPa, $U = ?$

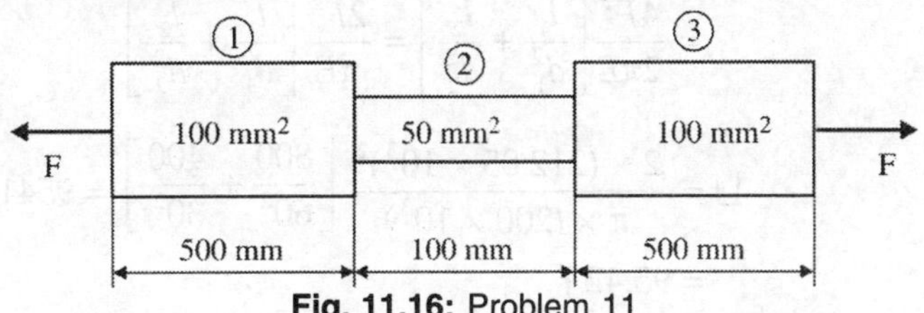

Fig. 11.16: Problem 11

Note: Maximum stress occurs in the section where the area is minimum.

$$\sigma_{max} = \sigma_2 = \frac{F_2}{A_2}$$

$$F_2 = 100 \times 50 = 5000 \text{ N}$$

Since the load acting on the bar is constant, we have $F_1 = F_2 = F_3 = 5000$ N

$$U = \sum \frac{F^2 l}{2AE} = \frac{F^2}{2E} \sum \frac{l}{A}$$

$$= \frac{F^2}{2E}\left[\frac{l_1}{A_1} + \frac{l_2}{A_2} + \frac{l_3}{A_3}\right]$$

$$U = \frac{5000^2}{2\times(2\times10^5)}\left[\frac{500}{100} + \frac{100}{50} + \frac{500}{100}\right]$$

$$U = 750 \text{ N-mm} = 0.75 \text{ J}$$

12. **Find the maximum strain energy that can be stored in a rod as shown in Fig. 11.17. The material used for the rod is steel having yield strength of 300 MPa and modulus of elasticity as 200 GPa.**

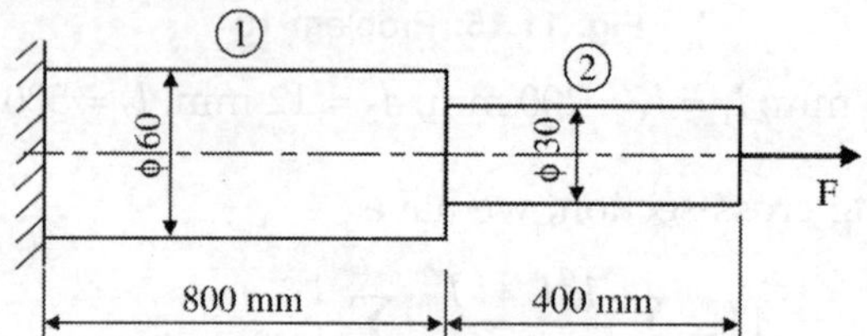

Fig. 11.17: Problem 12

Solution: $d_1 = 60$ mm, $l_1 = 800$ mm, $d_2 = 30$ mm, $l_2 = 400$ mm, $\sigma_y = 300$ MPa, $E = 200 \times 10^3$ MPa, $U = ?$

We know that
$$\sigma_y = \frac{F_y}{A} = \frac{F_y}{A_{min}} = \frac{F_y}{A_2}$$

$$300 = \frac{F_y}{\left(\pi \times 30^2/4\right)}$$

$$F_y = 212.05 \times 10^3 \text{ N}$$

Here F_y indicates the force applied at the end of the rod to cause yielding.
Since the load acting on the rod is constant, we have $F_1 = F_2 = 212.05 \times 10^3$ N

$$U = \sum\frac{F^2 l}{2AE} = \frac{F^2}{2E}\sum\frac{l}{A}$$

$$= \frac{4F^2}{2\pi E}\left[\frac{l_1}{d_1^2} + \frac{l_2}{d_2^2}\right] = \frac{2F^2}{\pi E}\left[\frac{l_1}{d_1^2} + \frac{l_2}{d_2^2}\right]$$

$$U = \frac{2\times(212.05\times10^3)^2}{\pi\times(200\times10^3)}\left[\frac{800}{60^2} + \frac{400}{30^2}\right] = 95419.12 \text{ N-mm}$$

$$= 95.42 \text{ J}$$

13. **The stepped bar having a square cross section with each side 10 mm and a circular cross section with diameter d is subjected to a pull of 20 kN as shown in Fig. 11.18. If the volume of circular portion alone is 24×10^3 mm³, find the dimensions of circular portion so that the total strain energy is minimum. Also find the strain energy. Take $E = 200$ GPa.**

Solution: *Let suffix '1' refers to circular bar and '2' refers to square bar.*
$d_1 = d = ?$, $l_1 = (200 - x)$, $A_2 = 10 \times 10 = 100$ mm², $l_2 = x$, $F = 20 \times 10^3$ N, $E = 200 \times 10^3$ MPa, $V_1 = 24 \times 10^3$ mm³, $U = ?$

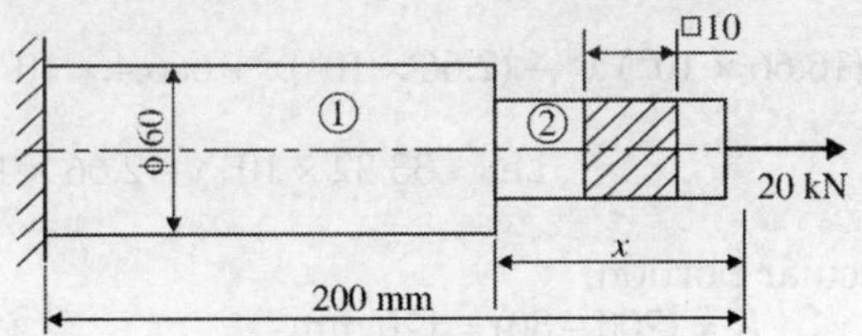

Fig. 11.18: Problem 13

We know that
$$U = \sum \frac{F^2 l}{2AE} = \sum \frac{\sigma^2 V}{2E} \qquad \text{... Eq. (i)}$$

$$\sigma_1 = \frac{F}{A_1} = \frac{20 \times 10^3}{\pi d^2/4} = \frac{25.46 \times 10^3}{d^3}$$

$$\sigma_2 = \frac{F}{A_2} = \frac{20 \times 10^3}{100} = 200 \, \text{MPa}$$

also $\qquad V_1 = 24 \times 10^3 \, \text{mm}^3$

i.e. $\quad (\pi d^2/4) \times (200 - x) = 24 \times 10^3$

$$d^2 = \left(\frac{30.56 \times 10^3}{200 - x} \right) \qquad \text{... Eq. (ii)}$$

Eq. (i) yields ...
$$U = \frac{1}{2E} \left[\left(\frac{25.46 \times 10^3}{d^2} \right)^2 \times 24 \times 10^3 + (200^2 \times 100 \times x) \right]$$

$$= \frac{1}{2E} \left[\frac{15.56 \times 10^{12}}{d^4} + (4 \times 10^6)x \right]$$

$$= \frac{1}{2E} \left[15.56 \times 10^{12} \left(\frac{200 - x}{30.56 \times 10^3} \right)^2 + (4 \times 10^6)x \right]$$
$$\text{... using Eq. (ii)}$$

$$= \frac{1}{2E} \left[16.66 \times 10^3 \times (200 - x)^2 + (4 \times 10^6)x \right]$$

$$= \frac{1}{2E} \left[16.66 \times 10^3 \times (40000 + x^2 - 400x) + (4 \times 10^6)x \right]$$

$$= \frac{1}{2E} \left[666.4 \times 10^6 + (16.66 \times 10^3) x^2 - (6.66 \times 10^6)x + (4 \times 10^6)x \right]$$

$$U = \frac{1}{2E} \left[(16.66 \times 10^3)x^2 - (2.66 \times 10^6)x + 666.4 \times 10^6 \right]$$
$$\text{... Eq. (iii)}$$

For strain energy to be minimum $\qquad \dfrac{dU}{dx} = 0$

$$\frac{d}{dx}\left\{\frac{1}{2E}[(16.66 \times 10^3)\,x^2 - (2.66 \times 10^6)x + 666.4 \times 10^6]\right\} = 0$$

i.e. $\quad 33.32 \times 10^3\,x - 2.66 \times 10^6 = 0$

$$x = 79.8\,\text{mm} \approx 80\,\text{mm} = l_2$$

Thus length of circular portion,

$$l_1 = (200 - 80) = 120\,\text{mm}$$

Eq. (ii) yields ... $\quad d^2 = \left(\dfrac{30.56 \times 10^3}{120}\right)$

$$d = 15.96\,\text{mm} \approx 16\,\text{mm}$$

Eq. (iii) yields ... $\quad \mathsf{U} = \dfrac{1}{2 \times (2 \times 10^5)}\,[(16.66 \times 10^3) \times 80^2 - (2.66 \times 10^6) \times 80$

$$+\, 666.4 \times 10^6]$$

$$\mathsf{U} = 1400.56\,\text{N-mm} = 1.4\,\text{J}$$

14. **The stepped bar having a square cross section with sides b and a circular cross section with diameter d is under an axial tensile force F as shown in Fig. 11.19. What is the ratio of d/b in order that the strain energy in both parts is the same? Also determine the total strain energy, for the above condition.**

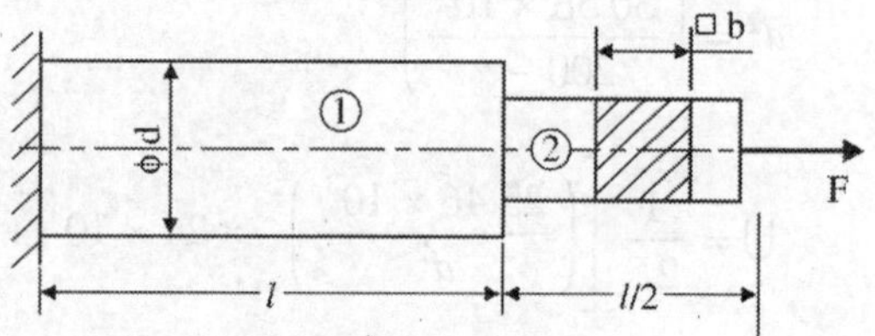

Fig. 11.19: Problem 14

Solution: *Let suffix '1' refers to circular bar and '2' refers to square bar.*
$d_1 = d\,?,\, l_1 = l,\, A_2 = b^2.\, l_2 = l/2,\, \mathsf{U}_1 = \mathsf{U}_2,\, d/b = ?$
Given $\qquad \mathsf{U}_1 = \mathsf{U}_2$

$$\left(\frac{F^2 l}{2AE}\right)_1 = \left(\frac{F^2 l}{2AE}\right)_2$$

Cancelling the common terms, we have

$$\frac{l_1}{A_1} = \frac{l_2}{A_2}$$

$$\frac{l}{\pi d^2/4} = \frac{l/2}{b^2}$$

$$\frac{4}{\pi d^2} = \frac{1}{2b^2}$$

$$2b^2 = \pi d^2/4 \qquad\qquad \text{... Eq. (i)}$$

$$\frac{d}{b} = \sqrt{\frac{8}{\pi}} \qquad\qquad \text{... Eq. (ii)}$$

Total strain energy
$$U = \sum \frac{F^2 l}{2AE} = \frac{F^2}{2E} \sum \frac{l}{A}$$

$$= \frac{F^2}{2E}\left[\frac{1}{\pi d^2/4} + \frac{l/2}{b^2}\right]$$

$$= \frac{F^2}{2E}\left[\frac{4l}{\pi d^2} + \frac{l}{2b^2}\right]$$

$$U = \frac{F^2 l}{2E}\left[\frac{4}{\pi d^2} + \frac{1}{2b^2}\right] \qquad \ldots \text{Eq. (iii)}$$

Substituting Eq. (i) in Eq. (iii)

$$U = \frac{F^2 l}{2E}\left[\frac{4}{\pi d^2} + \frac{1}{\pi d^2/4}\right]$$

$$U = \frac{F^2 l}{2E}\left[\frac{4}{\pi d^2} + \frac{4}{\pi d^2}\right]$$

$$U = \frac{4F^2 l}{\pi d^2 E} \qquad \ldots \text{Eq. (iv), in terms of diameter}$$

On similar lines, we have $U = \dfrac{F^2 l}{2b^2 E}$ $\qquad \ldots$ Eq. (v), in terms of b

15. **Derive an expression for strain energy stored in a bar as shown in Fig. 11.20. The modulus of elasticity of the material is E.**

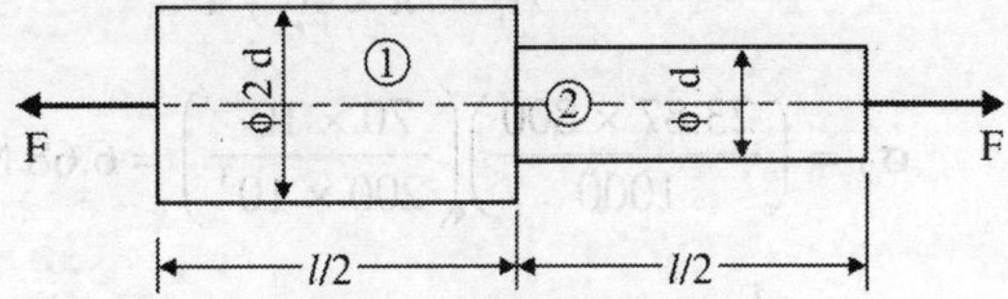

Fig. 11.20: Problem 15

Solution:

We know that
$$U = \sum \frac{F^2 l}{2AE} = \frac{F^2}{2E} \sum \frac{l}{A}$$

$$= \frac{4F^2}{2\pi E}\left[\frac{l/2}{(2d)^2} + \frac{l/2}{d^2}\right]$$

$$= \frac{F^2 l}{\pi E}\left[\frac{1}{4d^2} + \frac{1}{d^2}\right]$$

$$U = \frac{5F^2 l}{4\pi E d^2}$$

16. A composite rod made of steel and aluminium is to undergo same deformation under a tensile force of 30 kN, as shown in Fig. 11.21. Determine:
    (a) The diameter of aluminium rod
    (b) The total strain energy.
    Take E = 200 GPa and 70 GPa for steel and aluminium respectively

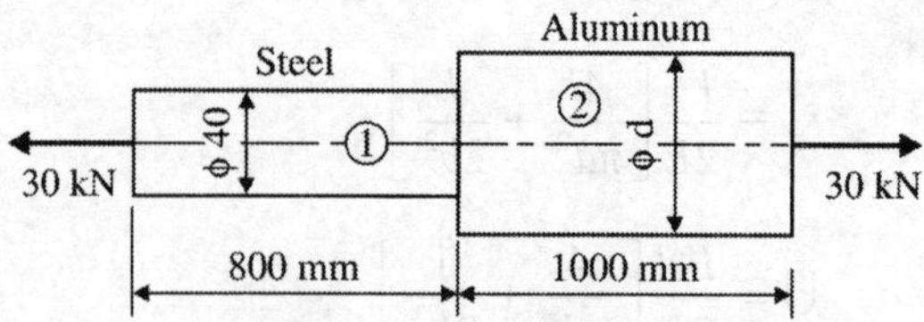

Fig. 11.21: Problem 16

Solution: *Let suffix '1' refers to steel and '2' refer to aluminum*
$F = 30 \times 10^3$ N, $\delta l_1 = \delta l_2$, $d_1 = 40$ mm, $l_1 = 800$ mm, $l_2 = 1000$ mm, $E_1 = 200 \times 10^3$ MPa, $E_2 = 70 \times 10^3$ MPa. a) $d_2 = ?$, b) $\cup = ?$

a. *Diameter of the rod:* For a composite bar

$$\delta l_1 = \delta l_2$$

$$\frac{F_1 l_1}{A_1 E_1} = \frac{F_2 l_2}{A_2 E_2} \qquad \text{(here } l_1 \neq l_2)$$

$$\frac{\sigma_1 l_1}{E_1} = \frac{\sigma_2 l_2}{E_2}$$

$$\sigma_2 = \left(\frac{\sigma_1 l_1}{E_2}\right) \frac{E_2}{E_1} \qquad \dots \text{ Eq. (i)}$$

But $\quad \sigma_1 = \dfrac{F}{A_1} = \dfrac{30 \times 10^3}{\pi \times 40^2 / 4} = 23.87$ MPa

Eq. (i) yields... $\quad \sigma_2 = \left(\dfrac{23.87 \times 800}{1000}\right)\left(\dfrac{70 \times 10^3}{200 \times 10^3}\right) = 6.68$ MPa

Also $\quad \sigma_2 = \dfrac{F}{A_2}$

$$6.68 = \frac{30 \times 10^3}{\pi d_2^2 / 4}$$

$$d_2 = 75.61 \text{ mm} \approx 76 \text{ mm}$$

b. *Total strain energy:*

$$\cup = \sum \frac{F^2 l}{2AE}$$

$$= \frac{4F^2}{2\pi}\left[\frac{l_1}{E_1 d_1^2} + \frac{l_2}{E_2 d_2^2}\right] = \frac{2F^2}{\pi}\left[\frac{l_1}{E_1 d_1^2} + \frac{l_2}{E_2 d_2^2}\right]$$

$$= \frac{2 \times (30 \times 10^3)^2}{\pi}\left[\frac{800}{(200 \times 10^3) \times 40^2} + \frac{1000}{(70 \times 10^3) \times 76^2}\right]$$

$$\cup = 2848.48 \text{ N-mm} = 2.85 \text{ J}$$

11.10.3 Problems on axial load: Tapered bars

17. A uniformly tapered rod of circular cross-section is subjected to a tensile load as shown in Fig. 11.22. Derive expression for strain energy stored in the bar.

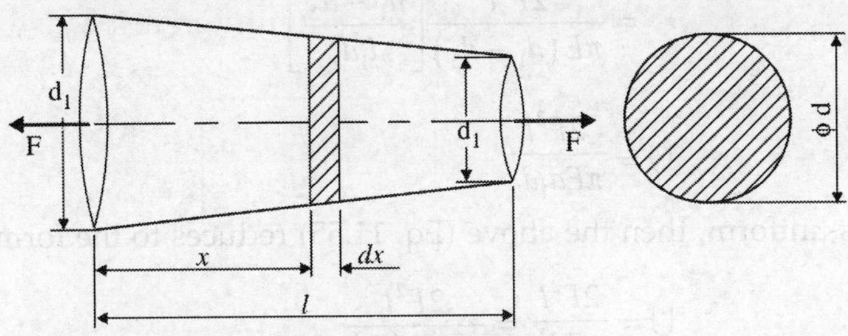

Fig. 11.22: Problem 17
(SE in a rod of uniform tapering circular c/s)

Fig. 11.21 shows a circular rod of uniform tapering section having diameter d_1 at one end and tapering down to a diameter d_2 at the other end, in length l and subjected to axial force F.

Consider a small element of length dx at a distance x from the larger diameter (d_1).

The rate of change of diameter in a length l is $= \dfrac{d_1 - d_2}{l}$

Therefore diameter at x is $d = d_1 - \left(\dfrac{d_1 - d_2}{l}\right) x$

$$\therefore \quad d = d_1 - kx \qquad \text{where } k = \left(\dfrac{d_1 - d_2}{l}\right) \qquad \text{... Eq. (a)}$$

Area of the element, $\quad A = \dfrac{\pi}{4} d^2 = \dfrac{\pi(d_1 - kx)^2}{4}$ ... Eq. (b)

Strain energy $\quad U = \displaystyle\int_0^l \dfrac{F^2 dx}{2AE}$ ... using (Eq. 11.5a)

$$= \int_0^l \dfrac{4F^2 dx}{2E\pi(d_1 - kx)^2} = \dfrac{2F^2}{\pi E} \int_0^l (d_1 - kx)^{-2} dx$$

$$= \dfrac{2F^2}{\pi E} \left[\dfrac{(d_1 - kx)^{-1}}{(-1).(-k)} \right]_0^l = \dfrac{2F^2}{\pi Ek} \left[\dfrac{1}{(d_1 - kx)} \right]_0^l$$

$$U = \dfrac{2F^2}{\pi Ek} \left[\dfrac{1}{d_1 - kl} - \dfrac{1}{d_1 - k(0)} \right] = \dfrac{2F^2}{\pi Ek} \left[\dfrac{1}{(d_1 - kl)} - \dfrac{1}{d_1} \right]$$

$$= \dfrac{2F^2}{\pi Ek} \left[\dfrac{1}{d_1 - \left(\dfrac{d_1 - d_2}{l}\right) l} - \dfrac{1}{d_1} \right] \qquad \text{... using Eq. (a)}$$

$$= \frac{2F^2}{\pi E k}\left[\frac{1}{d_2} - \frac{1}{d_1}\right] = \frac{2F^2}{\pi E k}\left[\frac{d_1 - d_2}{d_1 d_2}\right]$$

$$= \frac{2F^2 l}{\pi E (d_1 - d_2)}\left[\frac{d_1 - d_2}{d_1 d_2}\right] \qquad \text{... using Eq. (a)}$$

$$\therefore \quad U = \frac{2F^2 l}{\pi E d_1 d_2} \qquad \text{... (Eq. 11.55)}$$

If the rod is uniform, then the above (Eq. 11.55) reduces to the form,

$$U = \frac{2F^2 l}{\pi E d^2} = \frac{2F^2 l}{\pi E d^2 \left(\dfrac{2}{2}\right)}$$

$$\text{multiply and divide by 2 in denominator}$$

$$U = \frac{F^2 l}{2AE} \qquad \text{since } A = \frac{\pi}{4}d^2 \qquad \text{... same as (Eq. 11.5)}$$

18. **A uniformly tapered bar of rectangular cross-section is subjected to a tensile load as shown in Fig. 11.23. Derive expression for strain energy stored in the bar.**

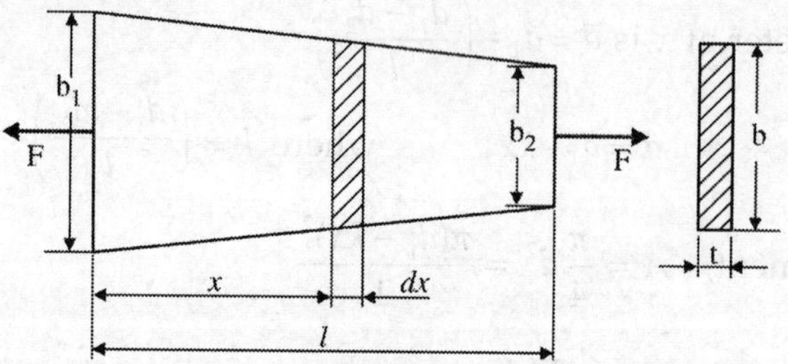

Fig. 11.23: Problem 18

Fig. 11.23 shows a rectangular bar of uniform tapering section having width b_1 at one end and tapering down to a width b_2 at the other end, in length l and subjected to axial force F.

Consider a small element of length dx at a distance x from the larger width (b_1).

The rate of change of diameter in a length l is $= \dfrac{b_1 - b_2}{l}$

Therefore diameter at x is $b = b_1 - \left(\dfrac{b_1 - b_2}{l}\right) x$

$$\therefore \quad b = b_1 - kx \qquad \text{where } k = \left(\frac{b_1 - b_2}{l}\right) \qquad \text{... Eq. (c)}$$

Area of the element, $\quad A = b \times t = (b_1 - kx) \times t \qquad \text{... Eq. (d)}$

Strain energy $\qquad U = \displaystyle\int_0^l \frac{F^2 dx}{2AE}$

$$= \int_0^l \frac{F^2 dx}{2E(b_1 - kx)t}$$

$$= \frac{F^2}{2tE} \int_0^l \frac{dx}{(b_1 - kx)} = \frac{F^2}{2tE}\left[\ln(b_1 - kx)\left(\frac{-1}{k}\right)\right]_0^l$$

$$= \frac{F^2}{2tEk}\left[-\ln(b_1 - kx)\right]_0^l$$

$$= \frac{F^2}{2tEk}\left\{-\ln\left[b_1 - \left(\frac{b_1 - b_2}{l}\right)x\right]\right\}_0^l \qquad \text{... using Eq. (c)}$$

$$= \frac{F^2}{2tEk}\left\{-\ln\left[b_1 - \left(\frac{b_1 - b_2}{l}\right)l\right] - \left[-\ln(b_1 - 0)\right]\right\}$$

$$= \frac{F^2}{2tEk}(-\ln b_2 + \ln b_1) = \frac{F^2}{2tEk}(\ln b_1 - \ln b_2)$$

$$U = \frac{F^2}{2tEk}\ln\left(\frac{b_1}{b_2}\right)$$

$$\therefore \quad U = \frac{F^2 l}{2tE(b_1 - b_2)}\ln\left(\frac{b_1}{b_2}\right) \qquad \text{... (Eq. 11.56), using Eq.(c)}$$

19. **A stepped bar is subjected to an external loading as shown in Fig. 11.24. Calculate the strain energy stored in the bar. Take $E = 200$ GPa for steel, $E = 70$ GPa for aluminum and $E = 100$ GPa for copper.**

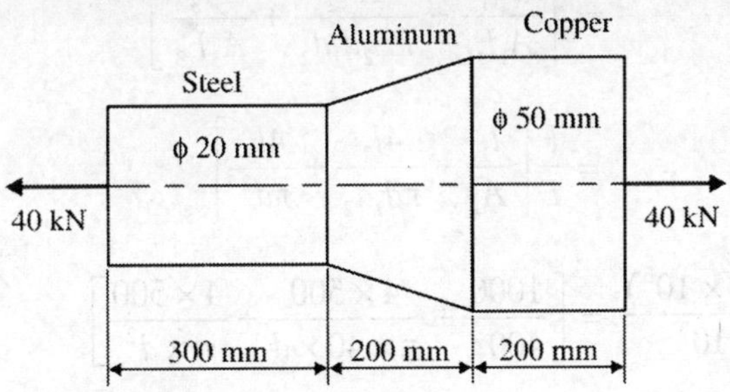

Fig. 11.24: Problem 19

Solution: *Let suffix '1' refers to steel, '2' refer to aluminum and '3' refer to copper materials respectively.*

$F = 40 \times 10^3$ N, $d_1 = 20$ mm, $l_1 = 300$ mm, $d_2 = d_3 = 50$ mm, $l_2 = l_3 = 200$ mm, $E_1 = 200 \times 10^3$ MPa, $E_2 = 70 \times 10^3$ MPa, $E_3 = 100 \times 10^3$ MPa. $U = ?$

We know that $\quad U = \sum \frac{F^2 l}{2AE} = \frac{F^2}{2E}\sum \frac{l}{A}$

$$= \left(\frac{F^2 l}{2AE}\right)_1 + \left(\frac{2F^2 l}{\pi E d_1 d_2}\right)_2 + \left(\frac{F^2 l}{2AE}\right)_3$$

$$= \frac{4F^2}{2\pi}\left[\frac{l_1}{E_1 d_1^2} + \frac{l_3}{E_3 d_3^2}\right] + \frac{2F^2 l_2}{\pi E_2 d_1 d_2} = \frac{2F^2}{\pi}\left[\frac{l_1}{E_1 d_1^2} + \frac{l_2}{E_2 d_1 d_2} + \frac{l_3}{E_3 d_3^2}\right]$$

$$= \frac{2 \times (40 \times 10^3)^2}{\pi}\left[\frac{300}{(200 \times 10^3) \times 20^2} + \frac{200}{(70 \times 10^3) \times 20 \times 50} + \frac{200}{(100 \times 10^3) \times 50^2}\right]$$

$\bigcup = 7544.85 \text{ N-mm} \approx 7.55 \text{ J}$

20. **A member is of total length 2 m its diameter is 40 mm for the first 1 m length. In the next 0.5 m length, its diameter gradually reduces from 40 mm to 'd' mm. For the remaining length of the member, the diameter remains 'd' mm uniform. When this member is subjected to axial tensile force of 150 kN, the total elongation observed is 2.39 mm. Determine the diameter 'd'. Assume $E = 2 \times 10^5 \text{ N/mm}^2$. Also find the strain energy stored.**

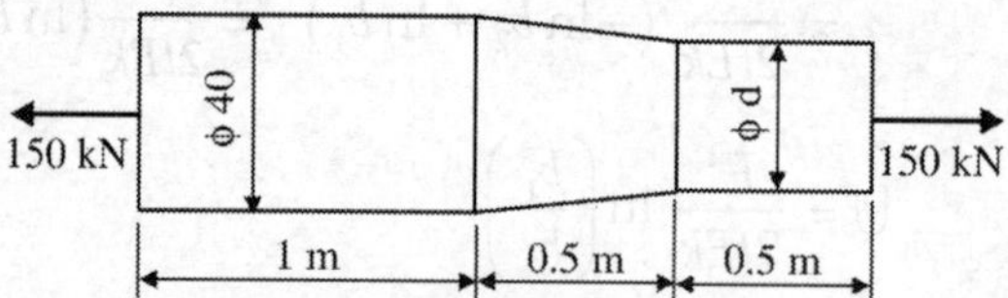

Fig. 11.25: Problem 20

Solution: Based on given data, the problem is represented in **Fig. 11.25**.

$d_1 = 40$ mm, $d_2 = d_3 = d$, $l_1 = 1000$ mm, $l_2 = 500$ mm, $l_3 = 500$ mm $\Delta = 2.39$ mm, $F = 150 \times 10^3$ N, $E = 2 \times 10^5 \text{ N/mm}^2$, $\bigcup = ?$

Total deformation, $\qquad \Delta = \delta l_1 + \delta l_2 + \delta l_3$

$$= \left[\frac{F l_1}{A_1 E_1} + \frac{4F l_2}{\pi E_2 d_1 d_2} + \frac{F l_3}{A_3 E_3}\right]$$

$$= \frac{F}{E}\left[\frac{l_1}{A_1} + \frac{4 l_2}{\pi d_1 d_2} + \frac{4 l_3}{\pi d^2}\right]$$

$$\frac{2.39 \times (2 \times 10^5)}{150 \times 10^3} = \left[\frac{1000}{400\pi} + \frac{4 \times 500}{\pi \times 40 \times d} + \frac{4 \times 500}{\pi \times d^2}\right]$$

$$3.186 = 0.7957 + \left[\frac{15.915}{d} + \frac{636.62}{d^2}\right]$$

$$2.3903 = \left[\frac{15.915}{d} + \frac{636.62}{d^2}\right]$$

$$2.3903 d^2 = 15.915\, d + 636.62$$

$$2.3903 d^2 - 15.915\, d - 636.62 = 0$$

$$\therefore \quad d = 19.98 \text{ mm} = d_2 = d_3 \approx 20 \text{ mm}$$

We know that $\quad U = \sum \dfrac{F^2 l}{2AE} = \dfrac{F^2}{2E}\sum \dfrac{l}{A}$

$$= \left(\dfrac{F^2 l}{2AE}\right)_1 + \left(\dfrac{2F^2 l}{\pi E d_1 d_2}\right)_2 + \left(\dfrac{F^2 l}{2AE}\right)_3$$

$$= \dfrac{4F^2}{2\pi}\left[\dfrac{l_1}{d_1^2} + \dfrac{l_3}{d_3^2}\right] + \dfrac{2F^2 l_2}{\pi E d_1 d_2} = \dfrac{2F^2}{\pi E}\left[\dfrac{l_1}{d_1^2} + \dfrac{l_2}{d_1 d_2} + \dfrac{l_3}{d_3^2}\right]$$

$$= \dfrac{2 \times (150 \times 10^3)^2}{\pi \times (2 \times 10^5)}\left[\dfrac{1000}{40^2} + \dfrac{500}{40 \times 20} + \dfrac{500}{20^2}\right]$$

$$U = 179.05 \times 10^3 \text{ N-mm} = 179.05 \text{ J}$$

11.10.4 Problems on axial load: Superposition

21. A steel bar of cross section 500 mm^2 is acted upon by forces shown in Fig. 11.26. Determine the total strain energy in the bar. Take $E = 200$ GPa.

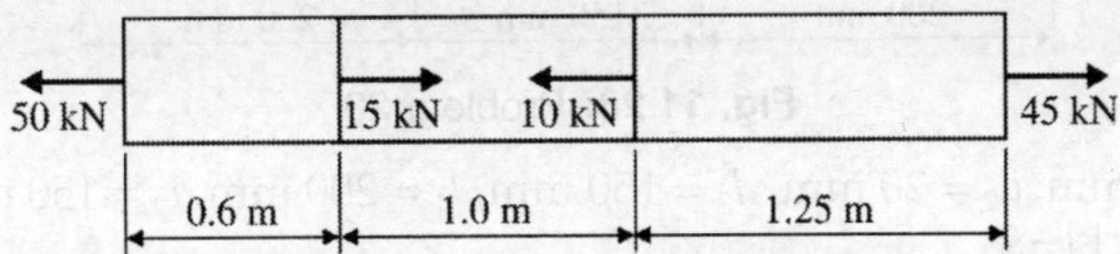

Fig. 11.26: Problem 21

Solution: $A = A_1 = A_2 = A_3 = 500$ mm^2, $l_1 = 600$ mm, $l_2 = 1000$ mm, $l_3 = 1250$ mm, $E = 105 \times 10^3$ N/mm^2, $U = ?$

Based on analysis, $\quad F_1 = 50$ kN, $F_2 = 35$ kN, $F_3 = 45$ kN

We know that $\qquad U = \sum \dfrac{F^2 l}{2AE} = \dfrac{1}{2AE}\left[F_1^2 l_1 + F_2^2 l_2 + F_3^2 l_3\right]$

$$= \dfrac{1}{2 \times 500 \times (2 \times 10^5)}\left[(50 \times 10^3)^2 \times 600 + (35 \times 10^3)^2\right.$$

$$\left. \times 1000 + (45 \times 10^3)^2 \times 1250\right]$$

$$U = 26.28 \times 10^3 \text{ N-mm} = 26.28 \text{ J}$$

22. A brass bar of uniform cross sectional area 300 mm^2 is subjected to a load as shown in Fig. 11.27. Find the total strain energy in the bar and the magnitude of load P if Young's modulus is 84 GPa.

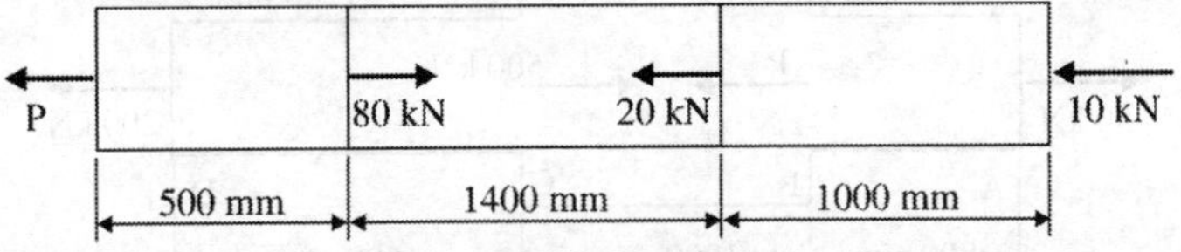

Fig. 11.27: Problem 22

Solution: $A = A_1 = A_2 = A_3 = 300$ mm^2, $l_1 = 500$ mm, $l_2 = 1400$ mm, $l_3 = 1000$ mm, $E = 84 \times 10^3$ N/mm^2, $U = ?$,

For equilibrium, $P + 20 + 10 = 80 \Rightarrow P = 50$ kN

Based on analysis, $F_1 = 50$ kN, $F_2 = -30$ kN, $F_3 = -10$ kN

We know that $U = \sum \dfrac{F^2 l}{2AE} = \dfrac{1}{2AE}\left[F_1^2 l_1 + F_2^2 l_2 + F_3^2 l_3\right]$

$$= \frac{1}{2 \times 300 \times (84 \times 10^3)}\,[(50 \times 10^3)^2 \times 500 + (-30 \times 10^3)^2$$

$$\times 1400 + (-10 \times 10^3)^2 \times 1000]$$

$$U = 51.79 \times 10^3 \text{ N-mm} = 51.79 \text{ J}$$

23. Determine the total strain energy in a circular bar of varying cross-section subjected to forces as shown in Fig. 11.28. Take $E = 210$ kN/mm^2.

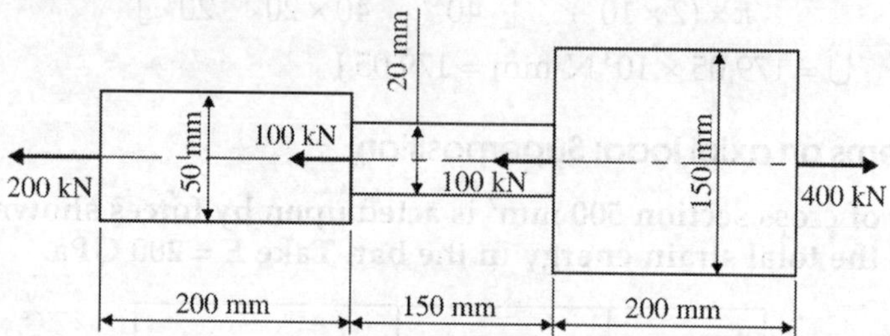

Fig. 11.28: Problem 23

Solution: $d_1 = 50$ mm, $d_2 = 20$ mm, $d_3 = 150$ mm, $l_1 = 200$ mm, $l_2 = 150$ mm, $l_3 = 200$ mm, $E = 210 \times 10^3$ MPa, $U = ?$

Based on analysis, $F_1 = 200$ kN, $F_2 = 300$ kN, $F_3 = 400$ kN

We know that $U = \sum \dfrac{F^2 l}{2AE} = \dfrac{1}{2E}\sum \dfrac{F^2 l}{A}$

$$= \frac{4}{2\pi E}\left[\frac{F_1^2 l_1}{d_1^2} + \frac{F_2^2 l_2}{d_2^2} + \frac{F_3^2 l_3}{d_3^2}\right] = \frac{2}{\pi E}\left[\frac{F_1^2 l_1}{d_1^2} + \frac{F_2^2 l_2}{d_2^2} + \frac{F_3^2 l_3}{d_3^2}\right]$$

$$= \frac{2}{\pi \times (210 \times 10^3)}\left[\frac{(200 \times 10^3)^2 \times 200}{50^2} + \frac{(300 \times 10^3)^2 \times 150}{20^2} + \frac{(400 \times 10^3)^2 \times 200}{150^2}\right]$$

$$U = 116.33 \times 10^3 \text{ N-mm} = 116.33 \text{ J}$$

24. A member ABCD is subjected to loads as shown in Fig. 11.29. Calculate the total strain energy in the bar. Take $E = 210$ GN/m^2.

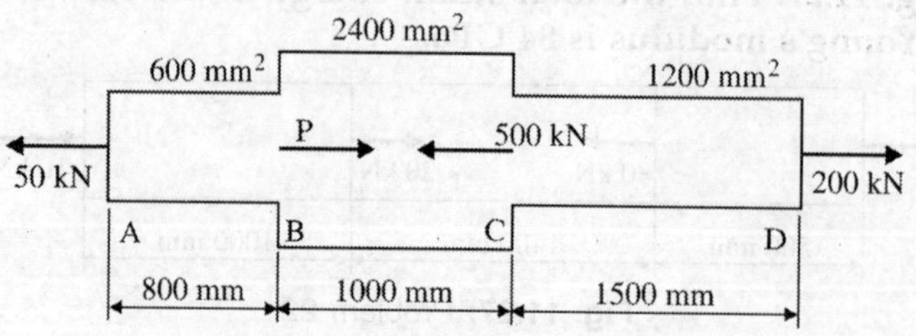

Fig. 11.29: Problem 24

Solution: $A_1 = 600$ mm^2, $A_2 = 2400$ mm^2, $A_3 = 1200$ mm^2, $l_1 = 800$ mm, $l_2 = 1000$ mm, $l_3 = 1500$ mm, $E = 210 \times 10^3$ N/mm^2, $U = ?$

For equilibrium, $50 + 500 = P + 200 \Rightarrow P = 350$ kN

Based on analysis, $F_1 = 50$ kN, $F_2 = -300$ kN, $F_3 = 200$ kN

We know that
$$U = \sum \frac{F^2 l}{2AE} = \frac{1}{2E} \sum \frac{F^2 l}{A}$$

$$= \frac{1}{2E}\left[\frac{F_1^2 l_1}{A_1} + \frac{F_2^2 l_2}{A_2} + \frac{F_3^2 l_3}{A_3} \right]$$

$$= \frac{1}{2 \times (210 \times 10^3)}\left[\frac{(50 \times 10^3)^2 \times 800}{600} + \frac{(-300 \times 10^3)^2 \times 1000}{2400} + \frac{(200 \times 10^3)^2 \times 1500}{1200} \right]$$

$$U = 216.27 \times 10^3 \text{ N-mm} = 216.27 \text{ J}$$

11.10.5 Problems on axial load: Determinate bars

25. Find the expression for strain energy stored in a bar as shown in Fig. 11.30. The bar has constant axial rigidity of *EA*.

Solution: $A = A_1 = A_2 = A_3, l = l_1 = l_2 = l_3 = l/3 , U = ?$, axial rigidity $= EA$

Let $R =$ be the reaction at the fixed end

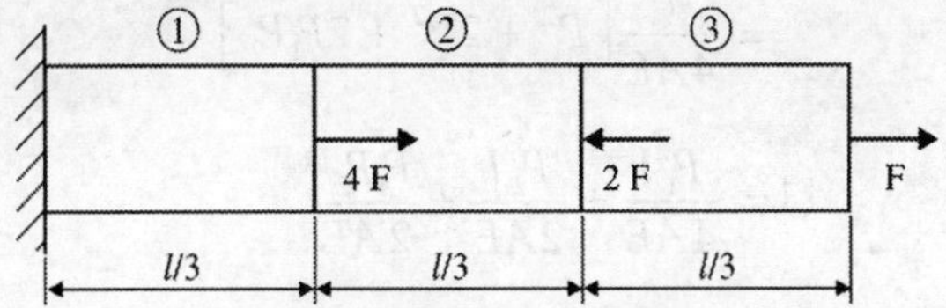

Fig. 11.30: Problem 25

Based on analysis, $F_1 = R = 3F, F_2 = -F, F_3 = F$

We know that
$$U = \sum \frac{F^2 l}{2AE} = \frac{1}{2AE}\left[F_1^2 + F_2^2 + F_3^2 \right]$$

$$= \frac{l/3}{2AE}\left[(3F)^2 + (-F)^2 + F^2 \right]$$

$$U = \frac{11 F^2 l}{6AE}$$

26. Fig. 11.31 represents a bar acted upon by two loads. If the bar has constant axial rigidity of *EA*. Determine the strain energy in the bar, if
(a) Force P_1 acts alone
(b) Force P_2 acts alone
(c) Force P_1 and P_2 acts simultaneously.

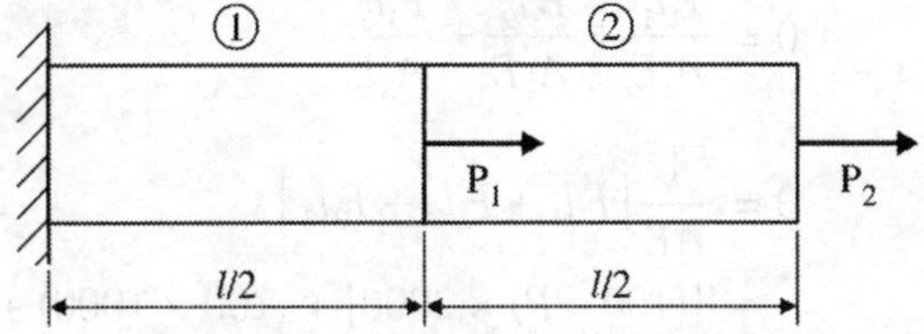

Fig. 11.31: Problem 26

Solution: $l = l_1 = l_2 = l/2$, axial rigidity $= EA$, $\mathsf{U} = ?$

a. *Strain energy due to P_1 alone:*

We know that $$\mathsf{U}_1 = \frac{F^2 l}{2AE} = \frac{P_1^2 (l/2)}{2AE} = \frac{P_1^2 l}{4AE}$$

b. *Strain energy due to P_2 alone:*

We know that $$\mathsf{U}_2 = \frac{F^2 l}{2AE} = \frac{P_1^2 (l/2 + l/2)}{2AE} = \frac{P_2^2 l}{2AE}$$

c. *Strain energy due to P_1 and P_2:*

Let $R =$ be the reaction at the fixed end

Based on analysis, $F_1 = R = P_1 + P_2$, $F_2 = P_2$

We know that

$$\mathsf{U} = \sum \frac{F^2 l}{2AE} = \frac{l}{2AE}\left[F_1^2 + F_2^2 \right]$$

$$= \frac{l/2}{2AE}\left[(P_1 + P_2)^2 + (P_2)^2 \right] = \frac{l}{4AE}\left[P_1^2 + P_2^2 + 2P_1 P_2 + P_2^2 \right]$$

$$= \frac{l}{4AE}\left[P_1^2 + 2P_2^2 + 2P_1 P_2 \right]$$

$$\mathsf{U} = \frac{P_1^2 l}{4AE} + \frac{P_2^2 l}{2AE} + \frac{P_1 P_2 l}{2AE}$$

27. **Determine the magnitude of load P necessary to produce no change in length of the bar shown in Fig. 11.32. Given c/s area $= 400$ mm^2 and $E = 2 \times 10^5$ MPa. Also find total strain energy in the member.**

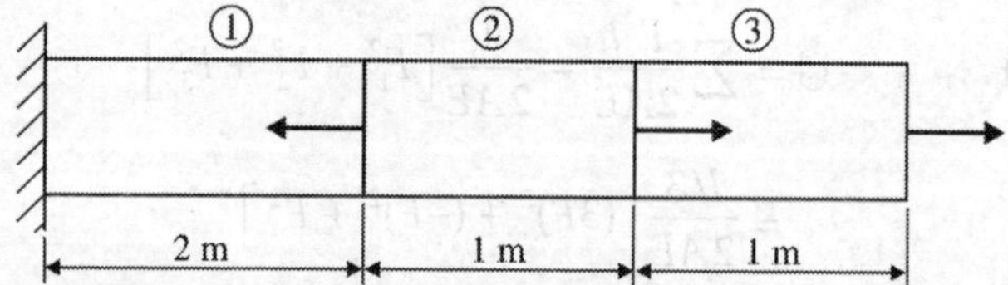

Fig. 11.32: Problem 27

Solution: $A = A_1 = A_2 = A_3 = 400$ mm^2, $l_1 = 2000$ mm, $l_2 = 1000$ mm, $l_3 = 1000$ mm, $E = 2 \times 10^5$ MPa, $\Delta = 0$, a) $P = ?$, b) $\mathsf{U} = ?$

Let $R =$ be the reaction at the fixed end

Based on analysis, $F_1 = R = (100 - P)$, $F_2 = 100$ kN, $F_3 = 40$ kN

a. *To find P:*

Total deformation, $\Delta = \delta l_1 + \delta l_2 + \delta l_3$

$$0 = \frac{F_1 l_1}{A_1 E} + \frac{F_2 l_2}{A_2 E} + \frac{F_3 l_3}{A_3 E}$$

$$0 = \frac{1}{AE}\left[F_1 l_1 + F_2 l_2 + F_3 l_3 \right]$$

$$= \{[(100 - P) \times 2000] + (100 \times 1000) + (40 \times 1000)\}$$

$$(P - 100) \times 2000 = 140000$$

$$\therefore \quad P = 170 \text{ kN}$$

Thus $F_1 = R = 100 - 170 = -70$ kN, $F_2 = 100$ kN, $F_3 = 40$ kN

b. *To find* U:

We know that
$$\mathsf{U} = \sum \frac{F^2 l}{2AE} = \frac{1}{2AE}\left[F_1^2 l_1 + F_2^2 l_2 + F_3^2 l_3\right]$$

$$= \frac{1}{2 \times 400 \times (2 \times 10^5)}\,[(-70 \times 10^3)^2 \times 2000 + (100 \times 10^3)^2$$

$$\times 1000 + (40 \times 10^3)^2 \times 1000]$$

$$\mathsf{U} = 133.75 \times 10^3 \text{ N-mm} = 133.75 \text{ J}$$

28. **Determine the total strain energy in a stepped bar as shown in Fig. 11.33. The bar is 20 mm in diameter for 200 mm length, 40 mm in diameter for 400 mm length and 60 mm in diameter for 350 mm. Take E = 200 GPa.**

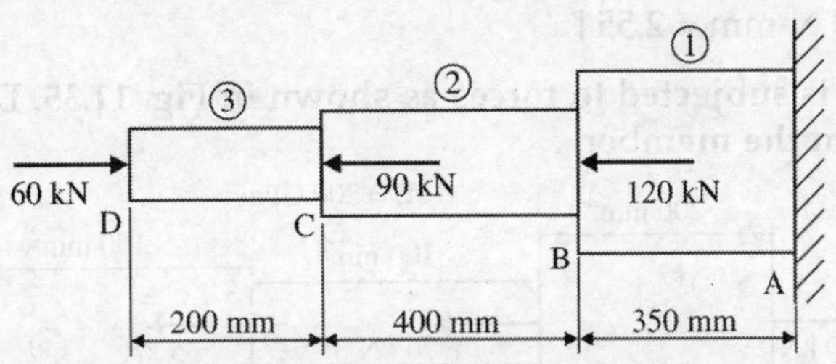

Fig. 11.33: Problem 28

Solution: d_1 = 60 mm, l_1 = 350 mm, d_2 = 40 mm, l_2 = 400 mm, d_3 = 20 mm, l_3 = 200 mm, $E = 200 \times 10^3$ N/mm^2. U = ?

Let R = be the reaction at the fixed end

Based on analysis, $F_1 = R$ = 150 kN, F_2 = 30 kN, $F_3 = -60$ kN

To find U:

We know that
$$\mathsf{U} = \sum \frac{F^2 l}{2AE} = \frac{1}{2E} \sum \frac{F^2 l}{A}$$

$$= \frac{4}{2\pi E}\left[\frac{F_1^2 l_1}{d_1^2} + \frac{F_2^2 l_2}{d_2^2} + \frac{F_3^2 l_3}{d_3^2}\right] = \frac{2}{\pi E}\left[\frac{F_1^2 l_1}{d_1^2} + \frac{F_2^2 l_2}{d_2^2} + \frac{F_3^2 l_3}{d_3^2}\right]$$

$$= \frac{2}{\pi \times (200 \times 10^3)}\left[\frac{(150 \times 10^3)^2 \times 350}{60^2} + \frac{(30 \times 10^3)^2 \times 400}{40^2} + \frac{(-60 \times 10^3)^2 \times 200}{40^2}\right]$$

$$\mathsf{U} = 13.41 \times 10^3 \text{ N-mm} = 13.41 \text{ J}$$

29. **A stepped bar is subjected to forces as shown in Fig. 11.34. Determine the total strain energy in the stepped bar. Take $E = 2 \times 10^5$ N/mm^2.**

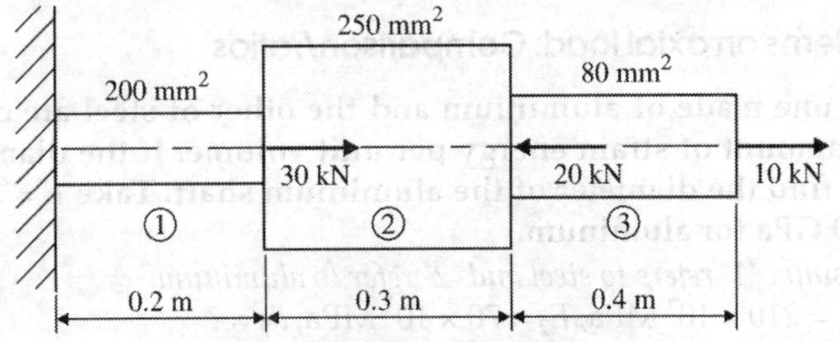

Fig. 11.34: Problem 29

Solution: A_1 = 200 mm^2, l_1 = 200 mm, A_2 = 250 mm^2, l_2 = 300 mm, A_3 = 80 mm^2, l_3 = 400 mm, $E = 2 \times 10^5$ N/mm^2, U = ?

Let R = be the reaction at the fixed end
Based on analysis, $F_1 = R = 20$ kN, $F_2 = -10$ kN, $F_3 = 10$ kN

We know that
$$U = \sum \frac{F^2 l}{2AE} = \frac{1}{2E} \sum \frac{F^2 l}{A}$$

$$= \frac{1}{2E}\left[\frac{F_1^2 l_1}{A_1} + \frac{F_2^2 l_2}{A_2} + \frac{F_3^2 l_3}{A_3} \right]$$

$$= \frac{1}{2 \times (2 \times 10^5)}\left[\frac{(20 \times 10^3)^2 \times 200}{200} + \frac{(-10 \times 10^3)^2 \times 300}{250} + \frac{(10 \times 10^3)^2 \times 400}{80} \right]$$

$$U = 2550 \text{ N-mm} = 2.55 \text{ J}$$

30. **A stepped bar is subjected to forces as shown in Fig. 11.35. Determine the total strain energy in the member.**

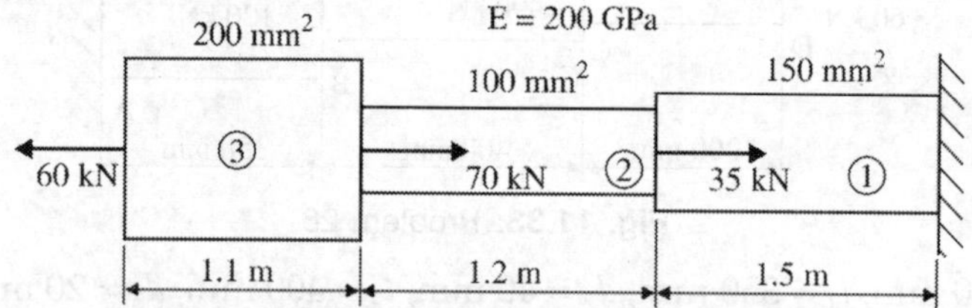

Fig. 11.35: Problems 30

Solution: $A_1 = 150$ mm², $l_1 = 1500$ mm, $A_2 = 100$ mm², $l_2 = 1200$ mm, $A_3 = 200$ mm², $l = 1100$ mm, $E = 2 \times 10^5$ N/mm².$U = ?$

Let R = be the reaction at the fixed end
Based on analysis, $F_1 = R = -45$ kN, $F_2 = -10$ kN, $F_3 = 60$ kN

We know that
$$U = \sum \frac{F^2 l}{2AE} = \frac{1}{2E} \sum \frac{F^2 l}{A}$$

$$= \frac{1}{2E}\left[\frac{F_1^2 l_1}{A_1} + \frac{F_2^2 l_2}{A_2} + \frac{F_3^2 l_3}{A_3} \right]$$

$$= \frac{1}{2 \times (2 \times 10^5)}\left[\frac{(-45 \times 10^3)^2 \times 1500}{150} + \frac{(-10 \times 10^3)^2 \times 1200}{100} + \frac{(60 \times 10^3)^2 \times 1100}{200} \right]$$

$$U = 103125 \text{ N-mm} = 103.125 \text{ J}$$

11.10.6 Problems on axial load: Comparison/ratios

31. **Two rods one made of aluminium and the other of steel are designed to store the same amount of strain energy per unit volume. If the diameter of steel rod is 60 mm, find the diameter of the aluminium shaft. Take $E = 210$ GPa for steel and $E = 70$ GPa for aluminum.**

Solution: *Let suffix '1' refers to steel and '2' refer to aluminum*
$d_1 = 60$ mm, $E_1 = 210 \times 10^3$ MPa, $E_2 = 70 \times 10^3$ MPa, $d_2 = ?$

Strain energy per unit volume, $u = \dfrac{\sigma^2}{2E} = \dfrac{F^2}{2A^2 E}$

Since the amount of strain energy per unit volume is same in both the rods, we have

$$u_1 = u_2$$

$$\left(\frac{F^2}{2A^2E}\right)_1 = \left(\frac{F^2}{2A^2E}\right)_2$$

$$\frac{1}{A_1^2 E_1} = \frac{1}{A_2^2 E_2}$$

$$\frac{1}{(\pi \times 60^2/4)^2 \times 210 \times 10^3} = \frac{1}{(\pi \times d_2^2/4)^2 \times 70 \times 10^3}$$

$$5.96 \times 10^{-13} = \frac{2.32 \times 10^{-5}}{d_2^4}$$

$$\therefore \quad d_2 = 78.95 \text{ mm}$$

32. Two elastic bars of the same material and length, one of circular section having a diameter of 100 mm and the other of square section, 100 mm side absorbs the same amount of strain energy delivered by axial forces. Compare the stresses in the two bars.

Solution: *Let suffix '1' refers to circular cross-section and '2' refer to square cross-section.*

Diameter $d = 100$ mm, side of square $= b = 100$ mm, $\sigma_1/\sigma_2 = ?$

Since the amount of strain energy is same in both the rods, we have

$$U_1 = U_2$$

$$\left(\frac{F^2}{2AE}\right)_1 = \left(\frac{F^2}{2AE}\right)_2$$

Cancelling the common terms, we have

$$\frac{F_1^2}{A_1} = \frac{F_2^2}{A_2}$$

$$\sigma_1^2 A_1 = \sigma_2^2 A_2$$

$$\frac{\sigma_1}{\sigma_2} = \sqrt{\frac{A_2}{A_1}} = \sqrt{\frac{100 \times 100}{(\pi \times 100^2/4)}} = \sqrt{\frac{4}{\pi}}$$

$$\therefore \quad \frac{\sigma_1}{\sigma_2} = 1.128$$

33. Compare the strain energies of two bars of the same material and length and carrying the same gradually applied compressive load if one is 25 mm diameter throughout and the other is turned down to 20 mm diameter over half its length, the remainder being 25 mm diameter.

Solution: $F_1 = F_2$, $U_1/U_2 = ?$

Case 1: Uniform bar: diameter $d = 25$ mm, length $= l$

Case 2: Stepped bar: diameter $d_1 = 25$ mm, $d_2 = 20$ mm, $l_1 = l_2 = l/2$.

For uniform bar:

Strain energy $\qquad U_1 = \dfrac{F^2 l}{2AE} = \dfrac{F^2 l}{2E \times (\pi \times 25^2/4)} = \dfrac{2F^2 l}{625\pi E}$

For Stepped bar:

Strain energy
$$U_2 = \sum \frac{F^2 l}{2AE} = \frac{F^2}{2E} \sum \frac{l}{A}$$

$$= \frac{F^2}{2E}\left[\frac{(l/2)}{(\pi \times 25^2/4)} + \frac{(l/2)}{(\pi \times 20^2/4)}\right] = \frac{F^2 l}{\pi E}\left[\frac{1}{625} + \frac{1}{400}\right]$$

$$U_2 = \frac{0.0041 F^2 l}{\pi E}$$

Ratio of strain energies, $\dfrac{U_1}{U_2} = \dfrac{2F^2 l/625\pi E}{0.0041 F^2 l/\pi E} = 0.78$

34. Two similar bars A and B are as shown in Fig. 11.36. Bar A receives an axial blow which produces a maximum stress of 200 MPa. Find the maximum stress produced by the same blow on bar B. If the bar is stressed to 200 MPa, determine the ratio of strain energy stored by the bars A and B.

Solution: $F_1 = F_2$, $\sigma_A = \sigma_{A1} = 200$ MPa, a) $\sigma_B = ?$, b) U_A/U_B = ?, if $\sigma_A = \sigma_B = 200$ MPa

Case 1 [Fig. 11.36(a)]: $d_1 = 20$ mm, $d_2 = 40$ mm, $l_1 = 100$ mm, $l_2 = 200$ mm, $\sigma_A = 200$ MPa,

Case 2 [Fig. 11.36(b)]: $d_1 = 20$ mm, $d_2 = 40$ mm, $l_1 = 200$ mm, $l_2 = 100$ mm

a. *Maximum stress in bar B:*

Case A: As per given data maximum stress occurs in 20 mm diameter of bar A. i.e. $\sigma_{A1} = 200$ MPa.

Since F is same, we have $F_{A1} = F_{A2}$

Therefore stress in 40 mm diameter portion **[Fig. 11.36(a)]** is found as
$$\sigma_{A1} A_1 = \sigma_{A2} A_2$$
$$\sigma_{A1} \times (\pi \times 20^2/4) = \sigma_{A2} \times (\pi \times 40^2/4)$$

$$\sigma_{A2} = 50 \text{ MPa} = \frac{\sigma_{A1}}{4} \qquad\qquad \ldots \text{Eq. (i)}$$

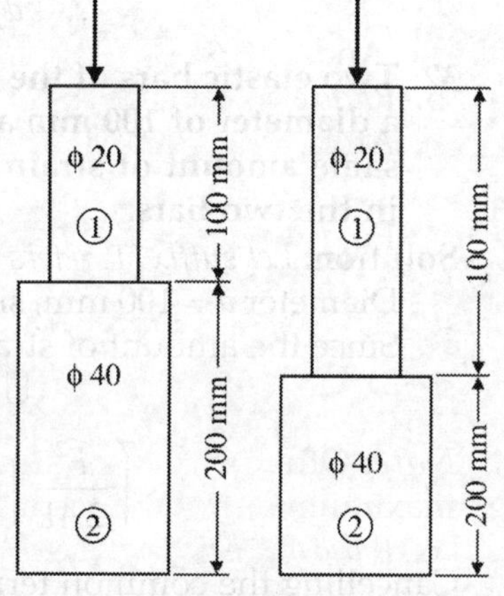

Fig. 11.36: Problem 34

Strain energy
$$U_A = \sum \frac{F^2 l}{2AE} = \sum \frac{\sigma^2 Al}{2E} = \frac{1}{2E}\Sigma(\sigma^2 Al)$$

$$= \frac{\pi}{8E}\left[\left(200^2 \times 20^2 \times 100\right) + \left(50^2 \times 40^2 \times 200\right)\right]$$

$$U_A = \frac{(300 \times 10^6)\pi}{E} \qquad\qquad \ldots \text{Eq. (ii)}$$

Case B: On similar lines to Eq. (i), we have

$$\sigma_{B2} = \frac{\sigma_{B1}}{4} \qquad\qquad \ldots \text{Eq. (iii)}$$

Strain energy $\qquad U_B = \sum \dfrac{F^2 L}{2AE} = \sum \dfrac{\sigma^2 Al}{2E} = \dfrac{1}{2E} \Sigma(\sigma^2 Al)$

$$= \dfrac{\pi}{8E} \left[\left(\sigma_{B1}^2 \times 20^2 \times 200\right) + \left(\sigma_{B1}/4\right)^2 \times 40^2 \times 100 \right]$$

$$\dots \text{using Eq. (iii)}$$

$$U_B = \dfrac{(11250) \times \sigma_{B1}^2 \pi}{E} \qquad\qquad \dots \text{Eq. (iv)}$$

Since blow on both bars are same (data), we have

$$U_A = U_B$$

$$\dfrac{(300 \times 10^6)\pi}{E} = \dfrac{(11250) \times \sigma_{B1}^2 \pi}{E}$$

$$\sigma_{B1} = 163.30 \text{ MPa} = \sigma_B$$

And $\qquad\qquad \sigma_{B2} = 163.30/4 = 40.83 \text{ MPa} \qquad\qquad \dots \text{using Eq. (i)}$

b. *Ratio of strain energies:*

At $\sigma_A = \sigma_B = 200 \text{ MPa}$,

Eq. (iv) yields... $\qquad U_B = \dfrac{(11250) \times 200^2 \times \pi}{E} = \dfrac{(450 \times 10^6)\pi}{E} \qquad \dots \text{Eq. (v)}$

$$\therefore \quad \dfrac{U_A}{U_B} = \dfrac{(300 \times 10^6)\pi/E}{(450 \times 10^6)\pi/E} = 0.667$$

Note: Other format of strain energy ratio is "find the ratio of strain enrgies if the maximum stress is same in both the cases"

c. *Ratio of strain energies per unit volume:*

Volume of bar A, $V_A = \Sigma(Al) = \dfrac{\pi}{4} \left[(20^2 \times 100) + (40^2 \times 200) \right] = 90000\,\pi \text{ mm}^3$

Volume of bar B, $V_B = \Sigma(Al) = \dfrac{\pi}{4} (20^2 \times 200) + (40^2 \times 100) = 60000\,\pi \text{ mm}^3$

For bar A $\qquad\qquad u_A = \dfrac{U_A}{V_A} = \dfrac{(300 \times 10^6)\pi/E}{90000\,\pi} = 3333.34/E$

For bar B $\qquad\qquad u_B = \dfrac{U_B}{V_B} = \dfrac{(450 \times 10^6)\pi/E}{60000\,\pi} = 7500/E$

$$\therefore \quad \dfrac{u_A}{u_B} = \dfrac{3333.34/E}{7500/E} = 0.44$$

35. **Two bars each of length *l* and of different material are each subjected to the same axial tensile force. The first bar has a uniform diameter of *d*. The second bar has a diameter of *d*/2 for a length of *l*/4 and a diameter *d* for the remaining length as shown in Fig. 11.37 (a) & (b).**
    (a) Compare the strain energies of the two bars.
    (b) Compare the amount of strain energy which the two bars can absorb in simple tension within the limits of proportionality, without exceeding a given stress or "find the ratio of strain energies if the maximum stress is same in both the cases"

(c) Compare the strain energy per unit volume if the maximum stress is to be same in both the cases.

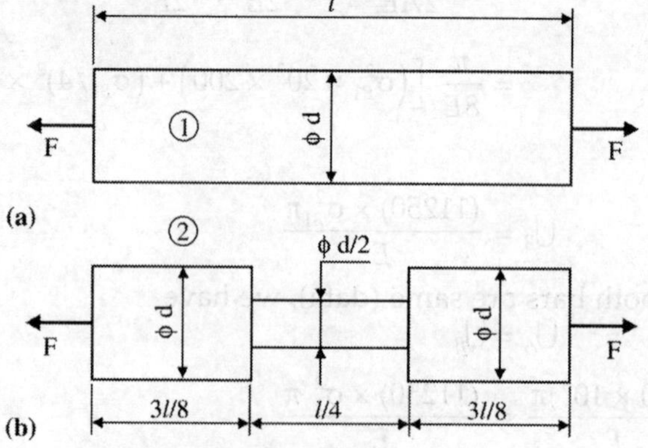

Fig. 11.37: Problem 35

Solution: *Let suffix '1' refers to uniform bar and '2' refer to stepped bar.* $F_1 = F_2$, a) U_1/U_2 = ? b) U_1/U_2 = ?, if $\sigma_A = \sigma_B$; c) u_1/u_2 = ?, if $\sigma_A = \sigma_B$

Case 1 [Fig. 11.37(a)]: Uniform rod: Diameter = d, length = l, Young's modulus = E_1.

Case 2 [Fig. 11.37(b)]: Stepped rod: Diameter $d_1 = d_3 = d$, $d_2 = 0.5d$, $l_1 = l_3 = 3l/8$, $l_2 = l/4$, Young's modulus = E_2

a. *Ratio of strain energies:*

For uniform bar:

Strain energy $\quad U_1 = \dfrac{F^2l}{2AE_1} = \dfrac{F^2l}{2E_1 \times (\pi \times d^2/4)} = \dfrac{2F^2l}{\pi E_1 d^2}$ ... Eq. (i)

For Stepped bar:

Strain energy $\quad U_2 = \sum \dfrac{F^2l}{2AE_2} = \dfrac{F^2}{2E_2} \sum \dfrac{l}{A}$

$$= \dfrac{2F^2}{\pi E_2}\left[\dfrac{(3l/8)}{d^2} + \dfrac{l/4}{(0.5d)^2} + \dfrac{(3l/8)}{d^2} \right]$$

$$= \dfrac{2F^2}{\pi E_2}\left[\dfrac{3l}{8d^2} + \dfrac{l}{d^2} + \dfrac{3l}{8d^2} \right]$$

$$U_2 = \dfrac{3.5F^2l}{\pi E_2 d^2} \qquad \text{... Eq. (ii)}$$

$$\therefore \quad \dfrac{U_1}{U_2} = \dfrac{2F^2l}{\pi E_1 d^2} \bigg/ \dfrac{3.5F^2l}{\pi E_2 d^2} = \dfrac{2/E_1}{3.5/E_2}$$

$$\therefore \quad \dfrac{U_1}{U_2} = \dfrac{2E_2}{3.5E_1} \qquad \text{... Eq. (iii)}$$

Multiplying and dividing with '2', we have

$$\dfrac{U_1}{U_2} = \dfrac{4E_2}{7E_1} \qquad \text{... Eq. (iv)}$$

If $E_1 = E_2,$ $\qquad \dfrac{U_1}{U_2} = 4/7$ $\qquad\qquad$ ... Eq. (v)

b. *Ratio of strain energies, if* $\sigma_A = \sigma_B$:

Stress in uniform bar $\qquad \sigma_A = \dfrac{4F}{\pi d^2}$

Stress in stepped bar $\qquad \sigma_{B2} = \dfrac{F}{A_{B2}} = \dfrac{16F}{\pi d^2}$

$\qquad\qquad$ [Maximum stress occurs in the section where the area is minimum]
Since the stress is same in both bars, we have

$$\sigma_A = \sigma_{B1} \qquad\qquad (\sigma_{B1} = \sigma_B)$$

$$\left(\dfrac{4F}{\pi d^2}\right)_A = \left(\dfrac{16F}{\pi d^2}\right)_B \qquad\qquad \text{... Eq. (vi)}$$

$$F_A = 4F_B$$

Hence replacing F with $4F$ in Eq. (i), we have

$$U_1 = \dfrac{32F^2 l}{\pi E_1 d^2} \qquad\qquad \text{... Eq. (vii)}$$

and $\qquad U_2 = \dfrac{3.5F^2 l}{\pi E_2 d^2}$ $\qquad$ ... same as before, using Eq. (ii)

$$\therefore \quad \dfrac{U_1}{U_2} = \dfrac{32F^2 l}{\pi E_1 d^2} \Big/ \dfrac{3.5F^2 l}{\pi E_2 d^2} = \dfrac{32/E_1}{3.5/E_2}$$

$$\therefore \quad \dfrac{U_1}{U_2} = (32 E_2)/(3.5 E_1) \qquad\qquad \text{... Eq. (viii)}$$

Multiplying and dividing with '2', we have

$$\dfrac{U_1}{U_2} = \dfrac{64 E_2}{7 E_1} \qquad\qquad \text{... Eq. (ix)}$$

If $E_1 = E$ $\qquad \dfrac{U_1}{U_2} = 64/7$ $\qquad\qquad$ ... Eq. (x)

c. Ratio of strain energies per unit volume, if $\sigma_A = \sigma_B$:

Volume of bar A, $\qquad V_A = \left(\dfrac{\pi d^2}{4}\right) l$

Volume of bar B, $\qquad V_B = \Sigma(Al) = \left(\dfrac{\pi d^2}{4}\right)\left(\dfrac{3l}{8}\right) + \left[\dfrac{\pi (d/2)^2}{4}\right]\left(\dfrac{l}{4}\right) + \left(\dfrac{\pi d^2}{4}\right)\left(\dfrac{3l}{8}\right)$

$$= \left(\dfrac{\pi d^2}{4}\right)\left[\left(\dfrac{3l}{8}\right) + \left(\dfrac{l}{16}\right) + \left(\dfrac{3l}{8}\right)\right]$$

$$= \left(\frac{\pi d^2}{4}\right)\left[\left(\frac{3l}{4}\right)+\left(\frac{l}{16}\right)\right]$$

$$V_B = \left(\frac{\pi d^2}{4}\right)\left(\frac{13l}{16}\right)$$

For bar A

$$u_A = \frac{U_A}{V_A} = \frac{32F^2 l/\pi E_1 d^2}{\pi d^2 l/4} = \frac{128F^2}{\pi^2 d^4 E_1} = \frac{128F^2}{\pi^2 d^4 E_1}$$

For bar B

$$u_B = \frac{U_B}{V_B} = \frac{3.5F^2 l/\pi E_2 d^2}{\left(\dfrac{\pi d^2}{4}\right)\left(\dfrac{13l}{16}\right)} = \frac{224F^2}{13\pi^2 d^4 E_2}$$

$$\therefore \quad \frac{u_A}{u_B} = \frac{128F^2}{\pi^2 d^4 E_1} \bigg/ \frac{224F^2}{13\,\pi^2 d^4 E_2}$$

$$\therefore \quad \frac{u_A}{u_B} = \frac{52E_2}{7E_1} \qquad\qquad \text{... Eq. (xi)}$$

If $E_1 = E_2$,

$$\frac{u_A}{u_B} = \frac{52}{7} \qquad\qquad \text{... Eq. (xii)}$$

11.10.7 Problems on axial load: Due to falling weight or load

36. An unknown weight falls through 10 mm on a collar rigidly attached to the lower end of a bar 3 m long and 600 mm² in section. If the maximum instantaneous extension is 2 mm, what are the corresponding stress and the value of unknown weight? Take $E = 200$ GPa.

Solution: $h = 10$ mm, $l = 3000$ mm, $A = 600$ mm², $\delta' = 2$ mm, impact stress $\sigma' = ?$, $F = ?$, $E = 2 \times 10^5$ MPa

To find σ':

Instantaneous deflection, $\delta l' = \dfrac{\sigma' l}{E}$

$$2 = \frac{\sigma' \times 3000}{2 \times 10^5}$$

$$\therefore \quad \sigma' = 133.34 \text{ MPa}$$

To find F:

We know that

$$\sigma' = \left(\frac{F}{A}\right)\left[1 + \sqrt{1 + \left(\frac{2AEh}{Fl}\right)}\right]$$

$$133.34 = \left(\frac{F}{600}\right)\left[1 + \sqrt{1 + \frac{2 \times 600 \times (2 \times 10^5) \times 10}{F \times 3000}}\right]$$

$$\frac{80 \times 10^3}{F} = 1 + \sqrt{1 + \left(\frac{8 \times 10^5}{F}\right)}$$

$$\frac{80 \times 10^3}{F} - 1 = \sqrt{1 + \left(\frac{8 \times 10^5}{F}\right)}$$

Squaring both sides, we have

$$\left(\frac{80 \times 10^3}{F} - 1\right)^2 = 1 + \left(\frac{8 \times 10^5}{F}\right)$$

$$\frac{6400 \times 10^6}{F^2} + 1 - \frac{160 \times 10^3}{F} = 1 + \left(\frac{8 \times 10^5}{F}\right)$$

$$\frac{6400 \times 10^6}{F^2} = \left(\frac{960 \times 10^3}{F}\right)$$

$$\therefore \quad F = 6.67 \text{ kN}$$

37. A rectangular bar 200 mm long is subjected to an impact load of 2 kN that falls from a height of 20 mm. Determine the dimensions of the bar if the allowable stress is 125 MPa. Assume the thickness as twice the width. Take E = 200 GPa.
Solution: l = 200 mm, impact load F = 2000 N, h = 20 mm, dimensions b, t = ?, if $t = 2b$, σ' = 125 MPa, $E = 2 \times 10^5$ MPa

We know that
$$\sigma' = \left(\frac{F}{A}\right)\left[1 + \sqrt{1 + \left(\frac{2AEh}{Fl}\right)}\right]$$

$$125 = \left(\frac{2000}{A}\right)\left[1 + \sqrt{1 + \frac{2A \times (2 \times 10^5) \times 20}{2000 \times 200}}\right]$$

$$0.0625\, A = \left[1 + \sqrt{1 + 20A}\right]$$

$$0.0625\, A - 1 = \sqrt{1 + 20A}$$

Squaring both sides, we have
$$(0.0625\, A - 1)^2 = 1 + 20\, A$$
$$(3.91 \times 10^{-3})\, A^2 + 1 - 0.125A = 1 + 20\, A$$
$$(3.91 \times 10^{-3})A^2 = 20.125\, A$$
$$A = 5147.05 \text{ mm}^2$$

But
$$A = bt = b(2b) \qquad\qquad \text{... (data)}$$
$$5147.05 = 2b^2$$
$$b = 50.73 \text{ mm} \approx 52 \text{ mm}$$

and
$$t = 2 \times 52 = 104 \text{ mm}$$

38. A steel rod 1.5 m long resists an impact load of 2 kN dropped through a distance of 50 mm along its axis. Limiting the maximum stress in the rod to 150 MPa, determine
(a) The diameter of the rod required.
(b) Impact factor. Use E = 200 GPa

Solution: $l = 1500$ mm, impact load $F = 2000$ N, $h = 50$ mm, $\sigma' = 150$ MPa, $E = 2 \times 10^5$ MPa, $d = ?$, impact factor = ?

a. *To find* δ:

We know that
$$\sigma' = \left(\frac{F}{A}\right)\left[1 + \sqrt{1 + \left(\frac{2AEh}{Fl}\right)}\right]$$

$$150 = \left(\frac{2000}{A}\right)\left[1 + \sqrt{1 + \frac{2A \times (2 \times 10^5) \times 50}{2000 \times 1500}}\right]$$

$$0.075\,A = \left[1 + \sqrt{1 + 6.67A}\right]$$

$$0.075\,A - 1 = \sqrt{1 + 6.67A}$$

Squaring both sides, we have
$$(0.075\,A - 1)^2 = 1 + 6.67A$$
$$(5.625 \times 10^{-3})\,A^2 + 1 - 0.15A = 1 + 6.67A$$
$$(5.625 \times 10^{-3})\,A^2 = 6.82\,A$$
$$A = 1212.44\ \text{mm}^2$$

But
$$A = \pi d^2/4$$
$$1212.44 = \pi d^2/4$$
$$d = 39.29\ \text{mm} \simeq 40\ \text{mm}$$

b. *Impact factor:*

We know that Impact factor $= \left[1 + \sqrt{1 + \left(\dfrac{2h}{\delta l}\right)}\right]$ ... Eq. (i)

But
$$\delta l = \frac{FL}{AE} = \frac{2000 \times 1500}{(\pi \times 40^2/4) \times 2 \times 10^5} = 0.0119\ \text{mm}$$

$\therefore$ Eq. (i) yields... impact factor $= \left[1 + \sqrt{1 + \left(\dfrac{2 \times 50}{0.0119}\right)}\right] = 92.53$

39. A mass of 500 kg is being lowered by means of a steel wire rope having cross sectional area of 250 mm². The velocity of weight is 0.5 m/sec. When the length of the extended rope is 20 m, the sheave gets stuck up. Determine the stresses induced in the rope due to sudden stoppage of the sheave. Neglect friction. Take $E = 190$ GPa

Solution: $m = 5$ kg, $A = 250$ mm², $v = 0.5$ m/s, $l = 20$ m, $\sigma = ?$, $E = 190$ GPa $= 190 \times 10^3$ MPa

Strain energy,
$$U = \frac{\sigma^2 V}{2E}$$

Volume $V = Al = 250 \times (20 \times 10^3) = 5 \times 10^6\ \text{mm}^3$

$$U = \frac{\sigma^2 \times (5 \times 10^6)}{2 \times (190 \times 10^3)} = 13.157\sigma^2\ \text{N-mm} = 0.013157\sigma^2\ \text{N-m} \qquad \text{... Eq. (i)}$$

Also Kinetic energy, $E_K = \dfrac{mv^2}{2} = \dfrac{500 \times 0.5^2}{2} = 62.5 \text{ N-m}$ ... Eq. (ii)

Equating Eqs (i) and (ii), we have
$$0.013157\sigma^2 = 62.5$$
$$\therefore \quad \sigma = 68.92 \text{ MPa.}$$

40. A wagon weighing 35 kN is attached to a wire rope and moving down an incline at 3.6 km/hr, when the rope jams and the wagon is suddenly brought to rest. If the length of the rope is 60 m at the time of sudden stoppage, calculate the maximum instantaneous stress and the maximum instantaneous elongation produced. Take the diameter of rope E = 30 mm and E = 200 GPa.

Solution: $F = 35$ kN, $v = 3.6$ km/hr $= 1$ m/s, $l = 60$ m, $\sigma = ?$, $\delta' = ?$, diameter of rope $d = 30$ mm, $E = 200$ GPa

Maximum instantaneous stress:

Strain energy, $\qquad\qquad U = \dfrac{\sigma^2 V}{2E}$

$$\text{Volume } V = Al = (\pi \times 30^2/4) \times (60 \times 10^3) = 42.41 \times 10^6 \text{ mm}^3$$

$$U = \frac{\sigma^2 \times (42.41 \times 10^6)}{2 \times (200 \times 10^3)} = 106.03 \, \sigma^2 \text{ N-mm} = 0.10603 \, \sigma^2 \text{ N-m}$$

$$\text{... Eq. (i)}$$

Also Kinetic energy, $E_K = \dfrac{Fv^2}{2g} = \dfrac{35000 \times 1^2}{2 \times 9.81} = 1783.89 \text{ N-m}$ ... Eq. (ii)

Equating Eqs (i) and (ii), we have
$$0.10603 \, \sigma^2 = 1783.89$$
$$\therefore \quad \sigma = 129.71 \text{ MPa.}$$

Maximum instantaneous deflection:

We know that $\delta l = \dfrac{\sigma l}{E} = \dfrac{129.71 \times 60000}{200 \times 10^3} = 38.91 \text{ mm}$

41. A weight of 5 kN is being lowered with a velocity of 2 m/s with the help of a wire rope and a sheave. When the sheave stops suddenly after the weight has reached a distance of 15 m, find the maximum stress in the rope. The area resisting the stress is 707 mm² and modulus of elasticity is 190 GPa. Neglect the inertia effect.

Solution: $F = 5$ kN, $v = 2$ m/s, $l = 15$ m, $\sigma = ?$, $A = 707$ mm², $E = 190$ GPa

Strain energy, $\qquad\qquad U = \dfrac{\sigma^2 V}{2E} \qquad\qquad \text{Volume } V = Al$

$$U = \frac{\sigma^2 \times (707 \times 15 \times 10^3)}{2 \times (190 \times 10^3)} = 27.91 \, \sigma^2 \text{ N-mm}$$

$$\therefore \quad U = 0.02791 \, \sigma^2 \text{ N-m} \qquad\qquad\qquad \text{... Eq. (i)}$$

Also Kinetic energy, $\quad E_K = \dfrac{Fv^2}{2g} = \dfrac{5000 \times 2^2}{2 \times 9.81} = 1019.37 \text{ N-m}$ ... Eq. (ii)

Equating Eqs (i) and (ii), we have

$$0.02791 \, \sigma^2 = 1019.37$$
$$\therefore \quad \sigma = 191.11 \text{ MPa.}$$

42. An elevator car carrying a load of 10 kN is descending by means of a steel rope at a speed of 1 m/sec. The cross section area of the rope is 400 mm^2. The rope is suddenly brought to rest by braking after 30 seconds of descent. Calculate the stress induced in the rope due to sudden stoppage if Young's modulus for the rope is 80000 MPa.

Solution: $F = 10$ kN, $v = 1$ m/s, $A = 400$ mm^2, $t = 30$ sec, $\sigma = ?$, $E = 80000$ MPa

Strain energy, $\qquad U = \dfrac{\sigma^2 V}{2E}$ ... Eq. (i)

But $\qquad$ volume $V = Al$ ... Eq. (ii)

Also $\qquad v^2 = u^2 + 2as$

Here $\qquad a = \dfrac{v}{t} = \dfrac{1}{30} = 0.0334 \text{ m/s}^2$ and $u = 0$ m/s

$$1^2 = 0 + (2 \times 0.0334 \times s)$$
$$s = 15 \text{ m}$$
$$\therefore \quad s = l = 15000 \text{ mm}$$

$\therefore$ Eq. (i) yields... $\quad U = \dfrac{\sigma^2 \times (400 \times 15 \times 10^3)}{2 \times 80000} = 37.5 \, \sigma^2 \text{ N-mm} = 0.0375 \, \sigma^2 \text{ N-m}$

... Eq. (iii)

Also kinetic energy, $E_K = \dfrac{Fv^2}{2g} = \dfrac{10000 \times 1^2}{2 \times 9.81} = 509.68 \text{ N-m}$ ... Eq. (iv)

Equating Eqs (iii) and (iv), we have

$$0.0375 \, \sigma^2 = 509.68$$
$$\therefore \quad \sigma = 116.58 \text{ MPa.}$$

43. A steel wire of 5 mm diameter is firmly held in clamp from which it hangs vertically. An anvil, the weight of which may be neglected is secured to the wire 2 m below the clamp. The wire is to be tested allowing a weight bored to the slide over the wire to drop freely from 1.5 m above the anvil. Calculate the weight required to stress the wire to 700 MPa, assuming the wire to be elastic up to this stress. Take $E = 210$ GPa.

Solution: Diameter of wire $d = 5$ mm, $l = 2$ m, $h = 1.5$ m, $F = ?$, $\sigma = 700$ MPa, $E = 210$ GPa

We know that $\qquad U = F \times (h + y')$ ... Eq. (i)

Also $\qquad U = \dfrac{\sigma^2 V}{2E}$ ... Eq. (ii)

Equating Eqs (i) and (ii), we have

$$F \times (h + y') = \dfrac{\sigma^2 V}{2E}$$ ... Eq. (iii)

But $\qquad y' = \dfrac{\sigma l}{E} = \dfrac{700 \times 2000}{210 \times 10^3} = 6.67 \text{ mm}$

$\therefore$ Eq. (iii) yields...

$$F \times (1500 + 6.67) = \frac{700^2 \times [(\pi \times 5^2/4) \times 2000]}{2 \times (210 \times 10^3)}$$

$$\therefore \quad F = 30.41 \text{ N}$$

44. A vertical steel rod of 20 mm diameter checks the fall on its end of weight 2 kN, which drops through a distance of 10 mm before it strikes the rod. Find the shortest length of the rod which will bear the impact, if the stress is not to exceed 150 MPa. Take E = 200 GPa.

Solution: Diameter of rod d = 20 mm, F = 2 kN, h = 10 mm, l = ?, σ = 150 MPa, E = 200 GPa

We know that $\qquad U = F \times (h + y')$ $\qquad\qquad$ ... Eq. (i)

Also $\qquad\qquad U = \dfrac{\sigma^2 V}{2E}$ $\qquad\qquad\qquad$ ... Eq. (ii)

Equating Eqs (i) and (ii), we have

$$F \times (h + y') = \frac{\sigma^2 V}{2E} \qquad\qquad \text{... Eq. (iii)}$$

But $\qquad\qquad y' = \dfrac{\sigma l}{E} = \dfrac{150 l}{200 \times 10^3} = (7.5 \times 10^{-4})\, l$

$\therefore$ Eq. (iii) yields... $2000 \times (10 + 7.5 \times 10^{-4}\, l) = \dfrac{150^2 \times [(\pi \times 20^2/4) \times l]}{2 \times (200 \times 10^3)}$

$$(10 + 7.5 \times 10^{-4}\, l) = 8.836 \times 10^{-3} l$$
$$10 = 8.086 \times 10^{-3} l$$
$$\therefore \quad l = 1236.71 \text{ mm} = 1.236 \text{ m}$$

45. A vertical tie rod fixed rigidly at the top consists of a steel rod 4 m long and 30 mm in diameter encased throughout in a brass tube 30 mm internal diameter and 40 mm external diameter. The casing and the rod are fixed together at both ends. The compound rod is suddenly loaded in tension by weight of 15 kN falling through 10 mm before being arrested by the tie. Determine the maximum stress in steel and brass. Take E = 200 GPa and 100 GPa for steel and brass respectively.

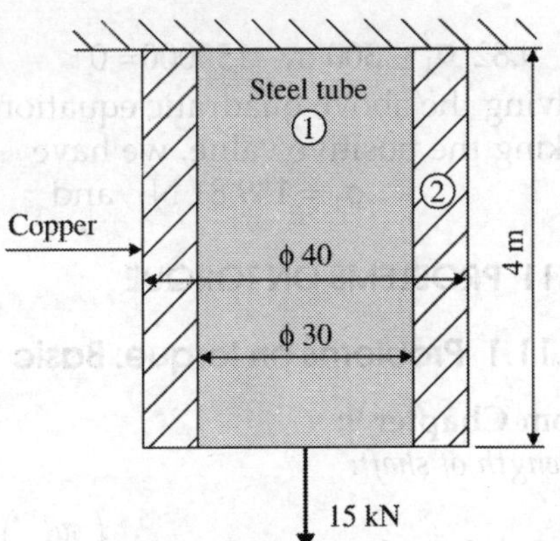

Fig. 11.38: Problem 45

Solution: *Let suffix '1' refers to steel and '2' refers to brass*

Based on given data, the problem is as shown in **Fig. 11.38**

d_1 = 30 mm, $(d_2)_o$ = 40 mm, $(d_2)_i$ = 30 mm, $l = l_1 = l_2$ = 4000 mm, F = 15 kN, E_1 = 200 × 10^3 MPa, E_2 = 100 × 10^3 MPa, h = 10 mm, σ_1 = ?, σ_2 = ?

For a composite bar we have

$$\frac{\sigma_1}{E_1} = \frac{\sigma_2}{E_2}$$

$$\frac{\sigma_1}{200 \times 10^3} = \frac{\sigma_2}{200 \times 10^3}$$

$$\sigma_2 = 0.5 \, \sigma_1 \qquad \qquad \text{... Eq. (i)}$$

Strain energy in steel $\quad U_1 = \dfrac{\sigma_1^2 V_1}{2E_1} = \dfrac{\sigma_1^2 \times [(\pi \times 30^2/4) \times 4000]}{2 \times 200 \times 10^3}$

$$U_1 = 7.07 \, \sigma_1^2 \qquad \qquad \text{... Eq. (ii)}$$

Strain energy in steel $\quad U_2 = \dfrac{\sigma_2^2 V_2}{2E_2} = \dfrac{(0.5\sigma_1) \times [\pi \times (40^2 - 30^2) \times 4000]}{2 \times 200 \times 10^3}$

$$U_2 = 2.75 \, \sigma_1^2 \qquad \qquad \text{... Eq. (iii)}$$

Total strain energy, $\quad U = U_1 + U_2$

$$= 7.07 \, \sigma_1^2 + 2.75 \, \sigma_1^2$$

$$U = 9.82 \, \sigma_1^2 \qquad \qquad \text{... Eq. (iv)}$$

Also strain energy stored = work done on the body

$$U = F(h + \delta l) \qquad \qquad \text{... Eq. (v)}$$

Since the length is same, for compatibility, we have

$$\delta l_1 = \delta l_2$$

$$\delta l_1 = \frac{\sigma_1 l_1}{E_1} = \frac{\sigma_1 \times 4000}{200 \times 10^3}$$

$$\delta l_1 = 0.02\sigma_1 = \delta l$$

Eq. (v) yields... $\qquad U = 15000 \times (10 + 0.02\sigma_1) \qquad \qquad \text{... Eq. (vi)}$

Equating Eqs (iv) and (vi), we have

$$9.82 \, \sigma_1^2 = 15000 \times (10 + 0.02\sigma_1)$$

$$9.82 \, \sigma_1^2 - 300 \, \sigma_1 - 150000 = 0$$

Solving the above quadratic equation, we have $\sigma_1 = 139.81, -109.26$ N

Taking the positive value, we have

$$\sigma_1 = 139.81 \text{ N} \quad \text{and} \quad \sigma_1 = 0.5 \times 139.81 = 69.91 \text{ N}$$

11.11 PROBLEMS ON TORQUE

11.11.1 Problems on torque: Basic

From Chapter 9:
Strength of shaft:

Solid shaft $\qquad T = \left(\dfrac{\pi d^3}{16}\right)\tau$

Hollow shaft $\qquad T = \left[\dfrac{\pi}{16}\left(\dfrac{d_o^4 - d_i^4}{d_o}\right)\right]\tau = \dfrac{\pi}{16} d_o^3 (1 - K^4)\tau; \ K = \dfrac{d_i}{d_o}$

Area $\qquad A = \dfrac{\pi d^2}{4} \qquad \qquad \text{... Solid shaft}$

Area $\qquad A = \dfrac{\pi}{4} d_o^2 (1 - K^2) \qquad \qquad \text{... Hollow shaft}$

Polar moment of inertia (J)

Solid shaft,
$$J = \frac{\pi d^4}{32}$$

Hollow shaft,
$$J = \frac{\pi}{32}(d_o^4 - d_i^4) = \frac{\pi}{32}d_o^4(1 - K^4)$$

Shafts in series (common torque)
$$T = T_1 = T_2 \quad \text{and} \quad \theta = \theta_1 + \theta_2$$

Shafts in parallel (shared torque)
$$T = T_1 + T_2 \quad \text{and} \quad \theta = \theta_1 = \theta_2 \text{ or } \Sigma = 0$$

46. Determine the strain energy stored in a solid shaft which will transmit 90 kW at 160 rpm. The length of the shaft is 900 mm and the maximum shear stress is limited to 60 MPa. Take the value of rigidity as 80 GPa.

Also find the energy stored per unit volume and the angle of twist from strain energy.

Solution: $P = 90 \times 10^3$ W, N = 160 rpm, $l = 900$ mm, $\tau = 60$ N/mm^2, $G = 80 \times 10^3$ MPa.
a) $\cup = ?$, b) $u = ?$, c) $\theta = ?$

a. *To find* $\cup$:

Strain energy
$$\cup = \frac{T^2 l}{2GJ} \qquad \text{... Eq. (i)}$$

But
$$P = \frac{2\pi NT}{60}$$

$$90 \times 10^3 = \frac{2\pi \times 160 \times T}{60}$$

$$T = 5371.48 \text{ N-m} = 5371.48 \times 10^3 \text{ N-mm}$$

Also
$$T = \left(\frac{\pi d^3}{16}\right)\tau \qquad \text{... Eq. (ii)}$$

$$5371.48 \times 10^3 = \left(\frac{\pi d^3}{16}\right) \times 60$$

$$d = 76.97 \text{ mm} \approx 78 \text{ mm}$$

Eq. (i) yields...
$$\cup = \frac{(5371.48 \times 10^3)^2 \times 900}{2 \times 80 \times 10^3 \times (\pi \times 78^4/32)} = 44.66 \times 10^3 \text{ N-mm}$$

$$= 44.66 \text{ N-m or J}$$

Method 2:

For a solid shaft
$$\cup = \frac{\tau^2 V}{4G} = \frac{\tau^2 Al}{4G} \qquad \text{... Eq. (iii)}$$

Based on round-off value of $d = 78$ mm, the shear stress is found from Eq. (ii) as

$$5371.48 \times 10^3 = \left(\frac{\pi \times 78^3}{16}\right) \times \tau$$

$$\tau = 57.65 \text{ MPa.}$$

Eq. (iii) yields... $\quad U = \dfrac{57.65^2 \times (\pi \times 78^2/4) \times 900}{4 \times 80 \times 10^3} = 44.66 \times 10^3$ N-mm

$$= 44.66 \text{ N-m or J}$$

b. *To find u:*

Energy stored per unit volume Strain energy density

$$u = \frac{U}{V} = \frac{44.66}{(\pi \times 78^2/4) \times 900} = 10.38 \times 10^{-6} \text{ N-m/mm}^3$$

$$= 10.38 \times 10^3 \text{ J/m}^3$$

c. *To find* θ:

Strain energy $\qquad U = \dfrac{1}{2}T\theta$

$$44.66 \times 10^3 = \frac{1}{2} \times (5371.48 \times 10^3) \times \theta$$

$$\theta = 0.0166 \text{ rad} = 0.95 \text{ deg}$$

47. A hollow circular steel shaft has to transmit 60 kW at 210 rpm such that the shear stress does not exceed 60 MPa. If the ratio of internal to external diameter is 3/4 and the value of rigidity modulus is 84 GPa, find the strain energy stored in the shaft. The length of the shaft is 3 m.

Also find the angle of twist from strain energy.

Solution: $P = 60 \times 10^3$ W, N = 210 rpm, $\tau = 60$ MPa, $K = \dfrac{d_i}{d_o} = \dfrac{3}{4}$, $G = 84 \times 10^3$ MPa,

$l = 3000$ mm. a) $d_o, d_i = ?$, b) $\theta = ?$

Method 1:

a. *To find* U:

Strain energy $\qquad U = \dfrac{T^2 l}{2GJ}$ $\qquad\qquad\qquad\qquad\qquad\qquad$ ... Eq. (i)

But $\qquad\qquad P = \dfrac{2\pi NT}{60}$

$$60 \times 10^3 = \frac{2\pi \times 210 \times T}{60}$$

$$T = 2728.37 \text{ N-m} = 2728.37 \times 10^3 \text{ N-mm}$$

Also $\qquad\qquad T = \dfrac{\pi}{16}\, d_o^3\,(1 - K^4)\tau$ $\qquad\qquad\qquad\qquad$ ... Eq. (ii)

$$2728.37 \times 10^3 = \left(\frac{\pi}{16}\right) d_o^3 \times [1 - (3/4)^4] \times 60$$

$$d_o = 69.71 \text{ mm} \approx 70 \text{ mm}$$

And $\qquad\qquad d_i = (3/4) \times 70 = 52.5 \text{ mm}$

$$J = \frac{\pi d_o^4}{32}\,(1 - K^4) = \frac{\pi \times 70^4}{32} \times [1 - (3/4)^4] = 1.61 \times 10^6 \text{ mm}^4$$

Eq. (i) yields...

$$U = \frac{(2728.37 \times 10^3)^2 \times 3000}{2 \times 84 \times 10^3 \times (1.61 \times 10^6)} = 82.56 \times 10^3 \text{ N-mm} = 82.56 \text{ J}$$

Method 2:

For a hollow shaft

$$U = \frac{\tau^2 V}{4G}(1 + K^2) = \frac{\tau^2 Al}{4G}(1 + K^2) \qquad \qquad \dots \text{Eq. (iii)}$$

Based on round-off value of diameters $d_o = 70$ mm and $d_i = 52.5$ mm, the shear stress is found from Eq. (ii) as

$$2728.37 \times 10^3 = \left(\frac{\pi \times 70^3}{16}\right)[1 - (3/4)^4] \times \tau \qquad \qquad (K = 52.5/70 = 3/4)$$

$$\tau = 59.26 \text{ MPa.}$$

Eq. (iii) yields...

$$U = \frac{59.26^2 \times [\pi \times 70^2 \,[1 - (3/4)^2]/4] \times 3000}{4 \times 84 \times 10^3} \times [1 + (3/4)^2]$$

$$= 82.49 \times 10^3 \text{ N-mm} = 82.49 \text{ N-m or J}$$

b. *To find* θ:

Strain energy

$$U = \frac{1}{2}T\theta$$

$$82.56 \times 10^3 = \frac{1}{2} \times (2728.37 \times 10^3) \times \theta$$

$$\theta = 0.06052 \text{ rad} = 3.48°$$

48. **Determine the strain energy stored in a solid shaft of diameter 50 mm and 1m length subjected to pure torsion at its ends. The maximum shear stress is limited to 75 MPa. Take the value of rigidity as 80 GPa.**

    Also calculate the angle of twist from the strain energy.

Solution: $d = 50$ mm, $l = 1000$ mm, $\tau = 75$ MPa, $G = 80 \times 10^3$ MPa. a) $U = ?$, b) $\theta = ?$

a. *To find* U:

Strain energy

$$U = \frac{T^2 l}{2GJ} \qquad \qquad \dots \text{Eq. (i)}$$

But

$$T = \left(\frac{\pi d^3}{16}\right)\tau$$

$$= \left(\frac{\pi \times 50^3}{16}\right) \times 75$$

$$T = 1.84 \times 10^6 \text{ N-mm}$$

Eq. (i) yields...

$$U = \frac{(1.84 \times 10^6)^2 \times 1000}{2 \times 80 \times 10^3 \times (\pi \times 50^4/32)} = 34.49 \times 10^3 \text{ N-mm} = 34.49 \text{ J}$$

b. *To find* θ:

Strain energy

$$U = \frac{1}{2}T\theta$$

$$34.49 \times 10^3 = \frac{1}{2} \times (1.84 \times 10^6) \times \theta$$

$$\theta = 0.0375 \text{ rad} = 2.15 \text{ deg}$$

11.11.2 Problems on series shafts: Known torque

49. Determine the strain energy stored for the shaft shown in Fig. 11.39(a). Take $G = 80$ GPa. The angle of twist is limited to 4°. Also find the diameter of the shaft.

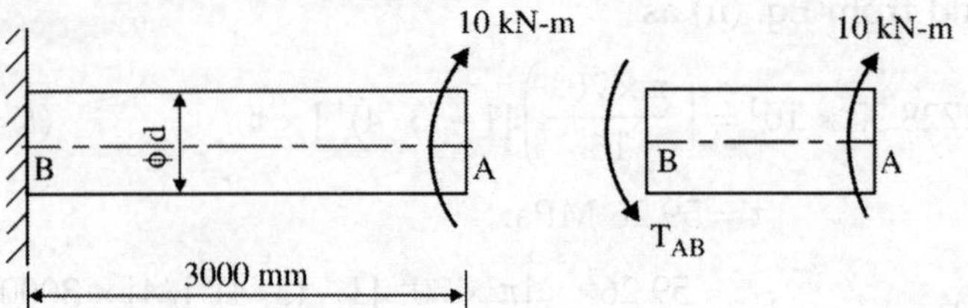

Fig. 11.39(a): Problem 49   **Fig. 11.39(b):** Problem 49: Free body diagram

Solution: $T = 10$ kN-m, $l = 3000$ mm, $\theta = 4° = 0.0698$ rad, $G = 80 \times 10^3$ MPa. a) $U = ?$ b) $d = ?$

The free-body diagram of the system is shown in **Fig. 11.39(b)**.

Assume that clockwise torques/moments are negative and counterclockwise torques/moments are positive.

Shaft AB: $\qquad \Sigma M = 0: T_{AB} - 100 = 0 \Rightarrow T_{AB} = 10$ kN-m $= 10 \times 10^6$ N-mm

Method 1:

a. *Strain energy:*

Strain energy $\qquad U = \dfrac{1}{2} T\theta$

$$= \frac{1}{2} \times (10 \times 10^6) \times 0.0698$$

$$U = 349000 \text{ N-mm} = 349 \text{ J}$$

b. *Diameter:*

For a solid shaft, $\qquad U = \dfrac{T^2 l}{2GJ}$

$$349000 = \frac{(10 \times 10^6)^2 \times 3000}{2 \times 80 \times 10^3 \times (\pi d^4 / 32)}$$

$$d = 86 \text{ mm}$$

Method 2:

a. *Diameter:*

For a solid shaft, $\qquad \theta = \left(\dfrac{Tl}{GJ}\right)_{AB}$

$$0.0698 = \frac{(10 \times 10^6) \times 3000}{80 \times 10^3 \times (\pi d^4 / 32)}$$

$$d = 86 \text{ mm}$$

b. *Strain energy:*

Strain energy

$$U = \frac{1}{2}\, T\theta = \frac{1}{2} \times (10 \times 10^6) \times 0.0698 = 349000 \text{ N-mm} = 349\text{ J}$$

OR

$$U = \frac{T^2 l}{2GJ} = \frac{(10 \times 10^6)^2 \times 3000}{2 \times 80 \times 10^3 \times (\pi \times 86^4/32)} = 349146 \text{ N-mm}$$

$$= 349.15\text{ J}$$

50. **A uniform sold shaft of diameter 45 mm carries two torques as shown in Fig. 11.40(a). Determine the strain energy stored in the shaft. Take $G = 78$ GPa.**

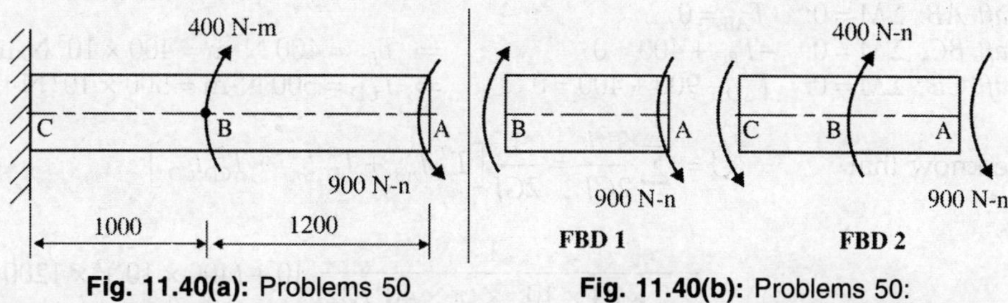

Fig. 11.40(a): Problems 50

Fig. 11.40(b): Problems 50: Free body diagrams

Solution: $d = 45$ mm, $T_1 = 900$ N-m, $T_2 = 400$ N-m, $l_{AB} = 1200$ mm, $l_{BC} = 1000$ mm, $G = 78 \times 10^3$ MPa, $U = ?$

The free-body diagram of the system is shown in **Fig. 11.40(b)**.

Assume that clockwise torques/moments are negative and counterclockwise torques/moments are positive.

Shaft AB: $\Sigma M = 0$: $-T_{AB} + 900 = 0$ $\Rightarrow T_{AB} = 900$ N-m $= 900 \times 10^3$ N-mm

Shaft BC: $\Sigma M = 0$: $T_{BC} - 400 + 900 = 0$ $\Rightarrow T_{BC} = 500$ N-m $= 500 \times 10^3$ N-mm

We know that

$$U = \sum \frac{T^2 l}{2GJ} = \frac{1}{2GJ}\left[T_{AB}^2 l_{AB} + T_{BC}^2 l_{BC} \right]$$

$$= \frac{1}{2 \times 78 \times 10^3 \times (\pi \times 45^4/32)} \left[(900 \times 10^3)^2 \times 1200 \right.$$

$$\left. + (500 \times 10^3)^2 \times 1000 \right]$$

$$U = 19.46 \times 10^3 \text{ N-mm} = 19.46\text{ J}$$

51. **Determine the strain energy stored in a shaft as shown in Fig. 11.41(a). Take $G = 84$ GPa.**

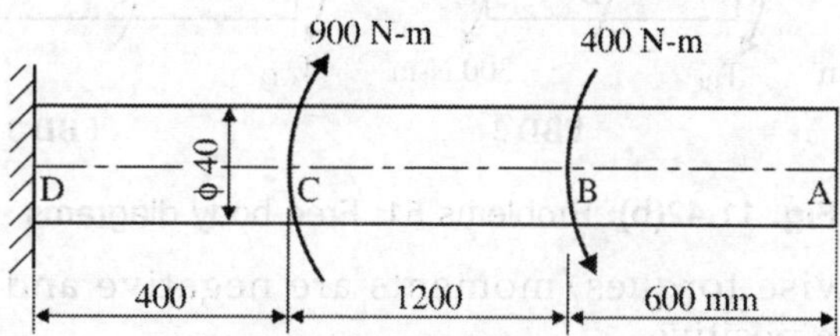

Fig. 11.41(a): Problem 50

Solution: $d = 40$ mm, $l_{AB} = 600$ mm, $l_{BC} = 1200$ mm, $l_{CD} = 400$ mm, $T_1 = 400$ N-m, $T_2 = 900$ N-m, $G = 84 \times 10^3$ MPa. $U = ?$

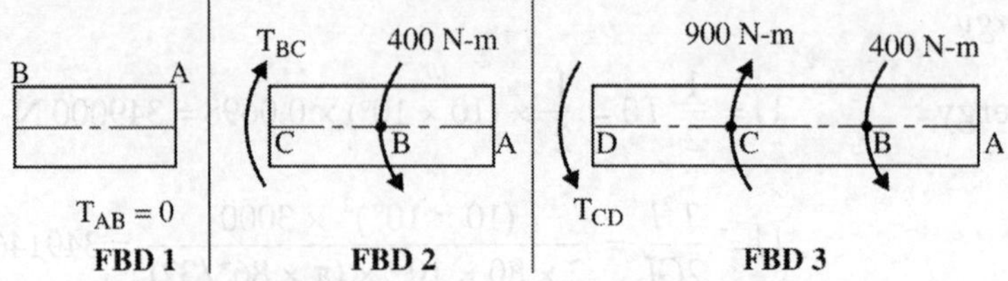

Fig. 11.41(b): Problem 51: Free body diagrams

The free-body diagram of the system is shown in **Fig. 11.41(b)**.
Assume that clockwise torques/moments are negative and counterclockwise torques/moments are positive.

Shaft AB: $\Sigma M = 0$: $T_{AB} = 0$

Shaft BC: $\Sigma M = 0$: $-T_{BC} + 400 = 0$ $\qquad \Rightarrow T_{BC} = 400$ N-m $= 400 \times 10^3$ N-mm

Shaft CD: $\Sigma M = 0$: $T_{CD} - 900 + 400 = 0$ $\qquad \Rightarrow T_{CD} = 500$ N-m $= 500 \times 10^3$ N-mm

We know that $\qquad U = \sum \dfrac{T^2 l}{2GJ} = \dfrac{1}{2GJ}\left[T_{AB}^2 l_{AB} + T_{BC}^2 l_{BC} + T_{CD}^2 l_{CD} \right]$

$$= \frac{1}{2 \times 84 \times 10^3 \times (\pi \times 40^4/32)} [0 + (400 \times 10^3)^2 \times 1200$$

$$+ (500 \times 10^3)^2 \times 400]$$

$$U = 6.92 \times 10^3 \text{ N-mm} = 6.92 \text{ J}$$

52. Determine the strain energy stored in a shaft as shown in Fig. 11.42(a). Take $G = 80$ GPa.

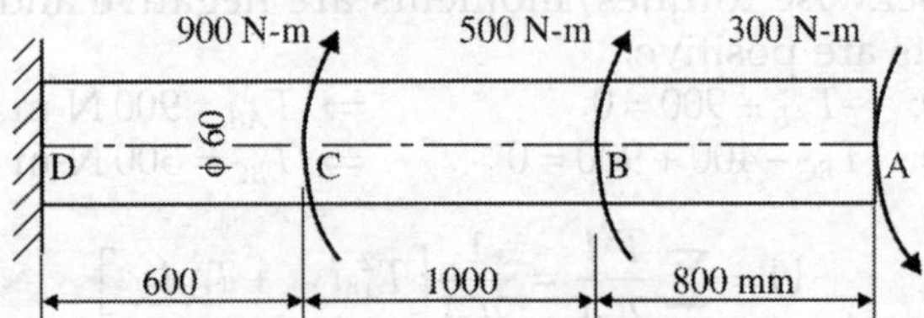

Fig. 11.42(a): Problems 52

Solution: $d = 60$ mm, $l_{AB} = 800$ mm, $l_{BC} = 1000$ mm, $l_{CD} = 600$ mm, $T_1 = 300$ N-m, $T_2 = 500$ N-m, $T_3 = 900$ N-m $G = 80 \times 10^3$ MPa. $U = ?$

The free-body diagram of the system is shown in **Fig. 11.42(b)**.

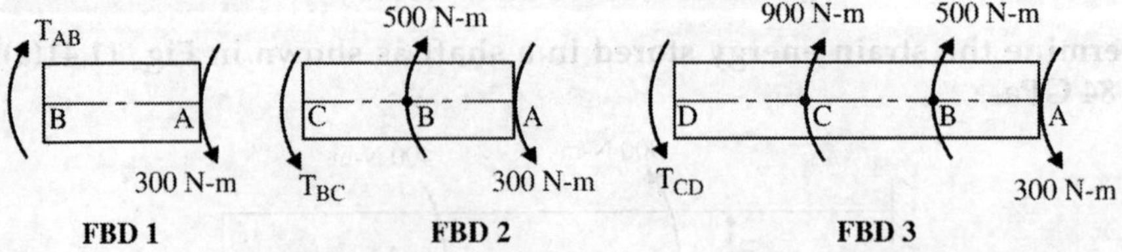

Fig. 11.42(b): Problems 51: Free body diagrams

Assume that clockwise torques/moments are negative and counterclockwise torques/moments are positive.

Shaft AB: $\Sigma M = 0$: $300 - T_{AB} = 0$ $\qquad \Rightarrow T_{AB} = 300$ N-m $= 300 \times 10^3$ N-mm

Shaft BC: $\Sigma M = 0$: $T_{BC} - 500 + 300 = 0$ $\qquad \Rightarrow T_{BC} = 200$ N-m $= 200 \times 10^3$ N-mm

Shaft CD: $\Sigma M = 0$: $T_{CD} - 900 - 500 + 300 = 0 \Rightarrow T_{CD} = 1100$ N-m $= 1100 \times 10^3$ N-mm

We know that
$$U = \sum \frac{T^2 l}{2GJ} = \frac{1}{2GJ}\left[T_{AB}^2 l_{AB} + T_{BC}^2 l_{BC} + T_{CD}^2 l_{CD}\right]$$

$$= \frac{1}{2 \times 80 \times 10^3 \times (\pi \times 60^4/32)}\,[(300 \times 10^3)^2 \times 800$$
$$+ (200 \times 10^3)^2 \times 1000 + (1100 \times 10^3)^2 \times 600]$$
$$U = 4.12 \times 10^3 \text{ N-mm} = 4.12 \text{ J}$$

53. Determine the strain energy stored in a shaft as shown in Fig. 11.43(a). Take $G = 80$ GPa.

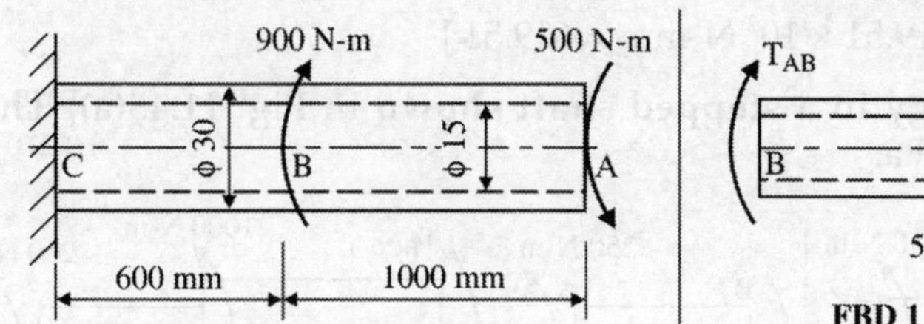

Fig. 11.43(a): Problem 53

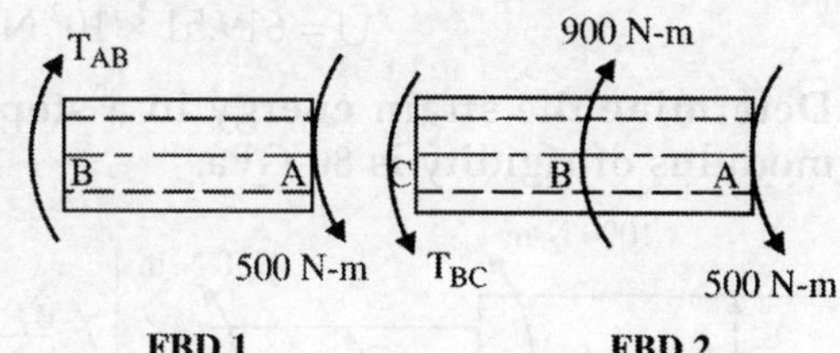

Fig. 11.43(b): Problem 53: Free body diagrams

Solution: $d_i = 15$ mm, $d_o = 30$ mm, $K = \dfrac{d_i}{d_o} = \dfrac{15}{30} = 0.5$, $l_{AB} = 1000$ mm, $l_{BC} = 600$ mm,

$T_1 = 500$ N-m, $T_2 = 900$ N-m, $G = 80 \times 10^3$ MPa. $U = ?$

The free-body diagram of the system is shown in **Fig. 11.43(b)**.

Assume that clockwise torques/moments are negative and counter clockwise torques/moments are positive.

Shaft AB: $\Sigma M = 0$: $500 - T_{AB} = 0$ $\Rightarrow T_{AB} = 500$ N-m $= 500 \times 10^3$ N-mm

Shaft BC: $\Sigma M = 0$: $500 - 900 + T_{BC} = 0$ $\Rightarrow T_{BC} = 400$ N-m $= 400 \times 10^3$ N-mm

We know that
$$U = \sum \frac{T^2 l}{2GJ} = \frac{1}{2GJ}\left[T_{AB}^2 l_{AB} + T_{BC}^2 l_{BC}\right]$$

$$= \frac{1}{2 \times 80 \times 10^3 \times [(\pi \times 30^4 \times (1 - 0.5^4))/32]}\,[(500 \times 10^3)^2$$
$$\times 1000 + (400 \times 10^3)^2 \times 600]$$
$$U = 29 \times 10^3 \text{ N-mm} = 29 \text{ J}$$

54. Two shafts are connected in series as shown in Fig. 11.44(a). Determine the strain energy stored in the shaft. Take $G = 85$ GPa.

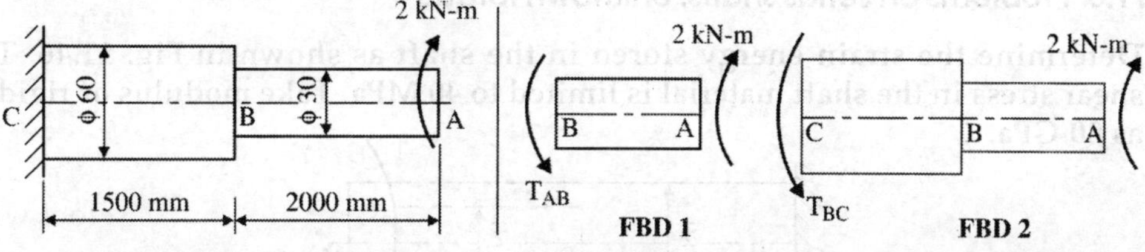

Fig. 11.44(a): Problem 54

Fig. 11.44(b): Problem 54: Free body diagrams

Solution: $d_{AB} = 30$ mm, $d_{BC} = 60$ mm, $l_{AB} = 2000$ mm, $l_{BC} = 1500$ mm, $T = 2$ kN-m, $G = 85 \times 10^3$ MPa. $U = ?$

The free-body diagram of the system is shown in **Fig. 11.44(b)**.

Assume that clockwise torques/moments are negative and counterclockwise torques/moments are positive.

Shaft AB: $\Sigma M = 0$: $T_{AB} - 2 = 0$ $\Rightarrow T_{AB} = 2$ kN-m $= 2 \times 10^6$ N-mm

Shaft BC: $\Sigma M = 0$: $T_{BC} - 2 = 0$ $\Rightarrow T_{BC} = 2$ kN-m $= 2 \times 10^6$ N-mm

We know that
$$U = \sum \frac{T^2 l}{2GJ} = \frac{T^2}{2G}\left[\frac{l_{AB}}{J_{AB}} + \frac{l_{BC}}{J_{BC}}\right]$$

$$= \frac{(2 \times 10^6)^2}{2 \times 85 \times 10^3}\left[\frac{2000}{(\pi \times 30^4 / 32)} + \frac{1500}{(\pi \times 60^4 / 32)}\right]$$

$$U = 619.51 \times 10^3 \text{ N-mm} = 619.51 \text{ J}$$

55. Determine the strain energy in a stepped shaft shown in Fig. 11.45(a). The modulus of rigidity is 80 GPa.

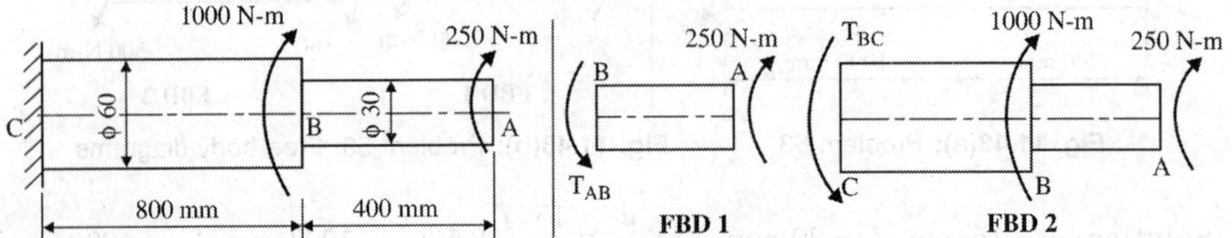

Fig. 11.45(a): Problem 55   **Fig. 11.45(b):** Problem 55: Free body diagrams

Solution: $d_{AB} = 30$ mm, $d_{BC} = 60$ mm, $l_{AB} = 400$ mm, $l_{BC} = 800$ mm, $T_1 = 250$ N-m, $T_2 = 1000$ N-m, $G = 80 \times 10^3$ MPa. $U = ?$

The free-body diagram of the system is shown in **Fig. 11.45(b)**.

Assume that clockwise torques/moments are negative and counterclockwise torques/moments are positive.

Shaft AB: $\Sigma M = 0$: $T_{AB} - 250 = 0$ $\Rightarrow T_{AB} = 250$ N-m $= 250 \times 10^3$ N-mm

Shaft BC: $\Sigma M = 0$: $T_{BC} - 1000 - 250 = 0$ $\Rightarrow T_{BC} = 1250$ N-m $= 1250 \times 10^3$ N-mm

We know that $U = \sum \dfrac{T^2 l}{2GJ} = \dfrac{1}{2G}\left[\dfrac{T_{AB}^2 l_{AB}}{J_{AB}} + \dfrac{T_{BC}^2 l_{BC}}{J_{BC}}\right]$

$$= \frac{1}{2 \times 80 \times 10^3}\left[\frac{(250 \times 10^3)^2 \times 400}{(\pi \times 30^4 / 32)} + \frac{(1250 \times 10^3)^2 \times 800}{(\pi \times 60^4 / 32)}\right]$$

$$U = 8.11 \times 10^3 \text{ N-mm} = 8.11 \text{ J}$$

11.11.3 Problems on series shafts: Unknown torque

56. Determine the strain energy stored in the shaft as shown in Fig. 11.46. The shear stress in the shaft material is limited to 40 MPa. Take modulus of rigidity as 80 GPa.

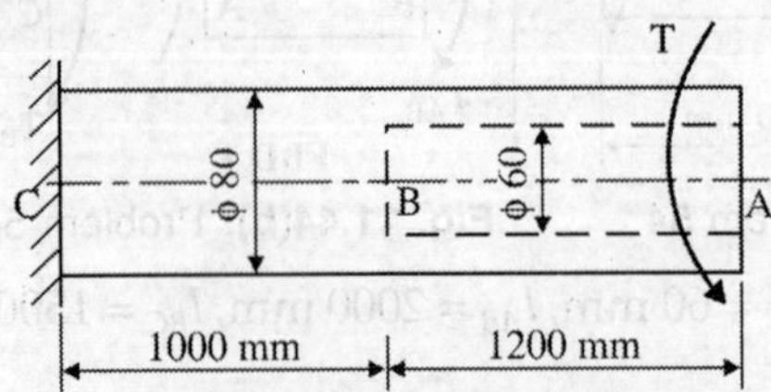

Fig. 11.46: Problem 56

Solution: $d_{AB})_i = 60$ mm, $d_{AB})_o = 80$ mm, $K = \dfrac{d_i}{d_o} = \dfrac{60}{80} = 0.75$, $d_{BC} = 80$ mm, $l_{AB} = 1200$ mm,

$l_{BC} = 1000$ mm, $\tau = 40$ MPa, $G = 80 \times 10^3$ MPa. $\mathsf{U} = ?$

To find T:

For a hollow shaft,
$$J = \frac{\pi}{32}\left(d_o^4 - d_i^4\right) = \frac{\pi}{32}\,d_o^4(1 - K^4) = \frac{\pi}{32} \times 80^4(1 - 0.75^4)$$
$$= 2.75 \times 10^6 \text{ mm}^4$$

For a solid shaft,
$$J = \frac{\pi d^4}{32} = \frac{\pi \times 80^4}{32} = 4.02 \times 10^6 \text{ mm}^4$$

Hence
$$T = \frac{\tau J_{\min}}{r} = \frac{40 \times 2.75 \times 10^6}{80/2} = 2.75 \times 10^6 \text{ N-mm}$$

To find U:

We know that
$$\mathsf{U} = \sum \frac{T^2 l}{2GJ} = \frac{T^2}{2G}\left[\frac{l_{AB}}{J_{AB}} + \frac{l_{BC}}{J_{BC}}\right]$$
$$= \frac{(2.75 \times 10^6)^2}{2 \times 80 \times 10^3}\left[\frac{1200}{2.75 \times 10^6} + \frac{1000}{4.02 \times 10^6}\right]$$
$$\mathsf{U} = 32.38 \times 10^3 \text{ N-mm} = 32.83 \text{ J}$$

57. **Two shafts are connected in series as shown in Fig. 11.47. Determine the strain energy stored in the shaft if shear stress is limited to 50 MPa. Take $G = 85$ GPa.**

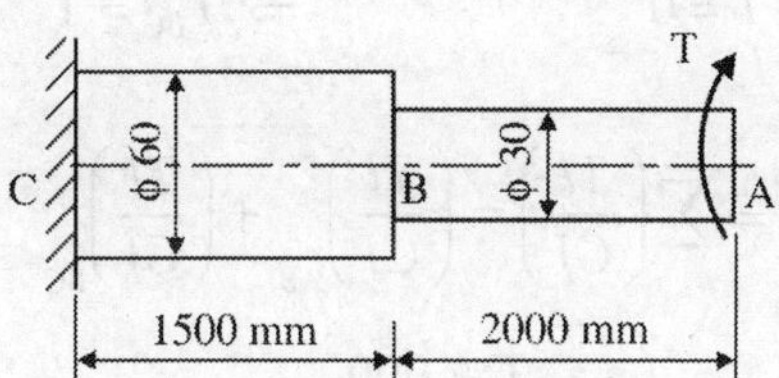

Fig. 11.47: Problem 57

Solution: $d_{AB} = 30$ mm, $d_{BC} = 60$ mm, $l_{AB} = 2000$ mm, $l_{BC} = 1500$ mm, $T = 2$ kN-m, $G = 85 \times 10^3$ MPa, $\tau = 50$ MPa, $\mathsf{U} = ?$.

To find T:

For shaft AB,
$$J = \frac{\pi d_{AB}^4}{32} = \frac{\pi \times 30^4}{32} = 79.52 \times 10^3 \text{ mm}^4$$

For shaft BC,
$$J = \frac{\pi d_{BC}^4}{32} = \frac{\pi \times 60^4}{32} = 1.27 \times 10^6 \text{ mm}^4$$

Hence
$$T = \frac{\tau J_{\min}}{r_{\min}} = \frac{50 \times 79.52 \times 10^3}{30/2} = 265.07 \times 10^3 \text{ N-mm}$$

To find U:

We know that
$$\mathsf{U} = \sum \frac{T^2 l}{2GJ} = \frac{T^2}{2G}\left[\frac{l_{AB}}{J_{AB}} + \frac{l_{BC}}{J_{BC}}\right]$$

$$= \frac{(265.07 \times 10^3)^2}{2 \times 85 \times 10^3}\left[\frac{2000}{79.52 \times 10^3} + \frac{1500}{1.27 \times 10^6}\right]$$

$$\mathsf{U} = 10.88 \times 10^3 \text{ N-mm} = 10.88 \text{ J}$$

58. Determine the strain energy in a stepped shaft as shown in Fig. 11.48(a), if rotation at the free end is limited to 4°. Take $G = 85$ **GPa.**

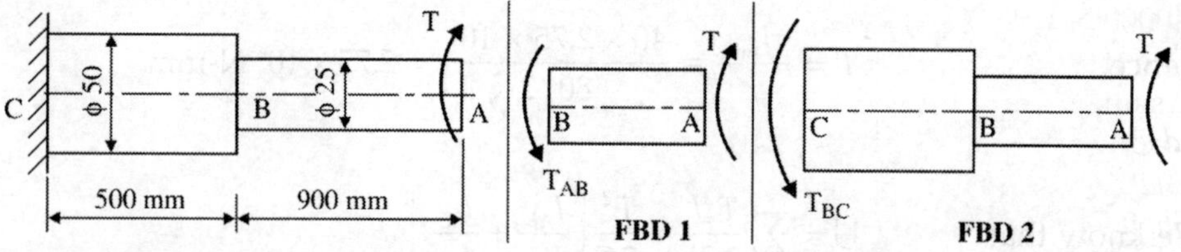

Fig. 11.48(a): Problem 55   Fig. 11.48(b): Problem 55: Free body diagrams

Solution: $d_{AB} = 25$ mm, $d_{BC} = 50$ mm, $l_{AB} = 900$ mm, $l_{BC} = 500$ mm, $G = 85 \times 10^3$ MPa, $\theta = 4° = 0.0698$ rad., $\mathsf{U} = ?$.

The free-body diagram of the system is shown in **Fig. 11.48(b)**.

Assume that clockwise torques/moments are negative and counterclockwise torques/moments are positive.

    Shaft AB: $\Sigma M = 0$: $T_{AB} - T = 0$ $\Rightarrow T_{AB} = \mathrm{T}$

    Shaft BC: $\Sigma M = 0$: $T_{BC} - T = 0$ $\Rightarrow T_{BC} = \mathrm{T}$

To find T:

Total angle of twist, $\theta = \sum\left(\frac{Tl}{GJ}\right) = \left(\frac{Tl}{GJ}\right)_{AB} + \left(\frac{Tl}{GJ}\right)_{BC}$

$$0.0698 = \frac{T \times 900}{85 \times 10^3 \times (\pi \times 25^4/32)} + \frac{T \times 500}{85 \times 10^3 \times (\pi \times 50^4/32)}$$

$$T = 244.33 \times 10^3 \text{ N-mm}$$

To find U:

We know that $\mathsf{U} = \dfrac{1}{2} T\theta = \dfrac{1}{2} \times (244.33 \times 10^3) \times 0.0698 = 8.53 \times 10^3$ N-mm

           $= 8.53$ J

OR $\mathsf{U} = \sum \dfrac{T^2 l}{2GJ} = \dfrac{T^2}{2G}\left[\dfrac{l_{AB}}{J_{AB}} + \dfrac{l_{BC}}{J_{BC}}\right]$

$$= \frac{(244.33 \times 10^3)^2}{2 \times 85 \times 10^3}\left[\frac{900}{(\pi \times 25^4/32)} + \frac{500}{(\pi \times 50^4/32)}\right]$$

$$\mathsf{U} = 8.53 \times 10^3 \text{ N-mm} = 8.53 \text{ J}$$

59. Determine the maximum torque that can be applied to the stepped shaft shown in Fig. 11.49(a) shaft if the elastic strain energy is to 40 J? Take $G = 80$ GPa.

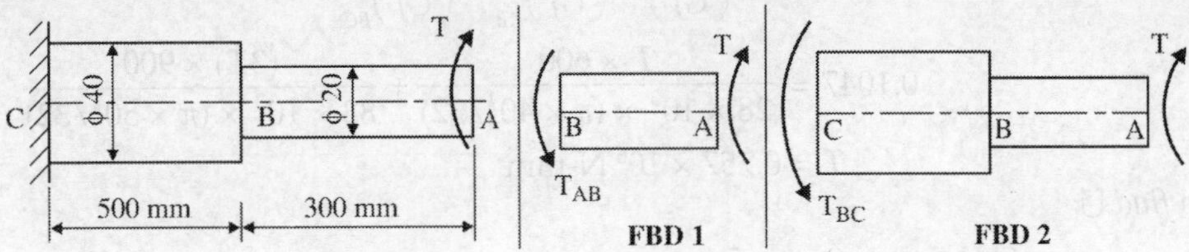

Fig. 11.49(a): Problem 55   **Fig. 11.49(b):** Problem 55: Free body diagrams

Solution: $d_{AB} = 20$ mm, $d_{BC} = 40$ mm, $l_{AB} = 300$ mm, $l_{BC} = 500$ mm, $G = 80 \times 10^3$ MPa, $U = 40000$ N-mm, $T = ?$.

The free-body diagram of the system is shown in **Fig. 11.49(b)**.

Assume that clockwise torques/moments are negative and counterclockwise torques/moments are positive.

Shaft AB: $\Sigma M = 0$: $T_{AB} - T = 0$ $\Rightarrow T_{AB} = T$

Shaft BC: $\Sigma M = 0$: $T_{BC} - T = 0$ $\Rightarrow T_{BC} = T$

OR
$$U = \sum \frac{T^2 l}{2GJ} = \frac{T^2}{2G}\left[\frac{l_{AB}}{J_{AB}} + \frac{l_{BC}}{J_{BC}}\right]$$

$$= \frac{T^2}{2 \times 80 \times 10^3}\left[\frac{300}{(\pi \times 20^4 / 32)} + \frac{500}{(\pi \times 40^4 / 32)}\right]$$

$$40000 = (1.32 \times 10^{-7})\ T^2$$

$$T = 550.9 \times 10^3 \text{ N-mm} = 550.9 \text{ N-m}$$

60. A compound shaft is as shown in Fig. 11.50(a). Determine the maximum permissible value of T if the angle of rotation of the free end is limited to 6°. Take $G = 83$ GPa for steel and $G = 28$ MPa for aluminum. Also find the strain energy stored in the shaft.

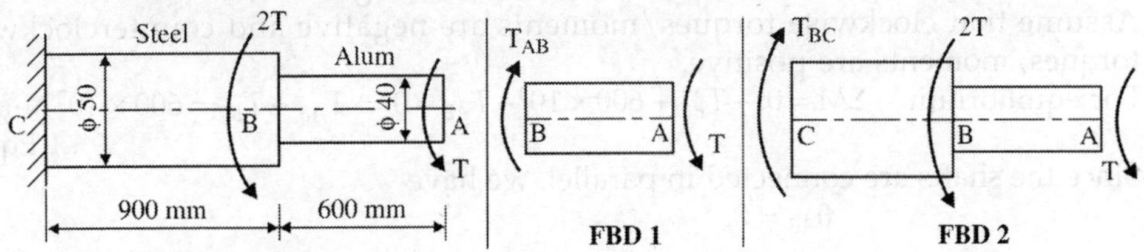

Fig. 11.50(a): Problem 60   **Fig. 11.50(b):** Problem 60: Free body diagrams

Solution: $d_{AB} = 40$ mm, $d_{BC} = 50$ mm, $l_{AB} = 600$ mm, $l_{BC} = 900$ mm, $\theta = 6° = 0.1047$ rad, $T_1 = T, T_2 = 2T, G_{AB} = G_{al} = 28 \times 10^3$ MPa, $G_{BC} = G_s = 83 \times 10^3$ MPa. $U = ?$

The free-body diagram of the system is shown in **Fig. 11.50(b)**.

Assume that clockwise torques/moments are negative and counterclockwise torques/moments are positive.

Shaft AB: $\Sigma M = 0: -T_{AB} + T = 0$ $\Rightarrow T_{AB} = T$

Shaft BC: $\Sigma M = 0: -T_{BC} + 2T + T = 0$ $\Rightarrow T_{BC} = 3T$

a. *To find T:*

Total angle of twist, $\quad \theta = \sum\left(\dfrac{Tl}{GJ}\right) = \left(\dfrac{Tl}{GJ}\right)_{AB} + \left(\dfrac{Tl}{GJ}\right)_{BC}$

$$0.1047 = \frac{T \times 600}{28 \times 10^3 \times (\pi \times 40^4/32)} + \frac{(3T) \times 900}{83 \times 10^3 \times (\pi \times 50^4/32)}$$

$$T = 0.757 \times 10^6 \text{ N-mm}$$

b. *To find* U:

$$U = \sum \frac{T^2 l}{2GJ} = \frac{1}{2}\left[\frac{(0.757 \times 10^6)^2 \times 600}{28 \times 10^3 \times (\pi \times 40^4/32)} + \frac{(3 \times 0.757 \times 10^6)^2 \times 900}{83 \times 10^3 \times (\pi \times 50^4/32)}\right]$$

$$= 70.06 \times 10^3 \text{ N-mm} = 70.06 \text{ J}$$

11.11.4 Problems on parallel shafts: Known torque

61. A steel shaft 1 m long, 30 mm diameter is rigidly fixed at its ends as shown in Fig. 11.50(a). If a torque of 600 N-m is applied at a distance of 250 mm from the left end, calculate:
    (a)   Reactions at the supports
    (b)   Strain energy stored in the shaft. Take $G = 84$ GPa

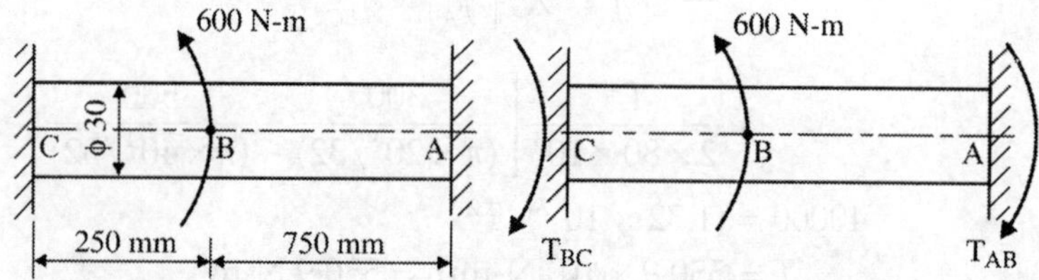

Fig. 11.51(a): Problem 61   **Fig. 11.51(b):** Problem 61: Free body diagrams

Solution: $d = 30$ mm, $l_{AB} = 750$ mm, $l_{BC} = 250$ mm, $T = 600$ N-m, $G = 84 \times 10^3$ MPa.
a) $T_{AB} = ?$, $T_{CD} = ?$ b) U = ?.

The free-body diagram of the system is shown in **Fig. 11.51(b)**.

Assume that clockwise torques/moments are negative and counterclockwise torques/moments are positive.

For equilibrium, $\quad \Sigma M = 0: -T_{BC} + 600 \times 10^3 - T_{AB} = 0 \Rightarrow T_{AB} + T_{BC} = 600 \times 10^3 \text{ N-mm}$

$$\dots \text{ Eq. (i)}$$

Since the shafts are connected in parallel, we have

$$\theta_{AB} = \theta_{BC}$$

$$\left(\frac{Tl}{GJ}\right)_{AB} = \left(\frac{Tl}{GJ}\right)_{BC}$$

Since J and G remain same, we have

$$T_{AB} \times 750 = T_{BC} \times 250$$

$$T_{BC} = 3\,T_{AB} \qquad\qquad \dots \text{ Eq. (ii)}$$

Substituting Eq. (ii) in Eq. (i), we have

$$600 \times 10^3 = T_{AB} + 3T_{AB}$$

$$T_{AB} = 150 \times 10^3 \text{ N-mm}$$

Eq. (ii) yields... $\quad T_{BC} = 3 \times (150 \times 10^3) = 450 \times 10^3 \text{ N-mm}$

a. *Reactions:*

$$T_{AB} = 150 \times 10^3 \text{ N-mm} \qquad T_{BC} = 450 \times 10^3 \text{ N-mm}$$

b. *To find* $\cup$:

We know that
$$\cup = \sum \frac{T^2 l}{2GJ} = \frac{1}{2GJ}\left[T_{AB}^2 l_{AB} + T_{BC}^2 l_{BC}\right]$$

$$= \frac{1}{2 \times 84 \times 10^3 \times (\pi \times 30^4/32)}\left[(150 \times 10^3)^2 \times 750\right.$$

$$\left. + (450 \times 10^3)^2 \times 250\right]$$

$$\cup = 5.05 \times 10^3 \text{ N-mm} = 5.05 \text{ J}$$

62. Determine the strain energy stored for the steel shaft shown in Fig. 11.52(a). Take $G = 84$ GPa.

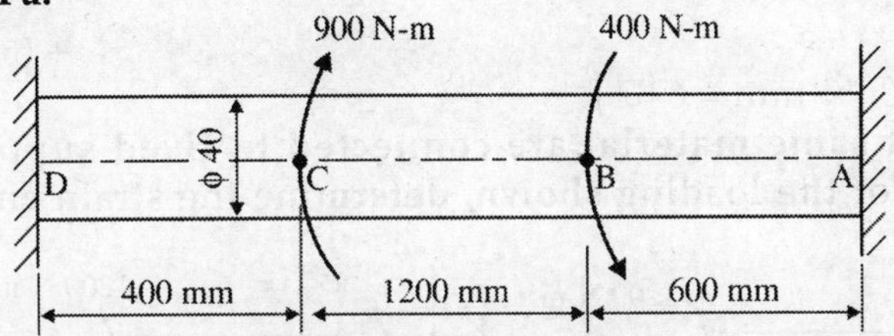

Fig. 11.52(a): Problem 62

Solution: $d = 40$ mm, $l_{AB} = 600$ mm, $l_{BC} = 1200$ mm, $l_{CD} = 400$ mm, $T_1 = 400$ N-m, $T_2 = 900$ N-m, $G = 84 \times 10^3$ MPa. $\cup = ?$

The free-body diagram of the system is shown in **Fig. 11.52(b)**.

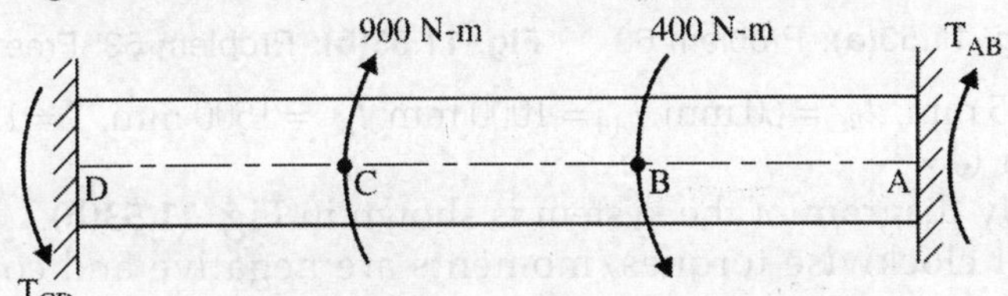

Fig. 11.52(b): Problem 62: Free body diagrams

Assume that clockwise torques/moments are negative and counterclockwise torques/moments are positive.

For equilibrium, $\Sigma M = 0$: $T_{CD} - T_2 + T_1 - T_{AB} = 0$

$$T_{CD} - T_{AB} = T_2 - T_1 = (900 \times 10^3) - (400 \times 10^3)$$

$$T_{CD} - T_{AB} = 500 \times 10^3 \text{ N-mm} \qquad \dots \text{Eq. (i)}$$

Since the shafts are connected in parallel, we have

$$\theta_{AB} = \theta_{BC} = \theta_{CD} \quad \text{or} \quad \Sigma\theta = 0$$

i.e. $\left(\dfrac{Tl}{GJ}\right)_{AB} + \left(\dfrac{Tl}{GJ}\right)_{BC} + \left(\dfrac{Tl}{GJ}\right)_{CD} = 0$

Here $T_{AB} = T_{AB}$; $T_{BC} = (T_{AB} - T_1)$; $T_{CD} = [T_{AB} - (T_1 + T_2)]$

Since J and G remain same, we have

$$[T_{AB} \times 600] + [T_{AB} - (400 \times 10^3)] \times 1200 + [T_{AB} - (-500 \times 10^3)] \times 400 = 0$$

$$(2200)\,T_{AB} - 480 \times 10^6 + 200 \times 10^6 = 0$$

$$(2200)\,T_{AB} = 280 \times 10^6$$

$$T_{AB} = 127.27 \times 10^3 \text{ N-mm}$$

Eq. (i) yields... $T_{CD} = 500 \times 10^3 + 127.27 \times 10^3 = 627.23 \times 10^3 \text{ N-mm}$

Reactions at the supports:
$$T_{AB} = 127.27 \times 10^3 \text{ N-mm}$$
$$T_{BC} = [T_{AB} - T_1] = [127.27 \times 10^3 - 400 \times 10^3] = -272.73 \times 10^3 \text{ N-mm}$$
$$T_{CD} = 627.23 \times 10^3 \text{ N-mm}$$

Check for equilibrium:
$$T_{CD} = [-T_{AB} + T_1 - T_2] = (-127.27 \times 10^3) + 400 \times 10^3 - 900 \times 10^3 = -627.23 \times 10^3 \text{ N-mm}$$

Opposite sign to obtained value, hence balanced

Strain energy:

$$U = \sum \frac{T^2 l}{2GJ} = \frac{1}{2GJ}\left[T_{AB}^2 l_{AB} + T_{BC}^2 l_{BC} + T_{CD}^2 l_{CD} \right]$$

$$= \frac{1}{2 \times 84 \times 10^3 \times (\pi \times 40^4/32)}[(127.27 \times 10^3)^2 \times 600 + (-272.73 \times 10^3)^2 \times 1200$$
$$+ (627.23 \times 10^3)^2 \times 400]$$

$$U = 6.07 \times 10^3 \text{ N-mm} = 6.07 \text{ J}$$

63. **Two shafts of same material are connected to fixed supports as shown in Fig. 11.53(a). For the loading shown, determine the strain energy stored. Take $G = 84$ GPa.**

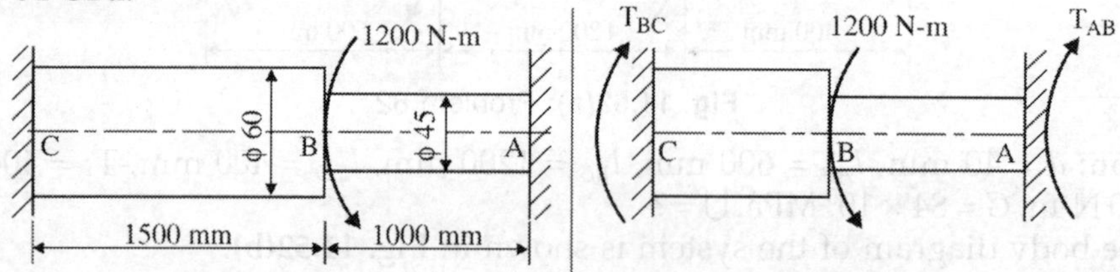

Fig. 11.53(a): Problem 63   **Fig. 11.53(b):** Problem 63: Free body diagrams

Solution: $d_{AB} = 45$ mm, $d_{BC} = 60$ mm, $l_{AB} = 1000$ mm, $l_{BC} = 1500$ mm, T = 1200×10^3 N-mm, $G = 84 \times 10^3$ MPa. $U = ?$

The free-body diagram of the system is shown in **Fig. 11.53(b)**.

Assume that clockwise torques/moments are negative and counterclockwise torques/moments are positive.

For equilibrium, $\Sigma M = 0$: $- T_{BC} + (1200 \times 10^3) - T_{AB} = 0 \Rightarrow T_{AB} + T_{BC} = 1200 \times 10^3$ N-mm
$$\dots \text{Eq. (i)}$$

Since the shafts are connected in parallel, we have
$$\theta_{AB} = \theta_{BC}$$

$$\left(\frac{Tl}{GJ}\right)_{AB} = \left(\frac{Tl}{GJ}\right)_{BC}$$

Since material is same, we have
$$\left(\frac{Tl}{J}\right)_{AB} = \left(\frac{Tl}{J}\right)_{BC}$$

$$\left[\frac{T_{AB} \times 1000}{(\pi \times 45^4/32)}\right] = \left[\frac{T_{BC} \times 1500}{(\pi \times 60^4/32)}\right]$$

$$T_{AB} = (0.4746)\, T_{BC} \qquad \dots \text{Eq. (ii)}$$

Substituting Eq. (ii) in Eq. (i), we have
$$1200 \times 10^3 = (0.4746)\, T_{BC} + T_{BC}$$

$$T_{BC} = 813.78 \times 10^3 \text{ N-mm}$$

Eq. (ii) yields... $\quad T_{AB} = (0.4746) \times (813.78 \times 10^3) = 386.22 \times 10^3 \text{ N-mm}$

Strain energy:

We know that $\displaystyle U = \sum \frac{T^2 l}{2GJ} = \frac{1}{2G} \times \sum \frac{T^2 l}{2J}$

$$= \frac{1}{2 \times 84 \times 10^3} \left[\frac{(386.22 \times 10^3)^2 \times 1000}{(\pi \times 45^4 / 32)} + \frac{(813.78 \times 10^3)^2 \times 1500}{(\pi \times 60^4 / 32)} \right]$$

$$U = 6.85 \times 10^3 \text{ N-mm} = 6.85 \text{ J}$$

11.11.5 Problems on parallel shafts: Unknown torque

64. **Obtain a relation of strain energy for a uniform shaft is as shown in Fig. 11.54(a). The material of the bar is the same throughout.**

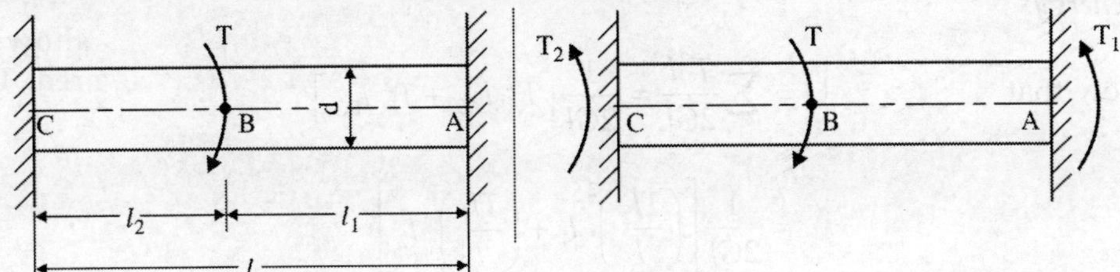

Fig. 11.54(a): Problem 64   **Fig. 11.54(b):** Problem 64: Free body diagrams

Solution: $l_{AB} = l_1,\ l_{BC} = l_2,\ G = G_{AB} = G_{BC}$

Let $\quad d = $ diameter of the shaft

$\quad T_{AB} = T_1$, be the reactive torque at support A

$\quad T_{BC} = T_2$, be the reactive torque at support C

$\quad J_{AB} = J_1$, be the polar modulus of portion AB

$\quad J_{BC} = J_2$, be the polar modulus of portion BC

The free-body diagram of the system is shown in **Fig. 11.54(b)**.

Assume that clockwise torques/moments are negative and counterclockwise torques/moments are positive.

For equilibrium, $\Sigma M = 0 : T_{BC} - T + T_{AB} = 0 \quad \Rightarrow T_{AB} + T_{BC} = T \quad$ i.e. $\quad T_1 + T_2 = T$

$$\text{... Eq. (i)}$$

Since the shafts are connected in parallel, we have

$$\theta_{AB} = \theta_{BC} \quad \text{or} \quad \Sigma \theta = 0$$

$$\left(\frac{Tl}{GJ} \right)_{AB} = \left(\frac{Tl}{GJ} \right)_{BC}$$

$$\left[\frac{T_1 l_1}{GJ_1} \right] = \left[\frac{T_2 l_2}{GJ_2} \right]$$

Since J and G remain same, we have

$$T_1 = T_2 \left(\frac{l_2}{l_1} \right) \qquad\qquad \text{... Eq. (ii)}$$

Or $\qquad\qquad T_2 = T_1 \left(\frac{l_1}{l_2} \right) \qquad\qquad \text{... Eq. (iii)}$

Substituting Eq. (iii) in Eq. (i) yields...

$$T = T_1 + T_1\left(\frac{l_1}{l_2}\right)$$

$$= \frac{T_1 l_2 + T_1 l_1}{l_2} = T_1\left[\frac{l_2 + l_1}{l_2}\right] = \left(\frac{T_1 l}{l_2}\right) \qquad (\because\ l = l_1 + l_2)$$

$$T_1 = \left(\frac{T l_2}{l}\right) \qquad \ldots \text{Eq. (iv)}$$

On similar lines, we have

$$T_2 = \left(\frac{T l_1}{l}\right) \qquad \ldots \text{Eq. (v)}$$

Strain energy:

We know that

$$U = \sum \frac{T^2 l}{2GJ} = \frac{1}{2GJ}\left[T_{AB}^2 l_{AB} + T_{BC}^2 l_{BC}\right]$$

$$= \frac{1}{2GJ}\left[\left(\frac{T l_2}{l}\right)^2 l_1 + \left(\frac{T l_1}{l}\right)^2 l_2\right]$$

$$= \frac{T^2}{2GJl^2}\left[l_2^2 l_1 + l_1^2 l_2\right]$$

$$= \frac{T^2 l_1 l_2}{2GJl^2}\left[l_2 + l_1\right]$$

$$U = \left(\frac{T^2 l_1 l_2}{2GJl}\right) \qquad (\because\ l = l_1 + l_2) \qquad \ldots \text{Eq. (vi)}$$

65. Obtain a relation of strain energy for a uniform shaft is as shown in Fig. 11.55(a). The material of the bar is the same throughout.

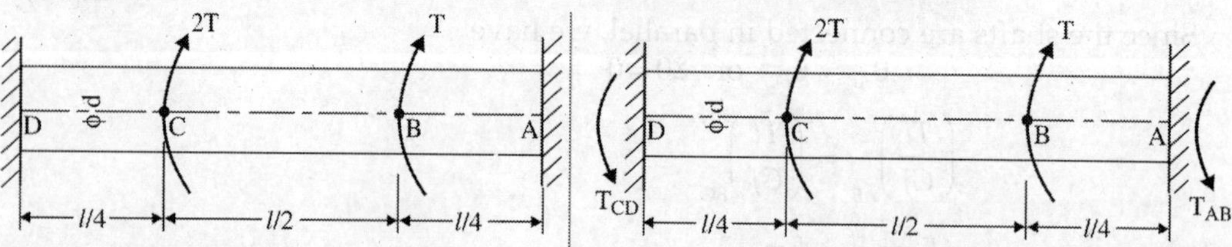

Fig. 11.55(a): Problem 65   **Fig. 11.55(b):** Problem 65: Free body diagrams

Solution: $l_{AB} = l/4 = l_{CD}$, $l_{BC} = l/2$, $T_1 = T$, $T_2 = 2T$, $G = G_{AB} = G_{BC} = G_{CD}$.

The free-body diagram of the system is shown in **Fig. 11.55(b)**.

Assume that clockwise torques/moments are negative and counterclockwise torques/moments are positive.

For equilibrium, $\Sigma M = 0$: $\quad T_{CD} - 2T - T + T_{AB} = 0 \qquad \Rightarrow T_{AB} + T_{CD} = 3T \ \ldots$ Eq. (i)

Since the shafts are connected in parallel, we have

$$\theta_{AB} = \theta_{BC} \quad \text{or} \quad \Sigma\theta = 0$$

$$\left(\frac{Tl}{GJ}\right)_{AB} + \left(\frac{Tl}{GJ}\right)_{BC} + \left(\frac{Tl}{GJ}\right)_{CD} = 0$$

Here
$$T_{AB} = T_{AB};$$
$$T_{BC} = (T_{AB} - T_1) = (T_{AB} - T);$$
$$T_{CD} = [T_{AB} - (T_1 + T_2)] = (T_{AB} - 3T) \qquad \text{... Eq. (ii)}$$

Since J and G remain same, we have

$$\left[\frac{T_{AB}(l/4)}{GJ}\right] + \left[\frac{(T_{AB} - T)(l/2)}{GJ}\right] + \left[\frac{(T_{AB} - 3T)(l/4)}{GJ}\right] = 0$$

$$T_{AB}(l/4) + (T_{AB} - T)(l/2) + (T_{AB} - 3T)(l/4) = 0$$
$$(l/4)[T_{AB} + 2(T_{AB} - T) + (T_{AB} - 3T)] = 0$$
$$4T_{AB} - 5T = 0$$
$$T_{AB} = 5T/4$$

Eq. (ii) yields...
$$T_{BC} = (5T/4 - T) = T/4$$
$$T_{CD} = (5T/4 - 3T) = -7T/4$$

Strain energy:

We know that
$$U = \sum \frac{T^2 l}{2GJ} = \frac{1}{2GJ}\left[T_{AB}^2 l_{AB} + T_{BC}^2 l_{BC} + T_{CD}^2 l_{CD}\right]$$

$$= \frac{1}{2GJ}\left[\left(\frac{5T}{4}\right)^2\left(\frac{l}{4}\right) + \left(\frac{T}{4}\right)^2\left(\frac{l}{2}\right) + \left(\frac{-7T}{4}\right)^2\left(\frac{l}{4}\right)\right]$$

$$= \frac{T^2 l}{2GJ}\left[\frac{25}{64} + \frac{1}{32} + \frac{49}{64}\right] = \frac{T^2 l^2}{2GJ}\left[\frac{25 + 2 + 49}{64}\right]$$

$$U = \frac{19T^2 l}{32GJ}$$

66. Obtain a relation of strain energy for a uniform shaft is as shown in Fig. 11.56(a). The material of the bar is the same throughout.

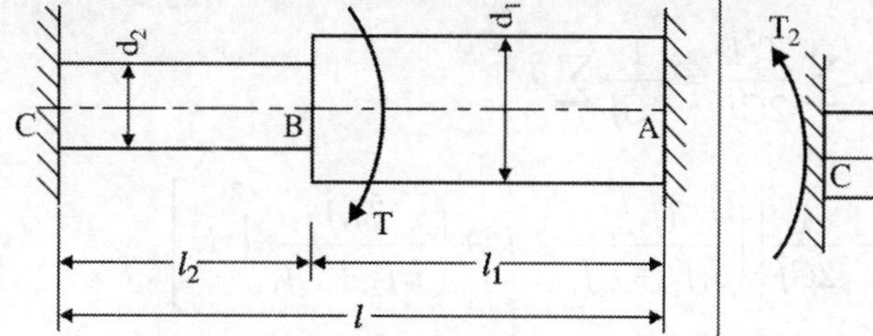

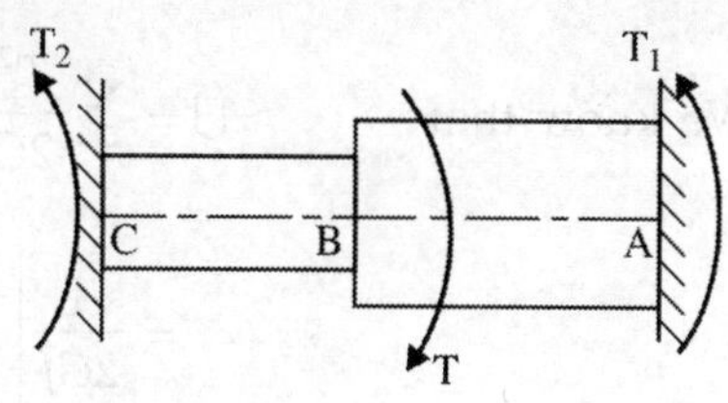

Fig. 11.56(a): Problem 66   **Fig. 11.56(b):** Problem 66: Free body diagrams

Solution: $d_{AB} = d_1$, $d_{BC} = d_2$, $l_{AB} = l_1$, $l_{BC} = l_2$, $G = G_{AB} = G_{BC}$

Let $T_{AB} = T_1$, be the reactive torque at support A

$T_{BC} = T_2$, be the reactive torque at support C

$J_{AB} = J_1$, be the polar modulus of portion AB

$J_{BC} = J_2$, be the polar modulus of portion BC

The free-body diagram of the system is shown in **Fig. 11.56(b)**.

Assume that clockwise torques/moments are negative and counterclockwise torques/moments are positive.

For equilibrium, $\Sigma M = 0$: $\quad T_{BC} - T + T_{AB} = 0 \quad \Rightarrow T_{AB} + T_{BC} = T \quad$ i.e. $\quad T_1 + T_2 = T$

$$\dots \text{Eq. (i)}$$

Since the shafts are connected in parallel, we have

$$\theta_{AB} = \theta_{BC} \quad \text{or} \quad \Sigma\theta = 0$$

$$\left(\frac{Tl}{GJ}\right)_{AB} = \left(\frac{Tl}{GJ}\right)_{BC}$$

$$\left[\frac{T_1 l_1}{GJ_1}\right] = \left[\frac{T_2 l_2}{GJ_2}\right]$$

$$T_1 = T_2 \left(\frac{l_2}{l_1}\right)\left(\frac{J_1}{J_2}\right) \qquad \dots \text{Eq. (ii)}$$

Or $\qquad\qquad T_2 = T_1 \left(\frac{l_1}{l_2}\right)\left(\frac{J_2}{J_1}\right) \qquad \dots \text{Eq. (iii)}$

Substituting Eq. (iii) in Eq. (i) yields...

$$T = T_1 + T_1 \left(\frac{l_1}{l_2}\right)\left(\frac{J_2}{J_1}\right)$$

$$= \frac{T_1 l_2 J_1 + T_1 l_1 J_2}{l_2 J_1} = T_1 \left[\frac{l_2 J_1 + l_1 J_2}{l_2 J_1}\right]$$

$$T_1 = T\left[\frac{l_2 J_1}{l_2 J_1 + l_1 J_2}\right] \qquad \dots \text{Eq. (iv)}$$

On similar lines, we have

$$T_2 = T\left[\frac{l_1 J_2}{l_1 J_2 + l_2 J_1}\right] \qquad \dots \text{Eq. (v)}$$

Strain energy:

We know that $\qquad U = \sum \dfrac{T^2 l}{2GJ} = \dfrac{1}{2GJ} \sum T^2 l$

$$= \frac{1}{2GJ}\left[\left(\frac{T l_2 J_1}{l_1 J_2 + l_2 J_1}\right)^2 l_1 + \left(\frac{T l_1 J_2}{l_1 J_2 + l_2 J_1}\right)^2 l_2\right]$$

$$= \frac{T^2 \left[l_1 l_2^2\, J_1^2 + l_2 l_1^2\, J_2^2\right]}{2GJ(l_1 J_2 + l_2 J_1)^2}$$

$$U = \frac{T^2 l_1 l_2 \left[l_2 J_1^2 + l_1 J_2^2\right]}{2GJ(l_1 J_2 + l_2 J_1)^2} \qquad \dots \text{Eq. (vi)}$$

If $J_1 = J_2$, then Eq. (vi) reduces to the form

$$U = \frac{T^2 l_1 l_2 J^2 [l_2 + l_1]}{2GJ^3 (l_1 + l_2)^2} = \frac{T^2 J^2 l_1 l_2 l}{2GJ^2 l^2}$$

$$U = \left(\frac{T^2 l_1 l_2}{2GJl}\right) \qquad (\because \ l = l_1 + l_2) \qquad \text{... Eq. (vii)}$$

The above equation is same as that derived in Problem 64 [Eq. (vi)].

11.11.6 Problems on torque: Comparison/ratios

67. A hollow shaft having the external diameter twice the internal diameter, subjected to a pure torque, attains a maximum shear stress τ. Show that the strain energy stored per unit volume of the shaft is $5\tau^2/16G$.

Such a shaft is required to transmit 4500 kW at 110 rpm with uniform torque, the maximum stress not exceeding 70 MPa. Calculate the shaft diameters and the energy stored per m^3 when transmitting this power. $G = 83$ GPa.

Solution: $d_o = 2d_i \Rightarrow K = \dfrac{d_i}{d_o} = 0.5$, $P = 4500$ kW, $N = 110$ rpm, $\tau = 70$ MPa, $G = 83 \times 10^3$ MPa, $d_o, d_i = ?, U = ?$

a. *Proof of $5\tau^2/16G$*

For a hollow shaft, $\quad u = \dfrac{U}{V} = \dfrac{\tau^2 (1 + K^2)}{4G}$ ... using (Eq. 11.26)

$$= \frac{\tau^2}{4G}(1 + 0.5^2) = \frac{\tau^2}{4G}\left(1 + \frac{1}{4}\right)$$

$$U = \frac{\tau^2}{4G}\left(\frac{5}{4}\right) = \frac{5\tau^2}{16G} = \frac{0.3125\tau^2}{G} \qquad \text{... Eq. (i)}$$

b. *To find diameters:*

For a hollow shaft, $\quad T = \dfrac{\pi}{16} d_o^3 (1 - K^4)\tau$ ... Eq. (ii)

But $\qquad P = \dfrac{2\pi NT}{60}$

$$4500 \times 10^3 = \frac{2\pi \times 110 \times T}{60}$$

$$T = 390.65 \times 10^3 \text{ N-m} = 390.65 \times 10^6 \text{ N-mm}$$

Eq. (ii) yields... $390.65 \times 10^6 = \left(\dfrac{\pi}{16}\right) d_o^3 \times [1 - 0.5^4] \times 70$

$$d_o = 311.82 \text{ mm} \simeq 312 \text{ mm}$$

and $\qquad d_i = 0.5 \times 312 = 156 \text{ mm}$

c. *To find u:*

$$u = \frac{\tau^2(1 + K^2)}{4G} = \frac{70^2 \times (1 + 0.5^2)}{4 \times (83 \times 10^3)} = 18.45 \times 10^{-3} \text{ N-mm/mm}^3$$

$$= 18.45 \text{ kJ/m}^3$$

Or
$$u = \frac{5 \times 70^2}{16 \times (83 \times 10^3)} = 18.45 \times 10^{-3}\ \text{N-mm/mm}^3$$

$$= 18.45\ \text{J/m}^3$$

68. A hollow shaft, subjected to a pure torque, attains a maximum shearing stress τ. Given that the strain energy stored per unit volume is $\tau^2/3G$, calculate the ratio of the shaft diameters.

Determine the actual diameters for such a shaft required to transmit 5000 kW at 150 rpm with uniform torque when the energy stored is 25 kJ/m^3 of material. $G = 80$ GPa.

Solution: $K = ?$, $P = 5000$ kW, $N = 150$ rpm, $u = 25$ kJ/m^3 = 0.025 N-mm/mm^3, $G = 80 \times 10^3$ MPa.

Given
$$u = \frac{\tau^2}{3G}$$

$$0.025 = \frac{\tau^2}{3 \times (80 \times 10^3)}$$

$$\tau = 77.46\ \text{MPa}$$

To find K:

$$u = \frac{\tau^2(1 + K^2)}{4G}$$

$$0.025 = \frac{77.46^2 \times (1 + K^2)}{4 \times (80 \times 10^3)}$$

$$K = 0.58$$

To find diameters:

For a hollow shaft,
$$T = \frac{\pi}{16}\, d_o^3 (1 - K^4)\tau$$

But
$$P = \frac{2\pi NT}{60}$$

$$5000 \times 10^3 = \frac{2\pi \times 150 \times T}{60}$$

$$T = 318.31 \times 10^3\ \text{N-m} = 318.31 \times 10^6\ \text{N-mm}$$

Eq. (i) yields...
$$318.31 \times 10^6 = \left(\frac{\pi}{16}\right) d_o^3 \times [1 - 0.58^4] \times 77.46$$

$$d_o = 286.84\ \text{mm} \approx 288\ \text{mm}$$

and
$$d_i = 0.58 \times 288 = 167.04\ \text{mm}$$

11.12 PROBLEMS ON MOMENT

11.12.1 Problems on bending: Cantilever beams

Note:
- In these problems, only the effect of normal stress is considered. The effect of shear stress is neglected.
- Concepts of shear force and bending moment are as explained in *Chapter 5*.

69. Derive an expression for strain energy stored and maximum deflection in a cantilever beam subjected to point load at free end. EI is constant.

Solution: Based on given data, the cantilever beam is as shown in **Fig. 11.57**.

Let W = Load at free end

L = Length of the beam

$y = y_{max}$ = Maximum deflection

Consider a section X-X at a distance x from free end A. Bending moment at X-X is given as

$$M = -W.x \qquad \text{(Negative because, hogging)}$$

Strain energy, $U = \displaystyle\int_0^L \dfrac{M^2 dx}{2EI}$

$$= \int_0^L \dfrac{(-W.x)^2 dx}{2EI} = \dfrac{W^2}{2EI} \int_0^L x^2 dx$$

$$= \dfrac{W^2}{2EI}\left(\dfrac{x^3}{3}\right)_0^L$$

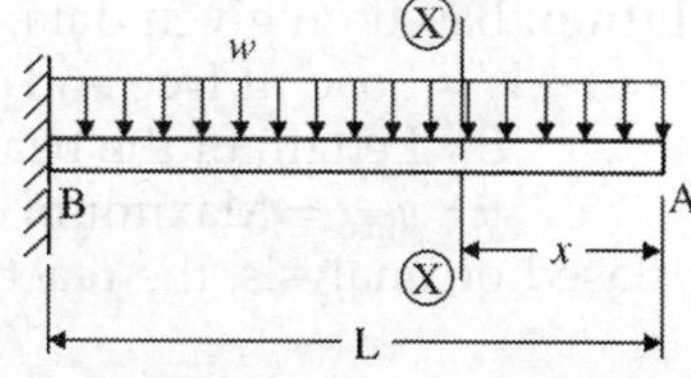
Fig. 11.57: Problem 69

$$U = \dfrac{W^2 L^3}{6EI} \qquad (F \text{ or } W) \qquad \dots \text{(Eq. 11.57)}$$

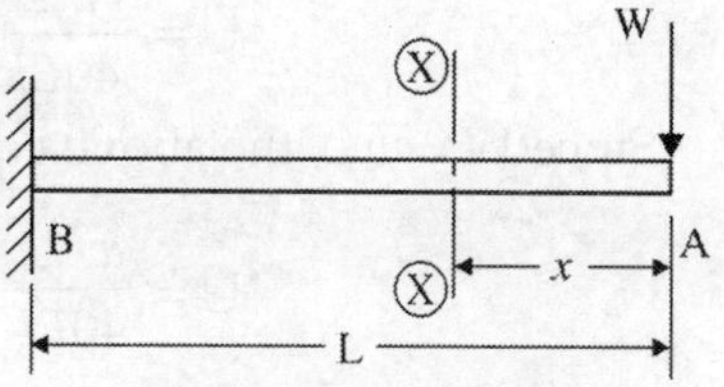

Since work done = strain energy, we have

$$\dfrac{1}{2}\, W.y_{max} = \dfrac{W^2 L^3}{6EI}$$

$$y_{max} = \dfrac{WL^3}{3EI} \qquad \text{(at free end)} \qquad \dots \text{(Eq. 11.58)}$$

70. Derive an expression for strain energy stored in a cantilever beam subjected to uniformly distributed load over the entire span. *EI* is constant.

If the cross-section is rectangular of $b \times h$ then prove that the maximum strain energy density due to bending is given by $u = \dfrac{15\, U}{V}$, where U = strain energy and V = volume of the beam

Solution: Based on given data, the cantilever beam is as shown in **Fig. 11.58**.

Let w = Uniformly distributed load per unit length

L = Length of the beam

$y = y_{max}$ = Maximum deflection

Consider a section X-X at a distance x from free end A. Bending moment at X-X is given as

$$M = -w.x\left(\dfrac{x}{2}\right) = -\left(\dfrac{wx^2}{2}\right)$$

Strain energy, $U = \displaystyle\int_0^L \dfrac{M^2 dx}{2EI}$

Fig. 11.58: Problem 70

$$= \frac{1}{2EI} \int_0^L \left(\frac{-wx^2}{2} \right)^2 dx$$

$$= \frac{w^2}{2EI} \int_0^L \frac{x^4}{4} dx = \frac{w^2}{8EI} \int_0^L x^4 dx$$

$$= \frac{w^2}{8EI} \left(\frac{x^5}{5} \right)_0^L$$

$$U = \frac{W^2 L^3}{40EI} \qquad\qquad\qquad \dots \text{(Eq. 11.59a)}$$

Since $W = w.L$, the above equation can also be written as

$$U = \frac{w^2 L^5}{40EI} \qquad\qquad (W \text{ or } F) \qquad\qquad \dots \text{(Eq. 11.59b)}$$

Strain energy density:

We know that $\quad u = \dfrac{U}{V} = \dfrac{\sigma^2}{2E} \qquad\qquad\qquad \dots \text{using (Eq. 11.8)}$

But $\qquad \sigma_b = \sigma = \dfrac{M}{Z} = \dfrac{Mc}{I}; M = -\left(\dfrac{wL^2}{2} \right); c = h/2; I = bh^3/12$

$$u = \frac{M^2 c^2}{2EI^2} = \frac{(-wL^2/2)^2 (h/2)^2}{2EI^2} = \frac{w^2 L^4 h^2}{32EI^2} \qquad \dots \text{(Eq. 11.60)}$$

$$\frac{U}{u} = \frac{w^2 L^5/40EI}{w^2 L^4 h^2/32EI^2}$$

$$= \frac{4LI}{5h^2} = \frac{4L(bh^3/12)}{5h^2}$$

$$\frac{U}{u} = \frac{Lbh}{15} = \frac{V}{15}$$

$$u = \frac{15\,U}{V} \qquad\qquad\qquad\qquad \dots \text{(Eq. 11.60a)}$$

11.12.2 Problems on bending: Simply supported beams

71. **Derive an expression for strain energy stored and maximum deflection in a simply supported beam subjected to point load at mid-span. *EI* is constant.**

Solution: Based on given data, the beam is as shown in **Fig. 11.59**.

Let $\quad W = $ Load at free end

$\qquad L = $ Length of the beam

$\qquad y = y_{max} = $ Maximum deflection

Based on analysis, the reactions at the supports are

$$R_A = R_B = \left(\frac{W}{2} \right)$$

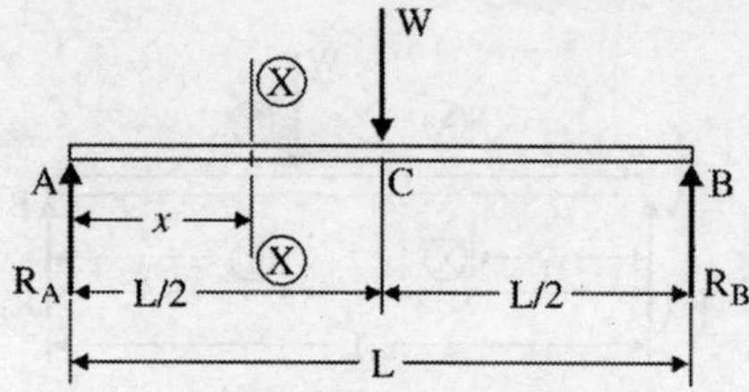

Fig. 11.59: Problem 71

Consider a section X-X at a distance x from end A. Bending moment at X-X is given as

$$M = R_A . x = \left(\frac{W}{2}\right)x$$

Due to symmetry, the above equation can also be used for segment BC with x originating from B

Total strain energy,

$$U = U_{AB} + U_{BC}$$

$$= \int_0^{L/2} \frac{M^2 dx}{2EI} + \int_{L/2}^{L} \frac{M^2 dx}{2EI}$$

$$= 2 \int_0^{L/2} \frac{M^2 dx}{2EI} = \frac{2}{2EI} \int_0^{L/2} \left(\frac{Wx}{2}\right)^2 dx$$

$$= \frac{W^2}{4EI} \int_0^{L/2} x^2 dx$$

$$= \frac{W^2}{4EI} \left(\frac{x^3}{3}\right)_0^{L/2}$$

$$U = \frac{W^2 L^3}{96EI} \qquad (W \text{ or } F) \qquad \dots \text{(Eq. 11.61)}$$

Since work done = strain energy, we have

$$\frac{1}{2} W.y_{max} = \frac{W^2 L^3}{96EI}$$

$$y_{max} = \frac{WL^3}{48EI} \qquad (\text{at mid-span}) \qquad \dots \text{(Eq. 11.62)}$$

72. Derive an expression for strain energy stored and maximum deflection in a simply supported beam carrying a point load in any position. _EI_ is constant. If _W_ = 50 kN, _a_ = 3 m, _b_ = 1 m, _EI_ = 25 MN-m², Find U.

Solution: Based on given data, the beam is as shown in **Fig. 11.60**.

Let W = Eccentric point load

      L = Length of the beam

     $y = y_{max}$ = Maximum deflection

Based on analysis, the reactions at the supports are

$$R_A = \left(\frac{Wb}{L}\right), R_B = \left(\frac{Wa}{L}\right)$$

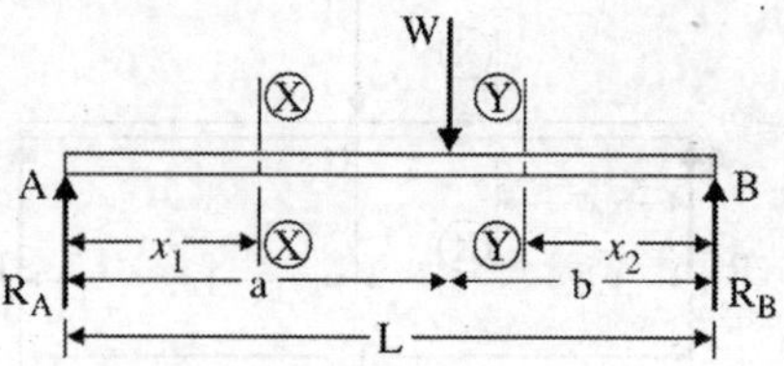

Fig. 11.60: Problem 72

Consider a section X-X at a distance x_1 from end A. Bending moment at X-X is given as

$$M_{AC} = R_A.x_1 = \left(\frac{Wb}{L}\right) x_1 \qquad \text{for } 0 < x_1 < a$$

Consider a section Y-Y at a distance x_2 from end B. Bending moment at Y-Y is given as

$$M_{BC} = R_B.x_2 = \left(\frac{Wa}{L}\right) x_2 \qquad \text{for } 0 < x_2 < b$$

Total strain energy, $U = U_{AB} + U_{BC}$

$$= \int_0^a \frac{M_{AC}^2}{2EI}\, dx_1 + \int_0^b \frac{M_{BC}^2}{2EI}\, dx_2$$

$$= \frac{1}{2EI} \int_0^a \left(\frac{Wbx_1}{L}\right)^2 dx_1 + \frac{1}{2EI} \int_0^b \left(\frac{Wax_2}{L}\right)^2 dx_2$$

$$= \frac{W^2b^2}{2EIL^2} \int_0^a x_1^2\, dx_1 + \frac{W^2a^2}{2EIL^2} \int_0^b x_2^2\, dx_2$$

$$= \frac{W^2b^2}{2EIL^2} \left(\frac{x_1^3}{3}\right)_0^a + \frac{W^2a^2}{2EIL^2} \left(\frac{x_2^3}{3}\right)_0^b$$

$$= \frac{W^2b^2a^3}{6EIL^2} + \frac{W^2a^2b^3}{6EIL^2}$$

$$= \frac{W^2a^2b^2}{6EIL^2} (a + b)$$

$$U = \frac{W^2a^2b^2}{6EIL} \qquad [\because L = a + b] \qquad \dots \text{(Eq. 11.63)}$$

Since work done = strain energy, we have

$$\frac{1}{2} W.y_{max} = \frac{W^2a^2b^2}{6EIL}$$

$$y_{max} = \frac{Wa^2b^2}{3EIL} \qquad \text{(at C)} \qquad \dots \text{(Eq. 11.64)}$$

Thus $\qquad U = \dfrac{(50 \times 10^3)^2 \times 3^2 \times 1^2}{6 \times 25 \times 10^6 \times 4} = 37.5\,\text{J}$

73. Derive an expression for strain energy stored in a simply supported beam subjected to uniformly distributed load over the entire span. *EI* is constant. If the cross-section is rectangular of b × h then prove that the maximum strain energy density due to bending is given by $U = \dfrac{45\,U}{8V}$, where U = strain energy and V = volume of the beam

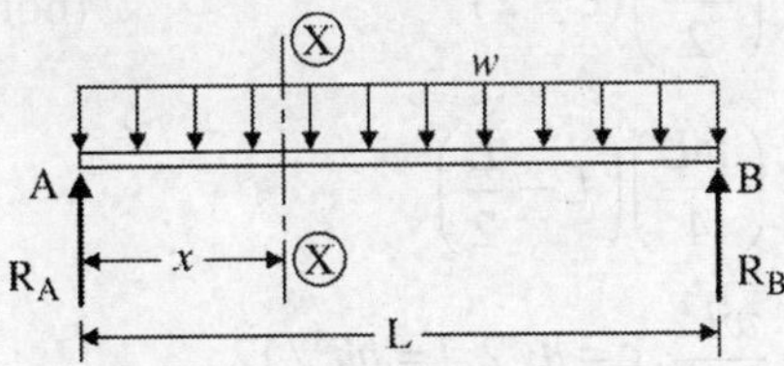

Fig. 11.61: Problem 73

Solution: Based on given data, the beam is as shown in **Fig. 11.61**.

Let $\qquad$ w = Uniformly distributed load per unit length

$\qquad$ L = Length of the beam

Based on analysis, the reactions at the supports are

$$R_A = R_B = \left(\frac{wL}{2}\right)$$

Consider a section X-X at a distance x from end A. Bending moment at X-X is given as

$$M = R_A.x - w.x\left(\frac{x}{2}\right)$$

$$= \left(\frac{wL}{2}\right)x - \left(\frac{wx^2}{2}\right)$$

$$M = \left(\frac{wx}{2}\right)(L-x)$$

Strain energy, $\quad U = \displaystyle\int_0^L \frac{M^2 dx}{2EI} = \frac{1}{2EI}\int_0^L \left[\left(\frac{wx}{2}\right)(L-x)\right]^2 dx$

$$= \frac{w^2}{8EI}\int_0^L \left[x^2(L-x)\right]^2 dx = \frac{w^2}{8EI}\int_0^L \left(x^2L^2 + x^4 - 2Lx^3\right)dx$$

$$= \frac{w^2}{8EI}\left[L^2\left(\frac{x^3}{3}\right) + \left(\frac{x^5}{5}\right) - 2L\left(\frac{x^4}{4}\right)\right]_0^L$$

$$= \frac{w^2}{8EI}\left[\left(\frac{L^5}{3}\right) + \left(\frac{L^5}{5}\right) - \left(\frac{L^5}{2}\right)\right]$$

$$U = \frac{w^2 L^5}{240EI} \qquad\qquad\qquad \text{... (Eq. 11.65)}$$

Strain energy density:

We know that $\quad u = \dfrac{U}{V} = \dfrac{\sigma^2}{2E}$ $\qquad\qquad$ ... using (Eq. 11.8)

But $\qquad \sigma_b = \sigma = \dfrac{M}{Z} = \dfrac{Mc}{I}$,

$$M = \left(\frac{wx}{2}\right)(L - x) \qquad\qquad (\text{here } x = L/2)$$

$$= \left(\frac{wL}{4}\right)\left(L - \frac{L}{2}\right)$$

$$M = \frac{wL^2}{8}, c = h/2, I = bh^3/12$$

$$u = \frac{M^2 c^2}{2EI^2} = \frac{(wL^2/8)^2(h/2)^2}{2EI^2} = \frac{w^2 L^4 h^2}{512 EI^2} \qquad ... \text{(Eq. 11.66a)}$$

$$\frac{U}{u} = \frac{w^2 L^5/240EI}{w^2 L^4 h^2/512 EI^2}$$

$$= \frac{32LI}{15h^2} = \frac{32L(bh^3/12)}{15h^2}$$

$$\frac{U}{u} = \frac{8Lbh}{45} = \frac{8V}{45}$$

$$u = \frac{45\, U}{8V} \qquad\qquad\qquad ... \text{(Eq. 11.66b)}$$

74. Derive an expression for strain energy stored in a prismatic beam as shown in Fig. 11.62(a). *EI* is constant. Also calculate the elastic strain energy if $P = 42$ kN, $L = 7$ m, $A = 1.5$ m and $EI = 3 \times 10^7$ N-m^2

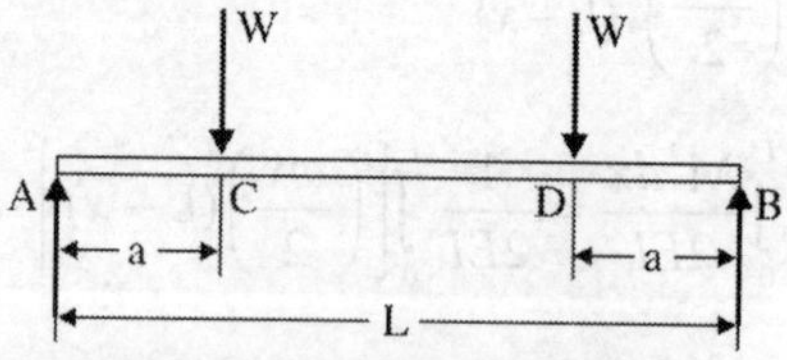

Fig. 11.62(a): Problem 74

Solution: Fig. 11.62(b) represents the reaction acting on the beam; **Fig. 11.62(c)** represents section X-X in portion AC.

Fig. 11.62(d) represents section Y-Y in portion CD

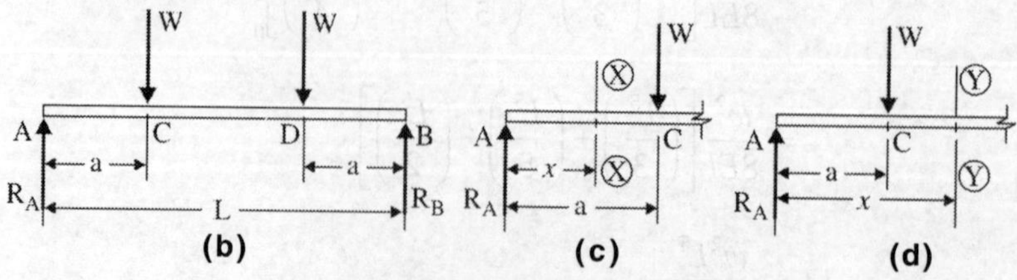

(b) $\qquad\qquad\qquad\qquad$ **(c)** $\qquad\qquad\qquad\qquad$ **(d)**

Fig. 11.62: Problem 74

Based on analysis, the reactions at the supports are
$$R_A = R_B = W$$
Consider a section X-X at a distance x from end A between A and C, as shown in **Fig. 11.62(c)**. Bending moment at X-X is
$$M_{AC} = R_A.x = Wx \qquad \text{for } 0 < x < a$$
From **Fig. 11.62(a)**, segment AC and segment BD have the same loading conditions, hence
$$M_{BD} = R_B.x = Wx \qquad \text{for } 0 < x < a$$
Consider a section Y-Y at a distance x from end A between C and D, as shown in **Fig. 11.62(d)**. Bending moment at Y-Y is
$$M_{CD} = R_A.x - W(x-a) = W.x - W(x-a) = Wa \quad \text{for } a < x < (L-a)$$
Total strain energy, $\mathsf{U} = \mathsf{U}_{AC} + \mathsf{U}_{CD} + \mathsf{U}_{DB} = 2\mathsf{U}_{AC} + \mathsf{U}_{CD}$

$$= 2\int_0^a \frac{M_{AC}^2 dx}{2EI} + \int_a^{L-a} \frac{M_{CD}^2 dx}{2EI}$$

$$= 2\int_0^a \frac{(Wx)^2 dx}{2EI} + \int_a^{L-a} \frac{(Wa)^2 dx}{2EI}$$

$$= \frac{W^2}{EI}\int_0^a x^2 dx + \frac{W^2 a^2}{2EI}\int_0^{L-a} dx$$

$$= \frac{W^2}{EI}\left(\frac{x^3}{3}\right)_0^a + \frac{W^2 a^2}{2EI}\left(\frac{x}{1}\right)_a^{L-a}$$

$$\mathsf{U} = \frac{W^2 a^3}{3EI} + \frac{W^2 a^2}{2EI}(L - 2a) \qquad\qquad \text{... (Eq. 11.67)}$$

Thus
$$\mathsf{U} = \frac{(42 \times 10^3)^2 \times 1.5^3}{3 \times (3 \times 10^7)} + \left[\frac{(42 \times 10^3)^2 \times 1.5^2}{2 \times (3 \times 10^7)}\right] \times (7 - 2 \times 1.5)$$

$$= 330.75 \text{ J}$$

11.13 CASTIGLIANO'S THEOREM

Castigliano's theorem is used to find deflection of an elastic structure based on strain energy of the structure. It is based on the assumption that the principle of superposition is applicable to the structure having constant temperature and that the material is linear-elastic. .

11.13.1 Castigliano's first theorem for deflection

It states that "For linearly elastic structure, if the total strain energy expressed in terms of the external loads is partially differentiated with respect to one of the loads, the result is the defection of the point of application of that load and in the direction of that load".

Or   The partial derivative of the strain energy of a structure with respect to any load is equal to the displacement corresponding to that load in the direction of its line of action.

$$\frac{\partial \mathsf{U}}{\partial F_n} = y_n \qquad\qquad \text{(F or W)}$$

Proof: Consider a beam subjected to any number of loads, F_1, F_2, F_3, ... F_n, as shown in **Fig. 11.63**. The deflections of the beam corresponding to the various loads are denoted are y_1, y_2, y_3, ... y_n. The total work done by the loads is equal to the strain energy stored in the beam.

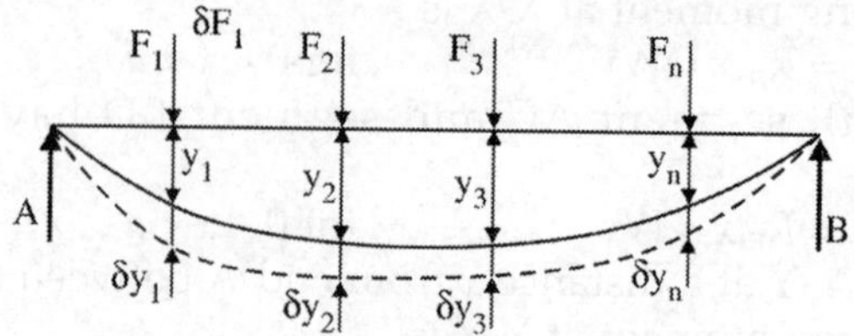

Fig. 11.63: Castigliano's first thorem

i.e.

$$W = U = \frac{1}{2} F_1.y_1 + \frac{1}{2} F_2.y_2 + \frac{1}{2} F_3.y_3 + \ldots \qquad \ldots \text{(Eq. a)}$$

If one of the loads say F_1 is increased to a value of δF_1 while the other loads are held constant, then changes in deflection will be δy_1, δy_2, δy_3, ... as shown in **Fig. 11.64**. In **Fig. 11.64(a)**, the increase in strain energy is represented by a small triangle and a rectangle, while **Fig. 11.64(b)** and **Fig. 11.64(c)** are just rectangles, since F_2 and F_3 are kept constant.

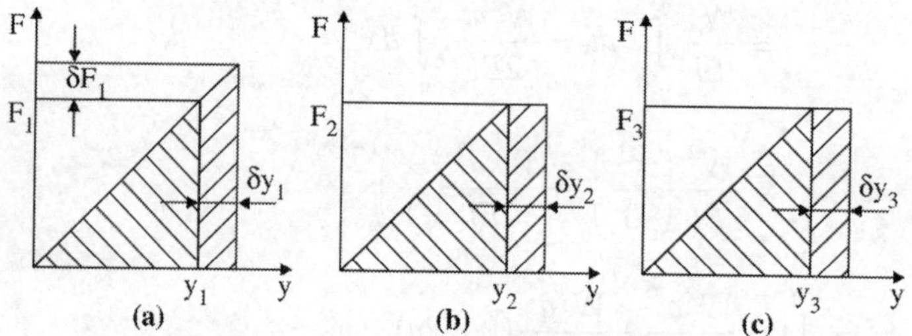

Fig. 11.64: Load extension curves

Increase in strain energy, $\quad \delta U = F_1.\delta y_1 + \frac{1}{2} \delta F_1.\delta y_1 + F_2.\delta y_2 + F_3.\delta y_3 + \ldots$

$$= \left(F_1 + \frac{1}{2} + \delta F_1 \right) \delta y_1 + F_2.\delta y_2 + F_3.\delta y_3 + \ldots \quad \ldots \text{(Eq. b)}$$

Neglecting the product of small quantities, we have

$$\delta U = F_1.\delta y_1 + F_2.\delta y_2 + F_3.\delta y_3 + \ldots \qquad \ldots \text{(Eq. c)}$$

If the same loads were applied gradually, then the total strain energy would be

$$U + \delta U = \frac{1}{2} (F_1 + \delta F_1)(y_1 + \delta y_1) + \frac{1}{2} F_2 (y_2 + \delta y_2) + \frac{1}{2} F_3 (y_3 + \delta y_3) + \ldots$$

$$= \frac{1}{2} F_1.y_1 + \frac{1}{2} F_1.\delta y_1 + \frac{1}{2} \delta F_1.y_1 + \frac{1}{2} \delta F_1.\delta y_1 + \frac{1}{2} F_2.y_2$$

$$+ \frac{1}{2} F_2.\delta y_2 + \frac{1}{2} F_3.y_3 + \frac{1}{2} F_3.\delta y_3 + \ldots$$

Neglecting the product of small quantities, we have

$$U + \delta U = \frac{1}{2} F_1.y_1 + \frac{1}{2} F_1.\delta y_1 + \frac{1}{2} \delta F_1.y_1 + \frac{1}{2} F_2.y_2 + \frac{1}{2} F_2.\delta y_2$$

$$+ \frac{1}{2} F_3.y_3 + \frac{1}{2} F_3.\delta y_3 + \ldots \qquad \ldots \text{(Eq. d)}$$

Thus the change in strain energy is obtained by subtracting (Eq. a) from (Eq. d)

$$(U + \delta U) - U = \left\{ \frac{1}{2} F_1.y_1 + \frac{1}{2} F_1.\delta y_1 + \frac{1}{2} \delta F_1.y_1 + \frac{1}{2} F_2.y_2 + \frac{1}{2} F_2.\delta y_2 \right.$$
$$\left. + \frac{1}{2} F_3.y_3 + \frac{1}{2} F_3.\delta y_3 + ... \right\} - \left\{ \frac{1}{2} F_1.y_1 + \frac{1}{2} F_2.y_2 \right.$$
$$\left. + \frac{1}{2} F_3.y_3 + ... \right\}$$

$$\delta U = \frac{1}{2} F_1.\delta y_1 + \frac{1}{2} \delta F_1.y_1 + \frac{1}{2} F_2.\delta y_2 + \frac{1}{2} F_3.\delta y_3 + ...$$

$$2\delta U = F_1.\delta y_1 + \delta F_1.y_1 + F_2.\delta y_2 + F_3.\delta y_3 + ... \qquad ... \text{(Eq. e)}$$

Subtracting (Eq. c) from (Eq. e), we have

$$2\delta U - \delta U = [F_1.\delta y_1 + \delta F_1.y_1 + F_2.\delta y_2 + F_3.\delta y_3 + ...]$$
$$- [F_1.\delta y_1 + F_2.\delta y_2 + F_3.\delta y_3 + ...]$$
$$\delta U = \delta F_1.y_1$$

$$y_1 = \frac{\delta U}{\delta F_1} \qquad ... \text{(Eq. f)}$$

(Eq. f) is obtained by keeping other forces constant. In the limits,

$$y_1 = \frac{\partial U}{\partial F_1} \qquad ... \text{(Eq. g)}$$

i.e. the partial differential of the strain energy U with respect to F_1 gives the deflection y_1 under that load and in the direction of F_1.

On similar lines if F_2 is changed while keeping other forces constant, we get

$$y_2 = \frac{\partial U}{\partial F_2}, \quad y_3 = \frac{\partial U}{\partial F_3} \qquad \text{and so on...}$$

Thus for a general case having n number of loads, (Eq. g) can be written as

$$y_n = \frac{\partial U}{\partial F_n} \qquad ... \text{(Eq. 11.68)}$$

Castigliano's theorem may also be used to determine the slope of a beam at the point of application of a couple

$$\theta_n = \frac{\partial U}{\partial M_n} \qquad ... \text{(Eq. 11.69)}$$

Similarly the angle of twist in a shaft may be found as

$$\phi_n = \frac{\partial U}{\partial T_n} \qquad ... \text{(Eq. 11.70)}$$

Applications:
In general, the strain energy of a bar subjected to combined loading is obtained by superimposing the contributions of axial loading, torsion, and bending

$$U = \int_0^l \frac{F^2 dx}{2AE} + \int_0^l \frac{T^2 dx}{2GJ} + \int_0^l \frac{M^2 dx}{2EI} \qquad ... \text{(Eq. 11.71a)}$$

The deflection $y_n = \dfrac{\partial U}{\partial F_n}$ is best evaluated by differentiating inside the integral signs before integrating. This procedure is permissible because F_n is not a function of x. With this simplification, we obtain

$$U = \frac{\partial U}{\partial F_n} = \int_0^l \left(\frac{F}{AE}\right)\left(\frac{\partial F}{\partial F_n}\right) dx + \int_0^l \left(\frac{T}{GJ}\right)\left(\frac{\partial T}{\partial F_n}\right) dx + \int_0^l \left(\frac{M}{EI}\right)\left(\frac{\partial M}{\partial F_n}\right) dx \qquad \text{... (Eq. 11.71b)}$$

If we wish to calculate displacement at a point or in a direction on a structure where there is no load, then a dummy *or fictitious or imaginary* load corresponding to the desired displacement must be added at that point.

Then, after differentiating but before integrating, we set the dummy load equal to zero. If we denote the dummy load by Q, the displacement in the direction of Q is given as

$$y_n = \left(\frac{\partial U}{\partial Q}\right)_{Q=0} = \int_0^l \left[\left(\frac{F}{AE}\right)\left(\frac{\partial F}{\partial Q}\right)\right]_{Q=0} dx + \int_0^l \left[\left(\frac{T}{GJ}\right)\left(\frac{\partial T}{\partial Q}\right)\right]_{Q=0} dx$$

$$+ \int_0^l \left[\left(\frac{M}{EI}\right)\left(\frac{\partial M}{\partial Q}\right)\right]_{Q=0} dx \qquad \text{... (Eq. 11.71c)}$$

Castigliano's method can also be used to find redundant reactions in statically indeterminate problems. Reaction forces at redundant supports on a beam can be found by setting the deflection at the redundant support to zero and solving for the force.

11.13.2 Castigliano's second theorem

Castigliano's first theorem is similar to his second theorem; however, it relates the load F_n to the partial derivative of the strain energy with respect to the corresponding displacement.

In any elastic structure having independent displacements corresponding to external forces along their lines of action, if strain energy is expressed in terms of displacements then equilibrium equations may be written as

$$F_n = \frac{\partial U}{\partial y_n} \qquad \text{... (Eq. 11.72)}$$

75. Using Castigliano's theorem, find the deflection and slope at free end of a cantilever beam subjected to concentrated load at free end.

Solution: Fig. 11.65(a) represents a cantilever beam subjected to point load at free end.

Let
$\qquad W$ = Point load at free end
$\qquad L$ = Length of the beam
$\qquad y_A$ = Deflection at A
$\qquad \theta_A$ = Slope at A

a. *Deflection:*
Consider a section X-X at a distance x from free end A. Bending moment at section X-X is given as

$$M = -W.x \qquad \text{(Negative because, hogging bending moment)}$$

and $\quad \dfrac{\partial M}{\partial W} = -x$

According to Castigliano's theorem,

Deflection at A, $y_A = \dfrac{\partial U}{\partial W}$

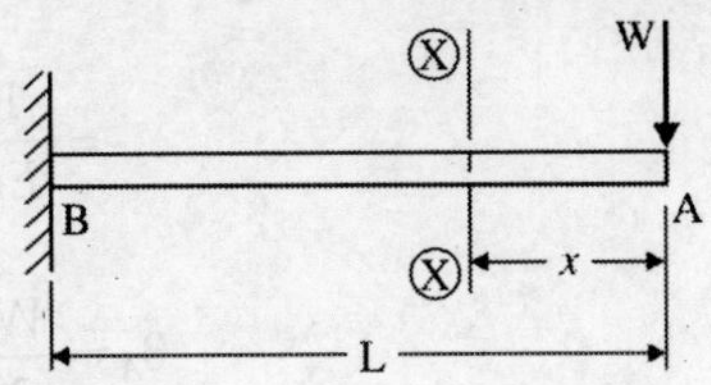

Fig. 11.65(a): Problem 75

$$= \int_0^L \left(\dfrac{M}{EI}\right)\left(\dfrac{\partial M}{\partial W}\right)dx = \dfrac{1}{EI}\int_0^L M\left(\dfrac{\partial M}{\partial W}\right)dx$$

$$= \dfrac{1}{EI}\int (-Wx)(-x)dx = \dfrac{W}{EI}\int_0^L x^2 dx$$

$$= \dfrac{W}{EI}\left(\dfrac{x^3}{3}\right)_0^L$$

$$y_A = \dfrac{WL^3}{3EI} \qquad \qquad \text{... (Eq. 11.73a)}$$

Method 2: From Problem 69, we have

$$U = \dfrac{W^2 L^3}{6EI} \qquad \qquad \text{... using (Eq. 11.57)}$$

Deflection at A, $y_A = \dfrac{\partial U}{\partial W}$

$$= \dfrac{\partial}{\partial W}\left(\dfrac{W^2 L^3}{6EI}\right)$$

$$y_A = \dfrac{WL^3}{3EI} \qquad \qquad \text{... (Eq. 11.73b)}$$

Eqs (11.73 a & b) are same as that obtained in (Eq. 11.58)

b. *Slope:* To find the slope at free end, apply a fictitious couple M_0 as shown in **Fig. 11.65(b)**. Consider a section X-X at a distance x from free end. Moment at X-X due to this couple alone is $= M_0$

Total moment at X-X $M = -Wx - M_0$.

and $\quad \dfrac{\partial M}{\partial W_0} = -1$

Substituting $M_0 = 0$ into the bending-moment equation, we get

$$M = -Wx$$

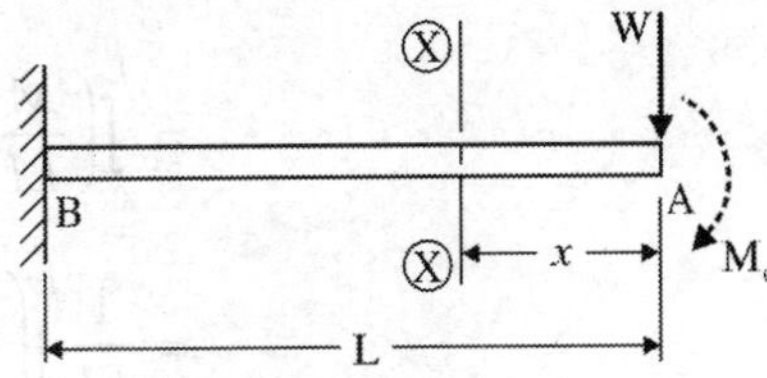

Fig. 11.65(b): Problem 75

Slope at A, $\quad \theta_A = \dfrac{\partial U}{\partial W_0}$

$$= \int_0^L \left(\dfrac{M}{EI}\right)\left(\dfrac{\partial M}{\partial M_0}\right)dx = \dfrac{1}{EI}\int_0^L M\left(\dfrac{\partial M}{\partial M_0}\right)dx$$

$$= \frac{1}{EI} \int_0^L (-Wx)(-1)dx = \frac{W}{EI} \int_0^L x.dx = \frac{W}{EI} \left(\frac{x^2}{2} \right)_0^L$$

$$\theta_A = \frac{WL^3}{2EI}$$

76. Using Castigliano's theorem, find the deflection and slope at free end of a cantilever beam subjected to uniformly distributed load over the entire span. EI is constant.

Solution:

Let

$$w = \text{Uniformly distributed load per unit length}$$
$$L = \text{Length of the beam}$$
$$y_A = \text{Deflection at A}$$
$$\theta_A = \text{Slope at A}$$

a. *Deflection:*

To determine the deflection of the cantilever beam, a dummy concentrated load (Q) is applied at A in the downward direction as shown in **Fig. 11.66(a)**.

Consider a section X-X at a distance x from free end A. Bending moment at any section X-X is given as

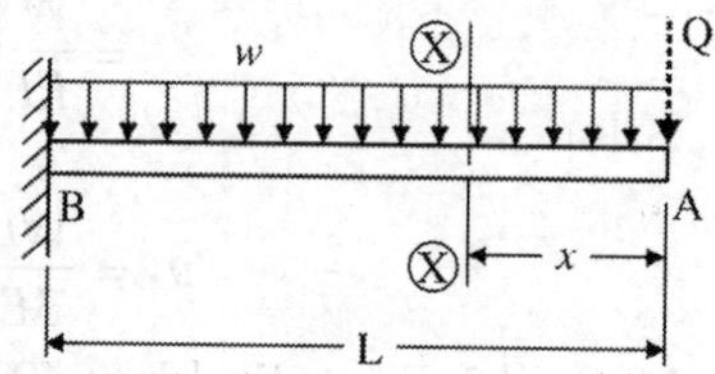

Fig. 11.66(a): Problem 76

$$M = -Qx - w.x \left(\frac{x}{2} \right) = -Qx - \left(\frac{wx^2}{2} \right) \qquad \text{for } 0 < x < L$$

and

$$\frac{\partial M}{\partial Q} = -x$$

Substituting $Q = 0$ into the bending-moment equation, we get

$$M = -\left(\frac{wx^2}{2} \right)$$

According to Castigliano's theorem,

Deflection at A, $y_A = \dfrac{\partial U}{\partial Q}$ \qquad (F or W)

$$= \int_0^L \left(\frac{M}{EI} \right) \left(\frac{\partial M}{\partial Q} \right) dx = \frac{1}{EI} \int_0^L M \left(\frac{\partial M}{\partial Q} \right) dx$$

$$= \frac{1}{EI} \int_0^L \left(-\frac{wx^2}{2} \right)(-x)dx$$

$$= \frac{w}{2EI} \int_0^L x^3 dx = \frac{w}{2EI} \left(\frac{x^4}{4} \right)_0^L$$

$$y_A = \frac{wL^4}{8EI}$$

b. *Slope:* To find the slope at free end, apply a fictitious couple M_0 as shown in **Fig. 11.66(b)**. Consider a section X-X at a distance x from free end. Moment at X-X due to this couple alone is $= M_0$

Total moment at X-X $M = -\left(\dfrac{wx^2}{2}\right) - M_0$

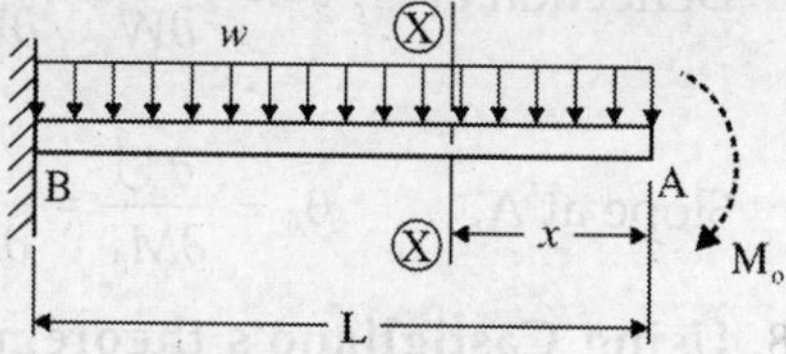

Fig. 11.66(b): Problem 76

and $\qquad \dfrac{\partial M}{\partial M_0} = -1$

Substituting $M_0 = 0$ into the bending-moment equation, we get

$$M = -\left(\frac{wx^2}{2}\right)$$

Slope at A, $\qquad \theta_A = \dfrac{\partial U}{\partial M_0} = \int_0^L \left(\dfrac{M}{EI}\right)\left(\dfrac{\partial M}{\partial M_0}\right)dx = \dfrac{1}{EI}\int_0^L M\left(\dfrac{\partial M}{\partial M_0}\right)dx$

$$= \frac{1}{EI}\int_0^L -\left(\frac{wx^2}{2}\right)(-1)dx = \frac{w}{2EI}\int_0^L x^2 dx$$

$$= \frac{w}{2EI}\left(\frac{x^3}{3}\right)_0^L$$

$$\theta_A = \frac{wL^3}{6EI}$$

77. **Using Castigliano's theorem, find the deflection and slope at free end of a cantilever beam subjected to combined action of concentrated load and end moment as shown in Fig. 11.67.**

Solution: Consider a section X-X at a distance x from free end.

Total moment at X-X $M = -Wx - M_0$.

We know that $\qquad U = \int_0^L \dfrac{M^2 dx}{2EI}$

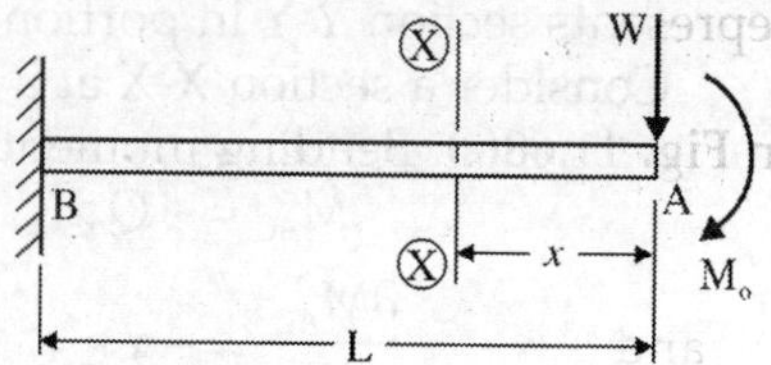

Fig. 11.67: Problem 77

$$\qquad\qquad \dots \text{ using (Eq. 11.32a)}$$

$$= \frac{1}{2EI}\int_0^L (-Wx - M_0)^2\, dx$$

$$= \frac{1}{2EI}\int_0^L \left(W^2 x^2 + M_0^2 + 2WM_0 x\right) dx$$

$$= \frac{1}{2EI}\left[\frac{W^2 x^3}{3} + M_0^2 . x + WM_0 x^2\right]_0^L$$

$$U = \frac{W^2 L^3}{6EI} + \frac{M_0^2 . L}{2EI} + \frac{WM_0 . L^2}{2EI} \qquad \dots \text{ Eq. (a)}$$

Deflection at A, $y_A = \dfrac{\partial U}{\partial W} = \dfrac{\partial}{\partial W}\left[\dfrac{W^2 L^3}{6EI} + \dfrac{M_0^2.L}{2EI} + \dfrac{WM_0 L^2}{2EI}\right] = \dfrac{WL^3}{3EI} + \dfrac{M_0 L^2}{2EI}$

Slope at A, $\qquad \theta_A = \dfrac{\partial U}{\partial M_0} = \dfrac{\partial}{\partial M_0}\left[\dfrac{W^2 L^3}{6EI} + \dfrac{M_0^2.L}{2EI} + \dfrac{WM_0 L^2}{2EI}\right] = \dfrac{M_0 L}{EI} + \dfrac{WL^2}{2EI}$

78. Using Castigliano's theorem, find the deflection at free end of a cantilever beam subjected to point load as shown in Fig. 11.68(a). EI is constant

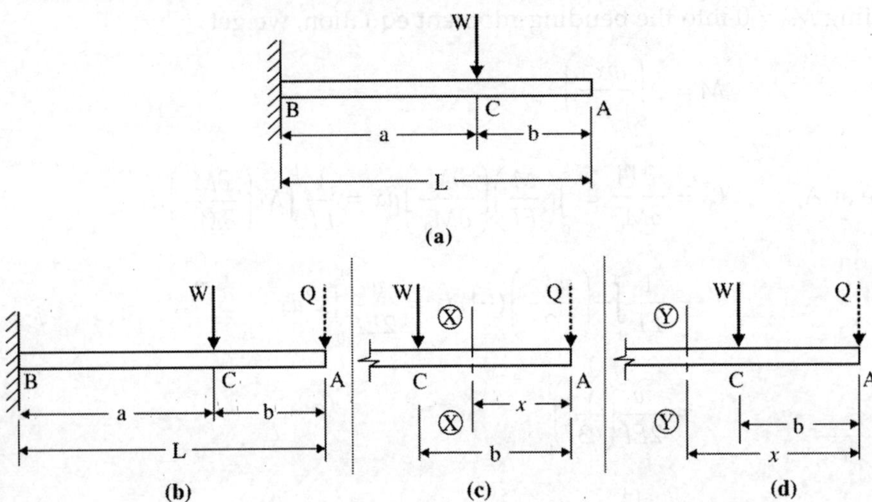

Fig. 11.68: Problem 78

Solution: To determine the deflection of the cantilever beam, a dummy concentrated load (Q) is applied at A in the downward direction as shown in **Fig. 11.68(b)**. **Fig. 11.68(c)** represents section X-X in portion AC. **Fig. 11.68(d)** represents section Y-Y in portion CB

Consider a section X-X at a distance x from end A between A and C, as shown in **Fig. 11.68(c)**. Bending moment at section X-X is

$$M_{AC} = -Q.x \qquad \text{for } 0 < x < b$$

and $\qquad \dfrac{\partial M_{AC}}{\partial Q} = -x$

Substituting $Q = 0$ into the bending-moment equation, we get

$$M = 0$$

Consider a section Y-Y at a distance x from end A between C and B, as shown in **Fig. 11.68(d)**. Bending moment at section Y-Y is

$$M_{CB} = -Q.x - W(x-b) \qquad \text{for } b < x < L$$

and $\qquad \dfrac{\partial M_{CB}}{\partial Q} = -x$

Substituting $Q = 0$ into the bending-moment equation, we get

$$M = -W(x-b)$$

According to Castigliano's theorem,

Deflection at A, $y_A = \dfrac{\partial U}{\partial Q} = \int_{0}^{b}\left(\dfrac{M_{AC}}{EI}\right)\left(\dfrac{\partial M_{AC}}{\partial Q}\right)dx + \int_{B}^{L}\left(\dfrac{M_{CB}}{EI}\right)\left(\dfrac{\partial M_{CB}}{\partial Q}\right)dx$

$$= \frac{1}{EI} \int_0^b 0 + \frac{1}{EI} \int_b^L [-W(x-b)](-x)dx$$

$$= \frac{W}{EI} \int_b^L (x^2 - bx)dx$$

$$= \frac{W}{EI} \left[\left(\frac{x^3}{3} \right)_b^L - b\left(\frac{x^2}{2} \right)_b^L \right]$$

$$= \frac{W}{6EI} \left[2(L^3 - b^3) - 3b(L^2 - b^2) \right]$$

$$= \frac{W}{6EI} \left[2L^3 - 2b^3 - 3bL^2 + 3b^3 \right]$$

$$y_A = \frac{W}{6EI} \left[2L^3 - 3bL^2 + b^3 \right]$$

79. **Using Castigliano's theorem, find the deflections at points A and C for a cantilever beam subjected to two point loads as shown in Fig. 11.69(a).**

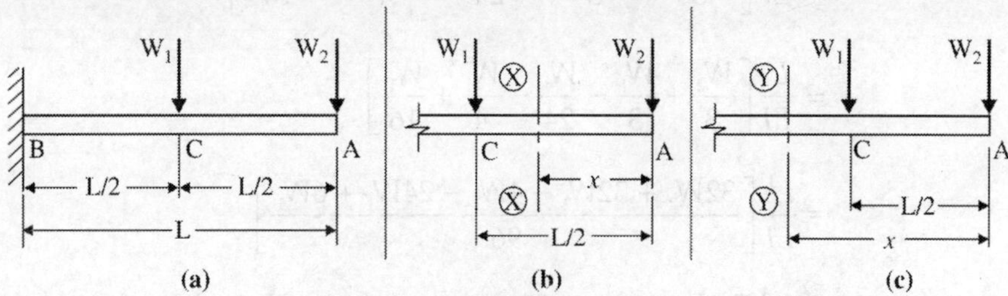

Fig. 11.69: Problem 79

Solution: Consider a section X-X at a distance x from end A between A and C, as shown in **Fig. 11.69(b)**. Bending moment at section X-X is

$$M_{AC} = - W_2 x \qquad\qquad \text{for } 0 < x < L/2$$

and $\qquad \dfrac{\partial M_{AC}}{\partial W_2} = -W_2, \quad \dfrac{\partial M_{AC}}{\partial W_1} = 0$

Consider a section Y-Y at a distance x from end A between C and B, as shown in **Fig. 11.68(c)**. Bending moment at section Y-Y is

$$M_{CB} = - W_2 x - W_1 \left(x - \frac{L}{2} \right) \qquad\qquad \text{for } L/2 < x < L$$

and $\qquad \dfrac{\partial M_{CB}}{\partial W_2} = -x, \quad \dfrac{\partial M_{CB}}{\partial W_1} = \left(-x + \dfrac{L}{2} \right) = \left(\dfrac{L}{2} - x \right)$

Deflection at A, $\quad y_A = \dfrac{\partial U}{\partial W_2} = \displaystyle\int_0^{L/2} \left(\dfrac{M_{AC}}{EI} \right) \left(\dfrac{\partial M_{AC}}{\partial W_2} \right) dx + \int_{L/2}^L \left(\dfrac{M_{CB}}{EI} \right) \left(\dfrac{\partial M_{CB}}{\partial W_2} \right) dx$

$$= \frac{1}{EI} \int_0^{L/2} M_{AC} \left(\frac{\partial M_{AC}}{\partial W_2} \right) dx + \frac{1}{EI} \int_{L/2}^L M_{CB} \left(\frac{\partial M_{CB}}{\partial W_2} \right) dx$$

$$= \frac{1}{EI}\int_0^{L/2}(-W_2 x)(-W_2)\,dx + \frac{1}{EI}\int_{L/2}^{L}\left[-W_2 x - W_1\left(x - \frac{L}{2}\right)\right](-x)\,dx$$

$$= \frac{W_2}{EI}\int_0^{L/2} x^2\,dx + \frac{1}{EI}\int_{L/2}^{L}\left[W_2 x^2 + W_1 x^2 - \left(\frac{W_1 L}{2}\right)x\right]dx$$

$$= \frac{W_2}{EI}\left(\frac{x^3}{3}\right)_0^{L/2} + \frac{W_2}{EI}\left(\frac{x^3}{3}\right)_{L/2}^{L} + \frac{W_1}{EI}\left(\frac{x^3}{3}\right)_{L/2}^{L} - \frac{W_1 L}{2EI}\left(\frac{x^3}{2}\right)_{L/2}^{L}$$

$$= \frac{W_2 L^3}{24EI} + \frac{W_2}{3EI}\left[L^3 - \left(\frac{L}{2}\right)^3\right] + \frac{W_1}{3EI}\left[L^3 - \left(\frac{L}{2}\right)^3\right] - \frac{W_1 L}{4EI}\left[L^2 - \left(\frac{L}{2}\right)^2\right]$$

$$= \frac{1}{EI}\left[\frac{W_2 L^3}{24} + \frac{W_2 L^3}{3} - \frac{W_2 L^3}{24} + \frac{W_1 L^3}{3} - \frac{W_1 L^3}{24} - \frac{W_1 L^3}{4} + \frac{W_1 L^3}{16}\right]$$

$$= \frac{1}{EI}\left[\frac{W_2 L^3}{3} + \frac{W_1 L^3}{3} - \frac{W_1 L^3}{24} - \frac{W_1 L^3}{4} + \frac{W_1 L^3}{16}\right]$$

$$= \frac{L^3}{EI}\left[\frac{W_2}{3} + \frac{W_1}{3} - \frac{W_1}{24} - \frac{W_1}{4} + \frac{W_1}{16}\right]$$

$$= \frac{L^3}{EI}\left[\frac{32W_2 + 32W_1 - 4W_1 - 24W_1 + 6W_1}{96}\right]$$

$$= \frac{L^3}{EI}\left[\frac{32W_2 + 10W_1}{48EI}\right]$$

$$y_A = \frac{(10W_1 + 32W_2)L^3}{48EI}$$

Deflection at C, $\displaystyle y_c = \frac{\partial U}{\partial W_1} = \int_0^{L/2}\left(\frac{M_{AC}}{EI}\right)\left(\frac{\partial M_{AC}}{\partial W_1}\right)dx + \int_{L/2}^{L}\left(\frac{M_{CB}}{EI}\right)\left(\frac{\partial M_{CB}}{\partial W_1}\right)dx$

$$= \frac{1}{EI}\int_0^{L/2} M_{AC}\left(\frac{\partial M_{AC}}{\partial W_1}\right)dx + \frac{1}{EI}\int_{L/2}^{L} M_{CB}\left(\frac{\partial M_{CB}}{\partial W_1}\right)dx$$

$$= \frac{1}{EI}\int_0^{L/2}(-W_2 x)(0)\,dx + \frac{1}{EI}\int_{L/2}^{L}\left[-W_2 x - W_1\left(x - \frac{L}{2}\right)\right]\left(\frac{L}{2} - x\right)dx$$

$$= \frac{1}{EI}\int_{L/2}^{L}\left[-W_2 x + W_1\left(\frac{L}{2} - x\right)\right]\left(\frac{L}{2} - x\right)dx$$

$$= \frac{1}{EI}\int_{L/2}^{L}\left[\left(\frac{-W_2 L}{2}\right)x + W_2 x^2 + W_1\left(\frac{L}{2} - x\right)^2\right]dx$$

$$= \frac{1}{EI} \int_{L/2}^{L} \left[\left(\frac{-W_2 L}{2} \right) x + W_2 x^2 + \left(\frac{W_1 L^2}{4} \right) + W_1 x^2 - W_1 L x \right] dx$$

$$= \frac{1}{EI} \left[\frac{-W_2 L}{2} \left(\frac{x^2}{2} \right)_{L/2}^{L} + W_2 \left(\frac{x^3}{3} \right)_{L/2}^{L} + \left(\frac{W_1 L^2}{4} \right) \left(\frac{x}{1} \right)_{L/2}^{L} + W_1 \left(\frac{x^3}{3} \right)_{L/2}^{L} - W_1 L \left(\frac{x^2}{2} \right)_{L/2}^{L} \right]$$

$$= \frac{1}{EI} \left[\frac{-W_2 L}{2} \left(L^2 - \frac{L^2}{4} \right) + \frac{W_2}{3} \left(L^3 - \frac{L^3}{8} \right) + \left(\frac{W_1 L^2}{4} \right) \left(L - \frac{L}{2} \right) \right.$$

$$\left. + \frac{W_1}{3} \left(L^3 - \frac{L^3}{8} \right) - \frac{W_1 L}{2} \left(L^2 - \frac{L^2}{4} \right) \right]$$

$$= \frac{1}{EI} \left[-\left(L^2 - \frac{L^2}{4} \right) \left(\frac{W_2 L}{4} + \frac{W_1 L}{2} \right) + \left(L^3 - \frac{L^3}{8} \right) \left(\frac{W_2}{3} + \frac{W_1}{3} \right) + \left(\frac{W_1 L^2}{4} \right) \left(L - \frac{L}{2} \right) \right]$$

$$= \frac{1}{EI} \left[-\left(\frac{3}{4} \right) \left(\frac{W_2 L^3}{4} + \frac{W_1 L^3}{2} \right) + \left(\frac{7}{8} \right) \left(\frac{W_2 L^3}{3} + \frac{W_1 L^3}{3} \right) + \frac{W_1 L^3}{8} \right]$$

$$= \frac{L^3}{EI} \left[\frac{W_1}{8} - \frac{3W_2}{16} - \frac{3W_1}{8} + \frac{7W_2}{24} + \frac{7W_1}{24} \right]$$

$$= \frac{L^3}{EI} \left[\frac{6W_1 - 9W_2 - 18W_1 + 14W_2 + 14W_1}{48} \right]$$

$$= \frac{L^3}{EI} \left[\frac{2W_1 + 5W_2}{48} \right]$$

$$y_C = \frac{(2W_1 + 5W_2) L^3}{48 EI}$$

80. Using Castigliano's theorem, find the maximum deflection in a simply supported beam carrying a point load in any position. *EI* is constant.

Solution: Referring to **Fig. 11.60** (Problem 72), the reactions at the supports are

$$R_A = \left(\frac{Wb}{L} \right), R_B = \left(\frac{Wa}{L} \right)$$

Bending moment at X-X is given as

$$M_{AC} = R_A . x_1 = \left(\frac{Wb}{L} \right) x_1 \qquad \text{for } 0 < x_1 < a$$

and $\qquad \dfrac{\partial M_{AC}}{\partial W} = \left(\dfrac{b}{L} \right) x_1$

Bending moment at Y-Y is given as

$$M_{BC} = R_B . x_2 = \left(\frac{Wa}{L}\right) x_2 \qquad \text{for } 0 < x_2 < b$$

and $\qquad \dfrac{\partial M_{BC}}{\partial W} = \left(\dfrac{a}{L}\right) x_2$

Deflection at C, $\quad y_c = \dfrac{\partial U}{\partial W} = \displaystyle\int_0^a \left(\frac{M_{AC}}{EI}\right)\left(\frac{\partial M_{AC}}{\partial W}\right) dx + \int_0^b \left(\frac{M_{CB}}{EI}\right)\left(\frac{\partial M_{CB}}{\partial W}\right) dx$

$$= \frac{1}{EI} \int_0^a \left(\frac{Wb}{L}\right) x_1 \times \left(\frac{b}{L}\right) x_1 dx_1 + \frac{1}{EI} \int_0^b \left(\frac{Wa}{L}\right) x_2 \times \left(\frac{a}{L}\right) x_2 dx_2$$

$$= \frac{W^2 b^2}{EIL^2} \int_0^a x_1^2 dx_1 + \frac{W^2 a^2}{EIL^2} \int_0^b x_2^2 dx_2$$

$$= \frac{W^2 b^2}{EIL^2} \left(\frac{x_1^3}{3}\right)_0^a + \frac{W^2 a^2}{EIL^2} \left(\frac{x_2^3}{3}\right)_0^b$$

$$= \frac{W^2 b^2 a^3}{3EIL^2} + \frac{W^2 a^2 b^3}{3EIL^2}$$

$$= \frac{W^2 a^2 b^2}{3EIL^2}(a + b)$$

$$y_c = \frac{W^2 a^2 b^2}{3EIL^2}$$

81. Using Castigliano's theorem, find the maximum deflection in a simply supported beam subjected to uniformly distributed load over the entire span. *EI* is constant.

Solution: Fig. 11.70(a) shows the beam subjected to uniformly distributed load over the entire span. To determine the maximum deflection of the beam, a dummy concentrated load (Q) is introduced at mid-span as shown in **Fig. 11.70(b)**.

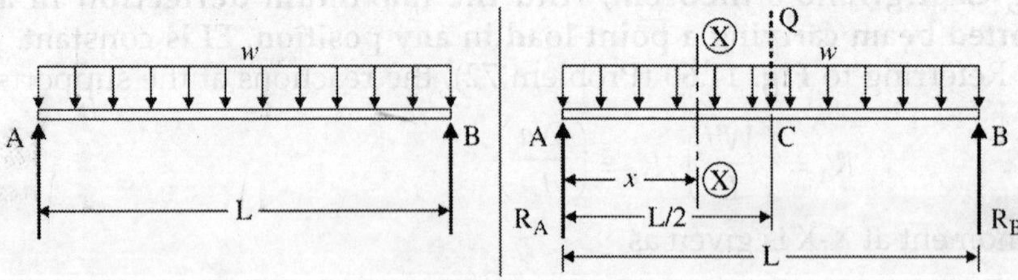

Fig. 11.70: Problem 81

Consider a section X-X at a distance x from free end A. Bending moment at any section X-X is given as

From **Fig. 11.70(b)**, we have

$$R_A + R_B = wL + Q$$

Due to symmetry of loading, the reactions at the supports are

$$R_A = R_B = \left(\frac{wL + Q}{2}\right)$$

Consider a section X-X at a distance x from end A. Bending moment at any section X-X is given as

$$M = R_A.x - w.x\left(\frac{x}{2}\right)$$

$$= \left(\frac{wL + Q}{2}\right) - \left(\frac{wx^2}{2}\right)$$

And $\quad \dfrac{\partial M}{\partial W} = \left(\dfrac{x}{2}\right)$

Substituting $Q = 0$ into the bending-moment equation, we get

$$M = \left(\frac{wL}{2}\right)x - \left(\frac{wx^2}{2}\right)$$

Deflection at C, $\quad y_C = \dfrac{\partial U}{\partial W} = 2\int_0^{L/2}\left(\dfrac{M}{EI}\right)\left(\dfrac{\partial M}{\partial W}\right)dx$

$$= \frac{2}{EI}\int_0^{L/2}\left[\left(\frac{wL}{2}\right)x - \left(\frac{wx^2}{2}\right)\right]\left(\frac{x}{2}\right)dx$$

$$= \frac{1}{2EI}\int^{L/2}\left(wLx^2 - wx^3\right)dx$$

$$= \frac{w}{2EI}\left[\left(\frac{Lx^3}{3}\right)_0^{L/2} - \left(\frac{x^4}{4}\right)_0^{L/2}\right]$$

$$= \frac{wL^4}{2EI}\left[\frac{1}{24} - \frac{1}{64}\right] = \frac{wL^4}{2EI}\left[\frac{8-3}{192}\right]$$

$$y_C = \frac{5wL^4}{384EI}$$

VTU QUESTION PAPERS

Dec. 2011 (10ME34)

1. a. Define work and strain energy. **(02 Marks)**

   b. A rectangular copper bar 50 mm × 75 mm in cross section is subjected to an axial energy input of 200 N-m. Determine the minimum length of the bar to limit the axial stress in the bar to 80 MPa. The modulus of elasticity of the bar is 1.15×10^5 N/mm^2. **(06 Marks)**

June 2012 (10ME34)

2. A cantilever of uniform section carries a point load at the free end. Find the strain energy stored by the cantilever and hence calculate the deflection at the free end.
(06 Marks)

Dec. 2012 (10ME34)

3. A simply supported beam of span L carries a point load W at mid-span. Find the strain energy stored by the beam.
(05 Marks)

June/July 2013 (10ME34)

4. a. State Castigliano's theorem. Where do you use it?
(03 Marks)
   b. The bar with circular cross section as shown in **Fig. U11.1** is subjected to a load of 10 kN. Determine the strain energy stored in it. Take $E = 2.1 \times 10^5 \, N/mm^2$
(07 Marks)

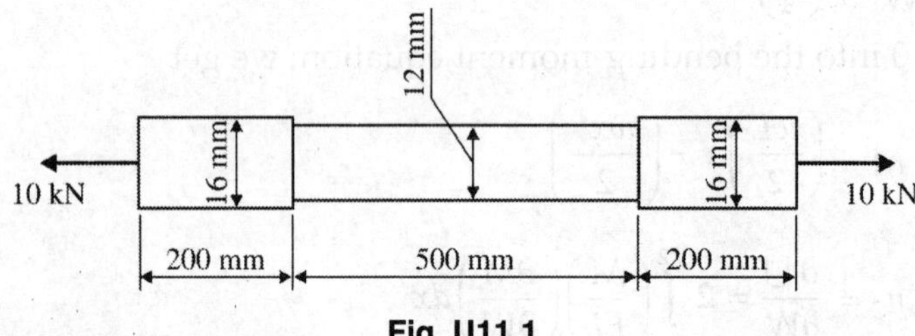

Fig. U11.1

Dec. 13/Jan. 14 (10ME34)

5. A beam of length l is simply supported at its ends. The beam caries a uniformly distributed load of w per unit run over the whole span. Find the strain energy stored by the beam.
(06 Marks)

June/July 2014 (10ME34)

6. Define: i. Strain energy   ii. Work.
(03 Marks)

Dec. 14/Jan. 15(10ME34)

7. The maximum stress produced by a pull in a bar of length 100 mm is $100 \, N/mm^2$. The area of cross section and length are as shown in **Fig. U11.2**. Calculate the strain energy stored in the bar if $E = 2 \times 10^5 \, N/mm^2$.
(10 Marks)

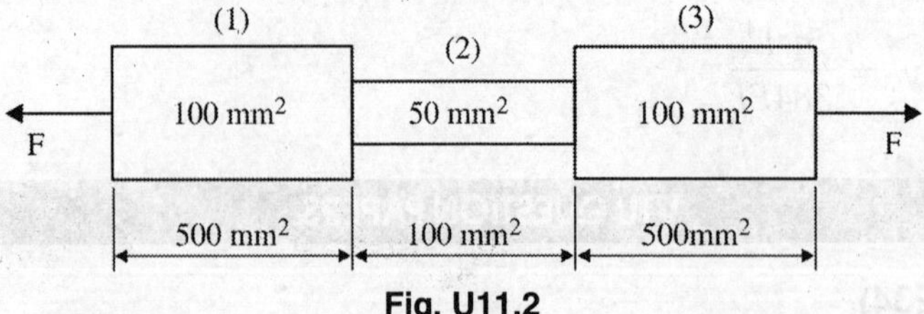

Fig. U11.2

June/July 15(10ME34)

8. Derive an expression for strain energy, when a member is subjected to impact loads.
(06 Marks)

Dec. 15/Jan. 16 (10ME/AU34)

9. Determine the strain energy in a cantilever beam of uniform cross section and length L subjected to a uniformly distributed load w kN/m over the entire span.

(04 Marks)

June/July 2016 (10ME/AU34)

10. Derive an expression for energy stored in a plain bar subjected to axial load F.

(05 Marks)

Dec. 16/Jan. 17 (15ME/MA34)

11. Write a note on the following:
   a. Castigliano's theorem I   **(04 Marks)**
   b. Modulus of resilience.   **(04 Marks)**
   c. Strain energy due to bending and torsion.   **(08 Marks)**

June/July 2017 (15ME/MA34)

12. Derive an expression for strain energy due to shear stress.   **(08 Marks)**

Dec. 17/Jan. 18 (15ME/MA34)

13. Explain: (i) Castigliano's first theorem   (ii) Castigliano's second theorem

(08 Marks)

Theories of Failure

Chapter Outline

12.1 INTRODUCTION

When a material is subjected to a single type of stress (i.e. axial, torsion or bending), it is very easy to predict when the failure is likely to occur. However if the material is subjected to a complex stress system (bi-axial or tri-axial) then it is difficult to predict the failure of the material.

Based on the behavior of the material, two types of failures are possible: yielding or elastic failure (ductile materials) and fracture (brittle materials). In ductile materials, elastic failure results in excessive deformation so that the component can no longer perform its intended function; while in brittle materials, fracture occurs and tears apart the component into two or more pieces.

Hence for *ductile materials*, the limiting strength is taken as the yield stress (tension or compression), while for *brittle materials*, the limiting strength is taken as the ultimate stress (tension or compression).

In order to predict the failure of material under combined stresses, the following theories of failure have been postulated

a. Maximum normal stress theory or Principal stress theory or Rankine's theory.

b. Maximum shear stress theory or Guest's or Tresca's theory or Shear difference theory (MSST).

c. Maximum normal strain theory or Principal strain theory or Saint Venant theory.

d. Maximum strain energy theory or Total strain energy theory or Haigh's theory.

e. Maximum shear strain energy theory or Distortion energy theory or Von-Mises theory (DET).

It is to be noted that, in static loading and ductile behavior, stress concentrations are harmless as they only create small localized yielding which do not lead to any objectionable dimensional changes.

12.2 FACTOR OF SAFETY

The term factor of safety is applied to a factor used to evaluate the safeness of a member. It is used separately for uncertainties that may occur in the strength of a part and uncertainties that might occur with loads acting on the part.

It is defined as the ratio of ultimate stress or load to the working stress or load.

$$\text{i.e.} \quad \text{Factor of safety} = \frac{\text{Ultimate stress}}{\text{Working stress}} \quad \text{i.e.} \; n = \frac{\sigma_u}{\sigma_d} \qquad \text{... (Eq. 12.1)}$$

Working stress is based on yield point stress for ductile materials and ultimate strength for brittle materials.

$$\text{For ductile materials,} \quad n = \frac{\text{Yield stress}}{\text{Working stress}} = \frac{\sigma_{yt}}{\sigma_d} \qquad \text{... (Eq. 12.2)}$$

$$\text{For brittle materials,} \quad n = \frac{\text{Ultimate stress}}{\text{Working stress}} = \frac{\sigma_u}{\sigma_d} \qquad \text{... (Eq. 12.3)}$$

σ_d = Working stress or design stress or allowable stress or applied stress

σ_{yt} = Yield or elastic strength of the material

12.3 MAXIMUM NORMAL STRESS THEORY OR PRINCIPAL STRESS THEORY OR RANKINE'S THEORY

According to this theory, "the failure of a machine component subjected to combined action of normal and shear stresses occurs whenever the maximum principal stress (σ_1) of the component becomes equal to the elastic strength (σ_e) of the material in simple tension test".

i.e.   Elastic strength = Maximum principal stress

$$\sigma_e = \sigma_1 \qquad \text{(in tension)} \qquad \text{... (Eq. 12.4)}$$

$$\sigma_e = \left(\frac{\sigma_x + \sigma_y}{2}\right) + \sqrt{\left(\frac{\sigma_x - \sigma_y}{2}\right)^2 + \tau_{xy}^2} \qquad \text{... (Eq. 12.5a)}$$

$$\text{Or} \qquad \sigma_e = \left(\frac{\sigma_x + \sigma_y}{2}\right) + \frac{1}{2}\sqrt{\left(\sigma_x - \sigma_y\right)^2 + 4\tau_{xy}^2} \qquad \text{... (Eq. 12.5b)}$$

If factor of safety is considered,

$$n = \frac{\sigma_e}{\sigma_1} \qquad \text{... (Eq. 12.6)}$$

$$\text{For design,} \qquad \frac{\sigma_e}{n} = \left(\frac{\sigma_x + \sigma_y}{2}\right) + \sqrt{\left(\frac{\sigma_x - \sigma_y}{2}\right)^2 + \tau_{xy}^2} \qquad \text{... (Eq. 12.7)}$$

The failure condition is

$$\sigma_1 \geq \frac{\sigma_e}{n} \qquad \qquad \text{... (Eq. 12.8)}$$

For a 3D case:

If the principal normal stresses are σ_1, σ_2 and σ_3, where $\sigma_1 \geq \sigma_2 \geq \sigma_3$

$$\sigma_e = \sigma_1 \qquad \text{(in tension)}$$
$$\sigma_e = |\sigma_3| \qquad \text{(in compression)} \qquad \text{... (Eq. 12.9)}$$

The failure condition is

$$\sigma_1 \geq \sigma_e/n \qquad \qquad \text{... same as (Eq. 12.8)}$$
$$|\sigma_3| \geq \sigma_e/n \qquad \qquad \text{... (Eq. 12.10)}$$

Applicable only for brittle materials. This theory disregards the effects of other principal stresses and the effects of shear stress on other planes and hence it is not used for ductile materials.

12.4 MAXIMUM SHEAR STRESS THEORY OR GUEST'S OR TRESCA'S THEORY OR SHEAR DIFFERENCE THEORY (MSST)

According to this theory, "the failure of a machine component subjected to combined action of normal and shear stresses occurs whenever the shear stress of the component becomes equal to the shear stress experienced by the material in simple tension test".

i.e. $$\tau_{max} = \tau_e \qquad \qquad \text{... (Eq. 12.11)}$$

Since the shear stress at yield point in a simple tension test is equal to one-half the yield stress in tension, we have

$$\tau_e = \frac{\sigma_e}{2} \qquad \qquad \text{... (Eq. 12.12)}$$

$$\therefore \quad \sqrt{\left(\frac{\sigma_x - \sigma_y}{2}\right)^2 + \tau_{xy}^2} = \frac{\sigma_e}{2} \qquad \qquad \text{... (Eq. 12.13a)}$$

$$\frac{1}{2}\sqrt{\left(\sigma_x - \sigma_y\right)^2 + 4\tau_{xy}^2} = \frac{\sigma_e}{2}$$

$$\sqrt{\left(\sigma_x - \sigma_y\right)^2 + 4\tau_{xy}^2} = \sigma_e \qquad \qquad \text{... (Eq. 12.13b)}$$

Or $$\sigma_1 - \sigma_2 = \sigma_e$$

$$\text{... (Eq. 12.14)}$$

If factor of safety is considered, then

$$n = \frac{\sigma_e}{\sigma_1 - \sigma_2} \qquad \qquad \text{... (Eq. 12.15)}$$

For design, $$\frac{\sigma_e}{n} = \sqrt{\left(\sigma_x - \sigma_y\right)^2 + 4\tau_{xy}^2} \qquad \qquad \text{... (Eq. 12.16)}$$

Or $$\frac{\sigma_e}{n} = \sigma_1 - \sigma_2 \qquad \qquad \text{... (Eq. 12.17)}$$

The failure condition is

$$\sqrt{\left(\sigma_x - \sigma_y\right)^2 + 4\tau_{xy}^2} \geq \frac{\sigma_e}{n} \qquad \text{... (Eq. 12.18)}$$

$$\text{Or } \sigma_1 - \sigma_2 \geq \frac{\sigma_e}{n} \qquad \text{... (Eq. 12.19)}$$

For a 3D case:

If the principal normal stresses are σ_1, σ_2 and σ_3, where $\sigma_1 \geq \sigma_2 \geq \sigma_3$, then

τ_{max} is the largest of: $\qquad \tau_{1-2} = \dfrac{\sigma_1 - \sigma_2}{2} \,;\, \tau_{2-3} = \dfrac{\sigma_2 - \sigma_3}{2} \,;\, \tau_{3-1} = \dfrac{\sigma_1 - \sigma_3}{2}$

i.e. $\qquad\qquad\qquad\qquad \sigma_e = \sigma_1 - \sigma_3 \qquad\qquad\qquad \text{... (Eq. 12.20)}$

If factor of safety is considered, then

$$\frac{\sigma_e}{n} = \sigma_1 - \sigma_3 \qquad \text{... (Eq. 12.21)}$$

The failure condition is

$$\sigma_1 - \sigma_3 \geq \frac{\sigma_e}{n} \qquad \text{... (Eq. 12.22)}$$

Applicable to ductile materials. The results are on the safer side.

Note: The principal stresses are found as

$$\sigma_{1,2} = \left(\frac{\sigma_x + \sigma_y}{2}\right) \pm \sqrt{\left(\frac{\sigma_x - \sigma_y}{2}\right)^2 + \tau_{xy}^2}$$

$$\text{(for 2D system)} \qquad \text{... (Eq. 12.23)}$$

12.5 MAXIMUM NORMAL STRAIN THEORY OR PRINCIPAL STRAIN THEORY OR SAINT VENANT THEORY

According to this theory, "the failure of a machine component subjected to combined action of normal and shear stresses occurs whenever the maximum principal strain of the component becomes equal to the maximum strain of the material in simple tension test".

i.e. $\qquad\qquad\qquad\qquad \varepsilon_e = \varepsilon_1 \qquad\qquad\qquad\qquad \text{... (Eq. 12.24)}$

The principal strains can be represented in terms of principal stresses as

$$\varepsilon_1 = \frac{1}{E}\left[\sigma_1 - \mu\sigma_2\right]$$

$$\varepsilon_2 = \frac{1}{E}\left[\sigma_2 - \mu\sigma_1\right] \qquad \text{... (Eq. 12.25)}$$

Substituting (Eq. 12.25) in (Eq. 12.24) yields

$$\varepsilon_e = \frac{1}{E}\left[\sigma_1 - \mu\sigma_2\right]$$

i.e. $\qquad \dfrac{\sigma_e}{E} = \dfrac{1}{E}\left[\sigma_1 - \mu\sigma_2\right] \qquad (\because E = \sigma/\varepsilon)$

$$\sigma_e = (\sigma_1 - \mu\sigma_2) \qquad \text{... (Eq. 12.26)}$$

If factor of safety is considered, then

$$n = \frac{\sigma_e}{(\sigma_1 - \mu\sigma_2)} \qquad \text{... (Eq. 12.27)}$$

For design, $\quad \dfrac{\sigma_e}{n} = (\sigma_1 - \mu\sigma_2) \qquad$ where μ = Poisson's ratio

$$\text{... (Eq. 12.28)}$$

The failure condition is

$$(\sigma_1 - \mu\sigma_2) = \frac{\sigma_e}{n} \qquad \text{... (Eq. 12.29)}$$

For a 3D case:

If the principal normal stresses are σ_1, σ_2 and σ_3, where $\sigma_1 \geq \sigma_2 \geq \sigma_3$

$$\varepsilon_1 = \frac{1}{E}\left[\sigma_1 - \mu(\sigma_2 + \sigma_3)\right]$$

$$\varepsilon_2 = \frac{1}{E}\left[\sigma_2 - \mu(\sigma_3 + \sigma_1)\right]$$

$$\varepsilon_3 = \frac{1}{E}\left[\sigma_3 - \mu(\sigma_1 + \sigma_2)\right] \qquad \text{... (Eq. 12.30)}$$

Substituting (Eq. 12.30) in (Eq. 12.24) yields

$$\varepsilon_e = \frac{1}{E}\left[\sigma_1 - \mu(\sigma_2 + \sigma_3)\right]$$

i.e. $\qquad \dfrac{\sigma_e}{E} = \dfrac{1}{E}\left[\sigma_1 - \mu(\sigma_2 + \sigma_3)\right]$

$$\sigma_e = \sigma_1 - \mu(\sigma_2 + \sigma_3) \qquad \text{... (Eq. 12.31)}$$

If factor of safety is considered, then

$$n = \frac{\sigma_e}{\sigma_1 - \mu(\sigma_2 + \sigma_3)} \qquad \text{... (Eq. 12.32)}$$

For design, $\quad \dfrac{\sigma_e}{n} = \sigma_1 - \mu(\sigma_2 + \sigma_3) \qquad \text{... (Eq. 12.33)}$

The failure condition is

$$\sigma_1 - \mu(\sigma_2 + \sigma_3) = \frac{\sigma_e}{n} \qquad \text{... (Eq. 12.34)}$$

This theory is not used in general.

12.6 MAXIMUM STRAIN ENERGY THEORY OR TOTAL STRAIN ENERGY THEORY OR HAIGH'S THEORY

According to this theory, "the failure of a machine component subjected to combined action of normal and shear stresses occurs whenever the strain energy per unit volume of the component becomes equal to the strain energy per unit volume of the material in simple tension test".

Consider a unit cube subjected to principal stresses σ_1, σ_2 and σ_3 as shown in **Fig. 12.1.** The corresponding strains are ε_1, ε_2 and ε_3. Thus the total strain energy (U)per unit volume is equal to the total work done by the system and is given as

$$U = \frac{1}{2}\Sigma\sigma\varepsilon \qquad \textit{(Chapter 11)}$$

i.e.
$$U = \frac{1}{2}(\sigma_1\varepsilon_1 + \sigma_2\varepsilon_2 + \sigma_3\varepsilon_3) \qquad \text{... (Eq. 12.35)}$$

From (Eq. 12.30), we have

$$\varepsilon_1 = \frac{1}{E}[\sigma_1 - \mu(\sigma_2 + \sigma_3)]; \; \varepsilon_2 = \frac{1}{E}[\sigma_2 - \mu(\sigma_3 + \sigma_1)];$$

$$\varepsilon_3 = \frac{1}{E}[\sigma_3 - \mu(\sigma_1 + \sigma_2)]$$

Substituting (Eq. 12.30) in (Eq. 12.35) yields

$$U = \frac{1}{2E}\{\sigma_1[\sigma_1 - \mu(\sigma_2 + \sigma_3)] + \sigma_2[\sigma_2 - \mu(\sigma_3 + \sigma_1)]$$

$$+ \sigma_3[\sigma_3 - \mu(\sigma_1 + \sigma_2)]\}$$

$$U = \frac{1}{2E}\left[\sigma_1^2 + \sigma_2^2 + \sigma_3^2 - 2\mu(\sigma_1\sigma_2 + \sigma_2\sigma_3 + \sigma_1\sigma_3)\right] \qquad \text{... (Eq. 12.36)}$$

The total strain energy in simple tension test is

$$U = \frac{1}{2}\sigma_e\varepsilon$$

$$= \left(\frac{\sigma_e}{2}\right)\left(\frac{\sigma_e}{E}\right) \qquad (\because E = \sigma/\varepsilon)$$

$$U = \left(\frac{\sigma_e^2}{2E}\right) \qquad \text{... (Eq. 12.37)}$$

Equating Eqs (12.36) and (12.37), we have

$$\left(\frac{\sigma_e^2}{2E}\right) = \frac{1}{2E}\left[\sigma_1^2 + \sigma_2^2 + \sigma_3^2 - 2\mu(\sigma_1\sigma_2 + \sigma_2\sigma_3 + \sigma_1\sigma_3)\right]$$

$$\sigma_e^2 = \sigma_1^2 + \sigma_2^2 + \sigma_3^2 - 2\mu(\sigma_1\sigma_2 + \sigma_2\sigma_3 + \sigma_1\sigma_3) \qquad \text{... (Eq. 12.38a)}$$

$$\sigma_e = \sqrt{\sigma_1^2 + \sigma_2^2 + \sigma_3^2 - 2\mu(\sigma_1\sigma_2 + \sigma_2\sigma_3 + \sigma_1\sigma_3)} \qquad \text{... (Eq. 12.38b)}$$

For design, $\qquad \dfrac{\sigma_e}{n} = \sqrt{\sigma_1^2 + \sigma_2^2 + \sigma_3^2 - 2\mu(\sigma_1\sigma_2 + \sigma_2\sigma_3 + \sigma_1\sigma_3)} \qquad \text{... (Eq. 12.39)}$

The failure condition is

$$\sqrt{\sigma_1^2 + \sigma_2^2 + \sigma_3^2 - 2\mu(\sigma_1\sigma_2 + \sigma_2\sigma_3 + \sigma_1\sigma_3)} \geq \frac{\sigma_e}{n} \qquad \text{... (Eq. 12.40)}$$

For a 2D case: Here $\sigma_3 = 0$

(Eq. 12.40) yields... $\sqrt{\sigma_1^2 + \sigma_2^2 - 2\mu\sigma_1\sigma_2} \geq \dfrac{\sigma_e}{n} \qquad \text{... (Eq. 12.41)}$

- Applicable to ductile materials. This theory yields good approximation.

12.7 MAXIMUM SHEAR STRAIN ENERGY THEORY OR DISTORTION ENERGY THEORY OR VON – MISES THEORY (DET)

According to this theory, "the failure of a machine component subjected to combined action of normal and shear stresses occurs whenever the shear strain energy (distortion energy) per unit volume of the component becomes equal to the shear strain energy (distortion energy) per unit volume of the material in simple tension test":

The total strain energy is given as

$$U = \frac{1}{2E}\left[\sigma_1^2 + \sigma_2^2 + \sigma_3^2 - 2\mu(\sigma_1\sigma_2 + \sigma_2\sigma_3 + \sigma_1\sigma_3)\right]$$

... using (Eq. 12.36)

The total strain energy consists of two components:
- Hydrostatic or Volumetric state of stress (U_h), which changes the volume of the component and
- Distortional or Deviatoric state of stress (U_d), which changes the shape of the component. (The strain energy due to this component is known as the shear strain energy or distortion energy)

Thus the total strain energy is given as

$$U = U_h + U_d$$

... (Eq. 12.42)

σ_2, σ_1, σ_3, σ_h, σ_h, σ_h, $\sigma_2 - \sigma_h$, $\sigma_1 - \sigma_h$, $\sigma_3 - \sigma_h$

(a) Triaxial stresses   (b) Hydrostatic component   (c) Distrotional component

Fig. 12.1: Components of distortion energy theory (DET)

Consider a unit cube subjected to principal stresses σ_1, σ_2 and σ_3 as shown in **Fig. 12.1(a)**, wherein $\sigma_1 > \sigma_2 > \sigma_3$. Each of the principal stresses can be expressed in terms of hydrostatic/volumetric component (σ_h) that is common to each face and a distortion component (σ_{id}), which is unique to each face as shown in **Figs 12.1(b) and (c)** respectively.

(suffix i represents the principal stress direction 1, 2 and 3)

i.e.
$$\sigma_1 = \sigma_h + \sigma_{1d}$$
$$\sigma_2 = \sigma_h + \sigma_{2d}$$
$$\sigma_3 = \sigma_h + \sigma_{3d}$$

... (Eq. 12.43)

Adding the three principal stresses in (Eq. 12.43), we have

$$\sigma_1 + \sigma_2 + \sigma_3 = 3\sigma_h + (\sigma_{1d} + \sigma_{2d} + \sigma_{3d})$$

... (Eq. 12.44)

For a volumetric change with no distortion, the term in the parenthesis on RHS of (Eq. 12.44) should be zero

i.e.
$$\sigma_1 + \sigma_2 + \sigma_3 = 3\sigma_h$$
$$\sigma_h = (\sigma_1 + \sigma_2 + \sigma_3)/3$$

... (Eq. 12.45)

Thus **hydrostatic** stress is the average of three principal stresses. Hydrostatic static stress is also called **spherical or dilatational** stress.

Replacing each principal stress with σ_h in (Eq. 12.36) yields

$$U_h = \frac{1}{2E}\left[\sigma_h^2 + \sigma_h^2 + \sigma_h^2 - 2\mu(\sigma_h\sigma_h + \sigma_h\sigma_h + \sigma_h\sigma_h)\right]$$

$$= \frac{1}{2E}\left[3\sigma_h^2 - 2\mu(3\sigma_h^2)\right]$$

$$U_h = \left(\frac{3\sigma_h^2}{2E}\right)[1 - 2\mu] \qquad\qquad \dots \text{(Eq. 12.46)}$$

Substituting (Eq. 12.45) in (Eq. 12.46) yields

$$U_h = \frac{3}{2}\left[\frac{1 - 2\mu}{E}\right]\left(\frac{\sigma_1 + \sigma_2 + \sigma_3}{3}\right)^2$$

$$U_h = \left[\frac{1 - 2\mu}{6E}\right]\left[\sigma_1^2 + \sigma_2^2 + \sigma_3^2 - 2(\sigma_1\sigma_2 + \sigma_2\sigma_3 + \sigma_3\sigma_1)\right]$$

$$\dots \text{(Eq. 12.47)}$$

Distortion component is calculated as...

$$U_d = U - U_h$$

$$= \left\{\frac{1}{2E}\left[\sigma_1^2 + \sigma_2^2 + \sigma_3^2 - 2\mu(\sigma_1\sigma_2 + \sigma_2\sigma_3 + \sigma_3\sigma_1)\right]\right\} -$$

$$\left\{\left[\frac{1 - 2\mu}{6E}\right]\left[\sigma_1^2 + \sigma_2^2 + \sigma_3^2 - 2(\sigma_1\sigma_2 + \sigma_2\sigma_3 + \sigma_3\sigma_1)\right]\right\}$$

Let

$$A = \left(\sigma_1^2 + \sigma_2^2 + \sigma_3^2\right) \text{ and } B = (\sigma_1\sigma_2 + \sigma_2\sigma_3 + \sigma_3\sigma_1)$$

$$\therefore \quad U_d = \frac{1}{2E}[A - 2\mu B] - \frac{(1 - 2\mu)}{6E}[A + 2B]$$

$$= \frac{1}{6E}[3A - 6B\mu - A - 2B + 2A\mu + 4B\mu]$$

$$= \frac{1}{6E}[2A - 2\mu B - 2B + 2A\mu]$$

$$= \frac{1}{6E}[2A(1 + \mu) - 2B(1 + \mu)]$$

$$= \frac{1}{3E}[A(1 + \mu) - B(1 + \mu)]$$

$$= \left(\frac{1 + \mu}{3E}\right)[A - B]$$

$$\therefore \quad U_d = \left(\frac{1 + \mu}{3E}\right)[\sigma_1^2 + \sigma_2^2 + \sigma_3^2 - (\sigma_1\sigma_2 + \sigma_2\sigma_3 + \sigma_3\sigma_1)]$$

$$\dots \text{(Eq. 12.48a)}$$

Since $[a^2 + b^2 + c^2 - (ab + bc + ca)] = \left[\dfrac{(a-b)^2 + (b-c)^2 + (c-a)^2}{2}\right]$, we have

$$U_d = \left(\frac{1+\mu}{6E}\right)[(\sigma_1 - \sigma_2)^2 + (\sigma_2 - \sigma_3)^2 + (\sigma_3 - \sigma_1)^2] \quad \text{... (Eq. 12.48b)}$$

For a uniaxial tensile test, $\sigma_1 = \sigma_e$ and $\sigma_2 = \sigma_3 = 0$, thus (Eq. 12.48a) and/or (Eq. 12.48b) reduces to

$$U_d = \sigma_e^2 \left(\frac{1+\mu}{3E}\right) \quad \text{... (Eq. 12.49)}$$

The failure condition is

$$\left[\frac{1+\mu}{3E}\right][\sigma_1^2 + \sigma_2^2 + \sigma_3^2 - (\sigma_1\sigma_2 + \sigma_2\sigma_3 + \sigma_3\sigma_1)] \geq \sigma_e^2 \left[\frac{1+\mu}{3E}\right] \quad \text{... (Eq. 12.50a)}$$

$$[\sigma_1^2 + \sigma_2^2 + \sigma_3^2 - (\sigma_1\sigma_2 + \sigma_2\sigma_3 + \sigma_3\sigma_1)] \geq \sigma_e^2 \quad \text{... (Eq. 12.50b)}$$

If factor of safety is considered, then the failure condition is

$$\sigma_1^2 + \sigma_2^2 + \sigma_3^2 - (\sigma_1\sigma_2 + \sigma_2\sigma_3 + \sigma_3\sigma_1) \geq \frac{\sigma_e^2}{n} \quad \text{... (Eq. 12.51a)}$$

Or

$$\frac{(\sigma_1 - \sigma_2)^2 + (\sigma_2 - \sigma_3)^2 + (\sigma_3 - \sigma_1)^2}{2} \geq \frac{\sigma_e^2}{n}$$

Or
$$(\sigma_1 - \sigma_2)^2 + (\sigma_2 - \sigma_3)^2 + (\sigma_3 - \sigma_1)^2 \geq \frac{2\sigma_e^2}{n} \quad \text{... (Eq. 12.51b)}$$

For a 2D case: Here $\sigma_3 = 0$

(Eq. 12.51a or 12.51b) yields,
$$\sigma_1^2 + \sigma_2^2 - \sigma_1\sigma_2 \geq \frac{\sigma_e^2}{n} \quad \text{... (Eq. 12.52a)}$$

Or
$$\sqrt{\sigma_1^2 + \sigma_2^2 - \sigma_1\sigma_2} \geq \frac{\sigma_e}{n} \quad \text{... (Eq. 12.52b)}$$

Note: Since $E = 2G[1 + \mu]$, (Eq. 12.48a) can also be written as

$$U_d = \left(\frac{1}{6G}\right)[\sigma_1^2 + \sigma_2^2 + \sigma_3^2 - (\sigma_1\sigma_2 + \sigma_2\sigma_3 + \sigma_3\sigma_1)] \quad \text{... (Eq. 12.53a)}$$

Or
$$U_d = \frac{1}{12G}[(\sigma_1 - \sigma_2)^2 + (\sigma_2 - \sigma_3)^2 + (\sigma_3 - \sigma_1)^2] \quad \text{... (Eq. 12.53b)}$$

Applicable to ductile materials. This theory gives satisfactory results.

12.8 FAILURE OF DUCTILE AND BRITTLE MATERIALS

For ductile materials the *distortion theory* gives accurate results. However *maximum shear stress theory* is also preferred as it gives results on safer side.

For brittle materials which fail by fracture, the *maximum normal or principal stress theory* and *distortion theory are preferred*. In majority of the cases, maximum normal stress theory is preferred.

1. **A bolt is designed to take up direct tensile load of 30 kN and a shear load of 16 kN with a factor of safety of 4. The yield strength of the materiel used is 400 MPa. Calculate the size of the bolt based on various theories of failure. Take μ = 0.3.**

Solution: $F = 30$ kN $= 30 \times 10^3$ N, $F_s = 16$ kN $= 16 \times 10^3$ N, factor of safety, $n = 4$, yield or elastic stress, $\sigma_e = 400$ MPa, $d = ?$, $\mu = 0.3$

- Axial stress, $\quad \sigma_D = \dfrac{F}{A} = \dfrac{30 \times 10^3}{\pi d^2/4} = \dfrac{38.20 \times 10^3}{d^2}$ MPa

- Shear stress, $\quad \tau = \dfrac{F_s}{A_s} \quad (A_s = A)$

$$\tau = \frac{16 \times 10^3}{\pi d^2/4} = \frac{20.37 \times 10^3}{d^2} \text{ MPa}$$

State of stress: Here $\sigma_x = \sigma_D = \dfrac{38.20 \times 10^3}{d^2}$ MPa; $\sigma_y = 0$; $\tau = \tau_{xy} = \dfrac{20.37 \times 10^3}{d^2}$ MPa

Principal stresses:

We know that $\quad \sigma_{1,2} = \left(\dfrac{\sigma_x + \sigma_y}{2}\right) \pm \sqrt{\left(\dfrac{\sigma_x - \sigma_y}{2}\right)^2 + \tau_{xy}^2}$

$$= \left(\frac{38.20 \times 10^3 + 0}{2d^2}\right) \pm \sqrt{\left(\frac{38.20 \times 10^3 - 0}{2d^2}\right)^2 + \left(\frac{20.37 \times 10^3}{d^2}\right)^2}$$

$$\sigma_{1,2} = \left(\frac{19.10 \times 10^3}{d^2}\right) \pm \left(\frac{27.92 \times 10^3}{d^2}\right)$$

Maximum principal stress, $\quad \sigma_1 = \left(\dfrac{47 \times 10^3}{d^2}\right)$

Minimum principal stress, $\quad \sigma_2 = \left(\dfrac{-8820}{d^2}\right)$

a. *Maximum normal stress theory:*

We know that $\quad \dfrac{\sigma_e}{n} = \sigma_1$

$$\frac{400}{4} = \left(\frac{47 \times 10^3}{d^2}\right)$$

$$100 = \left(\frac{47 \times 10^3}{d^2}\right)$$

$$\therefore \quad d = 21.68 \text{ mm}$$

b. *Maximum shear stress theory (MSST):*

We know that $\dfrac{\sigma_e}{n} = \sigma_1 - \sigma_2$

$$\frac{400}{4} = \left(\frac{47 \times 10^3}{d^2}\right) - \left(\frac{-8820}{d^2}\right)$$

$$100 = \left(\frac{55.84 \times 10^3}{d^2}\right)$$

$$\therefore \quad d = 23.63 \text{ mm}$$

c. *Maximum normal strain theory:*

We know that $\dfrac{\sigma_e}{n} = (\sigma_1 - \mu\sigma_2)$

$$\frac{400}{4} = \left(\frac{47 \times 10^3}{d^2}\right) - \left[0.3\left(\frac{-8820}{d^2}\right)\right]$$

$$100 = \left(\frac{49.67 \times 10^3}{d^2}\right)$$

$$\therefore \quad d = 22.28 \text{ mm}$$

d. *Distortion energy theory or Von-Mises theory (DET):*

We know that $\dfrac{\sigma_e}{n} = \sqrt{\sigma_1^2 + \sigma_1^2 - \sigma_1\sigma_2}$

$$\frac{400}{4} = \sqrt{\left(\frac{47 \times 10^3}{d^2}\right)^2 + \left(\frac{-8820}{d^2}\right)^2 - \left[\left(\frac{47 \times 10^3}{d^2}\right) \times \left(\frac{-8820}{d^2}\right)\right]}$$

$$100 = \left(\frac{52 \times 10^3}{d^2}\right)$$

$$\therefore \quad d = 22.80 \text{ mm}$$

e. *Strain energy theory:*

We know that $\dfrac{\sigma_e}{n} = \sqrt{\sigma_1^2 + \sigma_1^2 - 2\mu\sigma_1\sigma_2}$

$$\frac{400}{4} = \sqrt{\left(\frac{47 \times 10^3}{d^2}\right)^2 + \left(\frac{-8820}{d^2}\right)^2 - \left[2 \times 0.3\left(\frac{47 \times 10^3}{d^2}\right) \times \left(\frac{-8820}{d^2}\right)\right]}$$

$$100 = \left(\frac{52 \times 10^3}{d^2}\right)$$

$$\therefore \quad d = 22.44 \text{ mm}$$

2. **A bolt is subjected to an axial pull of 12 kN together with a transverse shear of 6 kN. Determine the diameter of the bolt using:**
   (a) Maximum principal stress theory   (b) Maximum shear stress theory.
   Take elastic limit in tension = 300 MPa, factor of safety = 3 and Poisson's ratio = 0.3

VTU – Dec. 16/ Jan. 17 – 16 Marks

Solution: $F = 12 \times 10^3$ N, $F_s = 6 \times 10^3$ N, yield or elastic stress, $\sigma_e = 300$ MPa, factor of safety, $n = 3$, $\mu = 0.3$, $d = ?$ a) MNST, b) MSST

- Axial stress, $\quad \sigma_D = \dfrac{F}{A} = \dfrac{12 \times 10^3}{\pi d^2/4} = \dfrac{15.28 \times 10^3}{d^2}$ MPa

- Shear stress, $\quad \tau = \dfrac{F_s}{A_s} \quad (A_s = A)$

$$\tau = \frac{6 \times 10^3}{\pi d^2/4} = \frac{7.64 \times 10^3}{d^2} \text{ MPa}$$

State of stress: Here $\sigma_x = \sigma_D = \dfrac{15.28 \times 10^3}{d^2}$ MPa; $\sigma_y = 0$; $\tau = \tau_{xy} = \dfrac{7.64 \times 10^3}{d^2}$ MPa

Method 1: Using stress components
a. *Maximum principal or normal stress theory:*

We know that $\quad \dfrac{\sigma_e}{n} = \left(\dfrac{\sigma_x + \sigma_y}{2}\right) + \sqrt{\left(\dfrac{\sigma_x - \sigma_y}{2}\right)^2 + \tau_{xy}^2}$

$$\frac{300}{3} = \left(\frac{15.28 \times 10^3 + 0}{2d^2}\right) + \sqrt{\left(\frac{15.28 \times 10^3 - 0}{2d^2}\right)^2 + \left(\frac{7.64 \times 10^3}{d^2}\right)^2}$$

$$100 = \left(\frac{7.64 \times 10^3}{d^2}\right) + \left(\frac{10.80 \times 10^3}{d^2}\right)$$

$$100 = \left(\frac{18.44 \times 10^3}{d^2}\right)$$

$$\therefore \quad d = 13.58 \text{ mm}$$

b. *Maximum shear stress theory (MSST):*

We know that $\quad \dfrac{\sigma_e}{n} = \sqrt{(\sigma_x - \sigma_y)^2 + 4\tau_{xy}^2}$

$$\frac{300}{3} = \sqrt{\left(\frac{15.28 \times 10^3 - 0}{d^2}\right)^2 + \left[4 \times \left(\frac{7.64 \times 10^3}{d^2}\right)^2\right]}$$

$$100 = \left(\frac{21.61 \times 10^3}{d^2} \right)$$

$$\therefore \quad d = 14.70 \text{ mm}$$

Method 2: Using principal stresses

We know that

$$\sigma_{1,2} = \left(\frac{\sigma_x + \sigma_y}{2} \right) \pm \sqrt{\left(\frac{\sigma_x - \sigma_y}{2} \right)^2 + \tau_{xy}^2}$$

$$= \left(\frac{15.28 \times 10^3 + 0}{2d^2} \right) \pm \sqrt{\left(\frac{15.28 \times 10^3 - 0}{2d^2} \right)^2 + \left(\frac{7.64 \times 10^3}{d^2} \right)^2}$$

$$\sigma_{1,2} = \left(\frac{7.64 \times 10^3}{d^2} \right) \pm \left(\frac{10.80 \times 10^3}{d^2} \right)$$

Maximum principal stress, $\sigma_1 = \left(\dfrac{18.44 \times 10^3}{d^2} \right)$

Minimum principal stress, $\sigma_2 = \left(\dfrac{-3160}{d^2} \right)$

a. *Maximum normal stress theory:*

We know that

$$\frac{\sigma_e}{n} = \sigma_1$$

$$\frac{300}{3} = \left(\frac{18.44 \times 10^3}{d^2} \right)$$

$$100 = \left(\frac{18.44 \times 10^3}{d^2} \right)$$

$$\therefore \quad d = 13.58 \text{ mm}$$

b. *Maximum shear stress theory (MSST):*

We know that

$$\frac{\sigma_e}{n} = \sigma_1 - \sigma_2$$

$$\frac{300}{3} = \left(\frac{18.44 \times 10^3}{d^2} \right) - \left(\frac{-3160}{d^2} \right)$$

$$100 = \left(\frac{21.60 \times 10^3}{d^2} \right)$$

$$\therefore \quad d = 14.70 \text{ mm}$$

3. **A mild steel shaft is subjected to 3500 N-m of bending moment at its critical point and transmits a torque of 2500 N-m. The shaft is made of steel having yield strength of 231 MPa. Estimate the size of the shaft based on various theories of failure and specify the final size. Take FOS = 2 and μ = 0.3.**

Solution: $M = 3.5 \times 10^6$ N-mm, $T = 2.5 \times 10^6$ N-mm, $\sigma_e = 231$ MPa, = ?, $n = 2$, $\mu = 0.3$

- Bending stress, $\quad \sigma_b = \dfrac{M}{Z} = \dfrac{M}{\pi d^3/32} = \dfrac{3.5 \times 10^6}{\pi d^3/32} = \dfrac{35.65 \times 10^6}{d^3}$

- Shear stress, $\quad \tau = \dfrac{16T}{\pi d^3} = \dfrac{16 \times (2.5 \times 10^3)}{\pi d^3} = \dfrac{12.73 \times 10^6}{d^3}$

State of stress: Here $\sigma_x = \sigma_b = \dfrac{35.65 \times 10^6}{d^3}$ MPa; $\sigma_y = 0$; $\tau = \tau_{xy} = \dfrac{12.73 \times 10^6}{d^3}$ MPa

Principal stresses:

a. Maximum normal stress theory:

We know that $\quad \dfrac{\sigma_e}{n} = \left(\dfrac{\sigma_x + \sigma_y}{2}\right) + \sqrt{\left(\dfrac{\sigma_x - \sigma_y}{2}\right)^2 + \tau_{xy}^2}$

$$\dfrac{231}{2} = \left(\dfrac{35.65 \times 10^6 + 0}{2d^3}\right) + \sqrt{\left(\dfrac{35.65 \times 10^6 - 0}{2d^3}\right)^2 + \left(\dfrac{12.73 \times 10^6}{d^3}\right)^2}$$

$$115.5 = \left(\dfrac{17.83 \times 10^6}{d^3}\right) + \left(\dfrac{21.90 \times 10^6}{d^3}\right)$$

$$115.5 = \left(\dfrac{39.73 \times 10^6}{d^3}\right)$$

$$\therefore \quad d = 70.06 \text{ mm}$$

b. Maximum shear stress theory (MSST):

We know that $\quad \dfrac{\sigma_e}{n} = \sqrt{(\sigma_x - \sigma_y)^2 + 4\tau_{xy}^2}$

$$\dfrac{231}{2} = \sqrt{\left(\dfrac{35.65 \times 10^6 - 0}{d^3}\right)^2 + \left[4 \times \left(\dfrac{12.73 \times 10^6}{d^3}\right)^2\right]}$$

$$115.5 = \left(\dfrac{43.80 \times 10^6}{d^3}\right)$$

$$\therefore \quad d = 72.38 \text{ mm}$$

c. Maximum normal strain theory:

We know that $\quad \dfrac{\sigma_e}{n} = (\sigma_1 - \mu\sigma_2)$

$$\sigma_{1,2} = \left(\dfrac{\sigma_x + \sigma_y}{2}\right) \pm \sqrt{\left(\dfrac{\sigma_x - \sigma_y}{2}\right)^2 + \tau_{xy}^2}$$

$$= \left(\frac{17.83 \times 10^6}{d^3} \right) \pm \left(\frac{21.90 \times 10^6}{d^3} \right)$$

$$\sigma_1 = \left(\frac{39.73 \times 10^6}{d^3} \right), \quad \sigma_2 = \left(\frac{-4.07 \times 10^6}{d^3} \right)$$

$$\frac{231}{2} = \left(\frac{39.73 \times 10^6}{d^3} \right) - \left[0.3 \left(\frac{-4.07 \times 10^6}{d^3} \right) \right]$$

$$115.5 = \left(\frac{40.95 \times 10^3}{d^3} \right)$$

$$\therefore \quad d = 70.78 \text{ mm}$$

d. *Distortion energy theory or Von-Mises theory (DET):*

We know that $\quad \dfrac{\sigma_e}{n} = \sqrt{\sigma_x^2 + \sigma_y^2 - \sigma_x \sigma_y + 3\tau_{xy}^2}$

$$\frac{231}{2} = \sqrt{ \left(\frac{35.65 \times 10^6}{d^3} \right)^2 + 0 - \left[\left(\frac{35.67 \times 10^6}{d^3} \right) \times 0 \right] + \left[3 \times \left(\frac{12.73 \times 10^6}{d^3} \right)^2 \right] }$$

$$115.5 = \left(\frac{41.92 \times 10^6}{d^3} \right)$$

$$\therefore \quad d = 71.33 \text{ mm}$$

e. *Strain energy theory:*

We know that $\dfrac{\sigma_e}{n} = \sqrt{\sigma_1^2 + \sigma_2^2 - 2\mu\sigma_1\sigma_2}$

$$\frac{231}{2} = \sqrt{ \left(\frac{39.73 \times 10^6}{d^3} \right)^2 + \left(\frac{-4.07 \times 10^6}{d^3} \right)^2 - \left[2 \times 0.3 \times \left(\frac{39.73 \times 10^6}{d^3} \right) \times \left(\frac{-4.07 \times 10^6}{d^3} \right) \right] }$$

$$115.5 = \left(\frac{41.13 \times 10^6}{d^3} \right)$$

$$\therefore \quad d = 70.89 \text{ mm}$$

Based on above theories, the maximum shaft diameter is $d = 72.38$ mm ≈ 75 mm

4. **A solid circular shaft is subjected to a bending moment of 9000 N-m and a twisting moment of 12000 N-m. In a simple uni-axial tensile test of same material, it gave the following particulars: stress at yield point = 300 MPa, E = 200 GPa. Estimate the least diameter required using:**
   (a) Maximum principal stress theory
   (b) Maximum shear stress theory.
   Take FOS = 3 and μ = 0.25

VTU – (CV) Dec. 16/ Jan. 17 – 12 Marks

Solution: $M = 9 \times 10^6$ N-mm, $T = 12 \times 10^6$ N-mm, $\sigma_e = 300$ MPa, $E = 200 \times 10^3$ MPa
$d = ?, n = 3, \mu = 0.25$

- Bending stress, $\sigma_b = \dfrac{M}{Z} = \dfrac{M}{\pi d^3/32} = \dfrac{9 \times 10^6}{\pi d^3/32} = \dfrac{91.67 \times 10^6}{d^3}$

- Shear stress, $\tau = \dfrac{16T}{\pi d^3} = \dfrac{16 \times (12 \times 10^6)}{\pi d^3} = \dfrac{61.12 \times 10^6}{d^3}$

State of stress: Here $\sigma_x = \sigma_b = \dfrac{91.67 \times 10^6}{d^3}$ MPa; $\sigma_y = 0$; $\tau = \tau_{xy} = \dfrac{61.12 \times 10^6}{d^3}$ MPa

Method 1: Using stress components

a. *Maximum principal or normal stress theory:*

We know that $\dfrac{\sigma_e}{n} = \left(\dfrac{\sigma_x + \sigma_y}{2}\right) + \sqrt{\left(\dfrac{\sigma_x - \sigma_y}{2}\right)^2 + \tau_{xy}^2}$

$$\dfrac{300}{3} = \left(\dfrac{91.67 \times 10^6 + 0}{2d^3}\right) + \sqrt{\left(\dfrac{91.67 \times 10^6 - 0}{2d^3}\right)^2 + \left(\dfrac{61.62 \times 10^6}{d^3}\right)^2}$$

$$100 = \left(\dfrac{45.84 \times 10^6}{d^3}\right) + \left(\dfrac{76.40 \times 10^6}{d^3}\right)$$

$$100 = \left(\dfrac{122.24 \times 10^6}{d^3}\right)$$

$$\therefore \quad d = 106.92 \text{ mm}$$

b. *Maximum shear stress theory (MSST):*

We know that $\dfrac{\sigma_e}{n} = \sqrt{(\sigma_x - \sigma_y)^2 + 4\tau_{xy}^2}$

$$\dfrac{300}{3} = \sqrt{\left(\dfrac{91.67 \times 10^6 - 0}{d^3}\right)^2 + \left[4 \times \left(\dfrac{61.62 \times 10^6}{d^3}\right)^2\right]}$$

$$100 = \left(\dfrac{152.79 \times 10^6}{d^3}\right)$$

$$\therefore \quad d = 115.18 \text{ mm}$$

Method 2: Using principal stresses

We know that $\sigma_{1,2} = \left(\dfrac{\sigma_x + \sigma_y}{2}\right) \pm \sqrt{\left(\dfrac{\sigma_x - \sigma_y}{2}\right)^2 + \tau_{xy}^2}$

$$= \left(\dfrac{91.67 \times 10^6 + 0}{2d^3}\right) \pm \sqrt{\left(\dfrac{91.67 \times 10^6 - 0}{2d^3}\right)^2 + \left(\dfrac{61.62 \times 10^6}{d^3}\right)^2}$$

$$\sigma_{1,2} = \left(\frac{45.84 \times 10^6}{d^3}\right) \pm \left(\frac{76.40 \times 10^6}{d^3}\right)$$

Maximum principal stress, $\quad \sigma_1 = \left(\frac{122.24 \times 10^6}{d^3}\right)$

Minimum principal stress, $\quad \sigma_2 = \left(\frac{-30.56 \times 10^6}{d^3}\right)$

a. *Maximum normal stress theory:*

We know that $\quad \dfrac{\sigma_e}{n} = \sigma_1$

$$\frac{300}{3} = \left(\frac{122.24 \times 10^6}{d^3}\right)$$

$$100 = \left(\frac{122.24 \times 10^6}{d^3}\right)$$

$$\therefore \quad d = 106.92 \text{ mm}$$

b. *Maximum shear stress theory (MSST):*

We know that $\quad \dfrac{\sigma_e}{n} = \sigma_1 - \sigma_2$

$$\frac{300}{3} = \left(\frac{122.24 \times 10^6}{d^3}\right) - \left(\frac{-30.56 \times 10^6}{d^3}\right)$$

$$100 = \left(\frac{152.8 \times 10^6}{d^3}\right)$$

$$\therefore \quad d = 115.18 \text{ mm}$$

5. **A mild steel shaft 60 mm diameter is subjected to a bending moment of 25×10^5 N-mm and torque T. If the yield point of steel in tension is 230 N/mm², find the maximum value of this torque without causing yielding of the shaft according to:**
   (a) Maximum principal stress theory of failure
   (b) Maximum shear stress theory of failure
   (c) Maximum distortion energy theory of failure.
   Adopt a factor of safety of 1.5

Solution: $d = 60$ mm, $M = 25 \times 10^5$ N-mm, $\sigma_e = 230$ MPa, $n = 1.5$, torque $T = ?$, (a) MNST, (b) MSST, (c) DET.

- Bending stress, $\quad \sigma_b = \dfrac{M}{Z} = \dfrac{M}{\pi d^3/32} = \dfrac{25 \times 10^5}{\pi \times 60^3/32} = 117.90$ MPa.

- Shear stress, $\quad \tau = \dfrac{16T}{\pi d^3} = \dfrac{16 \times T}{\pi \times 60^3} = (2.36 \times 10^{-5})T$ MPa

State of stress: Here $\sigma_x = \sigma_b = 117.90$ MPa; $\sigma_y = 0$; $\tau = \tau_{xy} = (2.36 \times 10^{-5})T$ MPa

a. *According to MNST:*

We know that

$$\frac{\sigma_e}{n} = \left(\frac{\sigma_x + \sigma_y}{2}\right) + \sqrt{\left(\frac{\sigma_x - \sigma_y}{2}\right)^2 + \tau_{xy}^2}$$

$$\frac{230}{1.5} = \left(\frac{117.90 + 0}{2}\right) + \sqrt{\left(\frac{117.90 - 0}{2}\right)^2 + \left(2.36 \times 10^{-5}T\right)^2}$$

$$153.33 = 58.95 + \sqrt{58.95^2 + \left(2.36 \times 10^{-5}T\right)^2}$$

$$94.38 = \sqrt{3475.10 + (5.57 \times 10^{-10})T^2}$$

$$\therefore \quad 94.38^2 = 3475.10 + (5.57 \times 10^{-10})T^2$$

$$T = 3.12 \times 10^6 \text{ N-mm} = 3.12 \text{ kN-m}$$

b. *According to MSST:*

We know that

$$\frac{\sigma_e}{n} = \sqrt{(\sigma_x - \sigma_y)^2 + 4\tau_{xy}^2}$$

$$\frac{230}{1.5} = \sqrt{117.90^2 + [4 \times \left(2.36 \times 10^{-5}T\right)^2]}$$

$$153.33 = \sqrt{13900.41 + (2.23 \times 10^{-9})T^2}$$

$$\therefore \quad 153.33^2 = 13900.41 + (2.23 \times 10^{-9})T^2$$

$$T = 2.08 \times 10^6 \text{ N-mm} = 2.08 \text{ kN-m}$$

c. *According to DET:*

We know that

$$\frac{\sigma_e}{n} = \sqrt{\sigma_x^2 + \sigma_y^2 - \sigma_x\sigma_y + 3\tau_{xy}^2}$$

$$\frac{230}{1.5} = \sqrt{117.90^2 + 0 - 0 + [3 \times (2.36 \times 10^{-5}T)^2]}$$

$$153.33 = \sqrt{13900.41 + (1.67 \times 10^{-9})T^2}$$

$$\therefore \quad 153.33^2 = 13900.41 + (1.67 \times 10^{-9})T^2$$

$$T = 2.40 \times 10^6 \text{ N-mm} = 2.40 \text{ kN-m}$$

6. **A round rod of diameter 30 mm is to sustain an axial compressive load of 20 kN and twisting moment of 1.5 kN-m. The rod is made of carbon steel having σ_{yt} = 328.6 MPa. Determine the factor of safety as per the following theories of failure:**
   (a) **Maximum principal strain theory**
   (b) **Maximum strain energy theory**
   (c) **Maximum shear stress theory of failure. Take FOS as 0.25**

Solution: $d = 30$ mm, $F = -20 \times 10^3$ N, $T = 1.5 \times 10^6$ N-mm, $\sigma_{yt} = \sigma_e = 328.6$ MPa, $n = ?$

- Axial stress, $\quad \sigma_D = \dfrac{F}{A} = \dfrac{-20 \times 10^3}{\pi \times 30^2/4} = -28.29 \text{ MPa}$

- Shear stress, $\quad \tau = \dfrac{16T}{\pi d^3} = \dfrac{16 \times (1.5 \times 10^6)}{\pi \times 30^3} = 282.94 \text{ MPa}$

State of stress: Here $\sigma_x = \sigma_D = -28.29 \text{ MPa}$; $\sigma_y = 0$; $\tau = \tau_{xy} = 282.94 \text{ MPa}$

Principal stresses:

$$\sigma_{1,2} = \left(\frac{\sigma_x + \sigma_y}{2}\right) \pm \sqrt{\left(\frac{\sigma_x - \sigma_y}{2}\right)^2 + \tau_{xy}^2}$$

$$= \left(\frac{-28.29 + 0}{2}\right) \pm \sqrt{\left(\frac{-28.29 - 0}{2}\right)^2 + 282.94^2}$$

$$\sigma_{1,2} = -14.15 \pm 283.30$$

Maximum principal stress, $\sigma_1 = 269.15 \text{ MPa}$

Minimum principal stress, $\sigma_2 = -297.44 \text{ MPa}$

a. *Maximum principal strain theory:*

We know that $\qquad \dfrac{\sigma_e}{n} = (\sigma_1 - \mu\sigma_2)$

$$\frac{328.6}{n} = 269.15 - [0.25 \times (-297.44)]$$

$$\frac{328.6}{n} = 343.51$$

$$n = 0.957$$

b. *Strain energy theory:*

We know that $\qquad \dfrac{\sigma_e}{n} = \sqrt{\sigma_1^2 + \sigma_2^2 - 2\mu\sigma_1\sigma_2}$

$$\frac{328.6}{n} = \sqrt{(269.15)^2 + (-297.44)^2 - [2 \times 0.25 \times (269.15) \times (-297.44)]}$$

$$\frac{328.6}{n} = 448.26$$

$$n = 0.733$$

c. *Maximum shear stress theory (MSST):*

We know that $\qquad \dfrac{\sigma_e}{n} = \sigma_1 - \sigma_2$

$$\frac{328.6}{n} = 269.15 - (-297.44)$$

$$\frac{328.6}{n} = 566.59$$

$$n = 0.580$$

7. **The state of stress in a two dimensional body for which the tensile yield strength is 250 MPa, is as shown in Fig. 12.2. Determine the factor of safety using various failure theories. Take μ = 0.3**

Solution: $\sigma_{yt} = \sigma_e = 250$ MPa, $n = ?$, $\sigma_x = 180$ MPa, $\sigma_y = 120$ MPa, $\tau_{xy} = 80$ MPa, $\mu = 0.3$.
Principal stresses:

$$\sigma_{1,2} = \left(\frac{\sigma_x + \sigma_y}{2}\right) \pm \sqrt{\left(\frac{\sigma_x - \sigma_y}{2}\right)^2 + \tau_{xy}^2}$$

$$= \left(\frac{180 + 120}{2}\right) + \sqrt{\left(\frac{180 - 120}{2}\right)^2 + 80}$$

$$\sigma_{1,2} = 150 \pm 85.44$$

Maximum principal stress, $\sigma_1 = 235.44$ MPa
Minimum principal stress, $\sigma_2 = 64.56$ MPa

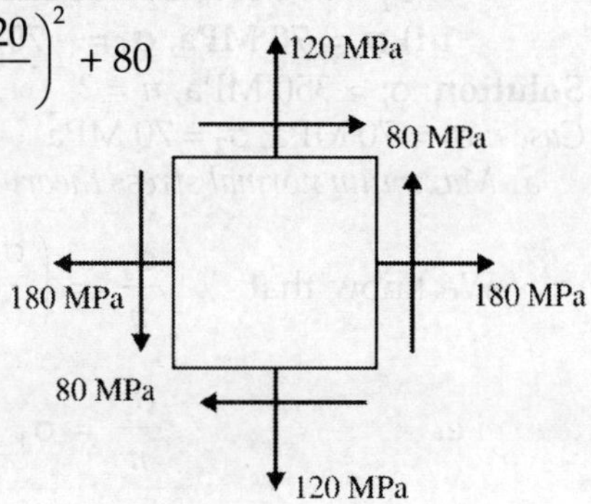

a. *Maximum normal stress theory:*

We know that $\quad \dfrac{\sigma_e}{n} = \sigma_1$

$$\frac{250}{n} = 235.44$$

$$n = 1.062$$

b. *Maximum shear stress theory (MSST):*

We know that $\quad \dfrac{\sigma_e}{n} = \sigma_1 - \sigma_2$

$$\frac{250}{n} = 235.44 - 64.56$$

$$n = 1.463$$

c. *Maximum normal strain theory:*

We know that $\quad \dfrac{\sigma_e}{n} = (\sigma_1 - \mu\sigma_2)$

$$\frac{250}{n} = 235.44 - (0.3 \times 64.56)$$

$$n = 1.157$$

d. *Distortion energy theory or Von-Mises theory (DET):*

We know that $\quad \dfrac{\sigma_e}{n} = \sqrt{\sigma_1^2 + \sigma_2^2 - \sigma_1\sigma_2}$

$$\frac{250}{n} = \sqrt{235.44^2 + 64.56^2 - (235.44 \times 64.56)}$$

$$n = 1.186$$

e. *Strain energy theory:*

We know that $\quad \dfrac{\sigma_e}{n} = \sqrt{\sigma_1^2 + \sigma_2^2 - 2\mu\sigma_1\sigma_2}$

Fig. 12.2: Problem 7

$$\frac{250}{n} = \sqrt{235.44^2 + 64.56^2 - [2 \times 0.3 \times (235.44 \times 64.56)]}$$

$$n = 1.113$$

8. **A machine member is statically loaded and has yield strength of 350 MPa. For each of the stress state indicated below. Find the factor of safety according to:**
   (a) Maximum normal stress theory
   (b) Maximum shear stress theory
   (c) Maximum distortion energy theory.

   i) $\sigma_1 = 70$ MPa, $\sigma_2 = 70$ MPa   ii) $\sigma_1 = 70$ MPa, $\sigma_2 = 35$ MPa

   iii) $\sigma_1 = 70$ MPa, $\sigma_2 = -70$ MPa   iv) $\sigma_1 = -70$ MPa, $\sigma_2 = 0$ MPa

Solution: $\sigma_e = 350$ MPa, $n = ?$.

Case i: $\sigma_1 = 70$ MPa, $\sigma_2 = 70$ MPa

a. *Maximum normal stress theory:*

We know that $\qquad \dfrac{\sigma_e}{n} = \left(\dfrac{\sigma_x + \sigma_y}{2}\right) + \dfrac{1}{2}\sqrt{\left(\sigma_x - \sigma_y\right)^2 + 4\tau^2} = \sigma_1$

i.e. $\qquad \dfrac{\sigma_e}{n} = \sigma_1$

$$\frac{350}{n} = 70$$

$$n = 5.0$$

b. *Maximum shear stress theory (MSST):*

We know that $\qquad \dfrac{\sigma_e}{n} = \sigma_1 - \sigma_2$

$$\frac{350}{n} = (70 - 70)$$

$$n = \infty \ (\text{infinity})$$

c. *Distortion energy theory (DET):*

We know that $\qquad \dfrac{\sigma_e}{n} = \sqrt{\sigma_1^2 + \sigma_2^2 - \sigma_1\sigma_2}$

$$\frac{350}{n} = \sqrt{70^2 + 70^2 - (70 \times 70)}$$

$$\frac{350}{n} = 70$$

$$n = 5.0$$

On similar lines, we have:

Case		Factor of safety (n)		
Stress arrangement: $\sigma_1 > \sigma_2$		MNST	MSST	DET
$\sigma_1 = 70$ MPa, $\sigma_2 = 35$ MPa		5.00	10.00	5.77
$\sigma_1 = 70$ MPa, $\sigma_2 = -70$ MPa		5.00	2.50	2.89
$\sigma_1 = 0$ MPa, $\sigma_2 = -70$ MPa				
(rearranged)		infinity	5.00	5.00

9. **A material has yield strength of 600 MPa. Compute the factor of safety for the following stress states using a) MSST b) DET.:**
   i) $\sigma_1 = 420$ MPa, $\sigma_2 = 410$ MPa, $\sigma_3 = 0$ MPa
   ii) $\sigma_1 = 420$ MPa, $\sigma_2 = 180$ MPa, $\sigma_3 = 0$ MPa
   iii) $\sigma_1 = 420$ MPa, $\sigma_2 = 0$ MPa, $\sigma_3 = -180$ MPa.
   iv) $\sigma_1 = 0$ MPa, $\sigma_2 = -180$ MPa, $\sigma_3 = -420$ MPa.

Solution: $\sigma_y = \sigma_e = 600$ MPa, = ?

Case i: $\sigma_1 = 420$ MPa, $\sigma_2 = 410$ MPa, $\sigma_3 = 0$ MPa (arrangement: $\sigma_1 > \sigma_2 > \sigma_3$)

  a. *According to MSST:*

We know that $\quad \dfrac{\sigma_e}{n} = \sigma_1 - \sigma_3$

$$\frac{600}{n} = (420 - 0)$$

$$n = 1.429$$

  b. *According to DET:*

We know that $\quad \dfrac{\sigma_e}{n} = \left[\sigma_1^2 + \sigma_2^2 + \sigma_3^2 - 2\mu(\sigma_1\sigma_2 + \sigma_2\sigma_3 + \sigma_1\sigma_3) \right]$

$$\dots \text{using (Eq. 2.32a)}$$

$$\frac{600}{n} = \sqrt{420^2 + 410^2 + 0 - [(420 \times 410) + 0 + 0]}$$

$$n = 1.445$$

On similar lines, we have:

Case	Factor of safety (*n*)	
Arrangement ($\sigma_1 > \sigma_2 > \sigma_3$)	MSST	DET
420,180,0	1.429	1.644
420,0,–180	1	1.125
0,–180,–420	1.429	1.644

10. **A material is tested under a state of stress $\sigma_1 = 3\sigma_2 = -2\sigma_3$. Yielding is observed at $\sigma_2 = 140$ MPa.**
    (a) **What is the yield stress in simple tension?**
    (b) **If the material is tested under the condition $\sigma_1 = -\sigma_3$, and $\sigma_2 = 0$, under what value of σ_3 will yielding occur?**

Solution: $\sigma_1 = 3\sigma_2 = -2\sigma_3$, $\sigma_2 = 140$ MPa. a). $\sigma_y = ?$, b). $\sigma_3 = ?$, if $\sigma_1 = -\sigma_3$ and $\sigma_2 = 0$

  a. *To find σ_e:*

According to DET, failure/yielding occurs when

$$(\sigma_1 - \sigma_2)^2 + (\sigma_2 - \sigma_3)^2 + (\sigma_3 - \sigma_1)^2 \geq 2\sigma_e^2 \qquad \dots \text{Eq. (i)}$$

From data, $\sigma_1 = 3\sigma_2 = -2\sigma_3$ and $\sigma_2 = 140$ MPa

i.e. $\sigma_1 = 3 \times 140 = 420$ MPa

and $\sigma_3 = -210$ MPa

Eq. (i) yields... $(420 - 140)^2 + (140 + 210)^2 + (-210 - 420)^2 = 2\sigma_e^2$

$$\sigma_e = 546.72 \text{ MPa}$$

  b. *To find σ_3, if $\sigma_1 = -\sigma_3$, and $\sigma_2 = 0$*

Eq. (i) yields... $(-\sigma_3 - 0)^2 + (0 - \sigma_3)^2 + (\sigma_3 + \sigma_3)^2 = 2\sigma_e^2$

$$6\sigma_3^2 = 2 \times 546.72^2$$

$$\sigma_3 = 315.65 \text{ MPa.}$$

11. **If the principal stresses at a point in an elastic material are 60 MPa tensile, 90 MPa tensile and 40 MPa compressive, find the stress at the limit of proportionality expected in a simple tensile test according to various theories of failure. Assume $\mu = 0.3$**

Solution: Principal stresses are 60 MPa, 90 MPa and -40 MPa. $\sigma_e = ?$, $\mu = 0.3$

Arrangement: $(\sigma_1 > \sigma_2 > \sigma_3)$ $\sigma_1 = 90$ MPa, $\sigma_2 = 60$ MPa, $\sigma_3 = -40$ MPa

a. *According to maximum principal stress:*

We know that $\dfrac{\sigma_e}{n} = \sigma_1$

$$\sigma_e = \sigma_1 = 90 \text{ MPa} \qquad\qquad \text{[Assume } n = 1, \text{ if not given]}$$

b. *According to MSST:*

We know that $\dfrac{\sigma_e}{n} = \sigma_1 - \sigma_3$

$$\sigma_e = [90 - (-40)]$$
$$\sigma_e = 130 \text{ MPa}$$

c. *According to maximum normal strain theory:*

We know that $\dfrac{\sigma_e}{n} = \sigma_1 - \mu(\sigma_2 + \sigma_3)$

$$\sigma_e = [90 - 0.3 \times (60 - 40)]$$
$$\sigma_e = 84 \text{ MPa}$$

d. *According to maximum strain energy theory:*

We know that $\dfrac{\sigma_e}{n} = \sqrt{\sigma_1^2 + \sigma_2^2 + \sigma_3^2 - 2\mu(\sigma_1\sigma_2 + \sigma_2\sigma_3 + \sigma_1\sigma_3)}$

$$\sigma_e = \sqrt{90^2 + 60^2 + (-40)^2 - [2 \times 0.3 \times \{(90 \times 60) + [60 \times (-40)] + [90 \times (-40)]\}]}$$
$$\sigma_e = 116.88 \text{ MPa}$$

e. *According to DET:*

We know that $\dfrac{\sigma_e}{n} = \sqrt{\sigma_1^2 + \sigma_2^2 + \sigma_3^2 - (\sigma_1\sigma_2 + \sigma_2\sigma_3 + \sigma_1\sigma_3)}$

$$\sigma_e = \sqrt{(90^2 + 60^2 + (-40)^2 - \{(90 \times 60) + [60 \times (-40)] + [90 \times (-40)]\})}$$
$$\sigma_e = 117.90 \text{ MPa}$$

12. **The stresses induced at a critical point in a machine component are as follows: $\sigma_x = 100$ MPa, $\sigma_y = 40$ MPa, $\tau_{xy} = 80$ MPa. The yield stress for the material is 350 MPa and Poisson's ratio is $\mu = 0.3$. Determine whether failure will occur or not according to various theories of failure**

Solution: $\sigma_x = 100$ MPa, $\sigma_y = 40$ MPa, $\tau_{xy} = 80$ MPa, $\sigma_e = 350$ MPa, $\mu = 0.3$. Failure = ?

Principal stresses:

We know that $\sigma_{1,2} = \left(\dfrac{\sigma_x + \sigma_y}{2}\right) \pm \sqrt{\left(\dfrac{\sigma_x - \sigma_y}{2}\right)^2 + \tau_{xy}^2}$

$$= \left(\dfrac{100 + 40}{2}\right) \pm \sqrt{\left(\dfrac{100 - 40}{2}\right) + 80^2}$$

$$\sigma_{1,2} = 70 \pm 85.44$$

Maximum principal stress, $\sigma_1 = 155.44$ MPa
Minimum principal stress, $\sigma_2 = -15.44$ MPa

a. *According to maximum principal stress:*

We know that $\dfrac{\sigma_e}{n} = \sigma_1$ $\qquad$ [Assume $n = 1$, if not given]

i.e. Failure occurs when
$$\sigma_1 \geq \sigma_e$$
$$155.44 \ngeq 350 \text{ MPa}.$$

Hence failure does not occur.

b. *According to MSST:*

We know that $\dfrac{\sigma_e}{n} = \sigma_1 - \sigma_2$

i.e. Failure occurs when
$$\sigma_1 - \sigma_2 \geq \sigma_e$$
$$[155.44 - (-15.44)] \geq 350$$
$$170.88 \ngeq 350 \text{ MPa}$$

Hence failure does not occur.

c. *According to maximum normal strain theory:*

We know that $\dfrac{\sigma_e}{n} = \sigma_1 - \mu\sigma_2$

i.e. Failure occurs when $\sigma_1 - \mu\sigma_2 \geq \sigma e$
$$[155.44 - 0.3 \times (-15.44)] \geq 350$$
$$160.07 \ngeq 350 \text{ MPa}$$

Hence failure does not occur.

d. *According to maximum strain energy theory:*

We know that $\dfrac{\sigma_e}{n} = \sqrt{\sigma_1^2 + \sigma_2^2 - 2\mu\sigma_1\sigma_2}$

i.e. Failure occurs when
$$\sqrt{\sigma_1^2 + \sigma_2^2 - 2\mu\sigma_1\sigma_2} \geq \sigma_e$$
$$\sqrt{155.44^2 + (-15.44)^2 - [2 \times 0.3 \times 155.54 \times (-15.44)]} \geq 350$$
$$160.75 \ngeq 350 \text{ MPa}$$

Hence failure does not occur.

e. *According to DET:*

We know that $\dfrac{\sigma_e}{n} = \sqrt{\sigma_1^2 + \sigma_2^2 - \sigma_1\sigma_2}$

i.e. Failure occurs when
$$\sqrt{\sigma_1^2 + \sigma_2^2 - \sigma_1\sigma_2} \geq \sigma_e$$
$$\sqrt{155.44^2 + (-15.44)^2 - [155.44 \times (-15.44)]} \geq 350$$
$$163.71 \ngeq 350 \text{ MPa}$$

Hence failure does not occur.

13. **The principal stresses at a point in an elastic material are 400 MPa, 140 MPa and $-$ 210 MPa. Determine whether failure will occur or not according to various theories of failure. The yield stress for the material is 550 MPa. Take $\mu = 0.3$**

Solution: Principal stresses are $\sigma_1 = 400$ MPa, $\sigma_2 = 140$ MPa, $\sigma_3 = -210$ MPa, $\sigma_e = 550$ MPa, $\mu = 0.3$. Failure = ?

    a. *According to maximum principal stress:*

We know that $\dfrac{\sigma_e}{n} = \sigma_1$ [Assume $n = 1$, if not given]

i.e. Failure occurs when
$$\sigma_1 \geq \sigma_e$$
$$400 \ngeq 550 \text{ MPa.}$$

Hence failure does not occur.

    b. *According to MSST:*

We know that $\dfrac{\sigma_e}{n} = \sigma_1 - \sigma_3$

i.e. Failure occurs when
$$\sigma_1 - \sigma_3 \geq \sigma_e$$
$$[400 - (-210)] \geq 550$$
$$610 \ngeq 550 \text{ MPa}$$

Hence failure occurs.

    c. *According to maximum normal strain theory:*

We know that $\dfrac{\sigma_e}{n} = \sigma_1 - \mu(\sigma_2 + \sigma_3)$

i.e. Failure occurs when
$$\sigma_1 - \mu(\sigma_2 + \sigma_3) \geq \sigma_e$$
$$[400 - 0.3 \times (140 - 210)] \geq 550$$
$$421 \ngeq 50 \text{ MPa}$$

Hence failure does not occur.

    d. *According to maximum strain energy theory:*

We know that $\dfrac{\sigma_e}{n} = \sqrt{\sigma_1^2 + \sigma_2^2 + \sigma_3^2 - 2\mu(\sigma_1\sigma_2 + \sigma_2\sigma_3 + \sigma_1\sigma_3)}$

i.e. Failure occurs when

$$\sqrt{\sigma_1^2 + \sigma_2^2 + \sigma_3^2 - 2\mu(\sigma_1\sigma_2 + \sigma_2\sigma_3 + \sigma_1\sigma_3)} = \sigma_e$$

$$\sqrt{400^2 + 140^2 + (-210)^2 - [2 \times 0.3 \times \{(400 \times 140) + [140 \times (-210)] + [400 \times (-210)]\}]}$$
$$\geq 550$$
$$508.07 \ngeq 550 \text{ MPa}$$

Hence failure does not occur.

    e. *According to DET:*

We know that $\dfrac{\sigma_e}{n} = \sqrt{\sigma_1^2 + \sigma_2^2 + \sigma_3^2 - (\sigma_1\sigma_2 + \sigma_2\sigma_3 + \sigma_1\sigma_3)}$

i.e. Failure occurs when

$$\sqrt{\sigma_1^2 + \sigma_2^2 + \sigma_3^2 - (\sigma_1\sigma_2 + \sigma_2\sigma_3 + \sigma_1\sigma_3)} \geq \sigma_e$$

$$\sqrt{400^2 + 140^2 + (-210)^2 - \{(400 \times 140) + [140 \times (-210)] + [400 \times (-210)]\}} \geq 550$$

$$530.19 \ngeq 550 \text{ MPa}$$

Hence failure does not occur.

14. **At a point in a steel member the major principal stress is 250 MPa, and the minor principal stress is compressive. If the tensile yield point of the steel is 350 MPa, find the value of the minor principal stress, according to:**
    (a) Maximum shearing stress
    (b) Maximum total strain energy;
    (c) Maximum shear strain energy. Take Poisson's ratio = 0.30.

Solution: $\sigma_1 = 250$ MPa, $\sigma_2 = ?$ (compressive), $\sigma_e = 350$ MPa, $\mu = 0.3$

a. *According to MSST:*

We know that $\dfrac{\sigma_e}{n} = \sigma_1 - \sigma_2$ [Assume n = 1, if not given]

$$350 = 250 - \sigma_2$$
$$\sigma_2 = -100 \text{ MPa (compressive)}$$

b. *Total strain energy theory or Haigh's theory:*

We know that $\dfrac{\sigma_e}{n} = \sqrt{\sigma_1^2 + \sigma_2^2 - 2\mu\sigma_1\sigma_2}$

$$350^2 = 250^2 + \sigma_2^2 - (2 \times 0.3 \times 250 \times \sigma_2)$$

$$60000 = \sigma_2^2 - 150\sigma_2$$

$$\sigma_2{}^2 - 150\sigma_2 - 60000 = 0$$

$$\sigma_2 = 331.17, -181.17$$
$$\sigma_2 = -181.17 \text{ MPa (compressive)}$$

c. *Maximum shear strain energy:*

We know that $\dfrac{\sigma_e}{n} = \sqrt{\sigma_1^2 + \sigma_2^2 - \sigma_1\sigma_2}$

$$350^2 = 250^2 + \sigma_2^2 - (250 \times \sigma_2)$$

$$60000 = \sigma_2^2 - 250\sigma_2$$

$$\sigma_2{}^2 - 250\sigma_2 - 60000 = 0$$

$$\sigma_2 = 400, -150$$
$$\sigma_2 = -150 \text{ MPa (compressive)}$$

15. **The principal stresses at a point in an elastic material are 90 MPa, 50 MPa both tensile and a compressive stress of 35 MPa. If Poisson's ratio = 0.3 and $E =$ 200 GPa, calculate:**
    (a) Total strain energy per unit volume
    (b) Volumetric strain energy per unit volume
    (c) Shear strain energy per unit volume

Solution: Arrangement: $(\sigma_1 > \sigma_2 > \sigma_3)$ $\sigma_1 = 90$ MPa, $\sigma_2 = 50$ MPa, $\sigma_3 = -35$ MPa, $\mu = 0.3$, $E = 2 \times 10^5$ MPa. Strain energy per unit volume = ?

a. *Total strain energy per unit volume:*

We know that $\quad U = \dfrac{1}{2E}[\sigma_1^2 + \sigma_2^2 + \sigma_3^2 - 2\mu(\sigma_1\sigma_2 + \sigma_2\sigma_3 + \sigma_1\sigma_3)]$

$$= \dfrac{1}{2\times(2\times10^5)}\,[90^2 + 50^2 + (-35)^2 - [2\times0.3\times\{(90\times50)$$

$$+ [50\times(-35)] + [90\times(-35)]\}]]$$

$$U = 0.03016 \text{ N-mm/mm}^3 = 30.16 \text{ kN-m/m}^3$$

b. *Volumetric strain energy per unit volume:*

We know that $\quad U_h = \left[\dfrac{1-2\mu}{6E}\right][\sigma_1^2 + \sigma_2^2 + \sigma_3^2 + 2(\sigma_1\sigma_2 + \sigma_2\sigma_3 + \sigma_3\sigma_1)]$

$$= \left[\dfrac{1-(2\times0.3)}{6\times(2\times10^5)}\right][90^2 + 50^2 + (-35)^2 + [2\times\{(90\times50)$$

$$+ [50\times(-35)] + [90\times(-35)]\}]]$$

$$U_h = 0.003675 \text{ N-mm/mm}^3 = 3.675 \text{ kN-m/m}^3$$

c. *Shear strain energy per unit volume:*

We know that $\quad U_d = \dfrac{1}{12G}\,[(\sigma_1 - \sigma_2)^2 + (\sigma_2 - \sigma_3)^2 + (\sigma_3 - \sigma_1)^2]$

But $\qquad\qquad E = 2G[1 + \mu]$

$$200\times10^5 = 2G[1 + 0.3]$$

$$G = 76.92\times10^3 \text{ MPa}$$

$$U_d = \dfrac{1}{12\times(76.92\times10^3)}\,\{(90-50)^2 + [50-(-35)]^2 + [90-(-35)]^2\}$$

$$U_d = 0.026488 \text{ N-mm/mm}^3 = 26.48 \text{ kN-m/m}^3$$

16. A material is subjected to a system of three mutually perpendicular stresses as follows: σ_o tensile, $2\sigma_o$ tensile and σ_o compressive. If this material failed in simple tension at a stress of 180 MPa, determine the value of σ_o, if the criterion of failure is:

(a) Maximum principal stress (b) Maximum shear stress;

(c) Maximum strain energy. (d) DET. Take Poisson's ratio $\mu = 0.3$.

Solution: Arrangement: $(\sigma_1 > \sigma_2 > \sigma_3)$ $\sigma_1 = 2\sigma_o$, $\sigma_2 = \sigma_o$, $\sigma_3 = -\sigma_o$, $\sigma_e = 180$ MPa, $\mu = 0.3$, $\sigma_o = ?$

a. *Maximum principal stress:*

We know that $\quad \dfrac{\sigma_e}{n} = \sigma_1$ $\qquad\qquad$ [Assume $n = 1$, if not given]

$$180 = 2\sigma_o$$

$$\sigma_o = 90 \text{ MPa}$$

b. *Maximum shear stress:*

We know that $\quad \dfrac{\sigma_e}{n} = \sigma_1 - \sigma_3$

$$180 = 2\sigma_o - (-\sigma_o)$$

$$\sigma_o = 60 \text{ MPa}$$

c. *Maximum strain energy:*

We know that $\dfrac{\sigma_e}{n} = \sqrt{\sigma_1^2 + \sigma_2^2 + \sigma_3^2 - 2\mu(\sigma_1\sigma_2 + \sigma_2\sigma_3 + \sigma_1\sigma_3)}$

$180 = \sqrt{(2\sigma_o)^2 + \sigma_o^2 + (-\sigma_o)^2 [2 \times 0.3 \times \{(2\sigma_o \times \sigma_o) + [\sigma_o \times (-\sigma_o)] + [2\sigma_o \times (-\sigma_o)]\}]}$

$180 = 2.57\sigma_o$

$\sigma_o = 70 \text{ MPa}$

d. *DET:*

We know that $\dfrac{\sigma_e}{n} = \sqrt{\sigma_1^2 + \sigma_2^2 + \sigma_3^2 - (\sigma_1\sigma_2 + \sigma_2\sigma_3 + \sigma_1\sigma_3)}$

$180 = \sqrt{(2\sigma_o)^2 + \sigma_o^2 + (-\sigma_o)^2 - [\{(2\sigma_o \times \sigma_o) + [\sigma_o \times (-\sigma_o)] + [2\sigma_o \times (-\sigma_o)]\}]}$

$180 = 2.65\sigma_o$

$\sigma_o = 68.03 \text{ MPa}$

VTU QUESTION PAPERS

Dec. 16/Jan. 17 (15ME/MA34)

1. A bolt is subjected to an axial pull of 12 kN together with a transverse shear of 6 kN. Determine the diameter of the bolt using:
   (a) Maximum principal stress theory
   (b) Maximum shear stress theory.
   Take elastic limit in tension = 300 N/mm^2, factor of safety = 3 and Poisson's ratio = 0.3 **(16 Marks)**

June/July 2017 (15ME/MA34)

2. Write a note on:
   (a) Maximum principal stress theory
   (b) Maximum shear stress theory. **(08 Marks)**
3. A solid circular shaft is subjected to bending moment of 40 kN-m and a torque of 10 kN-m. Design the diameter of the shaft according to
   (a) Maximum principal stress theory
   (b) Maximum shear stress theory.
   Take $\mu = 0.25$, factor of safety = 2 and stress at elastic limit as 200 MPa.

   (08 Marks)

Dec. 17/Jan. 18 (15ME/MA34)

4. Write a note on:
   (a) Maximum principal stress theory
   (b) Maximum shear stress theory. **(08 Marks)**
5. The plane state of stress at a point is given by $\sigma_x = 70$ MPa, $\sigma_y = 140$ MPa and $\tau_{xy} = -35$ MPa. If the yielding stress in tension is 175 MPa, check whether there is failure according to:
   (a) Maximum principal stress theory
   (b) Maximum shear stress theory
   If the material is safe then find the factor of safety. **(12 Marks)**